CURRENT THERAPY OF TRAUMA AND SURGICAL CRITICAL CARE

CURRENT THERAPY OF TRAUMA AND SURGICAL CRITICAL CARE

JUAN A. ASENSIO, MD, FACS, FCCM
Professor of Surgery
Director, Trauma Clinical Research, Training and Community Affairs
Director, Trauma Surgery and Surgical Critical Care Fellowship
Director, International Visiting Scholars/Research Fellowship
Medical Director for Education and Training, International Medicine Institute
Division of Trauma Surgery and Surgical Critical Care
Dewitt Daughtry Family Department of Surgery
University of Miami Miller School of Medicine
Ryder Trauma Center
Miami, Florida

DONALD D. TRUNKEY, MD, FACS
Professor and Chair
Department of Surgery
Oregon Health & Science University
Portland, Oregon

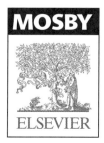

MOSBY

ELSEVIER

1600 John F. Kennedy Blvd.
Ste 1800
Philadelphia, PA 19103-2899

CURRENT THERAPY OF TRAUMA AND SURGICAL CRITICAL CARE ISBN: 978-0-323-04418-9

Notice

Knowledge and best practice in this field are constantly changing. As new research and experience broaden our knowledge, changes in practice, treatment, and drug therapy may become necessary or appropriate. Readers are advised to check the most current information provided (i) on procedures featured or (ii) by the manufacturer of each product to be administered, to verify the recommended dose or formula, the method and duration of administration, and contraindications. It is the responsibility of the practitioner, relying on his or her own experience and knowledge of the patient, to make diagnoses, to determine dosages and the best treatment for each individual patient, and to take all appropriate safety precautions. To the fullest extent of the law, neither the Publisher nor the Editors assume any liability for any injury and/or damage to persons or property arising out of or related to any use of the material contained in this book.

The Publisher

Library of Congress Cataloging-in-Publication Data
Current therapy of trauma and surgical critical care / [edited by] Juan A. Asensio, Donald D. Trunkey. — 1st ed.
    p. ; cm. — (Current therapy series)
  Includes bibliographical references and index.
  ISBN 978-0-323-04418-9
1. Wounds and injuries—Treatment. 2. Surgical intensive care. I. Asensio, Juan A. II. Trunkey, Donald D. III. Series.
[DNLM: 1. Wounds and Injuries—therapy. 2. Critical Care—methods. 3. Emergency Medical Services—organization & administration. 4. Emergency Treatment—methods. 5. Surgical Procedures, Operative—methods. 6. Trauma Centers—organization & administration. WO 700 C9766 2008]
  RD93.C776 2008
  617.1—dc22

2007043935

Acquisitions Editor: Scott Scheidt
Developmental Editor: Roxanne Halpine
Senior Project Manager: David Saltzberg
Design Direction: Steve Stave

Printed in the United States of America

Last digit is the print number: 9   8   7   6   5   4   3   2

Michel B. Aboutanos, MD, MPH, FACS
Assistant Professor of Surgery
Division of Trauma, Critical Care, and
Emergency Surgery
Department of Surgery
Virginia Commonwealth University Medical
Center
Medical College of Virginia Hospitals
Richmond, Virginia

*DIAGNOSTIC AND THERAPEUTIC ROLES OF
BRONCHOSCOPY AND VIDEO-ASSISTED
THORACOSCOPY IN TH E MANAGEMENT
OF THORACIC TRAUMA*

Roxie M. Albrecht, MD, FACS, FCCM
Associate Professor, Department of Surgery
University of Oklahoma College of Medicine
Medical Director, Trauma and Surgical
Critical Care
Medical Director, Surgical ICU
University of Oklahoma Medical Center
Oklahoma City, Oklahoma

*LOWER EXTREMITY VASCULAR INJURIES: FEM-
ORAL, POPLITEAL, AND SHANK VESSEL INJURY*

Preya Ananthakrishnan, MD
Resident
University of Medicine and Dentistry of New
Jersey—New Jersey Medical School
Newark, New Jersey

SEPSIS, SEPTIC SHOCK, AND ITS TREATMENT

John T. Anderson, MD, FACS
Associate Professor, Department of Surgery
Division of Trauma and Emergency Surgery
University of California, Davis
Sacramento, California

THE DIAGNOSIS OF VASCULAR TRAUMA

Michael Andreae, MD
Assistant Professor of Anesthesiology
University of Medicine and Dentistry of
New Jersey
Newark, New Jersey

*ANESTHESIA IN THE SURGICAL INTENSIVE
CARE UNIT—BEYOND THE AIRWAY: NEURO-
MUSCULAR PARALYSIS AND PAIN
MANAGEMENT*

John H. Armstrong, MD, FACS, FCCP
Division of Acute Care Surgery
Department of Surgery
University of Florida College of Medicine
Gainesville, Florida

TRIAGE

Juan A. Asensio, MD, FACS, FCCM
Professor of Surgery
Director, Trauma Clinical Research, Train-
ing and Community Affairs
Director, Trauma Surgery and Surgical
Critical Care Fellowship
Director, International Visiting Scholars/
Research Fellowship
Medical Director for Education and Train-
ing, International Medicine Institute
Division of Trauma Surgery and Surgical
Critical Care
Dewitt Daughtry Family Department of
Surgery
University of Miami Miller School of
Medicine
Ryder Trauma Center
Miami, Florida

*EMERGENCY DEPARTMENT THORACOTOMY;
CAROTID, VERTEBRAL ARTERY, AND JUGULAR
VENOUS INJURIES; OPERATIVE MANAGE-
MENT OF PULMONARY INJURIES: LUNG-
SPARING AND FORMAL RESECTIONS; CAR-
DIAC INJURIES; EXSANGUINATION: RELIABLE
MODELS TO INDICATE DAMAGE CONTROL;
LOWER EXTREMITY VASCULAR INJURIES:
FEMORAL, POPLITEAL, AND SHANK VESSEL
INJURY; ACUTE RESPIRATORY DISTRESS SYN-
DROME*

John A. Aucar, MD, MSHI, FACS
Professor and Chair
Department of Surgery
University of Texas Health Center at Tyler
Tyler, Texas

*DIAGNOSTIC PERITONEAL LAVAGE AND LAP-
AROSCOPY IN EVALUATION OF ABDOMINAL
TRAUMA*

Jeffrey S. Augenstein, MD, PhD, FACS
Professor of Surgery
Director, William Lehman Injury Research
Center
University of Miami Miller School of
Medicine
Director, Ryder Trauma Center
Jackson Memorial Hospital
Miami, Florida

*TRAUMA SYSTEMS AND TRAUMA TRIAGE
ALGORITHMS*

Michael M. Badellino, MD, FACS
Associate Professor of Surgery
Pennsylvania State University College of
Medicine
Hershey, Pennsylvania
Program Director, General Surgery Resi-
dency and Vice Chair, Educational Affairs
Department of Surgery
Division of Trauma/Surgical Critical Care
Lehigh Valley Hospital
Allentown, Pennsylvania

TRAUMA REHABILITATION

Philip S. Barie, MD, MBA, FCCM, FACS
Professor of Surgery and Public Health
Chief, Division of Critical Care and Trauma
Department of Surgery
Division of Medical Ethics
Department of Public Health
Weill Cornell Medical College
Chief, Trauma Service
Director, Anne and Max A. Cohen Surgical
Intensive Care Unit
New York-Presbyterian Hospital
Weill Cornell Center
New York, New York

*FUNDAMENTALS OF MECHANICAL
VENTILATION; ADVANCED TECHNIQUES IN
MECHANICAL VENTILATION; ANTIBACTERIAL
THERAPY: THE OLD, THE NEW, AND THE
FUTURE; FUNGAL INFECTIONS AND
ANTIFUNGAL THERAPY IN THE SURGICAL
INTENSIVE CARE UNIT*

Alexander Becker, MD
Trauma Surgery and Surgical Critical Care
Fellow
Division of Trauma and Critical Care
DeWitt Daughtry Family Department of
Surgery
Jackson Memorial Hospital
Leonard M. Miller School of Medicine
Miami, Florida
Attending Surgeon
Department of Surgery A
Haemek Medical Center
Afula, Israel

*BLAST INJURIES; ACUTE RESPIRATORY
DISTRESS SYNDROME*

Edward J. Bedrick, PhD
Professor of Biostatistics
Department of Mathematics and Statistics
and Department of Internal Medicine
University of New Mexico
Albuquerque, New Mexico

*INJURY SEVERITY SCORING: ITS DEFINITION
AND PRACTICAL APPLICATION*

Alfred F. Behrens, MD
Professor and Chair
Department of Orthopaedics
University of Medicine and Dentistry of
New Jersey—New Jersey Medical School
Newark, New Jersey
(deceased)

*UPPER EXTREMITY FRACTURES: ORTHOPE-
DIC MANAGEMENT*

Jay Berger, MD
Resident, Department of Anesthesiology
University of Medicine and Dentistry of
New Jersey
Newark, New Jersey

*ANESTHESIA IN THE SURGICAL INTENSIVE
CARE UNIT—BEYOND THE AIRWAY:
NEUROMUSCULAR PARALYSIS AND PAIN
MANAGEMENT*

John D. Berne, MD, FACS
Trauma Surgeon
East Texas Medical Center
Tyler, Texas

*TRACHEAL, LARYNGEAL, AND OROPHARYN-
GEAL INJURIES*

Charles D. Best, MD, FACS
Assistant Professor of Urology
University of Southern California
Chief of Service
Department of Urology
LAC/USC County Medical Center
Los Angeles, California

GENITOURINARY TRACT INJURY

Walter L. Biffl, MD, FACS
Associate Professor of Surgery
Denver Health Medical Center
University of Colorado
Denver, Colorado

*SCAPULOTHORACIC DISSOCIATION AND
DEGLOVING INJURIES OF THE EXTREMITIES*

F. William Blaisdell, MD, FACS
Professor, Department of Surgery
University of California, Davis
Sacramento, California

THE DIAGNOSIS OF VASCULAR TRAUMA

Grant V. Bochicchio MD, MPH, FACS
Associate Professor of Surgery
University of Maryland School of Medicine
Director of Clinical and Outcomes Research
R Adams Cowley Shock Trauma Center
Deputy Chief of Surgery and Chief of Sur-
gical Critical Care
Baltimore Veterans Affairs Medical Center
Baltimore, Maryland

*SURGICAL ANATOMY OF THE ABDOMEN
AND RETROPERITONEUM*

**Christopher T. Born, MD, FAAOS,
FACS**
Professor, Department of Orthopaedic
Surgery
The Warren Alpert Medical School of
Brown University
Chief of Orthopaedic Trauma
The Rhode Island Hospital
Providence, Rhode Island

*SCAPULOTHORACIC DISSOCIATION AND
DEGLOVING INJURIES OF THE EXTREMITIES*

Benjamin Braslow, MD
Assistant Professor of Surgery
Department of Surgery
University of Pennsylvania School of
Medicine
Assistant Professor of Surgery
Division of Traumatology and Surgical
Critical Care
University of Pennsylvania Medical Center
Philadelphia, Pennsylvania

TRAUMA IN THE ELDERLY

L. D. Britt, MD, MPH, FACS
Brickhouse Professor and Chair
Department of Surgery
Eastern Virginia Medical School
Norfolk, Virginia

*PENETRATING NECK INJURIES: DIAGNOSIS
AND SELECTIVE MANAGEMENT*

Susan I. Brundage, MD, MPH, FACS
Associate Professor, School of Medicine,
Department of Surgery
Associate Director of Trauma, Trauma
Services
Director, Trauma Quality Improvement
Program, Trauma Services
Stanford University Medical Center
Stanford, California

NOSOCOMIAL PNEUMONIA

Jon M. Burch, MD, FACS
University of Colorado School of Medicine
Department of Surgery
Denver Health Medical Center
Denver, Colorado

COLON AND RECTAL INJURIES

David G. Burris, MD, FACS, DMCC
Professor and Chair, Norman M. Rich
Department of Surgery
Uniformed Services University of the Health
Sciences
Staff General/Trauma/Critical Care Surgeon
National Naval Medical Center
Bethesda, Maryland
Staff General/Trauma/Critical Care Surgeon
Walter Reed Army Medical Center
Washington, DC

TRIAGE

Patricia M. Byers, MD, FACS
Professor, Department of Surgery
Miller School of Medicine at the University
of Miami
Chief of Intestinal Rehabilitation Service,
Faculty Trauma, Burns and Critical Care
Jackson Memorial Hospital
Miami, Florida

*PREOPERATIVE AND POSTOPERATIVE NUTRI-
TIONAL SUPPORT: STRATEGIES FOR ENTERAL
AND PARENTERAL THERAPIES*

Allan Capin, MD
Clinical Research Associate
Department of Surgery—Division of
Trauma and Critical Care
University of Miami Miller School of
Medicine
Ryder Trauma Center
Jackson Memorial Hospital
Miami, Florida

*EMERGENCY DEPARTMENT THORACOTOMY;
CARDIAC INJURIES; EXSANGUINATION:
RELIABLE MODELS TO INDICATE DAMAGE
CONTROL*

Guy J. Cappuccino, MD
Chief Resident
University of Medicine and Dentistry of
New Jersey—New Jersey Medical School
Newark, New Jersey

MAXILLOFACIAL INJURIES

Eddy H. Carrillo, MD, FACS
Clinical Assistant Professor of Surgery
University of Miami
Miami, Florida
Chief of Trauma Services
Division of Trauma Services
Memorial Regional Hospital
Hollywood, Florida

*DELIVERING MULTIDISCIPLINARY TRAUMA
CARE: CURRENT CHALLENGES AND FUTURE
DIRECTIONS*

Ricardo Castrellon, MD
Trauma Surgery and Surgical Critical Care
Fellow
DeWitt Daughtry Family Department
of Surgery
University of Miami
Ryder Trauma Center
Jackson Memorial Hospital
Miami, Florida

*OPERATIVE MANAGEMENT OF PULMONARY
INJURIES: LUNG-SPARING AND FORMAL
RESECTIONS*

David C. Chang, PhD, MPH, MBA
Assistant Professor, Department of Surgery
Johns Hopkins School of Medicine
Assistant Professor, Department of Health
Policy and Management
Johns Hopkins Bloomberg School of Public
Health
Baltimore, Maryland

*THE ROLE OF TRAUMA PREVENTION IN
REDUCING INTERPERSONAL VIOLENCE*

William C. Chiu, MD
Associate Professor of Surgery
Director, Surgical Critical Care Fellowship
Program
R Adams Cowley Shock Trauma Center
University of Maryland School of
Medicine
Baltimore, Maryland

TRAUMA IN PREGNANCY

Chee Kiong Chong, MD
Trauma Critical Care Fellow
Jackson Memorial Hospital
Miami, Florida

VASCULAR ANATOMY OF THE EXTREMITIES

A. Britton Christmas, MD
CMC General Surgery
Charlotte, North Carolina

TREATMENT OF ESOPHAGEAL INJURY

Danny Chu, MD
Assistant Professor of Surgery
Baylor College of Medicine
Staff Cardiothoracic Surgeon
Michael E. DeBakey Veterans Affairs
Medical Center
Division of Cardiothoracic Surgery
Houston, Texas

THORACIC VASCULAR INJURY

David J. Ciesla, MD, FACS
Associate Professor, Department of
Surgery
University of South Florida
Chief of Trauma, Emergency Surgery,
Surgical Critical Care
Tampa General Hospital
Tampa, Florida

COLON AND RECTAL INJURIES

William G. Cioffi, MD, FACS
J. Murray Beardsley Professor and Chair
Department of Surgery
The Warren Alpert Medical School of
Brown University
Surgeon-in-Chief
Department of Surgery
Rhode Island Hospital
Providence, Rhode Island

*SCAPULOTHORACIC DISSOCIATION AND
DEGLOVING INJURIES OF THE EXTREMITIES*

**Christine S. Cocanour, MD, FACS,
FCCM**
Professor of Surgery, Department of Surgery
University of Texas—Houston Medical
School
Medical Director, Shock/Trauma Intensive
Care Unit
Memorial Hermann Hospital
Surgical Critical Care Fellowship Director,
Department of Surgery
University of Texas—Houston Medical
School
Houston, Texas

THE IMMUNOLOGY OF TRAUMA

Mitchell J. Cohen, MD
Assistant Professor in Residence
Department of Surgery
University of California San Francisco
San Francisco, California

*CARDIAC HEMODYNAMICS: THE
PULMONARY ARTERY CATHETER
AND THE MEANING OF ITS READINGS*

Raul Coimbra, MD, PhD, FACS
Professor of Surgery
Department of Surgery
University of California, San Diego
Chief, Division of Trauma, Surgical
Intensive Care, and Burns
Department of Surgery
UCSD Medical Center
San Diego, California

*PREHOSPITAL AIRWAY MANAGEMENT:
INTUBATION, DEVICES, AND CONTROVERSIES*

**Edward E. Cornwell III, MD, FACS,
FCCM**
Professor of Surgery
Johns Hopkins University School of
Medicine
Chief, Adult Trauma Services
Johns Hopkins Hospital
Baltimore, Maryland

*THE ROLE OF TRAUMA PREVENTION IN
REDUCING INTERPERSONAL VIOLENCE*

C. Clay Cothren, MD, FACS
Assistant Professor of Surgery
University of Colorado School of Medicine
Program Director
Surgical Critical Care Fellowship
Department of Surgery
Denver Health Medical Center
Denver, Colorado

BLUNT CEREBROVASCULAR INJURIES

Thomas B. Cox, BS
President
Cox Business Consulting, Inc.
Hillsboro, Oregon

TRAUMA SCORING

Martin A. Croce, MD, FACS
Professor of Surgery
Chief, Trauma and Surgical Critical Care
Medical Director
Elvis Presley Memorial Trauma Center
Memphis, Tennessee

PANCREATIC INJURIES

Mark J. Dannenbaum, MD
Chief Resident
Department of Neurosurgery
Baylor College of Medicine
Houston, Texas

*TRAUMATIC BRAIN INJURY: PATHOPHYSIOL-
OGY, CLINICAL DIAGNOSIS, AND PREHOSPI-
TAL AND EMERGENCY CENTER CARE; TRAU-
MATIC BRAIN INJURY: IMAGING, OPERATIVE
AND NONOPERATIVE CARE, AND COMPLI-
CATIONS*

Ramazi O. Datiashvili, MD, PhD
Associate Professor, Department of Surgery
Division of Plastic Surgery
University of Medicine and Dentistry of
New Jersey—New Jersey Medical School
Newark, New Jersey

*EXTREMITY REPLANTATION: INDICATIONS
AND TIMING; TECHNIQUES IN THE MANAGE-
MENT OF COMPLEX MUSCULOSKELETAL
INJURY: ROLES OF MUSCLE, MUSCULOCUTA-
NEOUS, AND FASCIOCUTANEOUS FLAPS*

Daniel P. Davis, MD
Professor of Clinical Medicine
Department of Medicine
Division of Emergency Medicine
University of California San Diego
San Diego, California

*PREHOSPITAL AIRWAY MANAGEMENT: INTU-
BATION, DEVICES, AND CONTROVERSIES*

Kimberly A. Davis, MD, FACS
Associate Professor of Surgery
Vice Chair for Clinical Affairs
Chief of the Section of Trauma, Surgical
Critical Care, and Surgical Emergencies
Department of Surgery
Yale University School of Medicine
Trauma Director
Yale-New Haven Hospital
New Haven, Connecticut

*SURGICAL TECHNIQUES FOR THORACIC,
ABDOMINAL, PELVIC, AND EXTREMITY
DAMAGE CONTROL; BURNS*

Dan L. Deckelbaum, MD, CM, FRCSC
Trauma Surgery and Surgical Critical Care
Fellow
Fellow, Division of Trauma
Department of Surgery
University of Miami
Jackson Memorial Medical Center
Ryder Trauma Center
Miami, Florida

EMERGENCY DEPARTMENT THORACOTOMY

Edwin A. Deitch, MD, FACS
Chair, Department of Surgery
New Jersey Medical School
Chief of Surgery
University Hospital
Newark, New Jersey

*SYSTEMIC INFLAMMATORY RESPONSE
SYNDROME AND MULTIPLE-ORGAN
DYSFUNCTION SYNDROME: DEFINITION,
DIAGNOSIS, AND MANAGEMENT; SEPSIS,
SEPTIC SHOCK, AND ITS TREATMENT*

Ellise Delphin, MD
Professor and Chair
Department of Anesthesiology
University of Medicine and Dentistry of
New Jersey
Newark, New Jersey

*ANESTHESIA IN THE SURGICAL INTENSIVE
CARE UNIT—BEYOND THE AIRWAY:
NEUROMUSCULAR PARALYSIS AND PAIN
MANAGEMENT*

Rochelle A. Dicker, MD, FACS
Assistant Professor of Surgery
University of California, San Francisco
Attending Physician
Acute Care Surgery, Trauma, and Critical Care
Department of Surgery
San Francisco General Hospital
San Francisco, California

*CIVILIAN HOSPITAL RESPONSE TO MASS
CASUALTY EVENTS*

Lawrence N. Diebel, MD, FACS
Professor, Department of Surgery
Wayne State University
Attending Surgeon
Department of Surgery
Detroit Receiving Hospital
Detroit, Michigan

GASTRIC INJURIES

Jonathan M. Dort, MD, FACS
Clinical Associate Professor, Department of
Surgery
University of Kansas School of Medicine
Chair, Department of Surgery
Associate Medical Director, Trauma
Services
Medical Director, Pediatric Trauma
Services
Via Christi Regional Medical Center
Wichita, Kansas

COMMON ERRORS IN TRAUMA CARE

Therese M. Duane, MD, FACS
Assistant Professor of Surgery
Virginia Commonwealth University
Director of Infection Control STICU
Division of Trauma, Critical Care, and
Emergency Surgery
Virginia Commonwealth University Medical
Center
Richmond, Virginia

*DIAGNOSTIC AND THERAPEUTIC ROLES OF
BRONCHOSCOPY AND VIDEO-ASSISTED
THORACOSCOPY IN THE MANAGEMENT OF
THORACIC TRAUMA*

Wayne E. Dubov, MD
Clinical Assistant Professor of Medicine
Pennsylvania State University College of
Medicine
Hershey, Pennsylvania
Director of Acute Rehabilitation
Lehigh Valley Hospital
Allentown, Pennsylvania

TRAUMA REHABILITATION

Michael B. Dunham, MD, FRCSC
Clinical Assistant Professor, Department of
Surgery
University of Calgary
Calgary, Alberta, Canada

*THE ROLE OF FOCUSED ASSESSMENT WITH
SONOGRAPHY FOR TRAUMA: INDICATIONS,
LIMITATIONS, AND CONTROVERSIES*

Dominic J. Duran, BS
Surgical Critical Care and Trauma Surgery
Fellowship Coordinator
Assistant to Professor Asensio
University of Miami
Jackson Memorial Hospital
Jackson Health System
Ryder Trauma Center
Miami, Florida

*EMERGENCY DEPARTMENT THORACOTOMY;
OPERATIVE MANAGEMENT OF PULMONARY
INJURIES: LUNG-SPARING AND FORMAL
RESECTIONS; CARDIAC INJURIES*

Rodney M. Durham, MD, FACS
Professor of Surgery
Department of Surgery
University of South Florida
Tampa, Florida

*THE MANAGEMENT OF RENAL FAILURE: RE-
NAL REPLACEMENT THERAPY AND DIALYSIS*

Soumitra R. Eachempati, MD, FACS
Associate Professor of Surgery and Public
Health
Weill Cornell Medical College
Associate Attending Surgeon
New York-Presbyterian Hospital
New York, New York

*FUNDAMENTALS OF MECHANICAL VENTILA-
TION; ADVANCED TECHNIQUES IN MECHANI-
CAL VENTILATION; ANTIBACTERIAL THERAPY:
THE OLD, THE NEW, AND THE FUTURE; F
UNGAL INFECTIONS AND ANTIFUNGAL THER-
APY IN THE SURGICAL INTENSIVE CARE UNIT*

Brian John Eastridge, MD, FACS
Chief of Trauma, Burn, and Critical Care
Division
Brooke Army Medical Center
U.S. Army Institute of Surgical Research
Fort Sam Houston, Texas

*TRAUMA CENTER ORGANIZATION AND
VERIFICATION*

Thomas J. Ellis, MD
Associate Professor, Department of
Orthopaedic Surgery
Ohio State University
Ohio State University Medical Center
Columbus, Ohio

PELVIC FRACTURES

Michael Englehart, MD
Resident, General Surgery
Oregon Health & Science University
Portland, Oregon

*RESUSCITATION FLUIDS; ENDPOINTS OF
RESUSCITATION*

Thomas J. Esposito, MD, MPH, FACS
Professor, Department of Surgery
Director, Injury Analysis and Prevention
Programs
Loyola University Burn and Shock Trauma
Institute
Loyola University Stritch School of
Medicine
Director, Division of Trauma, Surgical
Critical Care, and Burns
Loyola University Medical Center
Maywood, Illinois

*THE ROLE OF ALCOHOL AND OTHER
DRUGS IN TRAUMA*

Timothy C. Fabian, MD, FACS
Harwell Wilson Alumni Professor and Chair
Department of Surgery
University of Tennessee Health Science Center
Staff Surgeon
Department of Surgery
Regional Medical Center/Presley Regional
Trauma Center
Memphis, Tennessee

*INTERVENTIONAL RADIOLOGY: DIAGNOSTICS
AND THERAPEUTICS*

Samir M. Fakhry, MD, FACS
Professor of Surgery
Virginia Commonwealth University—Inova
Campus
Chief, Trauma and Surgical Critical Care
Associate Chair for Research and Education
Trauma Services
Inova Fairfax Hospital
Falls Church, Virginia

*MANAGEMENT OF COAGULATION
DISORDERS IN THE SURGICAL INTENSIVE
CARE UNIT*

Anthony J. Falvo, DO
Clinical Assistant Professor, Department of
Osteopathic Surgical Specialties
Michigan State University
East Lansing, Michigan
Senior Staff Surgeon
Department of Surgery
Division of Trauma/Surgical Critical Care
Henry Ford Health System
Detroit, Michigan

*MANAGEMENT OF ENDOCRINE DISORDERS
IN THE SURGICAL INTENSIVE CARE UNIT*

Ara Feinstein, MD
Trauma Surgery and Surgical Critical Care
Fellow
Division of Trauma
Department of Surgery
University of Miami
Jackson Memorial Medical Center
Ryder Trauma Center
Miami, Florida

CARDIAC INJURIES

David V. Feliciano, MD, FACS
Professor of Surgery
Emory University School of Medicine
Chief of Surgery
Grady Memorial Hospital
Atlanta, Georgia
Adjunct Professor of Surgery
Uniformed Services University of the Health
Sciences
Bethesda, Maryland

ABDOMINAL VASCULAR INJURIES

**Luis G. Fernandez, MD, FACS, FASAS,
FCCP, FCCM, FICS**
Chair, Division of Trauma Surgery/Surgical
Critical Care
Chief of Combined Critical Care Units
Trinity Mother Francis Health System
Assistant Clinical Professor of Surgery/
Family Practice
University of Texas Health Science Center
Adjunct Clinical Professor of Medicine and
Nursing
University of Texas Arlington
Colonel, Texas State Guard, Medical Reserve
Corps, Texas Medical Rangers
Commander, TMR-Tyler
Tyler, Texas

*TRACHEAL, LARYNGEAL, AND OROPHARYN-
GEAL INJURIES*

Mitchell P. Fink, MD
President and Chief Executive Officer
Logical Therapeutics, Inc.
Waltham, Massachusetts

OXYGEN TRANSPORT

Lewis M. Flint, MD, FACS
Professor of Surgery
University of South Florida College of
Medicine
Tampa General Hospital
Tampa, Florida

*THE MANAGEMENT OF RENAL FAILURE: RE-
NAL REPLACEMENT THERAPY AND DIALYSIS*

William R. Fry, MD, FACS, RVT, RDMN
Trauma Director
Penrose St. Francis Healthcare Center
Colorado Springs, Colorado

*DIAGNOSTIC PERITONEAL LAVAGE AND
LAPAROSCOPY IN EVALUATION OF
ABDOMINAL TRAUMA*

Eric. R. Frykberg, MD, FACS
Professor of Surgery
University of Florida College of Medicine
Chief, Division of General Surgery
Shands Jacksonville Medical Center
Jacksonville, Florida

UPPER EXTREMITY VASCULAR TRAUMA

Richard L. Gamelli, MD, FACS
The Robert J. Freeark Professor and Chair
Department of Surgery
Loyola University Medical Center
Maywood, Illinois

BURNS

Parham A. Ganchi, PhD, MD
Medical Director
Ganchi Plastic Surgery
Wayne, New Jersey

HAND FRACTURES

George D. Garcia, MD
Chief Fellow, Trauma Surgery and Surgical
Critical Care
Division of Trauma, Critical Care, and
Burns
DeWitt Daughtry Family Department of
Surgery
Ryder Trauma Center
University of Miami
Jackson Memorial Hospital
Miami, Florida

*ACUTE RESPIRATORY DISTRESS SYNDROME;
DIAGNOSIS AND TREATMENT OF DEEP VE-
NOUS THROMBOSIS: DRUGS AND FILTERS*

Major Luis Manuel García-Núñez, MD
Assistant Professor, Department of
Surgery
Mexican Army and Air Force University
Staff Surgeon
Department of Surgery—Division of
Trauma Surgery
Central Military Hospital
National Defense Department
Distrito Federal, México

*EMERGENCY DEPARTMENT THORACOTOMY;
CAROTID, VERTEBRAL ARTERY, AND JUGULAR
VENOUS INJURIES; OPERATIVE MANAGE-
MENT OF PULMONARY INJURIES: LUNG-
SPARING AND FORMAL RESECTIONS; CAR-
DIAC INJURIES; EXSANGUINATION: RELIABLE
MODELS TO INDICATE DAMAGE CONTROL*

Robin Michael Gehrmann, MD
Director, Division of Sports Medicine and
Shoulder Surgery
Department of Orthopaedics
University of Medicine and Dentistry of
New Jersey—New Jersey Medical School
Newark, New Jersey

*UPPER EXTREMITY FRACTURES: ORTHOPE-
DIC MANAGEMENT*

Larry M. Gentilello, MD, FACS
Professor, Department of Surgery
University of Texas Southwestern Medical
Center
Parkland Memorial Hospital
Dallas, Texas
Adjunct Professor, Management, Policy, and
Community Health
University of Texas School of Public Health
Houston, Texas

*THE ROLE OF ALCOHOL AND OTHER
DRUGS IN TRAUMA; HYPOTHERMIA AND
TRAUMA*

Enrique Ginzburg, MD, FACS
Professor of Surgery
Division of Trauma and Surgical Critical
Care
DeWitt Daughtry Family Department of
Surgery
University of Miami Miller School of
Medicine
Attending Physician
Jackson Memorial Hospital
Attending Physician
University of Miami Hospital and Clinic
Miami, Florida

VASCULAR ANATOMY OF THE EXTREMITIES

Laurent G. Glance, MD
Associate Professor, Department of Anes-
thesiology
University of Rochester School of Medicine
and Dentistry
Strong Memorial Hospital
Rochester, New York

*INJURY SEVERITY SCORING: ITS DEFINITION
AND PRACTICAL APPLICATION*

Scott B. Gmora MD, FRCSC
Trauma Surgery and Surgical Critical Care
Fellow
Division of Trauma and Surgical Critical Care
Ryder Trauma Center
University of Miami School of Medicine
Miami, Florida

CARDIAC INJURIES

**Thomas J. Goaley Jr., MD, CDR MC
USN**
Trauma/Critical Care Fellow
Emory University School of Medicine
Grady Memorial Hospital
Atlanta, Georgia

ABDOMINAL VASCULAR INJURIES

Nestor R. Gonzalez, MD
Assistant Professor, Neurological Surgery
and Radiological Sciences
UCLA Medical Center
Los Angeles, California

*SPINE: SPINAL CORD INJURY, BLUNT AND
PENETRATING, NEUROGENIC AND SPINAL
SHOCK*

Roshini Gopinathan, MD
Assistant Clinical Professor of Surgery
Columbia University
Attending, Division of Plastic Surgery
Harlem Hospital Center
New York, New York

HAND FRACTURES

Vicente Gracias, MD, FACS
Division of Trauma
University of Pennsylvania Medical Center
Philadelphia, Pennsylvania

*PREHOSPITAL FLUID RESUSCITATION:
WHAT TYPE, HOW MUCH, AND
CONTROVERSIES*

Thomas S. Granchi, MD, MBA
Associate Professor, Department of Surgery
Baylor College of Medicine
Attending Surgeon
Ben Taub General Hospital
Houston, Texas

COMPARTMENT SYNDROMES

Mark S. Granick, MD, FACS
Professor of Surgery, tenured
Division of Plastic Surgery
Department of Surgery
University of Medicine and Dentistry of
New Jersey—New Jersey Medical School
Newark, New Jersey

*MAXILLOFACIAL INJURIES; HAND FRAC-
TURES; TECHNIQUES IN THE MANAGEMENT
OF COMPLEX MUSCULOSKELETAL INJURY:
ROLES OF MUSCLE, MUSCULOCUTANEOUS,
AND FASCIOCUTANEOUS FLAPS*

Eduard Grass, MD
Trauma Surgery and Surgical Critical Care
Fellow
University of Miami Miller School of
Medicine
Miami, Florida

BLAST INJURIES

Margaret Mary Griffen, MD, FACS
Surgeon
Trauma Services
Inova Fairfax Hospital
Falls Church, Virginia

UPPER EXTREMITY VASCULAR TRAUMA

Ronald I. Gross, MD, FACS
Assistant Professor, Traumatology and
Emergency Medicine
University of Connecticut School of Medicine
Farmington, Connecticut
Associate Director of Trauma
Traumatology and Emergency Medicine
Hartford Hospital
Hartford, Connecticut

*AIRWAY MANAGEMENT: WHAT EVERY
TRAUMA SURGEON SHOULD KNOW, FROM
INTUBATION TO CRICOTHYROIDOTOMY*

Joseph M. Gutmann, MD
University of South Florida
Tampa, Florida

*THE MANAGEMENT OF RENAL FAILURE:
RENAL REPLACEMENT THERAPY AND
DIALYSIS*

Fahim A. Habib, MD, FACS
Assistant Professor of Surgery
Division of Trauma and Surgical Critical Care
Co-Director, Injury Prevention Education
William Lehman Injury Research Center/
Medical Computer Systems Laboratory
DeWitt Daughtry Department of Surgery
University of Miami Miller School of Medicine
Miami, Florida

*DELIVERING MULTIDISCIPLINARY TRAUMA
CARE: CURRENT CHALLENGES AND FUTURE
DIRECTIONS*

**S. Morad Hameed, MD, MPH, FRCSC,
FACS**
Assistant Professor, Department of
Surgery
University of British Columbia
Vancouver, British Columbia, Canada

*PREOPERATIVE AND POSTOPERATIVE NUTRI-
TIONAL SUPPORT: STRATEGIES FOR ENTERAL
AND PARENTERAL THERAPIES*

Ola Harrskog, MD, DEAA
Assistant Professor, Department of
Anesthesiology and Perioperative Medicine
Oregon Health & Science University
Portland, Oregon

*AIRWAY MANAGEMENT IN THE TRAUMA
PATIENT: HOW TO INTUBATE AND MANAGE
NEUROMUSCULAR PARALYTIC AGENTS*

Robert A. Hart, MD
Associate Professor, Orthopaedics and
Rehabilitation
Oregon Health & Science University
Orthopaedic Spine Surgeon
Orthopaedics and Rehabilitation
Oregon Health & Science University
Hospital
Portland, Oregon

*CERVICAL, THORACIC, AND LUMBAR FRAC-
TURES*

Carl J. Hauser, MD, FACS, FCCM
Professor of Surgery
Harvard University
Attending Surgeon
New England Deaconess Medical Center
Boston, Massachusetts

*PULMONARY CONTUSION AND FLAIL
CHEST*

Sharon Henry, MD, FACS, FCCWS
Associate Professor of Surgery
University of Maryland School of Medicine
Director, Division of Wound Healing and
Metabolism
R.A. Cowley Shock Trauma Center
Baltimore, Maryland

SOFT TISSUE INFECTIONS

H. Mathilda Horst, MD, FACS, FCCM
Director of Surgical Critical Care
Department of Surgery
Henry Ford Hospital
Henry Ford Health System
Detroit, Michigan

*MANAGEMENT OF ENDOCRINE DISORDERS
IN THE SURGICAL INTENSIVE CARE UNIT*

Herman P. Houin, MD
Senior Staff Surgeon
Department of Plastic Surgery
Henry Ford Health System
Detroit, Michigan

*LOWER EXTREMITY AND DEGLOVING
INJURY*

David B. Hoyt, MD, FACS
John E. Connolly Professor and Chairman
Department of Surgery
University of California School of Medicine
Irvine, California
University of California Irvine Medical
Center
Orange, California

*PREHOSPITAL AIRWAY MANAGEMENT:
INTUBATION, DEVICES, AND
CONTROVERSIES*

Catherine A. Humphrey, MD
Assistant Professor, Orthopaedic Trauma,
Orthopaedic Surgery, and Rehabilitation
University of Rochester Medical Center
Rochester, New York

PELVIC FRACTURES

Felicia A. Ivascu, MD
Attending Surgeon
General Surgery, Trauma and Surgical
Critical Care
William Beaumont Hospital
Royal Oak, Michigan

*DIAGNOSIS AND TREATMENT OF DEEP
VENOUS THROMBOSIS: DRUGS AND FILTERS*

Rao R. Ivatury, MD, FACS
Professor of Surgery
Virginia Commonwealth University
Chief, Trauma, Critical Care, and Emergency Surgery
Virginia Commonwealth University Medical
Center
Richmond, Virginia

*DIAGNOSTIC AND THERAPEUTIC ROLES OF
BRONCHOSCOPY AND VIDEO-ASSISTED
THORACOSCOPY IN THE MANAGEMENT OF
THORACIC TRAUMA*

Lenworth M. Jacobs, MD, MPH, FACS
Professor and Chair
Department of Traumatology and Emergency Medicine
University of Connecticut
Farmington, Connecticut
Director, Trauma, Emergency Medicine,
LIFE STAR Helicopter, Rehabilitation,
Education Institute
Department of Trauma and Emergency
Medicine
Hartford Hospital
Director, Adult and Pediatric Trauma
Institute
Department of Trauma
Connecticut Children's Medical Center
Hartford, Connecticut

*AIRWAY MANAGEMENT: WHAT EVERY
TRAUMA SURGEON SHOULD KNOW, FROM
INTUBATION TO CRICOTHYROIDOTOMY*

Per-Olof Jarnberg, MD, PhD
Professor and Vice Chair
Clinical Affairs
Department of Anesthesiology and Perioperative Medicine
Oregon Health & Science University
Portland, Oregon

*AIRWAY MANAGEMENT IN THE TRAUMA PATIENT: HOW TO INTUBATE AND MANAGE
NEUROMUSCULAR PARALYTIC AGENTS*

Gregory J. Jurkovich, MD, FACS
Professor of Surgery
University of Washington
Seattle, Washington
Chief of Trauma
Department of Surgery
Harborview Medical Center
Seattle, Washington

*OPERATIVE MANAGEMENT OF PULMONARY INJURIES: LUNG-SPARING AND
FORMAL RESECTIONS; COMPLICATIONS OF
PULMONARY AND PLEURAL INJURY;
DUODENAL INJURIES*

Riyad Karmy-Jones, MD, FACS
Medical Director, Thoracic and Vascular
Surgery
Southwest Washington Medical Center
Vancouver, Washington

*OPERATIVE MANAGEMENT OF PULMONARY
INJURIES: LUNG-SPARING AND FORMAL
RESECTIONS; COMPLICATIONS OF
PULMONARY AND PLEURAL INJURY*

Tamer Karsidag, MD
Research Fellow
Division of Trauma Surgery and Surgical
Critical Care
University of Southern California
Los Angeles, California

*EXSANGUINATION: RELIABLE MODELS TO
INDICATE DAMAGE CONTROL*

Donald R. Kauder, MD, FACS
Associate Director, Trauma Services
Trauma and Emergency Surgery
Riverside Regional Medical Center
Newport News, Virginia

TRAUMA IN THE ELDERLY

Larry T. Khoo, MD
Assistant Professor, Division of
Neurosurgery
UCLA Medical Center
Los Angeles, California
Chief of Neurosurgery
UCLA Spine Center
Santa Monica, California

*SPINE: SPINAL CORD INJURY, BLUNT AND
PENETRATING, NEUROGENIC AND SPINAL
SHOCK*

Booker T. King, MD
Fellow, Trauma Surgery and Surgical
Critical Care
Leonard M. Miller School of Medicine at
University of Miami
Miami, Florida

BLAST INJURIES; ACUTE RESPIRATORY DISTRESS SYNDROME

David R. King, MD
Trauma Surgery and Surgical Critical Care
Fellow
Fellow, Trauma Surgery, Endovascular Surgery, and Surgical Critical Care
Division of Trauma
Department of Surgery
University of Miami Miller School of Medicine
Ryder Trauma Center
Jackson Memorial Medical Center
Miami, Florida

*OPERATIVE MANAGEMENT OF PULMONARY
INJURIES: LUNG-SPARING AND FORMAL
RESECTIONS*

Laszlo Kiraly, MD
Resident, General Surgery
Department of Surgery
Oregon Health & Science University
Portland, Oregon

RESUSCITATION FLUIDS

**Orlando C. Kirton, MD, FACS, FCCM,
FCCP**
Professor of Surgery and Vice Chair
Department of Surgery
University of Connecticut School of
Medicine
Farmington, Connecticut
Ludwig J. Pyrtek, MD Chair in Surgery
Director of Surgery
Department of Surgery
Hartford Hospital
Hartford, Connecticut

*PHARMACOLOGIC SUPPORT OF CARDIAC
FAILURE*

Michael F. Ksycki, DO
Surgery and Surgical Critical Care Fellow
Fellow, Trauma Critical Care
Ryder Trauma Center
Jackson Memorial Hospital
Miami, Florida
Trauma Fellow, Memorial Regional
Hospital
Hollywood, Florida

EMERGENCY DEPARTMENT THORACOTOMY

Anna M. Ledgerwood, MD, FACS
Professor, Department of Surgery
Wayne State University
Active Staff/Trauma Director
Detroit Receiving Hospital
Active Staff
Harper University Hospital
Detroit, Michigan

DIAPHRAGMATIC INJURY

**Guy Lin, MD, MA, Colonel
(IDF—reserve)**
Trauma and Critical Care Fellow
Ryder Trauma Center
Jackson Memorial Hospital
Miami, Florida

BLAST INJURIES

Edward Lineen, MD
Fellow, Trauma Surgery and Surgical
Critical Care
University of Miami
Jackson Memorial Hospital
Miami, Florida

*EXSANGUINATION: RELIABLE MODELS TO
INDICATE DAMAGE CONTROL*

David H. Livingston, MD, FACS
Wesley J. Howe Professor and Chief of
Trauma Surgery
Department of Surgery
New Jersey Medical School
Newark, New Jersey

*THORACIC WALL INJURIES: RIBS, STERNAL
SCAPULAR FRACTURES, HEMOTHORACES,
AND PNEUMOTHORACES; PULMONARY
CONTUSION AND FLAIL CHEST*

Charles E. Lucas, MD, FACS
Professor, Department of Surgery
Wayne State University
Active Staff, Detroit Receiving Hospital
Active Staff, Harper University Hospital
Detroit, Michigan

DIAPHRAGMATIC INJURY

Fred A. Luchette, MD, MS, FACS
Director, Division of Trauma, Critical Care,
and Burns
Ambrose and Gladys Bowyer Professor of
Surgery
Loyola University Stritch School of Medicine
Director of Trauma
Loyola University Medical Center
Maywood, Illinois

*SURGICAL TECHNIQUES FOR THORACIC,
ABDOMINAL, PELVIC, AND EXTREMITY
DAMAGE CONTROL*

Mauricio Lynn, MD
Associate Professor of Surgery
DeWitt Daughtry Family Department of
Surgery
University of Miami
Medical Director, Trauma Resuscitation Unit
Ryder Trauma Center
Jackson Memorial Medical Center
Miami, Florida

*TRAUMA SYSTEMS AND TRAUMA TRIAGE
ALGORITHMS; BLAST INJURIES*

Robert C. Mackersie, MD, FACS
Trauma/Critical Care
Department of Surgery
University of California San Francisco
San Francisco General Hospital
San Francisco, California

*CARDIAC HEMODYNAMICS: THE
PULMONARY ARTERY CATHETER
AND THE MEANING OF ITS READINGS*

Louis J. Magnotti, MD, FACS
Assistant Professor, Department of Surgery
University of Tennessee Health Science Center
Memphis, Tennessee

PANCREATIC INJURIES

John W. Mah, MD
Assistant Professor, Department of Surgery
University of Connecticut School of Medicine
Farmington, Connecticut
Associate Director, Surgical Intensive Care
Hartford Hospital
Hartford, Connecticut

*PHARMACOLOGIC SUPPORT OF CARDIAC
FAILURE*

George O. Maish III, MD, FACS
Assistant Professor, Department of Surgery
University of Tennessee Health Science Center
Assistant Professor, Department of Surgery
Regional Medical Center at Memphis
Memphis, Tennessee

*INTERVENTIONAL RADIOLOGY: DIAGNOSTICS
AND THERAPEUTICS*

Ajai K. Malhotra, MD
Assistant Professor, Department of Surgery
Virginia Commonwealth University
Richmond, Virginia

*DIAGNOSTIC AND THERAPEUTIC ROLES OF
BRONCHOSCOPY AND VIDEO-ASSISTED
THORACOSCOPY IN THE MANAGEMENT OF
THORACIC TRAUMA*

Matthew J. Martin, MD
Associate Professor, Department of Surgery
Uniformed Services University of Health
Sciences
Bethesda, Maryland
Chief, Trauma and Surgical Critical Care
Department of Surgery
Madigan Army Medical Center
Tacoma, Washington
Trauma Surgeon
Department of Surgery
Legacy Emanuel Hospital
Portland, Oregon

*NONOPERATIVE MANAGEMENT OF BLUNT
AND PENETRATING ABDOMINAL INJURIES*

Antonio Carlos C. Marttos Jr., MD
Assistant Professor of Surgery
Dewitt Daughtry Department of
Surgery—Division of Trauma and Surgical
Critical Care
University of Miami Miller School of
Medicine
Miami, Florida

*TRAUMA SYSTEMS AND TRAUMA TRIAGE
ALGORITHMS*

Kenneth Mattox, MD, FACS
Professor and Vice Chair
Michael E. DeBakey Department of Surgery
Baylor College of Medicine
Chief of Staff and Chief of Surgery
Ben Taub General Hospital
Houston, Texas

THORACIC VASCULAR INJURY

Kimball I. Maull, MD, FACS
Director of Trauma Services
Hamad General Hospital
Doha, Qatar
Consultant
International Services
University of Pittsburgh Medical Center
Pittsburgh, Pennsylvania

SMALL BOWEL INJURY

John C. Mayberry, MD, FACS
Associate Professor of Surgery
Trauma/Surgical Critical Care
Oregon Health & Science University
Portland, Oregon

*WOUND BALLISTICS: WHAT EVERY TRAUMA
SURGEON SHOULD KNOW; PERTINENT
SURGICAL ANATOMY OF THE THORAX AND
MEDIASTINUM*

Christopher A. McFarren, MD
Assistant Professor of Medicine
Division of Nephrology and Hypertension
Department of Internal Medicine
University of South Florida College of
Medicine
Tampa, Florida

*THE MANAGEMENT OF RENAL FAILURE:
RENAL REPLACEMENT THERAPY AND
DIALYSIS*

Mark G. McKenney, MD, FACS
Professor of Surgery and Chief
Trauma and Surgical Critical Care
DeWitt Daughtry Family Department of
Surgery
University of Miami Miller School of
Medicine
Miami, Florida

*THE ROLE OF FOCUSED ASSESSMENT WITH
SONOGRAPHY FOR TRAUMA: INDICATIONS,
LIMITATIONS, AND CONTROVERSIES*

Mario A. Meallet, MD
Assistant Professor, Ophthalmology
Doheny Eye Institute/LA County + USC
Medical Center
Los Angeles, California

TRAUMA TO THE EYE AND ORBIT

Mark M. Melendez, MD, MBA
Senior Resident
Clinical Assistant Instructor
Department of Surgery
Stony Brook University
Senior Resident
Clinical Assistant Instructor
Department of Surgery
Stony Brook University Medical Center
Stony Brook, New York

*ADVANCED TECHNIQUES IN MECHANICAL
VENTILATION*

J. Wayne Meredith, MD, FACS
Richard T. Myers Professor and Chair
Department of Surgery
Wake Forest University School of Medicine
Chief of Surgery
Wake Forest University Baptist Medical
Center
Winston Salem, North Carolina

*TRACHEAL AND TRACHEOBRONCHIAL TREE
INJURIES*

Christopher P. Michetti, MD, FACS
Medical Director, Trauma ICU
Inova Fairfax Hospital
Assistant Professor, Department of
Surgery
Virginia Commonwealth University School
of Medicine, Inova Campus
Falls Church, Virginia

*MANAGEMENT OF COAGULATION DISOR-
DERS IN THE SURGICAL INTENSIVE CARE
UNIT*

Preston Roy Miller, MD, FACS
Assistant Professor, Department of Surgery
Wake Forest University
Winston Salem, North Carolina

*TRACHEAL AND TRACHEOBRONCHIAL TREE
INJURIES*

Richard S. Miller, MD, FACS
Professor of Surgery
Department of Surgery/Trauma and
Surgical Critical Care
Director of the Trauma Intensive Care Unit
Vanderbilt University Medical Center
Nashville, Tennessee

*ABDOMINAL COMPARTMENT SYNDROME,
DAMAGE CONTROL, AND THE
POST-TRAUMATIC OPEN ABDOMEN*

Joseph P. Minei, MD, FACS
Professor and Vice Chair
Department of Surgery
University of Texas Southwestern Medical
Center
Medical Director, Surgical and Trauma Ser-
vices
Parkland Memorial Hospital
Dallas, Texas

*THE DIAGNOSIS AND MANAGEMENT OF
CARDIAC DYSRHYTHMIAS*

**Frank (Tres) Louis Mitchell III, MD,
MHA, FACS**
Medical Director, Trauma and Surgical Crit-
ical Care
St. John Medical Center
Tulsa, Oklahoma

*COMMON PREHOSPITAL COMPLICATIONS
AND PITFALLS IN THE TRAUMA PATIENT*

Alicia M. Mohr, MD, FACS
Associate Professor of Surgery
Department of Surgery
University of Medicine and Dentistry of
New Jersey—New Jersey Medical School
Newark, New Jersey

*EXSANGUINATION: RELIABLE MODELS TO
INDICATE DAMAGE CONTROL; SURGICAL
PROCEDURES IN THE SURGICAL INTENSIVE
CARE UNIT*

Ernest E. Moore, MD, FACS
Professor and Vice Chair, Surgery
University of Colorado Health Sciences
Center
Chief of Surgery
Denver Health
Bruce M. Rockwell Distinguished Chair in
Trauma Surgery
Rocky Mountain Regional Trauma Center
Denver Health Medical Center
Denver, Colorado

BLUNT CEREBROVASCULAR INJURIES

Boris Mordikovich, MD
Division of Plastic Surgery
Department of Surgery
University of Medicine and Dentistry of
New Jersey—New Jersey Medical School
Newark, New Jersey

*EXTREMITY REPLANTATION: INDICATIONS
AND TIMING*

Amanda J. Morehouse, MD, FACS
Surgical Critical Care Fellow
Department of Surgery
Division of Trauma and Surgical Critical
Care
Jackson Memorial Hospital
Miami, Florida

*EXSANGUINATION: RELIABLE MODELS TO
INDICATE DAMAGE CONTROL*

John A. Morris Jr., MD, FACS
Professor of Surgery
Vanderbilt University Medical Center
Nashville, Tennessee

*ABDOMINAL COMPARTMENT SYNDROME,
DAMAGE CONTROL, AND THE
POST-TRAUMATIC OPEN ABDOMEN*

Anne C. Mosenthal, MD, FACS
Associate Professor of Surgery
Department of Surgery
University of Medicine and Dentistry of
New Jersey—New Jersey Medical School
Newark, New Jersey

*PALLIATIVE CARE IN THE TRAUMA INTEN-
SIVE CARE UNIT; DEATH FROM TRAUMA—
MANAGEMENT OF GRIEF AND BEREAVE-
MENT AND THE ROLE OF THE SURGEON*

Patricia Murphy, PhD, APN, FAAN
Clinical Associate Professor of Surgery
New Jersey Medical School
APN Ethics/Bereavement
Patient Care Services
University of Medicine and Dentistry of
New Jersey—University Hospital
Newark, New Jersey

*DEATH FROM TRAUMA—MANAGEMENT OF
GRIEF AND BEREAVEMENT AND THE ROLE
OF THE SURGEON*

Nicholas Namias, MD, FACS
Associate Professor of Surgery
Division of Trauma and Surgical Critical
Care
DeWitt Daughtry Family Department
of Surgery
University of Miami Miller School of
Medicine
Miami, Florida

CARDIAC INJURIES

**Lena M. Napolitano, MD, FACS, FCCP,
FCCM**
Professor of Surgery
Division Chief, Acute Care Surgery
Associate Chair of Surgery for Critical Care
Director, Surgical Critical Care
University of Michigan Health System
Ann Arbor, Michigan

*TRANSFUSION: MANAGEMENT OF BLOOD
AND BLOOD PRODUCTS IN TRAUMA*

Mark A. Newell, MD, FACS
Assistant Professor, Department of Surgery
Brody School of Medicine at East Carolina
University
Attending Surgeon
Trauma and Surgical Critical Care
Pitt County Memorial Hospital
University Health Systems of Eastern
Carolina
Greenville, North Carolina

*PREHOSPITAL FLUID RESUSCITATION: WHAT
TYPE, HOW MUCH, AND CONTROVERSIES*

R. Joseph Nold, MD, FACS
Clinical Assistant Professor, Department of
Surgery—Trauma/Critical Care
University of Kansas School Of
Medicine—Wichita
Via Christi Regional Medical Center
Wesley Medical Center
Wichita, Kansas

COMMON ERRORS IN TRAUMA CARE

Scott H. Norwood, MD, FACS
Director, Trauma Services
East Texas Medical Center
Tyler, Texas

*TRACHEAL, LARYNGEAL, AND
OROPHARYNGEAL INJURIES*

Juan B. Ochoa, MD, FACS
Professor of Surgery and Critical Care
Associate Medical Director for UPMC
Trauma Services
University of Pittsburgh
Pittsburgh, Pennsylvania

OXYGEN TRANSPORT

Turner Osler, MD, MSc (Biostatistics)
Research Professor, Department of Surgery
University of Vermont
Research Professor, Department of Surgery
Fletcher Allen Hospital
Colchester, Vermont

*INJURY SEVERITY SCORING: ITS DEFINITION
AND PRACTICAL APPLICATION*

H. Leon Pachter, MD, FACS
The George David Stewart Professor and
Chair
New York University School of Medicine
New York, New York
LIVER INJURY

Manish Parikh, MD
Chief Surgical Resident
New York University School of Medicine
and The Bellevue Hospital Shock Trauma
Unit
New York, New York
LIVER INJURY

Michael D. Pasquale, MD, FACS
Associate Professor of Surgery
Pennsylvania State University College of
Medicine
Hershey, Pennsylvania
Senior Vice Chair, Department of Surgery
Division Chief
Trauma/Surgical Critical Care
Lehigh Valley Hospital
Allentown, Pennsylvania
TRAUMA REHABILITATION

Andrew B. Peitzman, MD, FACS
Executive Vice Chair
Chief General Surgery
University of Pittsburgh School of Medicine
Pittsburgh, Pennsylvania
*CURRENT CONCEPTS IN THE DIAGNOSIS
AND MANAGEMENT OF HEMORRHAGIC
SHOCK*

Antonio Pepe, MD, FRCSC
Assistant Professor of Surgery
Division of Trauma and Surgical Critical Care
University of Miami
Miami, Florida
*TRAUMA SYSTEMS AND TRAUMA TRIAGE
ALGORITHMS; BLAST INJURIES*

Patrizio Petrone, MD
Chief, International Fellows
Department of Surgery
USC+LAC Medical Center
Assistant Professor of Surgery
University of Southern California Keck
School of Medicine
Senior Research Associate
Department of Surgery
USC University Hospital
Los Angeles, California
*EMERGENCY DEPARTMENT THORACOTOMY;
CAROTID, VERTEBRAL ARTERY, AND JUGULAR
VENOUS INJURIES; OPERATIVE MANAGE-
MENT OF PULMONARY INJURIES: LUNG-
SPARING AND FORMAL RESECTIONS; CAR-
DIAC INJURIES; GYNECOLOGIC INJURIES;
EXSANGUINATION: RELIABLE MODELS TO
INDICATE DAMAGE CONTROL*

Louis R. Pizano, MD, FACS
Assistant Professor of Clinical Surgery
DeWitt Daughtry Family Department of
Surgery
University of Miami
Attending Physician, Department of
Trauma and Burns
Jackson Health System
Attending Physician, Department of Surgery
Veterans Administration Hospital
Attending Physician, Department of Surgery
University of Miami Hospital and Clinics
Miami, Florida
*OPERATIVE MANAGEMENT OF PULMONARY
INJURIES: LUNG-SPARING AND FORMAL
RESECTIONS; CARDIAC INJURIES*

Patricio M. Polanco, MD
Postdoctoral Fellow, Department of Surgery
Division of Trauma
University of Pittsburgh
General Surgery Resident
Department of Surgery
University of Pittsburgh
Pittsburgh, Pennsylvania
OXYGEN TRANSPORT

Juan Carlos Puyana, MD, FACS
Associate Professor of Surgery and Critical
Care Medicine
University of Pittsburgh
Chief Medical Officer
Innovative Medical Information
Technologies Center
University of Pittsburgh Medical Center
Pittsburgh, Pennsylvania
*CURRENT CONCEPTS IN THE DIAGNOSIS
AND MANAGEMENT OF HEMORRHAGIC
SHOCK; OXYGEN TRANSPORT*

Amritha Raghunathan, BS
Department of Surgery
Division of Trauma, Emergency, and
Critical Care Surgery
Stanford University Medical Center
Stanford, California
NOSOCOMIAL PNEUMONIA

R. Lawrence Reed II, MD, FACS
Professor of Surgery
Attending Surgeon
Department of Surgery
Loyola University Medical Center
Maywood, Illinois
Director, Surgical Intensive Care Unit
Department of Surgery
Edward Hines Jr. VA Hospital
Hines, Illinois
HYPOTHERMIA AND TRAUMA

**Peter M. Rhee, MD, MPH, FACS,
FCCM, DMCC**
Professor of Surgery
University of Arizona
Director of Trauma, Critical Care, and
Emergency Surgery
University Medical Center
Tucson, Arizona
*NONOPERATIVE MANAGEMENT OF BLUNT
AND PENETRATING ABDOMINAL INJURIES*

Samuel T. Rhee, MD
Assistant Professor
Division of Plastic Surgery
Department of Surgery
Weill Cornell Medical College
New York Presbyterian Hospital
New York, New York
Clinical Assistant Professor
Division of Plastic Surgery
Department of Surgery
University of Medicine and Dentistry of
New Jersey—New Jersey Medical School
Newark, New Jersey
MAXILLOFACIAL INJURIES

Michael Rhodes, MD, FACS
Professor of Surgery
Thomas Jefferson University
Philadelphia, Pennsylvania
Chair, Department of Surgery
Christiana Care Health System
Wilmington, Delaware
TRAUMA OUTCOMES

Norman M. Rich, MD, FACS
Department of Surgery
Uniformed Services University of Health
Sciences
Bethesda, Maryland
VASCULAR ANATOMY OF THE EXTREMITIES

J. David Richardson, MD, FACS
Professor and Vice Chair
Director Emergency Surgical Services
Department of Surgery
University of Louisville
Louisville, Kentucky
TREATMENT OF ESOPHAGEAL INJURY

Charles M. Richart, MD, FACS
Associate Professor, Department of Surgery
University of Missouri-Kansas City
Associate Director, Trauma Surgical Critical
Care
Director, Surgical Critical Care Research
and Surgical ANH Program
Saint Luke's Hospital of Kansas City
Kansas City, Missouri
*COMMON PREHOSPITAL COMPLICATIONS
AND PITFALLS IN THE TRAUMA PATIENT*

Donald Robinson, DO
Assistant Professor of Surgery and Director
Army Trauma Centre
Division of Trauma and Surgical Critical
Care
DeWitt Daughtry Family Department of
Surgery
University of Miami
Miami, Florida

*EMERGENCY DEPARTMENT THORACOTOMY;
OPERATIVE MANAGEMENT OF PULMONARY
INJURIES: LUNG-SPARING AND FORMAL RE-
SECTIONS; CARDIAC INJURIES; EXSANGUINA-
TION: RELIABLE MODELS TO INDICATE DAM-
AGE CONTROL*

Steven E. Ross, MD, FACS
Professor of Surgery, Department of
Surgery
University of Medicine and Dentistry of
New Jersey Robert Wood Johnson Medical
School—Camden
Head, Division of Trauma
Cooper University Hospital
Camden, New Jersey

*THE USE OF COMPUTED TOMOGRAPHY IN
INITIAL TRAUMA EVALUATION*

Michael F. Rotondo, MD, FACS
Professor and Chair, Department of Surgery
Brody School of Medicine
East Carolina University
Chief, Department of Surgery
Pitt County Memorial Hospital
Director, Center for Excellence for Trauma
and Surgical Critical Care
University Health Systems of Eastern
Carolina
Greenville, North Carolina

*PREHOSPITAL FLUID RESUSCITATION: WHAT
TYPE, HOW MUCH, AND CONTROVERSIES*

Vincent Lopez Rowe, MD, FACS
Assistant Professor of Surgery
Keck USC School of Medicine
Los Angeles, California

*CAROTID, VERTEBRAL ARTERY, AND JUGULAR
VENOUS INJURIES*

Francisco Alexander Ruiz Zelaya, MD
International Visiting Scholar and Trauma
Research Fellow
Department of Surgery, Trauma Surgery,
and Surgical Critical Care
University of Miami Miller School of
Medicine
Ryder Trauma Center
Miami, Florida

*EMERGENCY DEPARTMENT
THORACOTOMY*

Alisa Savetamal, MD
Bridgeport Hospital
Trauma, Burns, and Critical Care
Bridgeport, Connecticut

*THORACIC WALL INJURIES: RIBS, STERNAL
SCAPULAR FRACTURES, HEMOTHORACES,
AND PNEUMOTHORACES*

Thomas M. Scalea, MD, FACS
Physician-in-Chief
R. Adams Cowley Shock Trauma Center
Director, Program in Trauma
University of Maryland School of
Medicine
Baltimore, Maryland

*SURGICAL ANATOMY OF THE ABDOMEN
AND RETROPERITONEUM; MULTIDISCI-
PLINARY MANAGEMENT OF PELVIC FRAC-
TURES: OPERATIVE AND NON-OPERATIVE
HEMOSTASIS*

William P. Schecter, MD, FACS
Professor of Clinical Surgery
University of California, San Francisco
Chief of Surgery
San Francisco General Hospital
San Francisco, California

*CIVILIAN HOSPITAL RESPONSE TO MASS
CASUALTY EVENTS*

L. R. Tres Scherer III, MD, FACS
Professor, Department of Surgery
Indiana University School of Medicine
Director of Trauma
Riley Hospital for Children
Indianapolis, Indiana

PEDIATRIC TRAUMA

Paul Schipper, MD
Assistant Professor of Surgery
Section of General Thoracic Surgery
Division of Cardiothoracic Surgery
Oregon Health & Science University
Portland, Oregon

*PERTINENT SURGICAL ANATOMY
OF THE THORAX AND MEDIASTINUM*

Martin A. Schreiber, MD, FACS
Associate Professor of Surgery
Chief of Trauma and Surgical Critical Care
Oregon Health & Science University
Portland, Oregon

*RESUSCITATION FLUIDS; ENDPOINTS
OF RESUSCITATION*

Carl Schulman, MD, FACS
Assistant Professor of Surgery
Director, Injury Prevention Education
William Lehman Injury Research Center/
Medical Computer Systems Laboratory
University of Miami
Ryder Trauma Center
Miami, Florida

EMERGENCY DEPARTMENT THORACOTOMY

C. William Schwab, MD, FACS
Professor of Surgery
Department of Surgery
University of Pennsylvania School of Medicine
Chief, Division of Traumatology and
Surgical Critical Care
University of Pennsylvania Medical Center
Philadelphia, Pennsylvania

TRAUMA IN THE ELDERLY

Marc J. Shapiro, MD, FACS
Professor of Surgery and Anesthesiology
Department of Surgery
State University of New York—Stony Brook
Chief of General Surgery, Trauma, Critical
Care, and Burns
University Hospital—Stony Brook
Stony Brook, New York

*FUNDAMENTALS OF MECHANICAL
VENTILATION; ADVANCED TECHNIQUES IN
MECHANICAL VENTILATION; ANTIBACTERIAL
THERAPY: THE OLD, THE NEW, AND THE
FUTURE; FUNGAL INFECTIONS AND
ANTIFUNGAL THERAPY IN THE SURGICAL
INTENSIVE CARE UNIT*

David V. Shatz, MD, FACS
Professor of Surgery
Department of Surgery
Division of Trauma, Burns, and Surgical
Critical Care
University of Miami School of Medicine
Attending Trauma Surgeon
Jackson Memorial Hospital
Miami, Florida

*THE ROLE OF FOCUSED ASSESSMENT WITH
SONOGRAPHY FOR TRAUMA: INDICATIONS,
LIMITATIONS, AND CONTROVERSIES*

Ziad C. Sifri, MD
Assistant Professor of Surgery
Department of Surgery
Division of Trauma
University of Medicine and Dentistry of
New Jersey—New Jersey Medical School
Newark, New Jersey

*LOWER EXTREMITY VASCULAR INJURIES:
FEMORAL, POPLITEAL, AND SHANK VESSEL
INJURY; SURGICAL PROCEDURES IN THE
SURGICAL INTENSIVE CARE UNIT*

Amy C. Sisley, MD, MPH
R. Adams Cowley Shock Trauma Center
University of Maryland Medical Center
Baltimore, Maryland

TRAUMA IN PREGNANCY

L. Ola Sjoholm, MD
Attending Surgeon
Department of Surgery
Cooper University Hospital
Camden, New Jersey

*THE USE OF COMPUTED TOMOGRAPHY
IN INITIAL TRAUMA EVALUATION*

R. Stephen Smith, MD, RDMS, FACS
Professor of Surgery
University of Kansas School of Medicine
Wichita, Kansas

*DIAGNOSTIC PERITONEAL LAVAGE AND
LAPAROSCOPY IN EVALUATION OF
ABDOMINAL TRAUMA; COMMON ERRORS
IN TRAUMA CARE*

Eduardo Smith-Singares, MD
Department of Surgery
State University of New York
Stony Brook University Health Sciences
Center
Stony Brook, New York

*FUNGAL INFECTIONS AND ANTIFUNGAL
THERAPY IN THE SURGICAL INTENSIVE
CARE UNIT*

David A. Spain, MD, FACS
Professor, School of Medicine, Department
of Surgery
Chief of Trauma, Emergency and Critical
Care Surgery
Program Director, Surgical Critical Care
Fellowship, Department of Surgery
Associate Division Chief, Department of
Surgery
Stanford University Medical Center
Stanford, California

NOSOCOMIAL PNEUMONIA

Jason L. Sperry, MD, MPH
Assistant Professor of Surgery
Department of Surgery and Critical Care
Medicine
University of Pittsburgh Medical Center
Pittsburgh, Pennsylvania

*THE DIAGNOSIS AND MANAGEMENT OF
CARDIAC DYSRHYTHMIAS*

Kenneth D. Stahl, MD, FACS
Fellow, Trauma Surgery and Surgical Critical
Care
Division of Trauma and Surgical Critical Care
DeWitt Daughtry Family Department of
Medicine
University of Miami Miller School of Medi-
cine
Miami, Florida

EMERGENCY DEPARTMENT THORACOTOMY

Mithran S. Sukumar, MD
Assistant Professor of Surgery
Oregon Health & Science University
Section Head, General Thoracic Surgery
Division of Cardiothoracic Surgery
Portland VA Medical Center
Portland, Oregon

*PERTINENT SURGICAL ANATOMY OF THE
THORAX AND MEDIASTINUM*

Kenneth G. Swan, MD, FACS
Professor, Department of Surgery
University of Medicine and Dentistry of
New Jersey—New Jersey Medical School
Newark, New Jersey

*PREHOSPITAL CARE OF BIOLOGICAL
AGENT–INDUCED INJURIES*

Virak Tan, MD
Associate Professor, Department of
Orthopaedics
Fellowship Director—Hand, Upper Extrem-
ity, and Microvascular Surgery
University of Medicine and Dentistry of
New Jersey—New Jersey Medical School
Attending Surgeon, Department of
Orthopaedics
University Hospital
Newark, New Jersey
Attending Surgeon, Division of Orthopae-
dic Surgery—Department of Surgery
Overlook Hospital
Summit, New Jersey

*UPPER EXTREMITY FRACTURES:
ORTHOPEDIC MANAGEMENT*

Vartan S. Tashjian, MD, MS
Resident Surgeon
Division of Neurological Surgery
Resident Surgeon
Division of Neurosurgery
University of California, Los Angeles
Los Angeles, California

*SPINE: SPINAL CORD INJURY, BLUNT AND
PENETRATING, NEUROGENIC AND SPINAL
SHOCK*

Robert L. Tatsumi, MD
Chief Resident
Orthopaedics and Rehabilitation
Oregon Health & Science University
Portland, Oregon

*CERVICAL, THORACIC, AND LUMBAR
FRACTURES*

Tedla Tessema
Fellow, Trauma Surgery and Surgical
Critical Care
Department of Surgery
Division of Trauma Surgery
University of Miami Miller School of
Medicine
Miami, Florida

BLAST INJURIES

Erwin R. Thal, MD, FACS
Professor of Surgery
University of Texas Southwestern Medical
School
Dallas, Texas

*TRAUMA CENTER ORGANIZATION AND
VERIFICATION*

Brandon Tieu, MD
Resident, General Surgery
Oregon Health & Science University
Portland, Oregon

*RESUSCITATION FLUIDS; ENDPOINTS OF
RESUSCITATION*

Areti Tillou, MD
Associate Professor
UCLA David Geffen School of Medicine
Los Angeles, California

GYNECOLOGIC INJURIES

Glen H. Tinkoff, MD, FACS, FCCM
Clinical Associate Professor of Surgery
Thomas Jefferson University
Philadelphia, Pennsylvania
Medical Director of Trauma
Associate Director, Surgical Critical Care
Christiana Care Health Services
Newark, Delaware

TRAUMA OUTCOMES

Samuel A. Tisherman, MD, FACS
Associate Professor, Surgery and Critical
Care Medicine
University of Pittsburgh
Pittsburgh, Pennsylvania

*CURRENT CONCEPTS IN THE DIAGNOSIS
AND MANAGEMENT OF HEMORRHAGIC
SHOCK*

S. Rob Todd, MD, FACS
Assistant Professor of Surgery
General Surgery, Trauma, and Surgical
Critical Care
University of Texas Medical
School—Houston
Houston, Texas

THE IMMUNOLOGY OF TRAUMA

Peter G. Trafton, MD, FACS
Professor and Vice Chair
Department of Orthopaedic Surgery
Brown University School of Medicine
Providence, Rhode Island

LOWER EXTREMITY AND DEGLOVING INJURY

Matthew J. Trovato, MD
Fellow, Division of Plastic Surgery
University of Medicine and Dentistry of
New Jersey—New Jersey Medical School
Newark, New Jersey

*TECHNIQUES IN THE MANAGEMENT OF
COMPLEX MUSCULOSKELETAL INJURY:
ROLES OF MUSCLE, MUSCULOCUTANEOUS,
AND FASCIOCUTANEOUS FLAPS*

Donald D. Trunkey, MD, FACS
Professor and Chair
Department of Surgery
Oregon Health & Science University
Portland, Oregon

*THE DEVELOPMENT OF TRAUMA SYSTEMS;
WOUND BALLISTICS: WHAT EVERY TRAUMA
SURGEON SHOULD KNOW; LOWER
EXTREMITY AND DEGLOVING INJURY*

Glenn S. Tse, MD
Assistant Professor, Department of
Surgery
University of California, Davis
Sacramento, California

SPLENIC INJURIES

David W. Tuggle, MD, FACS
Chief, Pediatric Surgery
Vice Chair, Department of Surgery
Paula Milburn Miller/CMRI Chair in
Pediatric Surgery
University of Oklahoma College of
Medicine
Oklahoma City, Oklahoma

PEDIATRIC TRAUMA

Alex B. Valadka, MD, FACS
Professor and Vice Chair
Department of Neurosurgery
University of Texas Medical School at
Houston
Houston, Texas

*TRAUMATIC BRAIN INJURY:
PATHOPHYSIOLOGY, CLINICAL DIAGNOSIS,
AND PREHOSPITAL AND EMERGENCY
CENTER CARE; TRAUMATIC BRAIN INJURY:
IMAGING, OPERATIVE AND NONOPERATIVE
CARE, AND COMPLICATIONS*

Nicole M. VanDerHeyden, MD, PhD
Trauma Medical Director, Trauma Services
Salem Hospital
Salem, Oregon

TRAUMA SCORING

Alexander D. Vara
Undergraduate Student
Biology
University of Miami
Coral Gables, Florida
Research Assistant
Ryder Trauma Center
Jackson Memorial Hospital
Miami, Florida

*EMERGENCY DEPARTMENT THORACOTOMY;
OPERATIVE MANAGEMENT OF PULMONARY
INJURIES: LUNG-SPARING AND FORMAL
RESECTIONS; CARDIAC INJURIES;
EXSANGUINATION: RELIABLE MODELS TO
INDICATE DAMAGE CONTROL*

Ricardo Verdiner, MD
Resident, Department of Anesthesiology
University of Medicine and Dentistry of
New Jersey
Newark, New Jersey

*ANESTHESIA IN THE SURGICAL INTENSIVE
CARE UNIT—BEYOND THE AIRWAY:
NEUROMUSCULAR PARALYSIS AND PAIN
MANAGEMENT*

Matthew J. Wall Jr., MD, FACS
Professor, Michael E. DeBakey Department
of Surgery
Baylor College of Medicine
Deputy Chief of Surgery
Chief of Cardiothoracic Surgery
Ben Taub General Hospital
Houston, Texas

THORACIC VASCULAR INJURY

Anthony Watkins, MD
Resident, Department of Surgery and Burns
University of Medicine and Dentistry of
New Jersey—New Jersey Medical School
Newark, New Jersey

*SYSTEMIC INFLAMMATORY RESPONSE
SYNDROME AND MULTIPLE-ORGAN
DYSFUNCTION SYNDROME: DEFINITION,
DIAGNOSIS, AND MANAGEMENT*

Leonard J. Weireter Jr., MD, FACS
Professor of Surgery
Chief, Division of Trauma and Critical Care
Department of Surgery
Eastern Virginia Medical School
Norfolk, Virginia

*PENETRATING NECK INJURIES: DIAGNOSIS
AND SELECTIVE MANAGEMENT*

John S. Weston
Medical Student
University of Miami Miller School of
Medicine
Miami, Florida

*EMERGENCY DEPARTMENT THORACOTOMY;
OPERATIVE MANAGEMENT OF PULMONARY
INJURIES: LUNG-SPARING AND FORMAL
RESECTIONS; CARDIAC INJURIES; EXSANGUI-
NATION: RELIABLE MODELS TO INDICATE
DAMAGE CONTROL*

Harry E. Wilkins III, MD
Associate Professor, Department of Surgery
University of Missouri-Kansas City
Medical Director, Trauma and Surgical
Critical Care
Saint Luke's Hospital of Kansas City
Kansas City, Missouri

*COMMON PREHOSPITAL COMPLICATIONS
AND PITFALLS IN THE TRAUMA PATIENT*

D. Brandon Williams, MD
Department of Surgery
Division of Trauma, Emergency, and
Critical Care Surgery
Stanford University Medical Center
Stanford, California

NOSOCOMIAL PNEUMONIA

David H. Wisner, MD, FACS
Professor and Vice Chair
Department of Surgery
University of California, Davis
Chief of Trauma Surgery
University of California, Davis Medical
Center
Sacramento, California

SPLENIC INJURIES

FOREWORD

Current Therapy of Trauma has become the leading text for trauma management. *Current Therapy of Trauma and Surgical Critical Care,* a new volume in the *Current Therapy* series, builds on the infrastructure and credibility of the four previous volumes of *Current Therapy of Trauma,* and it includes critical care and aspects of rehabilitation as well. With these additions, Dr. Juan A. Asensio and Dr. Donald D. Trunkey now cover the full continuum of care—prevention, injury, prehospital treatment, triage, diagnosis, injury management, and postoperative care. The social consequences of trauma have been emphasized since the first edition of *Current Therapy of Trauma.* Unfortunately, traumatic injury is still the leading cause of lost years of productive life, surpassing cardiac disease, cancer, and stroke. However, no one young or old is immune to this disease. The ubiquitous, dramatic, and immediate nature of this medical malady means that this book will be valuable for many health care professionals, including emergency physicians, intensivists, residents, medical students, nurses, fire–rescue personnel—and not just surgeons.

Leading specialists who have busy clinical practices are the authors of the chapters, and they have contributed to this book because of its stature in the field of trauma care. Their emphasis has been on a practical approach to clinical problems following the principles of evidence-based medicine. Controversies are addressed, but the focus is on preferred treatment approaches. The evolving field of nonoperative management of blunt and penetrating trauma is critically reviewed and updated. The section on critical care is valuable and comprehensive in scope, but not overwhelming. There are even chapters on special issues, including trauma at the extremes of life and in pregnancy, palliative care in the intensive care unit, and management of grief.

Trauma and critical care have undergone rapid growth and maturation. The lessons taught in this book can be applied by everyone who treats trauma victims, and no one interested in their management could read it and not come away better prepared to take care of these patients. Dr. Trunkey has been one of the forces behind the *Current Therapy of Trauma* reference text since its inception, and the addition of Dr. Asensio represents a symbolic passing of the torch to the next generation of trauma surgeons dedicated to making a difference in this devastating and costly disease.

ALAN S. LIVINGSTONE, MD, FACS
DeWitt Daughtry Professor and Chair
Department of Surgery
University of Miami Miller School of Medicine

It is a privilege and an honor to serve as the editor of *Current Therapy of Trauma and Surgical Critical Care*. This book follows in the footsteps of the four previous volumes of *Current Therapy of Trauma*, borne out of the concerns of two of America's most distinguished trauma surgeons: Donald D. Trunkey, considered the dean of all trauma surgeons in the world, and Frank R. Lewis, who serves as executive director of the American Board of Surgery and guides the destinies of American surgery.

Stephen Ambrose, one of America's most distinguished historians, quoted Shakespeare's *Henry V* to describe Easy Company, 501 parachute infantry regiment (PIR), 101 Airborne Division as a "Band of Brothers," a symbol of what America has stood and stands for. Having the privilege of considering Frank Perconte, another Illinois boy of immigrant roots, a father figure, friend, and brother, I rise also to quote Shakespeare in describing America's trauma surgeons:

> That he which hath no stomach to this fight, let him depart; his passport shall be made and crowns for convoy put in his purse: we would not die in that man's company that fears his fellowship to die with us. From this day to the ending of the world, but we in it shall be remembered; we few we happy few, we Band of Brothers; for he that today sheds his blood with me shall be my brother ... (*Henry V*, Act IV, Scene 3)

America's trauma surgeons are an elite fraternity; as a Band of Brothers, we continue to uphold the highest of surgical traditions of a fraternity of surgeons that has never hesitated to use our God-given talents to attempt to save as many lives as possible, regardless of age, race, creed, color, or gender orientation.

It is my strong belief that the honor and the privilege of attempting to save a life not only in an operating room, but also by counseling patients is indeed a noble task in the effort to eliminate trauma as a disease. We continue to hold on to the dream that we as leaders will eventually see a world in which there will be no wars and there will be greater understanding and more time and effort dedicated to the improvement of the human condition. We continue to believe that with our dedication we will make a difference, hoping to create bridges among people, leading to greater understanding and cooperation in human relations and in the field of scientific research.

These ideals and goals remain lofty, but in speaking to my colleagues, this belief is strong and continues to motivate us all. I strongly believe that the alleviation of pain and suffering and the saving of a life remains a most important commitment for those who belong to this elite fraternity, this "Band of Brothers."

Once again I challenge, I urge, I beseech all of my colleagues in trauma surgery to go beyond the walls of academia to serve those who must be served, to use the power of our profession to exercise our consciences, to serve as leaders and advocates for human rights, to heal the wounded, and to teach the future generations of those who will be given the great gift to perform trauma surgery. We must be prepared to take forth the challenge to create peace and to heal wounds because it is us and those who have come before us who have been there, holding the hands of the wounded and injured, filled with pain and crying, often inwardly, when a life is lost, and continuing to struggle to save other lives.

There are many colleagues to thank for the knowledge that has been crystallized in these pages. The genuine effort by all of the contributors to share freely of their knowledge is to be admired and commended. Our gratitude and admiration goes to them. I would like to personally thank Dr. Donald D. Trunkey for his leadership and for the passing of the torch, a responsibility that I accept with the knowledge that it will be difficult to follow in the footsteps of one of the world's foremost trauma surgeons.

There are many people that I must personally thank, but to name them all would be impossible. As parting words, I would like to say that everything is possible if we possess the love and tenderness of women and children, the strong support of friends, the advice and kindness of our elders, the power of your sword and shield, the strength of your forefathers, and the faith of your people. I thank my people as well as the Virgin of Charity, patron saint of my birthplace, Cuba (Virgen de la Caridad, Santa Patrona de Cuba—Virgen Mambisa). As parting words, I leave you with these:

> To Live in the Light of Friendship
> To Walk in the Path of Chivalry
> To Serve for the Love of Service
> —Creed of Tau Epsilon Phi

For we are truly a Band of Brothers.

JUAN A. ASENSIO, MD, FACS, FCCM
PROFESSOR OF SURGERY
DIRECTOR, TRAUMA CLINICAL RESEARCH, TRAINING
AND COMMUNITY AFFAIRS
DIRECTOR, TRAUMA SURGERY AND SURGICAL CRITICAL CARE
FELLOWSHIP
DIRECTOR, INTERNATIONAL VISITING SCHOLARS/RESEARCH
FELLOWSHIP
MEDICAL DIRECTOR FOR EDUCATION AND TRAINING,
INTERNATIONAL MEDICINE INSTITUTE
DIVISION OF TRAUMA SURGERY AND SURGICAL CRITICAL CARE
DEWITT DAUGHTRY FAMILY DEPARTMENT OF SURGERY
UNIVERSITY OF MIAMI MILLER SCHOOL OF MEDICINE
RYDER TRAUMA CENTER
MIAMI, FLORIDA
DECEMBER 13, 2007
"PATRIA Y LIBERTAD"

CONTENTS

CRITICAL CARE II, SPECIAL ISSUES AND TREATMENTS

TRAUMA SYSTEMS

THE DEVELOPMENT OF TRAUMA SYSTEMS

Donald D. Trunkey

Modern trauma care consists of three primary components: prehospital care, acute surgical care or hospital care, and rehabilitation. Ideally, a society, through state (department, province, regional, etc.) government, should provide a trauma system that ensures all three components. The purpose of this chapter is to show how trauma systems have evolved, whether or not they work, and to define current problems.

From an historical viewpoint, it is an accepted concept that trauma care and trauma systems are inextricably linked to war. What is not appreciated is that trauma systems are not recent concepts. They date back to centuries before the Common Era. It is not known for certain whether the wounds of prehistoric humans were due primarily to violence or to accident. The first solid evidence of war wounds came from a mass grave found in Egypt and date to approximately 2000 BC. The bodies of 60 soldiers were found in a sufficiently well-preserved state to show mace injuries, gaping wounds, and arrows still in the body. The Smith Papyrus records the clinical treatment of 48 cases of war wounds, and is primarily a textbook on how to treat wounds, most of which were penetrating. According to Majno, there were 147 recorded wounds in Homer's *Iliad,* with an overall mortality of 77.6%. Thirty-one soldiers sustained wounds to the head, all of which were lethal. The surgical care for a wounded Greek soldier was crude at best. However, the Greeks did recognize the need for a system of combat care. The wounded were given care in special barracks *(klisiai)* or in nearby ships. Wound care was primitive. Barbed arrowheads were removed by enlarging the wound with a knife or pushing the arrowhead through the wound. Drugs, usually derived from plants, were applied to wounds. Wounds were bound, but according to Homer, hemostasis was treated by an *"epaoide,"* that is, someone sang a song or recited a charm over the wound.

The Romans perfected the delivery of combat care and set up a system of trauma centers throughout the Empire. These trauma centers were called *valetudinaria* and were built during the 1st and 2nd centuries ACE . The remains of 25 such centers have been found, but significantly, none were found in Rome or other large cities. Of some interest, there were 11 trauma centers in Roman Britannia, more than exist in this area today. Some of the *valetudinaria* were designed to handle a combat casualty rate of up to 10%. There was a regular medical corps within the Roman legions, and at least 85 army physicians are recorded, mainly because they died and earned an epitaph.

From elsewhere in the world came other evidence that trauma systems were provided for the military. India may well have had a system of trauma care that rivaled that of the Romans. The *Artasastra,* a book written during the reign of Ashoka (269–232 BC) documented that the Indian army had an ambulance service, with well-equipped surgeons and women to prepare food and beverages. Indian medicine was specialized, and it was the *shalyarara* (surgeon) who would be called upon to treat wounds. *Shalyarara* literally means "arrow remover," as the bow and arrow was the traditional weapon for Indians.

Over the next millennium, military trauma care did not make any major advances until just before the Renaissance. Two French military surgeons, who lived 250 years apart, brought trauma care into the Age of Enlightenment.

Ambrose Paré (1510–1590) served four French kings during the time of the French-Spanish civil and religious wars. His major contributions to treating penetrating trauma included his treatment of gunshot wounds, his use of ligature instead of cautery, and the use of nutrition during the postinjury period. Paré was also much interested in prosthetic devices, and designed a number of them for amputees.

It was Dominique Larrey, Napoleon's surgeon, who addressed trauma from a systematic and organizational standpoint. Larrey introduced the concept of the "flying ambulance," the sole purpose of which was to provide rapid removal of the wounded from the battlefield. Larrey also introduced the concept of putting the hospital as close to the front lines as feasible in order to permit wound surgery as soon as possible. His primary intent was to operate during the period of "wound shock," when there was an element of analgesia, but also to reduce infection in the postamputation period.

Larrey had an understanding of problems that were unique to military surgery. Some of his contributions can best be appreciated by his efforts before Napoleon's Russian campaign. Larrey did not know which country Napoleon was planning to attack, and there was even conjecture about an invasion of England. He left Paris on February 24, 1812, and was ordered to Mentz, Germany. Shortly thereafter, he went to Magdeburg and then on to Berlin, where he began preparations for the campaign, still not knowing precisely where the French army was headed. In his own words, "Previous to my departure from the capital, I organized six divisions of flying ambulances, each one consisting of eight surgeons. The surgeons-major exercised their divisions daily, according to my instructions, in the performance of operations, and the application of bandages. The greatest degree of emulation, and the strictest discipline, were prevalent among all the surgeons."

The 19th century may well be described as the century of enlightenment for surgical care in combat. This was partly because of better statistical reporting, but also because of major contributions of patient care, including the introduction of anesthesia. During the Crimean War (1853–1856), the English reported a mortality rate of 92.7% in cases of penetrating wounds of the abdomen, and the French had a rate of 91.7%. During the American War Between the States, there were 3031 deaths among the 3717 cases of abdominal penetrating wounds and a mortality rate of 87.2%.

The Crimean War was noteworthy in having been the conflict in which the French tested a number of local antiseptic agents. Ferrous chloride was found to be very effective against hospital-related gangrene, but the English avoided the use of antiseptics in wounds. It was also during the Crimean War that two further major contributions to combat medicine were introduced when Florence Nightingale emphasized sanitation and humane nursing care for combat casualties.

The use of antiseptics was continued into the American War Between the States. Bromine reduced the mortality from hospital gangrene to 2.6% in a reported series of 308 patients. This contrasted with a mortality of 43.3% among patients for whom bromine was not used. Strong nitric acid was also used as an antiseptic in hospital gangrene, with a mortality rate of 6.6%. Anesthetics were used by federal military surgeons in 80,000 patients. Tragically, mortality from gunshot wounds to the extremities remained high, paralleling that reported by Paré in the 16th century. The mortality from gunshot fractures of the humerus and upper arm was 30.7%; those of the forearm, 21.9%; of the femur, 31.7%; and of the leg, 14.4%. The overall mortality rate from amputation in 29,980 patients was 26.3%.

The Franco-Prussian War (1870–1874) was marked by terrible mortality and the reluctance of some surgeons to use the wound antiseptics advocated by Lister. The mortality rate for femur fractures was 65.8% in one series, and ranged from 54.2% to 91.7% in other series. Late in the conflict, surgeons finally accepted Lister's recommendations, and the mortality rate fell dramatically.

During the Boer War (1899–1902), the British advised celiotomy in all cases of penetrating abdominal wounds. However, early results were abysmal, and a subsequent British military order called for conservative or expectant treatment.

During the early months of World War I, abdominal injuries had an unacceptable 85% mortality rate. As the war progressed, patients were brought to clearing stations and underwent surgery near the front, with a subsequent decrease in mortality to 56%. When the Americans entered the conflict, their overall mortality from penetrating abdominal wounds was 45%. One of the major contributions to trauma care during World War I was blood transfusion.

Since World War II, many contributions to combat surgical care have led to reductions in mortality and morbidity. Comparative mortality rates for various conflicts are listed in Table 1. Surgical mortality is shown in Table 2. The introduction of antibiotics and improvements in anesthesia, surgical techniques, and rapid prehospital transport are just a few of the innovations that have led to better outcomes.

Table 2: Surgical Mortality for Head, Chest, and Abdominal Wounds in Soldiers from U.S. Army

	Head	Thorax	Abdomen
World War I			
Number of soldiers	189	104	1816
% Mortality	40	37	67
World War II			
Number of soldiers	2051	1364	2315
% Mortality	14	10	23
Korean Conflict			
Number of soldiers	673	158	384
% Mortality	10	8	9
Vietnam Conflict			
Number of soldiers	1171	1176	1209
% Mortality	10	7	9

MODERN TRAUMA SYSTEM DEVELOPMENT

Between the two world wars, some significant advances were made in civilian trauma care. Böhler formed the first civilian trauma system in Austria in 1925. Although initially directed at work-related injuries, it eventually expanded to include all accidents. At the onset of World War II, the Birmingham Accident Hospital was founded. It continued to provide regional trauma care until recently. By 1975, Germany had established a nationwide trauma system, so that no patient was more than 15–20 minutes from one of these regional centers. Due to the work of Tscherne and colleagues, this system has continued into the present, and mortality has decreased by over 60% (Figure 1).

In North America, foundations for modern trauma systems were being undertaken. In 1912, at a meeting of the American Surgical Association in Montreal, a committee of five was appointed to prepare a statement on the management of fractures. This led to a standing committee. One year later, the American College of Surgeons was founded, and in May 1922, the Board of Regents of the American College of Surgeons started the first Committee on Fractures with Charles Scudder, MD, as chair. This eventually became the Committee on Trauma. Another function begun by the college in 1918 was the Hospital Standardization Program, which evolved into the Joint Commission on Accreditation of Hospitals. One function of this

Table 1: Percentage of Wounded American Soldiers Who Died from Their Wounds

War	Year	Number of Wounded Soldiers	Percentage of Wounded Soldiers Who Died of Wounds
Mexican War	1846–1848	3,400	15
American War Between the States	1861–1865	318,200	14
Spanish-American War	1898	1,600	7
World War I (excluding gas)	1918	153,000	8
World War II	1942–1945	599,724	4.5
Korean Conflict	1950–1953	77,788	2.5
Vietnam Conflict	1865–1972	96,811	3.6

TRAUMA DEATHS

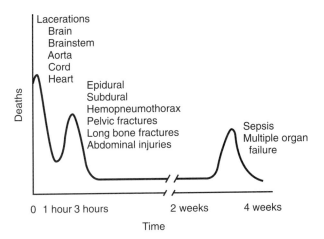

Figure 1 Trauma deaths have a trimodal distribution. The first death peak (approximately 50%) is within minutes of the injury. The second death peak (approximately 30%) occurs within a few hours to 48 hours. The third death peak occurs within 1 to 4 weeks (approximately 15%) and represents those patients who die from the complications of their injury or treatment. From a public health perspective, the first death peak can only be addressed by prevention, which is difficult, since part of this strategy means dealing with human behavior. The second death peak is best addressed by having a trauma system, and the third death peak by critical care and research.

standardization program was an embryonic start of a trauma registry with acquisition of records of patients who were treated for fractures. In 1926, the Board of Industrial Medicine and Traumatic Surgery was formed. Thus, it was the standardization program by the American College of Surgeons, the Fracture Committee appointed by the American College of Surgeons, the availability of patient records from the Hospital Standardization Program, and the new Board of Industrial Medicine in Traumatic Surgery that provided the seeds of the trauma system.

In 1966 the first two trauma centers were established in the United States: William F. Blaisdell at San Francisco General Hospital and Robert Freeark at Cook County Hospital in Chicago. Three years later, a statewide trauma system was established in Maryland by R. A. Cowley. In 1976, the American College of Surgeons Committee on Trauma developed a formal outline of injury care called Optimal Criteria for Care of the Injured Patient. Subsequently, the task force of the American College of Surgeons Committee on Trauma met approximately every 4 years and updated their optimal criteria, which are now used extensively, in establishing regional and state trauma systems, and have recently been exported to Australia. Other contributions by the American College of Surgeons Committee on Trauma include introduction of the Advanced Trauma Life Support courses, establishment of a national trauma registry (National Trauma Data Bank), and a national verification program. The latter is analogous to the old hospital standardization program, and "verifies" by a peer review process whether a hospital's trauma center meets American College of Surgeons guidelines.

ARE TRAUMA SYSTEMS EFFECTIVE?

Since 1984, more than 15 articles have been published showing that trauma systems benefit society by increasing the chances of survival when patients are treated in specialized centers. In addition, two

studies have shown that trauma systems also reduce trauma morbidity. In 1988, a report card was issued on the current status and future challenges of trauma systems. At that time, an inventory was taken of all state emergency medical service directors or health departments having responsibility over emergency and trauma planning. They were contacted via telephone survey in February 1987, and then were asked eight specific questions on their state trauma systems. Of the eight criteria, only two states, Maryland and Virginia, were identified as having all eight essential components of a regional trauma system. Nineteen states and Washington, DC, either had incomplete statewide coverage or lacked essential components. States or regions that did not limit the number of trauma centers was the most common deficient criterion.

In 1995, another report card was issued in the *Journal of the American Medical Association*. This report card was an update on the progress and development of trauma systems since the 1988 report. It was a more sophisticated approach, as it expanded the original eight criteria and was more comprehensive. According to the 1995 report, five states (Florida, Maryland, Nevada, New York, and Oregon) had all the components necessary for a statewide system. Virginia no longer limited the number of designated trauma centers. An additional 15 states and Washington, DC, had most of the components of a trauma system.

The 1995 report card was upgraded at the Skamania Conference in 1998. There are now 35 states across the United States actively engaged in meeting trauma system criteria. In addition to the report card, the Skamania Conference evaluated the effectiveness of trauma systems. The medical literature was searched and all available evidence was divided into three categories, including reports resulting from panel studies (autopsy studies), registry comparisons, and population-based research. Panel studies suffered from wide variation and poor inter-rater reliability, and the autopsies alone were deemed inadequate. This led to the general consensus that panel studies were only weak class III evidence. Despite these limitations, however, McKenzie concluded that when all panel studies are considered collectively, they do provide some face validity and support the hypothesis that treatment in a trauma center versus a non-trauma center is associated with fewer inappropriate deaths and possibly even disability. Registry evaluation was found to be useful for assessing overall effectiveness of trauma systems. Jurkovich and Mock concluded the data clearly did not meet class I evidence. Their critique of trauma registries included the following: there are often missing data, miscodings occur, there may be inter-rater reliability factors, the national norms are not population-based, there is little detail about the cause of death, and they do not take into account prehospital deaths. Despite these deficits, conference participants reached consensus, concluding that registry studies were better than panel studies but not as good as population studies. Finally, population-based studies were evaluated and found to comprise class II evidence. An advantage over registry studies is attributed to studying and evaluating a large population in all aspects of trauma care, including prehospital, hospital, and rehabilitation. Unfortunately, only a limited number of clinical variables can be evaluated, and it is difficult to adjust for severity of injury and physiologic dysfunction. Despite disadvantages with all three studies, the advantages may be applied to various individual communities to help influence public health policy with regard to trauma system initiation and evaluation.

Two recent studies document the effectiveness of trauma systems. The first is a comparison of mortality between Level I trauma centers and hospitals without a trauma center. The in-hospital mortality rate was significantly lower in trauma centers than in non-trauma centers (7.6% vs. 9.5%). This 25% difference in mortality was present 1 year postinjury with a 10.4% mortality rate connected to trauma centers and 13.8% to non-trauma centers. The second study was an assessment of the State of Florida's trauma system, and this study confirmed a 25% lower mortality rate in designated trauma centers.

WHAT ARE THE CURRENT PROBLEMS?

In the global burden of disease study by Murray and Lopez, the world is divided into developed regions or developing regions. They also examine various statistics on a global level. The most useful statistic or means of measuring disability is the disability-adjusted life year (DALY). This is the sum of life years lost due to premature mortality and years lived with disability adjusted for severity. By 2020, road traffic accidents will be the number three overall cause worldwide of DALYs. This does not include DALYs from war, which is number eight. In developed countries, road traffic accidents are the fifth highest cause of DALYs, and in developing regions, the second highest cause. One of the most difficult problems that we face in the next 15 years is how to provide reasonable trauma care and trauma system development in the developing regions of the world. Prehospital care is currently nonexistent in most of these developing countries. There are few, if any, trauma centers in the urban areas, and certainly not in the rural areas of the same countries. Even if there were such centers or a trauma system, rehabilitation is almost totally lacking, and therefore, the injured person would rarely be able to return to work or productivity after a severe injury.

As noted earlier, Europe has in the last century developed some statewide trauma systems. However, there is no concerted effort by the European Union (EU) to establish criteria for trauma systems or to coordinate trauma care between countries within the EU. Similarly, the EU does not have standards for prehospital care, nor is there a network of rehabilitation facilities that have standards and are peer reviewed. In theory, surgeons trained in one EU country should be able to cross the various national borders and to practice surgery, including trauma care, within these different countries. Again, there are no standards for what constitutes a trauma surgeon, and in fact, trauma surgery is a potpourri of different models. One model is exemplified by Austria, where trauma surgery is an independent specialty. Another model incorporates trauma surgical training into general surgery, and this includes France, Italy, The Netherlands, and Turkey. A third model is where the majority of trauma training is given with orthopedic surgery residency training. This would include Belgium and Switzerland. The largest model is where trauma surgery training is given to specific specialties without any single specialty having any major responsibility for trauma training, and this would include Denmark, Germany, Portugal, Estonia, Iceland, England, Norway, Finland, and Sweden.

Some of the most vexing problems in trauma surgery occur now in North America, particularly in the United States. This is in part due to changes in general surgery. It is predicted that there will be a *major* shortage of general surgeons in the United States within the next few years. General surgeons are now older, and more importantly, general surgeons are now subspecializing. We now have foregut surgeons, hepatobiliary surgeons, vascular surgeons, breast surgeons, and colorectal surgeons. The one thing they all have in common is they do not want to take trauma call. Our medical specialty colleagues' night call is now in transition and hospitals are hiring so-called "hospitalists," who are trained in family medicine or internal medicine. In many instances, the hospital will pay their salaries to provide 24/7 call, usually on a 12-hour shift basis. In some instances, possibly up to one third, various practice groups will pay these hospitalists to take their call in hospital. Another trend affecting general surgery is the rapid transition to nondiscrimination regarding gender. Over the past 2–3 years, at least 50% of entering medical students were female, but only 7% (approximately 500 individuals) applied to surgery. The reasons given are long hours and poor lifestyle, since these women wish to combine professional careers with parenting responsibilities. There is an overall decrease in applications to general surgery, and the reasons for this are complex and multifaceted. One important reason is that general surgeons' incomes are approximately 50% less than those of some specialty surgeons. A more concerning reason, however, is lifestyle perceptions. Younger

medical students and physicians tend to opt out of surgery, and they particularly abhor trauma surgery, because of the time commitment and related lifestyle issues. Another problem, which may be unique to the United States, is the decrease in operative cases in trauma. There has been a shift from penetrating trauma to blunt trauma and another shift to nonoperative management, particularly of liver and spleen injuries. General surgeons have compounded the problem by referring cases to surgeons who specialize in vascular surgery or chest surgery. Interventional radiologists also participate in management of certain traumatic injuries.

Another vexing problem in trauma care in the United States is the current demand for on-call pay by specialty surgeons. This is particularly true in orthopedics and neurosurgery. This on-call pay ranges from $1000 to $7000 a night. On average, a neurosurgeon in a Level I hospital would only be called in 33 times in the course of a year. In contrast, orthopedic surgeons average approximately 275 emergency cases during the year. Obviously, this could be shared between groups. Nevertheless, hospitals are being asked to pay on-call stipends to neurosurgeons that are quite large, considering the relatively low probability of being called in.

Other factors affecting trauma availability by specialty surgeons are freestanding ambulatory surgery centers where the surgeons can often avoid government regulations, do not have to take call, and have hospitalists care for their patients at night.

These problems will be accentuated in the next few years as the elderly population (aged 65 and older) reaches 30% of the total population. Studies in the United States show that mortality of people aged 65 and older in the intensive care unit is 3.5 times greater than that of younger people, and length of stay is longer. Unfortunately, the majority of these elderly patients who are seriously injured do not return to independent lifestyles following acute care.

SOLUTIONS

Fixing the problems in developing countries may be the most difficult. Most of these countries are totally lacking in the infrastructure for provision of a trauma system, including prehospital care, sufficient adequately trained surgeons, and rehabilitation services. International institutions such as the World Bank and World Health Organization would have to take a leading role in providing financial resources and training for prehospital care. This would be a potentially huge sum, since it would require creating and developing adequate communications, ambulances, and properly trained prehospital personnel. Similarly, provision of appropriately trained surgeons is equally problematic. Bringing surgeons to Western countries for training has been a problem, since many of them do not return to their countries of origin. In my opinion, the optimal way to train these individuals would be for surgical educators from countries with mature trauma systems to spend time educating surgeons in the appropriate medical schools in their home countries. This is also problematic, since the quality of medical schools varies tremendously in developing nations. Furthermore, in addition to surgeons, anesthesiologists, critical care physicians, and nurses would have to be educated as well. The third component of a trauma system, rehabilitation, is almost totally lacking in developing countries. This element may not be as resource-dependent or costly as other components, but it would have to be developed concomitantly with prehospital and acute care.

The fundamental problem in developing regions is setting priorities. If one accepts that DALYs are a reasonable approach to developing sound health care policy, then we can examine the 10 most common causes of DALYs. A rank order of the 10 most frequent DALYs in developing countries are unipolar major depression, road traffic accidents, ischemic heart disease, chronic obstructive pulmonary disease, cerebral vascular disease, tuberculosis, lower respiratory infections, war, diarrheal diseases, and HIV. I am biased, but I believe that road traffic accidents may be the most cost-effective DALY to try to address. Prevention would clearly play a major role in chronic obstructive pulmonary disease, ischemic heart disease, and cerebral vascular disease, if the United States (among others) simply quit making and exporting cigarettes. I would also argue that as the world economy becomes more globalized and developing countries become economic powers in their own right, it is important for us to be involved early on in providing the infrastructure for managing health care in general and trauma care in particular.

The solutions in Europe are also somewhat problematic. I believe it is safe to say there are no standards being developed by the EU to address what constitutes optimal prehospital care. I think it is also safe to say that medical education, and specifically surgical training, varies markedly from country to country. The same could be said regarding critical care standards. The current approach to training a trauma surgeon in the EU is variable, and various specialists tend to provide this training. This approach is not necessarily negative, but there should be some standards that constitute the bare minimum in order for surgeons to come and go across borders and meet this standard of care. Within the EU, rehabilitation is also variable. One of the best examples of an excellent trauma rehabilitation program exists in Israel, which might represent a model for the EU. The best place to start would be for the EU to develop a document similar to the American College of Surgeons Optimal Criteria that would apply to all countries. It cannot be overemphasized that some type of review and verification must be applied to all three components of a trauma system—prehospital, acute care, and rehabilitation.

The solutions for the United States may be even more problematic than for developing countries. The reason is quite simple: the U.S. health care system is broken. A system that was historically "not for profit" has become "for profit." Forty-four million individuals have no insurance, tens of millions are underinsured, and health care cost inflation is such that health care in the United States now accounts for a larger proportion of gross domestic product than in any other developed nation. Solving these issues obviously takes priority over solving the problems within trauma care, and yet they may be related.

There are many possible solutions to solve the health care problems in the United States from a global standpoint. Most economists argue that health care is a public good, similar to military, fire, and police services. Through a public good model, there could be direct provision of care by government, or it could be contracted to insurance companies. Some have argued that this arrangement would cost more, that there would be loss of incentives, and that the system would continue to be double-tiered, since people could still buy additional insurance or pay extra for their health care. Another solution would be a public utility model, where health care services would be regulated by local, state, or federal officials. The most positive aspect of this model is that there is public input. The disadvantage, particularly in the United States, is that given recent scandals associated with public utilities (e.g., Enron), there have been corruption and illegal activities.

In anticipation of growth in the global economy, it would be possible to reduce pharmaceutical costs by outsourcing to developing countries. For years, the United States has imported nurses to make up for deficiencies in the training of nurses in the United States. A similar effort could be made by importing health care professionals, such as surgeons. In many ways, this model is completely unrealistic, since it removes professionals from countries that need them the most.

The most reasonable model for the public would be to have universal health care with either a single payer or a multiple payer system. There would be a defined level of basic care, flexible co-payments, catastrophic care, and freedom of choice to select professionals and hospitals would be maintained. Such a system would also emphasize disease prevention, patient education, and oversight of insurers. Malpractice would be arbitrated, and overdiagnosis and overtreatment would be curtailed. Although this last

solution has merit, it is going to take time to bring about such changes.

The problems in trauma care in the United States are such that it is not possible to wait for a change in the overall health care system. Recently, a combined committee of the American College of Surgeons Committee on Trauma and the American Association for the Surgery of Trauma has recommended a set of solutions for trauma systems. They have proposed that the American Board of Surgery establish a primary board titled "The American Board of Emergency and Acute Care Surgery." The curriculum would comprise 4 years of general surgery, followed by 2 years of trauma surgery, including some of the specialties within trauma. It would include critical care and vascular and noncardiac thoracic surgery. Additional training could also include training in emergency orthopedics, neurosurgery, minor plastic surgery, and some interventional radiology as well. Essentially, the proposed curriculum would create a surgical hospitalist who would perform shift work and provide 24/7 coverage of nearly all surgical emergencies. One of the problems yet to be solved is how to provide continuity of care, particularly at shift change.

Prehospital care and rehabilitation are also problems that need to be solved. The committee has recommended that we develop optimal criteria standards for prehospital care that would include peer review and verification. Similarly, rehabilitation care needs development of optimal criteria standards with peer review and verification.

Trauma care and trauma systems in the Western Hemisphere are a microcosm of the rest of the world. Canada has provincial trauma systems and centers, but lacks a nationwide trauma system. Mexico, Central America, and South America have embryonic components of the trauma system, including trauma centers in many academic hospitals, but lack prehospital care, rehabilitation, and statewide trauma systems. This is particularly problematic for countries such as Colombia, where violence is a major contributor to trauma injuries. One could argue that as the economy becomes globalized, it will be important to have worldwide standards for trauma management and peer review. I consider this a challenge and an opportunity.

SUGGESTED READINGS

Bazzoli GJ: Community-based trauma system development: key barriers and facilitating factors. *J Trauma* 47(Suppl):S22–S25, 1999.

Bazzoli GJ, Madura KJ, Cooper GF, et al: Progress in the development of trauma systems in the United States. *JAMA* 273:395–401, 1995.

Cales RH, Trunkey D: Preventable trauma deaths: a review of trauma care system development. *JAMA* 254:1059–1063, 1985.

Cannon WB: *Traumatic Shock.* New York, Appleton & Company, 1923.

Comprehensive Assessment of the Florida Trauma System. University of Florida and University of South Florida. *J Trauma* 61:261, 2006.

Jurkovich GJ, Mock C: Systematic review of trauma system effectiveness based on registry comparisons. *J Trauma* 47(Suppl):S46–S55, 1999.

Loria FL: *Historical Aspects of Abdominal Injury.* Springfield, IL, Charles C. Thomas, 1968.

MacKenzie EJ: Review of evidence regarding trauma system effectiveness resulting from panel studies. *J Trauma* 47(Suppl):S34–S41, 1999.

MacKenzie EJ, Rivara FP, Jurkovich GJ, et al: A national evaluation of the effect on trauma center care on mortality. *N Engl J Med* 354:366–378, 2006.

Majno G: *The Healing Hand: Man and Wound in the Ancient World.* Cambridge, MA, Harvard University Press, 1975.

Murray JL, Lopez AD, editors: *The Global Burden of Disease.* Boston, Harvard University Press, 1996.

Trunkey DD: Trauma. *Sci Am* 249:28–35,1983.

Wangensteen OH, Wangensteen SD: *The Rise of Surgery: From Empiric Craft to Scientific Discipline.* Minneapolis, University of Minnesota Press, 1978.

West JG, Williams MJ, Trunkey DD, Wolferth CC: Trauma systems: current status—future challenges. *JAMA* 259:3597–3600, 1988.

Woodward JJ: *The Medical and Surgical History of the War of the Rebellion.* Washington DC, Government Printing Office, 1875.

Trauma Center Organization and Verification

Brian Eastridge   and   Erwin Thal

The development of trauma care has evolved from a synergistic relationship between the military and civilian medical environments for the past two centuries. During the Civil War, military physicians realized the utility of prompt attention to the wounded, early debridement, and amputation to mitigate the effects of tissue injury and infection, and evacuation of the casualty from the battlefield. World War I saw further advances in the concept of evacuation and the development of echelons of medical care. With World War II, blood transfusion and resuscitative fluids were widely introduced into the combat environment, and surgical practice was improved to care for wounded soldiers. In fact, armed conflict has always promoted advances in trauma care due to the concentrated exposure of military hospitals to large numbers of injured people during a relatively short span of time. Furthermore, this wartime medical experience fostered a fundamental desire to improve outcomes by improving practice. In Vietnam, more highly trained medics at the point of wounding and prompt aeromedical evacuation decreased battlefield mortality rate even further.

In 1966, the National Academy of Sciences (NAS) published *Accidental Death and Disability: The Neglected Disease of Modern Society,* noting trauma to be one of the most significant public health problems faced by the nation. Concomitant with advances on the battlefield and the conclusions of the NAS was the formal development of civilian trauma centers. This developmental evolution has continued over the last four decades. Ten years later, in 1976, the American College of Surgeons produced the first iteration of injury care guidelines, *Optimal Resources for the Care of the Injured Patient.* This concept rapidly evolved into the development of integrated trauma systems with a formal consultation and verification mechanism to assess trauma standards of care at the organizational level. As a result, trauma centers and trauma systems in the United States have had a remarkable impact on improving outcomes of injured patients.

TRAUMA SYSTEM AND TRAUMA CENTER ORGANIZATION

Trauma System Organization

The organization of trauma systems and trauma centers derives from efforts to match the supply of trauma services accessible to a population in a specific geographical area with the demand for these services in this area. In this process, resources tend to be concentrated in areas of higher patient volume and acuity. At the core of the system organization is the Level I trauma center. Most of these Level I facilities are located at tertiary referral centers within major urban environments. Along with the patient characteristics, these centers foster the development of trauma system infrastructure elements including trauma leadership, professional resources, information management, performance improvement, research, education, and advocacy. By virtue of their inherently academic disposition, Level I centers generally serve as the regional resource for injury care. In addition, due to their size and resourcing, most are capable of managing large numbers of injured patients and have immediate availability of in-house trauma surgeons.[1]

The next tier of trauma center organization is the Level II trauma center. Like the Level I center, many of these facilities tend to be located in communities of higher population density. The Level II centers aspire to similar standards as the Level I facilities with the exception that their accreditation is not contingent on having graduate medical education, research capacities, or specific volume requirements. Approximately 84% of U.S. residents have access to Level I or Level II trauma centers within 60 minutes of injury through the aeromedical evacuation system.[2] The benefits of this concentration of resources in Level I and II trauma centers are found in the association between trauma center volume and decreased average length of stay and improved patient mortality after injury.[3] Recent epidemiological studies of trauma patients show that mortality risk is significantly lower when care is provided in a trauma center rather than in a non-trauma center, which supports continued efforts at regionalization.[4] It has also been demonstrated that more severely injured patients, with an injury severity score of >15, have lower mortality rates when treated at Level I trauma centers as compared with lower-echelon centers.[5]

The Level III trauma centers comprise the vast majority of trauma centers, and are the last level of fully functional injury care. These hospitals serve smaller urban or suburban communities that do not have access to higher levels of trauma care. At Level III facilities, most injuries can be managed from resuscitation through operation and to rehabilitation. Level III facilities have the capacity to resuscitate, stabilize, and transport more severely injured patients to a higher level of definitive care.

Level IV trauma centers are generally located in rural environments with a paucity of resuscitative and surgical resources. The main capabilities of these hospitals are the recognition of injury and initial care phases. Due to their lack of acute injury care resources, many of these facilities have standing interfacility transfer agreements within the trauma system.

Trauma Center Organization

The development and success of a trauma center is contingent upon two basic building blocks: hospital organizational support and medical staff support. First, the hospital and its leadership must have a firm administrative and financial commitment to trauma center development, including incorporating the program into the formal organizational structure at a point commensurate with other clinical care departments of equal organizational stature. Second, medical staff support must be adequate for all levels and types of trauma patient care.[6] The basic organizational structure schematic is shown in Figure 1.

The core elements of a trauma center include the trauma team, the trauma service, and the trauma program, which has the overarching responsibility for the entire trauma center. The trauma team is the provider and ancillary support that responds to emergency department trauma activations.

Levels of response are guided by patient acuity and level of trauma center resources. Higher patient acuity with more robust resources, as in Level I and II trauma centers, encumbers response from the general/trauma surgeon, emergency physician, anesthesia provider, resident trainees, trauma/emergency nursing, respiratory therapy, radiology technician, security, and religious counsel. The team leader is the surgeon who is ultimately responsible for the patient's

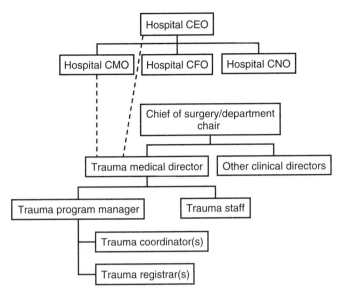

Figure I   Trauma center organizational structure.

Table I: Roles of Trauma Program Manager/Trauma Nurse Coordinator

Role	Definition
Clinical	Coordinating continuity and quality of trauma care in multidisciplinary environment
Administrative	Helps manage the operational and fiscal activities of the program as well as participates in various committee activities
Leadership liaison	Team building Promotes trauma program at local, regional, state, and national levels
Educational	Trains trauma program staff Provides resource plan to train local facilities Promotes outreach programs
Registry	Oversight of trauma registry data collection and accuracy
Performance improvement	Key proponent of trauma program performance improvement process from discovery through loop closure
Research	Promotes accurate and reliable data collection and analysis for performance improvement and facilitates clinical research endeavors
System advocate	Trauma system development, funding, patient advocate, injury prevention, public education, and outreach

disposition and care, but more importantly, all members of the team work together to streamline patient care according to Advanced Trauma Life Support® guidelines. The trauma service maintains the clinical responsibility for continuity of care in the multidisciplinary environment of injury care. In higher-echelon trauma centers, the trauma service is often a formal clinical service or services under the guidance of trauma staff surgeons. In Level II facilities, these trauma patients are often admitted to the primary surgeon of record and the continuity and oversight to maintain service integrity are provided by the trauma medical director.

The trauma program within a trauma center is a multidisciplinary effort that supports injury care from resuscitation through rehabilitation. Integral staff elements within the trauma program are the trauma medical director, trauma staff, physician specialty staff (orthopedics, neurosurgery, emergency medicine, anesthesia, radiology), trauma program manager/trauma nurse coordinator(s), and trauma registrar(s).[6] The key processes that distinguish a trauma center are performance improvement and multidisciplinary peer review.

Trauma Medical Director

The trauma medical director is usually a general surgeon with a specified interest or specialty training in trauma who functions as the key leader within the trauma medical staff. The trauma medical director should be learned in the field and proficient in the technical skills of the profession. More importantly, this individual should have authority over all aspects of the trauma program, including the development, alteration, and implementation of clinical practice guidelines; coordinating trauma and trauma specialty services; performance improvement monitoring and outcomes assessment; and providing strategic planning guidance for the program. Less tangible, although no less vital, requirements of this position include administrative and committee responsibility and team building responsibilities.

Trauma Program Manager/Trauma Nurse Coordinator

The position of trauma program manager and trauma nurse coordinator are dual positions or can be coalesced into a single position depending on the size and volume of the trauma program. This position is filled by a highly specialized registered nurse with advanced trauma training who is integral to the development, coordination, implementation, and evaluation of trauma care within the program. This position serves as a key leadership liaison between the staff and process elements within the program (Table 1).

Trauma Registrar

Trauma registry personnel are required in trauma programs on the basis of allocation of one registrar for every 500–1000 trauma admissions per year. The goal of maintaining such a record is to have a repository of trauma patient data that can be used for trauma program performance improvement or can be evaluated alone or in conjunction with other trauma registry databases in order to answer public health questions or provide trauma outcomes analysis. Registry databases are collected in standardized products to facilitate analysis and transfer of information between institutions, and to state and national repositories. Data are coded in standard formats and de-identified prior to analysis to safeguard individuals' protected health information.

TRAUMA PERFORMANCE IMPROVEMENT PROCESS

The trauma performance improvement process is perhaps the most important of all trauma program processes for ensuring that the highest quality of care is rendered to each injured patient. The importance of this process is vital from a functional and verification perspective. In fact, more than 50% of verification visit time is spent evaluating patient records and performance improvement. Trauma performance improvement begins with the definition of trauma (ICD-9 codes 800–959.9). This process is based on the tenets of program monitoring, which should be contemporary and based on reliable data. Outliers are identified that serve as indicators of deviation from the standard of care which require further review and discussion. A decision must be made as to whether no action is required or corrective action needs to be instituted in the form of individual counseling, education, policy review, peer review, or multidisciplinary trauma committee review. Once the corrective action has been implemented, the performance indicator returns to the monitoring phase. If performance measures are acceptable, the "loop" is closed (Figure 2).

Performance improvement measures can be categorized as process or outcome measures. Some commonly assessed performance measures follow:

Appropriate trauma activation
Track over-triage/under-triage
System delays
Response times
Trauma center diversion

ICU
Operating room

Emergency department capacity
Other

Delays to operating room
Time to computerized tomographic scan for altered level of consciousness

From the outcome perspective, frequently evaluated outcome measures include hospital and ICU length of stay, morbidity, and mortality. In particular, all trauma mortalities require review within the performance improvement process and each death classified as to whether it was preventable, possibly preventable, or nonpreventable.

TRAUMA CENTER VERIFICATION

The basic premise for trauma center verification is to ascertain whether a trauma center meets the guidelines outlined in the *Resources for the Optimal Care of the Injured Patient* published by the American College of Surgeons Committee on Trauma. Trauma center designation is a process that is geopolitical in origin, and is the ultimate responsibility of the local, regional, or state health care agency with which the trauma center is affiliated. In some states, trauma center designation tasks the regional provision of trauma care to particular hospital facilities, and is required to receive uncompensated care funding from governmental agencies and apply for governmental research grants and support. The designation and verification processes are complementary: designation recognizes capability, whereas verification confirms adherence to established guidelines. Effective trauma centers require both processes to affirm institutional and governmental commitment to the success of the trauma program.[7]

The verification visit is contingent on approval by the responsible designating authority or in the absence of such an agency, upon request of an individual hospital. Once this occurs, the facility completes the verification application for a site visit followed by completion of pre-review questionnaire (PRQ). A review team is selected, the composition of which may be dependent on the requirements of the designating authority. The verification review consists of a pre-review dinner meeting and an on-site review characterized by a tour of the facility followed by an in-depth chart review and performance improvement process analysis. Other aspects of the trauma program, including prevention,

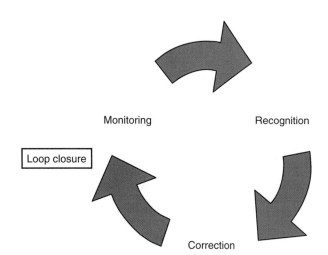

Figure 2 Performance improvement loop closure.

Table 2: Trauma Facilities Criteria

Trauma Center Level	Deficiencies by Level and Chapter
	1: Trauma Systems
I, II, III	1.1 There is insufficient involvement by the hospital trauma program staff in state/regional trauma system planning, development, and/or operation (see FAQs[a]).
	2: Description of Trauma Centers and Their Roles in a Trauma System
I, II, III	2.1 There is lack of surgical commitment to the trauma center.
I, II, III	2.2 All trauma facilities are not on the same campus.
I	2.3 The Level I trauma center does not meet admission volume performance requirements.
I, II, III	2.4 The trauma director does not have the responsibility or authority for determining each general surgeon's ability to participate on the trauma panel through the trauma POPS program and hospital policy.
I	2.5 General surgeon or appropriate substitute (PGY-4 or -5 resident) is not available for major resuscitations in-house 24 hours a day.
I, II	2.6 The PIPS program has not defined conditions requiring the surgeon's immediate hospital presence.
I, II, III	2.7 The 80% compliance of the surgeon's presence in the emergency department is not confirmed or monitored by PIPS (15 minutes for Levels I and II; 30 minutes for Level III).
I, II	2.8 The trauma surgeon on call is not dedicated to the trauma center while on duty.
I, II	2.9 A published backup call schedule for trauma surgery is not available.

Trauma Center Level	Deficiencies by Level and Chapter
III	2.10 A Level III center does not have continuous general surgical coverage.
III	2.11 The trauma panel surgeons do not respond promptly to activations, remain knowledgeable in trauma care principles whether treating locally or transferring to a center with more resources, or participate in performance review activities.
IV	2.12 The facility does not have 24-hour emergency coverage by a physician.
III, IV	2.13 Well-defined transfer plans are not present.
I, II, III	2.14 Trauma surgeons in adult trauma centers that treat more than 100 injured children annually are not credentialed for pediatric trauma care by the hospital's credentialing body.
I, II, III	2.15 The adult trauma center that treats more than 100 injured children annually does not have a pediatric emergency department area, a pediatric intensive care area, appropriate resuscitation equipment, and pediatric-specific trauma PIPS program.
I, II, III	2.16 The adult trauma center that treats children does not review the care of injured children through the PIPS program.
	3: Prehospital Trauma Care
I, II, III	3.1 The trauma director is not involved in the development of the trauma center's bypass protocol.
I, II, III	3.2 The trauma surgeon is not involved in the decisions regarding bypass.
I, II, III	3.3 The trauma program does not participate in prehospital care protocol development and the PIPS program.
	4: Interhospital Transfer
I, II, III	4.1 A mechanism for direct physician-to-physician contact is not present for arranging patient transfer.
I, II, III	4.2 The decision to transfer an injured patient to a specialty care facility in an acute situation is not based solely on the needs of the patient; for example, payment method is considered.
	5: Hospital Organization and the Trauma Program
I, II, III	5.1 The hospital does not have the commitment of the institutional governing body and the medical staff to become a trauma center.
I, II, III	5.2 There is no current resolution supporting the trauma center from the hospital board.
I, II, III	5.3 There is no current resolution supporting the trauma center from the medical staff.
I, II, III	5.4 The multidisciplinary trauma program does not continuously evaluate its processes and outcomes to ensure optimal and timely care.
I, II, III	5.5 The trauma medical director is neither a board-certified surgeon nor an American College of Surgeons fellow.
I, II, III	5.6 The trauma medical director does not participate in trauma call.
I, II, III	5.7 The trauma medical director is not current in Advanced Trauma Life Support®.
I, II	5.8 The trauma director is neither a member nor an active participant in any national or regional trauma organizations.
I, II, III	5.9 The trauma director does not have the authority to correct deficiencies in trauma care or exclude from trauma call the trauma team members who do not meet specified criteria.
I, II, III	5.10 The criteria for graded activation are not clearly defined by the trauma center and continuously evaluated by the PIPS program (see FAQs[a]).
I, II, III	5.11 Programs that admit more than 10% of injured patients to nonsurgical services do not demonstrate the appropriateness of that practice through the PIPS process (see FAQs[a]).
I, II	5.12 Seriously injured patients are not admitted to or evaluated by an identifiable surgical service staffed by credentialed trauma providers.
I, II	5.13 There is insufficient infrastructure and support to the trauma service to ensure adequate provision of care.
I, II	5.14 In teaching facilities, the requirements of the Residency Review Committee are not met.
III	5.15 The structure of the trauma program does not allow the trauma director to have oversight authority for the care of injured patients who may be admitted to individual surgeons.
III	5.16 There is no method to identify injured patients, monitor the provision of health care services, make periodic rounds, and hold formal and informal discussions with individual practitioners.
I, II	5.17 The trauma program manager does not show evidence of educational preparation (a minimum of 16 hours of trauma-related continuing education per year) and clinical experience in the care of injured patients.
I, II, III	5.18 There is no multidisciplinary peer review committee chaired by the trauma medical director or designee, with representatives from appropriate subspecialty services.
I, II, III	5.19 Adequate (>50%) attendance by general surgery (core group) at the multidisciplinary peer review committee is not documented.
I, II, III	5.20 The core group is not adequately defined by the trauma medical director.

Continued

Table 2: Trauma Facilities Criteria—cont'd

Trauma Center Level	Deficiencies by Level and Chapter
I, II, III	5.21 The core group does not take at least 60% of the total trauma call hours each month.
I, II, III	5.22 The trauma medical director does not ensure and document dissemination of information and findings from the peer review meetings to the noncore surgeons on the trauma call panel.
I, II, III	5.23 There is no Trauma Program Operational Process Performance Improvement Committee.

[a]Answers to FAQs can be viewed on the American College of Surgeons website at www.facs.org/trauma/faq_answers.html.
FAQ, Frequently asked questions; *PIPS,* performance improvement and patient safety.
Source: Adapted from Committee on Trauma, American College of Surgeons, *Resources for Optimal Care of the Injured Patient: 2006,* 5th ed. Chicago, American College of Surgeons, 2006, Chapter 16, pp. 139–141.

prehospital care, trauma service organization, educational activities, and rehabilitation programs are also evaluated. Trauma center criteria are shown in Table 2.

The preparation for verification and the verification process itself have demonstrated significant impact on trauma patient care and lowering of injury mortality.[8–10]

REFERENCES

1. Hoyt D, Coimbra R, Potenza B: *Trauma Systems, Triage, and Transport.* In Moore E, Feliciano D, Mattox K, editors: *Trauma.* New York, McGraw-Hill, pp. 57–85.
2. Branas CC, et al: Access to trauma centers in the United States. *JAMA* 293(21):2626–2633, 2005.
3. Nathens AB, et al: Relationship between trauma center volume and outcomes. *JAMA* 285(9):1164–1171, 2001.
4. MacKenzie EJ, et al: A national evaluation of the effect of trauma-center care on mortality. *N Engl J Med* 354(4):366–378, 2006.
5. Demetriades D, et al: Relationship between American College of Surgeons trauma center designation and mortality in patients with severe trauma (injury severity score >15). *J Am Coll Surg* 202(2):212–215, quiz A45, 2006.
6. Committee on Trauma, American College of Surgeons: *Resources for Optimal Care of the Injured Patient: 2006,* 5 ed. Chicago, American College of Surgeons, 2006.
7. Maull KI, et al: Trauma center verification. *J Trauma* 26(6):521–524, 1986.
8. DiRusso S, et al: Preparation and achievement of American College of Surgeons level I trauma verification raises hospital performance and improves patient outcome. *J Trauma* 51(2):294–299, discussion 299–300, 2001.
9. Ehrlich PF, et al: American College of Surgeons, Committee on Trauma Verification Review: does it really make a difference? *J Trauma* 53(5):811–816, 2002.
10. Sampalis JS, et al: Trauma center designation: initial impact on trauma-related mortality. *J Trauma* 39(2):232–237, discussion 237–239, 1995.

INJURY SEVERITY SCORING: ITS DEFINITION AND PRACTICAL APPLICATION

Turner M. Osler,   Laurent G. Glance,
and   Edward J. Bedrick

standards: the Injury Severity Score (ISS),[2] the Revised Trauma Score (RTS),[3] and their synergistic combination with age and injury mechanism into the Trauma and Injury Severity Score (TRISS).[4] We will then go on to examine the shortcomings of these methodologies and discuss two newer scoring approaches, the Anatomic Profile (AP) and the ICD-9 Injury Scoring System (ICISS), that have been proposed as remedies. Finally, we will speculate on how good prediction can be and to what uses injury severity scoring should be put given these constraints. We will find that the techniques of injury scoring and outcome prediction have little place in the clinical arena and have been oversold as means to measure quality. They remain valuable as research tools, however.

The urge to prognosticate following trauma is as old as the practice of medicine. This is not surprising, because injured patients and their families wish to know if death is likely, and physicians have long had a natural concern not only for their patients' welfare but for their own reputations. Today there is a growing interest in tailoring patient referral and physician compensation based on outcomes, outcomes that are often measured against patients' likelihood of survival. Despite this enduring interest the actual measurement of human trauma began only 50 years ago when DeHaven's investigations[1] into light plane crashes led him to attempt the objective measurement of human injury. Although we have progressed far beyond DeHaven's original efforts, injury measurement and outcome prediction are still in their infancy, and we are only beginning to explore how such prognostication might actually be employed.

In this chapter, we examine the problems inherent in injury measurement and outcome prediction, and then recount briefly the history of injury scoring, culminating in a description of the current de facto

INJURY DESCRIPTION AND SCORING: CONCEPTUAL BACKGROUND

Injury scoring is a process that reduces the myriad complexities of a clinical situation to a single number. In this process information is necessarily lost. What is gained is a simplification that facilitates data manipulation and makes objective prediction possible. The expectation that prediction will be improved by scoring systems is unfounded, however, since when ICU scoring systems have been compared to clinical acumen, the clinicians usually perform better.[4,5]

Clinical trauma research is made difficult by the seemingly infinite number of possible anatomic injures, and this is the first problem we must confront. Injury description can be thought of as the process of subdividing the continuous landscape of human injury into individual, well-defined injuries. Fortunately for this process, the human body tends to fail structurally in consistent ways. Le Fort[6] discovered that the human face usually fractures in only three patterns despite a wide variety of traumas, and this phenomenon is true for many other parts of the body. The common use of eponyms to describe apparently complex orthopedic injuries underscores the frequency with which bones fracture in predictable ways. Nevertheless, the total number of possible injuries is large. The Abbreviated Injury Scale is now in its fifth edition (AIS 2005) and includes descriptions of more than 2000 injuries (increased from 1395 in AIS 1998). The International Classification of Diseases, Ninth Revision (ICD-9) also devotes almost 2000 codes to traumatic injuries. Moreover, most specialists could expand by several-fold the number of possible injuries. However, a scoring system detailed enough to satisfy all specialists would be so demanding in practice that it would be impractical for nonspecialists. Injury dictionaries thus represent an unavoidable compromise between clinical detail and pragmatic application.

Although an "injury" is usually thought of in anatomic terms, physiologic injuries at the cellular level, such as hypoxia or hemorrhagic shock, are also important. Not only does physiologic impairment figure prominently in the injury description process used by emergency paramedical personnel for triage, but such descriptive categories are crucial if injury description is to be used for accurate prediction of outcome. Thus, the outcome after splenic laceration hinges more on the degree and duration of hypotension than on degree of structural damage to the spleen itself. Because physiologic injuries are by nature evanescent, changing with time and therapy, reliable capture of this type of data is problematic.

The ability to describe injuries consistently on the basis of a single descriptive dictionary guarantees that similar injuries will be classified as such. However, in order to compare different injuries, a scale of severity is required. Severity is usually interpreted as the likelihood of a fatal outcome; however, length of stay in an intensive care unit, length of hospital stay, extent of disability, or total expense that is likely to be incurred could each be considered measures of severity as well.

In the past, severity measures for individual injuries have generally been assigned by experts. Ideally, however, these values should be objectively derived from injury-specific data that is now available in large data bases. Importantly, the severity of an injury may vary with the outcome that is being contemplated. Thus, a gunshot wound to the aorta may have a high severity when mortality is the outcome measure, but a low severity when disability is the outcome measure. (That is, if the patient survives he or she is likely to recover quickly.) A gunshot wound to the femur might be just the reverse in that it infrequently results in death but often causes prolonged disability.

Although it is a necessary first step to rate the severity of individual injuries, comparisons between patients or groups of patients is of greater interest. Because patients typically have more than a single injury, the severity of several individual injuries must be combined in some way to produce a single overall measure of injury severity. Although several mathematical approaches of combining separate injuries into a single score have been proposed, it is uncertain which of these formulas is most correct. The severity of the single worst injury, the product of the severities of all the injuries a patient has sustained, the sum of the squared values of severities of a few of the injuries a patient has sustained, have all been proposed, and other schemes are likely to emerge. The problem is made still more complex by the possibility of interactions between injuries. We will return to this fundamental but unresolved issue later.

As noted, anatomic injury is not the sole determinant of survival. Physiologic derangement and patient reserve also play crucial roles. A conceptual expression to describe the role of anatomic injury, physiologic injury, and physiologic reserve in determining outcome might be stated as follows:

$$\text{Outcome} = \text{Anatomic Injury} + \text{Physiologic Injury} + \text{Patient Reserve} + \text{error}$$

Our task is thus twofold: First, we must define summary measures of anatomic injury, physiologic injury, and patient reserve. Second, we must devise a mathematical expression combining these predictors into a single prediction of outcome, which for consistency will always be an estimated probability of survival. We will consider both of these tasks in turn. However, before we can consider various approaches to outcome prediction, we must briefly discuss the statistical tools that are used to measure how well predictive models succeed in the tasks of measuring injury severity and in separating survivors from nonsurvivors.

TESTING A TEST: STATISTICAL MEASURES OF PREDICTIVE ACCURACY AND POWER

Most clinicians are comfortable with the concepts of sensitivity and specificity when considering how well a laboratory test predicts the presence or absence of a disease. Sensitivity and specificity are inadequate for the thorough evaluation of tests, however, because they depend on an arbitrary cut-point to define "positive" and "negative" results. A better overall measure of the discriminatory power of a test is the area under the receiver operation characteristic (ROC) curve. Formally defined as the area beneath a graph of sensitivity (true positive proportion) graphed against $1 - $ specificity (false positive proportion), the ROC statistic can more easily be understood as the proportion of correct discriminations a test makes when confronted with all possible comparisons between diseased and nondiseased individuals in the data set. In other words, imagine that a survivor and a nonsurvivor are randomly selected by a blindfolded researcher, and the scoring system of interest is used to try to pick the survivor. If we repeat this trial many times (e.g., 10,000 or 100,000 times), the area under the ROC curve will be the proportion of correct predictions. Thus, a test that always distinguishes a survivor from a nonsurvivor correctly has an ROC of 1, whereas a test that picks the survivor no more often than would be done by chance has an ROC of 0.5.

A second salutary property of a predictive model is that it has clarity of classification. That is, if a rule classifies a patient with an estimated chance of survival of 0.5 or greater to be a survivor, then ideally the model should assign survival probabilities near 0.5 to as few patients as possible and values close to 1 (death) or 0 (survival) to as many patients as possible. A rule with good discriminatory power will typically have clarity of classification for a range of cut-off values.

A final property of a good scoring system is that it is well calibrated, that is, reliable. In other words, a predictive scoring system that is well calibrated should perform consistently throughout its entire range, with 50% of patients with a 0.5 predicted mortality actually dying, and 10% or patients with a 0.1 predicted mortality actually dying. Although this is a convenient property for a scoring system to have, it is not a measure of the actual predictive power of the underlying model and predictor variables. In particular, a well-calibrated model does not have to produce more accurate predictions of outcome than a poorly calibrated model. Calibration is best thought of as a measure of how well a model fits the data, rather than how well a model actually predicts outcome. As an example of the malleability of calibration, Figure 2A and B displays the calibration of a single ICD-9 Injury Severity Score (ICISS) (discussed later), first as the raw score and then as a simple mathematical transformation of the raw score. Although the addition of a constant and a fraction of the score squared add no information and does not change the discriminatory power based on ROC, the transformed score presented in Figure 2B is dramatically better calibrated. Calibration is commonly evaluated using the Hosmer Lemeshow (HL) statistic. This statistic is calculated by first dividing the data set into 10 equal deciles (by count or value) and then comparing the predicted number of survivors in each decile to the actual number of survivors. The result is evaluated as a chi-square test. A high ($p > 0.05$) value implies that the model is well calibrated, that is, it is accurate. Unfortunately, the HL statistic is sensitive to the size of the data set, with very large data sets uniformly being declared "poorly calibrated."

Additionally, the creators of the HL statistic have noted that its actual value may depend on the arbitrary groupings used in its calculation,[7] and this further diminishes the HL statistic's appeal as a general measure of reliability.

In sum, the ROC curve area is a measure of how well a model distinguishes survivors from nonsurvivors, whereas the HL statistic is a measure of how carefully a model has been mathematically fitted to the data. In the past, the importance of the HL statistic has been overstated and even used to commend one scoring system (A Severity Characterization of Trauma [ASCOT]) over another of equal discriminatory power (TRISS). This represents a fundamental misapplication of the HL statistic. Overall, we believe much less emphasis should be placed on the HL statistic.

The success of a model in predicting mortality is thus measured in terms of its ability to discriminate survivors from nonsurvivors (ROC statistic) and its calibration (HL statistic). In practice, however, we often wish to compare two or more models rather than simply examine the performance of a single model. The procedure for model selection is a sophisticated statistical enterprise that has not yet been widely applied to trauma outcome models. One promising avenue is an information theoretic approach in which competing models are evaluated based on their estimated distance from the true (but unknown) model in terms of information loss. While it might seem impossible to compare distances to an unknown correct model, such comparisons can be accomplished by using the Akaike information criterion (AIC)[8] and related refinements.

Two practical aspects of outcome model building and testing are particularly important. First, a model based on a data set usually performs better when it is used to predict outcomes for that data set than other data sets. This is not surprising, because any unusual features of that data set will have been incorporated, at least partially, into the model under consideration. The second, more subtle, point is that the performance of any model depends on the data evaluated. A data set consisting entirely of straightforward cases (i.e., all patients are either trivially injured and certain to survive or overwhelmingly injured and certain to die) will make any scoring system seem accurate. But a data set in which every patient is gravely but not necessarily fatally injured is likely to cause the scoring system to perform no better than chance. Thus, when scoring systems are being tested, it is important first that they be developed in unrelated data sets and second that they be tested against data sets typical of those expected when the scoring system is actually used. This latter requirement makes it extremely unlikely that a universal equation can be developed, because factors not controlled for by the prediction model are likely to vary among trauma centers.

▣ MEASURING ANATOMIC INJURY

Measurement of anatomic injury requires first a dictionary of injuries, second a severity for each injury, and finally a rule for combining multiple injuries into a single severity score. The first two requirements were addressed in 1971 with the publication of the first AIS manual. Although this initial effort included only 73 general injuries and did not address penetrating trauma, it did assign a severity to each injury varying from 1 (minor) to 6 (fatal). No attempt was made to create a comprehensive list of injuries, and no mechanism to summarize multiple injuries into a single score was proposed.

This inability to summarize multiple injuries occurring in a single patient soon proved problematic and was addressed by Baker and colleagues in 1974 when they proposed the ISS. This score was defined as the sum of the squares of the highest AIS grade in each of the three (of six) most severely injured body areas:

$$\text{ISS} = (\text{highest AIS in worst area})^2 + (\text{highest AIS in second worst area})^2 + (\text{highest AIS in third worst area})^2$$

Because each injury was assigned an AIS severity from 1 to 6, the ISS could assume values from 0 (uninjured) to 75 (severest possible injury). A single AIS severity of 6 (fatal injury) resulted in an automatic ISS of 75. This scoring system was tested in a group of 2128 automobile accident victims. Baker concluded that 49% of the variability in mortality was explained by this new score, a substantial improvement over the 25% explained by the previous approach of using the single worst-injury severity.

Both the AIS dictionary and the ISS score have enjoyed considerable popularity over the past 30 years. The fifth revision of the AIS[9] has recently been published, and now includes over 2000 individual injury descriptors. Each injury in this dictionary is assigned a severity from 1 (slight) to 6 (unsurvivable), as well as a mapping to the Functional Capacity Index (a quality-of-life measure).[10] The ISS has enjoyed even greater success—it is virtually the only summary measure of trauma in clinical or research use, and has not been modified in the 30 years since its invention.

Despite their past success, both the AIS dictionary and the ISS score have substantial shortcomings. The problems with AIS are twofold. First, the severities for each of the 2000 injuries are consensus derived from committees of experts and not simple measurements. Although this approach was necessary before large databases of injuries and outcomes were available, it is now possible to accurately measure the severity of injuries on the basis of actual outcomes. Such calculations are not trivial, however, because patients typically have more than a single injury, and untangling the effects of individual injuries is a difficult mathematical exercise. Using measured severities for injuries would correct the inconsistent perceptions of severity of injury in various body regions first observed by Beverland and Rutherford[11] and later confirmed by Copes et al.[12] A second difficulty is that AIS scoring is expensive, and therefore is done only in hospitals with a zealous commitment to trauma. As a result, the experiences of most non-trauma center hospitals are excluded from academic discourse, thus making accurate demographic trauma data difficult to obtain.

The ISS has several undesirable features that result from its weak conceptual underpinnings. First, because it depends on the AIS dictionary and severity scores, the ISS is heir to all the difficulties outlined previously. But the ISS is also intrinsically flawed in several ways. By design, the ISS allows a maximum of three injuries to contribute to the final score, but the actual number is often fewer. Moreover, because the ISS allows only one injury per body region to be scored, the scored injuries are often not even the three most severe injuries. By considering less severe injuries, ignoring more severe injuries, and ignoring many injuries altogether, the ISS loses considerable information. Baker herself proposed a modification of the ISS, the new ISS (NISS[13]), which was computed from the three worst injuries, regardless of the body region in which they occurred. Unfortunately, the NISS did not improve substantially upon the discrimination of ISS.

The ISS is also flawed in a mathematical sense. Although it is usually handled statistically as a continuous variable, the ISS can assume only integer values. Further, although its definition implies that the ISS can at least assume all integer values throughout its range of 0 to 75, because of its curious sum-of-one (or two or three) square construction, many integer values can never occur. For example, 7 is not the sum of any three squares, and therefore can never be an ISS score. In fact, only 44 of the values in the range of ISS can be valid ISS scores, and half of these are concentrated between 0 and 26. As a final curiosity, some ISS values are the result of one, two, or as many as 28 different AIS combinations. Overall, the ISS is perhaps better thought of as a procedure that maps the 84 possible combinations of three or fewer AIS injuries into 44 possible scores that are distributed between 0 and 75 in a nonuniform way.

The consequences of these idiosyncrasies for the ISS are severe, as an examination of the actual mortality for each of 44 ISS scores in a large data set (691,973 trauma patients contributed to the National Trauma Data Bank [NTDB][14]) demonstrates. Mortality does not increase smoothly with increasing ISS, and, more troublingly, for many pairs of ISS scores, the higher score is actually associated with a lower mortality (Figure 1A). Some of these disparities are striking: patients

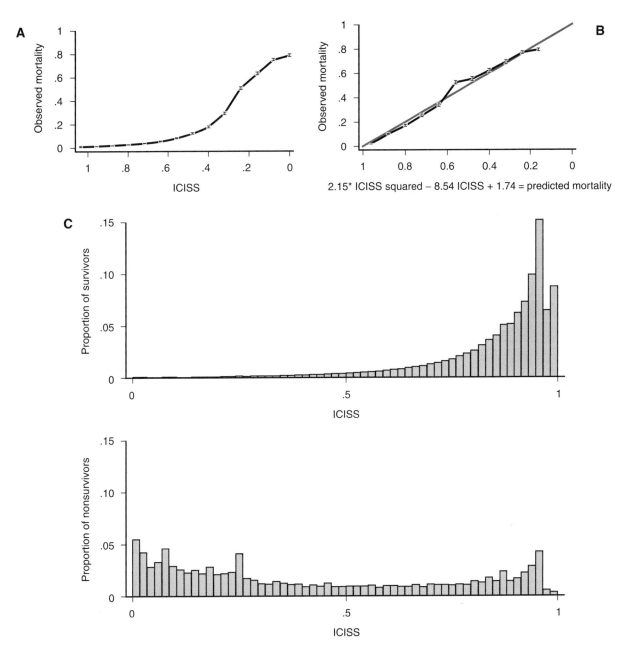

Figure 1 (**A**) Survival as a function of ICD-9 Injury Scoring System (ICISS) score (691,973 patients from the National Trauma Data Bank [NTDB]). (**B**) Survival as a function of ICISS score mathematically transformed by the addition of an ICISS² term (a "calibration curve"). Note that although this transformation does not add information (or change the discrimination [receiver operation characteristic value]) of the model, it does substantially improve the calibration of the model (691,973 patients from the NTDB). (**C**) ICISS scores presented as paired histograms of survivors (above) and nonsurvivors (691,973 patients from the NTDB).

with ISS scores of 27 are four times *less* likely to die than patients with ISS scores of 25. This anomaly occurs because the injury subscore combinations that result in an ISS of 25 (5,0,0 and 4,3,0) are, on average, more likely to be fatal than the injury subscore combinations that result in and ISS of 27 (5,1,1 and 3,3,3). (Kilogo et al.[15] note that 25% of ISS scores can actually be the result of two different subscore combinations, and that these subscore combinations usually have mortalities that differ by over 20%.)

Despite these dramatic problems, the ISS has remained the pre-eminent scoring system for trauma. In part this is because it is widely recognized, easily calculated, and provides a rough ordering of severity that has proven useful to researchers. Moreover, the ISS does

powerfully separate survivors from nonsurvivors, as matched histograms of ISS for survivors and fatalities in the NTDB demonstrate (Figure 1B), with an ROC of 0.86.

The idiosyncrasies of ISS have prompted investigators to seek better and more convenient summary measures of injury. Champion and coworkers[16] attempted to address some of the shortcomings of ISS in 1990 with the AP, later modified to become the modified AP (mAP).[17] The AP used the AIS dictionary of injuries, and assigned all AIS values greater than 2 to one of three newly defined body regions (head/brain/spinal, thorax/neck, other). Injuries were combined within body region using a Pythagorean distance model, and these values were then combined as a weighted sum. Although the discrimination of the AP and mAP improved upon the ISS, this success was purchased at the cost of substantially more complicated calculations, and the AP and mAP have not seen wide use.

Osler and coworkers in 1996 developed an injury score based upon the ICD-9 lexicon of possible injuries. Dubbed ICISS (ICD-9 Injury Severity Score), the score was defined as the product of the individual probabilities of survival for each injury a patient sustained.

$$ICISS = (SRR)_{Injury\ 1} \times (SRR)_{Injury\ 2} \times (SRR)_{Injury\ 3} \times ... \times (SRR)_{Injury\ Last}$$

These empiric "survival risk ratios" were in turn calculated from a large trauma database. ICISS was thus by definition a continuous predictor bounded between 0 and 1. ICISS provided better discrimination between survivors and nonsurvivors than did ISS, and also proved better behaved mathematically: The probability of death uniformly decreases as ICISS increases (Figure 1A), and ICISS powerfully separates survivors from nonsurvivors (Figure 1C). A further advantage of the ICISS score is that it can be calculated from hospital discharge data, and thus the time and expense of AIS coding are avoided. This coding convenience has the salutary effect of allowing the calculation of ICISS from administrative data sets, and thus allows injury severity scoring for all hospitals. A score similar to ICISS but based on the AIS lexicon, Trauma Registry Abbreviated

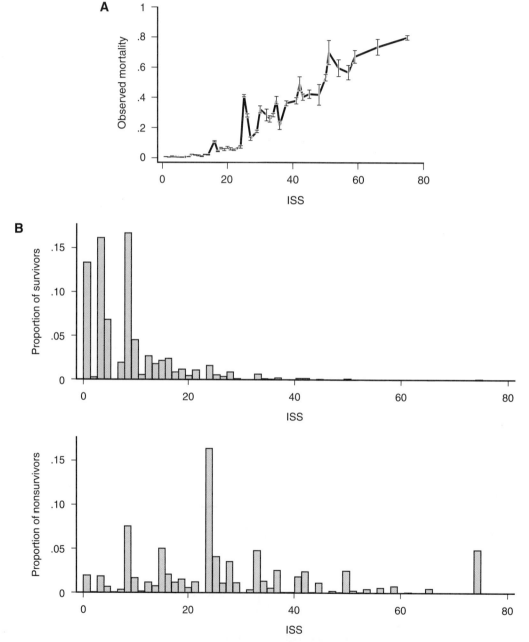

Figure 2 **(A)** Survival as a function of Injury Severity Scores (ISS). One-half of valid ISS score values are below 25 due to the sum of squares definition of ISS. Because the data set is spread over 44 ISS scores, and higher scores occur less often, error bars for higher ISS scores are wider than for lower ISS values (691,973 patients from the NTDB). **(B)** ISS presented as paired histograms of survivors (above) and nonsurvivors (below). Note that only the 44 possible ISS scores are represented. In general, survivors tend to have lower ISS scores. Some ISS scores are dramatically more common, in part because these scores result from two or more combinations of AIS severity scores (691,973 patients from the NTDB).

Injury Scale (TRAIS),[18] has been described and has performance similar to that of ICISS. Because ICISS and TRAIS share a common structure, it is likely that they will allow comparisons to be made between data sets described in the two available injury lexicons, AIS and ICD-9.

Other ICD-9-based scoring schemes have been developed which first map ICD-9 descriptors into the AIS lexicon,[19] and then calculate AIS-based scores (such as ISS or AP). In general, power is lost with such mappings because they are necessarily imprecise, and thus this approach is only warranted when AIS-based scores are needed but only ICD-9 descriptors are available.

Many other scores have been created. Perhaps the simplest was suggested by Kilgo and coworkers,[18] who noted that the survival risk ratio for the single worst injury was a better predictor of mortality than several other models they considered that used all the available injuries. This is a very interesting observation, because it seems unlikely that ignoring injuries should improve a model's performance. Rather, Kilgo's observation seems to imply that most trauma scores are miss-specified, that is, they use the information present in the data suboptimally. Much more complex models, some based on exotic mathematical approaches such as neural networks[20] and classification and regression trees have also been advocated, but have failed to improve the accuracy of predictions.

To evaluate the performance of various anatomic injury models, their discrimination and calibration must be compared using a common data set. The largest such study was performed by Meredith et al.,[21] who evaluated nine scoring algorithms using the 76,871 patients then available in the NTDB. Performance of the ICISS and AP were found to be similar, although ICISS better discriminated survivors from nonsurvivors while the AP was better calibrated. Both of these more modern scores dominated the older ISS, however. Meredith and colleagues[21] concluded that "ICISS and APS provide improvement in discrimination relative to . . . ISS. Trauma registries should move to include ICISS and the APS. The ISS . . . performed moderately well and (has) bedside benefits."

MEASURING PHYSIOLOGIC INJURY

Accurate outcome prediction depends on more than simply reliable anatomic injury severity scoring. If we imagine two patients with identical injuries (e.g., four contiguous comminuted rib fractures and underlying pulmonary contusion), we would predict an equal probability of survival until we are informed that one patient is breathing room air comfortably while the other is dyspneic on a 100% O_2 rebreathing mask and has a respiratory rate of 55. Although the latter patient is not certain to die, his chances of survival are certainly lower than those of the patient with a normal respiratory rate. Although obvious in clinical practice, quantification of physiologic derangement has been challenging.

Basic physiologic measures such as blood pressure and pulse have long been important in the evaluation of trauma victims. More recently, the Glasgow Coma Score (GCS) has been added to the routine trauma physical exam. Originally conceived over 30 years ago as measure of the "depth and duration of impaired consciousness and coma,"[22] the GCS is defined as the sum of coded values that describe a patient's motor (1–6), verbal (1–5), and eye (1–4) levels of response to speech or pain. As defined, the GCS can take on values from 3 (unresponsive) to 15 (unimpaired). Unfortunately, simply summing these components obscures the fact that the GCS is actually the result of mapping the 120 different possible combinations of motor, eye, and verbal responses into 12 different scores. The result is a curious triphasic score in which scores of 7, 8, 9, 10, and 11 have identical mortalities. Fortunately, almost all of the predictive power of the GCS is present in its motor component, which has a very nearly linear relationship to survival[23,24] (Figure 3C). It is likely that the motor component alone could replace the GCS with little or no loss of performance, and it has the clear advantage that such a score could be calculated for

intubated patients, something not possible with the three-component GCS because of its reliance on verbal response. Despite these imperfections, the GCS remains part of the trauma physical exam, perhaps because as a measure of brain *function*, the GCS assesses much more than simply the anatomic integrity of the brain. Figure 3B shows that GCS powerfully separates survivors from nonsurvivors.

Currently the most popular measure of overall physiologic derangement is the Revised Trauma Score. It has evolved over the past 30 years from the Trauma Index, through the Trauma Score to the RTS in common use today. The RTS is defined as a weighted sum of coded values for each of three physiologic measures: Glasgow Coma Scale (GCS), systolic blood pressure (SBP), and respiratory rate (RR). Coding categories for the raw values were selected on the basis of clinical convention and intuition (Table 1). Weights for the coded values were calculated using a logistic regression model and the Multiple Trauma Outcome Study (MTOS) data set. The RTS can take on 125 possible values between 0 and 7.84:

$$RTS = 0.9368\,GCS_{Coded} + 0.7326\,SBP_{Coded} + 0.2908\,RR_{Coded}$$

While the RTS is in common use, it has many shortcomings. As a triage tool, the RTS adds nothing to the vital signs and brief neurological examination because most clinicians can evaluate vital signs without mathematical "preprocessing." As a statistical tool, the RTS is problematic because its additive structure simply maps the 125 possible combinations of subscores into a curious, nonmonotonic survival function (Figure 4A). Finally, the reliance of RTS on the GCS makes its calculation for intubated patients problematic. Despite these difficulties, the RTS discriminates survivors from nonsurvivors surprisingly well (Figure 4B). Nevertheless, it is likely that a more rigorous mathematical approach to an overall measure of physiologic derangement would lead to a better score.

MEASURING PHYSIOLOGIC RESERVE AND COMORBIDITY RISK

Physiologic reserve is an intuitively simple concept that, in practice, has proved elusive. In the past, age has been used as a surrogate for physiologic reserve, and although this expedient has improved prediction slightly, age alone is a poor predictor of outcome. Using the example of two patients with four contiguous comminuted rib fractures and underlying pulmonary contusion, we would predict equal likelihood of survival until we are told that one patient is a 56-year-old triathlete, and the other is a 54-year-old with liver cirrhosis who is awaiting liver transplant and is taking steroids for chronic obstructive pulmonary disease (COPD). Although the latter patient is not certain to die, his situation is certainly more precarious than that of the triathlete. Remarkably, the TRISS method of overall survival prediction (see later) would predict that the triathlete is more likely to die. Although this scenario is contrived, it underscores the failure of age as a global measure of patient reserve. Not only does age fail to discriminate between "successful" and "unsuccessful" aging, it ignores comorbid conditions. Moreover, the actual effect of age is not a binary function as it is modeled in TRISS and is probably not linear either.

Although physiologic reserve depends on more than age, it is difficult to define, measure, and model the other factors that might be pertinent. Certainly compromised organ function may contribute to death following injury. Morris et al.[25] determined that liver cirrhosis, COPD, diabetes, congenital coagulopathy, and congenital heart disease were particularly detrimental following injury. Although many other such conditions are likely to contribute to outcome, the exact contribution of each condition will likely depend on the severity of the particular comorbidity in question. Because many of these illnesses will not be common in trauma populations, constructing the needed models may be difficult. Although the Deyo-Charlson scale[26] has been used in other contexts, it is at best an interim solution, with some researchers reporting no advantage to including it in trauma survival models.[27] As yet no general model for physiologic reserve following trauma is available.

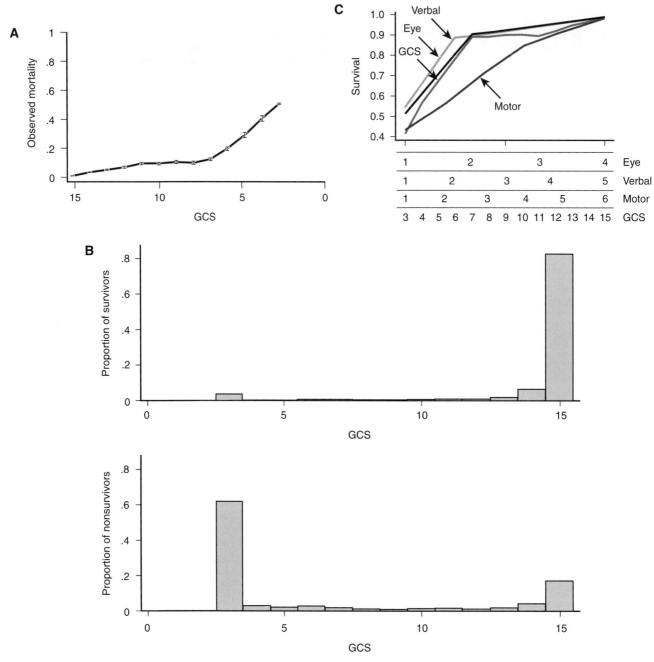

Figure 3 **(A)** Survival as a function of Glasgow Coma Score (GCS) (691,973 patients from the NTDB). **(B)** GCS scores presented as paired histograms of survivors (above) and nonsurvivors (below) (691,973 patients from the NTDB). **(C)** GCS scores (691,973 patients from the NTDB). Note that the eye and verbal subscores are not linear, and as a result the summed score GCS is also nonlinear. The motor score, by contrast, is quite linear.

MORE POWERFUL PREDICTIONS: COMBINING SEVERAL TYPES OF INFORMATION

The predictive power of models is usually improved by adding more relevant information and more relevant types of information into the model. This was recognized by Champion et al.[28] in 1981, as they combined the available measures of injury (ISS), physiologic derangement (RTS), patient reserve (age as a binary variable: age >55 or ≤55), and injury mechanism (blunt/penetrating) into a single logistic regression model. Coefficients for this model were derived from the MTOS data

set.[29] Called TRISS (TRauma score, Injury Severity Score age comorbidity index), this score was rapidly adopted and became the de facto standard for outcome prediction. Unfortunately, as was subsequently pointed out by its developers and others,[30] TRISS had only mediocre predictive power and was poorly calibrated. This is not surprising, because TRISS is simply the logit transformation of the weighted sum of three subscores (ISS, RTS, GCS), which are themselves poorly calibrated and in fact not even monotonically related to survival. Because of this "sum of subscores" construction, TRISS is heir to the mathematically troubled behavior of its constituent subscores, and as a result TRISS is itself not monotonically related to survival (Figure 5A). Although

Table 1: Coding Categories for Raw Values

Glasgow Coma Score	Systolic Blood Pressure	Respiratory Rate	Coded Value
13–15	89	10–29	4
9–12	76–89	.29	3
6–8	50–75	6–9	2
4–5	1–49	1–5	1
3	0	0	0

Source: "Categorical Scoring in Trauma Patients" Cambridge University Press.

TRISS was conceived in hopes of comparing the performance of different trauma centers, the performance of TRISS has varied greatly when it was used to evaluate trauma care in other centers and other countries,[31,32] suggesting that either the standard of trauma care varied greatly, or, more likely, that the predictive power of TRISS was greatly affected by variation in patient characteristics ("patient mix"). Still another shortcoming is that because TRISS is based on a single data set (MTOS), its coefficients were "frozen in time" (in the context of the likelihood that success of trauma care improves over time). When new coefficients are calculated for the TRISS model, predictions improve, but it is unclear how often such coefficients should be recalculated, or what data set they should be based on. Thus, as a tool for comparing trauma care at different centers, TRISS seems fatally deficient.

In an attempt to address the shortcomings of TRISS, Champion et al. proposed a new score, ASCOT.[16] ASCOT introduced a new

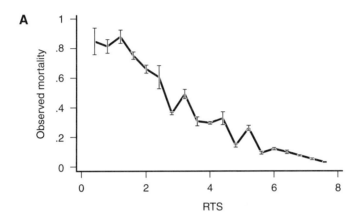

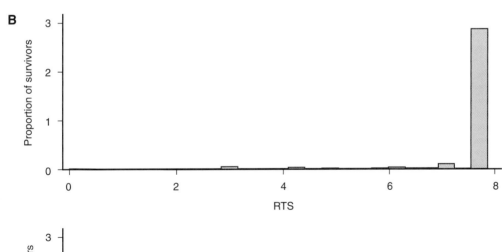

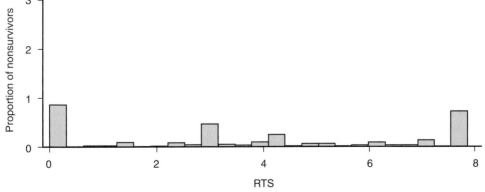

Figure 4 **(A)** Survival as a function of Revised Trauma Score (RTS) (691,973 patients from the NTDB). **(B)** RTS presented as paired histograms of survivors (above) and nonsurvivors (below) (691,973 patients from the NTDB).

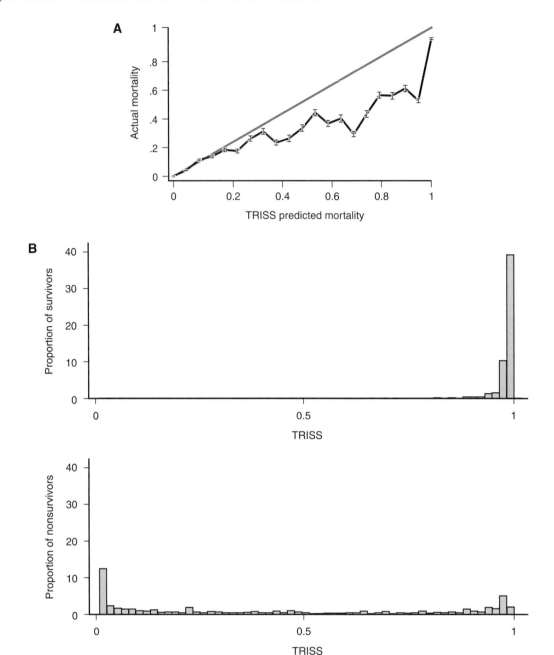

Figure 5 **(A)** Survival as a function of TRISS score. Note that survival is a nonmonotonic function of the Trauma and Injury Severity Score (TRISS), and further, that for TRISS scores greater than 0.2, TRISS uniformly greatly overpredicts mortality, an anomaly that results in most trauma centers evaluated using TRISS appearing to be "above average," a statistical impossibility (513,413 patients from the NTDB). **(B)** TRISS scores presented as paired histograms of survivors (above) and nonsurvivors (below) (513,413 patients from the NTDB).

measure of anatomic injury, the AP (see previous discussion), which was based on AIS severities of individual injuries, but summarized as the square root of the sum of squared injuries within three body regions, which were then weighed and summed. ASCOT also unbundled the RTS and included its newly coded components (GCS, RR, and SBP) as independent predictors in the model. Finally, age was modeled by decile over the age of 55. Despite these extensive and logical alterations, the discrimination of ASCOT only marginally improved over TRISS, and calibration was only slightly improved. Because ASCOT mixed anatomical and physiological measures of injury, the authors were unsure of the source of ASCOT's modest improvement. The substantial increase in computational complexity

further discouraged general adoption of ASCOT.[33] While some have advocated abandoning TRISS in favor of ASCOT, the data on which this view is based show no statistical difference in the discrimination of the two scores.[34] A difference in calibration was detected, but as we have argued, this is of less importance than discrimination.

STATISTICAL CONSIDERATIONS

Many statistical techniques are available to combine several predictor variables into a single outcome variable. Probably the best known is linear regression, which allows several linear predictor variables to be combined into a single continuous outcome measure. This technique might be appropriate for the prediction of such continuous outcome variables as hospital length of stay or total cost.

The outcome of overriding interest in injury severity scoring is the binary outcome survival/nonsurvival, however, and here logistic regression is the most commonly employed (although not necessarily optimal [Pepe et al.[35]]) approach. Logistic regression provides a formula that predicts the likelihood of survival for any patient given the values for his or her predictor variables, typically summary measures of anatomic injury, physiologic derangement, and physiologic reserve. This formula is of the form:

$$\text{Probability of Survival} = 1/(1 + e^{-b})$$

Here,

$$b = b_0 + b_{(anatomic\ injury)} \times \text{Anat Inj} + b_{(physiologic\ injury)} \times \text{Phys Inj} + b_{(physiologic\ reserve)} \times \text{Phys Res}$$

and Anat_Inj, Phys_Inj, and Phys_Res are summary measures of anatomic injury, physiologic injury, and physiologic reserve, respectively.

The values of the coefficients b_0, $b_{(anatomic\ injury)}$, $b_{(physiologic\ injury)}$, and $b_{(physiologic\ reserve)}$ are derived using a technique called maximum likelihood estimation. The details need not concern us, except to say that these coefficients are computed from a reference data set using an iterative procedure that requires a computer. The four coefficients thus capture much of the information present in the reference data set, including both the explicit information in the predictor variables and outcome, as well as implicit information included in other unmeasured variables of the data set. Logistic regression is extremely versatile, and can use both categorical and continuous variables as predictors. It does require that predictors be individually mathematically transformed to ensure that they are linear in the log odds of the outcome, however, and thus some statistical expertise is required to create and evaluate logistic models.

Despite the popularity and advantages of logistic regression, it is by no means the only approach to making a binary prediction from several predictor variables. Techniques such as neural networks and classification and regression trees have also been applied to medical prediction,[35,36] but in general prediction of mortality using these approaches is no better than standard logistic regression models.[37,38] These newer computer-intensive techniques have the further disadvantage that they are in general more difficult to implement and to explain. Occasional claims of remarkable success for such techniques[20] seem to be due to overfitting of the model under consideration rather than dramatically improved predictions. (Overfitting can be thought of as a technique's "cheating" by memorizing the peculiarities of a data set rather than generalizing the relationship present between predictors and the outcome of interest. An overfit model may perform extremely well with the reference data set, but perform poorly when confronted with new data.)

IMPROVED PREDICTION IN TRAUMA SCORING

As argued previously, it is unlikely that a different statistical modeling technique will substantially improve outcome prediction. Thus, improvement must come from better measures of anatomic injury, physiologic injury, and physiologic reserve. In effect, because the "recipe" for trauma scoring is unlikely to get better, we must concentrate upon improving the "ingredients," that is, the predictors used in our models. Fortunately, such improved measures are likely to be forthcoming, made possible by the advent of larger data sets and improved statistical methodology.

How Good Are Current Scoring Systems?

Outcome prediction can never be perfect. Not only are our descriptions of injured patients certain to be incomplete, but complications, which may occur weeks after injury and result in late mortality, will always be impossible to predict with certainty. Indeed, as noted previously, currently available scoring systems for ICU patients are generally no more accurate in their predictions of mortality than are clinicians. This level of accuracy may be difficult to improve upon, because the human brain itself can be considered a wonderfully powerful computer, optimized over eons to make accurate classifications.

The TRISS model for prediction following trauma is currently the most widely used, and has the theoretic advantage of using information about a patient's injuries (ISS, blunt/penetrating), physiologic derangement (RTS) and physiologic reserve (age) to reach a prediction. Although all of these inputs to the model are by today's statistical standards rather unsophisticated descriptions of the factors they are designed to quantify, the final prediction of TRISS on balance powerfully separates survivors from nonsurvivors (ROC = 0.95) (see Figure 5B). Unfortunately, TRISS is not only not linearly related to mortality, it is not even monotonically related to mortality (see Figure 5A), a defect that strongly suggests that TRISS can be improved upon.

The Uses of Injury Scoring

While it seems obvious that a uniform system of measurement is essential to the scientific study of trauma and the monitoring of trauma systems, the exact role of injury severity scoring in clinical trauma care, trauma research, and evaluation of trauma care is evolving. Certainly there is no role for injury scoring in the acute trauma setting: calculating such scores can be time consuming and error prone, and such mathematical preprocessing is a scant advantage for clinicians comfortable with assessing a patient's vital signs and physical exam. Trauma research, on the other hand, frequently requires a rough ordering of injury severity among patients, and here even statistically suboptimal scores (e.g., ISS, TRISS) can be very useful.

Trauma scoring has also been proposed as a way to evaluate the success of trauma care and thus compare trauma providers (physicians, centers, treatments, or systems). Although the trauma community has long been interested in assessing trauma care,[39] the recent claims of the Institute of Medicine[40] that as many as 90,000 Americans die yearly as a result of medical errors has accelerated the call for medical "report cards," and interest in "pay for performance" is building.[41] Initially it was hoped that simply comparing the actual mortality with the expected mortality (the sum of the expected mortalities for all patients based upon some outcome prediction model, such as TRISS) for groups of patients would provide a point estimate of the overall success of care provided. Unfortunately, summarizing the success of care has proved more complex than simply calculating the ratio of observed to expected deaths ("O to E ratio") because there is often substantial statistical uncertainty surrounding these point estimates. More problematic still, when confronted with data for several trauma providers (surgeons, centers, systems), it can be difficult or impossible to determine which, if any, providers actually have better outcomes.[42] Advanced statistical methods (e.g., hierarchal models[43]) are required to address these problems rigorously, but such procedures are not yet easily implemented or widely employed by medical researchers. Some of these difficulties are likely to be resolved by further research into the statistical properties of this kind of data, but currently some statistical researchers in this area recommend that tables of such data simply not be published because they are so likely to be misinterpreted by the public[42] or misused by government and other regulatory agencies.[44] The unintended consequences of such overzealous use of statistical methods, such as hospitals refusing to care for sicker patients,[45] may actually worsen patient care.

It can be argued that even statistically imprecise comparisons between providers can be usefully employed by committed groups of providers to foster discussion and help identify "best practices," and thus improve care.[46] This heuristic approach has occasionally been cited as the source of dramatic reductions in mortality.[47,48] However, the exact source of these improvements is uncertain, and it is difficult to guarantee how a ranking, once generated, will be subsequently employed. Tracking the performance of a single provider (surgeon, trauma center, etc.) over time may be a statistically more tractable problem.[49] This approach has recently been applied in cardiac surgery,[50] but has not yet been applied to trauma care.

Given the uncertainty inherent in comparing the success of trauma care among providers, the American College of Surgeons in its trauma center verification process has wisely eschewed assessment based on outcomes in favor of structure and process measures. This approach, first outlined by Donabedian[51] over 25 years ago, advocates the evaluation of structures that are believed necessary for excellent care (physical facilities, qualified practitioners, training programs, etc.) and of processes that are believed conductive to excellent care (prompt availability of practitioners, expeditious operating room access, and postsplenectomy patients' receipt of OPSI vaccines, among others). Although outcome measures were also included in Donabedian's[51] schema, he recognized that these would be the most difficult to develop and employ.

Thus, the early hope that something as complex as excellence in trauma care could be captured in a single equation (e.g., TRISS) now seems naïve. While the performance of local systems with consistent patient populations might be monitored using summary measures of past performance, the expectation that all trauma care can be objectively evaluated with a single equation seems not only unrealized, but unrealizable.

Recommendations

1. ICD-9 based scores (ICISS) should begin to supplement (and may supplant) AIS-based scores (ISS) because these ICD-9 based scores have better statistical properties and are less expensive to calculate. An ICISS-like score based on the AIS lexicon (TRAIS) has been described, and although AIS coding is required, TRAIS has the advantages of improved predictive power over ISS and allows the transparent comparison between ICISS scores and an AIS-based score.
2. Better measures of physiologic derangement and physiologic reserve must be developed and integrated into overall scoring systems.
3. Better understanding of the physiologic principles by which injuries combine to produce death is required to improve model specification.
4. The TRISS method for evaluation of trauma center performance is problematic, and is unlikely to ever be reliable. Careful case review by knowledgeable clinicians is a much more appropriate, albeit expensive, approach. Comparisons between trauma centers using scoring systems should be avoided except as research projects.

▪ CONCLUSIONS

Injury severity scoring is still in a prolonged infancy. Although over 30 years old, the first-generation summary predictors (ISS, GCS, RTS, and TRISS) are still the standard scores in general use. The development of large trauma databases (e.g., NTDB) and better statistical software have now allowed us to see clearly the

shortcomings of these early scoring techniques. In particular, the "summed subscores" approach to summary measures used in ISS, RTS, and GCS, as well as the overall survival predictor TRISS, uniformly results in probability of survival functions that are nonlinear, and, more problematically, often not monotonically related to mortality. Newer scoring systems that both better discriminate survivors from nonsurvivors and have better statistical properties have been developed (e.g., ICISS), but have failed to replace the first-generation scores. In part this is because the second generation of scores has not performed dramatically better than the older scores, and in part this is because the older scores are so firmly entrenched. Perhaps the most important reason for this inertia is that scores have as yet found no real use except in the arena of trauma research where scores that provide a rough ordering of injury severity have been adequate. However, if provider report cards, patient referrals, center certification, and revenue distribution come to depend on objective measures of the success of trauma care, it is likely that trauma scoring will elicit much greater interest. Even if reliable trauma scores are developed and adopted, the statistical challenge of comparing providers must not be underestimated.

We should continue to pursue improved trauma scores because we will learn much in the process, and substantially improved scoring systems may emerge. However, we must acknowledge that scoring systems cannot be perfect, and may never be powerful enough to be clinically useful or meet the perceived needs of monitoring organizations. We must have the courage to resist demands that injury severity scoring systems be extended into areas where they would detract from intelligent discourse or damage clinical practice until they are robust enough to perform reliably.

REFERENCES

1. DeHaven H: *The Site, Frequency and Dangerousness of Injury Sustained by 800 Survivors of Light Plane Accidents.* New York, Cornell University Medical College, 1952.
2. Baker SP, O'Neill B, Haddon W, et al: The injury severity score: a method for describing patients with multiple injuries and evaluating emergency care. *J Trauma* 14:187–196, 1974.
3. Champion HR, Sacco WJ, Copes WS, et al: A revision of the trauma score. *J Trauma* 29:623–629, 1989.
4. Kruse JA, Thill-Baharozian MC, Carlson RW: Comparison of clinical assessment with APACHE II for predicting mortality risk in patients admitted to a medical intensive care unit. *JAMA* 260:1739–1748, 1988.
5. Meryer AA, Messick WJ, Young P, et al: Prospective comparison of clinical judgment and APACHE II score in predicting the outcome in critically ill surgical patients. *J Trauma* 32:747–754, 1992.
6. Le Fort R: Etude experimental sur les fractures de la machoir supérieure. Parts I, II, III. *Revue de chirurgie, Paris* 23:201, 360, 479, 1901.
7. Hosmer DW, Lemeshow T, LeCessie S, et al: A comparison of goodness-of-fit tests for the logistic regression model. *Stat Med* 16:980–995, 1997.
8. Burnham KP, Anderson DR: *Model Selection and Multimodel Inference: A Practical Information-Theoretic Approach*, 2nd ed. New York, Springer, 2002.
9. Committee on Injury Scaling: *The Abbreviated Injury Scale 2005.* Des Plains, IL, Association for the Advancement of Automotive Medicine, 2005.
10. Mackenzie EJ, Damiano A, Miller T: The development of the Functional Capacity Index. *J Trauma* 41:799–807, 1996.
11. Beverland DE, Rutherford WH: An assessment of the validity of injury severity score when applied to gunshot wounds. *Injury* 16:19–22, 1973.
12. Copes WS, Champion HR, Sacco WJ, et al: The injury severity score revisited. *J Trauma* 28:69–77, 1988.
13. Osler TM, Baker SP, Long WB: A modification of the injury severity score that both improves accuracy and simplifies scoring. *J Trauma* 43:922–926, 1997.
14. Committee on Trauma, American College of Surgeons. *National Trauma Data Bank*, version 4.0. Chicago, American College of Surgeons, 2004.
15. Kilgo PD, Meredith JW, Hensberry R, Osler TM: A note on the disjointed nature of the injury severity score. *J Trauma Inj Infect Crit Care* 57:479–487, 2004.

16. Champion HR, Copes WS, Sacco WJ, et al: A new characterization of injury severity. *J Trauma* 30:539–546, 1990.

17. Sacco WJ, MacKenzie EJ, Champion HR, et al: Comparison of alternative methods for assessing injury severity based on anatomic descriptors. *J Trauma Inj Infect Crit Care* 47:441–448, 1999.

18. Kilgo PD, Osler TM, Meredith JW: The worst injury predicts mortality outcome the best: rethinking the role of multiple injuries in trauma outcome scoring. *J Trauma* 55:599–606, 2003.

19. MacKenzie EJ, Sacco WJ, et al: *ICDMAP-90: A Users Guide*. Baltimore, Johns Hopkins University School of Public Health and Tri-Analytics, Inc., 1997.

20. DiRusso SM, Sullivans T, Holly C, et al: An artificial neural network as a model for prediction of survival in trauma patients: validation for a regional trauma area. *J Trauma Inj Infect Crit Care* 49:212–223, 2000.

21. Meredith WJ, Evans G, Kilgo PD: A comparison of the abilities of nine scoring algorithms in predicting mortality. *J Trauma* 53:621–629, 2002.

22. Teasdale G, Jennett B: Assessment of coma and impaired consciousness: a practical scale. *Lancet* 11:81–83, 1974.

23. Jagger J, Jane JA, Rimel R: The Glasgow Coma Scale: to sum or not to sum? *Lancet* ii:97, 1983.

24. Healey C, Osler TM, Rogers FB, et al: Improving the Glasgow Coma Scale score: motor score alone is a better predictor. *J Trauma Inj Infect Crit Care*54:671–680, 2003.

25. Morris J, MacKenzie E, Edelstein S: The effect of preexisting conditions on mortality in trauma patients. *JAMA* 263:1942–1946, 1990.

26. Needham DM, Scales DC, Laupacis A: A systematic review of the Charlson comorbidity index using Canadian administrative databases: a perspective on risk adjustment in critical care research. *J Crit Care* 20:12–19, 2005.

27. Gabbe BJ, Magtengaard K, Hannaford AP, Camron PA: Is the Charlson Comorbidity Index useful for predicting trauma outcomes? *Acad Emerg Med* 12:318–321, 2005.

28. Champion HR, Sacco WJ, Carazzo AJ, et al: Trauma score. *Crit Care Med* 9:672–676, 1981.

29. Champion HR, Copes WS, Sacco WJ, et al: The Major Trauma Outcome Study: establishing national norms for trauma care. *J Trauma* 30:1356–1365, 1990.

30. Gabbe BJ, Cameron PA, Wolfe R: TRISS: does it get better than this? *Acad Emerg Med* 11:181–186, 2004.

31. Lane PL, Doid G, Stewart TC, et al: Trauma outcome analysis and the development of regional norms. *Accid Anal Prev* 29:53–56, 1997.

32. Bouillion B, Lefering R, Vorweg M: Trauma score systems: cologne validation study. *J Trauma* 42:652–658, 1997.

33. Markel J, Cayten CGT, Byrne DW, et al: Comparison between TRISS and ASCOT methods for controlling for injury severity. *J Trauma* 33:326–332, 1993.

34. Champion HR, Copes WS, Sacco WJ, et al: Improved predictions from A Severity of Characterization of Trauma (ASCOT) over Trauma and Injury Severity Score (TRISS): results of an independent evaluation. *J Trauma* 40:42–49, 1996.

35. Pepe MS: Evaluating technologies for classification and prediction in medicine. *Stat Med* 24:3687–3696, 2005.

36. Selker HP, Griffith JL, Patil S, et al: A comparison of performance of mathematical predictive methods for medical diagnosis: identifying acute cardiac ischemia among emergency department patients. *J Invest Med* 43:468–476, 1995.

37. Terrin N, Schmid CH, Griffith JL, et al: External validity of predictive models: a comparison of logistic regression classification trees and neural networks. *J Clin Epidemiol* 56:721–729, 2003.

38. DiRusso SM, Sullivan T, Golly C, et al: An artificial neural network as a model for prediction of survival in trauma patients: validation for a regional trauma area. *J Trauma Inj Infect Crit Care* 49:212–221, 2000.

39. Flora JD: A method for comparing survival of burn patients to a standard survival curve. *J Trauma* 18:701–705, 1978.

40. Institute of Medicine: *To Err is Human: Building a Safer Health System*. Washington, DC: National Academy Press, 2000.

41. Roland M: Linking physicians' pay to the quality of care—a major experiment in the United Kingdom. *N Engl J Med*;351:1448–1454, 2004.

42. Goldstein H, Spiegelhalter DJ: League tables and their limitations: statistical issues in comparisons of institutional performance. *J R Stat Soc A* 159:385–443, 1996.

43. Normand ST, Glickman ME, Gatsonis CA: Statistical methods for profiling providers of medical care: issues and applications. *J Am Stat Assoc* 92:803–814, 1997.

44. Lilford R, Mohammed MA, Spiegelhalter D, Thomson R: Use and misuse of process and outcome data in managing performance of acute medical care: avoiding institutional stigma. *Lancet* 363:1147–1154, 2004.

45. Burack JH, Impellizzeri P, Homel P, et al: Public reporting of surgical mortality: a survey of New York State cardiothoracic surgeons. *Ann Thorac Surg* 68:1195–1200, 1999.

46. Glance LG, Osler TM: Coupling quality improvement with quality measurement in the intensive care unit. *Crit Care Med* 33:1144–1146, 2005 (editorial).

47. O'Connor GT, Plume SK, Olmstead EM, et al: A regional intervention to improve the hospital mortality associated with coronary artery bypass graft surgery. The Northern New England cardiovascular Disease Study Group. *JAMA* 275:841–846, 1996.

48. Khuri SF, Daley J, Henderson WG: The comparative assessment and improvement of quality of surgical care in the Department of Veterans Affairs. *Arch Surg* 137:20–27, 2002.

49. Steiner SH, Cook RJ, et al: Monitoring surgical performance using risk-adjusted cumulative sum charts. *Biostatistics* 1(4):441–452, 2000.

50. Rogers CA, Reeves BC, Caputo M, et al: Control chart methods for monitoring cardiac surgical performance and their interpretation. *J Thorac Cardiovasc Surg* 128:811–819, 2004.

51. Donabedian A: *The Definition of Quality and Approaches to Its Assessment*. Ann Arbor, MI, Health Administration Press, 1980.

THE ROLE OF ALCOHOL AND OTHER DRUGS IN TRAUMA

Larry Gentilello and Thomas Esposito

Injury has been characterized as the neglected disease of modern society.[1] However, data suggest that for a significant number of trauma patients, injuries are an unrecognized symptom of an underlying alcohol or other drug use problem. Nearly 50% of injury deaths are alcohol related. Traumatic injury accounts for roughly the same number of alcohol-related deaths as cirrhosis, hepatitis, pancreatitis, and all other medical conditions caused by drinking, combined. A multicenter study that included data on more than 4000 patients admitted to six trauma centers demonstrated that 40% had some level of alcohol in their blood upon admission.[2] If drug use is included, up to 60% of patients test positive for one or more intoxicants.[2–4]

EFFECTS OF ALCOHOL AND DRUGS ON MANAGEMENT AND OUTCOME

The presence of alcohol significantly affects the initial management of trauma patients. Intoxicated patients are more likely to require intubation for airway control, intracranial pressure monitoring for neurological assessment, and more diagnostic tests such as CT scans to evaluate the abdomen.[5,6] Alcohol use may also increase the risk of death from serious injury. One study used data from more than 1 million drivers involved in a crash and controlled for the effects of variables such as safety belt use, vehicle deformation, speed, driver age, weather conditions, and vehicle weight, and found that intoxicated drivers were more than twice as likely to suffer serious injury or death compared with nondrinking drivers in a crash of equal severity.[7]

Patients with a history of chronic alcohol use are more likely to have underlying medical conditions such as cardiomyopathy, liver disease, malnutrition, osteoporosis, and immunosuppression. Acute, in addition to chronic, alcohol use may also affect outcome from trauma. Alcohol causes respiratory depression as well as vasodilatation that limits the ability to compensate for major blood loss. One study measured the amount of hemorrhage required to induce hypotension in dogs, and found that intoxication decreased this volume by one third.[8] Acute alcohol intoxication has also been shown to be immunosuppressive. One study analyzed infectious complications in patients with penetrating abdominal trauma and hollow viscus injury.[9] A blood alcohol concentration of 200 mg/dl or more was associated with a 2.6-fold increase in abdominal infectious complications, even after controlling for chronic use.

The effect of other drugs, alone or in combination with alcohol, has not been as rigorously studied. Heroin causes histamine release, which decreases systemic vascular resistance, and may potentiate the effect of blood loss. Cocaine, especially in its freebase form known as "crack," has the opposite effect, and causes peripheral vasoconstriction, pupillary dilation, tachycardia, and hypertension. These effects may mask or mimic the sequelae of injury.

ALCOHOL AND INJURY RECIDIVISM

Traumatic injury is a recurrent disease, especially in patients with alcohol or drug use disorders.[10] In a 5-year follow-up study of 263 alcohol intoxicated patients admitted to a level I trauma center, the readmission rate was 44%.[11] Although the mean age of the group was only 32 years, the injury-related mortality was 20%, with 70% of deaths attributed to continuing alcohol and other drug use. In a larger, more comprehensive study, over 27,000 patients discharged from a trauma center were followed using death certificate searches to detect postdischarge mortality. Patients who screened positive for an alcohol use disorder had a 35% injury-related mortality rate during the study period, which was significantly higher than patients who screened negative.[12]

WITHDRAWAL SYNDROMES: PROPHYLAXIS AND TREATMENT

Withdrawal is characterized by signs and symptoms that are the opposite of the pharmacologic effects of the drug involved. The four primary categories are alcohol, sedative hypnotics, opiates, and stimulants. The goals of prophylaxis and treatment of alcohol withdrawal syndromes are to minimize the risk of complications such as seizures, delirium tremens, and cardiovascular morbidity that occurs as a result of sympathetic overload.

Symptoms from cessation of short-acting drugs like alcohol may emerge within 24–48 hours, while withdrawal from long-acting drugs like chlordiazepoxide or methadone may not emerge for 3–5 days. Alcohol and sedative hypnotics have similar pharmacologic effects. Patients in the intensive care unit often receive benzodiazepines, leading to a delay in manifestations of alcohol withdrawal until after the patient is transferred to the floor. After 4 or 5 days it is no longer clear if symptoms should be attributable to alcohol or to benzodiazepine withdrawal, although treatment is similar.

Two main types of alcohol withdrawal prophylactic regimens exist. The first is symptom-triggered therapy, and the second is fixed-schedule dosing with a taper. Symptom-triggered therapy reduces the amount of medication administered, as many patients develop only mild symptoms that do not require therapy.[13] Symptoms are measured using a questionnaire such as the Clinical Institute Withdrawal Assessment–Alcohol Revised short form (CIWA–Ar), which measures 10 signs and symptoms of alcohol withdrawal on a 0–7 scale (nausea, tremor, autonomic hyperactivity, anxiety, agitation, tactile, visual and auditory disturbances, headache, and disorientation).[14] Treatment is titrated to maintain a score in the mild (8–10) range. Although the CIWA–Ar has been used in general medical settings, it requires training and experience, must be repeated at regular intervals, and is not feasible in critically injured patients. For these reasons, fixed-scheduled dosing is commonly practiced in most trauma intensive care units.

All currently existing guidelines recommend the use of benzodiazepines as a primary therapy for alcohol withdrawal.[15] Agents with a short to moderate half-life such as lorazepam are often used when frequent neurological assessments are needed, but may require increased overall dosage and more frequent administration in comparison to the longer-acting benzodiazepines such as diazepam and chlorodiazapoxide. Longer-acting drugs are preferred because slow elimination provides an intrinsic tapering effect.

The administration of alcohol for prophylaxis, either intravenously or orally, is no longer considered acceptable. Alcohol may block some of the autonomic effects of withdrawal, but it lowers the seizure threshold, is difficult to titrate, is highly toxic to tissues in the event of extravazation, increases the risk of gastric mucosal bleeding, may increase liver transaminase levels, and may precipitate acute liver failure in critically ill patients with reduced hepatic reserve.

There is a role for adjunctive agents such as beta blockers, clonidine, and neuroleptics, but none of these should be considered as primary therapy, and they should not be started until adequate doses of benzodiazepines have been administered. These agents do not prevent withdrawal syndromes, and may increase the incidence of delirium tremens by selectively reducing autonomic manifestations and agitation, causing delayed recognition of worsening withdrawal.

The principles of preventing and treating sedative-hypnotic withdrawal are similar to those used for alcohol. Management consists of substituting short-acting agents for longer-acting ones, and tapering the dose by 20% per day over 5 days. Cessation of stimulant use such as cocaine or methamphetamine is characterized by symptoms of depression and a substantial risk of suicidal behavior due to depressed cerebral dopamine levels.

Patients with opiate dependence may experience flu-like symptoms as the dose is tapered. Withdrawal from opiates may also be delayed in onset due to appropriate use of analgesics in trauma patients. Opiate withdrawal is highly stressful, but is not usually dangerous, as symptoms are much less severe than those seen with alcohol or benzodiazepine withdrawal. However, attempts to wean addicts on chronic methadone maintenance are inappropriate in an acute care setting. Their dose should be considered as maintenance, and additional opiates provided as needed for pain.

DEFINITION OF ALCOHOL PROBLEMS

Physicians typically identify patients with advanced or late-stage dependence, and ignore or fail to recognize less severe substance use problems. As a result, their primary experience is with patients who are least likely to quit or reduce their drinking. Alcohol problems exist across a broad spectrum of problem severity, from binge drinking to end-stage dependence. Classifying all patients who consume excessive amounts of alcohol as "alcoholic" is neither appropriate nor diagnostically accurate.

Some patients have a drinking problem that can be described as "risky" or "hazardous." They have not yet had any harm or consequences as a result of their drinking, but their level of consumption places them at high risk. In the United States this has been defined as more than seven drinks per week or more than three drinks on any one occasion for women, or more than 14 drinks per week or more than four on any one occasion for men.

Further along on the severity continuum are patients who meet diagnostic criteria for alcohol abuse. Alcohol abuse is defined as a pattern of repeated consequences involving health, relationships, employment, financial, or legal status that occur as a result of excessive alcohol intake. However, alcohol abusers are not addicted to alcohol. Alcohol dependence (alcoholism) is present in patients who have repeated consequences, but also experience loss of control, craving, and symptoms of withdrawal upon cessation of alcohol intake due to addiction.

The Institute of Medicine has recommended using the phrase "alcohol problems" as a more comprehensive term to describe patients with any type of abnormal drinking pattern.[16] Patients with less severe problems are responsible for the greatest proportion of the societal burden caused by alcohol use. Patients with severe dependence have a disproportionate share of alcohol-related consequences. However, most alcohol-related injuries occur in patients with mild to moderate problems because such patients constitute the greatest proportion of problem drinkers.

RATIONALE FOR BRIEF ALCOHOL INTERVENTIONS IN TRAUMA CENTERS

As a result of their intimate association with and influence on traumatic injury, alcohol use disorders are promising targets for injury prevention programs. Patients with an alcohol problem may not seek treatment for their problem, but they often receive treatment for medical conditions caused by their alcohol use. Injuries are the most common medical condition for which patients with an alcohol use disorder receive medical attention.[17]

A recent analysis of 12 randomized brief intervention trials, each of which was limited to one session and consisted of less than 1 hour of motivational counseling, demonstrated that brief interventions were associated with a reduction in hospital admissions, use of emergency department and trauma center resources, and medical costs.[18,19]

A randomized, prospective trial of brief interventions in injured adolescents demonstrated significant reductions in drinking and driving, moving violations, alcohol-related problems, and a greater than 50% reduction in alcohol-related injuries.[20] In a prospective, randomized trial conducted on adult trauma patients, at 1-year follow-up members of the intervention group decreased their alcohol intake by 22 drinks per week, compared to a two-drink reduction in the conventional care group.[21] There was a 47% reduction in new injuries requiring treatment in the emergency department, and a 48% reduction in injuries requiring hospital admission in the intervention group patients with up to 3 years follow-up. A recent cost-benefit analysis demonstrated a savings in direct injury-related medical costs of nearly four dollars for every dollar invested on screening and intervention programs conducted in trauma centers.[22]

Brief interventions may also be of use in patients with drug use disorders.[23] A recent randomized clinical trial conducted in an inner city teaching hospital compared brief interventions for cocaine and heroine use with standard care. At 6 months follow-up, hair was sampled for radioactive immunoassay to detect drug use. The intervention group had a greater than 50% increase in abstinence rate, and cocaine levels in the hair were reduced by 29% in the intervention group, compared to 4% in controls.

The provision of screening and brief interventions is consistent with the scope, mission, and responsibilities of trauma centers.

Trauma centers currently provide a variety of rehabilitative services, including physical and occupational therapy, nutrition services, and speech therapy. Resource allocation and staffing patterns should reflect the fact that the form of rehabilitative therapy most likely to be needed by a trauma patient is alcohol counseling.

Recognizing this, the Committee on Trauma of The American College of Surgeons, in the newest edition of its document on optimal resources for the care of trauma patients, has deemed the ability to screen for alcohol problems and the provision of brief interventions to patients who screen positive an essential service required to attain verification as a level I trauma center.[24] This is a major step toward raising the level of awareness of the importance and efficacy of treatment for alcohol use disorders in acute medical settings.

SCREENING FOR ALCOHOL PROBLEMS

Reliance on clinical judgment alone to detect alcohol problems has poor sensitivity and specificity, and is subject to discriminatory bias.[25] A study that examined the ability of trauma center staff to detect alcohol use disorders found that physicians and nurses were unable to detect alcohol intoxication in one third of significantly injured patients, and they failed to identify more than half of the patients who screened positive for a chronic alcohol problem. Thus, a formal method of screening using questionnaires and a blood alcohol concentration, and if indicated, a urine toxicology screen, is needed to maximize sensitivity and specificity.

The CAGE questionnaire is a widely used alcohol screening instrument. It takes its name from the four questions of which it is comprised. These questions inquire about the need to "Cut down on your drinking," being "Annoyed by people criticizing your drinking," "having felt bad or Guilty about drinking," and ever having "a drink in the morning (Eye-opener) to steady your nerves or get rid of a hangover."[26] Although widely used, brief, and easy to administer, the CAGE is useful primarily for the detection of severe problems such as dependence, and is relatively insensitive to mild problems, which limits its utility as a screening tool for trauma center use.

The AUDIT, or Alcohol Use Disorders Identification Test, is a 10-question screening instrument developed by the World Health Organization in 1992 as a brief screening tool.[27] It is specifically designed to be sensitive to at-risk drinking, as well as alcohol abuse and dependence. It takes approximately 5–10 minutes to administer, has been validated in trauma patients, and is currently the most widely recommended screening tool for use in trauma centers.

GOALS OF BRIEF INTERVENTIONS

Brief interventions typically target patients with hazardous drinking or abuse, rather than more severe disorders such as dependence. However, in the context of a trauma center, where the intervention is provided in an opportunistic manner by individuals who are usually not specialists in counseling, the focus should not be on establishing a specific diagnosis or severity level, but on capitalizing on the effect of the recent injury to increase the patient's awareness of the need to consider behavioral change. The recommended change would take into account the patient and interventionist's perception of the nature of the drinking problem, and the type of change that represents a realistic and achievable goal for the patient.

For patients with a mild problem, or a binge drinker, an appropriate goal might be to stay within recommended safe limits of consumption, avoiding certain activities (driving) while using alcohol, learning to pace drinks, and avoiding drinking on an empty stomach. On the other end of the spectrum, for patients with dependence, the recommendation provided may be for the patient to seek more formal treatment within the public or private sector, or change by means of self-help groups such as 12-Step programs.

Brief Intervention Techniques

Brief interventions are short, 15- to 30-minute counseling sessions, often utilizing motivational enhancement techniques, that are designed to increase the patient's level of awareness of the need for reducing or eliminating alcohol consumption. The interaction is patient centered, and intervention strategies are based on the patient's own expressed readiness to change. The counseling style emphasizes empathy, and eschews confrontational techniques.

The principles of brief motivational interviewing were developed by Miller and Rollnick,[28] and are encompassed in the acronym FRAMES. The interview is based on Feedback that reviews the problems experienced by the patient as a result of their use of alcohol, pointing out that it is the patient's Responsibility to change his or her alcohol use pattern, providing specific Advice to reduce or abstain from alcohol consumption, providing a Menu of options for changing behavior, using an Empathetic approach, and promoting Self-efficacy by encouraging patient optimism about their ability to change their behavior and the potential benefits of doing so.

Individuals who are not specialists in mental health, including trauma surgeons, emergency medicine physicians, nurses, students, social workers, and others, can deliver brief interventions after relatively little training.

▮ SUMMARY

Whether alcohol use is considered a comorbidity of trauma, or trauma is considered a comorbidity of alcohol use problems, the impact on society, the health care system, and the patient are significant. Regardless of whether alcohol use problems are considered a medical, behavioral, or legal problem, we know that like injury, there are clinical, educational, economic, and engineering strategies that can be used to control the prevalence and severity of these two entities. An injury requiring hospitalization creates a crisis that provides a unique opportunity to intervene and to motivate patients to alter their drinking behavior. Ignoring this important opportunity afforded to the health care provider represents a dis-service to the patient and society.

Key Points

■ Alcohol and drug use disorders are the leading risk factor for injury.
■ Alcohol problems exist across a broad spectrum of problem severity, ranging from occasional binge drinking to chronic dependence.
■ Optimal detection of alcohol problems requires combined use of a blood alcohol measurement and a screening questionnaire.
■ Brief alcohol interventions have been shown to significantly reduce subsequent alcohol intake, trauma center readmission, and health care costs.
■ Brief alcohol interventions are consistent with the time, financial and staffing constraints of a typical busy trauma center.

REFERENCES

1. Committee on Trauma and Committee on Shock: *Accidental Death and Disability: The Neglected Disease of Modern Society.* Public Health Service Publication 1071-A-13. Washington, DC, National Academy of Sciences, 1966.
2. Soderstrom CA, Dischinger PC, Smith GS, et al: Psychoactive substance dependence among trauma center patients. *JAMA* 267:2756–2759, 1992.
3. Madan AK, Yu K, Beech DJ: Alcohol and drug use in victims of life-threatening trauma. *J Trauma* 47:568–571, 1999.
4. Soderstrom CA, Dischinger PC, Kerns TJ, et al: Epidemic increases in cocaine and opiate use by trauma center patients: documentation with a large clinical toxicology database. *J Trauma* 51:557–564, 2001.
5. Gurney JG, Rivara FP, Mueller BA, et al: The effects of alcohol intoxication on the initial treatment and hospital course of patients with acute brain injury. *J Trauma* 33:709–713, 1992.
6. Jurkovich GJ, Rivara FP, Gurney JG, et al: Effects of alcohol intoxication on the initial assessment of trauma patients. *Ann Emerg Med* 21:704, 1992.
7. Waller PF, Stewart JR, Hansen AR: The potentiating effects of alcohol on driver injury. *JAMA* 256:1461–1466, 1986.
8. Moss LK, Chenault OW, Gaston EA: The effects of alcohol ingestion on experimental hemorrhagic shock. *Surg Forum* 10:390, 1959.
9. Gentilello LM, Cobean R, Wertz M, et al: Acute ethanol intoxication increases the risk of infection after penetrating abdominal trauma. *J Trauma* 34:669, 1993.
10. Rivara FP, Koepsell TD, Jurkovich GJ, et al: The effects of alcohol abuse on readmission for trauma. *JAMA* 270:1962–1964, 1993.
11. Sims DW, Bivins BA, Obeid FN, et al: Urban trauma: a chronic recurrent disease. *J Trauma* 29:940–947, 1989.
12. Dischinger PC, Mitchell KA, Kufera JA, et al: A longitudinal study of former trauma center patients: the association between toxicology status and subsequent injury mortality. *J Trauma* 51:877–886, 2001.
13. Saitz R, Mayo-Smith MF, Roberts MS, et al: Individualized treatment for alcohol withdrawal: a randomized double-blind controlled trial. *JAMA* 272:519–523, 1994.
14. Committee on Practice Guidelines, Working Group on Pharmacological Management of Alcohol Withdrawal: *Alcohol Withdrawal.* Bethesda, MD, American Society of Addiction Medicine, 2001.
15. Wesson DR: *Detoxification from Alcohol and Other Drugs.* DHHS Publication No. (SMA) 95:3046. Washington, DC: Treatment Improvement and Mental Health Services Administration, Center for Substance Abuse Treatment, 1995.
16. Institute of Medicine: *Broadening the Base of Treatment for Alcohol Problems.* Washington, DC: National Academy Press, 1990.
17. Blose JO, Holder HD: Injury-related medical care utilization in a problem drinking population. *Am J Public Health* 81:1571–1575, 1991.
18. Bien TH, Miller WR, Tonigan JS: Brief interventions for alcohol problems: a review. *Addiction* 88:315–335, 1993.
19. Wilk AI, Jensen NM, Havighurst TC: Meta-analysis of randomized control trials addressing brief interventions in heavy alcohol drinkers. *J Gen Intern Med* 12:274–283, 1997.
20. Monti PM, Colby SM, Barnett NP, et al: Brief intervention for harm reduction with alcohol-positive older adolescents in a hospital emergency department. *J Consult Clin Psychol* 67:989–994, 1999.
21. Gentilello LM, Rivara FP, Donovan DM, et al: Alcohol interventions in a trauma center as a means of reducing the risk of injury recurrence. *Ann Surg* 230:473–483, 1999.
22. Gentilello LM, Ebel BE, Wickizer TM, et al: Alcohol Interventions for trauma patients treated in emergency departments and hospitals: a cost benefit analysis. *Ann Surg* 241:541–550.
23. Bernstein J, Bernstein E, Tassiopoulo K, et al: Brief motivational intervention at a clinic visit reduces cocaine and heroin use. *Drug Alcohol Depend* 77:49–59, 2005.
24. American College of Surgeons Committee on Trauma: *Optimal Resources for the Care of the Injured.* Chicago, IL, American College of Surgeons, 2005.
25. Gentilello LM, Villaveces A, Ries RR, Nason KS, Daranciang E, et al: Detection of acute alcohol intoxication and chronic alcohol dependence by trauma center staff. *J Trauma* 47(6):1131–1139, 1999.
26. Mayfield D, McLeod G, Hall P: The CAGE questionnaire: validation of a new alcohol screening instrument. *Am J Psychiatry* 131:1121–1123, 1974.
27. Saunders J, Asland O, Babor T, De La Fuente J, Grant M: Development of the alcohol use disorders identification test (AUDIT). *Addiction* 88:791–804, 1993.
28. Miller WR, Rollnick S: *Motivational Interviewing: Preparing People to Change Addictive Behavior.* New York: Guilford Press, 1991.

The Role of Trauma Prevention in Reducing Interpersonal Violence

Edward E. Cornwell and **David Chang**

The issue of interpersonal violence as a public health problem gained a significant national spotlight through a workshop in October 1985 convened by the Surgeon General of the United States to address the problem.[1] A challenge went out to health care providers, administrators, and the public at large to consider violence as a public health problem, and to seek its causes and most effective treatment. In the ensuing 2 years, more Americans died from gunshot wounds than during the entire 8-½ years of war in Vietnam. By 1994, intentional injury was the 10th leading cause of death in America (20,000 per year) and the leading cause of premature mortality.[2]

The specter of violence has become increasingly prominent in the lives of American children and is one of our most pressing public health problems. Teenagers are more likely to die of gunshot wounds than all "natural" diseases combined. Furthermore, the physical and emotional consequences of nonfatal violence to children who are victims, witnesses, and perpetrators are staggering. Brain, spinal cord, and other debilitating injuries from interpersonal violence consume substantial health care resources through hospital readmissions and lifelong disability. Indeed, intentional injury is frequently referred to as a "chronic recurrent disease." An interesting phenomenon began to occur in the mid-1990s. Most major cities, and the United States overall, saw a gradual decrease in the rates of homicide and violent assault. Sadly, this trend was matched by the observation that the victims of violent assaults and penetrating injuries were becoming younger.

This chapter will describe the potential role of a trauma center in violence prevention, through the story of an urban, university-affiliated, Level I trauma center in an impoverished area.

UNDERSTANDING THE PROBLEM

Although the American College of Surgeons requires that a Level I trauma center be actively involved in injury control, the trauma surgeon dealing with resuscitation, operative intervention, and postoperative critical care requires guidance from a vast array of professionals to understand and prevent injuries due to interpersonal violence.[3] In 1991, Rosenburg and Mercy wrote, "Professionals from sociology, criminology, economics, law, public policy, psychology, anthropology, and public health must work together to understand the cause and solution" to the problem of intentional injuries. Intervention against intentional injuries requires consideration of the perpetrators, the victims, the assaulting weapons, and the environment and the circumstances of the event.

William Haddon devised an injury control approach, by considering factors related to trauma in three phases. These phases—pre-event, injury event, and post-event—were the basis for the development of the Haddon Matrix, which also considers the factors involved, such as the host, vehicle, and environment. In the parlance of Haddon Matrix, the experience of the trauma center at Johns Hopkins demonstrates that true injury prevention deals with factors in the pre-event phase.

IMPACT OF ENHANCED TRAUMA COMMITMENT ON PATIENT OUTCOMES

The result of several studies from the Division of Trauma at Johns Hopkins Hospital suggested the importance of violence prevention as the avenue for additional improvement in trauma patient outcome. It began with a study showing that, while the implementation of a multidisciplinary trauma program resulted in significant improvement in patient outcomes, no improvement was seen among patients with gunshot wounds, the majority of whom were youths (ages 15–24).[4] This observation was explained by a disturbing pattern showing an increasing prevalence of gunshot-wound patients arriving "in extremis" or dead on arrival (DOA) from multiple gunshot wounds to the head and/or chest. While 99% of patients leaving the emergency department (ED) alive ultimately survived their hospital visit, the ever-growing incidence of patients who are DOA suggests that the "glass ceiling" is being approached in terms of benefits in patient outcomes to be gained from in-hospital performance improvement endeavors. In 2005, 61 of the 88 trauma deaths (69%) seen at Johns Hopkins Hospital were declared dead in the ED in an average 6 minutes after arrival. Of the remaining 27 patients, 14 were declared dead in the intensive care unit from devastating brain injuries. This suggests that in an entire calendar year, at an urban, university-affiliated Level I trauma center, only 13 of 88 patients who died (15%) were even theoretically salvageable. This is perhaps the most compelling argument suggesting that further incremental improvement in injury outcomes are likely to be realized from prevention activities in the prehospital arena.

A second study involved a geographic analysis showing that the majority of trauma patients admitted to Johns Hopkins Hospital came from a 5-mile radius, incorporating some of Maryland's most impoverished neighborhoods, and confirmed the previously described predominance of youths (ages 15–24) among gunshot wound patients.[5] These data led to the conclusion that the injury prevention program should take the form of violence prevention activities for at-risk youths.

IN-HOSPITAL PREVENTION: SHORTCOMINGS

A third project sought to duplicate the experience with alcohol- and drug-abuse intervention described at other centers among predominantly blunt trauma populations.[6] Given the recognized comorbid incidence of alcohol and substance abuse among perpetrators and victims of interpersonal violence, a project was undertaken that sought to analyze introspection and readiness to change among young patients (ages 15–24) surviving an injury and demonstrating a positive toxicology screen. In contrast to other reports in the literature, this project demonstrated a depressingly low incidence of "readiness to change," and an even lower incidence in accessing available counseling services. This study suggests a major shortcoming of an in-hospital violence prevention program: The potential beneficiaries are random and are based on the trajectory of a bullet, rather than the presence of psychosocial risk factors.

EFFECTIVENESS OF A VIOLENCE PREVENTION PROGRAM

Baltimore is one of the most appropriate cities in America in which to pursue initiatives in youth violence prevention. It is the nation's 13th largest city, and the largest American city that did not enjoy the decrease in violence seen nationally in the mid-1990s. Baltimore ranks at or near the top of the nation in the following high-risk indicators: (1) rate of births to unwed teenage mothers, (2) episodes of assault and suspension among students in Baltimore City Elementary Schools (K–5), (3) dropout rate for Baltimore City Public High Schools (76% for black males), and (4) juvenile arrest rate for murder.

A project was undertaken evaluating the effectiveness of a violence-prevention initiative geared toward changing attitudes about interpersonal conflict among at-risk youths from a previously described catchment area.[7] Participants were given a package survey of six previously validated scales, both preintervention and postintervention, to assess their attitudes about interpersonal conflicts. This package included the following scales:

1. Beliefs Supporting Aggression
2. Attitude Toward Conflicts
3. Attitudes Toward School
4. Achievement Motivation
5. Likelihood of Violence and Delinquency
6. Violent Intentions from Teen Conflict Survey

After parental consent and the youths' consent, the children were administered the survey package as a preintervention test at their Police Athletic League (PAL) center. They were then brought to the hospital in groups on a day convenient for the officer at the PAL center to accompany them. The tour included video and slide presentations that graphically depicted the results of gun violence, followed by open discussions. The children would be given T-shirts on completion of their tour and their postintervention tests. Among the first 90 participants in the program, there was statistically significant reduction in the Beliefs Supporting Aggression scale, and a trend toward reduction in the Likelihood of Violence scale. This suggested a multidisciplinary violence-prevention program can produce short-term improvement in beliefs supporting aggression among at-risk youth.

CULTURE OF VIOLENCE

One might expect that this chapter would close with a description of a study of 90 young people demonstrating short-term improvements in attitudes toward conflict and aggression. However, recent visits by the authors to the executive offices of media production companies have emphasized the dominance of an American culture that glamorizes violence. Images that sensationalize violent acts reach millions of young people every day, while the previously

described outreach program reached only 90 kids over 1 year. Accordingly, it was decided to incorporate an approach that seeks to reach influential adults (journalists, TV/radio personalities, politicians, athletes, and entertainers) with a graphic message that describes the tragic consequences of trivializing interpersonal injuries.

A group has been formed to pursue the production of a professionally made educational video and/or public service announcement, titled "Hype vs Reality." The purpose of this project is to demonstrate the dramatic distinction between the glamorized concept of violence repeatedly offered by the entertainment media and the stark reality of violence in America as seen in EDs and trauma centers across the country.

With this effort, we join the growing cadre of surgeons and other physicians and public health professionals who have resolved to extend the sphere of their influence beyond the hospital and university walls, and interact with a larger audience beyond our typical professional societies and scientific publications. The process of changing a culture of violence will require a sustained generational effort from multiple disciplines, much as it took decades to reverse the notion among young people that cigarette smoking or casual cocaine use is "cool."

REFERENCES

1. Koop CE, Rosenberg ML, Mercy JA, et al: *Violence as a Public Health Problem*. Background papers prepared for the Surgeon General's Workshop on Violence and Public Health, October 27–29, 1985, Leesburg, VA. Atlanta, GA, Violence Epidemiology Branch, Center for Health Promotion and Education, Centers for Disease Control and Prevention, 1985.
2. Koop CE, Lundberg GD: Violence in America: a public health emergency. *JAMA* 267(22):3075, 1996.
3. Cornwell EE III, Jacobs D, Walker M, et al: National Medical Association Surgical Section position paper on violence prevention: a resolution of trauma surgeons caring for victims of violence. *JAMA* 273:1788, 1995.
4. Cornwell EE, Chang DC, Phillips J, Campbell KA: Enhanced trauma program commitment at a Level I trauma center: impact on the process and outcome of care. *Arch Surg* 138(8):838–843, 2003.
5. Chang DC, Cornwell EE, Phillips J, Baker D, Yonas M, et al: Community characteristics and demographic information as determinants for a hospital-based injury prevention outreach. *Arch Surg* 138(12):1344–1346, 2003.
6. Yonas M, Baker D, Cornwell EE, Chang DC, Phillips J, et al: Inpatient counseling for alcohol/substance abusing youths with major trauma. Ready or not? *J Trauma* 59(2):466–469, 2005.
7. Chang DC, Sutton ER, Cornwell EE, Allen F, Yonas M, et al: Evaluating the efficacy of a multi-disciplinary youth violence prevention initiative: changing attitudes regarding interpersonal conflict? *J Am Coll Surg* 201(5):721–723, 2005.

TRAUMA SCORING

Nicole VanDerHeyden and Thomas B. Cox

Trauma was the first medical specialty to regionalize health care delivery to specialized centers and to systematically measure health care outcomes. The first trauma scores were designed for a specific purpose: to standardize injury descriptions and rank injury severity to effectively triage injured patients to the appropriate

trauma center.[1] Since then trauma scores have evolved to serve two new purposes: to allow risk adjustment for comparisons of outcomes for research and quality performance, and to predict the probability of survival.[1–3] An additional purpose that trauma scores have only started to address is predicting functional impairment or disability.[4] Currently, trauma scores play a major role in quality improvement processes and patient safety by identifying unexpected deaths for peer review audit.[2,5,6] While existing scoring systems are reasonably predictive of survival, they are inadequate for measuring quality performance.[7–10]

Most trauma scoring is based on anatomical injury descriptors or physiological derangements. Current scoring systems have been modeled to address one principle outcome—mortality—while little attention has been paid to other quality performance outcomes such as functional impairment and quality of life issues.[11,12] Only recently have efforts been made to incorporate into scoring systems the impacts of demographics, comorbidities, and mechanism of injury. Unlike other medical scoring systems involving more uniform populations of patients and conditions (i.e., ischemic heart disease), it has proven extremely difficult to design a satisfactory scoring system in the heterogeneous trauma population. For example, there are a handful of ICD-9-CM descriptors that fully describe ischemic heart disease versus approximately 2000 descriptors for traumatic injuries. Patients with ischemic heart disease tend toward a uniform set of comorbidities and demographics, whereas trauma patients span the entire spectrum. Thus, scoring of traumatic injuries in a way that reduces the variables to a single numeric score, results in loss of detail, and generates similar or identical numeric scores for patients whose conditions are not comparable.

In the past, scoring systems were derived by consensus and did not undergo statistical modeling before release. During the last decade, much of trauma research has focused on the development, comparison, and validation of trauma scoring systems. In the future, to properly serve the new purpose of quality improvement, an ideal trauma scoring system must factor in the following:

- Severity of injury
- Physiologic derangements
- Patient demographics
- Mechanism of injury
- Comorbidities

Only by accounting for all significant variables can trauma scoring systems support accurate risk stratification for outcomes research and benchmarking performance.

ANATOMIC SCORING SYSTEMS

Anatomic scoring systems require a lexicon to describe the anatomy and severity of the large number of potential injuries that result from trauma. Traditionally, this was provided by the Abbreviated Injury Scale (AIS), but more recently descriptors from the ICD-9-CM (Clinical Modification of the 9th revision of International Classification of Disease) diagnosis codes have been used. The Injury Severity Scale (ISS), Anatomic Profile (AP), and New Injury Severity Scale (NISS) are based on AIS rubrics, whereas the ICD-9 Injury Severity Scale (ICISS) is based on ICD-9-CM injury codes. Despite an ever-increasing number of injury descriptors in both the AIS and ICD-9, there are still a number of injuries that are difficult to classify accurately. The soon-to-be-released ICD-10-CM has even a larger number of injury descriptors. A further limitation of anatomic scoring systems is the difficulty in identifying all of a patient's significant injuries, particularly in patients who die at the scene or early in their hospitalization and do not undergo autopsy.[13]

Abbreviated Injury Scale

In 1971, the American Medical Association Committee on Medical Aspects of Automotive Safety, later to become the Association for the Advancement of Automotive Medicine (AAAM), published the AIS, the first widely recognized anatomic injury scale.[14] The AIS rated the severity of tissue damage secondary to motor vehicle crashes, and provided standardized terminology to describe injuries. The AIS divides the body into nine regions: head, face, neck, thorax, spine, abdomen/pelvis, upper extremities, lower extremities, and unspecified. For each region a consensus-derived scale was developed for grading injuries from 1 (minor) to 6 (virtually unsurvivable). The AIS is not an interval scale; the increase in mortality from 4 to 5 is much higher than from 2 to 3. The first published AIS described 73 blunt injuries for five body regions. Since then the AIS has been

updated six times, most recently in 2005 (AIS 2005), and now includes descriptors for more than 1300 injuries covering blunt, penetrating, and pediatric injuries.[15] For the first time, AIS 2005 addressed the prediction of functional impairment or disability in its classification.[16] The AIS remains the foundation of most anatomic trauma scoring systems used by trauma registries as well as the National Highway Traffic Safety Administration (NHTSA) and other injury research and education organizations. The Organ Injury Scale (OIS) is a similar injury scaling system developed by the American Association for the Surgery of Trauma (AAST).[17] The OIS provides a common terminology and severity score to allow comparisons of equivalent injuries for clinical research. Unlike the AIS, the OIS is not used as part of any trauma scoring system.

Injury Severity Scale

The AIS failed to account for the cumulative effect of injury in different body regions, so in 1974 Baker proposed the ISS, an algorithm based on the AIS designed to improve the ability of the AIS to predict mortality.[1,18] The ISS divides injuries into six body regions compared to nine in the AIS. The ISS is calculated by taking the sum of the squares of the highest AIS from each of the three most severely injured body regions to achieve a score that ranges from 3 (least) to 75 (most) injured. By definition, an unsurvivable injury with an AIS of 6 is automatically given an ISS of 75. An ISS of 1–8 is considered minor, 9–15 moderate, 16–24 severe, and 25 and higher very severe. The ISS reduces the great variability of injury patterns to a much smaller range of values that can be used in outcomes research. Although the ISS score correlates well with mortality, the relationship is not linear and ISS methodology was not designed to predict disability or other outcomes.[19] The ISS is integral to most trauma registries, and is the basis for the anatomic component of TRISS (Trauma Injury and Severity Score) discussed later.

A significant limitation of the AIS and ISS is the cost, time, and training involved in capturing the data and calculating the scores (hand coding), particularly in hospitals that do not use a trauma registry.[20] Determination of the AIS requires abstraction of the injuries from the medical record and appropriate training of the trauma registrar or coder, and is dependent on the methodology used to assign the AIS codes and the version of AIS or algorithm used by the registry software to calculate the ISS. There can be significant differences in the calculation of the AIS and ISS due to registry software or personnel. These factors limit the ability to compare outcomes with data derived from varying institutional practices.[21] Commercial computerized applications (ICDMAP) are available that convert ICD-9-CM discharge diagnosis codes into AIS scores (ICD/AIS), which in turn can be used to calculate the ISS score.[22] The level to which injuries can currently be mapped by ICD-9-CM is crude compared to the AIS, as the detail of the injury descriptors is inadequate. AIS and ICDMAP are proprietary software, and this limits their availability. Despite these limitations, there is good correlation between AIS and ICD/AIS.[6,22] The most recent iteration of AIS (AIS 2005) was considered in developing the injury portion of the upcoming ICD-10-CM; thus, mapping between ICD-10-CM and AIS 2005 is likely to be even better once software becomes available.[16]

The ISS is statistically problematic because it is based on the sum of squares of triplets. As a result, it is nonlinear and nonmonotonic, which means that mortality does not necessarily increase with successive values of ISS. This characteristic is frequently not accounted for in outcomes research.[19] Of the 75 potential values, only 44 are represented by ISS scores and 11 of these scores are generated by pairs of triplets. Eight of these triplet pairs have mortality rates that are statistically different.[23] The reason that this difference exists is the variable maximal AIS scores within pairs of triplets. For example, an ISS score of 25 is generated both by the triplets 5,0,0 and 4,3,0. Intuitively, one would expect the ISS score based on the triplet containing the near lethal 5 AIS score to have a higher mortality. This was confirmed by Russell and colleagues,[24] who retrospectively calculated a mortality rate of 20.6% associated with the triplet 5,0,0 compared with 0% for the triplet 4,3,0. Thus, a trauma center with a higher percentage of the lethal triplets among its patients will have worse outcomes than expected if assessment is based on the ISS alone. Even for a single-value ISS triplet, one would expect significant variability in mortality rates depending on the body region affected. For example, the mortality rate for the same AIS of an isolated injury of the head would likely be more lethal than an isolated injury to the extremity. This was shown to be true when the mortality rate for an AIS of 4 of an isolated head injury was compared with an extremity injury and found to be 17.2% versus 0%.[19] And finally, at the highest ISS values of 75, there are unexpected survivors due to AIS 6 patients who do not die. The statistical problems of the ISS could potentially be improved by representing the numerical data as a categorical rather than a continuous variable in regression models; however, this does not correct the underlying problem with its methodology.

Anatomic Profile and New Injury Severity Score

Another problem with the ISS is that it underestimates mortality resulting from multiple injuries to a single body region or organ because only the single most severe injury in each region is considered.[25,26] The AP and NISS were designed specifically to address this limitation of the ISS. The AP score is a modification of the AIS and ISS that uses only four regions: brain and spinal cord, thorax and neck, all other serious injuries, and all other nonserious injuries. The AP score is calculated by taking the square root of the sum of the squares of all of the AIS scores within each region to give a summation score for each region, which is then used to calculate the ISS.[27] The AP performs better than the ISS in single-system injury.[27] The modified AP (mAP) only considers AIS values greater than 3, and coefficients derived from logistic regression analysis are then used to calculate the Anatomic Profile Score (APS) to predict survival.[27] The AP has found limited use as the anatomic component of ASCOT (A Severity Characterization of Trauma), detailed later in this chapter.[28] The NISS sums the squares of the three highest AIS score regardless of body region.[25] The NISS and APS predict mortality better than the ISS, especially in head injuries and higher injury-severity patients, but have not gained widespread use.[25,26,28–31]

The ideal number of injuries to include in trauma scoring is unknown. The ISS and NISS score up to three injuries per patient, while the AP includes all injuries in its score. Multiply injured patients are currently modeled as if the effects of their injuries are independent, not cumulative; some combinations of injuries are likely to be more lethal than predicted by individual models. However, including additional injuries in trauma scoring models has not improved performance. Indeed, it has been shown that regardless of scoring system, a patient's worst injury predicts survival best.[6,32] Accounting for multiple injuries may be more important when outcomes such as morbidity, length of stay, and disability rather than mortality are being evaluated.[33]

ICD-9 Injury Severity Score

The ICISS skirts all of the issues with the AIS and ISS by directly calculating the probability of survival (survival risk ratio [SRR]) from approximately 2000 individual trauma-related ICD-9-CM diagnoses.[33] The coefficients for the SRR are calculated from logistic regression from large databases. SRRs are only estimates of true survival and are database specific; however, they have been shown to be robust in terms of their application to other sets of injured patients from comparable populations.[33,34] In general, SRRs are not calculated independently of other injuries, and thus are not true representations of individual injury risk; however, independent SRRs based on single-injury cases are available.[35]

The original mortality tables for the ICISS SRRs are based on the non-trauma North Carolina Hospital Discharge Diagnosis (NCHDD) database.[36] The NCHDD is criticized for not being comparable to most populations of trauma patients with its overall low mortality, low numbers of trauma patients, and atypical injury patterns. Recalculated ICISS SRRs based on the National Trauma Data Bank (NTDB) and other databases have confirmed this, underscoring the need for adequate comparisons of SRRs from various sources.[7,36,37]

The ICISS carries the advantage that ICD-9-CM codes are readily available from hospital discharge codes; thus, no additional costs are incurred or trained personnel needed for capturing the data. Furthermore ICD-9-CM is universally available, and most medical personnel are familiar with ICD-based diagnosis coding in contrast to AIS coding. Another advantage of ICD-9 scoring is that risk stratification can easily be expanded to include coded comorbidities.[35] ICISS does not include physiologic data; however, it predicts mortality, costs, and length of stay as well as or better than risk adjustment models like TRISS and ASCOT that do.[35–40]

In ICD-9-CM, there are a limited number of rubrics for orthopedic, vascular, and solid organ injury descriptors, and severity of injury is not accounted for. Therefore, coding the best diagnosis with sufficient detail of the various potential injuries is problematic in ICD-9-CM. There has been an effort to correct these discrepancies in the ICD-10-CM, whose draft version is now available. ICD-10 is already in use in the United States for coding fatal injuries, but the clinical modification has not been finalized and approved yet. The number of injury descriptors in the ICD-10-CM is large and allows precise location of injuries, in particular of interest to researchers in transportation safety. A disadvantage that results when large numbers of descriptors are available is that the number of cases on which to base each SRR will be small, thus diminishing the accuracy of the SRRs. ICISS is rapidly becoming the trauma score of choice for mortality prediction and quality improvement processes and this trend will likely continue as ICD-10-CM becomes available.[37]

PHYSIOLOGIC SCORING SYSTEMS

Physiologic derangements including hypotension, tachypnea, and diminished mental status reflect the response of the patient to injury and have prognostic value. Physiologic scoring systems are hampered by the fact that physiologic parameters are constantly changing after injury and during resuscitation, and the timing and duration of these changes are not accounted for in existing systems. Typically, the ED admission or initial prehospital vital sign set is used for scoring, although there has always been a concern that prehospital vital signs may not be sufficiently accurate. Currently, there is no consensus on which data time point is the best predictor of outcome. Some patients with severe injury will not be identified by physiologic scores because they are able to compensate, or the field response is so rapid that physiologic compromise has not yet occurred. Physiologic scores overestimate injury severity when physiologic changes are the result of other factors such as drugs and alcohol rather than the consequences of trauma.[41]

Physiologic data are not captured by most inpatient administrative databases, and must be obtained by merging with prehospital or ED care databases or hand coding through trauma registries or chart review. As a result, patient records frequently have incomplete physiologic data, leading to substantial numbers of patients being excluded from outcome analysis.

Glasgow Coma Scale

The Glasgow Coma Scale (GCS) is a component of numerous trauma scoring systems since head injury and mental status carry significant prognostications. The GCS is the sum of three coded values: motor, verbal, and eye opening. However, the GCS may lead to overclassification of injury severity in patients with depression of the central nervous system secondary to drugs or alcohol or when the patient is intubated resulting in loss of the verbal score. It has been proposed that the best motor score of the GCS be used rather than the total GCS, as this tends to most accurately reflect true head injury and thus patient outcome.[41,42]

Revised Trauma Score

The Trauma Score (TS) and Revised Trauma Score (RTS) are physiologic trauma scores designed for field triage of patients who are significantly injured and require trauma center transfer. The TS is a simple sum of points based on the degree of derangement of the GCS, systolic blood pressure (SBP), respiratory rate (RR), respiratory expansion, and capillary refill time (CRT).[43] The RTS is a simplification of the TS that includes only the GCS, BP, and RR.[44] The RTS has been used as a tool for predicting survival by adding weighted coefficients based on logistic regression with values range from 0 (worst) to 7.84 (best). The RTS is heavily weighted toward the GCS to compensate for major head injury without significant physiological changes, and correlates well with survival.[44]

Acute Physiology and Chronic Health Evaluation

The Acute Physiology and Chronic Health Evaluation (APACHE II) is a widely used system to predict mortality in intensive care units, but has performed poorly in trauma patients most likely because it lacks an anatomical component.[35] APACHE III corrected this deficiency by including trauma-specific injury descriptors and equations, and accounting for head injury. However, this scoring system has not gained wide acceptance in part due to its proprietary nature, and it has not been validated in trauma patients.[45]

Physiologic Reserve

Physiologic reserve reflects a patient's ability to cope with injury, and is based on age, gender, comorbidities, and possibly genetic predisposition. Age has an effect on mortality in trauma patients gradually up to age 65 and increasing rapidly thereafter.[45] In-patient length of stay and discharge to long-term care are affected by age older than 55 and by some comorbidities.[45] The addition of an age factor improves the predictive ability for survival of most trauma scoring systems.[20] Comorbidities have a profound effect on individual patient outcome, even after controlling for age, anatomic and physiologic severity, and mechanism of injury.[46] Institutional outcomes may not be influenced by comorbidities, due to their low incidence in trauma patients.[47]

RISK-ADJUSTMENT SCORING SYSTEMS

Risk-adjustment scoring systems use regression analysis of large databases to determine probability of survival based on anatomical and physiological data and age. The addition of age or physiologic data to injury severity improves prediction of mortality in all trauma scoring models examined.[5]

Trauma and Injury Severity Score

The TRISS combines physiologic data from the RTS, anatomic data from the ISS, and age (less than or 55 years and older) and mechanism of injury to give a probability of survival or TRISS score.[2] A "pre-chart" analysis of RTS plotted against ISS can be used to calculate a survival probability of 0.5 based on regression analysis to identify patients with unexpected outcomes. These "TRISS unexpected survivors" are a widely used audit tool in identifying patients

for peer review to investigate prehospital and hospital factors that contribute to outcome.[10] The usefulness of this practice was recently called into question when a chart review of TRISS unexpected survivors revealed only 10% to be "unexpected survivors" based on clinical findings.[10]

Software to calculate TRISS is available and includes NATIONAL TRACS based on model coefficients derived from the MTOS (Major Trauma Outcome Study).[2] To determine the actual probability of survival, the calculated TRISS score is compared with the model data set using three statistics, W, Z, and M.[2,3] A positive W-statistic indicates that the institution has more survivors than predicted. The Z-statistic is used to assess whether the W-statistic is significantly different from zero, and hence whether the institution's performance is significantly different from that defined by the model data set. Z-statistics can be compared with a standard normal distribution. The M-statistic is used to examine the similarity in the case mix of the observed data, compared with the model data set. The value of M is between 0 and 1, with values close to 1 indicating a very similar mix of injury severities. A value of less than 0.88 has been deemed unacceptable for the purpose of comparison with the model database, and hence for interpretation of the W- and Z-statistics.[48] A relative outcome score (ROS) can be used to compare W-statistics against a perfect outcome of 100% survival. The ROS can be used as a benchmark to monitor improvement in institutional trauma care over time. An alternative to the Z- and W-statistics is the standardized mortality ratio (SMR). The SMR is defined as the ratio of the observed mortality rate (OMR) to the expected mortality rate (EMR) to identify hospital quality outliers. The SMR is the standard measure of quality used in critical care medicine.[9]

The TRISS has the best predictive value when studying patients with multiple injuries from blunt trauma. TRISS has poor predictive ability in isolated severe head trauma and multiple severe injuries to a single body region, and at the extremes of age. TRISS also does not distinguish between types of penetrating injuries, that is, stabbing versus gunshot, which are known to have disparate outcomes.[49] TRISS underestimates survival in the lowest predicted survival group because it is based on the ISS. TRISS methodology is currently advocated as the standard for benchmarking performance in the United States, and is widely accepted in many parts of the world.[50] Existing TRISS coefficients are based on MTOS data from U.S. trauma centers with a high percentage of penetrating trauma that is nearly 20 years old, and thus may not be applicable to foreign trauma centers and too outdated for current trauma systems. TRISS coefficients can be updated to reflect local databases, which should improve its predictive properties.[50]

A Severity Characterization of Trauma

To overcome the outcome limitations of TRISS, Champion and the American College of Surgeons Committee on Trauma proposed ASCOT, which uses AIS descriptors, physiologic data, mechanism, and age.[51] ASCOT incorporates all severe patient injuries in the prediction model via the AP, in contrast to TRISS, which considers only ISS injuries. ASCOT proved to be equivalent or better than TRISS in most studies, particularly penetrating trauma, but failed to be widely accepted, most likely because of the complex computations involved in deriving the score.[51] Like TRISS, the coefficients for ASCOT are based on the MTOS, which is biased toward severely injured and penetrating trauma patients.[3,52]

Risk-adjustment models like TRISS and ASCOT allow outcomes from different institutions to be adjusted for differences in injury severity, making it possible to compare hospital quality. Inaccurate risk adjustment may lead to some hospitals being labeled as poor quality and vice versa. However, a study comparing TRISS and ASCOT for identifying high-quality hospitals disagreed on the status of 35 of 69 hospitals studied.[9] A second study comparing trauma centers using TRISS found an unacceptably high misclassification rate in patients with severe trauma, further supporting the conclusion that currently these tools are unable to accurately provide benchmarking for quality improvement.[8] The addition of comorbidities was recently shown to improve TRISS performance for prediction of survival.[53]

Mechanism of Injury

The mechanism of injury, particularly blunt versus penetrating, is known to influence mortality. AIS, TRISS, and ASCOT all account for blunt and penetrating trauma in their methodology. More detailed data on mechanism of injury are collected by trauma registries or as external cause of injury codes (E-codes). E-codes refer to a supplemental code used to provide additional detail to injury ICD-9-CM codes within the range 800–999. Cause codes allow for the identification of excess morbidity and mortality associated with specific injury mechanisms for injury prevention programs.

SCORING SYSTEMS EVALUATION

Data Collection

The survival probability model is the most popular tool for evaluating trauma care.[54] Current models are based on linear logistic regression analysis of patient variables to identify those independently associated with mortality. Formulas are then derived to predict the probability of survival using weighted coefficients according to the effect of the variable on mortality. To be statistically sound, this multivariate analysis requires large databases of trauma patients. These databases must include data on a large number of variables, including patient demographics, comorbidities, injury type and severity, mechanism of injury, prehospital care, emergency department care, in-hospital care, and postdischarge follow-up. Complete and accurate data gathering into a database is dependent on operator input and data availability. Missing data are a particular problem with multivariate analysis, as often the entire patient record containing the missing piece of data must be discarded.

Databases

Trauma scores are derived from several types of databases: hospital administrative databases, trauma registries, and the NTDB. Administrative databases are derived from ICD-9-CM hospital discharge data that were collected for billing purposes.[46] They reflect the coding conventions of the institutions from which they were derived, and may be affected by reimbursement considerations. Furthermore, only the most significant injuries may be coded.[55] Administrative databases suffer from significant gaps in data, lacking such details as prehospital and emergency department care, physiologic data, and postdischarge follow-up. Trauma registries are designed to have no such gaps, capturing all phases of trauma care, but require dedicated personnel to administer. Trauma registries vary from hospital to hospital, mostly in the manner in which AIS and ISS are coded, which render comparisons between them difficult or even invalid.[21,48,56]

The NTDB functions as a national repository of trauma data to be used for epidemiology, injury prevention, clinical research, education, and resource allocation.[57] The NTDB voluntarily collects data from 565 U.S. hospitals, including 70% of the Level I trauma centers and 50% of the Level II trauma centers. It has a standardized data entry format that can be hand entered or automatically derived from existing trauma registry data. The NTDB collects data on a large number of variables felt to potentially impact quality of care in addition to patient demographics, complications, diagnosis, TRISS/ISS scores, and outcomes. It also documents the methodology used to determine AIS, ISS, TRISS, and diagnosis. The NTDB was created in 1989 by the American College of Surgeons, and participation by trauma centers has increased substantially in the past few years. The NTDB is nonproprietary, and its reports are available at no charge with a benchmark report for quality improvement processes provided annually to each participating hospital.

Outcome Measures

The most common outcome measured by trauma scores is mortality.[6] The timeframe for inclusion of mortality is not uniformly defined; thus, data on all fatalities may not be captured.[58–60] Mortality after injury may be variously defined as prehospital, in-hospital, 30- or 60-day postinjury, or all injury-related mortality identified postdischarge regardless of time period. For example, elderly patients are less able to survive mild to moderate injuries, and more likely to die of complications several weeks or months after the incident.[60] Such patients would not meet the mortality inclusion criteria of in-hospital or 30-day mortality definition. Postdischarge mortality is not captured by administrative databases, and is only sporadically captured by trauma registries.[61,62] Estimates of injury mortality substantially increase when using multiple independent databases to capture postdischarge fatalities.[63]

Prehospital deaths are not captured by trauma registries or administrative databases, but may affect mortality predictions for many injuries. Due to improved EMS, patients suffering fatal injuries that previously would have died, now make it to the hospital only to die soon after arrival.[58,64] In-hospital mortality is also affected by withdrawal of care practices. Hospitals with more liberal policies for withdrawal of care during the in-hospital period will report artificially higher in-hospital mortality. Lower in-hospital mortality rates will be reported by hospitals whose policy is to transfer early significantly disabled trauma patients to skilled nursing facilities. Withdrawal of care is usually documented in trauma registries but not in administrative databases.

Injury outcome is dependent on which outcome is measured, and may be impacted by factors not related to quality. Type of injury, age, and comorbidities affect various outcomes differently. For example, aortic injuries have a high mortality but low disability, compared with head injuries, which have moderate mortality and high disability. Young patients with head injuries have less disability and mortality than old patients.[65] Trauma patients with significant comorbidities are more likely to have complications. For example; diabetics are more likely to develop infections, obese patients are more likely to develop organ failure and patients with significant aortic stenosis have increased risk of death after injury.[66] The reported intensive care unit or hospital length of stay can be impacted by availability of ward beds or skilled nursing beds, and delay in discharge may be related to transportation and patient or family issues. Length of stay is increased in elderly patients and those with significant comorbidities. Length of stay is shorter when patients die early in their hospitalization, and these patients should be excluded from length-of-stay analysis. Trauma registries perform better than administrative databases for analyzing these situations.

Disability is a significant problem in trauma patients, and is an important outcome measure for quality improvement processes.[12] The Functional Capacity Index (FCI), Glasgow Outcome Scale score, and modified Functional Independence Measure (FIM) are all measures of functional impairment used in trauma research.[67,68] The predicted FCI ($pFCI_{12}$) is matched to descriptors in AIS-90 and measures the impact of injuries on function at 1 year. The original $pFCI_{12}$ did not discriminate well, and a consensus group was convened to address these issues. Those changes are currently being validated in the new version of AIS2005.[69] Hopefully, the $pFCI_{12}$ and other measures of functional impairment will prove useful in trauma research and quality improvement processes in the future.

SUMMARY

Trauma scoring systems are tools for ranking injury severity to allow risk adjustment for comparative analysis. The ideal trauma scoring system would accurately predict risk of death or functional disability, and provide a standard by which performance could be benchmarked for quality improvement processes.

Currently, there are no trauma scoring systems capable of fully supporting the quality improvement process because they fail to assess risk accurately enough to detect quality differences.

The AIS remains the foundation of most trauma scoring systems. Its widespread use in both the health care and transportation safety industries for injury description ensures its continued use. Furthermore, the availability of ICD mapping software and improved ICD injury descriptors will allow expanded use of the AIS by abstraction from non-trauma administrative databases. ISS functions well as a predictor of mortality, despite its statistical limitations. It will continue to find use in risk stratification of patients as a stand-alone function or as part of TRISS for trauma program quality improvement. Mortality, however, is best predicted by ICISS survival risk ratios derived from comparable databases. Furthermore, in most patients, the single worst injury predicts mortality the best.

Trauma scoring systems that only consider injury severity are useful, but insufficient for risk adjustment. It is not known which patient variables, in addition to injury severity, contribute most to accurate risk assessment. These variables are likely to differ depending on the outcome of interest. The design and validation of trauma scoring systems that can perform accurate risk adjustment will require access to large databases containing these variables of interest. These data are not available in administrative databases and are best captured through trauma databases. The NTDB fulfills that role in the United States. Data collection for the NTDB is dependent on trauma registries. To maximize accurate and complete data acquisition, an effort should be made to upgrade all trauma registries to a minimum standard including:

- Automatic data transfer to the NTDB
- Use of the latest version of AIS or ICD injury descriptors
- Accurate mapping software to convert ICD to AIS
- A method by which older data can be upgraded into the new system
- Well-defined quality outcome measures

Standardization would also allow trauma registry data to be easily meshed with other relevant databases for injury research, treatment, and prevention.

The ultimate goal of risk adjustment for quality improvement is to separate outcomes due to patient injury and reserve from issues of patient care. Trauma scoring systems must be developed that can support accurate risk adjustment, a vital component to continual quality improvement in trauma care.

REFERENCES

1. Baker SP, O'Neill B, Haddon W, Long WB: The injury severity score: a method for describing patients with multiple injuries and evaluating emergency care. *J Trauma* 14:167–196, 1974.
2. Boyd CR, Tolson MA, Copes WS: Evaluating trauma care: the TRISS method. Trauma Score and the Injury Severity Score. *J Trauma* 27:370–378, 1987.
3. Champion HR, Copes WS, Sacco WJ, Lawnick MM, et al: The Major Trauma Outcome Study: establishing national norms for trauma care. *J Trauma* 30:1356–1365, 1990.
4. MacKenzie EJ, Damiano A, Miller T, Luchter S: The development of the Functional Capacity Index. *J Trauma* 41:799–807, 1996.
5. Hannan EL, Hicks Waller C, Szypulski Farrell L, Cayten GC: A comparison among the abilities of various injury severity measures to predict mortality with and without accompanying physiologic information. *J Trauma* 58:244–251, 2005.
6. Meredith JW, Evans G, Kilgo PD, MacKenzie E, et al: A comparison of the abilities of nine scoring algorithms in predicting mortality. *J Trauma* 53:621–628, 2002.
7. Meredith JW, Kilgo PD, Osler TM: Independently derived survival risk ratios yield better estimates of survival than traditional survival risk ratios when using the ICISS. *J Trauma* 55:933–938, 2003.
8. Demetriades D, Chan L, Velmanos GV, Sava J, et al: TRISS methodology: an inappropriate tool for comparing outcomes between trauma centers. *J Am Coll Surg* 193:250–254, 2001.
9. Glance LG, Osler TM, Dick AW: Evaluating trauma center quality: does the choice of the severity-adjustment model make a difference? *J Trauma* 56:1265–1271, 2005.
10. Norris R, Woods R, Harbrecht B, Fabian T, et al: TRISS unexpected survivors: an outdated standard? *J Trauma* 52:229–234, 2002.
11. Jones JM: An approach to the analysis of trauma data having a response variable of death or survival. *J Trauma* 38:123–128, 1995.
12. Glance LG, Dick A, Osler TM, Mukamel D: Judging trauma center quality: does it depend on the choice of outcomes? *J Trauma* 56:165–172, 2004.
13. Harviel JD, Landsman I, Greenberg A, Copes WS, et al: The effect of autopsy on injury severity and survival probability calculations. *J Trauma* 29:766–772, 1989.
14. Committee on Medical Aspects of Automotive Safety: Rating the severity of tissue damage—1. The Abbreviated Injury Scale. *JAMA* 215:277–280, 1971.
15. Copes WS, Lawnick M, Champion HR, Sacco WJ: A comparison of abbreviated injury scale 1980 and 1985 versions. *J Trauma* 28:78–86, 1988.
16. Gennarelli T, Wodzin E: The Abbreviated Injury Scale–2005. Des Plaines, IL, Association for the Advancement of Automotive Medicine, 2005.
17. Moore EE, Cogbill TH, Malangoni MA, Jurkovich GJ, et al: Organ injury scaling. *Surg Clin North Am* 75:293–303, 1995.
18. Baker SP, O'Neill B: The injury severity score: an update. *J Trauma* 16:882–885, 1976.
19. Copes WS, Champion HR, Sacco WJ, Lawnick MM, et al: The injury severity score revisited. *J Trauma* 28:69–77, 1988.
20. Stephenson SCR, Langley JD, Civil ID: Comparing measures of injury severity for use with large databases *J Trauma* 53:326–332, 2002.
21. Garthe E, State JD, Mango NK: Abbreviated Injury Scale Unification: the case for unified injury system for global use. *J Trauma* 47:309–323, 1999.
22. MacKenzie EJ, Steinwachs DM, Shankar B: Classifying trauma severity based on hospital discharge diagnoses. Validation of an ICD-9CM to AIS-85 conversion table. *Med Care* 27:412–422, 1989.
23. Kilgo PD, Meredith JW, Hensberry R, Osler TM: A note on the disjointed nature of the injury severity score. *J Trauma* 57:479–485, 2004.
24. Russell RM, Halcomb BN, Caldwell BA, Sugrue M: Differences in mortality predictions between injury severity score triplets: a significant flaw. *J Trauma* 56:1321–1324, 2004.
25. Osler TM, Baker SP, Long W: A modification of the injury severity score that both improves accuracy and simplifies scoring. *J Trauma* 43:922–926, 1997.
26. Brenneman FD, Boulanger BR, McLellan BA, Redelmeier DA: Measuring injury severity: time for a change? *J Trauma* 44:580–582, 1998.
27. Copes WS, Champion HR, Sacco WJ, Lawnick MM, et al: Progress in characterizing anatomic injury. *J Trauma* 30:1200–1207, 1990.
28. Champion HR, Copes WS, Sacco WJ, Lawnick MM, et al: A new characterization of injury severity. *J Trauma* 30:539–545, 1990.
29. Tay SY, Sloan EP, Zun L, Zaret P: Comparison of the New Injury Severity Score and the Injury Severity Score. *J Trauma* 56:162–164, 2004.
30. Frankema SPG, Steryerberg EW, Edwards MJR, vanVugt AB: Comparison of current injury scales for survival chance estimation: an evaluation comparing the predictive performance of the ISS, NISS, and AP scores in a Dutch local trauma registration. *J Trauma* 58:596–604, 2005.
31. Lavoie A, Moore L, LeSage N, Liberman M, Sampalis JS: The New Injury Severity Score: a more accurate predictor of in-hospital mortality than the injury severity score. *J Trauma* 56;1312–1320, 2004.
32. Kilgo PD, Osler TM, Meredith W: The worst injury predicts mortality outcome the best: rethinking the role of multiple injuries in trauma outcome scoring. *J Trauma* 55:599–607, 2003.
33. Osler T, Rutledge R, Deis J, Bedrick E: ICISS: an international classification of disease-9 based injury severity score. *J Trauma* 41:380–386, 1996.
34. Meredith JW, Kilgo PD, Osler T: A fresh set of survival risk ratios derived from incidents in the National Trauma Data Bank from which the ICISS may be calculated. *J Trauma* 55:924–932, 2003.

35. Osler TM, Rogers FB, Glance LG, Cohen M, et al: Predicting survival, length of stay, and cost in the surgical intensive care unit: APACHE II versus ICISS. *J Trauma* 45:234–237, 1998.
36. Rutledge R, Osler T, Kromhout-Schiro S: Illness severity adjustment for outcomes analysis: validation of the ICISS methodology in all 821,455 patients hospitalized in North Carolina in 1996. *Surgery* 124:187–194, 1998.
37. Clarke JR, Ragone AV, Greenwald L: Comparisons of survival predictions using survival risk ratios based on International Classification of Diseases, Ninth Revision and Abbreviated Injury Scale trauma diagnosis codes. *J Trauma* 59:563–569, 2005.
38. Osler TM, Cohen M, Rogers FB, Camp L, et al: Trauma registry injury coding is superfluous: a comparison of outcome prediction based on trauma registry International Classification of Diseases-Ninth Revision (ICD-9) and hospital information system ICD-9 codes. *J Trauma* 43(2):253–256, 1997.
39. Rutledge R, Osler T, Emery S, Kromhout-Schiro S: The end of the Injury Severity Score (ISS) and the Trauma and Injury Severity Score (TRISS): ICISS, an International Classification of Diseases, ninth revision–based prediction tool, outperforms both ISS and TRISS as predictors of trauma patient survival, hospital charges, and hospital length of stay. *J Trauma* 44:41–49, 1998.
40. Rutledge R, Osler T: The ICD-9-based illness severity score: a new model that outperforms both DRG and APR-DRG as predictors of survival and resource utilization. *J Trauma* 45:791–799, 1998.
41. Healey C, Osler TM, Rogers FB, Healey MA, et al: Improving the Glasgow coma scale: motor score alone is a better predictor. *J Trauma* 54:671–680, 2003.
42. Offner PJ, Jurkovich GJ, Gurney J, Rivara FP: Revision of TRISS for intubated patients. *J Trauma* 32:32–35, 1992.
43. Champion HR, Sacco WJ, Carnazzo AJ, Copes W, Fouty WJ: Trauma Score. *Crit Care Med* 9:672–676, 1981.
44. Champion HR, Sacco WJ, Copes WS, Gann DS, et al: A revision of the Trauma Score. *J Trauma* 29:623–629, 1989.
45. Vassar MJ, Lewis FR Jr, Chambers JA, Mullins RJ, et al: Prediction of outcome in intensive care unit trauma patients: a multicenter study of Acute Physiology and Chronic Health Evaluation (APACHE), Trauma and Injury Severity Score (TRISS), and a 24-hour intensive care unit (ICU) point system. *J Trauma* 47(2):324–329, 1999.
46. Clark DE, Winchell RJ: Risk adjustment for injured patients using administrative data. *J Trauma* 57:130–140, 2004.
47. Sacco WJ, Copes WS, Bain LW Jr, MacKenzie EJ, et al: Effect of preinjury illness on trauma patient survival outcome. *J Trauma* 35:538–542, 1993.
48. Joosse P, Goslings JC, Luitse JSK, Ponsen KJ: M-study: arguments for regional trauma databases. *J Trauma* 58:1272–1276, 2005.
49. Cayton CG, Stahl WM, Murphy JG, Agarwal N, Byrne DW: Limitations of the TRISS method for interhospital comparisons: a multihospital study. *J Trauma* 31:471–482, 1991.
50. Clark DE: Comparing institutional trauma survival to a standard: current limitations and suggested alternatives. *J Trauma* 47:S92–S98, 1999.
51. Champion HR, Copes WS, Sacco WJ, Frey CF, et al: Improved predictions from a severity characterization of trauma (ASCOT) over Trauma and Injury Severity Score (TRISS): results of an independent evaluation. *J Trauma* 40:42–48, 1996.
52. Hannan EL, Medeloff J, Farrell LS, Cayten CG, Murphy JG: Validation of TRISS and ASCOT using a non-MTOS trauma registry. *J Trauma* 38:94–95, 1995.
53. Bergeron E, Rossignol M, Osler T, Clas D, Lavoie A: Improving the TRISS methodology by restructuring age categories and adding comorbidities *J Trauma* 56:760–767, 2004.
54. Jones JM, Redmond AD, Templeton J: Uses and abuses of statistical models for evaluating trauma care. *J Trauma* 38:89–93, 1995.
55. Hunt JP, Cherr GS, Hunter C, Wright MJ, et al: Accuracy of administrative data in trauma: splenic injuries as an example. *J Trauma* 49:679–686, 2000.
56. Jurkovich GJ, Mock C: Systematic review of trauma system effectiveness based on registry comparisons. *J Trauma* 47:S46–S55, 1999.
57. American College of Surgeons: National Trauma Data Bank Report 2005. Available at www.facs.org/trauma/ntdb.html.
58. Demetriades D, Murray J, Charalambides K, Alo K, et al: Trauma fatalities: time and location of hospital deaths. *J Am Coll Surg* 198:20–26, 2004.
59. Lucas CE, Buechter KJ, Coscia RL, Hurst JM, et al: The effect of trauma program registry on reported mortality rates. *J Trauma* 51:1122–1126, 2001.
60. Olson CJ, Brand D, Mullins RJ, Harrahill M, Trunkey DD: Time to death of hospitalized injured patients as a measure of quality of care. *J Trauma* 55:45–52, 2003.
61. Mullins RJ, Mann NC, Hedges JR, Worrall W, et al: Adequacy of hospital discharge status as a measure of outcome among injured patients. *JAMA* 279:1727–1731, 1998.
62. Mullins RJ, Mann NC, Brand DM, Lenfesty BS: Specifications for calculation of risk-adjusted odds of death using trauma registry data. *Am J Surg* 173:422–425, 1997.
63. Mann NC, Knight S, Olson LM, Cook LJ: Underestimating injury mortality using statewide databases. *J Trauma* 58:162–167, 2005.
64. Riddick L, Long WB, Copes WS, Dove DM, Sacco W: Automated coding of injuries from autopsy reports. *Am J Forensic Med Pathol* 19:269–274, 1998.
65. Demetriades D, Kuncir E, Murray J, Velmahos GC, et al: Mortality prediction of head Abbreviated Injury Score and Glasgow Coma Scale: analysis of 7,764 head injuries. *J Am Coll Surg* 199(2):216–222, 2004.
66. Neville AL, Brown CV, Weng J, Demetriades D, Velmahos GC: Obesity is an independent risk factor of mortality in severely injured blunt trauma patients. *Arch Surg* 139:983–987, 2004.
67. Livingston DH, Lavery RF, Mosenthal AC, Knudson MM, et al: Recovery at one year following isolated traumatic brain injury: a Western Trauma Association prospective multicenter trial. *J Trauma* 59:1298–1304, 2005.
68. MacKenzie EJ, Sacco WJ, Luchter S, Ditunno JF, et al: Validating the Functional Capacity Index as a measure of outcome following blunt multiple trauma. *Qual Life Res* 11:797–808, 2002.
69. Gotschall CS: The Functional Capacity Index, second revision: morbidity in the first year post injury. *Int J Inj Contr Saf Promot* 12:254–256, 2005.

TRAUMA SYSTEMS AND TRAUMA TRIAGE ALGORITHMS

Antonio Pepe, Antonio Marttos, Mauricio Lynn, and Jeffrey A. Augenstein

Trauma is a major national health care problem that affects one of four U.S. citizens annually. Traumatic injury, both accidental and intentional, is the leading cause of death in the United States for people aged 1 to 34 years. There are as many as 150,000 trauma deaths and approximately 80,000 others who sustain long-term disability each year with annual costs of more than $260 billion for trauma injury and treatment when loss of future productivity is considered. The most common fatal injuries in the country result form motor vehicle crashes, followed closely by gunshot wounds. Driving while impaired by alcohol is the most frequent cause of fatal motor vehicle crashes and accounts for 40% of traffic fatalities. The causes of traumatic death vary considerably depending on demographics. Urban and politically unstable areas typically have a higher incidence of penetrating trauma, whereas rural and stable communities have a predominance of blunt injuries, usually vehicular accidents. Nonetheless, causes of death after injury are remarkably similar. Central nervous system injury accounts for approximately half of all fatalities; hemorrhage for 35%; and sepsis, multiple organ failure, and pulmonary embolism combine for approximately 15%. With the introduction of trauma systems during the last three decades, the incidence of preventable death has dropped from approximately 25% to less than 5%. This is the result of improvements in care both for acute head injuries and for control of hemorrhage. In addition, the incidence of late death attributable to sepsis and multiple organ failure has diminished, possibly as a result of better and early resuscitation. The responsibility of the trauma surgeon encompasses the early recognition of injury, resuscitation, and then definitive care of the patient. As we improve the operative and intensive care rendered to trauma patients, we are beginning to reach the flat portion of the outcome curve. The area of injury prevention is still open to substantial improvement. To reduce the morbidity and mortality from trauma, surgeons must take a more active role in the prevention of trauma at the community level. Studies have shown the effect of these systems on the improvement of trauma care, with outcomes better than those predicted for some study populations. The necessary elements of a trauma system have been defined. These include four primary patient needs—access to care, prehospital care, hospital care, and rehabilitation. In addition, five issues require social and political solutions to supplement medical efforts: prevention, disaster medical planning, patient education, research, and rational financial planning. Recent federal legislation (The Trauma Care Systems Planning and Development Act) authorized planning, implementation, and development of statewide trauma care systems.

Data show, however, that only 23 states in the United States have functional, statewide trauma systems, and eight states have no trauma system at all. In the United States, as many as 35% of trauma patients who die do so because optimal acute care is not available. Despite the evidence that trauma care systems save lives, existing systems serve only one fourth of the U.S. population.

TRAUMA SYSTEMS

A trauma system is an organized, coordinated effort in a defined geographic area that delivers the full range of care to all injured patients and is integrated with the local public health system. The true value of a trauma system is derived from the seamless transition between each phase of care, integrating existing resources to achieve improved patient outcomes. Success of a trauma system is largely determined by the degree to which it is supported by public policy. The development of civilian regional trauma systems has provided the single most significant improvement in the care of injured patients in the last three decades.

Numerous regional and statewide systems have been created to optimize quality of care and outcomes for severely injured patients. An essential component of a trauma system involves the evaluation of patients at the scene by emergency medical technicians to determine if their injuries meet specified trauma triage criteria that indicated they would be best served by being transported to a trauma center, thereby integrating the prehospital, transport, and trauma center settings. Triage is the process whereby the patient's medical needs are matched with the available medical resources and can occur in the field and at the hospital. Field triage identifies those patients needing transport to the most appropriate trauma center rather than the nearest hospital and also identifies the type of transport needed. The trauma patient is an injured person who requires timely diagnosis and treatment of actual or potential injuries by a multidisciplinary team of health care professionals. Supported by the appropriate resources, the goal is to diminish or eliminate the risk of death or permanent disability. Injuries occur across a broad spectrum and a trauma system must determine the appropriate level of care for each type of injury. The goal of triage criteria is to closely match patients' needs to the appropriate resources.

With respect to hospital triage, both the available level of hospital resources and time/distance factors are considered in making triage and destination decisions. Level III/IV hospital triage should serve to identify those patients who require initial stabilization and rapid transfer to the next highest level of care, and those patients that can be safely held in a Level III/IV center for further evaluation and serial observations. Level I/II hospital triage identifies patients who require a full trauma team approach as well as those who can be initially evaluated by identified members of the trauma team with subsequent consultation by either a trauma surgeon or the appropriate subspecialist.

Many areas of the country already have resources in place to provide appropriate trauma care. To provide optimal care of the seriously injured with maximum efficiency and minimal cost in terms or lives, disability, and dollars, these resources must be organized using a systems approach to plan for the rapid decisions required for initial treatment or all injured patients—an inclusive system. A proper systems approach requires a regional triage system with identified trauma centers capable of providing trauma care to major trauma patients. Patients must be identified and delivered or transferred based on clinical need to the appropriate level of care in a timely fashion. An optimal trauma care system is designed to care for all injured patients with specific attention focused on major trauma patients.

Major trauma patients are those with either a severe injury or a risk for severe injury. A severe injury is one that could result in morbidity or mortality, and is classically defined as an injury with an Injury Severity Score (ISS) of 16 or higher. On initial evaluation, these patients typically have abnormal vital signs or a significant anatomical injury. However, triage is often inexact due to patients' variable physiological responses to trauma. In some patients, minor injuries can result in morbidity or mortality due to the patient's age and/or comorbid factors, and some patients may have a delayed physiological response to trauma. Patients involved in a high-energy event are at risk for severe injury. Five to 15% of these patients, despite normal vital signs and no apparent anatomical injury on initial evaluation, will have a severe injury discovered after full trauma evaluation with serial observations (Figure 1).

Current systems ("exclusive systems") often rely on overtriage to trauma centers, and often an exaggerated and unnecessary response from trauma professionals. Such systems may cause overtreatment of certain patients, unnecessary expenses, burnout of participants, and underutilization of certain health care resources, including personnel. In spite of these excesses, such systems may still run the risk of not treating all injured patients, including not appropriately treating all major trauma patients. Undertriage runs the obvious risk of excluding some major trauma patients from receiving appropriate care. An inclusive system uses a tiered response to provide appropriate delivery, evaluation, and care for all patients, including the major trauma patient, in a cost-effective manner. One example of an inclusive trauma system is patient triage designed to care for major trauma patients by matching patient severity to facility in a timely manner. Considerations in triage include injury severity, injury severity risk, time and distance from site of injury to definitive care, inter-hospital transfers considering guidelines for immediate versus postintervention transports, and factors that activate the regional system (Figure 2).

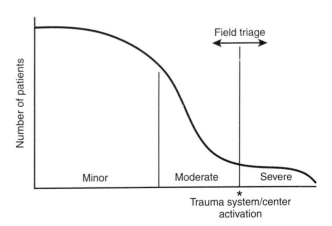

Figure 1   Triage in trauma care system.

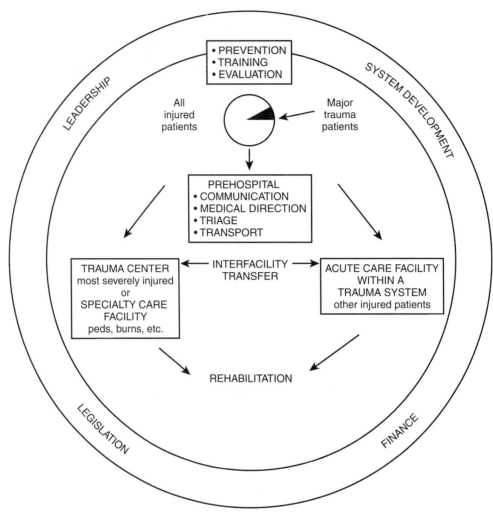

Figure 2 Components of an inclusive trauma care system. The components in this model are based on the components described in several trauma care resources. *(Adapted from Trauma Care Systems, a position paper from the Third National Injury Control Conference, "Setting the National Agenda for Injury Control in the 1990's," p. 388.)*

TRAUMA SYSTEMS SUMMARY

A systems approach to the provision of trauma care, including appropriate guidelines for the triage of patients, is essential. The triage protocols should be reasonable and inclusive, considering such factors as time and distance to designated trauma centers and appropriate utilization or resources at these centers. In order for a systems approach to work, appropriate protocols that are well thought out and supported by all members of the trauma system should be in place and followed unless clinical judgment dictates a valid reason otherwise.

By combining triage algorithms with an appropriate quality improvement monitoring system, optimal and cost-effective care can be provided. Continuous quality improvement and research are essential to evaluate an algorithm's applicability in a given trauma care system. The result should be protocols with the sensitivity to identify major injury, yet specific enough to not overburden the system, allowing for optimal and cost-effective care using existing resources. Identification of the major trauma patient is fundamental to trauma system design because it describes the patient who will benefit the most from regionalized care, and indirectly determines the level and intensity of resources needed to provide definitive care.

Triage criteria should provide a basis for the establishment of protocols for patient identification, delivery decisions, and appropriate response at acute care facilities for all trauma patients in an inclusive care system. They should recognize the requirements of individual trauma systems, as well as the importance of clinical judgment. Patients can then be delivered, depending on degree of injury in addition to time and distance from site of injury to definitive care.

SUPPORT FOR REGIONALIZED TRAUMA CARE

Although regionalization of trauma care has the inevitable consequence of increased prehospital transport times, particularly in rural areas removed from large trauma centers, some states have designed inclusive systems in which a large number of smaller centers have been designated as lower-level trauma centers. One of the primary functions of a statewide trauma system is to oversee the initiation of standardized protocols intended to ensure the timely triage and transfer of severely injured patients to facilities with appropriate therapeutic resources. Several studies document increased trauma center use and enhanced patient outcomes among metropolitan trauma centers after implementation of a regionalized trauma system.

In 1987, Shackford et al. examined the impact of a trauma system on the survival of patients and attributed the improved survival to the integration of prehospital and hospital care and subsequent expeditious surgery. In 1999, Mullins and Mann reviewed published studies that used population-based data in evaluating the effectiveness of trauma systems in North America. They found that data for eight of nine trauma systems evaluated demonstrated improve outcomes (15%–20%), principally measured as hospital survival, after the establishment of a trauma system or some component of a trauma system. In the National Study on the Costs and Outcomes of Trauma (2006), MacKenzie et al. examined the effect of care in a trauma center on the risk of death and costs associated with treatment at hospitals with a Level 1 trauma center and at hospital without a trauma team. They concluded that, with the 25% lower overall risk of death noted when care was provided at a trauma center versus a non-trauma center, efforts for continued regionalization should be supported.

INITIAL APPROACH TO THE CRITICALLY INJURED PATIENT

Salvage of the critically injured patient is optimized by a coordinated team effort in an organized trauma system. Management of life-threatening trauma must be prioritized according to physiologic necessity for survival—that is, active efforts to support airway, breathing, and circulation (the ABCs) are usually initiated before specific diagnoses are made. A systematic approach to the severely injured patient within the "golden hour" is critical. The initial approach to the critically injured patient can be divided into prehospital care and emergency department (ED) management; the ED component is further divided into (1) primary survey with initial resuscitation, (2) evaluation and continued resuscitation, and (3) secondary survey with definitive diagnosis and triage.

Prehospital Care: Intervention at Injury Site

Resuscitation and evaluation of the trauma patient begins at the injury site. The goal is to get the right patient to the right hospital at the right time for definitive care. First responders (typically, firefighters and police) provide rapid basic trauma life support (BTLS) and are followed by paramedics and fight nurses with advanced trauma life support (ATLS) skills. Medical control is ensured by pre-established field protocols, radio communication with a physician at the base hospital, and subsequent trip audits. Management priorities of BTLS on the scene are (1) to access and control the scene for the safety of the patient and the prehospital care providers, (2) to tamponade external hemorrhage with direct pressure, (3) to protect the spine after blunt trauma, (4) to clear the airway of obstruction and provide supplemental inspired oxygen, (5) to extricate the patient, and (6) to stabilize long-bone fractures. Whereas the benefits of BTLS are undisputed, the merits of the more advanced interventions remain controversial.[1,2] Airway access, once considered a major asset of the care provided by paramedics and flight nurses, has now been questioned, not only because missed tracheal intubation is a concern but also because unintentional hyperventilation (hypocarbia) is detrimental in the setting of traumatic brain injury (TBI) and during cardiopulmonary resuscitation (CPR).[3–5] Moreover, the value of intravenous fluid administration remains controversial.[6,7]

Field Triage

Prehospital trauma scores have been devised to identify critically injured trauma victims, who represent about 10%–15% of all injured patients. When it is geographically and logistically feasible,

critically injured patients should be taken directly to a designated Level I trauma center or to a Level II trauma center if a Level I trauma center is more than 30 minutes away. The currently available field trauma scores, however, are not entirely reliable for identifying critically injured patients[8]: to capture a sizable majority of patients with life-threatening injuries, a 50% overtriage is probably necessary. Advance transmission of key patient information to the receiving trauma center facilitates the organization of the trauma team and ensures the availability of ancillary services[9] (Figures 3 and 4).

Declaration of Death at Scene

The determination that care is futile during prehospital evaluation is best made on the basis of the cardiac rhythm. Asystole justifies declaration of death at the scene, and recent profound bradycardia (heart rate <40 beats/min) has been shown to signal an unsalvageable situation.

GUIDELINES FOR WITHHOLDING OR TERMINATION OF RESUSCITATION IN PREHOSPITAL CARDIOPULMONARY ARREST

Injury is the leading cause of death for Americans between age 1 and 44 years. The EMS system is the portal into the medical system for many of the most seriously injured trauma victims. Some of these patients will be unsalvageable due to the extent of their injuries. In order to preserve dignity and conserve precious human and financial resources, as well as to minimize risks to the health care workers involved, patients who can be predicted to be unsalvageable should not be transported emergently to the emergency department (ED) or trauma center. The National Association of EMS Physicians (NAEMSP) and the American College of Surgeons Committee on Trauma (COT) support out-of-hospital withholding or termination of resuscitation for adult traumatic cardiopulmonary arrest (TCPA) patients who meet specific criteria. The literature review of prehospital TCPA is extrapolated from emergency thoracotomy research. This research is retrospective in nature, therefore limiting the validity of the conclusions. The guidelines appear in Table 1.

Initial Electrocardiographic Rhythm

There is some evidence that the initial ECG rhythm obtained at the scene by EMS may be predictive of survival. All of the studies combined by Batistella et al.,[10] Fulton et al., Esposito et al.,[9] and Aprahamian suggest that the presence of an ECG rhythm such as asystole, idioventricular rhythm, or severe bradycardia is indicative of an unsalvageable patient. Patients with a sinus-based pulseless electrical activity may represent a potentially salvageable subset of TCPA patients. Given that the TCPA is a critical event, the presence of any abnormal ECG pattern as an indicator of survival has limited significance. Blunt and penetrating injury as the cause of the TCPA was not distinguished in these studies, and given that blunt injury causing TCPA is associated with a very poor survival rate, it may be that survivors of TCPA may have penetrating trauma as their inciting event.

Resuscitation Duration

The data collectively suggest that a patient with TCPA and more than a 15-minute transport time while in arrest will not survive, regardless of the aggressiveness of the care delivered.

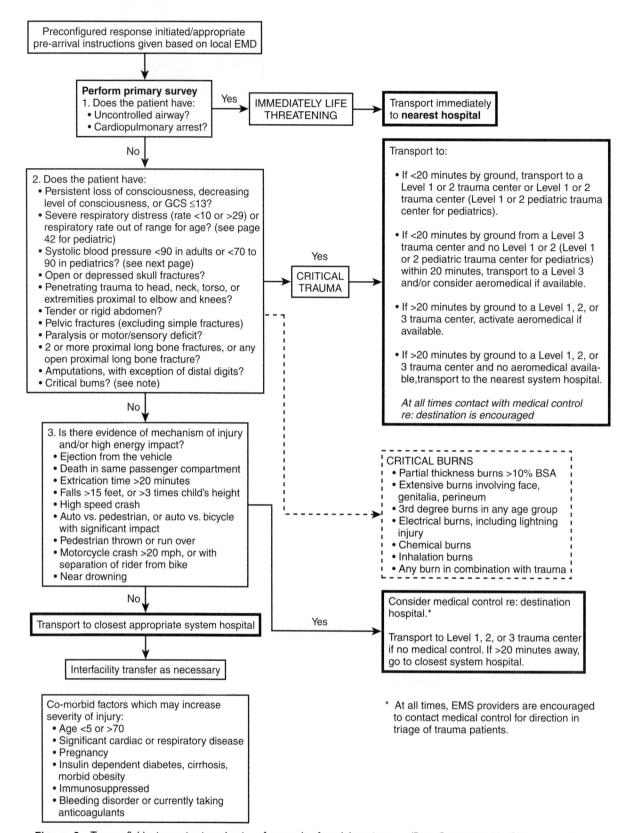

Figure 3 Trauma field triage criteria and point-of-entry plan for adult patients.   *(From Commonwealth of Massachusetts, Department of Public Health.)*

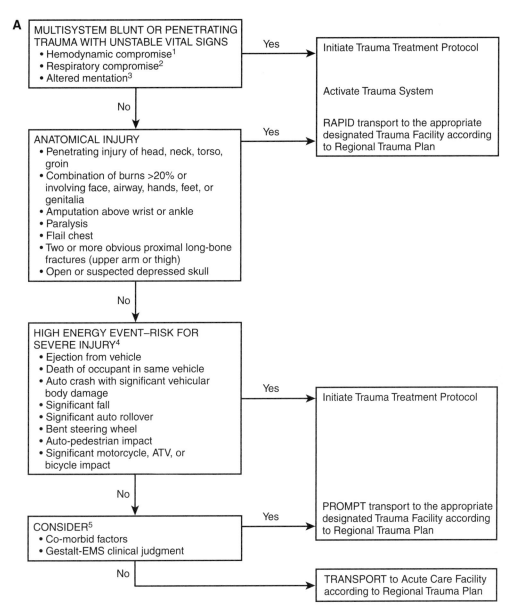

Figure 4 Adult triage, transport, and transfer guidelines: Oklahoma model trauma triage algorithms for **(A)** prehospital, **(B)** Level I/II trauma center, and **(C)** Level III/IV trauma center. For prepubescent patients, refer to the pediatric trauma algorithm (Figure 5). 1. In addition to hypotension, other early signs of hypovolemia may include pallor, tachycardia, or diaphoresis. 2. Tachypenia (hyperventilation) alone will not necessarily initiate this level of response. 3. Altered sensorium secondary to sedative-hypnotic will not necessarily initiate this level of response. 4. High-energy event signifies a large release of uncontrolled energy. Patient is assumed injured until proven otherwise, and multisystem injuries might exist. Determinants to be considered by medical professionals are direction and velocity of impact, patient kinematics and physical size, and the residual signature of energy release (e.g., major vehicle damage). 5. Clinical judgment must be exercised and may upgrade to a high level of response and activation. Age and comorbid conditions should be considered in the decision. 6. Isolated blunt or penetrating trauma not associated with a high-energy event with a potential for multisystem injury. *(Based on American College of Emergency Physicians Guidelines. Approved by the Triage, Transport, and Transfer Committee of the Oklahoma State Trauma Advisory Council, October 27, 1995, and the Oklahoma Emergency Medical Services Advisory Council on January 24, 1997.)*

Continued

Emergency Department Thoracotomy

The prehospital implications of these studies are significant. At the scene of blunt injury, patients without vital signs (reported survival rates less than 2%) or in the case of penetrating trauma, patients without vital signs or other significant signs of life will not survive even with the most aggressive of therapies. Therefore, resuscitation and emergent transport of these TCPA victims are not warranted. Of patients who sustain TCPA, data suggest that penetrating trauma isolated to the thorax is the most salvageable subset of patients and any signs of life at the time of EMS arrival may reflect a potential survivor.

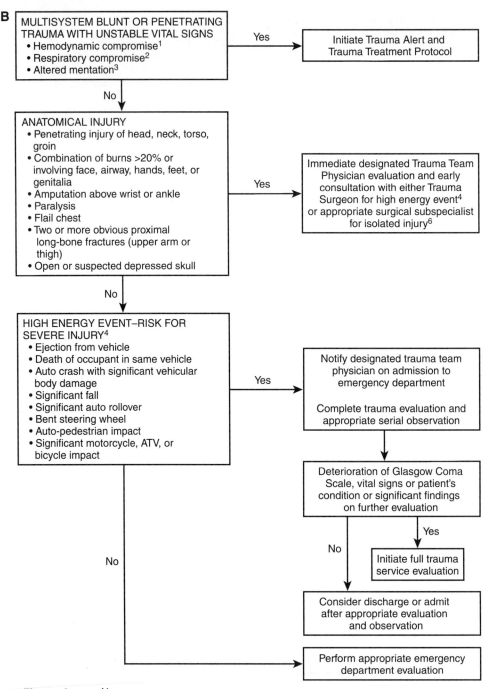

Figure 4, cont'd.

Rapid Transport versus Field Stabilization

The question of which patients with severe traumatic injuries should be transported without delay, and which patients might benefit from on-scene stabilization has spurred debate for many years. Despite conflicting reports and recommendations, some generalizations can be made based on the available evidence. Consistent with data from the ET literature, in the case of TCPA, expeditious transportation of a patient deemed to be potentially salvageable to a trauma center for definitive treatment is crucial. In addition to the need for expedient transport, TCPA patients appear to benefit from interventions such as intubation and IV line insertion. Time is critical, and TCPA lasting more than 10–15 minutes in the field is a lethal event. It appears that,

at least in urban settings with short EMS transport times, ATLS interventions may be lifesaving if they can be performed in a timely fashion.

Air Medical Transport

Studies by Wright et al. and Margolin et al. have specifically addressed the transport of TCPA patients in their respective studies. Although retrospective and influenced by selection bias, the results from theses studies may indicate that for a select group of patients who are resuscitated successfully, prompt transfer to a trauma center may confer a survival benefit.

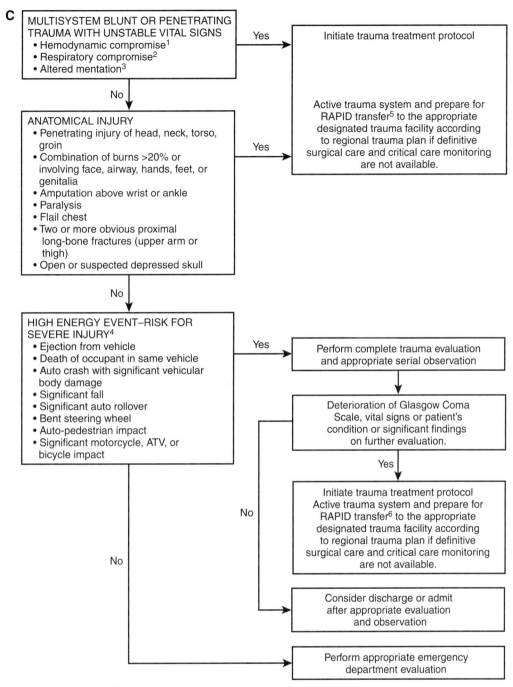

Figure 4, cont'd.

Exceptions

Situations in which trauma is complicated by significant hypothermia should not be included in these recommendations. Profound hypothermia below 32° C will cause progressive bradycardia, decreased cardiac output, loss of consciousness, and, ultimately, loss of brainstem reflexes—effectively mimicking death, but with the potential for successful resuscitation with appropriate medical treatment and rewarming. Examples of hypothermia complicating trauma may include cold-water submersion (particularly in children), avalanche burial, and minor trauma with subsequent environmental exposures. In these situations, patients should be aggressively resuscitated and transported to a center capable of aggressively rewarming the victims.

PREHOSPITAL CARE CONTROVERSIES

Advanced Trauma Life Support

The growing sophistication of emergency medical services has expanded the scope of prehospital care, but the extent of prehospital interventions remains a highly controversial issue. In trauma, advocates of the so-called scoop-and-run philosophy argue that resuscitative efforts in the field unnecessarily delay provision of definitive care and have detrimental effects on physiology and survival when overzealously applied. At present, there is little evidence to support the use of ATLS in prehospital management

Table 1: Guidelines for Withholding or Termination of Resuscitation in Prehospital Cardiopulmonary Arrest

Resuscitation efforts may be withheld in any blunt trauma patient who, based on out-of-hospital personnel's thorough primary patient assessment, is found apneic, pulseless, and without organized ECG activity upon the arrival of EMS at the scene.

Victims of penetrating trauma found apneic and pulseless by EMS, based on their patient assessment, should be rapidly assessed for the presence of other signs of life, such as papillary reflexes, spontaneous movement, or organized ECG activity. If any of these signs are present, resuscitation should be performed and the patient transported to the nearest emergency department or trauma center. If these signs of life are absent, resuscitation efforts may be withheld.

Resuscitation efforts should be withheld in victims of penetrating or blunt trauma with injuries obviously incompatible with life, such as decapitation or hemi-corpectomy.

Resuscitation efforts should be withheld in victims of penetrating or blunt trauma with evidence of a significant time lapse since pulseless-ness, including dependent lividity, rigor mortis, and decomposition.

Cardiopulmonary arrest patients in whom the mechanism of injury does not correlate with clinical condition, suggesting a nontraumatic cause of the arrest, should have standard resuscitation initiated.

Termination of resuscitation efforts should be considered in trauma patients with EMS-witnessed cardiopulmonary arrest and 15 minutes of unsuccessful resuscitation and cardiopulmonary resuscitation (CPR).

Traumatic cardiopulmonary arrest patients with transport time to an emergency department or trauma center of more than 15 minutes after the arrest is identified may be considered nonsalvageable, and termination of resuscitation should be considered.

Guidelines and protocols for TCPA patients who should be transported must be individualized for each EMS system. Consideration should be given to factors such as the average transport time within the system, the scope of practice of the various EMS providers within the system, and the definitive care capabilities (trauma centers) within the system. Airway management and intravenous line placement should be accomplished during transport when possible.

Special consideration must be given to victims of drowning and lightning strike and in situations where significant hypothermia may alter prognosis.

EMS providers should be thoroughly familiar with the guidelines and protocols affecting the decision to withhold or terminate resuscitative efforts.

All termination protocols should be developed and implemented under the guidance of the system EMS medical director. On-line medical control may be necessary to determine the appropriateness of terminating resuscitation.

Policies and protocols for terminating resuscitation efforts must include notification of the appropriate law enforcement agencies and notification of the medical examiner or coroner for final disposition of the body.

Families of the deceased should have access to resources, including clergy, social workers, and other counseling personnel, as needed. EMS providers should have access to resources for debriefing and counseling as needed.

Adherence to policies and protocols governing termination of resuscitation should be monitored through a quality review system.

of urban trauma patients. ATLS skills may be of value in rural areas where transport time exceeds 30 minutes, but unfortunately, the limited volume of serious trauma in such areas makes it difficult to gain the experience necessary to maintain this expertise.

Airway Management

The current recommendation—orotracheal intubation with in-line manual stabilization of the head and neck—has proved safe in clinical series to date. When orotracheal intubation fails, the laryngeal mask airway (LMA) is a rapid, safe, and effective technique for maintaining temporary airway control until definitive medical care becomes available. For patients with extensive maxillofacial trauma that precludes oral intubation, cricothyroidotomy has been the traditional alternative, but this procedure has some risks, particularly in children.

Prehospital Intubation of Patients with Traumatic Brain Injury

Because hypoxia has been associated with increased mortality in patients with TBI, aggressive prehospital airway protocols that include rapid sequence intubation have been instituted. This practice may, however, be associated with worse outcomes.[3]

Prehospital Volume Resuscitation

Hypotensive patients with penetrating torso injuries, survival improved when fluid resuscitation was delayed until surgical intervention had controlled the source of hemorrhage. Although this clinical trial had some methodologic flaws, it is important because it emphasizes that source control of hemorrhage is an overriding priority in hemodynamically unstable patients. At present, the rational compromise between these two approaches is hypotensive resuscitation with moderate volume loading. Whereas this approach is becoming the standard of care for penetrating trauma, its application to blunt trauma is not as clear. Some 20% of patients with major torso trauma have a serious concomitant TBI; if they are inadequately resuscitated, reduced cerebral perfusion pressure may lead to devastating secondary brain injury.

Resuscitation with Hypertonic Saline

Small-volume hypertonic saline (HS) has been shown to be as effective as large volume crystalloid in expanding plasma volume and enhancing cardiac output. HS increases perfusion of the microcirculation by inducing selective arteriolar vasodilation and by reducing the swelling of red blood cells and endothelium, at the expense of possibly increasing bleeding. HS combined with HS dextran (HSD) may have improved resuscitative effects. Trials comparing HS to HSD have shown inconsistent results with respect to improved survival, yet confirming that a bolus of either fluid was safe. Subgroup analysis of these studies showed that patients who presented with shock and concomitant severe TBI benefited the most from HSD. In comparison to isotonic saline, both HS and HSD raised cerebral perfusion pressure, lowered intracranial pressure, and reduced brain edema.

PEDIATRIC TRAUMA SYSTEM

Injury is the leading cause of death in children older than 1 year. In 2001, more than 5500 children younger than 15 years died as a result of injuries. Another 1000 died because of violent deaths, the result of homicide or suicide. With respect to nonfatal injuries, in 2002, more than 100,000 children were hospitalized, and more than 6 million children were evaluated in emergency departments after sustaining an injury. Falls are the most common mechanism of injury and motor vehicle crashes are the most deadly, accounting for 30%–60% of traumatic pediatric deaths. Trauma systems, pediatric trauma centers (PTCs), and caregivers who are specifically trained to treat children are all components of a system of care designed to provide better outcomes for patients. Regional PTCs were established to optimize the care of injured children. However, because of the relative shortage of PTCs, many injured children continue to be treated in adult trauma centers (ATCs). It is well known that the geographic distribution of trauma centers results in a significant number of children being treated in adult centers with various ACS designations.[15] As a result, growing controversy has evolved regarding the impact of PTCs and ATCs on outcome for injured children. Many medical facilities are not adequately staffed or equipped with the necessary resources to optimally care for severely injured pediatric trauma victims.

An EMSC sponsored APSA study published in 2005 demonstrated that injured children have better outcomes when trauma care is received at a designated children's hospital. Densmore et al.[17] used the 2000 Kid's Inpatient Database (part of the Health Care Cost and Utilization Project sponsored by the Agency for Health Care Research and Quality) to describe pediatric trauma patient allocation to hospitals and associated injury outcomes. Approximately 80,000 pediatric trauma cases from 27 states were analyzed. The authors concluded that younger and more severely injured children have improved outcomes in children's hospitals.

Potoka et al.[12] analyzed 13,351 injured children from the Pennsylvania Trauma Outcome Study between 1993 and 1997. With mortality as the major outcome variable, cases were evaluated and compared based on type of trauma center: PTC, Level I ATC (ATC I), Level II ATC, or an ATC with added qualification to treat children (ATC AQ). They reported that most injured children were treated at a PTC or an ATC AQ and that most children younger than 10 years were admitted to a PTC. Overall survival was significantly better at a PTC and an ATC AQ compared with an ATC I and a Level II ATC. Survival for head, spleen, and liver injuries was significantly better at a PTC compared with all other destinations combined. Children who sustained moderate or severe head injuries were most likely to undergo neurosurgical intervention and have a better outcome when treated at a PTC. Despite similar mean AISs for spleen and liver trauma, significantly more children underwent surgical exploration (especially splenectomy) for spleen and liver injuries at an ATC compared with a PTC. Nonoperative management of splenic and hepatic injuries decreases the potential morbidities of surgical therapy and postsplenectomy sepsis. They concluded that pediatric commitment in a Level I trauma center results in nonoperative treatment of injured children commensurate with that established in regional PTCs. The authors concluded that children treated at a PTC or ATC-AQ have significantly better outcomes compared to those treated at an ATC. In addition, ACS-verified centers had significantly higher survival rates compared with unverified centers. Severely injured children (ISS >15) with head, spleen, or liver injuries had the best overall outcome when treated at a PTC. This difference in outcome may be attributable to the approach to operative and nonoperative management of head, liver, and spleen injuries at PTCs.

Three studies, two retrospective and one prospective, provided evidence (class 3) of the influence of trauma systems and pediatric trauma centers on mortality rates for children who sustain moderate to severe TBI as well as evaluating the influence of a PTC on the number of neurosurgical procedures. Conclusions from the studies follow:

- Pediatric patients with severe TBI are more likely to survive if treated in PTCs or ATC AQs, rather than in Level I or Level II ATCs.
- The pediatric patient with severe TBI who requires neurosurgical procedures has a lower chance of survival in Level II ATCs versus the other centers.
- In 2001, Osler et al.[19] reviewed 53,113 pediatric trauma cases from 22 PTCs and 31 ATCs included in the National Pediatric Trauma Registry to evaluate survival rates. They reported the overall mortality rate to be lower at PTCs (1.81% of 32,554 children) than at ATCs (3.88% of 18,368 children). The authors concluded that although PTCs have higher overall survival rates compared with ATCs, the difference disappears when the analysis controls for ISS, Pediatric Trauma Score, age, mechanism, and ACS verification status.
- In 1994, Bensard et al.[18] sought to critically evaluate the outcome of injured children treated in an ATC I by adult trauma surgeons. The probability of survival was calculated using TRISS methodology. They found that the observed survival (98.0%) in children compared favorably with the TRISS-predicted survival (97.7%), and showed no difference in relative risk for acutely injured children (+0.47) compared with young adults (+0.45) or national norms such as the Major Trauma Outcomes Study (MTOS) reference set. They concluded that the triage of injured children to an ATC I does not adversely affect outcome. However, there are limitations when applying the TRISS methodology to children which include very few pediatric patients in the original data set, elements of the physiological data which use adult norms and not pediatric norms, and finally, the MTOS-derived data from 1982 to 1989 may be questionable, as injury rates declined from 1990 to 2005. These data support the continued triage of acutely injured children to regional trauma centers regardless of pediatric or adult designation.

Conclusions

Over the past decade, there has been much debate regarding to pediatric trauma outcomes and their association with different types of trauma centers. There appears to be sufficient data, however, to support continued development of formalized pediatric systems despite the lack of definitive evidence on the effectiveness of PTCs and pediatric trauma systems. Several recent studies have concluded that injured children treated at PTCs have better outcomes and are more likely to survive compared with those treated at ATCs. Other studies concluded that children treated at a PTC or an ATC AQ have significantly better outcomes compared with those treated at ATCs. Studies on the management of blunt pediatric trauma suggest that trauma centers have lower rates of pediatric splenectomy after blunt trauma compared with nontrauma centers. Designated PTCs should spearhead the development of an effective field triage system that would guarantee that the most severely injured children undergo treatment at a trauma center with commitment to the care of the injured child.

With the regionalization of designated pediatric subspecialty and trauma care centers and the triaging of injured children to appropriate designations, pediatric trauma systems in the United States are becoming valuable tools in the optimum care of injured children. However, with the specialization of pediatric trauma care systems still in its infancy, the triage of all injured children to regional PTCs may be impractical and may unnecessarily exclude Level I ATCs from the care of acutely injured children. Ongoing studies on pediatric trauma, including measures of morbidity and functional outcomes, are needed to further define the optimal models and systems for trauma care. PTCs are the only institutions with the pediatric trauma volumes necessary for the study of outcome measures, and with the capabilities to take the initiative in the study injury prevention (Figure 5 and Table 2).

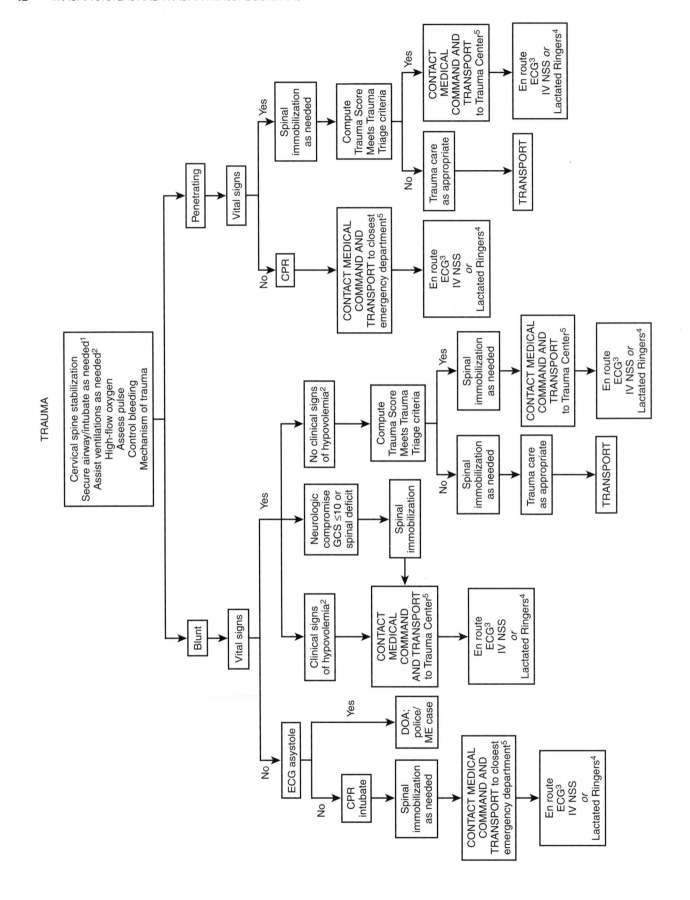

Figure 5 Pediatric trauma algorithm. This protocol refers to all pediatric major trauma victims. One of the greatest causes of death and permanent morbidity in children is hypoxia secondary to central nervous system or airway injury. Any child with neurologic compromise (Glasgow Coma Scale [GCS]≤10 or spinal deficit) should have a secure airway, adequate ventilation, and spinal immobilization, and then immediate transport to an accredited pediatric trauma center. As a goal, time on scene must not exceed 10 minutes for patients meeting physiologic (vital signs, GCS) or anatomy-of-injury trauma-triage criteria. Life-threatening injuries occur less frequently in patients who meet mechanism-of-injury criteria only. Therefore, if it is necessary to complete patient immobilization and packaging, prehospital providers may extend on-scene time to 20 minutes. Circumstances such as prolonged extrication, which result in on-scene time intervals exceeding those stated above, must be documented. 1. Confirm and document endotracheal tube placement with $ETCO_2$ detector. Listen for and document equal bilateral breath sounds in the chest and an absence of sounds over the epigastrium. 2. Clinical signs of hypoperfusion: (i) tachycardia, thready pulse; (ii) diaphoresis, peripherally cold and clammy; (iii) decreased capillary nail bed filling; (iv) lightheadedness, vertigo; (v) altered mental state; (vi) pallor, mottled, cyanotic; (vii) weakness, fatigue. 3. Organized ECG activity without vital signs (pulseless electrical activity [PEA]) indicates the need for immediate transport to a receiving facility that is determined appropriate by medical command authority. Ventricular fibrillation should be treated in accordance with the pediatric ventricular fibrillation protocol while en route. 4. For hypotensive trauma patients, an intravenous line of normal saline or lactated Ringer's, as per trauma center protocols, may be started while en route to an accredited trauma center. If unable to obtain IV access, place an intraosseous (IO) line. Once established, the IO line replaces the IV line as the primary route of administration for fluid and medications. 5. Notify medical command. *(From Delaware County EMS Medical Intervention Procedures: Pediatric Protocols 2002.)*

Table 2: Average Pediatric Vital Signs

Temperature	Age	Pulse	Blood Pressure[a]	Respirations
36°–37° C	Newborn	140–160	80/50	Infant: 40
	1 year	120	82/54	Preschool: 30
	2 years	110	84/56	School age: 20
	4–6 years	100	90/60–110/76	
	8–10 years	90	116/78	
	12 years	80	120/80	

[a]Hypotension implies a systolic blood pressure 10 mm Hg less than the average value for age.
Adapted from *Delaware County EMS Medical Intervention Procedures: Pediatric Protocols 2002.*

PRACTICE MANAGEMENT GUIDELINES FOR GERIATRIC TRAUMA

Advanced age is a well-recognized risk factor for adverse outcomes following trauma. A substantial body of literature demonstrates increased morbidity and mortality in geriatric trauma patients compared to their younger counterparts. Whether this outcome difference is due to the deceased physiologic reserve that accompanies aging, a higher incidence of pre-existing medical conditions in the geriatric patient, or to other factors yet to be identified, remains unclear. It is clear, however, that good outcomes can be achieved in this patient with survivable injuries. Implicit in the above statement is the need to identify, as soon as possible following injury, patients who will benefit from aggressive resuscitation, timely injury management, and posttrauma rehabilitation. It is equally important, however, to limit these intensive and expensive treatment modalities to patients whose injuries are not only survivable, but are compatible with an acceptable quality of life.

Triage Issues in Geriatric Trauma

Statement of the Problem

The process of triage, as it relates to the geriatric trauma patient, is an attempt to provide the patient with the appropriate intensity of medical resources, taking into account the severity of illness, the cost and availability of medical resources, the prognosis for functional survival and, if known, the expressed desires of the patient. For the geriatric trauma patient this process begins in the prehospital phase of care where decisions must be made regarding the appropriate patient destination, trauma center versus non-trauma center. Throughout the hospital phase of care, the patients must be "triaged" toward or away from operative procedures, invasive and expensive critical care therapies, and powerful, yet potentially dangerous pharmacologic treatment options, decisions which, again, must be based upon the likelihood of achieving a good, long-term outcome for the patient.

Issues to define include the following:

1. Appropriate criteria for triage of geriatric trauma patients to trauma centers
2. Clinical variables that would be useful in predicting the need for intensive care resources for geriatric trauma patients
3. Clinical circumstances in which a nonaggressive approach from the outset could be justified (Table 3)

Scientific Foundation

For the geriatric trauma patient, the process begins in the prehospital arena, where prehospital providers must decide on the basis of relatively scant clinical information whether a patient should bypass the local hospital in favor of a trauma center. The American College of Surgeons Committee on Trauma (ACS-COT), among other medical organizations, in its manual "Optimal Resources for the Care of the Trauma Patient," has published a set of triage

Table 3: Triage Recommendations for the Geriatric Patient

Level I	There are insufficient class I and class II data to support any standards regarding triage of geriatric trauma patients.
Level II	Advanced patient age should lower the threshold for field triage directly to a trauma center.
Level III	Advanced patient age is not predictive of poor outcomes following trauma, and therefore should *not* be used as the sole criterion for denying or limiting care in this patient population.
	The presence of pre-existing medical conditions in elderly trauma patients adversely affects outcome.
	In patients 65 years of age and older, a Glasgow Coma Scale (GCS) <8 is associated with a dismal prognosis. If substantial improvement in GCS is not realized within 72 hours of injury, consideration should be given to limiting further aggressive therapeutic interventions.
	Postinjury complications in the elderly trauma patient negatively impact survival and contribute to longer lengths of stay in survivors and nonsurvivors compared to younger trauma patients.
	With the exception of patients who are moribund on arrival, an initial aggressive approach should be pursued with the elderly trauma patient, as the majority will return home, and up to 85% will return to independent function.
	In patients 55 years of age and older, an admission base deficit <6 is associated with a 66% mortality. Patients in this category may benefit from inpatient triage to a high-acuity nursing unit.
	In patients 65 years of age and older, a Trauma Score <7 is associated with a 100% mortality. Consideration should be given to limiting aggressive therapeutic interventions.
	In patients 65 years of age and older, an admission respiratory rate <10 is associated with a 100% mortality. Consideration should be given to limiting aggressive therapeutic interventions.
	Compared to younger trauma patients, patients 55 years of age and older are at considerably increased risk for undertriage to trauma centers even when these older patients satisfy appropriate triage criteria. The factors responsible for this phenomenon must be identified and strategies developed to counteract it.

criteria to aid prehospital providers in identifying appropriate patients for direct transport to trauma centers.[1] Within this document, it is suggested that patients aged over 55 should be "considered" for direct transport to a trauma center, apparently without regard to the severity of injury. This recommendation is based on a substantial medical literature that demonstrates significantly worse outcomes for geriatric trauma patients compared to their nongeriatric counterparts.

The MTOS, sponsored by the ACS-COT. Data from 3833 patients 65 years and older were compared with data from of 42,944 patients aged under 65. Mortality rose sharply between age 45 and 55 and doubled at 75. This age-dependent survival decrement occurred at all ISS values, for all mechanisms of injury, and for all body regions. Numerous other studies have supported the findings that the effect of trauma on the elderly is more serious than on younger patients.

Predictors of Mortality in Geriatric Population

Age and Outcome

The ISS was found to be the best predictor of mortality in trauma patients, but age, gender, and pre-existing medical conditions (PECs) were also found to be *independent* predictive factors of mortality. Mortality was defined as in-hospital death.

Can the age of a geriatric patient, then, be used to predict outcome following trauma? While age appears to have some value in mortality projections for a *population* of geriatric trauma patients, there is certainly no literature support for a specific age above which geriatric trauma *in-hospital mortality* can be predicted with any degree of confidence.

The preponderance of available literature, however, suggests more favorable long-term outcomes, with up to 85% of survivors functioning independently at home at follow-up intervals as long as 6 years postinjury. Thus, given reasonable long-term functional outcomes for geriatric trauma patients surviving hospitalization, and the inability of patient age, by itself, to predict in-hospital mortality, advanced patient age should not be used as the sole

criteria for denying or limiting care in the geriatric trauma population.

Pre-Existing Conditions and Outcome

Since the frequency of PECs does increase with age, it may be difficult to separate these two factors and their relationships to adverse outcomes in geriatric trauma. The literature addressing the prognostic value of PECs in geriatric trauma outcome is inconclusive.

Severity of Injury Scoring and Outcome

A number of physiologic and anatomic "scores" have been shown to correlate with geriatric outcome. However, from the perspective of field or ED triage, many of these scores have little value in that they are not derivable at the moment that these particular triage decisions need to be made. These indices may have some value in the prediction of lethal outcomes in geriatric trauma, and, therefore, may be valuable triage tools in the intensive care unit.

On the other hand, measures of *physiologic* derangement, whether obtained via physical examination or chemical analysis, may help to identify patients who will perhaps benefit from aggressive resuscitation strategies (and should therefore be triaged to an intensive care unit), as well as those in which further resuscitated efforts are futile (thus facilitating earlier termination of resuscitation). Only the base deficit has been subjected to sufficient scientific study, and is sufficiently relevant to geriatric trauma resuscitation.

Measurement of arterial base deficit may provide useful information regarding the extent of shock and the adequacy of resuscitation in trauma patients, and may therefore be useful in early decision making and resource allocation. Elderly patients with severe base deficits had a high mortality as high as 80% in some series. However, geriatric trauma mortality was still markedly elevated at 60% in patients with only moderate base deficits. Even a "normal" base deficit carried a mortality of 24%. Thus, early determination of admission base deficit in geriatric trauma patients may facilitate early identification of "occult shock," and identify a subgroup of patients who may benefit from more intensive monitoring and resuscitation.

The ISS is probably the most widely studied anatomic or physiologic severity of illness score yet to be correlated with geriatric trauma outcome. Its use as a predictor of outcome and mortality in geriatric are inconclusive. ISS is severely limited in its prognostic capability due to significant delays in obtaining sufficient data to calculate the score.

Complications and Outcome

It is generally acknowledged that when the geriatric trauma patient sustains complications during the initial hospitalization that overall outcome is adversely affected. Comparing elderly survivors with nonsurvivors, a statistically higher incidence of cardiac and septic complications and respiratory complications occurs in nonsurvivors. Other authors, employing logistic regression statistical methodology, have identified cardiac, infectious, and pulmonary complications as independent predictors of poor outcome following geriatric trauma. The *number* of complications sustained by a given geriatric trauma patient has been identified as a risk factor for poor outcomes. Smith, in a study of 456 trauma patients aged 65 and over, reported 5.4% mortality for patients with no complications, 8.6% for those with one complication, and 30% for those with more than one complication. Similar results have been noted for geriatric patients sustaining TBIs.

Outcome from Geriatric Head Injury

The topic of geriatric head injury has received more attention in the literature than has any other aspect of geriatric trauma. Unfortunately, all of it is retrospective in nature and, therefore, suffers from many of the same methodological shortcomings. "Low" admission GCS is clearly associated with poor outcomes in elderly head-injured patients. The available scientific literature, however, does not support the use of a specific GCS that will reliably identify patients destined for poor outcomes. Thus, it seems that, while "low" GCS scores are indeed associated with poor outcomes, it does not seem possible, or advisable, based on the existing literature, to make triage decisions in head-injured geriatric patients based solely upon the *admission* GCS. It does seem reasonable to conclude that head-injured patients aged 65 years and older have very poor outcomes when the admission GCS is less than 7 or 8.

It is recommended that aggressive treatment for 24 hours only for those patients *without* space-occupying lesions. Aggressive treatment, then, is continued only in those patients who show "significant" improvement within this timeframe. Thus, in geriatric head injury, it seems reasonable to adopt an initial course of aggressive treatment (with the possible exception of the patient who is moribund upon arrival), followed by a re-evaluation of the patient's neurologic status at 72 hours postadmission. The intensity of the subsequent care provided can then be based on the initial response to therapy.

Parameters for Resuscitation of the Geriatric Trauma Patient

In the United States, the elderly, defined as individuals aged 65 years and older, are the fastest-growing segment of the population. Trauma is the seventh leading cause of death in the elderly with a death rate significantly higher compared to younger cohorts. Several studies have indicated that shock, respiratory failure, decreasing trauma score (TS), increasing injury severity score (ISS), increasing base deficit, and infectious complications portend a poor outcome. The multiply injured geriatric patient may appear stable, yet may have a significant perfusion deficit due to low cardiac output. The early use of invasive monitoring may improve survival. Although mortality may be increased compared to younger patients, an aggressive treatment program will allow many geriatric patients to regain function at or near their preinjury independence.

The evidence-based recommendations in Table 4 will provide the trauma practitioner a guide to decision making in the resuscitation phase of care of the geriatric patient.

Summary

While multiple clinical and demographic factors have demonstrated an association with outcome following trauma in geriatric patients, the ability of any specific factor alone, or in combination with other factors, to predict an unacceptable outcome for any individual geriatric trauma patient is quite limited. An initial course of aggressive therapy seems warranted in all geriatric trauma patients, regardless of age or injury severity, with the possible exception of those patients who arrive in a moribund condition. Geriatric trauma patients who do not respond to aggressive resuscitative efforts within a timely fashion are likely to have poor outcomes even with continued aggressive treatment. Modification of the intensity of treatment provided to these "nonresponders" should be considered. For geriatric trauma patients who do respond favorably to aggressive resuscitative efforts, the prognosis, not only for

Table 4: Evidence-Based Recommendations for Decision Making in Resuscitation Phase of Care of the Geriatric Patient

Level I recommendations:	There are insufficient data to support a Level I recommendation for endpoints of resuscitation in the elderly patient as a standard of care.
Level II recommendations:	Any geriatric patient with physiologic compromise, significant injury (Abbreviated Injury Scale [AIS] >3), high-risk mechanism of injury, uncertain cardiovascular status, or chronic cardiovascular or renal disease, should undergo invasive hemodynamic monitoring using a pulmonary artery catheter.
	There are insufficient data to support a Level I recommendation for endpoints of resuscitation in the elderly patient as a standard of care.
Level III recommendations:	Attempts should be made to optimize to a cardiac index ≥4 l/min/m² and/or an oxygen consumption index of 170 cc/min/m².
	Base deficit measurements may provide useful information in determining status of resuscitation and risk of mortality.

survival but also for return to their preinjury level of function, is quite good, and certainly justifies the effort.

CONCLUSION

The development of a trauma system in a geographic area provides for access to trauma care and rapid transport of major trauma victims to specific hospitals in that region. The development of trauma systems has resulted in a significant reduction in patient mortality rates within the first hours after injury. Trauma centers have concentrated resources and expertise to treat severely injured patients immediately and effectively throughout their care. Trauma systems, when fully implemented throughout the United States, will enhance community health through an organized system of injury prevention, acute care, and rehabilitation that is fully integrated with the public health system in a community. Trauma systems will possess the distinct ability to identify risk factors and related interventions to prevent injuries, and will maximize the integrated delivery of optimal resources for patients who ultimately need acute trauma care. Trauma systems will address the daily demands of trauma care and form the basis for disaster preparedness. The resources required for each component of a trauma system will be clearly identified, deployed, and studied to ensure that all injured patients gain access to the appropriate level of care in a timely, coordinated, and cost-effective manner. Experience gained from the development of trauma systems has demonstrated the importance of the commitment required from surgeons to meet the specific problems encountered in the process. Regardless of the number of injured or the source of injury, advanced planning, preparation, and coordination are essential for optimal response and care.

The benefits of successful implementation of this plan include the following:

- Reduction in deaths caused by trauma
- Reduction in the number and severity of disabilities caused by trauma
- Increase in the number of productive working years seen in the United States through reduction of death and disability
- Decrease in the costs associated with initial treatment and continued rehabilitation of trauma victims
- Reduced burden on local communities as well as the federal government in support of disabled trauma victims
- Decrease in the impacts on "second trauma" victims—families.

Suggested Readings

Aprahamian C, Thompson BM, Gruchow HW, Mateer JR, Tucker JF, Stueven HA, Darin JC: Decision-Making in pre-hospital sudden cardiac arrest. *Ann Emerg Med* 15(4):445–449, 1986.

Batistella FD, et al: Trauma patients 75 years and older: long-term follow-up results justify aggressive management. *J Trauma* 44:618–624, 1998.

Bensard DD, et al: A critical analysis of acutely injured children managed in an adult Level 1 trauma center. *J Pediatr Surg* 29:11–18, 1994.

Delaware County EMS Medical Intervention Procedures II: Pediatric Protocols. Rev. December 15, 2002.

Densmore et al: Outcomes and delivery of care in pediatric injury. *J Pediatr Surg* 41:92–98, 2006.

EAST Practice Management Guidelines Work Group: *Practice Management Guidelines for Geriatric Trauma.* East Northport, NY, Eastern Association for the Surgery of Trauma, 2001.

Esposito TH, et al: Do pre-hospital trauma center triage criteria identify major trauma victims? *Arch Surg* 130:171–176, 1995.

Fulton RL, Voigt WJ, Hilakos AS: Confusion surrounding the treatment of traumatic cardiac arrest. *J Am Coll Surg* 181:209–214, 1995.

Gaines BA: Pediatric trauma care: an ongoing evolution. *Clin Pediatr Emerg Med* 6:4–7, 2005.

Hannan EL, Farrell LS, Cooper A, Henry M, et al: Physiologic trauma triage criteria in adult trauma patients: are they effective in saving lives by transporting patients to trauma centers? *J Am Coll Surg* 200:584–592, 2005.

Hopson LR, Hirsh E, Delgado J, Domeier RM, et al: *Guidelines for Withholding or Termination of Resuscitation in Prehospital Traumatic Cardiopulmonary Arrest: Joint Position Statement of the National Association of EMS Physicians and the American College of Surgeons Committee on Trauma.* Lenexa, KS: National Association of EMS Physicians, 2003.

Hoyt DB, Coimbra R: Trauma systems. In Greenfield LJ, editor: *Surgery: Scientific Principles and Practice,* 3rd ed. Philadelphia, Lippincott, Williams & Wilkins, 2001, pp. 280–283.

Junkins EP, O'Connell KJ, Mann NC: Pediatric trauma systems in the United States: do they make a difference? *Clin Pediatr Emerg Med* 7(2): 76–81, 2006.

Khan CA, et al: National Highway Traffic Safety Administration (NHTSA) Notes. *Ann Emerg Med* 41(6):212, 2003.

MacKenzie EJ, et al: A national evaluation of the effect of trauma-center care on mortality. *N Engl J Med* 354:366–378, 2006.

Margolin DA, Johan DJ, Fallon WF: Response After Out of Hospital Cardiac Arrest in the Trauma Patient Should Determine Aeormedical Transport to a Trauma Center.

Mullins RJ, Mann NC: Population-based research assessing the effectiveness of trauma systems. *J Trauma* 47:S34–S41, 1999.

Osler TM, et al: Do pediatric trauma centers have better survival rates than adult trauma centers? An examination of the National Pediatric Trauma Registry. *J Trauma* 50:96–101, 2001.

Peterson TD, Vaca F: Commentary: trauma systems: a key factor in homeland preparedness. *Ann Emerg Med* 41(6):799–801, 2003.

Potoka DA, et al: Blunt abdominal trauma in the pediatric patient. *Clin Pediatr Emerg Med* 6:23–31, 2005.

Reilly JJ, et al: Use of a statewide administrative database in assessing a regional trauma system: the New York City experience. *J Am Coll Surg* 198(4):509–518, 2004.

Scalea TM, et al: Geriatric blunt multiple trauma: improved survival with invasive monitoring. *J Trauma* 30:129–136, 1990.

Smith DP, Enderson BL, Maull KI: Trauma in the elderly: determinants of outcome. *South Med J* 83:171–177, 1990.

Trauma Systems, Pediatric Trauma Centers, and the Neurosurgeon. Pediatr Crit Care Med 4(3)(Suppl), 2003.

Wright SW, Dronen SC, Combs TJ, Storer D: Aeormedical transport of patients with posttraumatic cardiac arrest. *Ann Emerg Med* 18:721–726, 1989.

PREHOSPITAL TRAUMA CARE

DELIVERING MULTIDISCIPLINARY TRAUMA CARE: CURRENT CHALLENGES AND FUTURE DIRECTIONS

Fahim Habib and **Eddy H. Carrillo**

The origins of trauma care delivery are deeply rooted in the major military conflicts of the last century. During the Napoleonic Wars, Dominique Larrey established the concepts of field hospitals, the use of the "flying ambulances" and the principles of triage.[1] In World War I, rapid and timely evacuation of the injured from the battlefield through echelons of treatment facilities, each with increasing surgical capabilities, became the standard of care.[2] During World War II, in addition to reducing the time from evacuation to treatment, the principle of "resuscitation" or treatment of shock prior to transport evolved. When combined with the other advances in transfusion technology, surgical technique, antibiotics, and so on, this systematic approach to trauma care resulted in a significant decrease in mortality. This approach was further refined in the Korean conflict and the Vietnam War, when wounded soldiers were rapidly transported within minutes by helicopter to fully capable hospitals, where the entire spectrum of trauma care from initial resuscitation to definitive surgical management was delivered.[3] Experience gained in the battlefield allowed large, urban medical centers to develop similar paradigms of trauma care for victims of "urban warfare." However, in spite of extensive training, these same trauma surgeons were unable to provide the same level of care outside these urban hospitals. Therefore, it became clear that the system, and not the individuals, were responsible for the observed successes, and the need for trauma systems, not just trauma surgeons, became recognized.

The publication of the seminal report, *Accidental Death and Disability: The Neglected Disease of Modern Society*, in 1966 became the catalyst in changing the delivery of trauma care. This report highlighted the magnitude of the problem in both human and economic terms and lack of an organized public or governmental response to the problem. As this became a major political issue, Congress responded by enacting the National Highway Safety Act of 1966. The resultant funding spurred the development of trauma systems in the states of Maryland, Florida, and Illinois. Additional federal funding followed passage of Titles 18 and 19 of the Medicare and Medicaid Act, the Emergency Medical Services Systems Act of 1973, and the Emergency Medical Services Amendments of 1976. Prompted by

perceived financial gains, a large number of hospitals sought designation as "trauma centers." With the sharp decline in funding following the Omnibus Budget Reconciliation Act of 1981, the exodus of participating institutions was as rapid as their entry into the system. The specialty care of trauma then became the purview of centers that retained an interest in caring for victims of traumatic injury in spite of the disadvantages that are associated with doing so.[4]

Over the ensuing years, trauma systems have matured with the trauma center as their cornerstone. Adequately addressing the issue of traumatic injury is recognized to include a spectrum beginning with injury prevention and education, throughout the immediate acute care phase, and extending into the rehabilitation. The success of these systems is recognized in the ability of trauma centers, in the context of trauma systems, to reduce mortality and morbidity. Further, lessons learned are being applied in the theater of war. Medical teams on the front lines of battle in Iraq and Afghanistan are receiving training prior to deployment at select trauma centers and employing principles refined in the civilian sector (Figure 1).

In spite of this compelling evolution, the delivery of trauma care continues to face significant challenges (Table 1). Technological advances of the last decade have increased the complexity of care, and require a multidisciplinary approach for an optimal outcome. Such an approach is associated with increasing costs, which in the face of skyrocketing malpractice premiums and declining reimbursements, challenges the financial health of trauma centers. Increased involvement of multiple specialists makes the logistics of providing adequate emergency room coverage and coordination of care a potentially daunting task. The workforce of trained trauma surgeons is shrinking as new graduates from general surgery training programs see trauma, in all but select programs, as a predominantly nonoperative specialty.

Trauma surgeons are essentially viewed as specialists who prepare injured patients for surgical procedures conducted by other specialists. Mandated reductions in resident work hours have limited their ability to maintain the traditional continuity of care that until recently was the hallmark of a surgical residency program. Such reductions have also raised concerns regarding the operative experience of current trainees. Additionally, in contrast to elective surgical patients, trauma patients pose unique challenges including the need to address nutritional concerns, issues of substance abuse, need for neuropsychological support, rehabilitation, and requirement for social support after resolution of the acute event. Further, additional considerations need to be entertained when managing special populations including children, pregnant women, and the elderly. Finally, educational outreach activities and continued research are an integral part of the efforts to improve outcomes. Unfortunately, despite the magnitude of its impact as the leading cause of death and disability in the first four decades of life, funding for trauma sadly trails that of diseases such as cancer and heart disease.

In order to overcome these challenges, we need to redefine the philosophy of trauma surgery and trauma surgeons. The purpose of

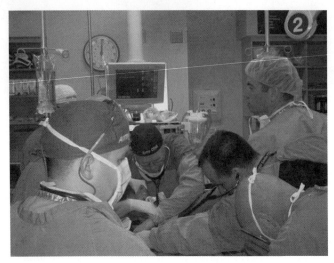

Figure 1 The forward surgical team of the Army Trauma Training Center receives hands-on training at the Ryder Trauma Center of the University of Miami/Jackson Memorial Hospital.

this review is to describe efforts that are currently under way and other potential solutions currently being entertained to optimize patient care.

ORGANIZING THE INITIAL CARE OF TRAUMA PATIENTS

Prehospital Communication

Direct communication between the trauma center and emergency medical personnel is key.[5] The heads-up on the nature and number of arriving trauma victims along with the estimated time of arrival allows for better preparation of required personnel and equipment. This becomes more relevant when multiple casualties are involved, and team members of varying levels of experience are designated

Table 1: Key Challenges to Multidisciplinary Delivery of Trauma Care

Financial	Increasing costs
	Skyrocketing malpractice premiums
	Declining reimbursements
Multispecialty care	Emergency room coverage
	Coordination of care
Shrinking workforce	Limited trained trauma surgeons
	Restricted resident work hours
	Reduced operative experience
Special considerations	Nutritional support
	Substance abuse
	Neuropsychological support
	Rehabilitation
	Placement
Special populations	Children
	Pregnant women
	Elderly
Funding	Educational outreach activities
	Research

according to patients' severity of injuries. In specific circumstances, it also allows certain specialists to be called in even before the patient arrives (e.g., the neurosurgeon for a traumatic quadriplegia). Activation of "surge capacity" procedures for mass casualty events can be done with the maximum lead time.[6] In addition, medical direction can be provided to prehospital personnel in cases outside the realm of those in standard operating procedures.

Tiered Trauma Team Activation

Patients meeting trauma criteria result in activation of a trauma alert. The full complement of providers arrives at the resuscitation bay after being notified. The time before actual patient arrival is utilized to determine what is known about the patient, the likely interventions required, and to reaffirm roles. Members of such a team include the trauma surgeon, trauma fellow/senior surgical resident, junior surgical resident, trauma nurses, physician assistant (PA) anesthesiologists, respiratory technician, and radiology technician. Our current criteria for a trauma alert are enumerated in Table 2. Evaluation and management then follows the principles of the Advanced Trauma Life Support (ATLS) protocols.

For patients with traumatic injuries who do not meet trauma criteria, the designation "high index" is applied. These patients are taken directly to the emergency department (ED). They undergo a similar and thorough trauma work-up under the direction of the ED

Table 2: Trauma-Alert and High-Index Criteria

Adult Trauma Alert Criteria	
Red criteria	Active airway assistance required
	Blood pressure <90 systolic *or* no radial pulse with sustained heart rate >120
	Multiple long-bone fractures
	2nd- or 3rd-degree burns ≥body surface area, amputation proximal to wrist or ankle, penetrating injury to head, neck, torso
	Glasgow Coma Scale <12
	Paramedic judgment
Blue criteria	Sustained respiratory rate ≥30
	Sustained heart rate ≥120 with radial pulse
	Single long-bone fracture due to motor vehicle accident or fall ≥10 feet
	Major degloving, flap avulsion >5 inches, gunshot wound to extremities
	Best motor response = 5
	Ejection from vehicle (excluding open vehicles) or deformed steering wheel
	Age 55 or older
High-Index Criteria	
	Falls ≥12 feet in adults, and ≥6 feet in children
	Extrication time >15 minutes
	Rollover
	Death of an occupant in the same vehicle
	Major intrusion
	Ejection from a bicycle
	Pedestrian struck by a vehicle
	Age 55 or greater
	Paramedic judgment

Note: Presence of one red or two blue criteria constitutes a trauma alert.

physician. Once the work-up has been completed, a consultation with the trauma service is obtained. The team reviews findings and the plan of care, and arranges for the necessary follow-up.

On occasion, a high-index patient will be found to have significant injuries or comorbidities that exceed the abilities of the ED physician or the capabilities of the ED. On such occasions, an in-house trauma alert is called, the patient transferred to the resuscitation bay, and the entire team rapidly assembled. Availability of this safety net allows the ED to increasingly participate in the management of the injured. It also reduces the workload imposed on an already busy trauma service, and decreases the costs of an otherwise full activation. It is, however, associated with a more prolonged ED stay, but does not result in suboptimal outcome.[7,8]

In-House Trauma Attending

It is being increasingly recognized that trauma outcomes are directly related to institutional commitment and not just to the experience of the individual surgeon.[9,10] As such, the need for the presence of the trauma attending has been challenged. Attending presence, however, has certain definite advantages. Patient disposition can be more rapid, with real-time interpretation of diagnostic studies and front-end decision making, bypassing the traditional approach of communication along progressive echelons of command. Coordination with other specialists becomes easier with direct attending-to-attending discussions. In institutions where trauma patients may be admitted to services other than the trauma service (e.g., the orthopedic service for isolated orthopedic injuries or the neurosurgical service of isolated neurological injury), the patient may be appropriately arbitrated to the service that will serve the patients interest best. Presence of an in-house trauma attending allows this arbitration to be made after careful consideration of the patient's trauma burden, preventing admission of trauma patients to nonsurgical services. Finally, attending presence allows for the provision of billing for services, including the initial evaluation and management, surgeon-performed ultrasonography, tube thoracostomy, vascular access lines, and so on.

Captain of the Ship Concept

Over the last two decades, there has been explosive increase in the modalities available for the management of complex injuries.[11] The emphasis has been on the development of nonoperative and minimally invasive strategies that involve interventional radiologists and endovascular surgeons, among others.[12] Additionally, nontraditional stakeholders such as anesthesiologists (e.g., epidural catheters for pain management in rib fractures) and endoscopists (e.g., endoscopic retrograde cholangiopancreatography/papillotomy for complex liver trauma with bile leaks) are now becoming key players in delivering care.[13,14] It is of paramount importance, therefore, to have strong leadership in the trauma service serving as the "captain of the ship," guiding the patient's care through the nuances of the various available options, while at the same time, protecting the patient from the need or desire to "push the envelope."

Trauma Coverage by Specialists

The provision of emergency coverage by specialists has been, and continues to be a major challenge.[15,16] On the one hand, tertiary hospitals must provide specialist coverage or risk potential loss of substantial federal and state funding for their trauma centers. At the same time, use of hospitalists to relieve specialists of admissions and the development of alternative venues of practice (e.g., ambulatory surgery centers) have encouraged some specialists, once dependent

on hospitals, to reduce or drop their clinical privileges. Change of privilege status from active to courtesy is becoming an increasingly popular option in avoiding provision of emergency coverage. This is further compounded by the skyrocketing malpractice premiums.

Radical changes will be necessary to overcome this problem. Some of the potential solutions to improving emergency coverage by specialists are enumerated in Table 3. Another alternative is to incorporate training of basic emergency procedures used in these specialties into the core trauma curriculum. The dependence on specialties may be reduced with an orthopedic trauma rotation focused on irrigation and debridement of open fractures and application of external fixators, along with a neurosurgical rotation focusing on placement of intracranial monitoring devices, decompressive craniotomies, and evacuation of space occupying lesions, such as subdural or epidural hematomas.[17] The ability to provide trauma care on a more elective basis may be appealing and result in increased involvement. It is also our experience that maintaining the care of the patient on the trauma service serves as a strong incentive to motivate participation.

ORGANIZING SUBSEQUENT CARE OF TRAUMA PATIENTS

Role of Tertiary Survey

Despite due diligence, the potential for missed injuries exists.[18–20] The presence of a low Glasgow Coma Scale (GCS) on admission, or the need for pharmacologic paralysis, limits the accuracy of the physical examination, significantly increasing this risk. The most common reason for a missed injury is an inadequate clinical examination. The majority of missed injuries can be identified on repeat clinical assessment with the appropriate imaging studies, especially when a high index of suspicion is maintained. When present, these injuries add to the morbidity and mortality with a less than optimal outcome. It is our routine for the trauma attending to perform a tertiary survey for all patients admitted for more than 24 hours. The task may alternatively be delegated to the trauma surgery fellow or senior surgical resident. It must, however, be performed in all admitted patients, at the prescribed time and in a

Table 3: Potential Solutions to Improve Emergency Coverage by Surgical Specialists

Outsource coverage to corporations of multispecialty groups.

Pay emergency availability stipend to specialists.

Work together at local, state, and federal levels to obtain funding for uninsured or partly insured patients.

Establish working networks with hospitals within the jurisdiction to minimize unnecessary transfers and prevent EMTALA violations.

Make community leaders aware of the crisis in emergency specialist coverage to facilitate a designated tax increase for provision of stipends.

Establish a fair on-call schedule among the different specialists.

Hospitals need to recognize that the days for free emergency coverage in lieu of maintaining clinical privileges are over.

Emergency coverage needs to be a key part when negotiating managed care contracts.

Increase the number of hospitalists to reduce the admission burden for specialists.

Create additional sources of funding for trauma centers (red light violations, speeding tickets, dedicated taxes, etc.).

EMTALA, Emergency Medical Treatment and Labor Act.

thorough manner. It includes a complete physical examination and review of all radiological studies.[21] Any detected abnormality can be addressed appropriately, with the necessary interventions taken.

Communication

The Accreditation Council for Graduate Medical Education (ACGME) has mandated that resident duty hours be limited to a maximum 80 hours per week, in-hospital call no more frequent than every third night, and 1 day free of clinical responsibilities for every 7 worked, each averaged over a 4-week period. Since the attending coverage of the service is similarly in blocks of time, usually 24 hours, this results in an increase in the frequency of hand-offs, incurring the risk of communication errors, translating ultimately to medical errors. While computerized medical records are becoming more common, they are not universally available. Current strategies to maintain patient data ranges from pen and paper, to computerized data sheets and the use of personal digital assistants.[22] We employ a Microsoft® Excel spreadsheet containing the patient list, key clinical points, and pending tasks. The list is updated several times a day by the surgical resident or the PA and serves as the template for communication during the various rounds. As a means to overcome potential deficiencies in communication we have instituted mandatory group rounds, fostering the exchange of patient information ensuring the continuity of care. These include the morning report, check-out rounds, and the biweekly multidisciplinary rounds (Figure 2).

Morning Report

Every morning at 8 AM, all members of the previous night's on-call team, the team coming on-call, and other members of the trauma service not engaged in other clinical activities, gather for the morning report. All patients still in the resuscitation area are discussed first. The work-up thus far and pending studies, along with ongoing consultations, are presented and discussed. The senior resident then presents all interesting trauma cases and all trauma cases requiring operative intervention. The emergency surgery consultations are then reviewed in a similar manner. The faculty also utilizes this opportunity to teach, with the use of digitally captured images of injuries and operative findings, as well as computerized radiology imaging software (Figure 3). The use of these multimedia presentations allows for enhanced educational value.[23]

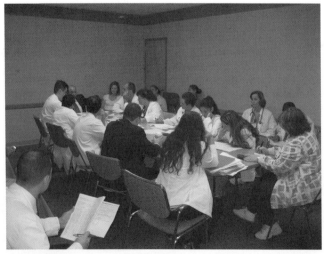

Figure 2 Morning sign-out: In addition to improving communication between the trauma teams coming on and going off, it serves as a key educational opportunity.

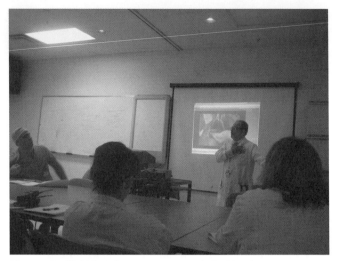

Figure 3 Multidisciplinary trauma rounds: Led by the senior trauma surgeon and attended by the various members of the trauma service, these rounds allow direct multidisciplinary communication, reducing lag time and increasing efficiency.

Check-Out Rounds

On weekdays, check-out rounds are performed daily at 2 PM. Again, consistency in time and location is key to maximizing participation. All members of the trauma service are expected to participate, with special emphasis on those who are on-call that day. On weekends, the check-out is performed once all ICU and floor patients have been seen. These rounds focus on any significant change in patient condition, results of interventions/studies, pending issues, and anything special that the on-call team must watch out for. The goal of these daily check-out rounds is to better coordinate the daily disposition of patients and *not* to sign out tasks to the on-call members of the team.

Multidisciplinary Rounds

In addition to multispecialty medical care, trauma patients present with unique social, financial, and psychological needs. Optimal care and eventual disposition therefore require the active participation of social workers, neuropsychologists, and rehabilitation specialists, among others. It is therefore our practice to conduct biweekly multidisciplinary rounds. Consistency in timing and location of the rounds allows increased participation across the various disciplines. The rounds are led by the most senior trauma attending. Over the course of about 1 hour, all patients on the service are reviewed, issues addressed, and care coordinated. The emphasis is not on therapeutic decisions, but rather on the steps necessary to achieve optimal care and early discharge planning. Issues regarding other disciplines are directly addressed with the representative of that service. Such an approach streamlines care, reduces length of stay, and ultimately decreases the cost of caring for these patients.[24] The usual participants in these rounds are listed in Table 4. The trauma performance improvement nurse uses the presentations to identify potential complications and departures from standard of care. Identified issues are then followed up and clarifications sought from the responsible person.

Role of Physician Extenders

Physician extenders, including nurse practitioners and PAs, have taken on a more significant role since the implementation of the 80-hour work-week rule by the ACGME in 2003.[25] As previously

Table 4: Participants of Multidisciplinary Rounds

Trauma services
Senior trauma attending
Trauma attendings
Trauma fellows
Residents
Physician assistants
Trauma program manager
Performance improvement nurse
Trauma research coordinator
Students
Rehabilitation
Physiatrist
Physical therapists
Nursing staff
ICU charge nurse
Trauma floor charge nurse
Pharmacists
Registered dietitian
Infection control nurse
Social/case workers
Neuropsychologists/addiction specialists
Hospital administration representative

discussed, with these new requirements, residents are no longer able to provide the same continuity of care as in the past. The incorporation of physician extenders into our practice has allowed us to maintain the necessary continuity.[26] When well-trained and properly supervised, they function as mid-level residents. In addition to assisting with patient care, they are able to orient new fellow/residents to the routines and the protocols of the service. They act as liaisons with the various services coordinating care and executing decisions made at rounds. They secure supplies, obtain consents, and assist with the performance of procedures such as placement of lines, feeding tubes, tracheotomies, vena caval filters, percutaneous endoscopic gastrostomies, and so on. By virtue of their consistent presence in the unit, or on the floor, they are able to provide families with frequent updates on the status of the patient. The rapport established with the family has been found to be extremely beneficial during family meetings regarding the care of complex, critically ill patients. Their consistent presence expedites patient disposition, translating into a shorter ICU and hospital length of stay. The resultant streamlining of care results in cost savings that offset the expenditures of hiring physician extenders. Further, their schedule can be arranged to complement that of the residents on the service. This leads to team members always being available, reducing the potential for medical errors that otherwise result from a failure to review studies and obtain appropriate follow-up. Their incorporation into a given setting is dependent on state law, level of training, experience, and especially, the level of supervision.

Next Generation of Trauma Surgeons

A significant shortage of fellowship trained trauma surgeons reflects the current attitudes of graduating general surgery residents toward the specialty.[27,28] The most common reasons cited for this include heavy workload, decreasing number of operative cases, nonoperative nature of the surgical critical care fellowship, night work, the perception of increased exposure to viral infections, and litigation.[17]

Working Hours

The workload of practicing trauma surgeons has significantly increased since the adoption of the 80-hour work-week rule for residents, the increase in trauma incidence, and a greater need for documentation. The increased time spent on routine clinical care has come at the cost of the pursuit of academic activities, such as research and publications, and often impacts the quality of personal lives.[29] Potential solutions include the incorporation of physician extenders to assist with delivery of routine clinical care, adoption of computerized mobile documentation technologies, and the addition of additional faculty members. The coupling of trauma with surgical critical care is a financially viable option. In addition to the critical care for trauma patients, the service must strive to provide the critical care needs of all surgical patients at their institution. This is beneficial in several ways. First, the higher reimbursements would augment the financial viability of the service. Second, there is physiologic similarity between the severely injured and the critically ill surgical patients; management of these patients is not only intellectually stimulating, but also lessons learned from one group to be applied to the other. Finally, a period of time dedicated to the ICU allows recovery from the time spent on a busy trauma rotation, potentially reducing burnout.

Workload reduction can also be achieved by the fair distribution of trauma patients.[30] Patients with multisystem trauma clearly belong on the trauma service, under the care of the trauma surgeon. Patients with injuries isolated to a single system may, however, be adequately managed by subspecialty services after a complete and comprehensive trauma evaluation. This has been made possible by the availability and aggressive use of whole-body computed tomography (CT) scanning. Examples include isolated skeletal injuries; isolated traumatic brain or spinal cord injury; and isolated facial fractures that may be admitted to orthopedic, neurosurgical, and maxillofacial services, respectively. All patients must, however, undergo a complete trauma work-up to rule out other injuries, and the trauma service must always remain available to assist with care when requested. Minor injuries to other organ systems do not preclude admission to the subspecialty service. As a measure to reduce missed injuries, all patients admitted to subspecialty services are re-evaluated with a tertiary survey performed by the trauma service at 24–48 hours. In addition, these patients are separately flagged and their outcomes reviewed at the monthly trauma quality management and performance improvement meeting.

On occasion, patients are brought to the trauma center after having been "found down," without a clear mechanism of injury. When on work-up, they are found to have medical conditions such as cerebrovascular events, myocardial infarctions, and complications of diabetes, they are transferred to the medical emergency room. These strategies may help in maintaining acceptable service loads.

Trauma as a Nonoperative Specialty

The incidence of penetrating trauma is on the decline. In all but a handful of select trauma centers, the majority of trauma is blunt and can be managed nonoperatively. Often when patients do require surgical intervention, it is by other specialties (orthopedics, neurosurgery, reconstructive surgery, etc.). The dwindling true surgical opportunities have resulted in career dissatisfaction among current trauma surgeons. It is also having a negative impact on current graduates of general surgical residency programs. First, residents are graduating with only nominal operative trauma experience. Second, other specialists perceive trauma as a nonoperative specialty or surgical internists who prepare patients for operative procedures.[31]

The emergence of the field of acute care surgery and redefinition of the trauma surgeon and the acute care surgeon may help overcome the lack of operative opportunity.[32,33] The balance achieved will allow for an adequate number of cases that maintain operative skills and career satisfaction. Also, patients seen in the acute setting after evaluation may be found to be candidates for elective surgery for either related or unrelated procedures. Development of collaborations may also serve to increase the opportunity for elective surgery. Close relations with the hospitalists have made the trauma service the routine provider of all general surgery services for this group at our institution. The field, however, needs to be clearly defined. In its current vague form, we run the risk of being given ownership of cases that the elective services do not wish to be involved with. This may be on the basis of the patient's insurance status, the nature of the disease, or the time of day. We need to remain vigilant for the potential of becoming the "dumping ground."[34] Another alterative is to include within the trauma fellowship advanced training in a defined field of general surgery that would allow for the development of a limited elective general surgical practice. Focused advanced laparoscopy, endocrine surgery, and endovascular surgery are potential fields that may be explored.

Operative Trauma Education

Over the past two decades, the incidence of penetrating trauma has sharply declined. Also, with better imaging techniques such CT, adoption of modalities such as ultrasonography, adoption of nonoperative strategies for solid organ injuries, and the development of minimally invasive techniques, the management of blunt trauma is essentially nonoperative. General surgery residents are graduating with progressively decreasing operative trauma experience. Innovative educational strategies are therefore of paramount importance. The advanced trauma operative management (ATOM) course is one such useful tool.[35,36] Developed by Lenworth Jacobs at the University of Connecticut, Hartford, the course has been enthusiastically adopted at the University of Miami, where it has been regularly offered since 2004. Held over the course of a single day, it begins with six didactic lectures on operative techniques for the various organs of the abdomen and thorax. The subsequent live laboratory section involves the use of approximately 50-kg swine as the trauma model. One instructor and one student are assigned to each animal to maximize the learning experience (Figure 4). After performance of a trauma laparotomy where the anatomical differences between the swine and human are pointed out, the student leaves the table. The instructor then creates a standard defined set of injuries. On return of the student, they are given a mechanism and must explore the

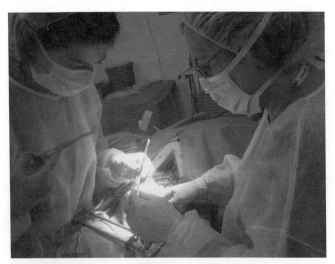

Figure 4 One of the trauma fellows receiving one-on-one instruction in operative trauma management during an advanced trauma operative management course at the University of Miami.

animal, identify the injuries and perform the appropriate operative repair. Throughout this process, the instructor quizzes the student on various aspects of the particular injury. The course is currently offered to all senior (PGY-4, PGY-5) surgical residents and trauma fellows. While enthusiasm for the course is uniform, it is greatest among the critical care fellows who have been out of the operative arena for a time and appreciate the opportunity to practice prior to their return to the trauma service.

The nonoperative nature of the surgical critical care fellowship becomes even more emphasized when one considers that the resident's maximal operative experience, both in terms of the number and type of cases, comes in their year as chief resident. The abrupt deterioration to the "nonoperating intensivist" can therefore have a profound impact. In recent years, we have encountered a small number of fellows who elect to discontinue their critical care fellowship and pursue fellowships in other operative disciplines. The development of a curriculum that allows for periodic return to operative services may help overcome this deficiency. Alternatively, change in regulations that allow for trauma or emergency general surgery call, while on critical care rotations may be feasible. The approach, however, must be tailored to the critical care load and needs of the individual institution, as it is certain that a one-size-fits-all approach will not meet the best interests of the trainee and the patient.[37]

Unlike elective general surgery, where one has relative control over the type of patients one treats, the trauma patient arrives unsolicited. Unsavory characters are often the rule rather than the exception. It must be in the character of the trauma surgeon to have a greater degree of altruism, providing the best care without regard to the nature of the person. The ability to provide care for even the so-called dregs of society must be viewed as a reason for pride and not a shortcoming of the field.

OTHER CHALLENGES IN ORGANIZING TRAUMA CARE

In addition to medical care, trauma patients often have other needs that must be adequately addressed to optimize outcome. They have a higher frequency of alcohol and substance abuse and social and financial issues that impede discharge planning, and often have rehabilitative needs that go beyond the realm of acute care.

Alcohol and Substance Abuse

Use, abuse, or dependence on alcohol lies at root of many traumatic injuries and complicates management resulting in poor outcomes.[38] In addition, the resulting abrupt cessation of drinking that results from hospitalization may precipitate alcohol withdrawal syndrome. It may range from anxiety and increased irritability in its mild form to seizures or delirium tremens when severe. The symptoms most commonly begin 48–72 hours after abrupt cessation and usually peak at 5 days. Patients who develop alcohol withdrawal syndrome have more ICU days, ventilator days, and hospital days, develop more morbidities, and ultimately incur greater hospital costs.[39] Recognition of the pervasive presence of alcohol in our patient population has led us to incorporate a neuropsychologist specializing in addiction disorders into our trauma service. At initial evaluation, all patients are screened for potential alcohol or substance abuse. High-risk patients are placed on short-acting benzodiazepines, clonidine, and their maintenance intravenous fluids are supplemented with thiamine and folate. The neuropsychologist performs a formal evaluation and administers a brief intervention.[40,41] They also assist with tailoring the narcotic medication needs of this group of patients, which can often be challenging. The entry of patients into support and detoxification programs on discharge is also coordinated. We have also identified issues with substance abuse in patients who have become habituated to narcotics used to treat injuries during their current hospitalization. These patients do not have a history of pre-injury drug use and have been fully functional prior to the event. Neuropsychological intervention in addition to strategies such as gradual tapering, use of drugs with lesser narcotic potency, and use of non-narcotics are generally successful.

Social and Financial Issues

A good proportion of trauma patients are designated self-pay, which in essence translates into "unable to pay." The frequency of self-pay patients has been noted to be higher in pedestrians hit by motor vehicles and victims of penetrating trauma. These patients are often more severely injured and cost more to care for. At the same time, they often lack the social and financial support necessary to fully recover from the injury after discharge from the acute care setting. Questionable immigration status further compounds the problem, limiting the rehabilitation facilities that are able to accept these patients. To alleviate some of these issues, an experienced case worker is assigned to each patient immediately after admission. Case workers serve as patient advocates, assisting them with obtaining the best postdischarge support possible. Also, during each multidisciplinary round, the eventual disposition of each patient is addressed. Barriers to discharge can therefore be identified early and alternatives sought.[42]

REHABILITATION AND FURTHER DISPOSITION

With improvements in trauma care, the focus has sifted from mere survival to an optimal functional recovery from the traumatic event.[43] This functional recovery often requires months or even years of rehabilitation as in the case of traumatic brain injury or spinal cord injury. The costs of such therapy are therefore substantial, and may in cases even exceed those of the acute phase of care. Several measures to evaluate functional outcome have been validated and include the Functional Independence Measure (FIM), Glasgow Outcome Scale (GOS), the Short Form Health Survey (SF-36), and the modified FIM. Periodic analysis of these outcome measures serves as a useful benchmark for the quality of trauma care being delivered. Although poor follow-up by trauma patients is a recognized limitation, we utilize the SF-36 to monitor functional outcome.

NUTRITIONAL SUPPORT

Multisystem trauma is a highly catabolic state; resultant nutritional deficiencies compound the systemic immunosuppression that results due to the injury itself.[44] The situation is made worse by pre-existing malnutrition that is not uncommon in the trauma population. Certain groups are especially at risk, including those who abuse alcohol or use drugs, the elderly, and patients with open abdomens following damage control operations.[45] While several aspects of nutritional support remain controversial, such as the use of immunonutrition, several generalizations can be made. Nutritional support is best started early, once resuscitation has been completed. Enteral nutrition is the preferred route when a functional gastrointestinal tract is available.[46] Total parenteral nutrition is employed when the gastrointestinal tract is not available and function is not expected to return for over a week. While the best parameter to monitor the adequacy of nutritional support is still debatable, prealbumin remains our current choice. The influence of an elevated C-reactive protein level that is almost invariably present in critically ill trauma patients needs to be determined. A pharmacist specialized in nutrition is an integral part of our trauma team. The pharmacist determines initial nutritional requirements, assists with selection of the best formulation to use, and monitors nutritional parameters.

POPULATIONS AT RISK

Additional considerations need to be addressed when treating special subgroups of trauma patients. These include the elderly, pregnant women, and children.

Geriatric Population

The elderly are the fastest-growing segment of the population. Additionally, improvement in general well-being has allowed this group to participate in activities beyond that which were customary. This will likely result in a significant increase in elderly trauma patients who will require care. The American College of Surgeons Committee on Trauma (ACS-COT) recommends that patients over 55 years of age should be considered for transport to a trauma center. This recommendation is based on the finding that there is a sharp increase in mortality that occurs at this age independent of injury severity, mechanism, and body region involved. The basis for this disproportionate mortality has not been clearly elucidated. Postulated factors that may be responsible include decreased physiologic reserve, presence of pre-existing medical conditions, use of certain medications, and the greater degree of injury sustained in impacts of lesser severity. It is our practice to have a very low threshold to admit these patients to the ICU, to use invasive hemodynamic monitoring, and to obtain subspecialty medical consultations.[47] The reduced functional capabilities impede the functional recovery from the traumatic event. A rehabilitation service consultation is obtained early in the hospital course to assess needs. Social services are also recruited early to assess the family support structure. Disposition in the majority of cases is to a rehabilitation or long-term care facility.

Obstetric Trauma Patients

On receiving report of an incoming pregnant trauma patient, in addition to the trauma team, the in-house obstetric resident and attending are paged. The trauma team manages initial resuscitation. Special emphasis is placed on administering supplemental oxygen and tilting the long spine board to take pressure off the inferior vena cava in gestations of over 20 weeks. Once the primary survey has been performed according to guidelines, a secondary survey is performed. In addition to assessing for nonobstetric injury, the fetal heart tones are assessed and a speculum examination performed. In the absence of fetal heart tones, no further fetal resuscitation is indicated. When fetal heart tones are present, the duration of gestation is estimated. If less than 24 weeks, routine maternal trauma care is provided. If more than 24 weeks, electronic fetal monitoring is instituted, and after completion of the trauma work-up the patient is admitted to the obstetric unit for continued observation. The speculum examination is performed to assess for spontaneous rupture of membranes and vaginal bleeding. The trauma service continues to follow the patient for the entire duration of their hospitalization. For patients requiring emergent nonobstetric operative interventions, intraoperative electronic fetal monitoring is carried out during the entire procedure with an obstetric nurse in attendance for gestations that have reached viability. The obstetric team remains on alert should fetal decelerations develop. For gestations that have not reached viability, fetal heart tones are documented before and after the operation.[48] To reduce radiation exposure, magnetic resonance imaging (MRI) is used to clear the spine when this cannot be safely achieved clinically.

Pediatric Population

Children are not little adults. They have unique anatomic physiologic and anatomic features that must be recognized when delivering trauma care.[48] The outcome of pediatric trauma is therefore best when the injured child is cared for in centers with the necessary capabilities. In addition to the trauma team, the senior pediatric surgery resident and pediatric intensive care fellow are paged on receipt of the trauma alert. Once the primary survey and initial resuscitation have been completed, further work-up is delegated to the senior pediatric surgery resident, under the supervision of the pediatric surgery attending. Admission when necessary is made to the pediatric floor or pediatric ICU (PICU). In centers lacking a residency program, a pediatric emergency room physician and PICU nurses are useful resources to enlist in providing pediatric trauma care.

FUNDING FOR EDUCATIONAL OUTREACH AND RESEARCH

In spite of being the leading cause of death between ages 1 and 44, and resulting in the greatest loss in years of productive life, trauma education and research sadly lags behind that for cancer, heart disease, and stroke. Also, largely as a result of the poor payer mix, increased use of sophisticated technologies, and improvements in critical care science that allow more critically injured trauma patients to survive, most trauma center are in the middle of a financial crisis. Meager resources are directed toward providing patient care. As a consequence, providing educational outreach activities and performing research have become even more challenging.[49] Innovative funding sources need to be identified. Potential sources include revenues generated from red-light violations and speeding tickets, dedicated taxes, and grants from corporations and foundations. Additionally, the public needs to be educated on the enormity of the problem, the value of trauma centers and systems, and the needs of the future. Strong public opinion may sway lawmakers to give the trauma system its due.

SUMMARY

Organizing trauma care in today's health care environment is a real challenge for surgeons administrating trauma units. Imagination, creativity, and better utilization of human and other resources are three elements that should be utilized by the physician leader to face those challenges. Multidisciplinary rounds and other instituted forums for communication work toward improving continuity of care as well as the outcome of the patient. It is clear that the trauma surgeon of the future should be a master technician, an astute clinician, and a strong leader with a business perspective. Other innovative strategies, such as ATOM, or the development of a curriculum that allows for periodic return to operative services, may give the trauma fellow additional surgical experience. Development of a defined field of acute care surgery may serve to decrease the perception of trauma as a nonsurgical specialty.

REFERENCES

1. Skandalakis PN, Lainas P, Zoras O, Skandalakis JE, Mirilas P: "To afford the wounded speedy assistance": Dominique Jean Larrey and Napoleon. *World J Surg* 30(8):1392–1399, 2006.
2. Hawk R: Military medicine comes of age. The First World War. *J Fla Med Assoc* 79(5):309–313, 1992.
3. King B, Jatoi I: The mobile Army surgical hospital (MASH): a military and surgical legacy. *J Natl Med Assoc* 97(5):648–656, 2005.
4. Mullins RJ: A historical perspective of trauma system development in the United States. *J Trauma* 47(Suppl 3):S8–S14, 1999.
5. Gerndt SJ, Conley JL, Lowell MJ, Holmes J, et al: Prehospital classification combined with an in-hospital trauma radio system response reduces cost and duration of evaluation of the injured patient. *Surgery* 118(4):789–794, 1995.
6. Doyle CJ: Mass casualty incident. Integration with prehospital care. *Emerg Med Clin North Am* 8(1):163–175, 1990.
7. Eastes LS, Norton R, Brand D, Pearson S, Mullins RJ: Outcomes of patients using a tiered trauma response protocol. *J Trauma* 50(5):908–913, 2001.
8. Tinkoff GH, O'Connor RE, Fulda GJ: Impact of a two-tiered trauma response in the emergency department: promoting efficient resource utilization. *J Trauma* 41(4):735–740, 1996.
9. Durham R, Shapiro D, Flint L: In-house trauma attendings: is there a difference? *Am J Surg* 190(6):960–966, 2005.
10. Helling TS, Nelson PW, Shook JW, Lainhart K, Kintigh D: The presence of in-house attending trauma surgeons does not improve management or outcome of critically injured patients. *J Trauma* 55(1):20–25, 2003.
11. Pilgrim CH, Usatoff V: Role of laparoscopy in blunt liver trauma. *ANZ J Surg* 76(5):403–406, 2006.
12. Kawamura S, Nishimaki H, Takigawa M, Lin ZB, et al: Internal mammary artery injury after blunt chest trauma treated with transcatheter arterial embolization. *J Trauma* 61(6):1536–1539, 2006.
13. Bajaj JS, Spinelli KS, Dua KS: Postoperative management of noniatrogenic traumatic bile duct injuries: role of endoscopic retrograde cholangiopancreaticography. *Surg Endosc* 20(6):974–977, 2006.
14. Lubezky N, Konikoff FM, Rosin D, Carmon E, et al: Endoscopic sphincterotomy and temporary internal stenting for bile leaks following complex hepatic trauma. *Br J Surg* 93(1):78–81, 2006.
15. McConnell KJ, Johnson LA, Arab N, Richards CF, et al: The on-call crisis: a statewide assessment of the costs of providing on-call specialist coverage. *Ann Emerg Med* 13(1):727–735, 2007.
16. Glabman M: Specialist shortage shakes emergency rooms: more hospitals forced to pay for specialist care. *Physician Exec* 31(3):6–11, 2005.
17. Spain DA, Miller FB: Education and training of the future trauma surgeon in acute care surgery: trauma, critical care, and emergency surgery. *Am J Surg* 190(2):212–217, 2005.
18. Biffl WL, Harrington DT, Cioffi WG: Implementation of a tertiary trauma survey decreases missed injuries. *J Trauma* 54(1):38–43, 2003.
19. Houshian S, Larsen MS, Holm C: Missed injuries in a level I trauma center. *J Trauma* 52(4):715–719, 2002.
20. Brooks A, Holroyd B, Riley B: Missed injury in major trauma patients. *Injury* 35(4):407–410, 2004.
21. Hoff WS, Sicoutris CP, Lee SY, Rotondo MF, et al: Formalized radiology rounds: the final component of the tertiary survey. *J Trauma* 56(2):291–295, 2004.
22. Van Eaton EG, Horvath KD, Lober WB, Rossini AJ, Pellegrini CA: A randomized, controlled trial evaluating the impact of a computerized rounding and sign-out system on continuity of care and resident work hours. *J Am Coll Surg* 200(4):538–545, 2005.
23. Cohn S, Dolich M, Matsuura K, Namias N, et al: Digital imaging technology in trauma education: a quantum leap forward. *J Trauma* 47(6):1160–1161, 1999.
24. Dutton RP, Cooper C, Jones A, Leone S, et al: Daily multidisciplinary rounds shorten length of stay for trauma patients. *J Trauma* 55(5):913–919, 2003.
25. Oswanski MF, Sharma OP, Raj SS: Comparative review of use of physician assistants in a level I trauma center. *Am Surg* 70(3):272–279, 2004.
26. Christmas AB, Reynolds J, Hodges S, Franklin GA, et al: Physician extenders impact trauma systems. *J Trauma* 58(5):917–920, 2005.
27. Chiu WC, Scalea TM, Rotondo MF: Summary report on current clinical trauma care fellowship training programs. *J Trauma* 58(3):605–613, 2005.
28. Shackford SR: The future of trauma surgery—a perspective. *J Trauma* 58(4):663–667, 2005.
29. Esposito TJ, Leon L, Jurkovich GJ: The shape of things to come: results from a national survey of trauma surgeons on issues concerning their future. *J Trauma* 60(1):8–16, 2006.
30. Rogers F, Shackford S, Daniel S, Crookes B, et al: Workload redistribution: a new approach to the 80-hour workweek. *J Trauma* 58(5):911–914, discussion 914–916, 2005.
31. Fakhry SM, Watts DD, Michetti C, Hunt JP, EAST Multi-Institutional Blunt Hollow Viscous Injury Research Group: The resident experience on trauma: declining surgical opportunities and career incentives? Analysis of data from a large multi-institutional study. *J Trauma* 54(1):1–7, discussion 7–8, 2003.
32. Ciesla DJ, Moore EE, Moore JB, Johnson JL, et al: The academic trauma center is a model for the future trauma and acute care surgeon. *J Trauma* 58(4):657–661, discussion 661–662, 2005.
33. Austin MT, Diaz JJ Jr, Feurer ID, Miller RS, et al: Creating an emergency general surgery service enhances the productivity of trauma surgeons, general surgeons and the hospital. *J Trauma* 58(5):906–910, 2005.
34. Ciesla DJ, Moore EE, Cothren CC, Johnson JL, Burch JM: Has the trauma surgeon become house staff for the surgical subspecialist? *Am J Surg* 192(6):732–737, 2006.

35. Jacobs LM, Burns KJ, Kaban JM, Gross RI, et al: Development and evaluation of the advanced trauma operative management course. *J Trauma* 55(3):471–479, 2003.

36. Jacobs LM, Burns KJ, Luk SS, Marshall WT 3rd: Follow-up survey of participants attending the Advanced Trauma Operative Management (ATOM) Course. *J Trauma* 58(6):1140–1143, 2005.

37. Richardson JD, Franklin GA, Rodriguez JL: Can we make training in surgical critical care more attractive? *J Trauma* 59(5):1247–1248; discussion, 1248–1249, 2005.

38. Walsh JM, Flegel R, Cangianelli LA, Atkins R, et al: Epidemiology of alcohol and other drug use among motor vehicle crash victims admitted to a trauma center. *Traffic Inj Prev* 5(3):254–260, 2004.

39. Bard MR, Goettler CE, Toschlog EA, Sagraves SG, et al: Alcohol withdrawal syndrome: turning minor injuries into a major problem. *J Trauma* 61(6):1441–1445, 2006.

40. Sommers MS, Dyehouse JM, Howe SR, Fleming M, et al: Effectiveness of brief interventions after alcohol-related vehicular injury: a randomized controlled trial. *J Trauma* 61(3):523–531, 2006.

41. Gentilello LM, Rivara FP, Donovan DM, Jurkovich GJ, et al: Alcohol interventions in a trauma center as a means of reducing the risk of injury recurrence. *Ann Surg* 230(4):473–480, 1999.

42. FitzPatrick MK, Reilly PM, Laborde A, Braslow B, et al: Maintaining patient throughput on an evolving trauma/emergency surgery service. *J Trauma* 60(3):481–486; discussion 486–488, 2006.

43. Cameron PA, Gabbe BJ, McNeil JJ: The importance of quality of survival as an outcome measure for an integrated trauma system. *Injury* 37(12): 1178–1184.

44. Hasenboehler E, Williams A, Leinhase I, Morgan SJ, et al: Metabolic changes after polytrauma: an imperative for early nutritional support. *World J Emerg Surg* 1:29, 2006.

45. Cheatham ML, Safcsak K, Brzezinski SJ, Lube MW: Nitrogen balance, protein loss, and the open abdomen. *Crit Care Med* 35(1):127–131, 2007.

46. Kozar RA, McQuiggan MM, Moore EE, Kudsk KA, et al: Postinjury enteral tolerance is reliably achieved by a standardized protocol. *J Surg Res* 104(1): 70–75, 2002.

47. Jacobs DG: Special considerations in geriatric injury. *Curr Opin Crit Care* 9(6):535–539, 2003.

48. Kuczkowski KM: Trauma in the pregnant patient. *Curr Opin Anaesthesiol* 17(2):145–150, 2004.

49. Nagel RW, Hankenhof BJ, Kimmel SR, Saxe JM: Educating grade school children using a structured bicycle safety program. *J Trauma* 55(5): 920–923, 2003.

TRIAGE

John Armstrong   and   David G. Burris

Triage is the process of prioritizing patient care based on patient need and available resources. In daily practice, triage decisions link individual patients with resources appropriate for their injuries, with the goal being "the greatest good for the patient." In the setting of ubiquitous resources, these are "life or life" decisions. Triage occurs at each level along the pathway of care, from prehospital and emergency room; through the operating room, intensive care unit, and ward; to discharge and rehabilitation.

In a mass casualty incident, the needs of a population of patients exceed available resources. Triage decisions in this situation work to promote "the greatest good for the greatest number." With scare resources, these are tough decisions because the paradigm of care shifts from bringing all available resources to bear on the individual patient to managing resources for the greatest effect on a population of patients. Triage is not a static process—it is a dynamic sequence of decisions that change depending on the nature of the patient, resources, and event situation. Triage in a mass casualty event works to identify and separate the most critically injured patients from the mass of less injured casualties. As such, mass casualty triage systems must be error tolerant through repetitive cycles of reevaluation along the care pathway.

A common link between effective daily and mass casualty triage is situational awareness of system resources for daily and surge capacity. Many systems experience "chronic surge capacity" challenges in meeting the regular health care needs of their populations.

FIELD TRIAGE

Field triage identifies severely injured trauma patients at the point of injury in the "field" and triggers a decision to transport severely injured patients to a hospital that has resources commensurate with patient needs. A common field triage decision scheme assesses the injured patient in four steps, each step linked to a determination about patient need for a level of care at a trauma center. The field triage decision scheme presented here (Figure 1), originally developed by the American College of Surgeons Committee on Trauma, was revised through an evidence-based review by an expert panel representing emergency medical services, emergency medicine, trauma surgery, and public health. The panel was convened by the Centers for Disease Control and Prevention (CDC), with support from the National Highway Traffic Safety Administration (NHTSA). Its contents are those of the expert panel and do not necessarily represent the official views of CDC and NHTSA.

Step 1 assesses physiology; step 2, anatomy of the injury; step 3, mechanism of injury and high-energy impact; and step 4, special patient or system considerations. Effective implementation of a triage decision scheme is enhanced by simplicity within relevant steps. In other words, scheme complexity harms good triage.

Steps 1 and 2 are screens of the severity of physiologic and anatomic injury, respectively, and rapidly identify the most critically injured patients requiring transport to higher levels of care within the trauma system. The initial physiologic assessment of the patient measures vital signs (systolic blood pressure and respiratory rate) and level of consciousness (Glasgow Coma Scale). Anatomic assessment emphasizes readily visualized or identifiable anatomic injuries, to include centrally located penetrating injuries, severe musculoskeletal injuries, and consequent paralysis. Patients without apparent life-threatening physiologic or anatomic issues are then screened in step 3 for further evidence of high-energy mechanisms that increase the risk for significant injury. Certain characteristics of falls, automobile crashes, pedestrian/bicyclist crashes, and motorcycle crashes are associated with a higher risk of injury that is less obvious, and yet merits further evaluation at a facility within the trauma system. Step 4 looks for patient characteristics antecedent to the traumatic event that exacerbate the consequences of injury (extremes of age, bleeding diatheses, end-stage renal disease, and pregnancy), isolated limb or eyesight-threatening injuries, and burns. The presence of patient characteristics or characteristic injuries prompts consideration for patient transport to specific centers within a trauma system.

The field triage decision scheme emphasizes the importance of explicitly defining the capabilities of facilities within the system of care and matching the patient to the facility with the most appropriate level of care. An *inclusive* trauma system brings all local prehospital agencies and acute care facilities together as a network for the focused application of system capabilities to the care of each acutely

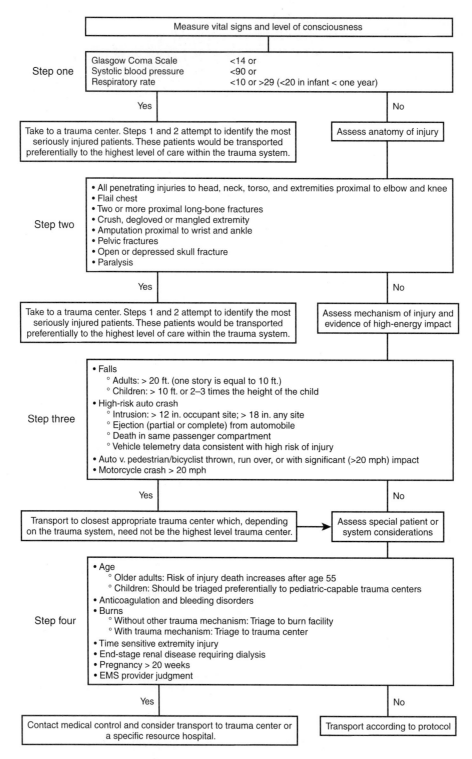

Figure 1   Field triage decision scheme.

injured patient. The idea is to get the right patient to the right place within the right time. Underestimation of patient injuries can lead to *undertriage* to facilities without adequate resources for patient needs, and overestimation of patient injuries can lead to *overtriage* to facilities with resources far greater than patient needs. Effective triage requires an integrated and defined shared mental model of triage across all settings of care.

MASS CASUALTY TRIAGE

Mass casualty incidents are distinguished from multiple casualty situations by available resources: with mass casualties, resources for each patient are limited, whereas with multiple casualties, full resources can be brought to bear on each individual patient. Mass casualty triage begins with recognition that an event has occurred that has generated casualties exceeding available resources.

Triage in a mass casualty incident seeks to put order into chaos by sifting out noncritically injured casualties in order to find those casualties who need acute attention. Triage begins at the scene, following scene risk assessment and implementation of first responder safety and security measures. The "second-hit" phenomenon, whether by secondary building collapse, chemical contamination, or intentional sequential explosives, is real. Failure to pay attention to scene safety can result in secondary casualties, which can include first responders, and the magnitude of the event increases.

The MASS technique is a useful method for limited first responders to separate acute and nonacute care casualties within a large casualty population: Move, Assess, Sort, Send. First, casualties who can walk are directed to move to an easily identified area with a visible care giver; these are the "walking wounded." Next, the remaining casualties who cannot walk are instructed to raise an arm or leg, indicating that they have cerebral perfusion and anatomic injuries; these are "delayed" in priority. The remaining casualties then fall into one of three areas: those who require immediate attention, those who have injuries incompatible with survival, and those who are dead. Simple airway, breathing, and circulation assessments are conducted through this population using common field triage instruments to identify the primary casualties who need immediate/acute care.

Triage categories help to prioritize the care of casualties and guide the timing of intervention and evacuation. They include immediate, delayed, minimal, expectant, and dead. Following an intervention, the casualty is reassessed and re-triaged based on the result.

Immediate casualties have emergent, life-threatening consequences of injury and require rapid intervention for primary airway, breathing, and circulation issues. Airway compromise, tension pneumothorax, and uncontrolled external hemorrhage are classic examples in which relatively simple interventions can be life-saving. Delayed casualties have stable major wounds without uncontrolled hemorrhage, and include nonhemorrhagic penetrating torso injuries and long-bone fractures. Minimal casualties have non–life-threatening, nonurgent injuries, such as superficial soft tissue wounds and stress responses. Expectant casualties have injuries that are unsalvageable regardless of circumstances, or that are unsalvageable given resource limitations. Examples include severe head injury and high-percentage body surface area burns. This category has been largely unused in the American experience, and represents a potential siphon of resources in a bona fide mass casualty incident. "Dead" is listed as a triage category to prevent inappropriate use of resuscitation resources. External identifiers include missing body parts, open head wounds, and massive open torso wounds. The reality is that the mechanisms underlying mass casualty incidents carry a high scene mortality.

Triage occurs at every level of care and is designed to prevent missed casualties with life-threatening injuries. Transitions between care settings are ideal opportunities for reassessment and re-triage. At each care location, it is important that there is adequate space for casualty disposition, forward casualty flow without backtracking, separate places for expectant and dead, an identified place with care for minimal casualties, a decontamination area preceding the initial care area, and a control point.

Usually, a facility has a designated triage officer at the control point to make initial casualty disposition. This position should be preassigned in the facility's mass casualty plan. The essential characteristics of the triage officer are experience within the system, ability to make decisions, and ability to communicate. Although there is one

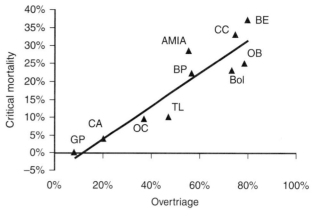

Figure 2 Graphic relation of overtriage to critical mortality rate in 10 terrorist bombing incidents from 1969 to 1995. Linear correlation coefficient $(r) = 0.92$. AMIA, Buenos Aires; BE, Beirut; Bol, Bologna; BP, Birmingham pubs; CA, Cragavon; CC, Cu Chi; GP, Guildford pubs; OB, Old Bailey; OC, Oklahoma City; TL, Tower of London. *(From Frykberg ER: Medical management of disasters and mass casualties from terrorist bombings: how can we cope? J Trauma 53:201–212, 2002.)*

formal triage officer at point-of-facility entry, it bears emphasizing that across a system of triage, there are many caregivers performing triage, even within a facility.

Sequential triage as casualties move along the care pathway creates an efficient, error-tolerant system that minimizes the consequences of persistent undertriage and overtriage. Overtriage keeps "distracting" casualties within the care pathway and increases the critical mortality rate, a more appropriate measure of casualty population outcome than overall mortality (Figure 2). Adequate documentation is essential for casualty tracking and re-triage. As patients move across care levels, pertinent documentation provides the developing story to the next caregivers in line.

COMMENTS

Effective triage is a unifying thread through a functioning trauma system. Systems that perform daily care and train disciplines together provide the best preparation for mass casualty incidents—surge capacity and capability are practiced regularly. The Institute of Medicine's 2006 *Report on The Future of Emergency Care* offers a cautionary assessment of the current state of emergency and trauma care in the United States: the current situation of overcrowding, fragmentation, and resource shortages must be replaced with system planning, coordination, and financing, so that the needs of acutely injured patients are met individually and as a population.

SUGGESTED READINGS

American College of Surgeons: *Resources for the Optimal Care of the Injured Patient.* Chicago, American College of Surgeons, 1999.

Frykberg ER: Triage: principles and practice. *Scan J Surg* 94:272–278, 2005.

Institute of Medicine: *The Future of Emergency Care in the United States Health Care System Report Brief.* Washington, DC, Institute of Medicine, 2006, www.iom.edu.

MacKersie RC: History of trauma field triage development and the American College of Surgeons Criteria. *Prehosp Emerg Care* 10(3): 287–294, 2006.

Prehospital Airway Management: Intubation, Devices, and Controversies

Raul Coimbra, Daniel P. Davis, and David Hoyt

Prehospital trauma airway management is probably the biggest challenge faced by prehospital providers. These professionals must not only acquire but also maintain essential skills to adequately manage airway problems at the scene and during transport of trauma victims to trauma centers.

Endotracheal intubation is the definitive method of airway management. However, to acquire such skill requires significant training and practice. Although the emergency medical technician-basic (EMT-B) curriculum contains an advanced airway module, the low frequency of these procedures makes it difficult for these professionals to maintain proficiency. In most systems, paramedics and flight nurses are the only professionals allowed to perform rapid sequence intubation (RSI). Therefore, there is a need for simpler ways to maintain a patent airway by emergency medical technicians, until the patient is delivered to a hospital. Several devices are now available and have been used by prehospital personnel when endotracheal intubation is not practical or possible. These alternate methods include bag-valve-mask with oral or nasopharyngeal airway, the laryngeal mask, and the esophageal-tracheal double lumen tube, popularized as the Combitube.

In this chapter, the indications for airway management in the prehospital arena, the different modalities, devices and techniques, the recognition of a difficult airway, and associated pitfalls will be discussed.

WHO NEEDS AN AIRWAY?

Before we define who needs an airway in the prehospital arena, it is important to clarify that few studies to date have shown efficacy of advanced airway management in trauma prior to arrival at a trauma center.

The goal of airway management is to provide adequate oxygenation and ventilation as part of the overall resuscitation effort. Candidates include those with decreased or absent respiratory movements, signs of airway obstruction, and cardiopulmonary resuscitation (CPR) in progress. Severe traumatic brain injury (TBI) as an indication for prehospital intubation will be discussed later.

In trauma, it has been shown that moribund patients would benefit from an airway, particularly those who are candidates for a resuscitative thoracotomy upon arrival at the hospital.[1]

DIFFICULT AIRWAY

The Mallampati classification has been used for many years by anesthesiologists during preoperative evaluations for the identification of a difficult airway and to predict difficult intubation[2] (Figure 1). It compares tongue size with the oropharyngeal space, and its reliability has been questioned because it does not take into account other factors that may make intubation difficult or impossible in the prehospital setting. However, if the patient is still able to follow simple commands, direct visualization of the oropharynx by asking the patient to open the mouth will give additional and important information to the astute prehospital provider. Rich[3] described the 6-D methods of airway assessment: disproportion; distortion; decreased thyromental distance; decreased interincisor gap; decreased range of motion in any or all of the joints—atlanto-occipital, temporomandibular, and cervical spine, always present in trauma; and dental overbite.

Identifying a difficult airway prevents patient deterioration or death. Alternative devices and strategies should be used when the diagnosis of a difficult airway is made. These include the laryngeal mask airway (LMA), Combitube, or bag-valve-mask.

WHICH STRATEGY SHOULD BE USED?

The strategies described as follows are alternatives to conventional bag-valve-mask with either a nasopharyngeal or an oropharyngeal airway.

Laryngeal Mask Airway

The LMA is one alternative to endotracheal intubation (Figure 2). Its use is particularly important in patients with difficult airways (defined later) and in patients treated in "unfriendly" environments (rain, dark, prolonged extrication, etc.). It also can be used as a rescue strategy following a failed RSI. Additionally, it can be used to facilitate intubation, which is obtained by passing the endotracheal tube through the LMA.

The insertion of the LMA is done blindly into the oropharynx, and it is usually tolerated without the need of neuromuscular blockade. The LMA lies in the hypopharynx in the supraglottic position. The successful placement of the LMA is independent of the Mallampati score, presence of a C-collar, or in-line immobilization of the neck. Spontaneous ventilation through the LMA is possible, and manual ventilation through the LMA is superior to bag-valve-mask ventilation, because the latter requires two hands to maintain a good seal. Studies comparing the success rates have shown that paramedics achieve higher levels of successful placement with the LMA compared to endotracheal intubation.[4] The LMA may be particularly useful in patients with a difficult airway, since direct visualization of the cords is not required and neuromuscular blocking agents are not necessary. The advantages of the LMA over the Combitube (described next) include lower risk of malpositioning, no risk of esophageal intubation, and less trauma to the oropharynx. A major disadvantage of the LMA is that it does not protect against aspiration, which may carry significant risk in patients with intact airway reflexes. Another limitation of LMA is related to the difficulty in generating high airway pressures, which may lead to ineffective ventilation.[5]

Combitube

The Combitube consists of a device with two lumens. One of the lumens has an open distal end similar to an endotracheal tube, whereas the other lumen has a closed distal end, with several holes proximal to its balloon cuff. A second balloon of higher volume is located more proximally to the side holes, and it is used to secure the tube in position. The Combitube is inserted blindly and allows ventilation through either lumen. Following blind insertion, the distal tip is usually

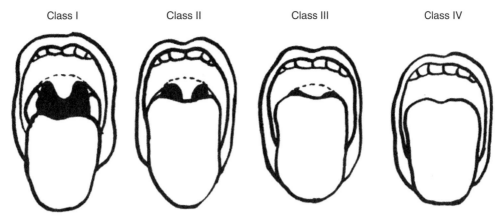

Figure 1   Difficult airway—the Mallampati score modified by Samsoon and Young.   *(From Mallampati SR, et al: A clinical sign to predict difficult tracheal intubation: a prospective study.* Can Anaesth Soc J *32:429–435, 1985.)*

located in the esophagus. After inflating the oropharyngeal balloon, the esophageal cuff is inflated. Attempts to ventilate through the pharyngeal lumen will determine whether the distal tip is in the esophagus or trachea. If there is no change in the colorimetric, end-tidal carbon dioxide detector, or if breath sounds are absent, then the distal tip is in the trachea and the patient should be ventilated through the tracheal lumen (Figures 3 and 4).

The Combitube is a useful alternative to endotracheal intubation when an airway is not obtained after multiple attempts, when the airway is considered a difficult one, when direct visualization of the vocal cords by laryngoscopy is not possible at the scene, or when prehospital providers are not trained to perform orotracheal intubation. The great majority of patients brought to trauma centers after insertion of a Combitube will be ventilating and oxygenating well, and there is no need for immediate removal of the Combitube and orotracheal intubation. The Combitube is also useful in patients with significant maxillofacial trauma and cervical spine injuries. Because the esophageal cuff is immediately inflated after tube insertion, the Combitube offers protection against aspiration of gastric contents.

The Combitube is contraindicated in patients with intact gag reflex, or when upper airway obstruction is suspected. The Combitube is not available in pediatric sizes. Potential complications include injury to the pharynx and esophagus, and failure to recognize the exact location of the distal end and attempting to oxygenate and ventilate through the wrong lumen.

Orotracheal Intubation

Endotracheal intubation (ETI) is the gold standard of airway management. In the prehospital setting, endotracheal intubation without the use of sedatives or neuromuscular blockade is only achievable in obtunded patients. Because few systems allow paramedics to use RSI,

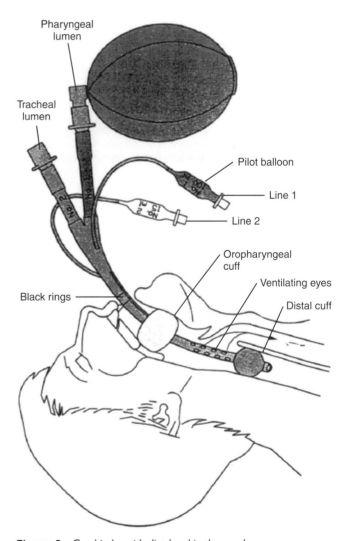

Figure 3   Combitube with distal end in the esophagus.

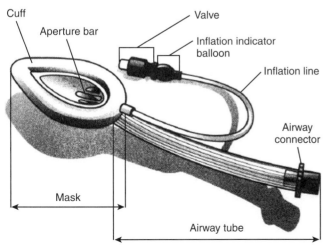

Figure 2   Laryngeal mask airway.

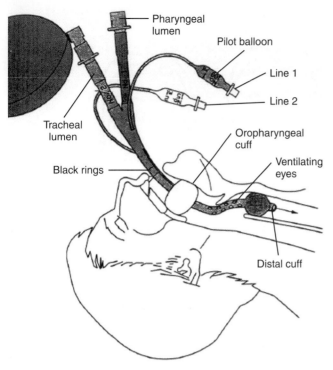

Figure 4 Combitube with the distal end in the trachea.

the esophagus or when the stomach has been insufflated with expired gas during bag-valve-mask ventilation.

Another way to determine proper placement of endotracheal tubes is the syringe aspiration technique. If the tube is properly placed in the trachea, the provider should not feel any resistance when attempting to aspirate air from the endotracheal tube (ETT) with a 60-cc syringe. If the tube is in the esophagus, upon negative pressure generated by the syringe, the wall of the esophagus collapses and resistance is felt by the provider.

CONTROVERSIES IN PREHOSPITAL INTUBATION

Prehospital Intubation in Traumatic Brain Injury

While an aggressive approach to airway management including ETI is standard-of-care for patients with severe TBI, it is notable that there is little evidence to support this approach.[7] In fact, several recent studies have demonstrated an increase in mortality associated with prehospital intubation.[8–10] It is not clear whether this represents a selection bias or a true detrimental effect of invasive airway management on outcome. The purported benefits of early intubation include reversal of hypoxia and airway protection from aspiration. However, the morbidity and mortality associated with these secondary insults may not be preventable or reversible with invasive airway management 10–15 minutes after the initial injury.[11] In addition, there has been a recent increase in awareness of the adverse effects of positive-pressure ventilation on outcome, especially with hyperventilation and hypocapnia.

This makes patient selection for early intubation extremely important so as to maximize the benefit of the procedure. The use of the Glasgow Coma Scale (GCS) score alone to select patients to undergo prehospital intubation has several limitations. An early GCS score appears to have only moderate specificity in identifying severe TBI.[12] In addition, the relationship between GCS score and aspiration is indirect at best. Aspiration events may occur prior to arrival of EMS personnel or with manipulation of laryngeal structures during intubation.[11] Furthermore, hypoxemia may be reversible with noninvasive airway maneuvers, and oxygen saturation (SpO_2) values with supplemental oxygen may be an important factor in considering prehospital intubation.[13] While no study has clearly defined a subgroup of head-injured patients who should undergo early intubation, neural network analysis using data from our trauma registry suggests that the most critically injured patients, as defined by GCS score and the presence of hypotension, benefit from the procedure. In addition, intubation does provide additional benefit with regard to the reversal of hypoxemia in some patients.[3,13]

Who Should Perform Prehospital RSI?

The San Diego Paramedic RSI Trial prospectively enrolled severe TBI patients who could not be intubated without medication. The primary outcome analyses compared trial patients with non-intubated historical controls matched for age, gender, mechanism, trauma center, and body region Abbreviated Injury Scores. Despite a substantial increase in the percentage of patients arriving with an invasive airway, trial patients had higher mortality and a lower incidence of good outcomes.[14] Subsequent analyses suggest that suboptimal performance of the procedure, including hyperventilation and deep desaturations, accounts for at least part of the mortality increase.[13] This may reflect the inexperience of paramedics in that system with regard to RSI and the limitations of a single, 8-hour training session.

Other systems providing more intensive training have documented improved success rates, although the link between experience and performance of RSI remains unclear.[15] In the San Diego study, the only subgroup with improved outcomes versus matched historical controls was the group undergoing RSI by paramedics then transported by air

and based on the fact that obtunded patients carry a poor prognosis, endotracheal intubation in those situations may cause more harm than good. Without ideal conditions, endotracheal intubation may be accompanied by an increased number of complications, including hypoxemia, esophageal intubation, and intubation of the mainstem bronchus, with subsequent complete lung collapse, injury to the oropharynx, regurgitation, exacerbation of a potential spinal cord injury, circulatory compromise, increased intracranial pressure, and delay in transport to a trauma center, just to name a few. Inability to recognize a difficult airway may make the intubation impossible and if preceded by RSI may lead to devastating complications and eventually death. Common pitfalls of endotracheal intubation will be discussed.

Confirmation of Orotracheal Tube Placement

Several factors contribute to endotracheal tube malpositioning and include poor lighting, limited access to the patient, insufficient suctioning, difficult airway, intraoral bleeding, vomiting, facial trauma, and airway swelling.

The gold standard for confirmation of adequate placement of an endotracheal tube is the direct visualization of the tube passing through the vocal cords. This is obviously not always possible considering less than ideal conditions at the scene. Auscultation of breath sounds also may be difficult at the scene, particularly in a noisy and chaotic environment.

The colorimetric, end-tidal carbon dioxide detector has been used by prehospital personnel to confirm endotracheal tube placement. In the presence of high levels of carbon dioxide, the device changes color from purple to yellow. The device has been deemed reliable; however, it lacks sensitivity in the setting of cardiopulmonary arrest due to the lack of pulmonary blood flow limiting carbon dioxide delivery. Therefore, approximately 15% of patients properly intubated in that setting would have their endotracheal tubes removed based on the lack of color change in the device.[6] The opposite is also true, and a color change may be observed in patients who have ingested large volumes of carbonated liquids (beer, sodas, etc.), when the tube is in medical crews.[13,14] The low incidence of hyperventilation in this cohort may explain this somewhat unexpected finding. Subsequent analyses from San Diego and from Pennsylvania document worse outcomes with paramedic intubation but improved outcomes with air medical RSI as compared to emergent intubation in the ED.[8,16] Together, these studies suggest that prehospital RSI may be efficacious when performed by experienced, highly trained individuals. The extent and frequency of initial and ongoing training remains to be defined.

Role of Capnometry in Prehospital Intubation

Quantitative capnometry has several advantages in the management of brain-injured patients. First, capnometry offers accurate confirmation of endotracheal tube placement, both at the time of initial intubation and continuously throughout the prehospital course. Clearly, early recognition of a misplaced endotracheal tube can avoid serious morbidity and mortality. Systems that have instituted quantitative capnometry as the "gold standard" for endotracheal tube placement have reported unrecognized esophageal intubation rates approaching zero.[17]

Perhaps equally important to the TBI patient is the ability of capnometry to guide ventilation. Data from the San Diego Paramedic RSI Trial established the importance of avoiding hyperventilation and demonstrated the ability of quantitative capnometry to avoid hyperventilation based on arrival pCO_2 value.[13,18] There does appear to be a

learning curve, however, as air medical crews who had used capnometry to guide ventilation for many years had better end-tidal carbon dioxide and arrival pCO_2 values than paramedics using capnometry.[18] It is our belief that quantitative capnometry should be the standard of care for management of intubated patients in the prehospital environment, especially those with TBI who are especially susceptible to secondary insults.

Use of Positive End-Expiratory Pressure

While avoiding hyperventilation may be the most important lesson of the San Diego Paramedic RSI Trial, it is possible that invasive airway management is inherently detrimental due to a combination of barotrauma and "atelectrauma," which results from complete alveolar closure with each breath when positive end-expiratory pressure (PEEP) is not applied. Experimental data suggest detrimental immunologic and structural effects with "injurious" ventilation, defined as 10–12 cc/kg without PEEP.[19] In addition, PEEP may enhance alveolar recruitment and improve oxygenation, making it preferable to the use of hyperventilation to reverse hypoxemia. However, PEEP also appears to result in adverse hemodynamic effects in hypovolemic patients.[18] This is an area requiring additional study before a final verdict on the use of PEEP can be rendered.

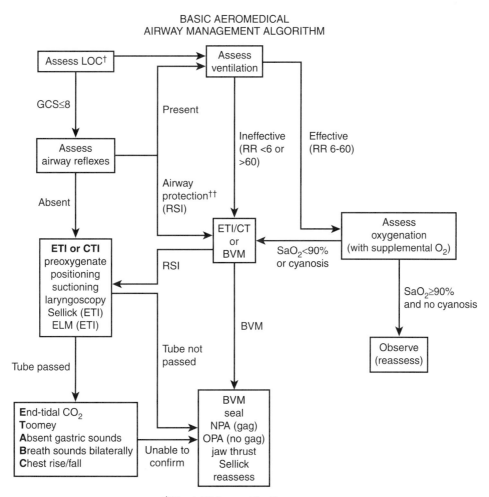

BASIC AEROMEDICAL
AIRWAY MANAGEMENT ALGORITHM

†Check FSG, consider Narcan
††Severe TBI, warning LOC, weak airway reflexes,
limited ability to continually reassess

Figure 5   Basic aeromedical airway algorithm.

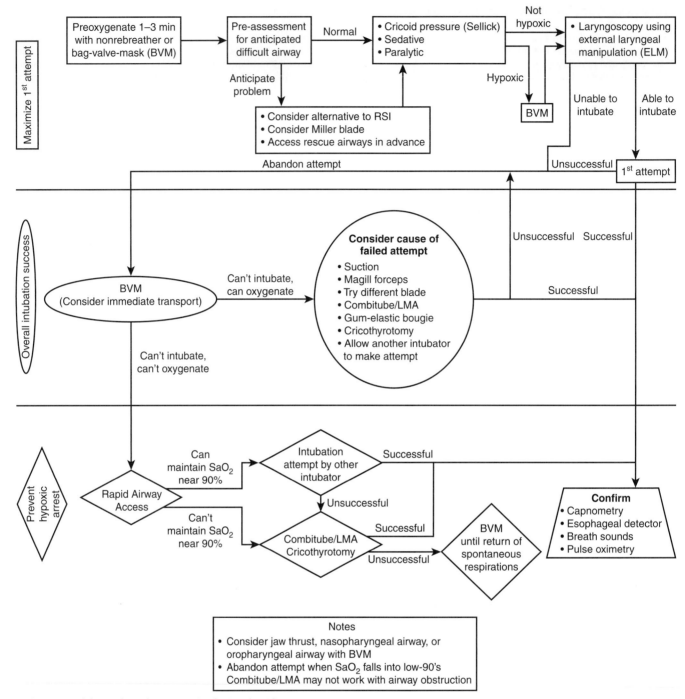

Figure 6   Advanced rapid-sequence intubation algorithm.

FINAL COMMENTS

Prehospital airway management is a difficult task that requires training and skills. Endotracheal intubation remains the gold standard of airway management. Specific strategies need to be in place for basic and advanced units (Figures 5 and 6). Higher success rates will be achieved if endotracheal intubation is attempted after the use of rapid sequence analgesia and paralysis; however, most ground units are not prepared and are not allowed to use such strategy. On the other hand, most aeromedical transport units are facile with RSI and employ this strategy with marked success. A successful RSI program requires medical direction and supervision, training and continuing education, resources for patient monitoring, drug storage and delivery, conformation and

monitoring of endotracheal tube placement, standardized protocols, back-up airway methods, and continuing quality assurance and performance review.[20]

REFERENCES

1. Durham LA, Richardson RJ, Wall MJ, et al: Emergency center thoracotomy: Impact of prehospital resuscitation. *J Trauma* 32:775–779, 1992.
2. Samsoon GLT, Young JRB: Difficult tracheal intubations. *Anesthesia* 42: 487–490, 1987.
3. Rich JM: Recognition and management of the difficult airway with special emphasis on the intubating LMA-Fastrach/whistle technique: a brief review with case reports. *Baylor Univ Med Ctr Proc* 18:220–227, 2005.

4. Deakin CD, Peters R, Tomlinson P, et al: Securing the pre-hospital airway: a comparison of laryngeal mask insertion and endotracheal intubation by UK paramedics. *Emerg Med J* 22:64–67, 2995.

5. Hulme J, Perkins GD: Critical injured patients, inaccessible airways, and laryngeal mask airways. *Emerg Med J* 22:742–744, 2005.

6. Bhende MS, Thompson AE: Evaluation of an end-tidal carbon dioxide detector during pediatric cardiopulmonary resuscitation. *Pediatrics* 95:395–399, 1995.

7. Walls RL: Rapid-sequence intubation in head trauma. *Ann Emerg Med* 22(6):1008–1013, 1993.

8. Wang HE, Peitzman AD, Cassidy LD, et al: Out-of-hospital endotracheal intubation and outcome after traumatic brain injury. *Ann Emerg Med* 44(5):439–450, 2004.

9. Davis DP, Peay J, Sise MJ, et al: The impact of prehospital endotracheal intubation on outcome in moderate-to-severe traumatic brain injury. *J Trauma* 58:933–939, 2005.

10. Bochicchio GV, Ilahi O, Joshi M, et al: Endotracheal intubation in the field does not improve outcome in trauma patients who present without lethal traumatic brain injury. *J Trauma* 54(2):307–311, 2003.

11. Atkinson JLD: The neglected prehospital phase of head injury: apnea and catecholamine surge. *Mayo Clin Proc* 75:37–47, 2000.

12. Bazarian JJ, Eirich MA, Salhanick SD: The relationship between pre-hospital and emergency department Glasgow coma scale scores. *Brain Inj* 17(7):553–560, 2003.

13. Davis DP, Dunford JV, Poste JC, et al: The impact of hypoxia and hyperventilation on outcome after paramedic rapid sequence intubation on severely head-injured patients. *J Trauma* 57:1–10, 2004.

14. Davis DP, Hoyt DB, Ochs M, et al: The effect of paramedic rapid sequence intubation on outcome in patients with severe traumatic brain injury. *J Trauma* 54(3):444–453, 2003.

15. Wayne MA, Friedland E: Prehospital use of succinylcholine: a 20-year review. *Prehosp Emerg Care* 3(2):107–109, 1999.

16. Davis DP, Peay J, Serrano JA, et al: The impact of aeromedical response to patients with moderate-to-severe traumatic brain injury. *Ann Emerg Med* 46(1):1–8, 2005.

17. Silvestri S, Ralls GA, Krauss B, et al: The effectiveness of out-of-hospital use of continuous end-tidal carbon dioxide monitoring on the rate of unrecognized misplaced intubation within a regional emergency medical services system. *Ann Emerg Med* 45:497–503, 2005.

18. Davis DP, Dunford JV, Ochs M, et al: The use of quantitative end-tidal capnometry to avoid inadvertent severe hyperventilation in patients with head injury after paramedic rapid sequence intubation. *J Trauma* 56:808–814, 2004.

19. Slutsky AS, Ranieri VM: Mechanical ventilation: lessons from the ARDSNet trial. *Respir Res* 1:73–77, 2000.

20. Swanson ER, Fosnocht DE, Barton ED: Air medical rapid sequence intubation: how can we achieve success? *Air Med J* 24:40–46, 2005.

PREHOSPITAL FLUID RESUSCITATION: WHAT TYPE, HOW MUCH, AND CONTROVERSIES

Mark Newell, Vincente Gracias, and Michael Rotondo

Fluid resuscitation is a vital treatment in the care of hypotensive trauma patients. Restoration of effective circulating blood volume improves oxygen delivery, thereby diminishing the untoward effects of shock at the cellular and organ level. However, fluid resuscitation, in and of itself, is not a panacea. Whereas restoration of effective circulating blood volume is essential, the method of supplying fluid is more controversial and complicated by several confounding factors. The inability to deliver definitive care in the field, the heterogeneity of patient populations, the variability in mechanism of injury, and the level of in-field hemorrhage control make precise study of the topic challenging. Therefore, the debate persists concerning the type, the amount, and the timing of fluid administration. The purpose of this chapter is to provide insight in the use of fluid resuscitation of trauma patients in the prehospital setting.

EPIDEMIOLOGY

If trauma is the leading cause of civilian death in Americans aged less than 45 years and the fourth leading cause of death in the United States for all ages,[1] hemorrhagic shock is the primary physiologic defect leading to death. Volume deficits develop not only as a result of blood loss, but also due to diffuse capillary-endothelial leak and fluid shifts from the intravascular to the interstitial space.[2] These deficits, and the attendant hypoperfusion, potentially lead to multiple organ dysfunction, failure, and death.[2]

Aggressive fluid administration has been mainstay therapy in trauma patients for over 40 years. Estimates of the numbers of trauma patients in the United Kingdom given prehospital intravenous fluid range from 8.6 to 65 patients per 100,000 population per year.[3] However, for the last 15 years this practice, especially in the setting of uncontrolled hemorrhage, has been questioned.

CAUSES OF SIGNIFICANT HEMORRHAGE

The causes of hemorrhage vary depending on the mechanism of injury. In blunt trauma, bleeding usually emanates from solid organs such as the spleen and liver, mesenteric blood vessel tears, pelvic and femur fractures, thoracic bleeding from lung lacerations or intercostal vessel bleeding from rib fractures, or external causes such as scalp lacerations. Uncontained bleeding from aortic transection and cardiac rupture usually leads to exsanguination at the scene. When the wounding mechanism is secondary to penetrating trauma, uncontrolled major vascular injury usually is the source of the hemorrhage.

DIAGNOSIS/ASSESSMENT

In the prehospital setting, emergency medical technicians perform an immediate assessment of the trauma victim in the form of a primary and secondary survey. This assessment includes an evaluation of the patient for life-threatening conditions that need to be promptly addressed. The patency of the airway is initially evaluated. This is followed by auscultation of breath sounds assessing for pneumothoraces or hemothoraces. Attention is then turned to the circulation. Central and peripheral pulses are assessed. Obvious sources of external bleeding are controlled. The patient's blood pressure is measured. Because definitive care cannot be rendered at the scene, a "scoop and run" rather than a "stay and stabilize" philosophy should be evoked. Attempts at intravascular cannulation should not delay transfer to the trauma center.

CLASSES OF HEMORRHAGIC SHOCK

Hemorrhage is the most common cause of shock in the injured patient.[4] Shock is defined as the presence of inadequate organ perfusion and tissue oxygenation.[4] In the presence of inadequate oxygen for normal aerobic metabolism, anaerobic metabolism occurs leading to lactic acidosis. If this process continues, cellular membranes lose their integrity leading to cellular swelling, progressive cellular damage, and ultimately, cellular death.[4]

Hemorrhage, an acute loss of circulating blood volume, is classified based on the percentage of blood volume loss. Specific hemodynamic, respiratory, central nervous system, urinary, and integumentary changes occur given the degree of shock (Table 1). Whereas class I hemorrhage is associated with minimal clinical symptoms and requires little, if any, volume replacement, class IV hemorrhage is immediately life-threatening, necessitates blood transfusion, and usually calls for surgical intervention to halt ongoing bleeding.[4]

MANAGEMENT

Access

The basic management principles to follow in hemorrhagic shock are to stop the bleeding and replace the volume loss. Establishing a patent airway with adequate ventilatory exchange and oxygenation is the first priority. Supplemental oxygen is supplied while external bleeding is controlled. Two large-caliber (minimum of 16-gauge) peripheral intravenous catheters are inserted, preferably in the antecubital veins.[4] Intravenous access should not delay transport of the patient to the trauma center.

Types of Fluid

Crystalloid

A crystalloid is a solution of small nonionic or ionic particles. They are freely permeable to the vascular membrane and are distributed mainly in the interstitial space. As such, only one-third of the volume of crystalloid infused expands the intravascular space. This accounts for the need to provide at least three times more volume of crystalloid than the volume of blood lost. Because of decreased colloid osmotic pressure secondary to decreased serum protein concentration from hemorrhage, capillary leaks, and crystalloid replacement, this ratio of volume of crystalloid infused to blood volume lost may even approach 7–10:1.[5]

Depletion of both the interstitial fluid volume and the intravascular space following severe injury may be a reason to use crystalloids for fluid resuscitation, which restore volume to both spaces.[6] Animal and human studies demonstrating improved survival from shock when utilizing isotonic fluid and blood versus blood transfusion alone support this view. Other advantages of crystalloid use in prehospital fluid resuscitation include its negligible cost in comparison to other resuscitative fluids, immediate availability, and long-term storage capacity.

Given the predilection of crystalloid to primarily fill the interstitial space, tissue edema is common and may have deleterious effects. In head-injured patients, increased brain edema may adversely affect outcome. Gas exchange may be impaired secondary to pulmonary edema. Endothelial and red cell edema impair microcirculation and tissue oxygen exchange, potentially contributing to multiple organ dysfunction.[5]

According to Advanced Trauma Life Support (ATLS) guidelines, fluid resuscitation of the trauma patient begins with a 2-L bolus of crystalloid, usually lactated Ringer's (LR) solution. LR is an isotonic fluid that contains L-lactate and D-lactate in a 50:50 mixture. The L-lactate is metabolized in the liver to bicarbonate, thereby providing additional buffer. Although the D-lactate isomer is thought to be a cause of acidosis, studies have shown that resuscitation with LR does not lead to increased lactic acid levels.[7] However, normal saline (NS), another isotonic crystalloid, can induce a hyperchloremic acidosis when given in large volumes because of its concentration of chloride ions (154 mEq/l).[6] Healey et al.[7] suggest, in their animal model of massive hemorrhage, increased survival rate in animals resuscitated with LR and blood relative to those animals that received NS and blood. This difference was thought to be secondary to the profound acidosis occurring in the NS/blood group.

Because LR has a lower osmolality than plasma (273 mOsm/l vs. 285–295 mOsm/l), large volumes of LR can reduce serum osmolality and contribute to cerebral edema. For this reason, NS may be the preferred resuscitative fluid in head-injured patients.[6]

Hypertonic sodium chloride (HS) in concentrations ranging from 3% to 7.5% has been used for the treatment of hypovolemic shock.[2] Because of its elevated osmolality (2400 mOsm/l in 7.5%), HS produces an increase in intravascular volume that far exceeds the infused volume[6] (Table 2). The cardiovascular effects of HS include improved myocardial contractility, decreased systemic and pulmonary vascular resistance, mobilization of tissue edema into the blood compartment, and reduction in venous capacitance.[2,6] These effects are transient, however, so HS has been mixed with colloids (dextran or hydroxyethyl starch) to prolong its efficacy, especially when used for small volume resuscitation.

HS decreases intracranial pressure (ICP), primarily in areas of the brain with an intact blood-brain barrier.[8] Cooper et al.,[9] in a double-blind, randomized controlled trial of hypotensive patients with severe traumatic brain injury, studied the effects of prehospital resuscitation with hypertonic saline versus Ringer's lactate on neurological outcome. These investigators did not find a significant difference in 3- or 6-month extended Glasgow Outcome Scores between the two groups.

Immunomodulatory effects of HS, either immunostimulatory or immunosuppressive depending on the concentration, have been described. HS affects nuclear activation, protein synthesis and proliferation, polymorphonuclear leukocyte function, and cytoskeleton polymerization. In animal models of hemorrhage, these effects have

Table 1: Classification of Hemorrhagic Shock

	Class 1	Class 2	Class 3	Class 4
Blood loss (%)	<15	15–30	30–40	>40
Blood loss (ml)	<750	750–1500	1500–2000	>2000
Systolic blood pressure	Unchanged	Normal	Reduced	Very low
Diastolic blood pressure	Unchanged	Raised	Reduced	Very low
Pulse	<100	>100	>120	>140

Source: Adapted from Advanced Trauma Life Support (ATLS).

Table 2: Effect on Plasma Volume Expansion of Various Solutions

Volume Infused (ml)	Fluid Infused	Plasma Volume Expansion (ml)
1000	D$_5$W	100
1000	Lactated Ringer's	250
250	7.5% hypertonic saline	1000
500	5% albumin	375
100	25% albumin	450
500	6% hetastarch	750

Modified from Rizoli SB: Crystalloids and colloids in trauma resuscitation: a brief overview of the current debate. *J Trauma* 54:S82–S88, 2003.

been associated with reduced organ dysfunction and improved survival.[8]

Despite its benefits, a meta-analysis evaluating the effect of HS compared to isotonic crystalloid on 30-day outcome in trauma patients failed to show a survival advantage.[1] As such, the role of HS in prehospital fluid resuscitation has yet to be defined.

Colloid

Nonbiologically active

Colloids seemingly have many advantages as resuscitative fluids over crystalloids. Their ability to effectively expand plasma volume exceeds that of crystalloids. Endpoints of resuscitation are met using smaller volumes of colloid, which in turn reduce tissue edema.[5] However, some investigators suggest that colloids potentiate tissue edema. The capillary-endothelial cell leak that develops after severe injury may allow the colloid to pass into the interstitium and exacerbate swelling.[6]

Albumin, a natural colloid, is synthesized in the liver and is responsible for 80% of the oncotic pressure of the plasma.[5] The molecular weight of albumin is approximately 69 kD. Infusion of the 25% solution expands plasma volume four to five times the volume infused[5] (see Table 2). Derived from pooled human plasma, its risk of transmitting infectious diseases is low because of stringent heating and sterilization. Aside from its volume replacing properties, albumin also possesses a transport function for drugs and endogenous substances and may have a beneficial effect on membrane permeability secondary to free radical scavenging. These theoretical effects have not been proven clinically.[2]

Disadvantages of albumin include its cost, short supply, and potential disease transmission.[5] Additionally, albumin's use for the resuscitation of critically ill patients has demonstrated either a trend toward or a significant increase in mortality.[5] Therefore, the use of albumin can not be recommended as a resuscitative fluid for hypotensive trauma patients.

Synthetic colloids include dextran, hydroxyethyl starch (HES), and mixtures of dextran and HES with hypertonic saline solutions. Dextran is a glucose polymer available as 6% dextran 70 (70 kD) and 10% dextran 40 (40 kD) solutions. Increase of plasma volume after infusion of 1000 ml of dextran 70 ranges from 600 to 800 ml.[2] Dextran reduces blood viscosity, reduces platelet adhesiveness, and enhances fibrinolysis,[6] resulting in increased bleeding tendency.[2] Severe, life-threatening anaphylactic reactions are also well described.[2,6] The use of dextran as an exclusive fluid resuscitant is limited by these side effects.

As mentioned previously, dextran has been added to hypertonic saline (HSD) to extend its intravascular presence. Its use as a resuscitative fluid was compared with isotonic crystalloid and analyzed via a meta-analysis of several randomized controlled trials of hypotensive trauma patients. Although HSD was safe, demonstrated higher increases in blood pressure, and decreased early fluid and blood requirements, no statistically significant survival benefit was attributed to its use.[1] Conversely, in a study by Wade et al.,[10] survival to discharge was significantly improved in patients resuscitated with 250 ml of HSD that sustained penetrating torso trauma requiring surgical intervention. This suggests a subset of trauma patients may benefit from HSD in the prehospital setting.

HES solutions are modified natural polymers of amylopectin.[6] The pharmacokinetic properties of each formulation are determined by its molecular weight, the pattern of hydroxyethylation, and the ratio of C2:C6 hydroxyethylation.[2,5,6] These properties influence the plasma expansion, degradation, and side effect profile of HES.

Side effects associated with HES include pruritis and increased bleeding due to reduction of factor VIII and von Willebrand factor.[6] However, most recent studies using modern HES preparations demonstrated no impairment of hemostasis or increased bleeding propensity.[2]

Still, despite the apparent advantages of colloids, meta-analyses suggest a trend toward increased mortality when they are used for the resuscitation of trauma patients.[5] Although the methodology of these studies can be questioned, until better designed clinical trials provide irrefutable evidence suggesting improved outcome with the use of colloids for fluid resuscitation, these agents cannot be recommended.

Biologically active

When considering an ideal resuscitative fluid in hemorrhagic shock, its properties would include volume expansion, oxygen-carrying capacity, universal compatibility, immediate availability, long-term storage capacity, and the absence of vasoactive properties and disease transmission.[11] Although blood transfusion effectively improves volume deficits and provides oxygen delivery, its use in the prehospital setting is limited by expense, short shelf-life, short supply, risk of disease transmission, and need for cross-matching. Allogenic red blood cells (RBCs) may have adverse immunoinflammatory effects that increase the risk of postinjury multiple organ failure (MOF).[12]

Hemoglobin-based oxygen carriers (HBOC) are attractive in the prehospital setting, then, for several reasons. Because HBOC can be heat treated, their risk of disease transmission is low. They have a shelf-life of up to 3 years and have oxygen-carrying, as well as volume-expansion properties. They are universally compatible, thus eliminating the need for cross-matching.[13] Phase II clinical trials, as well as in vitro and in vivo work, suggest that resuscitation with a HBOC—in lieu of stored RBCs—attenuates the systemic inflammatory response invoked in the pathogenesis of MOF.[12]

Clinical trials with HBOC have shown mixed results. When diaspirin cross-linked hemoglobin (DCLHb) was studied against normal saline in a U.S. multicenter trial for the treatment of severe traumatic hemorrhagic shock, the 28-day mortality was 46% for DCLHb compared to 17% for NS. An increase in systemic and pulmonary vascular resistance leading to decreased cardiac output was felt to be responsible for the higher mortality rate.[12] However, polymerized hemoglobin solutions have shown more promise. In a prospective, randomized trial comparing the therapeutic benefits of Poly-Heme with that of allogenic RBCs in the treatment of acute blood loss, the Poly-Heme group demonstrated similar total hemoglobin concentration after infusion as the RBC group with less RBC transfusion required through the first day of treatment and without serious or unexpected adverse consequences resulting from Poly-Heme.[11] In time, it is possible that one or more HBOC may be routinely used in the resuscitation of hemorrhagic shock.

Resuscitation Targets

Delayed

Studies have begun to scrutinize the potential detrimental effects of raising the blood pressure during uncontrolled hemorrhage.[14-18] Whereas early work utilizing controlled hemorrhage models was used to support the use of fluid resuscitation of post-traumatic hemorrhage, these models of resuscitation do not mimic the actual life situation of uncontrolled bleeding and concurrent treatment.[16] In the setting of uncontrolled hemorrhage, fluid administration may disrupt thrombus formation, induce coagulopathy by diluting clotting factors, and lead to increased bleeding.[14] In 1918, Cannon observed increased bleeding induced by rapid fluid infusion prior to hemorrhage control.[19] More recently, in a study of penetrating torso trauma, hypotensive patients were randomized to immediate versus delayed fluid resuscitation with isotonic crystalloid.[14] Prehospital fluid resuscitation was started in the immediate group, but held in the delayed group until control of hemorrhage in the operating room. Compared to patients in the delayed group, patients in the immediate resuscitation group had higher mortality and higher rates of postoperative complications. Although the results of this study have been argued,[16] the study rekindled interest and stimulated thought concerning approaches of management for the treatment of uncontrolled hemorrhage.

Hypotensive

This strategy of resuscitation attempts to maintain adequate vital organ perfusion while minimizing further bleeding.[20] A mean arterial pressure (MAP) of 60 mm Hg has been used as a resuscitation target. It is regarded as the lowest safe level because it is the lowest MAP of active autoregulation of cerebral blood flow.[19] No lower limit of hypotensive resuscitation, however, has been firmly established.

Using blood pressure as a guideline simulates prehospital scenarios in which this variable is one of the only hemodynamic parameters available.[19] Dutton et al.[18] randomized hypotensive blunt and penetrating trauma patients to a systolic blood pressure (SBP) of 70 mm Hg (hypotensive) or more than 100 mm Hg (normotensive). Crystalloid or blood products were administered to maintain the intended SBP for each group. There was no difference in survival between the two cohorts. This was partly attributed to the difficulty in maintaining the targeted blood pressures. The average SBP for the hypotensive and normotensive groups were 100 mm Hg and 114 mm Hg, respectively. This response suggests spontaneous reduction of bleeding due to inherent hemostatic mechanisms and may validate use of this resuscitation strategy in certain scenarios of uncontrolled hemorrhage.[18]

Normotensive

The traditional approach to the resuscitation of trauma patients in hemorrhagic shock has been to normalize blood pressure by administering large volumes of crystalloid followed by transfusion of blood products. This method of resuscitation developed from animal models of controlled hemorrhage. Restoration of vital organ perfusion improved survival, whereas untreated animals developed organ dysfunction and succumbed. In situations of uncontrolled hemorrhage, animal studies revealed decreased splanchnic perfusion and greater blood loss.[21] In situations in which bleeding has spontaneously resolved, the standard approach to resuscitation is reasonable. It is difficult to predict, however, whether bleeding has spontaneously ceased or may be exacerbated by aggressive resuscitation.

MORBIDITY AND COMPLICATIONS

Prehospital fluid resuscitation is not without its own complications. Exacerbated bleeding, dilution of clotting factors, and dislodgement of thrombi, among other problems, have already been mentioned, and may act to decrease survival of hemorrhagic shock. Additionally,

a balance needs to be achieved between under-resuscitation and over-resuscitation, as both of these concerns contribute to increased morbidity and mortality. Whereas the goal of prehospital fluid resuscitation is to preserve blood flow to vital organs (brain, heart) without incurring significant, irreversible damage to other organ systems (renal, splanchnic), excess crystalloid resuscitation may contribute to the development of the abdominal compartment syndrome.

Hypothermia develops commonly after traumatic shock and is exacerbated with the administration of cold fluids. Adverse consequences of hypothermia include impaired coagulation function, reduction of oxygen delivery, and increased rate of infection.[22] The importance of administering warm fluids to avoid the untoward effects of hypothermia cannot be overstated.

SUMMARY

The clinical study of massive hemorrhage and resuscitation is complicated by small numbers, urgency of care, varying goals and endpoints, and patient heterogeneity with respect to age, comorbidity, mechanism of injury, prehospital time and therapy, and complications of resuscitation. Some definite conclusions can be drawn from the vast literature. The rapid transport of the trauma patient to a center where definitive care can be rendered is paramount. Second, the importance of hemorrhage control prior to aggressive fluid resuscitation cannot be overstated. Despite the number of options of resuscitation strategies and fluids, no single choice is perfectly applicable in every trauma scenario. Until human studies can be performed utilizing particular strategies for particular injuries with proven improved outcomes, ATLS guidelines should continue to be practiced.

REFERENCES

1. Wade CE, Kramer GC, Grady JJ, et al: Efficacy of hypertonic 7.5% saline and 6% dextran-70 in treating trauma: a meta-analysis of controlled clinical studies. *Surgery* 122:609–616, 1997.
2. Boldt J: Fluid choice for resuscitation of the trauma patient: a review of the physiological, pharmacological, and clinical evidence. *Can J Anesth* 51:500–513, 2004.
3. Dretzke J, Sandercock J, Bayliss S, Burls A: Clinical effectiveness and cost-effectiveness of prehospital intravenous fluids in trauma patients. *Health Technol Assess* 8(23)1–103, 2004.
4. American College of Surgeons Committee on Trauma: *Advanced Trauma Life Support Manual*. Chicago, American College of Surgeons, 2001.
5. Rizoli SB: Crystalloids and colloids in trauma resuscitation: a brief overview of the current debate. *J Trauma* 54:S82–S88, 2003.
6. Nolan J: Fluid resuscitation for the trauma patient. *Resuscitation* 48:57–69, 2001.
7. Healey MA, Davis RE, Liu FC, et al: Lactated Ringer's is superior to normal saline in a model of massive hemorrhage and resuscitation. *J Trauma* 45:894–899, 1998.
8. Hoyt DB: Fluid resuscitation: the target from an analysis of trauma systems and patient survival. *J Trauma* 54:S31–S35, 2003.
9. Cooper DJ, Myles PS, McDermott FT, et al: Prehospital hypertonic saline resuscitation of patients with hypotension and severe traumatic brain injury. *JAMA* 291:1350–1357, 2004.
10. Wade CE, Grady JJ, Kramer GC: Efficacy of hypertonic saline dextran fluid resuscitation for patients with hypotension from penetrating trauma. *J Trauma* 54:S144–S148, 2003.
11. Gould SA, Moore EE, Hoyt DB, et al: The first randomized trial of human polymerized hemoglobin as a blood substitute in acute trauma and emergent surgery. *J Am Coll Surg* 187:113–122, 1998.
12. Moore EE, Johnson JL, Cheng AM, et al: Insights from studies of blood substitutes in trauma. *Shock* 24:197–205, 2005.
13. Philbin N, Rice J, Gurney J, et al: A hemoglobin-based oxygen carrier, bovine polymerized hemoglobin (HBOC–201) versus hetastarch (HEX) in a moderate severity hemorrhagic shock swine model with delayed evacuation. *Resuscitation* 66:367–378, 2005.
14. Bickell WH, Wall MJ, Pepe PE, et al: Immediate versus delayed fluid resuscitation for hypotensive patients with penetrating torso injuries. *N Engl J Med* 331:1105–1109, 1994.

15. Martin RR, Bickell WH, Pepe PE, et al: Prospective evaluation of preoperative fluid resuscitation in hypotensive patients with penetrating truncal injury: a preliminary report. *J Trauma* 33:354–362, 1992.
16. Fowler R, Pepe P: Prehospital care of the patient with major trauma. *Emerg Med Clin North Am* 20:953–974, 2003.
17. Pepe P, Mosesso VN, Falk JL: Prehospital fluid resuscitation of the patient with major trauma. *Prehosp Emerg Care* 6:81–91, 2002.
18. Dutton RP, Mackenzie CF, Scalea TM: Hypotensive resuscitation during active hemorrhage: impact on in-hospital mortality. *J Trauma* 52:1141–1146, 2002.
19. Friedman Z, Berkenstadt H, Preisman S, et al: A comparison of lactated Ringer's solution to hydroxyethyl starch 6% in a model of severe hemorrhagic shock and continuous bleeding dogs. *Anesth Analg* 96:39–45, 2003.
20. Revell M, Greaves I, Porter K: Endpoints for fluid resuscitation in hemorrhagic shock. *J Trauma* 54:S63–S67, 2003.
21. Varela JE, Cohn SM, Diaz I, et al: Splanchnic perfusion during delayed, hypotensive, or aggressive fluid resuscitation from uncontrolled hemorrhage. *Shock* 20:476–480, 2003.
22. Gentiello LM: Advances in the management of hypothermia. *Surg Clin North Am* 75:243–256, 1995.

CIVILIAN HOSPITAL RESPONSE TO MASS CASUALTY EVENTS

Rochelle A. Dicker and William P. Schecter

On February 20, 1993, six people were killed and more than 1000 injured when a bomb exploded at the World Trade Center in New York City. Two years later, on April 19, 1995, 168 people died and 850 were injured when a bomb destroyed the Alfred P. Murrah Building in Oklahoma City. On September 11, 2001, 2986 people lost their lives when the Twin Towers of the World Trade Center collapsed after two hijacked civilian airliners were piloted into the towers by Islamic fundamentalists. These events served as a stimulus to the medical community to better prepare for mass casualty events caused by attacks with both conventional and unconventional weapons. The tsunami that destroyed coastal areas in Southern Asia on December 26, 2004 and the flooding of New Orleans after hurricane Katrina in September 2005 demonstrated inadequate responses to loss of infrastructure caused by natural disasters. A thoughtful and well-rehearsed disaster plan is essential to an effective response.

KEY DEFINITIONS

A mass casualty event is defined as a situation in which the number of patients and the severity of their injuries exceed the capability of the facility to deliver care in a routine fashion. The appropriate initial response is to treat patients sustaining major injuries with the greatest chance of survival first so that valuable resources are not expended on patients with little hope of survival.

A multiple casualty event is defined as a situation in which the facility can mobilize additional resources in response to a large number of patients so as to continue to deliver care in a relatively routine fashion. The optimal field management of a mass casualty event is to convert it into a multiple casualty event for each receiving hospital. If appropriate distribution of victims to facilities occurs, the number of patients and the severity of their injuries will not exceed the ability of a facility to render care.

Triage refers to the medical sorting of patients according to their need for treatment and the available resources. In a mass casualty event, conventional standards of medical care cannot be delivered to all victims. The goal of triage is to optimize care for the maximum number of salvageable patients.

Patients are triaged into four categories at the scene: minor, delayed, immediate, and dead. In military triage systems, a fifth category, expectant care, is used for patients with a small chance of survival who would use scarce resources to such an extent as to adversely affect the chance of survival of other more salvageable patients. This category is rarely used in civilian situations as mobilization of additional personnel resources is usually possible. Numbers, colors, or symbols may be used to denote the categories (Table 1). "Undertriage" refers to assignment of patients to a level of care inadequate for their level of injury. An under-triage rate greater than 5% is unacceptable as it may lead to unnecessary morbidity and mortality in severely injured patients. "Overtriage" refers to assignment of patients to a level of care greater than required for their level of injury. An overtriage rate of 50% is considered acceptable to minimize undertriage. Excessive overtriage at the scene threatens the response of the entire system due to expenditure of limited resources on the wrong patients.

PREHOSPITAL CARE IN MASS CASUALTY EVENT

The response to a mass casualty event requires the coordinated effort of many agencies with disparate cultures, command structures, and even communications equipment (Figure 1). Appropriate agencies should submit to the authority of the incident field commander at the scene. Prior joint training can break down these barriers and improve overall response to the event.

Whether the event is caused by an accident, an intentional attack, or a natural disaster, the area of the event must be secured. In the event of a terrorist or military attack with conventional weapons, additional enemy operatives must be identified and neutralized. The area must be searched for additional unexploded ordinance and if found it must be either disarmed or exploded in a safe area. If these principles are not followed, the probability of a "second hit" is significantly increased.

Victims must be extracted, concentrated in a safe area, and triaged. Immediate care patients should be transported first, but often require management of airway, breathing, and circulation problems.

Transportation of victims from the scene to the hospital does not always occur in formal ambulances. Buses and private vehicles are sometimes used. Worried well persons and patients with minor injuries sometimes self-triage to hospitals without the knowledge of the incident field commander, leading to increased confusion and inundating the receiving hospitals.

Crowd control at the scene is a major problem. Multiple volunteers with various skills arrive to help and hinder. The triage area should optimally be secured and individuals inserted to help at the discretion of the triage commander.

HOSPITAL TRIAGE

If either a large number of casualties suddenly arrive without warning, or the hospital is informed of their impending arrival, the hospital should initiate its mass casualty plan. In a true mass

Table 1: The Four Colors of Triage

Minor—Green	Delayed care/can delay up to 3 hours
Delayed—Yellow	Urgent care/can delay up to 1 hour
Immediate—Red	Immediate care/life-threatening
Dead—Black	Victim is dead/no care required

Adapted from Los Angeles Community Emergency Response Team.

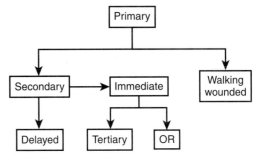

Figure 2 Initial triage stations.

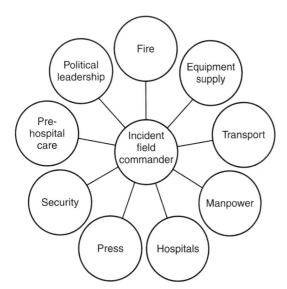

Figure 1 Components of disaster response.

casualty event, all area hospitals must participate in the care of victims to avoid exhaustion of the resources of any one facility. The common goal is salvaging as many lives as possible. A contingency plan for patients not involved in the mass casualty event must be in place as part of emergency preparedness. This plan permits the hospital to convert to mass casualty mode in a short period of time.

In preparation to receive and care for multiple victims, all elective surgery must be cancelled. Rapid disposition of pre-existing patients in the emergency department (ED) is required. Depending on the size of the event, hospitalized patients who are fit may be discharged and patients transferred within the hospital if required to maximize the availability of surgical beds.

The initial hospital triage (Figure 2) should occur outside the ED as patients arrive by ambulance. Ideally, ambulances should pass through a security checkpoint prior to entrance to the hospital grounds to identify terrorists or ordinance that may be on board. Initial triage need not be done by a surgeon, but should be done by a highly experienced clinician. If possible, the walking wounded should be escorted through a separate entrance.

As soon as stretcher patients enter the ED, a senior surgeon should triage each patient to either immediate or delayed care (see Figure 2). The immediate treatment area should be reserved for salvageable patients with life-threatening problems. This area should have enough space for equipment and provide a one-way flow of traffic. The following personnel should be present at each bed in the immediate care area: a senior surgeon for decision making, an anesthesiologist to provide airway control, two ED or critical care nurses, and a junior surgeon for vascular access and tube thoracostomy as necessary.

Treatment in the immediate care area is based upon the principles of advanced trauma life support. The goals of therapy in the immediate care area are airway control, ventilation, cessation of external hemorrhage, vascular access, and rapid transfer of the patient to the next appropriate treatment station, usually the intensive care unit (ICU) or the operating room (OR), for completion of the primary and secondary surveys and further diagnostic or therapeutic interventions. Factors affecting the decision as to where to perform the secondary survey and the patient's ultimate disposition include the patient's condition and the number of immediate care patients (Figure 3). This decision should be made by a senior surgeon.

Prior arrangements should be made to expand the ICU. The postanesthesia care unit is an ideal venue for expansion of ICU services. Since most victims do not require immediate access to the OR (unless they have penetrating trauma due to shrapnel, or traumatic amputations), even empty ORs could be used to temporarily manage critically ill patients in an unusual situation.

Patients with significant but non–life-threatening injuries are triaged to delayed care. A junior surgeon and nurse should be assigned to each of these delayed care patients. A senior surgeon, however, should be in charge of the delayed care area and the area designated for the walking wounded in order to provide advice and correct any errors in triage that may have been made.

Many of the walking wounded from a mass casualty event are not transported by emergency medical services. Civilian transport can make up as much as 80% of victims arriving at hospitals, often causing overtriage at the closest hospitals to the event. Most of the walking wounded patients can be discharged from the ED. Many of these patients require psychological counseling and support and should be screened for psychological trauma.

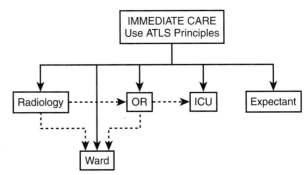

Figure 3 Intra-hospital traffic flow.

HOSPITAL EMERGENCY INCIDENT COMMAND SYSTEM

The Incident Command System in the United States was developed in the 1980s in order to improve command and control of firefighters in complex operations. An adaptation of that system, the Hospital Emergency Incident Command System (HEICS), is quickly becoming the standard for hospital disaster management. The goal of any disaster management scheme is to create an efficient system of care that will both save lives and return the hospital to routine function as soon as possible. The advantages of the HEICS include a predictable chain of command and a common language to facilitate communication among disparate agencies coordinating the response to the event.

The basic principle of HEICS is that one individual supervises no more than five people and reports to only one person. A senior surgeon is the ideal incident commander. This system allows for efficient and manageable lines of communication and easy accountability. There are four main section chiefs: planning, logistics, finance, and operations. The operations chief has overall responsibility for the triage of victims and their clinical care, and potential coordination with other area hospitals (Figure 4).

In order for HEICS to be effective, it must be incorporated into a hospital's disaster plan and training exercises. Implementation of such a vast network plan requires that each individual be familiar with his or her role prior to the incident and have a working knowledge of the organizational chart.

Disaster Preparedness through Simulation

Hospitals and first responders disaster drills, although useful, have limitations. They are often treated with complacency, do not always give detailed information for improvement strategies, and occur within unrealistic timeframes. Technical and nontechnical skills training in a variety of medical fields has been augmented with the use of simulation. Simulation techniques including computer models, tabletop exercises, and patient care simulators are helpful for

both the development of hospital disaster plans and the improvement of individual staff skills required in mass casualty events.

CAUSES OF MASS CASUALTY EVENTS

Conventional Weapons/Blast Injury

The majority of terrorist attacks and unintentional mass casualty events involve "conventional" weapons. Bombings were responsible for almost 70% of terrorist attacks in the United States and its territories between 1980 and 2001. Many terrorist bombs contain intentionally placed fragments, such as nails, bolts, and tacks, in an effort to increase bodily harm. Some bombs, such as Molotov cocktails, cause burns.

Injury patterns from explosions are dependent on several factors: materials involved, surrounding environment (open versus closed space), distance of the victim from the explosion, and presence of protective barriers.

Physics of Blast Wave

Energy is transferred from the explosion to the atmosphere generating a supersonic blast wave that rapidly slows to the speed of sound (Figure 5). In an open space, the blast wave dissipates rapidly. In a closed space, however, the blast wave reverberates against a solid wall increasing the force of the wave. For this reason, the mortality rate and severity of injuries of the victims are significantly higher in closed-space as opposed to open-space explosions.

A primary blast injury occurs when the pressure wave directly hits the body surface. Gas-filled organs are particularly susceptible to injury, such as the lungs, intestines, and ears. Damage to the eye and brain may also occur. Specific injuries are summarized in Table 2. A secondary blast injury occurs as a result of flying debris and bomb fragments. It can cause both blunt and penetrating injury and can affect any part of the body. Tertiary blast injury occurs as a result of blunt trauma as victims are thrown against solid objects by the blast impulse. A quaternary blast injury encompasses miscellaneous explosion-related injuries such as burns, crush injuries, and impalements. Illnesses directly related to the blast such as post-traumatic stress disorder, asthma exacerbations, angina, infection, or other complications secondary to inhalation of toxic fumes are also classified as quaternary blast injuries.

Blast lung injury, the most serious common primary blast injury, is a direct result of injury to the pulmonary parenchyma due to barotrauma. Many victims of blast lung injury are dead at the scene. The

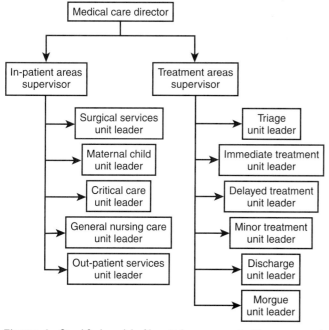

Figure 4 Simplified model of hospital emergency incident command system.

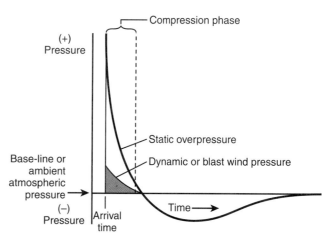

Figure 5 Physics of a blast wave.

Table 2: Spectrum of Explosive Related Injuries

Organ System	Effect
Auditory	Ruptured tympanic membrane (almost always seen with blast lung), ossicular disruption, foreign body
Eye, orbit, face	Ruptured globe, foreign body, fracture, air embolus
Respiratory	Blast lung, pulmonary contusion, pneumothorax, left-sided air embolism, aspiration
Circulatory	Myocardial contusion, myocardial infarction (air embolism), hemorrhagic shock
Central nervous system	Closed or open head injury, stroke or spinal cord injury from air embolism, spinal cord injury from blunt trauma
Renal	Contusion, laceration, acute renal failure from hypotension or rhabdomyolysis
Gastrointestinal	Bowel perforation, hemorrhage, solid organ injury, mesenteric ischemia (air embolus)
Extremity	Amputation, crush, fracture, compartment syndrome, burns, vascular injury. Most common system needing operative intervention

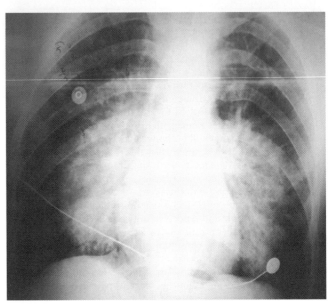

Figure 6 Blast lung.

clinical presentation is similar to pulmonary contusion. The most common symptoms and signs are hemoptysis and hypoxia leading to dyspnea, tachypnea, and poor compliance. Unlike pulmonary contusion, blast lung injury does not usually have associated rib fractures. Typical chest radiographic findings (Figure 6) include a "butterfly" pattern of infiltrates, pneumomediastinum, hemothorax, and pneumothorax.

Intraparenchymal hemorrhage causes a V/Q mismatch that may be significant, requiring mechanical ventilation and judicious fluid resuscitation. For victims requiring mechanical ventilation, care includes avoidance of ventilator associated lung injury and further barotrauma by limiting tidal volumes and levels of PEEP. On occasion, a patient with blast lung injury can develop left-sided air embolism due to rupture of the alveolar capillary membrane. Neurologic symptoms are most common, but the patient can also develop coronary artery obstruction due to air embolism. Tidal volumes, peak inspiratory pressures, and PEEP levels should be kept as low as possible to decrease the risk of both left-sided air embolism and ventilator-associated barotrauma.

Biological Agents

Unlike a conventional mass casualty event, the full effects of a bioterror attack may not be known for some time, given the insidious nature of this type of attack. Many victims may initially be unaware that they are infected and contagious. Health care facilities may become contaminated prior to recognition of the attack.

The United States categorizes agents based on their risk to national security and the safety of its citizens. Category A agents, the highest risk category, can be easily disseminated, have a high mortality rate, may cause panic, and require a major public health effort to contain the spread of disease. The four major agents in Category A, their characteristics, and management strategies are listed in Table 3.

Category B diseases are defined as moderately easy to disseminate and have a moderate morbidity and mortality potential. Included in this category are brucellosis, *Clostridium perfringens*, *Salmonella*, *Escherichia coli*, *Shigella*, glanders, ricin, typhus, streptococcus enterotoxin B, Q fever, psittacosis, water safety threats, and viral encephalitis.

Category C diseases are emerging pathogens that could be engineered as biologic weapons in the future. They have a high potential for morbidity and mortality.

Health Care and Hospital Response to Bioterrorism

In an attack with a Category A biologic weapon, there is no initial scene. The patient's first contact with the health care system may be a doctor's office, a free-standing clinic, or an emergency room. Multiple health care facilities, including hospitals and their staff, will be exposed to the pathogen and may well be infected. Viral hemorrhagic fevers such as the Ebola and Marburg viruses are particularly infectious.

The principles of management of a biologic weapons attack are similar to those for management of an epidemic: (1) rapid detection and strict isolation of patients; (2) identification and treatment of contacts; (3) strict hospital infection control, possibly including hospital lockdown depending on the nature of the infection; and (4) avoidance of funeral practices allowing close contact with the bodies. These public health measures are essential but difficult to achieve.

Patients injured in a biologic weapon attack will most likely acquire infection via the inhalation route. Routine reverse isolation suffices for all of these patients except those with highly contagious, viral hemorrhagic fevers who require strict isolation and care by individuals wearing Level A protective clothing. Lack of experience with biologic weapons, lack of functional personal protective equipment and a doctrine for its use, and lack of experience with large-scale quarantine are limiting factors to an effective response to a biologic weapon attack. Surgeons are least likely to be directly involved in the management of these patients.

Table 3: Category A Diseases/Agents

Agent	Etiology	Incubation	Transmission	Presentation	Treatment	Prevention
Anthrax	Bacillus anthracis	1 day to 8 weeks	Inhalation, skin contact, ingestion	Flu-like symptoms, then respiratory failure, wide mediastinum on chest x-ray	Fluoroquinolones or doxycycline	Inactivated vaccine, limited availability
Botulism	7 toxins produced by Clostridium botulinum	12–72 hours	Ingestion, inhalation of spores (no person-to-person transmission)	Symmetric cranial neuropathies, descending weakness proximal to distal, respiratory dysfunction	Mechanical ventilation can be for 2–3 months while neurologic function recovers	Investigational pentavalent vaccine
Plague	Yersinia pestis	2–8 days (may be shorter if inhaled)	Infected fleas, with bioterror, likely aerosolized	Fever, cough, hemoptysis, chest pain	Doxycycline, second choice is ciprofoxacin	Not available in United States
Smallpox	Variola virus	7–17 days	Inhalation, can be person to person, or contact with skin lesion	Fever, myalgias, then rash mostly to face and extremities	Vaccination except if pregnant or immunocompromised	Live-virus vaccine, may not confer lifetime immunity

Viral hemorrhagic fevers such as filovirus and arenavirus are also now being considered potential Category A threats.

Chemical Agents

Four types of chemical weapons can potentially be used in a terrorist attack: nerve agents, cyanide, vesicants, and pulmonary agents. The most likely weapons to be employed are nerve agents and cyanide.

Nerve Agents

Nerve agents are organophosphate compounds that inhibit cholinesterase at the synaptic and neuromuscular junctions causing an excess of acetylcholine leading to a cholinergic crisis. Five nerve agents have been produced as weapons: tabun, sarin, soman, GF, and VX.

Acetylcholine binds to receptors on the post synaptic cell membrane, the smooth muscle end plates and secretory glands causing the muscarinic effects of acetylcholine. The muscarinic effects include bronchospasm, low pulmonary compliance, nausea, vomiting, diarrhea, miosis, blurred vision, bradycardia, and hypersecretions of the oropharynx, conjunctivae, tracheobronchial tree, and gastrointestinal tract.

Acetylcholine also binds to skeletal muscle end-plates and synaptic ganglia causing the nicotinic effects. The nicotinic effects of acetylcholine include fasciculations, flaccid paralysis, tachycardia, and hypertension. Heart rate during a cholinergic crisis is variable due to the opposing actions of the nicotinic and muscarinic effects. Patients may experience initial tachycardia progressing to bradycardia as the severity of the cholinergic crisis increases.

The severity of nerve agent poisoning is classified as mild, moderate, or severe. Patients who are comatose, seizing, or apneic are classified as severely injured, and will require admission to an intensive care environment with ventilatory support. Patients who are supine with wheezing, fasciculations, and incontinence are classified as moderately injured. The ambulatory patient with cholinergic symptoms is classified as having a mild injury.

There are two separate antidotes for a cholinergic crisis. Atropine is a very effective antidote for the muscarinic effects but has no influence on the nicotinic effects. Atropine competitively binds at the postsynaptic muscarinic receptor, thereby displacing acetylcholine.

Atropine should be given until secretions abate and pulmonary compliance improves.

The antidote for the nicotinic effects of acetylcholine is a class of drugs called oximes. In the United States, pradiloxime chloride is the oxime of choice. Oximes act as a "molecular crowbar" separating the nerve agent from the cholinesterase, thereby allowing acetylcholine breakdown at the nicotinic receptors. Unfortunately, the oximes must be given before irreversible binding of the nerve agent and the cholinesterase occurs, a phenomenon known as aging. The aging half-life varies from 2 minutes for soman to several hours for sarin.

The recommended initial treatment for mild to moderate nerve agent injury is atropine, 2 mg IM; and pradiloxime chloride, 600 mg IM. For severe injury, atropine, 6 mg IM; and pradiloxime chloride, 1200 mg IM, are recommended.

Cyanide

Cyanide is a highly effective chemical weapon when employed in closed spaces as demonstrated by the criminal efficiency of the gas chambers in Nazi concentration camps during World War II. The high volatility of cyanide makes it an ineffective weapon when employed in open spaces because of rapid dissemination. The explosive device used in the first World Trade Center bombing in New York in 1993 contained enough cyanide to contaminate the entire building, but fortunately it was destroyed by the force of the blast.

Moderate exposure causes a bright red appearance to the skin and venous blood, metabolic acidosis, and the odor of bitter almonds. Severe exposure causes coma, apnea, and cardiac arrest.

Patients with cyanide poisoning should be treated by inhalation of a 0.3-ml ampule of amyl nitrite or 10 ml of 3% sodium nitrite (300 mg) IV over 3 minutes to produce methemoglobin. Methemoglobin has a high affinity for the cyanide ion. Subsequently, 50 ml of 25% sodium thiosulfate (12.5 g) should be given IV over a 10-minute period to convert the cyanomethemoglobin complex to the metabolically inactive thiocyanate ion, which is excreted in the urine.

Vesicants

The mustards are liquid chemical weapons that cause burns to the skin and mucous membranes and induce bone marrow suppression. Treatment involves decontamination, management of the burn wounds, and treatment of hematologic abnormalities. At least 40,000 Iranian casualties sustained vesicant injuries when Iraq employed mustard agents during the Iran–Iraq War in the 1980s. Terrorist use of a vesicant chemical weapon is less likely than a nerve agent or cyanide because of the large volumes required.

Pulmonary Agents

Chlorine and later phosgene were employed as chemical weapons causing pulmonary edema and respiratory insufficiency during World War I. Patients exposed to these agents developed chest tightness progressing to cough, hoarseness, stridor, and hypoxia over a period of 2–4 hours depending on the degree of exposure. The pulmonary parenchymal injury resembles an inhalation injury resulting from exposure to smoke and burning plastic.

Implications of Chemical Weapon Attack for Scene Management and Hospital Disaster Plan

If a chemical agent is suspected, individuals providing care at the scene should don protective clothing. Ideally, victims should be decontaminated at the scene before leaving the "hot zone" (Figure 7).

Experience from the Aum Shinrikyo Japanese sarin attacks demonstrates that nerve agents are more of a "mass hysteria" weapon than a "mass destruction" weapon. Most of the severe cases will be dead in the field. A large number of worried well or mildly exposed patients will flood the hospital. Hospital security and early lockdown is essential to prevent contamination of the facilities and staff, as happened in the Tokyo sarin attack. There most likely will not be time to employ a decontamination facility prior to arrival of the first patient. At San Francisco General Hospital, it takes a minimum of 1 hour to deploy the decontamination tent during prearranged drills occurring in daylight with all key personnel assembled in advance.

Decontamination is a critical part of the treatment. Early decontamination protects the patient from further exposure. Late decontamination protects the medical team. Simple removal of clothing results in decontamination of approximately 80% of a liquid nerve agent. Decontamination showers should be part of a hospital mass casualty event plan in case of a terrorist nerve agent attack. The prob-

lem of hypothermia during decontamination in cold climates has yet to be solved.

Patients in severe cholinergic crisis will require resuscitation by health care personnel in the decontamination zone wearing personal protective equipment. The idea that efficient resuscitation of large numbers of patients with cholinergic crisis due to nerve agent poisoning by staff unpracticed in this procedure wearing bulky unwieldy protective clothing is naïve. Surgeons and anesthesiologists should be aware of the potentiating effect of nerve agents on neuromuscular blockade as well as the effect of hypersecretions and bronchospasm on general anesthesia in the event that surgery is required to treat a trauma patient exposed to nerve agents.

Radiation Injuries

There are three types of possible exposure to radiation. The first is exposure due to radiation dispersal devices (dirty bombs), which results in a pattern of conventional blast injury. Radiation levels are not typically high enough to cause acute radiation syndrome (see below). Eighty-five percent of decontamination occurs when clothing is removed; therefore, radiation exposure to health care personnel is minimal. The second type of exposure occurs after either unintentional or intentional damage to nuclear power plant reactors. Victims suffer both blast and radiation injury. First responders would be at risk for severe radiation exposure and contamination of the surrounding region would be likely. The third scenario, a nuclear detonation, would cause massive destruction and large numbers of victims dead and injured at the scene.

The immediate effects of radiation exposure are hair loss, burns, acute radiation sickness (ARS), or death. Three syndromes are associated with major exposure: hematopoietic, gastrointestinal, and neurologic/cardiovascular. The initial symptoms of the hematopoietic syndrome are nausea, vomiting, and anorexia. In the latent phase, stem cells in the bone marrow die. Patients with significant exposure (over 120 rads) may die within a few months. Less severely affected individuals can make a full recovery.

The initial symptoms of the gastrointestinal syndrome are similar to the hematopoietic syndrome with the addition of diarrhea. The LD 100 for this syndrome is about 1000 rads, with individuals dying secondary to infection and dehydration. The cardiovascular/central nervous system syndrome is seen at exposures greater than 2000 rads. Initial symptoms include those described previously with the addition of mental status changes. Convulsions and coma may occur within hours.

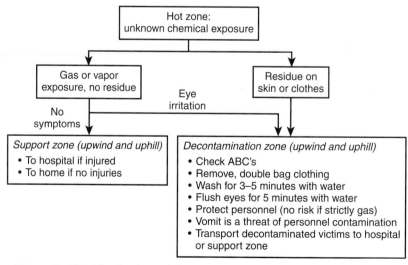

Figure 7 Algorithm for chemical decontamination at the scene.

The response to release of radiation should include protection of first responders and hospital personnel. At the scene, all efforts should be made to put emergency equipment and decontamination zones upwind and uphill. Responders should wear full masks and protective garments. Individuals without life-threatening blast injuries should be decontaminated at the scene prior to being transported to a hospital.

Hospitals should be equipped with a radiation survey device and a separate decontamination area outside of the ED should be established. As with chemical exposure, decontamination consists of removal of all clothing and thorough washing with water. Open wounds should be washed first. Symptoms consistent with ARS should be addressed. Treatment consists of supportive care. It is important to emphasize that after the patient has been decontaminated, health care workers are not at risk for radiation injury. The patient is suffering the effects of radiation exposure but is not radioactive. Additional help can be obtained from the Radiation Emergency Assistance Center/Training Site (Oak Ridge Institute for Science and Education) and the Medical Radiobiology Advisory Team (Armed Forces Radiobiology Research Institute, Bethesda, MD).

CONCLUSION

Surgeons should take an active role in preparation for disasters and mass casualty events. A well–thought out plan with elements of efficient triage and resource allocation is critical in order to maximize the number of lives saved and provide protection to personnel. Mass casualty events secondary to terrorist attacks most likely involve conventional explosive devices. However, hospital disaster plans should be prepared in the event that chemical, biologic, or radioactive agents are components of the attack.

SUGGESTED READINGS

California Emergency Medical Services Authority: Hospital Incident Command System, 1998. Available at www.HEICS.com/.
Centers for Disease Control and Prevention: Available at www.cdc.gov/.
Community Emergency Response Team—Los Angeles. Available at: www.cert-la.com/triage/.
Einav S, Feigenberg Z, et al: Evacuation priorities in mass casualty terror-related events. Implications for contingency planning. *Ann Surg* 39(3):304–310, 2004.
Frykberg ER: Principles of mass casualty management following terrorist disasters. *Ann Surg* 239:319–321, 2004.
Hirshberg A, Holcomb J, Mattox K: Hospital trauma care in multiple-casualty incidents: a critical review. *Ann Emerg Med* 37:647–652, 2001.
Kennedy K, Aghbabian RV, et al: Triage: techniques and applications in decision making. *Ann Emerg Med* 28(2):136–144, 1996.
Klein JS, Weigelt JA: Disaster management: lessons learned. *Surg Clin North Am* 71:257–266, 1991.
Lee S, Morabito D, et al: Trauma assessment training with a patient simulator: a prospective, randomized study. *J Trauma* 55(4):651–657, 2003.
Leibovici D, Gofrit O, et al: Blast injuries: bus versus open air bombings-a comparative study of injuries in survivors of open-air versus confined-space explosions. *J Trauma* 41:1030–1035, 1996.
U.S. Department of Defense: Available at www.defenselink.mil/.
U.S. Department of Health and Human Services: Available at www.hhs.gov/.
U.S. Department of Homeland Security: Available at www.dhs.gov/dhspublic/.
Waeckerle JF: Disaster planning and response. *N Engl J Med* 324:815–821, 1991.

BLAST INJURIES

Antonio Pepe, Booker T. King, Alexander Becker, Guy Lin, Tedla Tessema, Mauricio Lynn, and Eduard Grass

Blast injury is unique in that it combines the mechanisms of several categories of injury, including blunt, penetrating, and thermal. This results in a wide range of overt and occult injury patterns making the diagnosis and treatment of specific injuries difficult.[1] However, like most problems in medicine, a basic knowledge of and methodical approach to the problem can save lives. The use of explosives can be traced to the use of black powder by the Chinese in the 10th century. In the 1800s other explosive substances were invented, including nitroglycerin, trinitrotoluene (TNT), and dynamite. Explosives have been used in every major conflict by the United States since the American Revolution. Blast injury was first described in World War I and at that time was primarily thought to involve the lung. In World War II, blast injury to the bowel was seen due to an increase in casualties of underwater explosions. The treatment of blast injury advanced during the Korean War. In Vietnam, blast injuries were seen, but the predominant injuries were due to high-velocity gunshot wounds.[2,3]

The Israelis had the greatest experience with blast injury during the latter quarter of the 20th century, and have reported extensively on the subject.[4] Examples of recent domestic terrorist attacks that resulted in significant destruction and casualties include the 1993 bombing of the World Trade Center, the 1995 bombing of the Alfred P. Murrah Federal Building in Oklahoma City, and the bombing of the Centennial Park in Atlanta (1996).[5,6] Many casualties of the September 11, 2001 attacks occurred as result of blast effect and structural collapse.[7]

The use of improvised explosive devices (IEDs) by insurgents has become the predominant weapon against coalition troops in Iraq. A recent article reviewed the injuries of wounded soldiers returning to Walter Reed Army Medical Center from March to July 2003. Of 294 casualties seen, 31% sustained blast injuries.[8] Another study focused on 18 blast-injured patients evaluated at a forward resuscitative surgical hospital. A significant proportion of these casualties presented with penetrating head injuries, severe lung injuries, and multiple open fractures. This study characterizes the lethal effects of blast.[1]

MECHANISMS OF INJURY AND INJURY PATTERNS IN EXPLOSIONS

Explosions produce specific injury patterns and the potential to cause life-threatening multisystem or multidimensional injuries. These patterns are the result of the composition and type of bomb, the delivery method, the distance between the victim and the blast, whether the blast occurred in a closed or open space[2] and surrounding environmental barriers or hazards. Blast injury is a general term that refers to the biophysical and pathophysiological events and the clinical syndromes that occur when a living body is exposed to blast of any origin. Explosions are caused by a rapid chemical conversion of a solid or liquid into a gas with resultant energy release. Explosives are either high or low order. High-order explosives are designed to detonate quickly, generate heat and loud noise, fill the space with high-pressure gases in 1/1000th second, and produce a supersonic overpressurization shock (the increased pressure above normal atmospheric pressure from a blast) that expands from the point of detonation outward in a pressure pulse. The level of overpressure depends on the following: (1) the energy of the explosion, (2) the distance from the point of detonation, (3) the elapsed time since the explosion, and (4) the measurement technique. Blast strength is described as the ratio of overpressure to ambient pressure. The blast wave (positive wave) moves in all directions away form the explosion, exerting pressures of up to 700 tons (Figure 1). Shock waves possess the quality of brisance (shattering effect). The displaced air then compresses and forms a vacuum returning to the point of detonation (negative wave). The negative phase is not considered to result in blast injury. High-order explosives include TNT, C-4, Semtex, nitroglycerin, dynamite, and ammonium nitrate fuel oil. Low-order explosives produce a subsonic explosion without overpressurization wave. Energy is released slowly and burns by a process of deflagration. Low-order explosives include pipe bombs, gun powder, Molotov cocktails, and pure petroleum-based bombs. Explosives have several effects: the blast pressure wave as described previously, the fragmentation effect, the blast wind, the incendiary thermal effect, secondary blast pressure effects, and ground and water shocks for explosions that occur below ground or water.[9]

Fragmentation effect occurs from projectiles included in the container, projectiles produced from the destruction of the container, and from objects surrounding the detonator and target. These projectiles can travel up to 2700 feet per second. The blast wind is created by the motion of air molecules responding to pressure differentials generated by the blast. These winds may be as high as those seen in hurricanes but are not sustained. The incendiary thermal effect is different for high- and low-order explosives. High-order explosives produce higher temperatures for shorter periods of time, usually resulting in a fireball at the time of the detonation. Low-order explosives have a longer thermal effect and cause secondary fires. Secondary blast pressure effects are caused by the blast wave's reflection off surfaces prolonging and magnifying the effect, particularly in enclosed spaces. Greater transfer of energy to the body occurs. Underground and underwater explosions propagate the shock waves farther and with more force than air.[10]

Bombs are weapons and defined as any container filled with explosive material whose explosion is triggered by a clock or other timing device. Terrorist bombs, IEDs, are usually custom-made, may use a number of designs or explosives, and are of two types: conventional (filled with chemical explosives containing the compounds of hydrogen, oxygen, nitrogen, and carbon) or dispersives (filled with chemical or other projectiles such as nails, steel pellets, screws, and nuts) designed to disperse. Nuclear devices rely on nuclear fission or fusion. Explosions can produce unique patterns of injury. They have the potential to inflict multisystem life-threatening injuries on many persons simultaneously. The injury patterns following such events are a product of the composition and amount of the materials involved, the surrounding environment, and the delivery method, the distance between the victim the blast, and any intervening protective barriers or environmental hazards. Because explosions are relatively infrequent, blast-related injuries can present unique triage, diagnostic, and management challenges to providers or emergency care personnel.[11]

BLAST INJURY: CLINICAL ASPECTS

Blast-related injuries are now very common and have become a threat for populations all over the world. Powerful explosions that result in different tissue and air interactions have the potential to inflict complex and unique injuries. Severely injured patients from explosions often sustain combined blunt, penetrating, and burn injuries.[12] Therefore, knowledge of the mechanisms of blast effect and early recognition of the potential injuries are of paramount importance in the management of blast-injured patients. The injury patterns vary depending on setting (open or closed space), amount of explosive, and chemical properties of the explosive.[13] Explosions in confined spaces are significantly more deadly and associated with high incidence of primary blast injuries than those in open air. Improvised explosive devices are accompanied by heavy shrapnel that result in various injury patterns involving more body regions and increase severity. This makes management of blast injuries more challenging.[4] According to their underlying mechanisms, blast injury is classified into four categories: primary, secondary, tertiary, and quaternary (Table 1).[14] Quinary blast injury also has recently been described.

Primary Blast Injury

Primary blast injury causes barotrauma. The organs most vulnerable to primary blast injury are the gas-filled, namely the ear, lung, and gastrointestinal tract. The eardrum, the most frequently injured structure, may rupture at pressure as low as 2 psi (pounds/square inch).[15] High overpressure may cause more significant injury to the ear such as dislocation and fracture of the ossicles of the middle ear, cochlear damage, and traumatic disruption of the oval or round window and subsequent permanent hearing loss.

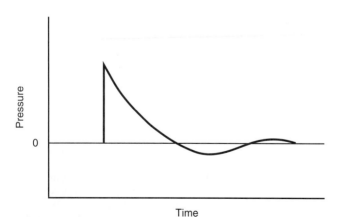

Figure 1 Propagation of blast wave over time. *(Data from Jensen JH, Bonding P: Experimental pressure induced rupture of the tympanic membrane in man.* Acta Otolaryngol *113:62–67, 1993.)*

Table 1: Categories of Blast Injury

Type of Blast Injury	Features
Primary	Caused by barotrauma Affects gas-filled structures including tympanic membrane, lungs, bowel
Secondary	Caused by flying debris and fragments Responsible for most of casualties Causes multiple injuries
Tertiary	Caused by collapse and fragmentation of buildings Causes severe fractures and amputations
Quaternary	Includes all explosion-related injuries Affected by patient's premorbidities
Quinary	Hyperinflammatory state Toxins in explosives

The most common manifestations of ear blast injury are tinnitus, deafness, and vertigo. The fact that tympanic membrane injury occurs at low pressure and much more pressure is needed to damage other structures make tympanic membrane perforation an indicator of blast injury.

The anatomical structure of the lungs is characterized by large surface area with low tensile strength. This makes the lung very susceptible to primary blast injury, and injury to the lung may be the most fatal. The incidence of blast lung injury is unknown. In a study by Brismar and Bergenwald,[16] 8.4% of patients admitted after a blast were diagnosed with lung injury. Hadden et al.[17] in a study from Northern Ireland reported that only 2 of 250 admitted patients (0.8%) suffered from primary blast lung injury; on the other hand, histopathologic evidence consistent with primary blast lung injury was found in 45% of the victims who died at the scene. A high proportion of primary blast lung injury occurs in explosions in enclosed space. In a study of 55 survivors after a terrorist bus bombing, Katz et al.[18] found that 38% of patients had primary blast lung injury. Primary blast lung injury occurs at air pressure of 1100 kpcal (kilopascals) (Figure 2). The pressure differentials disrupt the alveolar walls and the alveolar-capillary membrane, and damage airway epithelium, producing a stripped-epithelium lesion. This results when bronchiolar epithelium is stripped from the basal membrane.[19] As a result of these widespread structural disturbances, hemorrhage, pulmonary contusion, pneumothorax, hemothorax, pneumomediastinum, and subcutaneous emphysema can occur. Intrapulmonary hemorrhage and edema are major factors in the development of initial respiratory insufficiency from primary blast lung injury.[20] Some experience apnea, bradycardia, and hypotension as immediate responses to blast injury of the lung. The diagnosis of primary blast lung injury is based on clinical manifestations, such as dyspnea, hypoxia, and hemoptysis. A chest x-ray may show the characteristic bihilar "butterfly" pattern representing underlying pulmonary contusion.[21,22] A tear that may occur between the alveoli and the wall of the venule can create alveolo-venous fistulae, the major prerequisite for another life-threatening condition—arterial air embolism. This is a principal cause of early mortality.[18]

The blast lung severity score was introduced to estimate the severity of blast lung injury. The score is based on hypoxemia (PO₂/FiO₂ ratio), chest x-ray abnormalities, and presence of bronchopleural fistulae or pneumothorax. Severe blast lung injury is defined as a PO_2/FiO_2 ratio of less than 60 mm Hg, bilateral lung infiltrates, and bronchopleural fistu-lae, moderate as a PO_2/FiO_2 ratio of 60–200 mm Hg, diffuse lung infiltrates with or without pneumothorax; and mild blast lung injury as a PO_2/FiO_2 ratio of more than 200 mm Hg, localized lung infiltrates, and no pneumothorax.[23] Pizov et al.[20] studied 15 survivors of a bus explosion diagnosed with blast lung injury. Ten patients were intubated for respiratory failure within 2 hours after the explosion. Six patients with a moderate blast lung injury severity score required mechanical ventilation. Four patients who sustained severe lung injuries were managed with positive pressure ventilation immediately after the event. Out of the four with blast injury to the lung, three died. In conclusion, primary blast lung injury is life-threatening. The treatment of blast lung injury is challenging. Symptoms can manifest early resulting in immediate onset of pulmonary dysfunction, or the patient may have a less dramatic course of pulmonary insufficiency developing several days after the explosion.

Exposure to extreme blast overpressure may produce injury to the abdominal viscera. The colon is the organ most commonly affected by primary blast injury. Intestinal damage may present as free bowel perforation, hemorrhage, serosal hematoma, and mesenteric shear injuries. Intestinal perforation may occur immediately after blast exposure or develop as a result of mesenteric ischemia, infarct, and bowel contusion in hours to days after the event.[17,21] Insidious manifestations of symptoms and the presence additional life-threatening injuries make abdominal injury difficult to recognize. Blast abdominal injury should not be overlooked in patients with abdominal pain, nausea, vomiting, and hematemesis. Lacerations and hemorrhage of solid organs such as liver, kidney, and spleen may occur with powerful explosions. Other injuries caused by primary blast effect include facial fractures, brain concussion, cerebral air embolism, and eye trauma. Traumatic limb amputations from blast phenomena are a hallmark of severe blast injury.[24] The blast waves run along the long bones, creating a powerful shearing force. The long bones fracture into multiple fragments and then soft tissue is avulsed by the primary blast wave.[25] Mellor et al.[26] reported on 52 victims who sustained traumatic limb amputations, of whom only nine survived.

Secondary Blast Injury

Secondary blast injuries are caused by flying debris, and bomb fragments penetrating multiple body regions are responsible for a great proportion of casualties. Mallonee and colleagues[27] studied

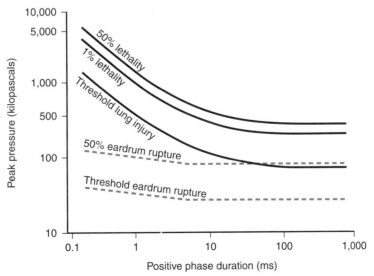

Figure 2   Tolerance and lethality of blast wave.   *(Data from Jensen JH, Bonding P: Experimental pressure induced rupture of the tympanic membrane in man. Acta Otolaryngol 113:62–67, 1993.)*

the Murrah Building explosion in Oklahoma City, and reported that most common injuries were penetrating injuries to the extremities (74%), head and neck (48%), face (45%), and chest (35%). Penetrating injuries from fragments of the weapon and debris are the leading cause of death and injury. Suicide bombs used by terrorists contain large amounts of metal objects. It has been shown that missiles with irregular shapes have inherent ballistic instability and tend to have greater kinetic energy, causing more severe tissue destruction than symmetric missiles.[28] These factors explain why multiple body regions are involved in a large number of casualties.

Tertiary Blast Injury

Tertiary blast injuries are caused by collapse and fragmentation of buildings, vehicles, and other objects. The collapse of buildings and other structures is characterized a large number of casualties and carries a high fatality rate. During the terrorist bombing of the Murrah Building in Oklahoma City, 88% of 361 people who were inside the building were injured. People located at the sites of structural collapse were significantly more likely to die (153/175, 87%) than those in the noncollapsed region of the building (10/186, 5%). Survivors who were located in the collapsed region of the building were significantly more likely to require hospitalization (82%), than those in the noncollapsed area. Collapse and fragmentation of these structures cause a wide range of blunt trauma injuries, multiple penetrating injuries, and crush syndrome.[5]

Tertiary blast injuries can also occur when the victims themselves become airborne by the blast wave and collide with nearby objects. These blast victims usually are very close to the explosion source and therefore sustain multiple injuries. Any body part may be affected and open fractures, traumatic limb amputations, and brain injuries may occur.[29]

Quaternary Blast Injury

Quaternary blast injuries may affect any part of the body and include all explosion-related injuries and conditions not due to primary, secondary, and tertiary blast effects. Quaternary blast injuries include burns, inhalation lung injury, and asphyxia caused by inhalation of incomplete combustion of explosion materials (e.g., carbon monoxide, cyanide), toxic dust, gas, and radiation exposure. Quaternary blast injury may involve exacerbation of chronic disease (including asthma, diabetes, hypertension, coronary artery disease, mental health issues, and substance abuse) as well as new behavioral problems. Materials used in incendiary bombs can cause severe burns. Burns sustained by victims of confined-space explosions affect a larger body surface area than those of open-space explosions.[24]

Quinary Blast Injury

A fifth category of blast injury has recently been described in blast injury victims. It occurs commonly after attack with incendiary devices. This type of blast injury is characterized by a "hyperinflammatory state" similar to systemic inflammatory response syndrome. This hyperinflammatory state cannot be explained by injuries that result from the other types of blast injury.[4] Some clinicians hypothesize that quinary blast injury is due to toxic substances that are liberated by explosives which are inhaled or absorbed by skin and mucus membranes. Pentaerythritoltetranitrate (PETN), a vasodilator, is implicated as one such toxin. This form of blast injury is poorly understood but is increasingly identified in this cohort.[30]

Multidimensional Injury Pattern

The classical approach to managing blast injury patients has changed, and patients are now viewed as having a "multidimensional injury pattern." This new concept was adopted largely from the experience of trauma surgeons treating victims of blast injury in Israel.[30] The multidimensional injury pattern view relates different types of blast injury (primary, secondary, tertiary, etc.) with various mechanisms of injury (blunt, penetrating, thermal, radiation, etc.) and the organs injured (lung, ear, brain, gastrointestinal tract, etc.). Studies have shown that these types of injuries have higher morbidity and mortality when compared with non–blast-related trauma. The majority of these patients have multiple severe injuries and require management in an intensive care setting.[4] The management of these patients requires a multidisciplinary approach, and can easily overwhelm local medical resources in a mass casualty situation.

TREATMENT OF BLAST INJURIES

The rate-limiting step in the management of blast injuries is the diagnosis of each specific injury, while treatment is straightforward. Patients found to have pneumothorax or hemothorax that result from a blast will often require chest tube thoracostomy. The presentation may be more subtle, and patients may present with subcutaneous emphysema, mediastinal air on chest radiograph, or delayed pneumothorax. Pulmonary contusion can be treated with supplemental oxygen and incentive spirometry; but patients with severe blast lung injury and hypoxemia need mechanical ventilation. The mode of ventilation should be tailored, and depends on the degree of hypoxia, presence of the bronchopleural fistulae, and injuries to the other organs. Generally, ventilation should use limited peak inspiratory pressure because of high risk of air embolism and pneumothorax. High-frequency ventilation provides adequate oxygenation with low airway pressure, and is recommended for ventilation of patients with bronchopleural fistulae.[31]

Clinical signs of arterial air embolism include air seen on retinoscopy, cardiac dysrhythmias or signs of ischemia, neurologic defects, livedo reticularis, and blanching tongue. Air emboli form when air escapes from a pulmonary laceration into the arterial tree. The treatment for air emboli is largely supportive. The patient should be monitored for signs of cerebral and cardiac ischemia. Hyperbaric oxygen therapy has been shown to be beneficial in animal studies, but its efficacy in humans has yet to be determined.[12]

Significant blast injury to the gastrointestinal tract will almost always require exploration. These injuries may be obvious on presentation or can be detected by CT scan or diagnostic peritoneal lavage. Bowel injuries resulting in perforation and extensive mesenteric and intramural hematomas will require resection. The amount of bowel destruction can be impressive.[32] All blast injury victims should be screened for hearing loss. Debris and foreign material must be removed from the external auditory canal. Small to moderate perforations of the tympanic membrane should heal spontaneously. Large perforations may require patching or tympanoplasty.[33]

Explosions in closed spaces or that result in structural collapse have higher mortality and injury rates.[9] Arnold and colleagues,[34] in an epidemiological review of terrorist bombings that produced 30 or more casualties, found that 1 in 4 victims died immediately in structural collapse, 1 in 12 in confined-space bombings, and 1 in 25 in open-air bombings. Bus bombings in the Israeli experience resulted in the highest mortality rate.

There is a triphasic distribution of mortality related to blast injury: (1) high immediate mortality rate, (2) a low early emergency department mortality rate, and (3) a late (in-hospital) mortality rate. Injury patterns causing death can be classified as the following: complete disruption of bodies, 14%; multiple injuries, 39%; head and chest injuries, 21%; head injuries, 12%; and chest injuries, 11%. Hidden injuries such as air emboli and cardiac dysrhythmias may account for fatalities in which no other cause of death is found. Injury patterns are varied as well. Structural collapse victims sustained more inhalational and crush injuries (secondary, quaternary injuries) and fewer primary blast injuries. Confined-space bombings resulted in more primary and quaternary blast injuries, while open-air bombing led to higher rates of ballistic soft tissue injuries or more secondary blast injuries.[35]

Blast injuries and casualty numbers caused by terrorist bombings have been constantly increasing. They have devastating consequences and can overwhelm medical resources. The combination of multiple and complex injuries, involvement of multiple body regions, and mass-casualty situations are challenging to prehospital personnel, emergency physicians, and surgeons. Knowledge of the potential mechanisms, clinical aspects, and triage-related issues are of great importance for trauma surgeons and all personnel involved in the management of blast-injured patients.

REFERENCES

1. Nelson TJ, Wall DB, Stedje-Larsen ET, et al: Predictors of mortality in close proximity blast injuries during Operation Iraqi Freedom. *J Am Coll Surg* 202:418–422, 2006.
2. Oxendine H: The history of explosives. University of Vermont, Environmental Safety Website, January 13, 2000. Available at: www.esf.uvm.edu\sirippt\blast1\index.htm.
3. Thall E: Explosives. Florida Community College at Jacksonville. Available at: www.mooni.fccj.org\~ethall\explode\explode.htm.
4. Kluger Y, Peleg K, Daniel-Aharonson L, et al: The special injury pattern in terrorists bombing. *J Am Coll Surg* 199(6):875–879, 2004.
5. Teague DC: Mass casualties in the Oklahoma City bombing. *Clin Orthop Relat Res* 422:78–81, 2004.
6. Felicano DV, Anderson GV, Rozycki GS, et al: Management of casualties from the bombing of the Centennial Olympics. *Am J Surg* 176:538–543, 1998.
7. Quenemoen LE, Davis YM, Malilay J, et al: The World Trade Center bombing: injury prevention strategies for high rise buildings. *Disasters* 20(2):125–132, 1996.
8. Montgomery SP, Swiecki CW, Shriver CD: The evaluation of casualties from Operation Iraqi Freedom to return to continental United States from March to June 2003. *J Am Coll Surg* 201:7–13, 2005.
9. Avidan V, Hersch M, Armon Y, et al: Blast lung injury: clinical manifestations, treatment and outcome. *Am J Surg* 190(6):927–931, 2005.
10. Arnold JL, Halpern P, Tsai MC, Smithline H: Mass casualty terrorist bombings: epidemiological outcomes, resource utilization and the time course of emergency needs. *Prehosp Disaster Med* 18(3):220–260, 2003 (review).
11. Lucci EB: Civilian preparedness and counter-terrorism: conventional weapons. *Surg Clin N Am* 86:579–600, 2006.
12. Stuhmiller JH, Phillips YY, Richmond DR: The physics and mechanisms of primary blast injury. In Bellamy RF, Zajtchuk R, eds. *Textbook of Military Medicine Part I. Conventional Warfare: Ballistic, Blast and Burn Injuries*. Washington, DC, Office of the Surgeon General, 1989.
13. Horrocks CL: Blast injuries: biophysics, pathophysiology and management principles. *J R Army Med Corps* 147(1):28–40, 2001 (review).
14. Burris DG, Fitzhrans JB, Holcomb JB, et al, editors: *Emergency War Surgery. The Third United States Revision*. Washington, DC, Borden Institute, 2004.
15. Phillips YY: Primary blast injuries. *Ann Emerg Med* 15:1446–1450, 1986.
16. Brismar B, Bergenwald L: The terrorist bomb explosion in Bologna, Italy, 1980: an analysis of the effects and injuries sustained. *J Trauma* 22:216–220, 1982.
17. Hadden MA, Rutherford WH, Merrett JD: The injuries of terrorist bombing: a study of 1532 consecutive patients. *Br J Surg* 65:525–531, 1978.
18. Katz E, Ofek B, Adler J, et al: Primary blast injury after a bomb explosion in civilian bus. *Ann Surg* 209:484–488, 1989.
19. Brown R, Cooper G, Maynard R: The ultrastructure of rat lung following acute primary blast injury. *Int J Exp Pathol* 74: 151–162, 1993.
20. Pizov R, Oppenheim-Eden A, Mator I, et al: Blast injury from explosion on a civilian bus. *Chest* 115:165–172, 1999.
21. Gutierrez de Ceballos JP, Fuentes FT, Diaz DP, et al: Casualties treated at the closest hospital in the Madrid, March 11, terrorist bombings. *Crit Care Med* 33:S107–S112, 2003.
22. de Candole CA: Blast injury. *CMAJ* 96:207–214, 1967.
23. Bernard GR, Artigas A, Brigham KL et al: The American-European Consensus Conference on ARDS: definitions, mechanisms, relevant outcomes, and clinical trial coordination. *Am J Respir Crit Care Med* 149: 818–824, 1994.
24. Leibovici D, Gofrit O, Stein M et al: Blast injuries: bus versus open-air bombings—a comparative study of injuries in survivors of open-air versus confined-space explosions. *J Trauma* 41(6):1030–1035, 1996.
25. Hull JB: Traumatic amputation by explosive blast: pattern of injury in survivors. *Br J Surg* 79:1303–1306, 1992.
26. Mellor SG, Cooper GJ: Analysis of 828 servicemen killed or injured by explosion in Northern Ireland 1970–1984: the Hostile Action Casualty System. *Br J Surg* 77:1006–1010, 1989.
27. Mallonee S, Shariat S, Stenies G, et al: Physical injuries and fatalities resulting from the Oklahoma City bombing. *JAMA* 276:382–387, 1996.
28. Cooper GJ, Maynard RL, Cross NL: Casualties from terrorist bombing. *J Orthop Trauma* 23:955–967, 1983.
29. DePalma RG, Burris DG, Champion HR, et al: Blast injuries. *N Engl J Med* 352(13):1335–1342, 2005 (review).
30. Mayo A, Kluger Y: Terrorist bombing. *World J Emerg Surg* 1:33, 2006. Available at www.wjes.org/content/1/1/33.
31. Wanek S, Mayberry JC: Blunt thoracic trauma: flail chest, pulmonary contusion, and blast injury. *Crit Care Clin* 20(1):171–181, 2004 (review).
32. Sharma OP, Oswanski MF, White PW: Injuries to the colon from blast effect and penetrating extraperitoneal thoraco-abdominal trauma. *Injury* 35(3):320–324, 2004.
33. Cripps NP, Glover MA, Guy RJ: The pathophysiology of primary blast injury and its implications for treatment. Part II: The auditory structures and the abdomen. *J R Nav Med Serv* 85(1):13–24, 1999 (review).
34. Arnold JL, Halpern P, Tsai MC, et al: Mass casualty terrorist bombing: a comparison of outcomes by bombing type. *Ann Emerg Med* 43(2): 263–273.
35. Jensen JH, Bonding P: Experimental pressure induced rupture of the tympanic membrane in man. *Acta Otolaryngol* 113:62–67, 1993.

Prehospital Care of Biological Agent–Induced Injuries

Kenneth G. Swan

On a busy Baghdad bridge spanning the great Tigris River coursing Iraq from north to south, a crowd of people intermingled in their bidirectional flow. Most were hurrying to and from the nearby market on the east side of the river below. Some were carrying parcels, others infant children in their arms or on their backs. Someone shouted something; it was never determined who or what, but those within hearing interpreted the alarm as a warning, presumably of an improvised explosive device (IED) on the bridge. The reaction among the already apprehensive civilians was instant panic and they scattered in all directions. Some attempted to cross to the other side; others tried to retreat from where they were headed, some jumped into the waters below. A herd mentality eliminated all sense of proportion; flight with presumed escape dominated the thought processes of the terrified populace. In the aftermath of the incident, almost 1000 were dead and many more were injured. The causes of death included suffocation, exsanguination from blunt trauma to torso, head injuries, and multiple long-bone fractures. Many drowned. The alleged IED never detonated, nor was it ever identified. The date was August 31, 2005. The inciting event remains a mystery.[1] The inciting event, however, exemplifies two phenomena pertinent to the trauma surgeon.

Acts of civilian terrorism (ACTs) can result from many instruments or have unknown etiologies. Equally important, if perpetrated in the setting of heightened anxiety or apprehension, they can have devastating consequences of panic, stampede, and resultant blunt trauma. An explosive device need not be the inciting event. Just the threat of one or of any number of alternative hazards to personal safety may have the same result. Such alternatives include the agents of bioterrorism. Ignorance and superstition, primarily the former, cloud rationality when their presence is suspected. Thus, two forms of trauma must be considered by prehospital caregivers under such circumstances, the biohazard itself and the trauma that ensued from the panic that it produced.

Prehospital care is provided by the most medically sophisticated at the scene and en route to a medical treatment facility (MTF). Such caregivers may be emergency medical technicians (EMTs), paramedics, and even physicians.[2] They will be required, by necessity, to perform patient assessment, threat assessment, triage, and first aid until additional help arrives.

Patient assessment proceeds along standardized guidelines established by the American College of Surgeons and its Advanced Trauma Life Support program as modified to complement varying skill levels (Prehospital Trauma Life Support), such as those relevant to nurses, paramedics, and EMTs. Included in the patient assessment is the threat assessment. What caused the panic? Was it explosive, radioactive, chemical, or biological and does it still pose a threat? Answers to these questions may not be readily apparent, initially; nevertheless, answers will be essential to successful triage, patient resuscitation, stabilization, and transport, as well as notification and protection of those not yet exposed to the dangers presented.

Triage is patient-location dependent.[3] Casualties from biological agent–induced injuries may be encountered in the field or at the scene of agent exposure. At this level the term "field triage," as distinguished from "hospital triage," is appropriate. The word is derived from the French verb "trier," which means to sort, and dates back to the 15th century and European marketplaces where fur and fiber were sorted according to quality and price. Any number of categories can be designated, but perhaps the simplest is three tiers. Most "patients" are apprehensive, bordering on hysteria. They need to be conveniently relocated and comforted by a minimal number of caregivers. This category may comprise the largest percentage of patients at the scene. A small percentage of the remainder are in extremis or agonal. They are termed "expectant," and cannot be helped other than to allow them to die with a minimum of discomfort and as much dignity as can be provided under the circumstances. The remainder are "priority," and they all need transport to an MTF. These patients are bleeding, have airway problems, head injuries, burns, chest or abdominal pain, or evidence of spine or long-bone fracture. This latter category may represent only 20% of the casualties, but it is the most important.

Principles of triage[3] that must be understood include the fact that patients are triaged and re-triaged, not only at all levels of patient care, but also within levels of patient care. The triage officer does not treat, assuming there is more than one caregiver present. The triage officer only sorts patients according to injury and probable outcome. The latter is dependent on available resources—time, personnel, and equipment—and their presumed efficient use. Weather, communications, and available transportation will all play critical roles in determining anticipated outcome. Assuming that explosive ordinance, radiation, and chemical threats have been eliminated, but a biological agent has not, what steps should be taken by the first responder or caregiver present at the scene of an ACT?[4]

The ranking medical caregiver must establish communications, ascertain the risk of additional threat to the immediate area, and in addition to providing first aid to those most in need, attempt to identify the biological agent responsible for the mass casualties and the probable time of onset of exposure.

At present, there are five specific agents considered likely sources of bioterrorism. They have several general characteristics in common that make them preferable to alternative agents. These characteristics include relative ease of production, packaging, transport, and delivery, as well as not only lethality, but also morbidity. Agents that kill rapidly may be less inducive of panic and terror than those that cause large numbers to be extremely ill for prolonged periods of time, their condition apparently communicable. The five agents most commonly cited, as potential threats, are those associated with anthrax, smallpox, botulism, plague, and tularemia. The characteristics of each will be presented with emphasis placed on detection, diagnosis, treatment, precautions, prophylaxis, quarantine, decontamination, and necrology (Tables 1, 2, and 3). Other less likely agents, such as the encephalitides, the Ebola virus, and so on, will be mentioned, but only in passing, because of their much lower probability of encounter.

Anthrax[5] has a long history as a disease among animals, but is much less commonly encountered in humans. Spores of *Bacillus anthracis* have been weaponized by the governments of many countries and individuals have been exposed accidentally in Russia as well as targeted by attacks in Japan and more recently the United States. While the number of deaths from these exposures is relatively small, the potential is impressive. The World Health Organization (WHO) estimated that aerial release of 50 kg of anthrax spores over an urban population of 5 million, would cause 250,000 casualties, almost half of whom would die without treatment. Similar scenarios have compared an aerosolized attack with anthrax spores to the effects of a hydrogen bomb attack on a large city.

Table 1: Five Most Frequently Cited Bioterrorism Agents: Characteristics, Associated Disease, Recognition, and Identification

Disease	Organism	Aerosol	Onset	Symptoms	Distinction	Identification
Anthrax	*Bacillus anthracis*	Spore	2 days	Acute onset, flu-like illness	Mediastinal widening	Large Gram-positive rods, blood
Smallpox	DNA orthopoxvirus	Virus	12–14 days	Severe febrile illness	Rash	Viruses (EM), pustular fluid
Plague	*Yersinia pestis*	Bacterium	1–6 days	Severe pneumonia, sepsis	Hemoptysis	Bipolar ("safety pin") Gram-negative coccobacilli, sputum
Botulism	*Clostridium botulinum*	Toxin	Hours–days	Paralysis	No fever	Mouse bioassay, blood
Tularemia	*Francisella tularensis*	Bacterium	3–5 days	Acute onset, febrile illness, nonspecific	Slower progression	Small Gram-negative coccobacilli, sputum

Table 2: Five Most Frequently Cited Bioterrorism Agents: Treatment, Prevention, Cause of Death, and Necrology

Disease	Treatment		Prevention	Cause of Death	Necrology
	Antibiotics (q12h)		Vaccination, antitoxin		
	Parenteral	Oral			
Anthrax	Ciprofloxacin 400 mg	Ciprofloxacin 500 mg	6-dose series, U.S. military	Respiratory failure, sepsis	Burial, cremation
Smallpox	For secondary infections		None available	Sepsis	Cremation
Plague	Streptomycin 1.0 g, gentamycin	Doxycycline 100 mg, ciprofloxacin	None available	Sepsis	Burial
Botulism	For secondary infections		Antitoxin	Respiratory failure	Burial
Tularemia	Streptomycin 1.0 g, gentamycin	Doxycycline 100 mg, ciprofloxacin	None available	Respiratory failure, sepsis	Burial

Table 3: Five Most Frequently Cited Bioterrorism Agents: Prophylaxis, Infection Control, and Decontamination

Disease	Prophylaxis	Infection Control	Decontamination
Anthrax	Same as "therapy," 60 days	No H-HT, SP	1°, 2° aerosolization without direct contact, soap and water
Smallpox	Vaccination	Isolation and vaccination of all patients plus their contacts	Spontaneous, 6–24 hours
Plague	Same as "therapy," all contacts plus anyone with fever or cough	Respiratory droplet precaution (RP) until 48 hours ABT	Spontaneous, 1 hour
Botulism	Close observation, antitoxin scarce	Standard precautions	Toxin easily destroyed, bleach 1/10, soap and water
Tularemia	Same as "therapy," any exposed	No H-HT, SP	Short half-life, soap and water, bleach 1/10, alcohol 70%

ABT, Antibiotic therapy; *H-HT,* human-to-human transmission; *RP,* respiratory droplet precautions (with masks); *SP,* standard precautions (without masks).

Three forms of anthrax infection delivery occur in humans: inhalation, cutaneous, and gastrointestinal. Anthrax spores are 1.0 mcm, extremely hardy, and, when aerosolized, odorless, tasteless, colorless, and invisible. Obviously bioterrorists would most likely attempt inhalation exposure via an aerosolized release of spores from an aerial source. A two-stage illness ensues. In the primary phase, which lasts hours to days, the victim experiences fever, dyspnea, cough, headache, nausea, vomiting, chills, weakness, and pain in the chest and abdomen within days to weeks of exposure, depending on number and size of spores inhaled. The second phase begins with an abrupt increase in severity of symptoms, which coincides with massive lymphadenopathy, bacteremia, hypotension, and death, if untreated.

The massive hilar lymphadenopathy presents radiographically as a "widened mediastinum." Mediastinitis, meningitis, and cyanosis are common in the second phase. Clues to the diagnosis are the sudden appearance, in large numbers, of previously healthy city dwellers with an overwhelming flu-like illness. Differential diagnosis includes pneumonic plague. Treatment includes parenteral antibiotics (penicillin, etc.), ventilator and pressors if patients can be hospitalized, and if not, oral antibiotics. Blood cultures before antibiotic therapy are confirmatory, but case fatality rates approach 80% and most of those occur within the first 2 days of symptoms.

Prophylaxis consists of vaccination (six-dose series),[6] which has been administered to all U.S. service personnel. Since there is no threat of patient-to-patient transmission of anthrax, patient contacts do not require treatment; however, the dead should be cremated because of spore hardiness. Decontamination of all suspected victims of inhalation anthrax is necessary to avoid secondary aerosolization of spores that remain on clothing, etc. Health care workers must wash their hands after contact with anthrax victims for the same reason.

Should first responders and health care providers at the scene suspect an anthrax aerosolization as the source of the ensuing scene of fear and panic, several important measures need immediate attention. As in all cases of suspected bioterrorism, appropriate local, state, and federal reporting centers must be notified. Local hospitals need also to be alerted and appropriate steps taken to maximize availability of ventilators since those who do sustain inhalation anthrax will likely require endotracheal intubation and respiratory support. Numbers may overwhelm resource availability in such situations. Triage is also considered.

When relatively large numbers of burn victims require triage for resource management, a 50% total body burn (TBB) is considered sufficiently lethal to designate expectancy under such circumstances. Since there often are associated injuries in burn victims, additional trauma is added to the burn percentage. For example, if a person jumped from a burning building and fractured his femur, his burn percentage (50%) would be increased to 55%, or 5% for each long-bone fracture. Similarly, the trauma patient who was injured while attempting to flee an anthrax attack that exposed him or her to inhalation of the agent, might be more likely declared expectant because of an inevitably poor prognosis. Because of unpredictable timing of disease onset, this set of circumstances would be very challenging to the triage officer.

Perhaps the most feared of the biological agents on the top five lists for likely agents of bioterrorism is smallpox.[7] It is especially threatening for several reasons. Since global eradication through vaccination was declared almost 30 years ago, vaccination has been terminated. Thus, no one today is protected from a smallpox attack even though the only known sources of the virus are in state-controlled laboratories in the United States and Russia. In addition, there is no known treatment for smallpox. Person-to-person contact enables aerosol transmission of body secretions, and contaminated clothing, as well as bedding, readily holds as well as transmits the virus from patient to contacts. Only a few viruses are necessary for infection to progress to viremia, which lasts a few days. The hemopoietic and reticuloendothelial systems are inoculated, and a secondary, heavier viremia results within 8 days. Victims exhibit high fever, malaise, headache, prostration, backache, and abdominal pain. A characteristic vesicular skin eruption progresses centrifugally and involves the palms of the hands and soles of the feet, which distinguishes smallpox (variola) from chicken pox (varicella). The former lesions conform to a single stage, whereas those of varicella appear in crops and also occur centripetally. Treatment of smallpox consists of supportive measures, including antibiotics, but case fatality is in excess of 30%. Contacts need vaccination, and this of course includes all exposed health care workers, including all those who have had contact with the victim. Patients must be isolated and can be confined to a designated hospital, and even their home where possible. The incubation period is 12–14 days, and the subsequent viremia progresses as outlined

previously. Since the patients remain heavily infective, even in death, cremation is necessary as with victims of anthrax.

Although perhaps most feared as an agent for bioterrorism, world condemnation of smallpox use for such purposes coupled with the very difficult, virtually impossible access to sufficient stores of the virus make it extremely impractical. Nonetheless, because Russia remains somewhat unpredictable, and because Russia and the United States may not be the only repositories for the virus,[8] the threat remains and so must the registration of smallpox in all bioterrorism training programs in the United States and elsewhere.

Plague has its own history of bioterrorist use, and rivals any other biological agent in terms of numbers killed, certainly as a percentage of world population, including the Great Influenza of 1918.[9] Plague is high on the list of choices for current bioterrorists because of ready availability, ease of production, and applicability to aerosolization. It is estimated that 50 kg of *Yersenia pestis*, the causative organism, aerosolized over an urban population of 5 million, would result in pneumonic plague in 150,000, of whom 36,000 would die. The organisms would be expected to survive within the area for 1 hour and remain a threat during that time. Because pneumonic plague can be transmitted from one person to another, panic and flight could readily spread the initial infection. The disease presents as a severe respiratory illness 1–6 days following exposure. Since actual exposure may not be known, the clue to recognition of pneumonic plague is its nearly simultaneous presentation in a relatively large number of previously healthy individuals with negligible risk factors. Historically, plague was anticipated in the wake of large numbers of dead and dying rats in an urban population, causing the fleas carrying the bacilli to turn to humans as hosts. In a terrorist attack, however, this phase of the life cycle would be obviated. The disease in humans became known as the "Black Death" from the acral cyanosis associated with digital vasospasm and gangrene associated with septicemic plague, a complication of any form of infection with *Y. pestis*. Others attribute the term to the intense, generalized cyanosis coincident with pneumonic plague and its resultant hypoxia. Since the prodroma of pneumonic plague include coryza, a sneeze in the 14th century was greeted with "God bless you" by those in attendance who quickly scurried away because the presumption was that the person who sneezed was about to come down with the plague, for which there was no treatment and death almost a certainty.

Because of its similarity to anthrax, several distinguishing features are mentioned. Hemoptysis is more suggestive of pneumonic plague than the pneumonia caused by anthrax. Sputum from patients with plague reveals Gram-negative coccobacilli that have been likened to "safety pins" in appearance because of their bipolar nuclei.[10] Treatment is with parenteral antibiotics (tetracycline, gentamycin) preferably; but, faced with large numbers of patients and limited hospital space, oral tetracycline, doxycycline, or ciprofloxacin is recommended. A vaccine was developed for prevention against bubonic plague, but offers little protection against pneumonic plague contracted from aerosalization, and in fact, it is no longer manufactured. Once the organism is identified, health care providers should isolate patients because they remain infective and those in attendance should implement standard respiratory droplet precautions (SRDP), which include mask and eye screens in addition to gown and gloves. Patients who do not survive can be buried because the organisms will not survive. Environmental precautions are usually not a concern because the organisms have a limited life expectancy following release (1 hour).

A fourth agent for bioterrorism is botulinum toxin,[11] considered the most poisonous substance known to mankind. Aerosolization of 1 g of the toxin, if adequately dispersed and inhaled by those exposed, could kill 1 million people. One-tenth of 1 mcg, intravenously, is sufficient to kill an adult. The toxin blocks acetylcholine release at neuromuscular junctions, and it does so by binding irreversibly with the cholinergic synapse. The clinical picture then is a classic triad of symptoms: (1) symmetric, descending flaccid paralysis with prominent bulbar palsies, in (2) an afebrile patient, with (3) a clear sensorium. The bulbar palsies are often referred to as "the 4Ds": diplopia, dysphoria, dysarthria, and dysphagia. Recovery from inhalation botulism requires intensive care and ventilatory and nutritional support, and may take weeks to months because neural regeneration is required to displace the previously blocked synapses at myoneural junctions. For this reason alone—the prolonged disability and delayed recovery of so many victims—the toxin is a highly prized agent of bioterrorism. In fact, prior to the outbreak of the Gulf War in 1991, Iraq is said to have stockpiled and weaponized enough botulinum toxin to kill three times the world's population. The toxin is easily produced, and readily stored and transported, as well as delivered, to a target.

Recognition of botulism without a history of a terrorist attack will be dependent on the prerequisite of a high index of suspicion. Otherwise, healthy individuals, who do not have a history suggestive of alternative forms of the disease, such as food poisoning or wound abscess, but present with the neurological symptoms mentioned previously, progressing in a descending fashion to involve upper and then lower extremities symmetrically, must be suspect. Appropriate notification must be initiated while confirmatory evidence is sought from serum bioassay, in the case of inhalation botulism, and stool samples in the case of intestinal botulism. Since ventilatory support will be required to avoid death from respiratory paralysis, hospital preparedness is critical to successful management of any significant number of victims from such an attack. Large numbers of prolonged, ventilator-dependent patients could exhaust the resources of even a large medical community. Thus, the value of an antitoxin, which can ameliorate the paralysis and shorten the recovery time, has increased. Currently there is such treatment available through the Centers for Disease Control in Atlanta, Georgia, but supply is limited and the antitoxin is released for clinical use only and on a case-by-case basis.

What might be expected at the prehospital phase of the bioterrorist attack with aerosolized botulinum toxin? The agent, like anthrax spores, even in large volume and concentration, is colorless, odorless, tasteless, and invisible. Hence, its detection would go unnoticed, at least initially. Symptoms might not appear for an hour and for obvious reasons. Experience with human inhalation botulism is very limited.[12] In its only delivery against civilians, Japanese terrorists failed on three occasions in the early 1990s to injure anyone, presumably for technical reasons. Nonetheless, word of the attacks did terrorize those in attendance. Many who fled the scene sustained injuries, but the final report concluded "non-toxin casualties were light." Had the population been forewarned of a possible attack or, like the Iraqi civilians on the bridge mentioned earlier, been subjected to potential terror attacks for several years before, the ensuing panic could have been infinitely more injurious to those present. Add to that possibility the likelihood that symptoms occurred more rapidly and word spread among the crowd that death was imminent unless the victims could reach a major treatment facility. Pandemonium would ensue and nearby hospitals would be inundated and overwhelmed within a matter of minutes. Such examples point to the need for education of the populace, and those who care for them in the field and at the MTF. The former need to know that they should avoid panic, await instructions, leave the area, and listen to the radio and other media for further information and instructions. Similarly, hospital and field staff must be notified of probable patient surge and agent, and the latest diagnostic treatment and reporting algorithms to follow. Prehospital teams—EMTs, paramedics, and first responders—should assess the scene for symptomatic victims who need to be transported expeditiously to the MTF.

The toxin is readily decontaminated with a variety of solutions, including soap and water or 0.1% hypochlorite bleach. Without attention, the toxin decays at a rate of 1% per minute in a neutral environment.

Francisella tularensis,[13] a small, nonmotile, aerobic, Gram-negative coccobacillus, is responsible for tularemia in humans and is one of the most infectious pathogenic bacteria known to human-kind. Inoculation or inhalation of as few as 10 organisms is sufficient to cause disease. For this reason, its extreme infectivity, the ease of its dissemination, and its capacity to cause severe illness, even death, *F. tularensis* is a likely agent for use in bioterrorism. WHO estimated that 50 kg of live organisms, aerosolized over an urban population center of 5 million, would cause 250,000 casualties including 19,000 deaths.

The bacterium is ubiquitous, its vectors are arthropods, and its reservoirs are small mammals. It can be transmitted to humans by insect bite; direct contact with animal carcasses; ingestion of contaminated water, food, or soil; and inhalation. The latter would be the method of choice for terrorism. Person-to-person transmission does not occur; hence, human infection would not spread the disease as in smallpox.

The result of an aerosolized release of *F. tularensis* would be a large number of patients with an unusual respiratory disease 3 to 5 days after inhalation. A high index of suspicion is again needed to distinguish tularemia from community-acquired infections such as influenza or atypical pneumonia. If a bioterrorist attack is suspected, the differential diagnosis includes other agents of bioterrorism such as plague, anthrax, and, yet to be discussed, Q-fever. Tularemia generally has a slower progression of symptoms and a lower case fatality rate. Plague progresses to hemoptysis, respiratory failure, sepsis, and shock, which are not usually seen in tularemia. Anthrax has a characteristic radiographic appearance (widened mediastinum), which is not seen in tularemia. Culture from sputum establishes the diagnosis, although light microscopy of sputum may reveal the Gram-negative coccobacilli. Treatment consists of parenteral antibiotics, such as streptomycin or gentamycin, under ideal conditions.[14] When mass casualties exceed, numerically, the facilities for parenteral antibiotics, oral doxycycline or ciprofloxacin are substituted. Vaccination is not useful because of the very short incubation period of the organism in humans. Patients need not be isolated since person-to-person transmission does not occur. Standard precautions are all that is necessary for patient care providers. Environmental decontamination is minimally problematic because of the presumed short half-life of the organism exposed to environmental factors such as desiccation and solar radiation. Alcohol, soap and water, and household bleach (dilute) are decontaminants if there is concern about additional potential contamination of equipment or other materials.

Other agents are available and the list of possibilities is extensive. We will conclude, as indicated earlier, with a brief presentation of other agents that are often mentioned, but thought less likely to be deployed than "the big five" discussed previously. Included here are Q-fever, Staphylococcal enterotoxin B, the equine encephalitides, and the hemorrhagic fever viruses.[15] Each has a special characteristic that makes it attractive to bioterrorists, but also at least one that makes it less likely to be used than one of the big five.

Q-fever is the cause of a flu-like illness that results from inhalation of the etiologic agent, *Coxiella burnetii.*[15] The latter has been called a rickettsia by some, and a bacterium by others. It is for this reason that the resultant disease derives its name. "Q" stands for "query," indicating the enigma surrounding its definition. The terrorist appeal relates to the organism's high infectivity. This "asset" is countered by a relatively low lethality and self-limited clinical course. Diagnosis is problematic, a high index of suspicion is necessary, and confirmation requires serological testing. Treatment, if necessary, is antibiotic (doxycycline).

Staphylococcal enterotoxin B is an exotoxin that can be aerosolized, and when inhaled results in sepsis. Its appeal is its ability to produce an incapacitating illness that would persist long enough to spread terror, even panic, among a large number (essentially all) of those exposed. Theoretically, the living can more readily dramatize the threat than can the dead because the former remain vocal. The "disadvantage" of the agent for bioterrorists is its very low lethality and ease of therapy, which is largely supportive. Diagnosis again depends on a high index of suspicion, and identification is based upon serological confirmation. Of concern is the potential mixture of agents for aerosolization that would cause obvious confusion among caregivers and heighten the terror and panic.

The equine encephalitides include three viruses that have special interest to bioterrorists. These RNA viruses are highly infectious, and the Eastern form is especially lethal, but none is of significant risk for human-to-human transmission. The diagnosis is based on the appearance of a viral illness that progresses to encephalitis. Treatment is supportive, and identification is based on culture of the organism from throat swabs or blood samples.

The hemorrhagic fever viruses include a final agent of probable interest to bioterrorists, the Ebola virus. The latter is the one most often mentioned because of its case fatality rate, which approaches 100%. This group of viruses also includes those responsible for dengue fever and yellow fever. The viruses attack endothelial cells, and for this reason the resultant diseases are characterized by bleeding among other symptoms. Human-to-human transmission is especially problematic, and complicates its use by bioterrorists, who have, apparently, not attempted its use. Most likely all of these agents would be delivered by aerosolization.

Since victims of bioterrorism may seek different treatment facilities and because onset of symptoms may not always be synchronous, health care deliverers must have surveillance systems in place so that any "flu-like illness," unusual in number or presentation, is reported to all regional health care facilities. This practice is essential for early detection of an otherwise silent bioterrorist attack.[16,17] What else can be done in preparation for such an event?

As of this writing, President Bush has announced the commitment of $7.1 billion to prepare for an anticipated pandemic of so called "bird flu." A significant percentage of those monies will be earmarked for research concerning vaccine production. Most bioterrorist agents lack vaccines for victims, and mass producing, as well as stockpiling, vaccines for a variety of agents is a daunting and ambitious project. Until the threat actually becomes realistic, there will be insufficient funding and resource commitment. We probably have time to prepare for the bird flu pandemic; we would not have time to prepare for a bioterrorist attack. Bird flu or its threat may provide for a more efficient process of future vaccine production.

REFERENCES

1. BBC, *World News*, 31 August 2005.
2. Clements BW, Evans RG: The doctor's role in bioterrorism. *Lancet* 364: 26–27, 2004.
3. Swan KG, Swan KG Jr: Triage: the past revisited. *Mil Med* 8:448–452, 1996.
4. Fry DE, Schecter WP, Parker JS, et al: The surgeon and acts of civilian terrorism: biologic agents. *J Am Coll Surg* 200:291–302, 2005.
5. Inglesby TV, Henderson DA, Bartlett JG, et al: Anthrax as a biological weapon. *JAMA* 281:1735–1745, 1999.
6. Fowler RA, Saunders GD, Bravata DM, et al: Cost effectiveness of defending against bioterrorism: a comparison of vaccination and antibiotic prophylaxis against anthrax. *Ann Intern Med* 42:601–610, 2005.
7. Henderson DA, Inglesby TV, Bartlett JG, et al: Smallpox as a biological weapon. *JAMA* 281:2127–2137, 1999.
8. Beeching NJ, Dance DAB, Miller ARO, Spencer RC: Biological warfare and bioterrorism. *BMJ* 324:336–339, 2002.
9. Inglesby TV, Dennis DT, Henderson DA: Plague as a biological weapon. *JAMA* 283:2281–2290, 2000.
10. Franz DR, Zajtchuk R: Biological terrorism: understanding the threat, preparation and medical response. *Dis Mon* 48:489–564, 2002.
11. Arnon SS, Schechter R, Inglesby TV, et al: Botulinum toxin as a biological weapon. *JAMA* 285:1059–1070, 2001.
12. Karwa M, Currie B, Kvetan V: Bioterrorism: preparing for the impossible or the improbable. *Crit Care Med* 33:575–595, 2005.
13. Dennis DT, Inglesby TV, Henderson DA, et al: Tularemia as a biological weapon. *JAMA* 285:2763–2773, 2001.
14. Eachempati SR, Flomenbaum N, Barie PS: Biological warfare: current concerns for the health care provider. *J Trauma* 52:179–186, 2002.
15. Gosden C, Gardener D: Weapons of mass destruction—threats and responses. *BMJ*, 331:397–400, 2005.
16. Moran GJ, Talon DA: Update on emerging infections: news from the Centers for Disease Control and Prevention. *Ann Emerg Med* 41:414–418, 2003.
17. Bravata DM, McDonald KM, Smith WM, et al: Systemic review: surveillance systems for early detection of bioterrorism-related diseases. *Ann Intern Med* 140:910–922, 2004.

WOUND BALLISTICS: WHAT EVERY TRAUMA SURGEON SHOULD KNOW

John C. Mayberry   and   **Donald D. Trunkey**

Although most trauma centers in the past two decades have experienced a reduction in the volume of firearm-related injuries, trauma and general surgeons still have an obligation to be familiar with the basic principles of ballistics and the management of the varieties of wounds that projectiles produce. Wounds caused by firearms will not only be encountered in urban "high-crime" areas, but will also be seen in rural areas where hunting accidents occur. Wounds encountered in a military environment have unique characteristics that are clinically important and distinct from those seen in the civilian sector. The study of wound ballistics is an essential part of the general and trauma surgeon's training.

FIREARM AND PROJECTILE DESIGN

Although there are many variables, the muzzle velocity (speed of the bullet as it leaves the barrel) and the bullet characteristics such as mass and deformability are the most important determinants of the wound that a particular weapon will produce (Table 1). The muzzle velocity is determined by the caliber of the bullet, the capacity of the casing (amount of powder), and gun barrel length. The bullet's velocity rapidly increases as it travels down the barrel, but gradually slows upon meeting air resistance once it has exited. Handguns generally accept smaller bullets with less powder and have shorter barrels than rifles, and therefore produce projectiles of considerably less velocity (Table 2).

The mass of the bullet is determined by its caliber (diameter), length, and the density of its metal components. Because of its heavier mass, and therefore its increased energy per given velocity, lead is the principal element of most bullets. Lead, however, is a relatively soft metal that deforms readily during high-velocity flight. "Jacketed" bullets have a lead body covered with metal alloys that prevent deformation during flight, and therefore help the bullet retain speed and accuracy over a long distance. Conventionally jacketed bullets will deform when they strike dense tissue, but bullets with thicker jackets are intended to retain their shape and therefore penetrate deeply into large game animals such as elephants (Figure 1). Bullets that deform upon striking the body will cause considerably more collateral tissue damage by direct contact,

Table 1: Factors Involved in Wound Ballistics

Bullet Design

Caliber (diameter)
Mass
Shape (profile)
Jacket
Pellets
Powder (amount and type)

Weapon Design

Barrel length
Rifling
Single shot
Automatic
Semi-automatic
Portability (weight and size)

Victim

Position
Distance from weapon
Location of wound
Tissue characteristics (bone, muscle, vessel, organ)

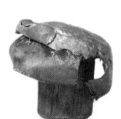
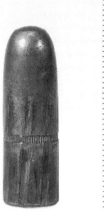

Figure 1 Full-metal-jacket .308 caliber rifle bullet that has opened upon impact with a game animal (left) compared with same caliber bullet with a thicker jacket that has passed undeformed through the animal (right). Notice the grooves on the base of each bullet caused by the internal rifling of the barrel. *(Bullets courtesy of Gerald Warnock, MD, Portland, OR.)*

cavitation, and shock waves than nondeformable bullets. Fragmentation of bullets will also occur when the bullet strikes bone and will add to the damage by shredding surrounding tissue (Figure 2).

According to The Hague Declarations of 1899, military rifle bullets "which expand or flatten easily in the human body, such as bullets with a hard envelope which does not entirely cover the core" are banned. This prohibition was designed to reduce the severity of wounds, and therefore the suffering of soldiers on the battlefield, but does not apply to combatants of noncontracting organizations and does not apply to bullets commonly used for hunting. In fact, "full-metal-jacket" (FMJ) bullets are prohibited for game hunting in many jurisdictions. For this reason, hunting rifle wounds may be more severe than those resulting from an equivalent military rifle. The exception to this principle is the assault rifle, which although its bullet is jacketed, causes severe wounds from the bullet's tendency to tumble in tissue.

Table 2: Muzzle Velocity by Gun and Bullet Type

Handguns	M/sec
.38 special	290
.44	305
9 mm	315
.44 magnum	420
Rifles	
.22 long	380
30.06	890
.308 (7.62 mm)	860
Military	
.223 (M-16)	950
.30 (AK-47)	720
.50 (Browning)	850

HANDGUNS

Handguns are commonly used in urban areas because they are lightweight and can be concealed. Fortunately, handguns cannot produce as highly accelerated and accurate a projectile as rifles. The amount of gunpowder packed into a handgun bullet casing must be limited to avoid barrel damage and permit the shooter to fire the weapon supported only by their arms and hands. Experienced marksmen can master the handgun under controlled circumstances, but both police and criminals probably strike their target less than half the time in the field. Accuracy is dramatically decreased with distance. The majority of handgun wounds, therefore, are generated from 10 yards or less.

The immediate danger of a handgun wound stems from direct injury to vital organs such as are found in the head, neck, or chest. The probability of proximity injury to vasculature is less with handgun wounds than it is with rifle or automatic weapon injuries, but should still be considered. Because the velocity of a handgun bullet is less as the bullet strikes the tissue, the bullet is less likely to deform or fragment and tissue cavitation may be slight. Jacketed handgun bullets cause even less collateral damage than the nonjacketed, and in some cases may penetrate the tissue and subsequently exit the body with much of their destructive potential intact.

Nonetheless, several measures designed to increase the wounding potential or "stopping-power" of handguns are available and will be encountered. These include "hollow-point" bullets designed to expand (Figure 3, right) and Glaser Safety Slugs® designed to disintegrate into tiny pellets after impact (Figure 4). The Glaser Safety Slug® is marketed to law enforcement and security personnel who need to immobilize a human target in a crowded environment such as an airport or an airplane without concern of overpenetration or ricochet into innocent bystanders. "Magnum" handguns have extra powder and longer barrels that will produce a devastating wound at close range. Fortunately, magnum editions are not as commonly seen as regular handguns because they are expensive, heavy, and difficult to master.

Indications for operation of handgun wounds of the neck, chest, and abdomen would include mandatory exploration for Zone II neck injuries, selective exploration of the chest based on hemorrhage, and mandatory exploration of all abdominal penetrations except tangential injuries that do not penetrate the fascia and selective liver injuries. Patients with bullet entrance sites below the nipple on the chest require abdominal exploration if the

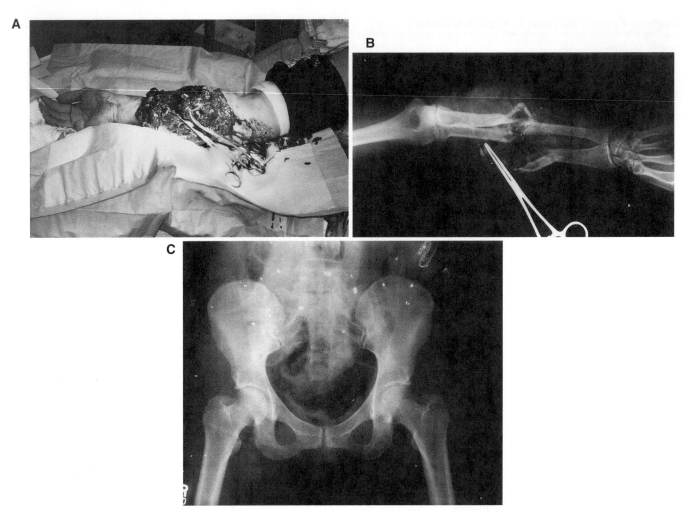

Figure 2   **(A)** Close range .30-06 hunting rifle wound to the right forearm. **(B)** Radiograph of same injury showing extensive bony comminution and bullet fragmentation. **(C)** Radiograph of same patient's pelvis demonstrating extensive fragmentation of the bullet. This patient required lower abdominal wall reconstruction.

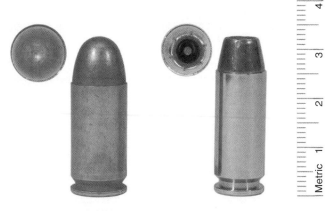

Figure 3   .45 caliber full-metal-jacket handgun bullet (left) and 10-mm "hollow-point," partially jacketed bullet (right)   *(Bullets courtesy of Bruce Ham, MD, and Gerald Warnock, MD, Portland, OR.)*

abdomen is tender, a diagnostic peritoneal lavage is suspicious, or the diaphragm is not well visualized on radiograph. Stable patients with right upper quadrant wounds may be selectively evaluated by CT scan and managed nonoperatively if the bullet clearly injures only the liver. Laparoscopy may be used to evaluate the diaphragm

in stable, nontender patients with chest wounds or as an adjunct to nonoperative management of liver penetrations that result in bile leaks.

HUNTING RIFLES

Civilian rifle wounds, such as those resulting from hunting accidents, are among the most destructive injuries seen by surgeons. The increased amount of gunpowder contained in the bullet case and the enhanced length of the barrel that exposes the bullet to the force of the powder blast for a longer distance leads to dramatically more projectile acceleration than is possible with a handgun (Figure 5). Rifling, the barrel's internal spiraling grooves, causes the bullet to spin and consequently improves distance and accuracy. The average muzzle velocity of a 30-06 hunting rifle is 890 m/sec and may maintain up to 90% of its kinetic energy at 100 m. A rifle wound to an extremity, whether close range or distant, will destroy soft tissue, bone, and vessels, and cause dramatic hemorrhage that may need to be controlled with direct pressure or a tourniquet at the scene (see Figure 2).

Because of the potential for extensive damage to an extremity struck by a rifle bullet, plain radiographs looking for fractures, operative wound exploration with debridement, and intraoperative angiograms are highly recommended. Even if the overlying skin is uninjured, the soft tissue hidden beneath may be irreversibly damaged. All devascularized tissue and pieces of clothing should be removed. Serial

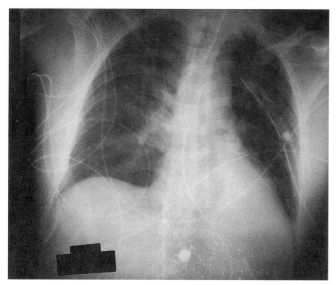

Figure 4 Radiograph of chest and upper abdomen of patient shot with a Glaser Safety Slug®. Note the midline larger projectile with multiple accompanying pellets in the right upper quadrant. This patient sustained colon, gastric, renal, splenic, diaphragmatic, and pancreatic injuries as well as paraplegia from the main projectile striking the spinal cord. Since the main projectile passed through the colon, it was electively removed posteriorly.

debridements at daily intervals may be necessary to identify all devascularized tissue. Abdominal gunshot wounds from hunting rifles are best managed by open abdomen techniques with second-look operations if several organs are simultaneously injured.

ASSAULT RIFLES

The M-16 (United States), AK-47 and AK-74 (Russia), Uzi and Galil (Israel), Fal (Belgium), and their variations are relatively lightweight, short-barreled military rifles that fire rapidly sequential, high-velocity bullets that tumble and yaw shortly after striking tissue. Military actions that rely on these weapons seek to rapidly disable as many combatants as possible. Although these rifles and their ammunition are no longer sold on the civilian market in most Western countries, rifles that the owner possessed prior to 1994 can be legally fired in the United States, such as in target practice. These are the most common assault rifles that will be encountered in military actions; it is estimated that tens of millions of AKs and Uzis have been manufactured and distributed around the world. The caliber of bullet used in assault rifles ranges from the smaller 5.45-mm (0.21-inch) AK-74, to the 0.223-inch M-16, to the 7.62-mm (0.3-inch) AK-47, to the 9-mm (0.35-inch) Uzi.

In general, these bullets will produce severe wounds that will require soft tissue debridement; however, surgeons who have operated on injuries caused by assault rifles have occasionally noted their surprise that more injury is not apparent. This is because both the M-16 and the AK-74 deliver an FMJ bullet not much larger than a .22-caliber small-game rifle. If a single bullet passes cleanly through an extremity, the surrounding tissue damage will not be as dramatic as what a deformable, larger-caliber hunting rifle bullet would cause.

The salient point for surgeons to remember about automatic or semi-automatic assault rifles is the difficulty there can be in determining the bullet's trajectory after it strikes the victim. Abdominal wounds may contain several areas of bowel injury as well as solid organ disruptions. Thoracic penetrations need ultrasonic visualization of the pericardial space and esophageal contrast radiography if nonoperative therapy is chosen. Extremity wounds may require operative exploration and debridement and an angiogram is indicated if the ankle-brachial index (ABI) is 0.9 or less.

SHOTGUNS

Shotguns and their shells come in four main sizes: .410 juvenile, 20-gauge, 12-gauge, and the 10-gauge (Figure 6). Pellets are of variable sizes and are made of lead or steel. Heavier lead pellets scatter less than steel pellets, but are illegal for shooting waterfowl. Slugs are also available for shotguns and are commonly used for game hunting in some states, such as New Jersey (Figure 7). The shotgun is ineffective against humans at distances greater than 10 or 15 yards (30–45 feet), but close range (<4 feet) blasts are 85% fatal. These wounds are extremely morbid and often require several operations and multidisciplinary management. Pellets spread in every direction and strike multiple types of tissue, but fortunately because of their small mass the damage potential of the shot dissipates quickly. Pellets may enter arteries and veins and embolize peripherally or centrally. A search for the plastic insert dispelled from the shell and pieces of the patient's clothing hidden in the wound is advised in close-range cases. There is no indication to remove all the pellets—lead poisoning does not occur from pellets or bullets left permanently in human tissue.

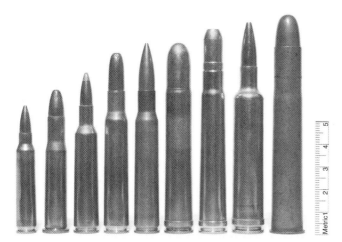

Figure 5 Various rifle bullets compared. Left to right: .223 caliber FMJ (M-16 assault rifle), 30-30 soft point, 6-mm soft point, 30-06 soft point, .308 caliber military-style FMJ (7.62 mm NATO), .458 caliber FMJ magnum, .375 caliber FMJ magnum, .378 caliber FMJ hollow tip, World War II–era .47 caliber FMJ. FMJ, full metal jacket. *(Bullets courtesy of Bruce Ham, MD, and Gerald Warnock, MD, Portland, OR.)*

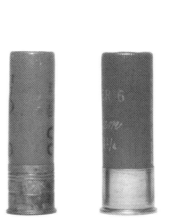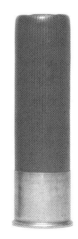

Figure 6 20-gauge, 12-gauge, and 10-gauge shotgun shells compared (left to right). *(Bullets courtesy of Gerald Warnock, MD, Portland, OR.)*

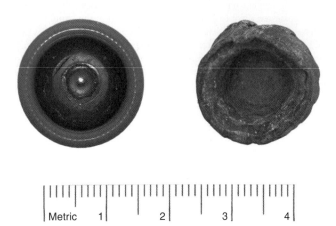

Figure 7 Shotgun shell loaded with lead slug instead of pellets (left). Same type of slug removed from game animal. Note deformity of central zone from flight and contact. *(Bullets courtesy of Gerald Warnock, MD, Portland, OR.)*

Thoracic wounds created by close-range shotgun blasts may be challenging to cover if part of the chest wall is lost—diaphragm transposition or emergent muscular flaps have been described. Abdominal wounds are best managed with serial operations and debridement through an open abdomen mesh prosthesis. Extremity shotgun blasts usually require wound exploration and debridement with intraoperative angiograms.

PROTECTIVE VESTS

There are many varieties of "bullet-proof" vests manufactured with successive layers of synthetic materials such as Kevlar® (Dupont), which is a lightweight aramid fiber with extreme tensile strength. These vests are categorized according to their level of protection: Level I will protect the wearer from a .38 handgun at 259 m/sec, Level II from a 9-mm FMJ at 332 m/sec, and Level III from a 9-mm FMJ (assault rifle) at 427 m/sec. Protection from rifle bullets at higher velocities requires the addition of a ceramic plate to the vest. No vest is 100% effective, however. Even if the bullet does not penetrate, chest wall and pulmonary contusions can occur from the blunt force that is dissipated into the vest and onto the chest wall. Many varieties of "armor-piercing" bullets are manufactured for both handguns and rifles, and may be encountered in both military and nonmilitary situations, even though they are illegal for civilian use. These projectiles are jacketed and have a lead inner shell and a hardened steel or tungsten interior core. As the conventional portion of the projectile strikes the vest, it deforms and "softens up" the barrier. The hardened cores of these bullets pass through their softer shells to penetrate body and vehicular armor and even, in some cases, concrete walls.

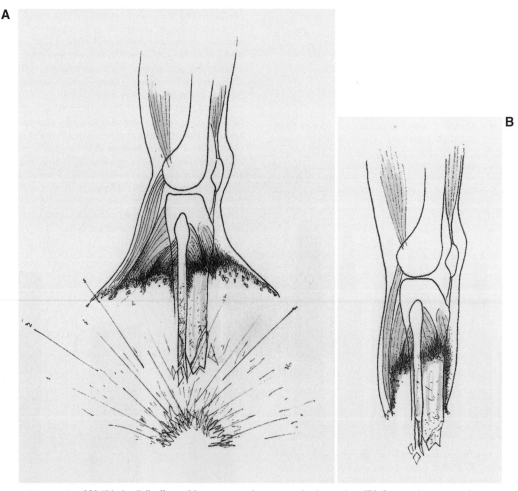

Figure 8 **(A)** "Umbrella" effect of foot-triggered mine on the lower leg. **(B)** Severe damage to the compartments of the lower leg may be concealed by overlying skin. *(From Coupland RM: War Wounds of Limbs: Surgical Management. Oxford, Butterworth-Heinemann, Ltd., 1993, with permission of the author and the International Committee of the Red Cross.)*

LANDMINES AND IMPROVISED EXPLOSIVE DEVICES

The detonation of a concealed explosive device such as a conventional landmine or an improvised explosive device (IED) usually results in the immediate amputation or at least partial amputation of the triggering extremity. Exsanguination from major vessel injury is possible, and therefore a field tourniquet may be necessary. Fragments of metal and debris will also shower the contralateral extremity, perineum, torso, and face. The current military standard for operative management is damage control—repeated debridements of devascularized tissue and the use of external fixators for bone stability are recommended. Conventional landmines triggered by the foot will cause an umbrella effect that spares the skin and subcutaneous tissue of the lower leg while destroying underlying muscle and bone (Figure 8A). The overlying skin will hide significant destruction and contamination beneath (Figure 8B). Aggressive debridement to prevent infection tracking along the popliteal vessels and neural sheaths is advised. Robin Coupland of the International Red Cross makes an argument, however, to conserve the partially protected gastrocnemius muscle for reconstruction.

RED CROSS WOUND CLASSIFICATION

Classification of wounds has merit since in practical terms it may be difficult to determine the exact type of weapon used. The International Committee of the Red Cross has adopted Coupland's wound description method. There are six main criteria that are used to divide wounds into three grades and four types. At first glance the system seems formidable, but surgeons of the Red Cross, who classify about 4000 wounds per year, have accepted the system and are developing guidelines based on it. Wounds are scored on initial assessment or after surgery by entry size (centimeters), exit size (centimeters), cavity size (fingers), fractures, vital structures (brain, viscera, major vessels), and metallic body (intact bullet vs. fragments). The categories are E, X, C, F, V, and M, respectively (Figure 9). The advantages of uniform classification of wounds for research purposes are multiple.

BULLET REMOVAL

Bullet removal is generally unnecessary and ideally would not be used as the only indication for a surgical procedure. An occasional patient is symptomatic enough from an irritating focus to tempt the surgeon to remove the projectile. Many a surgeon, however, has searched subcutaneous tissue in vain looking for a foreign body that seems to be just beneath the skin. Radiographic localization may be necessary.

The only risk of lead poisoning seems to be from bullets in contact with synovial fluid and by extrapolation, spinal cord fluid. Bullets that pass through colon and subsequently lodge in bone are at risk to cause osteomyelitis. Controversy exists as to the magnitude of the risk, but at our center we favor removal if possible. The alternative is irrigation of the tract and a minimum of 10 days of broad-spectrum intravenous antibiotics. Other true indications for bullet removal include removing bullet emboli in arteries and veins and bullets lodged in cardiac chambers.

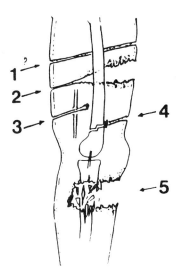

EXAMPLES OF WOUND SCORES

	E	X	C	F	V	M
WOUND 1	1	1	0	0	0	0
WOUND 2	1	4	1	0	0	0
WOUND 3	1	0	0	0	1	1
WOUND 4	1	0	0	1	0	1
WOUND 5	6	0	1	2	0	1

Figure 9 Examples of wound scores obtained under International Red Cross Wound Classification. *(From Coupland RM: War Wounds of Limbs: Surgical Management. Oxford, Butterworth-Heinemann, Ltd., 1993, with permission of the author and the International Committee of the Red Cross.)*

SUGGESTED READINGS

Barach E, Tomlanovich M, Nowak R: Ballistics: a pathophysiologic examination of the wounding mechanisms of firearms (part I). *J Trauma* 26:225–235, 1986.

Bender JS, Lucas CE: Management of close-range shotgun injuries to the chest by diaphragmatic transposition: case reports. *J Trauma* 30:1581–1584, 1990.

Coupland RM: *War Wounds of Limbs: Surgical Management.* Oxford, Butterworth-Heinemann, Ltd., 1993.

Coupland RM, Loye D: The 1899 Hague Declaration concerning expanding bullets: a treaty effective for more than 100 years faces complex contemporary issues. *Int Rev Red Cross* 849:135–142, 2003.

Fackler ML: Wound ballistics: a review of common misconceptions. *JAMA* 259:2730–2736, 1988.

Fackler ML, Surinchak JS, Malinowski JA, Bowen RE: Bullet fragmentation: a major cause of tissue disruption. *J Trauma* 24:35–39, 1984.

Long D: *AK47: The Complete Kalashnikov Family of Assault Rifles.* Boulder, CO, Paladin Press, 1988.

Marshall TJ: Combat casualty care: the Alpha Surgical Company experience during Operation Iraqi Freedom. *Mil Med* 170:469–472, 2005.

COMMON PREHOSPITAL COMPLICATIONS AND PITFALLS IN THE TRAUMA PATIENT

Frank L. Mitchell, Charles M. Richart, and Harry E. Wilkins

The evolution of prehospital care in this country has an interesting and continually evolving record. Although there is recorded history of wagons and carts being used to transport the sick and injured as early as 900 ACE, the term "ambulance" was not used until introduced by Queen Isabella of Spain in the early 15th century. Even at that time, it referred more to military field hospitals and tents for the wounded than to a means of transporting wounded and dead from battlefields. Not until the time of Baron Larrey would the term "ambulance" take up its more current meaning of "a specially equipped motor vehicle, airplane, or ship for carrying sick or injured people, usually to a hospital."[1]

Baron Dominique-Jean Larrey was Napoleon Bonaparte's surgeon and developed what was known as "flying ambulances." Prior to 1792, there was very little organized transportation of the wounded from the battlefield. As is the case with most medical advances, advances in ambulance transportation occurred as a result of military conflict. Throughout the remainder of the 1800s and the conflicts of the early 20th century, ambulances and other means of transporting individuals from the field of battle were employed.

During the 1950s through the 1970s, helicopters were employed to transport the injured from battlefields to MASH (mobile army surgical hospital) units attaining particular effectiveness in the Korean and Vietnam conflicts. Throughout the first several decades of the 20th century, civilian transport for the injured continued to lag behind advances established in the military.

One of the prime factors identified as contributing to the continued reduction in battlefield casualties from 8% in World War I to less than 2% in the Vietnam War was reducing the time from injury to initiation of medical care. On this backdrop, the mid-1960s and early 1970s sought to improve prehospital care, education, equipment, and processes. The early 1960s called for an extension of basic and advanced first aid training to greater numbers of the lay population, and preparation of nationally accepted texts, training aids, and courses of instruction for rescue squad personnel, policemen, firefighters, and ambulance attendants.[2] Ambulance services in the 1960s was very piecemeal and adequate at best. In a few major cities, there were specially equipped ambulances prepared to care for the injured and sick, and trained professional prehospital personnel were available. However, approximately 50% of the country's ambulance services at that time were provided by over 12,000 morticians mainly because their vehicles were able to accommodate transportation of patients on gurneys or stretchers.

In the mid-1960s, the National Traffic and Motor Safety Act and the Highway Safety Act[3] provided for the establishment of national standards for used motor vehicles, motor vehicle inspections, and emergency services. Communications were also problematic. At a time when the United States had just placed a man on the moon, it was easier in most instances to communicate with that extraterrestrial individual than it was for prehospital providers to communicate with the emergency department where they were headed.

Over the next several decades, the education and provision of specifically equipped vehicles progressed until the mid-1980s when *Injury in America: a Continuing Public Health Problem* was published.[4] Although the report found that there had been significant progress in the credentialing and education of prehospital care providers, more than 2.5 million Americans died from injuries in the 1966–1985 period. This prompted the expenditure of more federal dollars to study the continuing public health problem, as the report noted and called for the institution of more systems of communication and transportation of the injured to facilities specially equipped for managing critically injured patients.

In 1992, the Model of Trauma Care Systems Plan, developed by Health Resources and Services Administration under the Authority of the Trauma Systems Planning and Development Act of 1990,[5] marked the next major step in the evolution of health policy related to trauma care. This plan emphasized the need for a fully inclusive trauma care system that involved not only trauma centers, but also all health care facilities according to availability of trauma resources, including prehospital providers. As a result, the numbers of dedicated trauma centers and state trauma systems developed, although at a still-less-than-adequate pace. Trauma centers were charged with becoming resource facilities for emergency medical response agencies. Educational programs such as Prehospital Trauma Life Support (PHTLS), Basic Trauma Life Support (BTLS), and others were developed with states being empowered to license and credential prehospital providers at various levels.

Today, the initial care of the injured patient continues to reside primarily with trained prehospital providers. Emergency medical technician, basic, intermediate, and paramedic levels of instruction, with police and fire departments also being trained in basic life support, as well as increased communication and education with the lay public with regard to cardiac arrest, seat belt usage, wearing of helmets, and other prevention initiatives are in place to continue to try to combat the unacceptably high level of death and disability in this country from intentional and unintentional injury.

Along with the ever evolving technologies available to the prehospital provider come the unintended risk of complications associated with the implementation of these devices and processes. This chapter addresses some of the more common prehospital complications.

INCIDENCE

According to the National Highway Traffic Safety Administration, the leading cause of death in the United States in 2002 for people aged 4–34 is overwhelmingly motor vehicle traffic crashes (Table 1). In terms of years of life lost, motor vehicle crashes ranks third, after malignant neoplasms and heart disease, at 5% of total years of life lost for the entire population.

A total of 37% of trauma deaths are caused by motor vehicle crashes and motorcycle crashes. Other important causes of trauma deaths are gunshot wounds, stabbings, and falls. Today's prehospital provider is in a position to be the first responder to the vast majority of these injuries at or shortly after the time they occur.

The major causes of death in the prehospital period are secondary to severe head injury, respiratory compromise, and exsanguinating hemorrhage. Initial and emergent prehospital treatment focuses on the treatment and prevention of these eventualities.

The foundation of Advanced Trauma Life Support® of the American College of Surgeons[6] stresses an ABC (airway, breathing, and circulation) approach. Much of the emphasis on prehospital care and subsequent care involves appropriate management of the airway, providing for ventilation by breathing for the patient, and control of circulation consisting of hemorrhage control and restoration of intravascular volume. Not surprisingly, the most common prehospital complications occur in these three areas.

AIRWAY

Ensuring that the trauma victim has a patent airway is the highest management priority.[7] If manual maneuvers (clearing the airway of foreign bodies, jaw thrust, or chin lift) or basic adjuncts (oropharyngeal or nasopharyngeal airways) are not adequate to maintain the airway, then alternate, more invasive methods are required.

Current prehospital techniques used for airway management and ventilation include (1) bag-valve-mask (BVM), (2) laryngeal mask airways (LMA), (3) dual lumen tubes (i.e., Combitubes), (4) endotracheal intubation (with or without the use of paralytics), and (5) emergency cricothyroidotomy.

BVM can be a temporizing method for providing adequate oxygenation and ventilation of the injured patient, but can occasionally be problematic related to obtaining an adequate seal at the mouth, potential for aspiration, problems with bleeding from soft tissue injury, patient cooperation, and the lack of satisfactory ventilation and oxygenation depending on the specific clinical situation. Acute gastric dilatation from overzealous ventilation can also lead to ventilatory impairment from increased intra-abdominal pressure, and, in extreme cases, gastric rupture.

The prehospital use of LMAs and dual lumen tubes has an advantage over conventional endotracheal intubation related to ease of technique and maintenance of insertion skill. LMAs and dual lumen tubes are beneficial in an unconscious patient who cannot be adequately ventilated with a BVM device and/or cannot be successfully intubated. However, because the trachea is not completely protected, the use of an LMA may result in aspiration. The use of dual lumen tubes may also result in aspiration if the gag reflex is intact, and there is also potential for damage to the esophagus, and the possibility for hypoxia if the wrong lumen is used.

The identification of patients requiring definitive airway management may sometimes be problematic based on the patient's injuries, mental status (secondary to injury, alcohol, and/or drugs), underlying medical conditions, and the experience of the prehospital provider. Delay of intubation until respiratory arrest increases morbidity and mortality and should be avoided if at all possible. Early recognition of the need for intubation is of paramount importance for the prehospital provider.

Late endotracheal intubation may result because of a false sense of security by the provider, the inability to obtain an airway, and lack of recognition of likely deterioration in a patient's ventilatory status (secondary to airway and chest injuries, traumatic brain injury [TBI], alteration in mental status, or the overall complexity of the injuries). Patients with facial burns and maxillofacial trauma may have progression of their underlying injury, and may deteriorate secondary to edema or hematoma formation, causing airway obstruction. Intubation of these patients can be a difficult challenge with the potential for disastrous results if proactive intubation is not accomplished. This is especially true if paralytic agents have been used and the vocal cords can not be easily visualized. Anticipation of this problem along with early intubation may prevent a catastrophe.

The use of paralytic agents for intubation in the prehospital setting results in a quicker and higher success rate of intubation. However many prehospital providers do not have access to use these agents. Additionally, if paralytic agents are used, it is critical that adequate analgesia and sedation are also administered, so that the injured patient is not chemically paralyzed, while awake and hurting. At the time of hand-off of the trauma patient from the prehospital provider to the trauma team in the emergency department, it is important that all of the medications that have been administered to the patient prior to arrival are reviewed, so that the emergency physician and trauma surgeon will ensure adequate pain management and sedation, even when the patient is chemically paralyzed.

Successful endotracheal intubation is beneficial for the trauma patient whose airway needs to be secured, but there are potential complications and pitfalls that may occur during the process of intubation, regardless of the expertise of the provider. Prehospital personnel should be aware of these potential complications and how to clinically recognize them if they occur.

Esophageal intubation is a known complication of intubation, and should be quickly recognized by the prehospital provider if it occurs. The difficulty of the intubation and in visualizing the vocal cords should increase concerns of an esophageal intubation, and warrants aggressive evaluation to ensure adequate placement of the endotracheal tube. The placement of an esophageal endotracheal tube should be clinically evident by routine chest auscultation immediately after intubation. The routine use of end-tidal CO_2 detectors ($ETCO_2$) is beneficial in rapidly detecting the presence of CO_2 in the exhaled air. The calorimetric devices have a chemically treated indicator strip that reflects the CO_2 level. If there is a question of the exact location, visualization of the ETT location should be repeated and appropriate location confirmed.

Right main-stem intubation is an occasional complication of intubation that occurs up to 30% of the time in pediatric trauma patients, and should be detected by physical exam at the time of intubation, and with frequent routine clinical reassessments, or urgent reassessment if the patient clinically deteriorates. The distance of the tip of the ETT should be evaluated, relative to the size of the patient and the expected appropriate distance of ETT. Repositioning of the ETT while auscultating the chest helps in determining the appropriate location of the ETT. Other possible traumatic injuries that may lead to similar clinical findings must also be considered in severely injured patients, including a pneumothorax, hemothorax, pulmonary contusion, or ruptured hemidiaphragm.

Surgical airways are occasionally needed when endotracheal intubation cannot be successfully achieved secondary to facial trauma, anatomic difficulties, and soft tissue injuries. While the use of surgical airways in the prehospital setting is controversial, local protocols should outline the specific indications and circumstances for their use.

Complications of needle cricothyroidotomy include inadequate ventilation resulting in hypoxia and death, esophageal laceration, hematoma formation, posterior tracheal wall perforation, thyroid laceration, and bleeding.

Complications of surgical cricothyroidotomy include false passage into the tissues, hemorrhage or hematoma formation, esophageal laceration, vocal cord paralysis, and potential subglottic stenosis/edema. If a surgical airway is needed, a surgical cricothyroidotomy should be performed. A formal tracheostomy should not be performed by prehospital providers because of the difficulty and length of time to successfully accomplish the procedure.

BREATHING

A tension pneumothorax is a life-threatening situation as a result of an injury to the lung causing a pneumothorax that results in air leaking into the pleural space, causing increased pressure that results in difficult ventilation and decreased venous return. Typically it is recognized by a variety of signs and symptoms, including tachypnea, dyspnea, decreased breath sounds or unilateral absence of breath sounds, air hunger, respiratory distress, tachycardia, hypotension, tracheal deviation, neck vein distention, and cyanosis (late). Hyperresonant percussion tone and absent breath sounds are typical of a significant pneumothorax. While there are many signs and symptoms that are

Table 1: Deaths, Top 10 Causes by Age Group, United States, 2002[a]

Rank	Infants under 1	Toddlers 1–3	Young Children 4–7	Children 8–15	Youth 16–20	Young Adults 21–24
1	Perinatal period 14,106	Congenital anomalies 474	MV traffic crashes 495	MV traffic crashes 1,584	MV traffic crashes 6,327	MV traffic crashes 4,446
2	Congenital anomalies 5,623	MV traffic crashes 410	Malignant neoplasms 449	Malignant neoplasms 842	Homicide 2,422	Homicide 2,650
3	Heart disease 500	Accidental drowning 380	Congenital anomalies 180	Suicide 428	Suicide 1,810	Suicide 2,036
4	Homicide 303	Homicide 366	Accidental drowning 171	Homicide 426	Malignant neoplasms 805	Accidental poisoning 974
5	Septicemia 296	Malignant neoplasms 285	Exposure to smoke/fire 151	Congenital anomalies 345	Accidental poisoning 679	Malignant neoplasms 823
6	Influenza/pneumonia 263	Exposure to smoke/fire 163	Homicide 134	Accidental drowning 270	Heart disease 449	Heart disease 518
7	Nephritis/nephrosis 173	Heart disease 144	Heart disease 73	Heart disease 258	Accidental drowning 345	Accidental drowning 238
8	MV traffic crashes 120	Influenza/pneumonia 92	Influenza/pneumonia 41	Exposure to smoke/fire 170	Congenital anomalies 254	Congenital anomalies 186
9	Stroke 117	MV non-traffic crashes[c] 69	Septicemia 38	Chr. lower respiratory disease 131	MV nontraffic crashes[c] 121	Accidental falls 134
10	Malignant neoplasms 74	Septicemia 63	Benign neoplasms 36	MV nontraffic crashes[c] 115	Accidental discharge of firearms 113	HIV 130
ALL[d]	28,034	4,079	2,586	6,760	16,239	15,390

[a]When ranked by specific ages, MV crashes are the leading cause of death for ages 3 through 33.

[b]Number of years calculated based on remaining life expectancy at time of death; percents calculated as a proportion of total years of life lost due to all causes of death.

[c]A motor-vehicle nontraffic crash is any vehicle crash that occurs (entirely) in any place other than a public highway.

[d]Not a total of top 10 causes of death.

MV, Motor vehicle.

associated with a tension pneumothorax, some may be difficult to recognize in the prehospital setting, and some may not be present in all situations. In a patient who has required intubation and positive pressure ventilation, a minimal lung injury may develop into a clinically significant tension pneumothorax, and should be anticipated if a patient in this type of setting suddenly deteriorates.

The management of a tension pneumothorax in the prehospital setting includes the recognition of the presence of a clinically significant pneumothorax, and then prompt needle decompression with a large-bore needle, classically inserted into the pleural space in the second intercostal space, midclavicular line. This location minimizes the risk of injuring underlying internal structures; however, the development of a hematoma or lung laceration is possible. There is also the possibility of the needle not being placed deep enough to reach the pleural cavity, thus not relieving the tension pneumothorax. Placement of the needle in the lateral aspect of the affected chest cavity has also been shown to be of benefit in resolving tension pneumo-

thoraces. Once a pleural cavity has been decompressed with a needle, a definitive chest tube should be placed. The lack of recognition of a tension pneumothorax, and a delay in its management may result in a life threatening situation. In a patient who is intubated, the location of the endotracheal tube should be determined to make sure that it is not in a main-stem bronchus as the cause of absent breath sounds, prior to needle decompression of the chest cavity.

CIRCULATION

One of the most common prehospital complications related to circulation is the failure to detect and address ongoing hemorrhage. Control of external hemorrhage is best controlled by applying direct pressure to the bleeding site. Common areas that are missed that are sources of external hemorrhage include the posterior scalp, axillae, perineum, and posterior trunk. Bulky dressings,

	Other Adults		Elderly ≥65	All Ages	Years of Life Lost[b]
25–34	**35–44**	**45–64**			
MV traffic crashes 6,933	Malignant neoplasms 16,085	Malignant neoplasms 143,028	Heart disease 576,301	Heart disease 696,947	Malignant neoplasms 23% (8,686,782)
Suicide 5,046	Heart disease 13,688	Heart disease 101,804	Malignant neoplasms 391,001	Malignant neoplasms 557,271	Heart disease 22% (8,140,300)
Homicide 4,489	MV traffic crashes 6,883	Stroke 15,952	Stroke 143,293	Stroke 162,672	MV traffic crashes 5% (1,766,854)
Malignant neoplasms 3,872	Suicide 6,851	Diabetes 15,518	Chronic lower respiratory disease 108,313	Chronic lower respiratory disease 124,816	Stroke 5% (1,682,465)
Heart disease 3,165	Accidental poisoning 6,007	Chronic. lower respiratory disease 14,755	Influenza/ pneumonia 58,826	Diabetes 73,249	Chronic lower respiratory disease 4% (1,466,004)
Accidental poisoning 3,116	HIV 5,707	Chronic liver disease 13,313	Alzheimer's 58,289	Influenza/pneumonia 65,681	Suicide 3% (1,109,748)
HIV 1,839	Homicide 3,239	Suicide 9,926	Diabetes 54,715	Alzheimer's 58,866	Perinatal period 3% (1,099,767)
Diabetes 642	Chronic liver disease 3,154	MV traffic crashes 9,412	Nephritis/ nephrosis 34,316	MV traffic crashes 44,065	Diabetes 3% (1,050,798)
Stroke 567	Stroke 2,425	HIV 5,821	Septicemia 26,670	Nephritis/nephrosis 40,974	Homicide 2% (822,762)
Congenital anomalies 475	Diabetes 2,164	Accidental poisoning 5,780	Hypertension renal disease 17,345	Septicemia 33,865	Accidental poisoning 2% (675,348)
41,355	91,140	425,727	1,811,720	2,443,387	All causes 100%

Source: NHTSA (National Highway Traffic Safety Administration), U.S. Department of Transportation Technical report (DOT HS 809 843), June 2005, National Center for Statistics and Analysis. Available at http://www-nrd.nhtsa.dot.gov/pdf/nrd-30/NCSA/Rpts/2005/809843.pdf. Data from National Center for Health Statistics, Centers for Disease Control and Prevention, mortality data, 2002.
Note: The cause of death classification is based on the National Center for Statistics and Analysis (NCSA) Revised 68 Cause of Death Listing. This listing differs from the one used by the NCJS for its reports on leading causes of death by separating out unintentional injuries into separate causes of death, i.e., motor vehicle traffic crashes, accidental falls, motor vehicle nontraffic crashes, etc. Accordingly, the rank of some causes of death will differ from those reported by the NCHS. This difference will mostly be observed for minor causes of death in smaller age groupings.

particularly applied to the scalp, may be dangerous for a number of reasons. First, they can hide posterior scalp hemorrhage from view of the providers while providing a false sense of security that the bleeding has been controlled. Failure to recognize signs and symptoms of intrathoracic, intra-abdominal and pelvic bleeding is another potential prehospital complication related to circulatory insufficiency.

Prehospital intravenous fluid therapy is an area of continued controversy. A thorough discussion of the types and amount of fluid to be administered in the prehospital setting is beyond the scope of this chapter. In general, there are very few complications in the prehospital setting related to fluid excess. There is also evidence that subsets of patients—particularly trauma patients who have suffered penetrating trauma—may do better with no prehospital fluid or limited prehospital fluid than those who receive prehospital fluid.[8] There is general agreement among providers

of trauma care that extra time spent in the field trying to obtain intravenous access is detrimental to efforts to get the patient to definitive care and attempts to obtain access should be limited in most situations.[9] In the case of significant intracavitary bleeding, fluid cannot be administered in adequate amounts in the prehospital setting to restore effective intravascular volume. Therefore, efforts should be directed toward expeditious transfer to definitive care.

Other causes of circulatory insufficiency must be kept in mind. Pericardial tamponade manifested by Beck's triad of hypotension, jugular venous distension, and muffled heart tones may be difficult to discern in the frenetic prehospital setting. A temporizing measure for this rare prehospital occurrence it pericardiocentesis. Complications related to this procedure are significant and include, but are not limited to, inadvertent ventricular laceration/ puncture, laceration of the coronary arteries or vein, injury to the thoracic or upper abdominal great vessels, pneumothorax, or injury to the upper abdominal viscera. Prehospital attempts at pericardiocentesis are discouraged except by the most experienced providers and then in only the most dire of circumstances. Restoration of intravascular volume may temporarily offset the negative circulatory effects of pericardial tamponade, but, again, rapid transport to definitive care is the best approach in this situation.

DISABILITY

The major goal during the resuscitation of patients with traumatic neurologic injury is to avoid or minimize secondary brain injury and spinal cord damage. Avoiding hypoxemia and shock are also major priorities. Management of ventilation and maintenance of cerebral perfusion pressure can and should be addressed, altered, and optimized in the prehospital setting. Maintaining adequate perfusion and oxygenation in order to prevent secondary brain injury makes a positive difference in morbidity and mortality from TBI. The ABCs are important in the management of TBI in order to prevent secondary brain injury. The goals should be to maintain systolic blood pressure greater than 90 mm Hg, oxygenation saturations of at least 95%, and provide ventilation to maintain $ETCO_2$ of 30–35 mm Hg.[10]

There are multiple reasons for the development of altered mental status in trauma patients other than TBI (hypoxia, hypotension, alcohol, and other mind-altering drugs). However, in the prehospital setting the patient with an altered mental status and a mechanism of injury consistent with a TBI should be assumed to have suffered a significant brain injury until proven otherwise and treated aggressively in order to prevent secondary brain injury. Severity of the TBI may not be readily apparent in the prehospital setting. A high index of suspicion should be maintained based on the mechanism of injury and the patient's initial neurologic exam.

Historically, prehospital intubation has been the highest priority for patients with TBI with an associated coma (GCS ≤8), but recent evidence has shown that prehospital intubation may worsen outcomes for patients with TBI.[11] This has been somewhat controversial and has been refuted based on the variability of the expertise of prehospital providers, and the use of neuromuscular blockade agents (rapid-sequence intubation [RSI]) as an aid to intubation, which varies based on prehospital protocols. These results appear to be related to the expertise of the prehospital provider and the use of neuromuscular blockade agents (RSI). Intubation with pharmacologic agents is thought to lessen the "struggling" and difficulty in intubation. Without adequate sedation or paralytics, the intubation time may be prolonged, resulting in hypoxia, which may be the reason for the worsened outcomes, versus providers that have full pharmacologic agents available. Additionally, some prehospital providers have more expertise in intubation techniques, based on frequency of intubation. Therefore, it likely depends on the expertise and ease of intubation whether intubation is beneficial or harmful in the prehospital setting for patient outcomes with TBI.[12] Using the BVM technique and maintaining adequate minute ventilation and oxygenation is preferred compared to a prehospital provider with less proficiency at endotracheal intubation and the potential for the patient to have significant (degree and duration) hypoxemia and/or hypercarbia while attempting to accomplish endotracheal intubation. The use of intravenous lidocaine (1 mg/kg) may blunt an increase in intracranial pressure (ICP) during intubation.

The use of mannitol for severe head injuries should only be used for patients with localizing signs or evidence of elevated intracranial hypertension, when the patient is adequately volume resuscitated. Otherwise, the patient's volume status may be worsened, producing hypovolemia, and contribute to secondary brain injury and thus further worsening cerebral perfusion. Patients should be maintained in a euvolemic state.

Controlled hyperventilation—mild therapeutic hyperventilation ($ETCO_2$ of 25–30 mm Hg)—may be utilized in situations with acute neurologic deterioration with signs of herniation or obvious increase in ICP. Hyperventilation should be stopped if the signs of intracranial hypertension resolve (i.e., dilated pupil responds). Prophylactic hyperventilation should not be used in the prehospital management of TBI. Overaggressive hyperventilation produces cerebral vasoconstriction that in turn leads to a decrease in cerebral oxygen delivery. Routine prophylactic hyperventilation has been shown to worsen neurologic outcomes and should not be used.[10]

The use of benzodiazepines for treating seizures should be used with caution (titrated) because of the potential for developing hypotension and ventilatory depression.

Patients with TBI should be taken to the appropriate facility, one that cares for patients with TBI. If the transport time to a facility is prolonged, sedation, analgesia, chemical paralysis, controlled hyperventilation, and treatment with mannitol (osmotherapy) should be utilized as indicated. Prolonged attempts at intubation should be avoided—especially if a short transport time—as an oropharyngeal airway with BVM ventilations is a reasonable alternative.

Patients with suspected TBI should be placed in spinal immobilization, because of the significant incidence of cervical spine fractures. A tight C-collar may impede venous drainage from the head, thereby increasing ICP.

TRANSPORT

Upon arrival at the scene of injury, it is of paramount importance that the prehospital provider have a good understanding of the local resources available in terms of transport times, the transport environment, the transport vehicle, and the receiving facility. It is also very important that information gathered at the time of the initial evaluation be transmitted to the receiving facility in order to facilitate the receiving facility's ability to properly prepare for the patient's arrival. At the scene of a crash or injury incident, the paramedic must make a decision based on his or her resources as to which of the patients (if there are multiple patients) requires the first and most resources. Ideally, the most critically injured patient would be attended to first and sent out of the scene toward definitive care in the most expeditious fashion. Toward this end most health providers who care for the injured patient advocate a rapid transport team rather than spending additional time on the scene employing other modalities of advanced access, advanced airway techniques, or any other attempts at what would be definitive control at the scene. Put in another way, there's more of a desire by health care providers for a "scoop-and-run" than a "stay-and-play" approach. Subsequently, prehospital complications surrounding this include too much time on the scene allowing for the patient with potential intracavitary bleeding to deteriorate beyond the ability to provide definitive control. Second, there is the tendency to perform too many procedures at the scene that may be provided more effectively in the hospital setting.

Finally, there may be a tendency to employ protocol over what may in fact be better for the patient. An example is forcing patients with massive maxillofacial injury, who may otherwise be stable, into a supine position where they may choke on their own secretions. These patients may need to be transported in the decubitus position with cervical spine control or even transported in the sitting position to allow gravity to help secretions fall away from the airway. Similarly, patients who have potential tracheal injuries may actually do worse with repeated attempts at endotracheal intubation, when in fact their airway may be adequate and patent for transfer. Another factor is intravenous access.

COMORBIDITIES

With advances in medicine and medical care, Americans are living longer with chronic medical illnesses. Failure to recognize the underlying chronic medical condition in the victim of trauma is a common prehospital complication.

With advancement of age of the general population, the use of anticoagulants (warfarin, clopidogrel, aspirin) is becoming more common. Failure to recognize the patient who is fully medically anticoagulated may lead to a delay in recognizing significant intracranial, intrathoracic, or intra-abdominal bleeding. Alternatively, recognition of the medically anticoagulated state can lead to a higher index of suspicion on the part of prehospital providers as to the potential for significant injury, despite what might otherwise be considered minor trauma.

Chronic medical conditions that must be considered include chronic cardiopulmonary, renal, hepatic, and endocrine systems.

Patients with chronic congestive heart failure are often on a number of medications that may blunt their ability to mount a response to trauma. Beta-blocking drugs, for instance, may prevent these patients from mounting a tachycardiac response to acute hemorrhage. Chronic diuretic therapy may cause these patients to be chronically intravascularly depleted. These patients are often severely dyspneic, precluding their ability to lay supine on a transport gurney and, finally, their chronic congestive failure may predispose them to easy fluid overload with relatively minimal amounts of intravenous fluid therapy.

Patients with chronic obstructive pulmonary disease (COPD) may be difficult to assess, as they have chronically diminished breath sounds to auscultation. This makes it difficult, if not impossible, to clinically detect a condition such as pneumothorax, hemothorax, and pericardial tamponade. In addition, patients with severe COPD may be dependent on relative hypoxemia to promote respiratory efforts, and too much supplemental oxygen administration may acutely blunt this drive resulting in acute respiratory arrest.

Patients with chronic renal and hepatic insufficiency may manifest diminished clearing of administered intravenous medications used in the prehospital setting. Choice and dosage of these medications such as benzodiazepines and opioids must be made carefully with the patient's estimated hepatic and renal clearances in mind.

Patients with diabetes, adrenal insufficiency, and thyroid disorders may also manifest altered physiologic responses to acute trauma and the ability to elicit this history from the patient or guardian may be helpful in the acute and subsequent management of these patients. Many of these disorders can be ascertained from a review of the medications that the patient is taking. Eliciting this history from a family member, caregiver, or the patient him or herself is extremely useful in helping to manage the patient in the prehospital setting and beyond.

CONCLUSION

The initial management of the trauma victim is a challenging endeavor that lends itself readily to the application of an ordered approach to care. Following the ABCs of care, prioritizing the injuries with which a patient presents, and prioritizing rapid transport to definitive care yield the best possible outcome for the patient. Errors in the prehospital arena, as in others, include those of omission and those of commission. Both types of errors are avoidable with careful attention to defined principles of the approach to the patient.

REFERENCES

1. Ortiz JM: *U.S. Army Medical Department Journal*, October–December 1998, pp. 17–25.
2. National Research Council: *Accidental Death and Disability: The Neglected Disease of Modern Society*. Washington, DC, National Academy Press, 1996.
3. Highway Safety Act 1966 (PL 89-564), September 9, 1966.
4. National Research Council: *Injury in America: A Continuing Public Health Problem*. Washington, DC, National Academy Press, 1985.
5. Trauma Systems Planning and Development Act of 1990 (PL 101-590), November 16, 1990.
6. American College of Surgeons: *Advanced Trauma Life Support® Program for Physicians*. Chicago, American College of Surgeons Committee on Trauma, 1993.
7. Prehospital Trauma Life Support Committee of the National Association of Emergency Medical Technicians in cooperation with the Committee on Trauma of the American College of Surgeons: *PHTLS—Basic and Advanced Prehospital Trauma Life Support*, 5 ed. St. Louis, MO, Mosby, 2003.
8. Bickell WH, Wall MJ, Pepe PE, et al: Immediate versus delayed fluid resuscitation for hypotensive patients with penetrating torso injuries. *N Engl J Med* 331:1105–1109, 1994.
9. Sampalis JS, Tammim H, Davis R, et al: Ineffectiveness of on-site intravenous lines: is prehospital time the culprit? *J Trauma* 43:608–615, 1997.
10. Vincent J-L, Bené J: Primer on medical management of severe brain injury. *Crit Care Med* 33(6):1392–1399, 2005.
11. Davis DP, Hoyt DB, Ochs M, et al: The effect of paramedic rapid sequence intubation on outcome in patients with severe traumatic brain injury. *J Trauma* 54(3):444–453, 2003.
12. Cascio AN: Letter to the editor. *J Trauma* 56(2):454, 2004.

INITIAL ASSESSMENT AND RESUSCITATION

AIRWAY MANAGEMENT: WHAT EVERY TRAUMA SURGEON SHOULD KNOW, FROM INTUBATION TO CRICOTHYROIDOTOMY

Ronald I. Gross   and   Lenworth M. Jacobs

The concept of immediate and appropriate airway management spans all disciplines of medicine. Achieving, protecting, and maintaining the airway have been well recognized as the initial steps necessary in resuscitation of the critically ill and/or injured patient. The basic premise of the *Advanced Trauma Life Support for Doctors Course* (ATLS®) is that all resuscitations should follow the mnemonic "ABCDE." This mnemonic "defines the specific, ordered evaluations and interventions that should be followed in all injured patients,"[1] where the "A" stands for airway, and the "B" for breathing.

The optimal airway is the airway that the awake patient can maintain without assistance, while the worst-case scenario is an airway that can only be achieved with surgical intervention. The success or failure to achieve an adequate and protected airway is dependent on many factors. Techniques available to the clinician range from the simple to the complex. The concept of tracheal intubation is by no means a new one. In fact, the first documented report of tracheal intubation dates back to 1543, and actually refers to a tracheostomy. In his atlas *On the Fabric of the Human Body*, the Renaissance anatomist Anreas Vesalius observed, "Life may, in a manner of speaking, be restored. An opening must be attempted in the trunk of the trachea into which a reed or cane should be put; you will then blow into this so that the lung may rise again."[2]

From the clinician's standpoint, the appropriate management of the airway can be, and occasionally is, the most stressful part of a patient's initial care. This chapter will deal with the anatomic aspects of the head, neck, and respiratory system that one must know and understand to successfully manage the airway. It will also address how these anatomic variations, in association with the clinical situation faced by the clinician, will affect the clinician's choice of airway management. The chapter will describe the techniques available to the clinician to obtain and maintain an airway.

AIRWAY ANATOMY

Successful execution of any procedure demands a thorough understanding of the procedure: indications, technical requirements, and necessary equipment to complete the task. In addition, the operator must be cognizant of potential complications and their management. Obtaining an airway, whether by conventional or surgical means, is no different than any other procedure.[3,4] The anatomy and normal functions of the structures that comprise the upper airway are complex. The surgeon must recognize the essential anatomic structures to effectively manage the airway.

The nose and mouth are the two natural external openings to the airway. The nasal cavity is separated by the nasal septum into two pyramids containing bone, cartilage, and sinus orifices. The roof of the nose is formed by the nasal and frontal bones, the ethmoid cribiform plate, and the body of the sphenoid bone. The floor is formed by the maxilla and palatine bones, and the medial wall by septal cartilage, the vomer, and the perpendicular plane of the ethmoid. Laterally, the wall contains a portion of the ethmoid bone along with the superior, middle, and inferior turbinate bones. In addition, it contains the openings to the paranasal sinuses and the nasolacrimal duct. The nerve supply to the nasal cavities is from the olfactory and the trigeminal nerves (cranial nerves I and V, respectively). The blood supply is from the anterior and posterior branches of the ophthalmic artery, as well as branches of the maxillary and facial arteries.

The mouth is defined by the lips and cheeks externally; the gingiva, teeth, and palate superiorly; and mucosa and tongue inferiorly. The palate forms the roof of the mouth and the floor of the nasal cavity. The hard palate forms the anterior four-fifths of the palate and is a bony framework covered with a mucus membrane. The soft palate, comprising the posterior one-fifth of the palate, is a fibromuscular fold that moves posteriorly against the pharyngeal wall to close the oropharyngeal cavity when swallowing or speaking.

Although separated anteriorly by the palate, the mouth and nasal cavities join posteriorly at the end of the soft palate to form the pharynx. The pharynx is separated into the nasopharynx and the oropharynx. The pharynx extends to the inferior border of the cricoid cartilage anteriorly and the inferior border of the body of C6 posteriorly. The wall of the pharynx is composed of two layers of pharyngeal muscles: the external circular layer consists of the constrictor muscles and the internal longitudinal layer consists of muscles that elevate the larynx and pharynx during swallowing and speaking. The nasopharynx follows directly from the nasal cavity at the level of the soft palate, and communicates with the nasal cavities through the nasal choanae and with the tympanic cavity through the Eustachian tube. It contains the pharyngeal tonsils in its posterior wall. The oropharynx begins at the soft palate and continues to the tip of the epiglottis. It contains the palatine tonsils, important landmarks in the Mallampati airway classification.[5]

The epiglottis is a spoon-shaped plate of elastic cartilage that lies behind the tongue. It prevents aspiration by covering the glottis—the opening of the larynx—during swallowing. The laryngopharynx/hypopharynx extends from the upper border of the epiglottis to the lower border of the cricoid cartilage. It is separated laterally from the larynx by the arytenoepiglottic folds, which contain the piriform recesses. The piriform sinuses are found at each side of the opening of the larynx, in which the inferior laryngeal nerve lies and swallowed foreign materials may be lodged.

The laryngeal skeleton consists of several cartilages connected by ligaments and muscles: the thyroid, cricoid, epiglottic, and (in pairs) the arytenoid, corniculate, and cuneiform. The larynx serves as a sphincter to prevent the passage of food and drink into the trachea and lungs during swallowing. It also contains the vocal cords and regulates the flow of air to and from the lungs for phonation. It is through the abducted vocal cords of the larynx that an endotracheal tube is advanced during endotracheal intubation.

The thyroid cartilage is a large anterior structure that consists of right and left laminae that meet in the midline, forming the thyroid notch and thyroid prominence. The right and left superior projections (horns) of the thyroid cartilage connect to the hyoid bone, and the cricothyroid membrane connects the inferior edge to the cricoid cartilage. This latter anatomic relationship is of particular importance when an emergency surgical airway must be obtained.

Unlike the thyroid cartilage, which does not project posteriorly, the cricoid cartilage is a complete signet-shaped cartilaginous ring connected to both the thyroid cartilage and the first tracheal ring. This anatomic relationship was used by Sellick,[6] who described the prevention of passive regurgitation of gastric contents by posterior pressure on the cricoid cartilage during the induction of general anesthesia, a technique that has since become the accepted standard of care.

The epiglottis is an elastic cartilaginous structure covered by a mucous membrane. The reflection of this mucous membrane forms a slight depression known as the vallecula. It is at this point that the tip of the laryngoscope blade is placed so as to elevate the epiglottis and visualize the vocal cords. The epiglottis is anteriorly attached, superiorly to the hyoid bone by the hypoepiglottic ligament, and inferiorly to the thyroid cartilage by the thyroepiglottic ligament. The quadrangular ligament extends between the lateral aspects of the arytenoid and epiglottic cartilages. Its free inferior edge is the vestibular ligament, and, covered with mucosa, it forms the vestibular fold, which lies above the vocal cord (fold) and extends from the thyroid to the arytenoid cartilage. The arytenoids articulate with the superolateral aspect of the cricoid, and each has an anterior vocal cord process that attaches to the vocal cords via the cord ligament. The free superior margin forms the aryepiglottic ligament, and its mucosal covering forms the aryepiglottic fold. It is within the posterior aspects of aryepiglottic folds that the cuneiform and corniculate cartilages can be seen. These cartilages rest on the apex of the arytenoids. Their elastic properties facilitate the return of the arytenoid cartilages to their anatomic position of rest after abduction, and can usually be seen during direct laryngoscopy. They can, therefore, be used as a landmark for the tracheal opening when it is difficult to visualize the vocal cords (Figure 1).

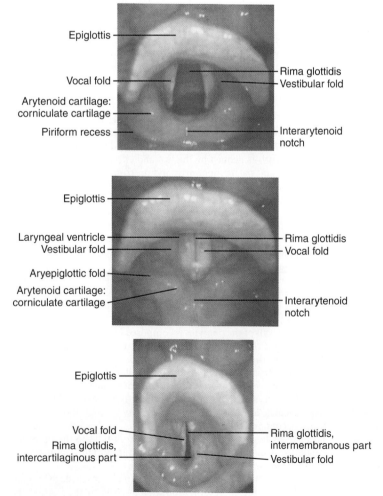

Figure 1 Landmarks of the tracheal opening. *(From Putz R, Pabst R, editors: Sobotta Atlas of Human Anatomy, 13 ed Baltimore, Williams & Wilkins, 2001, with permission.)*

The glottis is contained within the larynx, and is the narrowest part of the adult airway. It is composed of the vocal cords (or folds) and the space between them is called the rima glottides. Because the true vocal cords are covered by stratified epithelium, they have the characteristic pearly white color when illuminated. The cords are innervated by the recurrent laryngeal nerves, and the musculature of the larynx receives its innervation from branches of the vagus nerve (cranial nerve X). The larynx is inclusive of the structures noted previously.

The trachea extends from the inferior border of the cricoid cartilage for a variable distance, dividing into the right and left mainstem bronchi at the carina, which anatomically corresponds to the T4-T5 junction posteriorly and the sternal notch anteriorly. Like the thyroid cartilage, the sixteen to twenty tracheal cartilages form incomplete C-shaped rings that open posteriorly, allowing for variability in the tracheal diameter needed for normal airway functional changes. The trachea is in direct apposition posteriorly to the esophagus. This may be of significance in patients who have esophageal tumors, mediastinal hematomas (either traumatic or postoperative in origin), or have ingested large foreign bodies. All of these can cause upper (tracheal) airway obstruction.

ASSESSING THE AIRWAY

A thorough but rapid initial assessment of the trauma patient begins with the airway and breathing as the first priorities. This must be done with the understanding that, unless the cervical spine has already been "cleared" clinically, every patient has a cervical spine injury until proven otherwise. Breathing and speech are impossible without an intact airway. As such, one of the easiest determinants of an intact airway is the patient's ability to respond to the simple question, "My name is Dr. Jones, who are you?" If the patient is unable to answer in a normal voice because of a compromised airway or depressed mental status, then the clinician knows that an airway must be secured immediately.

Any patients with a Glasgow Coma Scale (GCS) of 8 or less, regardless of etiology, will need to be intubated to protect their airway. Intoxication and use of illicit substances are frequent causes of an altered mental status, as are closed head injuries and hypoxia. One must, therefore, err on the side of caution, and always assume that the depressed GCS is injury related, and that intubation will be needed to protect the airway. Hoarseness, shortness of breath, or, in the case of burn victims, carbonaceous sputum, should alert the clinician that an airway may be in jeopardy even if the patient can respond appropriately at that time. These patients must have careful and frequent interval reevaluations, with a low threshold for intubation. In addition, these patients may pose particularly difficult challenges to intubation, and underscore to the need to understand the need for a rapid and careful assessment of each individual airway.

Patient anatomy, both inherent and as altered by injury, is an important factor that requires careful assessment by the clinician prior to attempting intubation, whether nasal, orotracheal, or surgical. In the trauma patient, the clinician must always be cognizant of the potential for cervical spine injury. This is particularly important in the patient whose physical exam is compromised by an altered mental status, regardless of the cause. The presence of maxillofacial trauma or injuries of the soft tissues of the neck must also be considered when deciding the best way to secure and protect the airway. In the absence of injury or pathologic conditions, the ability to ventilate and control the supraglottic airway is a function of the size of the airway and the compliance of the supralaryngeal tissues. It should be remembered that under normal conditions air flow through the nasal cavity is not usually a concern in that this portion of the airway is usually supported by rigid elements in its walls. Conversely, the pharynx does not have a rigid support system, and therefore, it is predisposed to collapse. It can also be obstructed by the tongue in obtunded or comatose

patients; in most cases this collapse and/or obstruction can initially be dealt with effectively with the use of the oral airway.[7]

A more ominous situation arises when the airway is compromised in the immediate vicinity of the laryngeal inlet because of the size of the base of the tongue or the epiglottis. Air flow in this region will be inversely proportional to the size of these structures, as well as the condition of the perilaryngeal tissues. Trauma to the neck causing anatomic disruption and/or tissue edema, prior irradiation to the neck, head and neck tumors, or redundant fatty tissue in the perilaryngeal area secondary to obesity will all restrict normal air flow. These conditions may lead to the "cannot-ventilate-and-cannot-intubate scenario," a potentially lethal situation in even the most competent intubators.[7]

As with any other medical procedure, it is always prudent to perform a methodical evaluation of the situation, and determine the preferable approach and equipment needed to perform the task efficiently. In addition to factors previously discussed, one must also assess for scarring and fibrosis to the airway and surrounding tissues, injury to the trachea; congenital anomalies; acute inflammatory or neoplastic diseases of the airway; and finally gingival, mandibular, and dental anomalies/disease.[8] Short, muscular individuals with very short necks and obese patients tend to be difficult to intubate. Morbidly obese patients can compromise the airway with excessive redundant tissue in the paratonsillar and paraglottic areas, masking visualization and accessibility of the glottis during laryngoscopy. Anatomic factors that should be assessed include mandibular mobility at the temporomandibular joints; mobility of the head at the atlanto-occipital joint (when cervical spine injury has been ruled out); the length, size, and muscularity of the neck; size and configuration of the palate; the proportionate size of the mandible in relation to the face; and the presence of an overbite of the maxillary teeth.

Difficulty in laryngoscopic visualization varies in accordance with the extent of anatomic variation or pathologic conditions. The Mallampati classification is routinely used by anesthesiologists to evaluate the airway in elective cases (see Figure 1 on page 59).

In order to classify a patient, the patient is asked to open the mouth as widely as possible and protrude the tongue out as far as possible while seated, with the head in the neutral position,[8] something that is almost impossible to accomplish in the trauma setting. Evaluation of the atlanto-occipital extension is another tool that is used by anesthesiologists in the elective setting. Because this requires an awake patient who can sit upright and flex and extend the neck, it is not useful in the trauma setting. However, a clinician familiar with the Mallampati classification can perform a cursory evaluation of the oropharynx using a tongue blade or laryngoscope, which provides the clinician some idea as to the potential for difficulty in intubation. It will also demonstrate the existence of any evidence of injury to the oropharynx, the presence of foreign bodies, blood, or vomitus.

Because one cannot always rely on the anesthesiologist to secure the airway, all clinicians caring for the trauma patient must have the ability to provide immediate and effective airway protection and ventilation. Clinicians must, therefore, be able to recognize limitations to airway access, and must possess techniques to overcome these limitations. There are many tools and techniques available to the anesthesiologist in the elective setting, and while many of these may not be practical in the emergent trauma setting, several can be used, and these will be the focus of the rest of this discussion.

CONTROLLING THE AIRWAY

The best airway is the airway that the patient can safely maintain without any external intervention. The Eastern Association for the Surgery of Trauma has sited the need for emergency tracheal intubation in trauma patients with airway obstruction, hypoventilation, severe hypoxia in spite of supplemental oxygen administration, severe cognitive impairment (GCS score <8), cardiac arrest, and severe hemorrhagic shock.[9] Once it has been decided that the airway is not adequate, or that the patient is unable to protect the airway, then intubation must be accomplished in an efficient and safe manner. It is important to remember that all trauma patients must be intubated with one person maintaining in-line cervical immobilization throughout the procedure to protect the possibly injured cervical spine.

As with all other procedures, a successful outcome depends on the operator's experience and on having immediate access to all of the correct equipment. Most emergency departments have airway carts that contain all of the equipment that will routinely be needed for emergency intubations, as well as specialty carts designed for the "difficult airway." While the contents of these carts will vary from institution to institution, they will usually be standardized within each hospital. Examples of stocking lists for the standard airway cart (Figure 2) and the difficult airway cart appear in Tables 1 and 2, respectively.

Once the decision to intubate has been made, all patients should be preoxygenated with 100% oxygen. The jaw thrust and chin lift can be done without endangering the cervical spine, and should be performed in an attempt to open an airway that may be obstructed by the tongue, which tends to fall posteriorly in the obtunded patient. The chin lift is accomplished by placing one's fingers under the mandible and gently lifting the mandible upward. The thumb of the same hand is used to depress the lower lip and open the mouth. Care must be taken to prevent hyperextension of the neck while performing the chin lift. The jaw thrust can be performed alone or used in conjunction with bag-valve-mask (BVM) ventilation of the obtunded, but breathing patient, and the respiratory efforts are assisted with compression of the bag. By grasping both mandibular angles and displacing the mandible forward, one is able to simultaneously open the airway and obtain and maintain an effective seal with the mask during assisted bag mask ventilation.

Oropharyngeal and nasopharyngeal airways (see Figure 2) are useful, but must be inserted with care. While neither one is well tolerated by the awake patient, the nasopharyngeal airway is better tolerated in the semiresponsive patient, and is less likely to stimulate gagging and vomiting.[10] They can both be used to help maintain a patent upper airway in the obtunded patient. In the adult, the oral airway is inserted with the convexity facing down initially, and then rotated 180 degrees once in the oropharynx. It must be placed carefully, so that it does not push the tongue posteriorly, but rather, is seated posterior to the tongue displacing the tongue anteriorly. In children, the oral airway must always be placed with the convex surface facing cephalad initially to avoid injury to the soft tissues of the mouth and pharynx. It is important to remember that in patients with a persistent (intact) upper airway gag reflex, the insertion of the oral airway can precipitate laryngospasm and bronchospasm, as well as coughing, gagging, vomiting, and ultimately, aspiration.[11]

DOCUMENTATION OF PROPER ENDOTRACHEAL TUBE PLACEMENT

Once tracheal intubation has been accomplished, it is imperative that proper tube position is ascertained and documented. The best confirmation of proper tube placement is the direct visualization of the tube passing through the vocal cords during laryngoscopy. Since this is not always the case, tube placement can be tentatively confirmed by physical exam. Observation and auscultation of the chest is a valuable clinical tool. In the absence of chest wall disruption due to rib fractures, the clinician will see symmetric chest wall motion upon ventilation with appropriate tube placement.

Auscultation of the chest is done both anteriorly and in the axillae, and is useful when breath sounds are heard bilaterally and are equal. This is not always the case, even with appropriate tube placement, because of the presence of pneumothoraces or hemo-

Table 1: Respiratory/Airway Cart

Top of Airway Cart
Stat respiratory rx box
2 x 2's
Hurricane spray
Benzoin (1)
2% xylocaine jelly (1)
Surgilube (1)
EID (1)
#7, 7.5, 8 ETT (1 @)
Stylette (1)
12-cc syringe (1)
#18 NG tube (1)
60-cc catheter tip syringe (1)
Magill forceps (1)
Green, yellow, red oral airway (1 @)
Laryngoscope handle
#2, 3, 4 Mac blades (1 @)
#2, 3 Wis/Miller blades (1 @)

Top Drawer
#6, 6.5, 7, 7.5, 8, 8.5, 9 ETT (2 @)
Stylette (2)
#2, 3 Miller blades (1 @)
#2, 3, 4 Miller blades (1 @)

Drawer 2
PEEP valves (2)
Nasal cannulas (2)
ETCO$_2$ sensors (2)
Adult O$_2$ sensors (2)
Green, yellow, red oral airways (2 @)
#28, 30, 32 nasal airways (1 @)
Tube holders, IV tubing, tape, Dale holders

Drawer 3
Luekens trap (2)
#18, 14 NG tube (2 @)
Surgilube
2% xylocaine jelly
Yankauer (2)
Suction catheters (2)

Drawer 4
Transtrach jet (1)
Bag-in aerosol setups with meds (2)
Rebreather masks (2)
Venti masks (2)

Drawer 5
BVM (2)
Cross-vent circuits (2)
Extra vent sheets

Left Side Facing Front
Waste bin
BVM

Right Side Facing Front
Sterile gloves

Table 2: Difficult Intubation Cart

Outside of Cart

Jet ventilator present and connected to 50-psi regulator

Jet vent tank, regulator attached, >1500 psi (50 psi/1–15 lpm regulator)

Portable CO_2 monitor with line attached and charger (in top drawer) *or*

CO_2 clip colormetric detector

Drawer 1

Intubation stylette 6 Fr., 10 Fr., 14 Fr. (1 @)

2% lidocaine jelly (1 @)

Cetacaine spray (1 @)

4% lidocaine solution (1 @)

Nasal spray (1 @)

14 Fr. Jelco (5 @)

Magill forceps, pediatric (1 @)

Magill forceps, adult (1 @)

Bite block (1 @)

Fiberoptic bronchoscope adapter swivel (2 ea)

Ovasappian airway (2 ea)

Sampling elbow (1 @ch)

Sampling tee (1 @ch)

Sample tubing for CO_2 monitor (2 @ch)

MAD (mucosal atomization device) (1 @)

Drawer 2

Fiberoptic laryngoscope handle standard size ((1 @)

Fiberoptic laryngoscope handle penlight size (1 @)

Fiberoptic laryngoscope handle stubby size (1 @)

Fiberoptic laryngoscope blade Miller 1, 2, 3, 4 (1 @)

Fiberoptic laryngoscope blade Mac 2, 3 (1 @)

Fiberoptic CLM laryngoscope blade size 3, 4 (1 @)

Drawer 3

Endotracheal tube cuffed 4.0, 5.0, 5.5, 6.0, 6.5, 7.0, 7.5, 8.0, (2 @)

Endotrol endo tube 6.0, 7.0 (2 @)

MLT endotracheal tube 6.0 (2 @)

Drawer 4

Endotracheal tube uncuffed w/monitoring lumen 2.5, 3.0, 3.5, 4.0, 4.5, 5.0, 5.5 (1 @)

Drawer 5

Sheridan Combitube© 41 Fr., 37 Fr. (1 @)

Mask size child (1 @)

Mask size small adult (1 @)

Mask size large adult (1 @)

Drawer 6

LMA size 3 (1 @)

LMA size 4 (1 @)

Duoflex long guidewire (1 @)

Hyperinflation bag 3 liter (1 @)

Retrograde intubation kit (Cook) (1 @)

Cook airway exchange catheter 3 mm, 4 mm, 5 mm, 6 mm, 7 mm (1 @)

Cook "Frova Catheter" (1 @)

Cook "Melker" emergency cricothyrotomy catheter sets size 3.5, 4.0 (1 @)

Fastrach intubating LMA size 4 with endotracheal tubes and pusher (1 @)

Tissue spreader (1 @)

Bougie (1 @)

Olympus LF-GP

Cabinet for FOB

Cric Set

2 Army Navy retractors

2 thyroid retractors

1 needle holder

2 curved hemostats

2 straight hemostats

1 trach spreader

2 Jackson tracheal hooks

2 disposable scalpels

2 sutures

Check

Satisfactory batteries in laryngoscope

Outdates on drugs and supplies

---

thoraces seen in the trauma patient population. It is incumbent on the clinician to immediately treat the pneumothorax and/or hemothorax, and then confirm tube placement by both physical exam and chest radiograph. Auscultation over the left upper quadrant of the abdomen is important; with appropriate placement of the endotracheal tube, there will be no gurgling in the stomach during ventilation.

The cuffed portion of the endotracheal tube should be at least 1–2 cm below the cords, and in the average patient, the endotracheal tube will be taped in position at the 21–23-cm mark. Lastly, a chest radiograph should be performed to confirm proper placement of the endotracheal tube after every intubation.[10] The tip of an appropriately placed endotracheal tube should be approximately 5 cm above the carina in the average adult.[12]

Cyanosis as an indicator of a fall in oxygen concentration is a late event, and is influenced by factors such as room lighting, anemia, and hemoglobin anomalies. Resolution of hypoxia is a reliable sign of proper tube placement, but minutes may elapse before

a patient shows desaturation by pulse oximetry, especially in patients who have been properly preoxygenated.[12] Identification of carbon dioxide (CO_2) in exhaled gas has become the standard for verification of appropriate placement of an endotracheal tube in the elective or emergent setting. This can be accomplished with capnography (the instantaneous display of the CO_2 waveform during ventilation) or capnometry, which is the measurement of CO_2 in the expired gas. The latter has become the method of choice in the emergent setting because of the availability of colorimetric CO_2 detectors.[10,12] Colorimetric CO_2 detectors are routinely inserted into the respiratory circuit between the end of the endotracheal tube and the ventilator tubing or Ambu-bag, and will detect the presence of CO_2 as soon as ventilation begins after intubation. It must be remembered that although useful, the presence of CO_2 is not, by itself, absolute assurance of proper tube placement. The endotracheal tube could be improperly positioned in a mainstem bronchus and one would still detect CO_2. CO_2 will not be detected in patients who are in cardiac arrest. In patients who

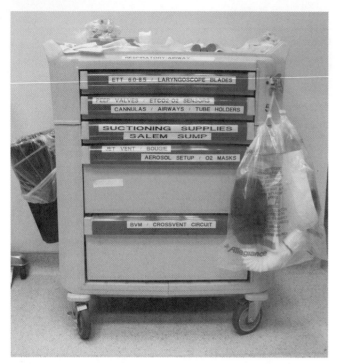

Figure 2 Standard respiratory/airway cart.

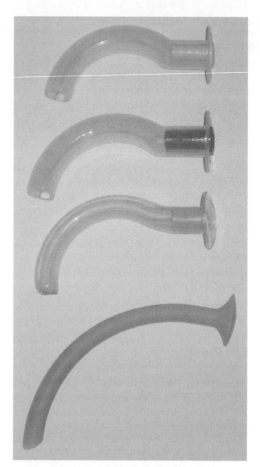

Figure 3 Oral airways (upper three) and nasal airway.

have been actively ventilated prior to intubation, CO_2 can be detected in gas from the stomach when the endotracheal tube is improperly placed in the esophagus. This will clear with several breaths, however, and indicate to the clinician that the tube is improperly placed.[10]

Even with all of the equipment and technical advances available to the clinician, clinical judgment, the physical exam, and attention to detail is essential in management of the airway.

COMBITUBE©

The inability to intubate can be a lethal event due to the hypoxia resulting from the inability to ventilate and, therefore, oxygenate the critically ill or injured patient. There are certain "rescue" techniques available, and one such technique involves the use of the dual lumen esophagotracheal tube, known as the Combitube© (Tyco Healthcare Group LP, 2001). This redesigned tube, which comes in a regular and small adult size, has minimized the problems that had been seen with the use of the esophageal obturator airway as an airway rescue technique.[13] The disposable Combitube© has a longer blue tube (No. 1) with a blind distal end and pharyngeal side holes, and a shorter clear tube (No. 2) with an open distal end (Figure 4). While Wissler[13] recommends using the laryngoscope for placement of the tube under direct vision, the tube can be inserted blindly through the mouth.

While the tip of the tube can end up in the trachea (Figure 4), it will enter the esophagus 99% of the time.[14] Once the tube is successfully placed, the balloons are inflated with air, 100 ml in the pharyngeal balloon to occlude the pharynx, and 15 ml in the distal balloon occluding either the esophagus or the trachea. Ventilation is now begun using tube no. 1. If the tip of the tube is positioned in the esophagus (the preferred position), one will hear breath sounds bilaterally, capnography will be positive for carbon dioxide, and auscultation over the left upper quadrant of the abdomen will be negative for gastric insufflation. At this point, a gastric tube can be placed through tube no. 2.

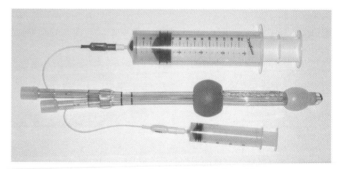

Figure 4 Combitube© with both balloons inflated. Larger syringe inflates the blue tube (No. 1) balloon.

If the tip of the tube is in the trachea, no breath sounds will be heard in the chest, and capnography will be negative for CO_2. Ventilation should immediately be switched to tube no. 2, and the exam repeated to confirm breath sounds by auscultation and CO_2 by capnography.

The Combitube© has been shown to be an effective alternative to prehospital cricothyroidotomy after failed rapid sequence intubation (RSI) attempts in patients with severe maxillofacial trauma. In fact, Blostein et al.[15] studied 10 such patients who failed in-field intubation. The Combitube© was successfully replaced by an orotracheal tube in 7 of the 10 patients, and only 3 required a surgical airway. It must be remembered that the Combitube© must be replaced with a definitive airway as soon as the clinical situation permits. Furthermore, it should be remembered that contraindications to use of a Combitube© include patients who (1) are younger than 16 years, (2) are responsive with an intact gag reflex, (3) have known esophageal disease, and (4) have a known ingestion of a caustic substance.[4]

ENDOTRACHEAL INTUBATION

In the adult, the placement of a cuffed tube within the trachea is considered to be the definitive airway. This definitive airway can be achieved nasally, orally, or surgically (cricothyroidotomy or tracheostomy). The indications for each of these techniques will be determined by the level of clinical urgency for airway control, and the skill level of the clinician performing the intubation. Some of the indications for establishment of a definitive airway in the trauma patient include apnea, a GCS of less than 8 (and therefore the need to protect the airway), inability to oxygenate with face mask,[10] massive facial trauma with hemorrhage, and trauma to the neck resulting in airway disruption and/or compression from hematoma.

Nasal Intubation

Nasal intubation is a well-accepted technique for intubation in the obtunded patient, but the patient must be breathing, and not in extremis. Because injured patients can be, and often are, in extremis, and cannot protect their airway, nasal intubation is rarely performed on the multiple-trauma patient. In addition, this technique is not routinely used in the trauma setting because of the possibility of occult and as yet unrecognized facial bony fractures. Lastly, because most trauma patients have not been fasting, and are at risk for vomiting and aspiration, intubation is most often performed using the RSI technique. This technique renders the patient apneic, and nasal intubation is, therefore, not possible.

Orotracheal Intubation

Orotracheal intubation is the mainstay for definitive airway control in the emergent setting. When performed by an anesthesiologist in the elective setting, orotracheal intubation is completed with the patient's head in extension. In the trauma patient with a potential cervical spine injury, extension of the neck is contraindicated. It is important to remember that in the trauma population, orotracheal intubation is a *two-person* procedure, with one person performing the intubation and a second person maintaining constant in-line cervical spine immobilization.

Trauma patients who require intubation often have a variety of anatomic and physiologic derangements that make intubation difficult. These patients frequently have varying degrees of hypoxia, acidosis, and hemodynamic instability. Compromised cardiac or pulmonary function, especially in the elderly patient, further increase the risk of myocardial or cerebral ischemia when attempts at intubation are prolonged. Associated conditions related to the traumatic event, such as intracranial hypertension, myocardial ischemia or dysfunction, upper airway bleeding, inhalation injury, and vomiting can actually be exacerbated by the physical manipulation required to intubate the patient.[16] These factors necessitated the development of a standardized approach when emergency intubation is warranted. The advent of RSI has provided this standardized approach to those caring for the critically ill patient.

Rapid sequence intubation is the almost simultaneous administration of an induction agent (sedative, anxiolytic, amnesic) and a paralyzing dose of a neuromuscular blocking agent. The goal of RSI is to obtain a secure airway while avoiding complications such as vomiting and aspiration, cardiac arrhythmias, or the reflex sympathetic response caused by laryngoscopy. Relative contraindications include those situations where BVM ventilation will most likely be ineffective or impossible. When used appropriately, RSI has been shown to decrease complications associated with intubation while increasing the intubation success rate to 98%.[16] The most commonly used RSI medications include lidocaine, the induction agents midazolam or etomidate, and the neuromuscular blocking agents (NMBAs) succinylcholine or rocuronium.

Lidocaine is commonly used to decrease the hypertensive response and airway reactivity of laryngoscopy, to prevent or minimize intracranial hypertension, and to decrease the incidence of cardiac arrhythmias during intubation. To be effective, however, 1.5 mg/kg should be administered intravenously 3 minutes prior to intubation.

Induction agents will facilitate intubation by rapidly rendering the patient unconscious. Both midazolam and etomidate are rapidly effective and have a similar elimination half-life. Given parenterally, midazolam (1–2.5 mg/kg) has a greater propensity to precipitate hypotension, and etomidate (0.15–0.3 mg/kg) does not affect blood pressure, and has a cerebral protective effect in that it reduces cerebral blood flow and cerebral oxygen uptake. It is, therefore, favored for use in the trauma patient with hypotension.[12,16]

Succinylcholine, a depolarizing agent, is the most commonly used NMBA. It has a rapid onset (30–60 seconds) and relatively short duration of effect (5–15 minutes) that will allow for effective ventilation after 9–10 minutes. About 10–15 seconds after administration of succinylcholine, fasciculations occur that are associated with brief increase in intracranial, intraocular, and intragastric pressures. However, the potential increase in intracranial pressure is so small that its effects are outweighed and offset by the avoidance of hypoxia seen with an improved success rate of intubation.[17] Succinylcholine cannot be used in patients with penetrating globe injuries, pseudocholinesterase deficiency, any history of myopathy or muscular dystrophy. In addition, patients who have, or are at risk for hyperkalemia, such as patients with thermal (burn) injuries more than 24 hours old, or crush syndromes with myonecrosis or rhabdomyolysis, should not receive succinylcholine.[16] Rocuronium, a nondepolarizing NMBA, also has a short onset of action (30–60 seconds) after a dose of 1.0 mg/kg, but a longer recovery time (45–60 minutes) than succinylcholine.[17] It does not have any of the deleterious side effects of succinylcholine, and according to Perry et al.,[18] the success of intubation is similar with rocuronium and succinylcholine under all study conditions.

Rapid sequence intubation can be used in the pediatric patient, but dosing is different than that recommended in the patient over age 10 years. Pediatric patients have increased vagal tone and a decreased functional residual capacity. Bradycardia during intubation can result from both vagal stimulation and hypoxia. In addition, succinylcholine can cause bradycardia in the pediatric population. Table 3 shows the protocol used at our institution when dealing with the pediatric patient.

Table 3: Rapid-Sequence Intubation Medications in the Pediatric Population

Patients Up to Age 2 Years	Patients Aged 2–10 Years
Atropine 0.02 mg/kg IV (Minimum dose 0.1 mg, maximum dose 0.5 mg)	Atropine 0.02 mg/kg IV (Minimum dose 0.1 mg, maximum dose 0.5 mg)
Lidocaine 1.5 mg/kg IV	Lidocaine 1.5 mg/kg IV
Midazolam 0.15 mg/kg IV	Etomidate 0.3 mg/kg IV
Rocuronium 1.0 mg/kg IV *or*	Rocuronium 1.0 mg/kg *or*
Succinylcholine 2.0 mg/kg (1.5 mg/kg if patient >12 kg)	Succinylcholine 1.5 mg/kg IV (2.0 mg/kg for patient <12 kg)

From LIFE STAR Standards of Practice, Hartford, CT, Hartford Hospital, April 2007, with permission.

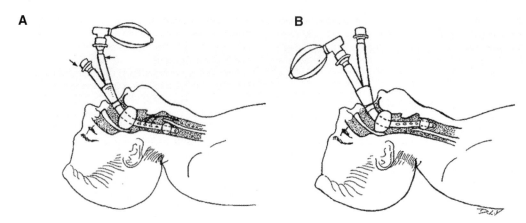

Figure 5   Placement of the Combitube© with the tip in the esophagus, both balloons inflated. **(A)** Ventilate through tube no. 1 (blue) placement of the Combitube© with the tip in the trachea. Both balloons are inflated. **(B)** Ventilate through tube no. 2 (clear).   *(From Shoemaker et al, editors: Textbook of Critical Care, 4th ed. Philadelphia, W.B. Saunders, 2000, p. 1241, with permission.)*

Intubation must be preceded by preoxygenation with 100% oxygen by mask until the oxygen saturation (SO_2) by pulse oximetry is either at 100% or has reached a maximal level. BVM ventilation can be used to assist the breathing patient, and is used to control the airway in the apneic patient prior to intubation. The Sellick maneuver should be performed whenever possible to reduce the possibility of aspiration. The stomach may be insufflated during BVM ventilation, and an orogastric or nasogastric tube must be inserted after the patient is successfully intubated.

In the comatose and apneic patient, no medication is needed, and the patient can be intubated upon laryngoscopic visualization of the cords. There are several different laryngoscope blades for use (Figure 5). The appropriate shape and size should be selected for intubation. The laryngoscope is inserted into the mouth with care taken not to injury the lips or teeth. The blade of the laryngoscope is advanced posteriorly, sweeping the tongue upward and to the left. Once the tonsillar pillars are visualized, the tip of the blade is placed into the vallecula, exposing the larynx and the triangular glottic opening, which is formed and bordered by the vocal cords. If the epiglottis is seen to overhang the larynx, the blade is advanced farther into the vallecula, exposing the cords. Once the cords are visualized, the endotracheal tube is gently placed through the cords into the trachea. The use of an endotracheal tube stylette is common, but not mandatory. Endotracheal tubes vary in size, and those used for children are uncuffed. In the adult, the cuffed tube size will be determined by the size of the opening between the cords. Most adults will tolerate an endotracheal tube with an internal diameter of 7, 7.5, or 8 mm, placed to a depth of about 21–24 cm at the lip. In the child, the endotracheal tube should be uncuffed, and about the same size as the child's nostril or little (fifth) digit of the hand. Placement should not be any further than 2 cm past the cords.[1] The endotracheal tube should never be forced through the cords, but rather, should be gently guided through the glottis (Figure 6).

It is in these patients that securing a difficult airway can be fraught with difficulty. Complications related to hemodynamic alterations, as well as difficulties in oxygenation and ventilation have been shown to be significant issues in the patient population requiring emergent intubation outside the elective operating room (OR) setting.[17–19] One study has shown that difficult intubations requiring more than three attempts account for almost 10% of all out-of-OR intubations, and that airway-related and hemodynamic-related complications were "relatively common."[18] This points to the fact that anyone dealing with the emergent airway must always have a secondary or backup plan. This backup plan should include what Mort referred to as "rescue operations."[17] These rescue plans

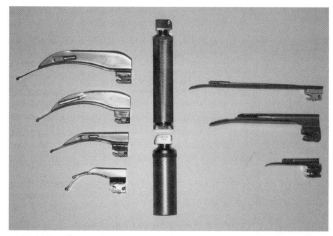

Figure 6   Left: Macintosh curved blades (from top to bottom, nos. 4, 3, 2, and 1). Center: Laryngoscope handles. Right: Miller straight blades (from top to bottom nos. 3, 2, and 0).

should include the Combitube© (discussed earlier), flexible bougies, laryngeal mask airways (LMAs), intubating LMAs, and finally, the emergency cricothyroidotomy. In addition, whenever possible, additional assistance by those proficient in intubation must be readily available if one hopes to avoid complications that include death when dealing with the difficult airway.

Bougies are semi-rigid, gum-elastic stylette-like devices with a bent tip. They should be a standard piece of equipment on any difficult airway cart, and should be immediately available whenever a difficult airway is anticipated. They are used most often when only the arytenoids or the epiglottis can be visualized. During laryngoscopy, the bougie is advanced into the larynx and through the cords, into the trachea. As the bougie moves down the trachea, the tip of the bougie rubs against the tracheal rings. This is transmitted up the bougie and one can experience what has been referred to as the "washboard effect." Care must be exercised so as not to advance the bougie too far; this has the possibility of creating a bronchial injury. Once in position, the bougie position is maintained by one clinician as a second clinician advances a lubricated endotracheal tube over the bougie, through the cords, and into position in the trachea under laryngoscopic visualization (whenever possible). The bougie is then removed, and the steps to confirm ET tube placement are performed as mentioned earlier (Figure 7).

Originally introduced by Brain in 1983,[20,21] the LMA is now routinely used for airway management in the elective anesthesia setting. The LMA (Laryngeal Mask Company Ltd) and the LMA Fastrach™ are also now becoming valuable additions to the armamentarium of emergency airway management (Figure 8).

The LMA is a large-bore tube that is attached to an ovoid or elliptical silicone cuff that, once well lubricated, is inserted blindly into the airway as far as it will go. Once properly positioned, and the cuff is inflated with 20–30 ml of air, the leading edge or tip of the cuff will obstruct the esophageal lumen while the cuff provides a low pressure seal around the entrance to the larynx, allowing for ventilation in an emergent setting. It is important to remember that the LMA will not be well tolerated in any patient with an existing gag reflex, and may precipitate vomiting and aspiration in these patients.[18] The LMA comes in several sizes, and can be used in the pediatric and adult populations. As with endotracheal intubation, successful insertion will require the appropriate size selection. Indications for the emergent placement of the LMA in trauma patients include a GCS of 3 after rapid-sequence drug administration and attempted orotracheal intubation has failed.[9]

Although the LMA has been used to secure the airway in the trauma patient, it is, indeed, more suited for elective airway management situations. The LMA Fastrach (Figure 9), or intubating LMA, on the other hand, has been shown to be effective when used in the trauma center setting. The pharyngeal orifice of the LMA Fastrach is different that that of the regular LMA (Figures 10 and 11) and it allows the passage of a specifically designed and compatible endotracheal tube once the LMA Fastrach is appropriately placed. The maximal size endotracheal tube that the LMA Fastrach will allow is an 8-mm internal diameter. As with the LMA, the LMA Fastrach is placed in trauma patients when attempts to place an orotracheal tube with RSI have failed, the patient has a GCS of 3, and an airway must be controlled immediately.[9] Placement of the intubating LMA is done in the same manner as with the LMA, but passage of the endotracheal tube is usually done as a two-person technique, with one person controlling the LMA and a second passing the very well-lubricated endotracheal tube. Once placement of the endotracheal tube is confirmed, the LMA can carefully be removed while maintaining the position of the endotracheal tube.

SURGICAL AIRWAY

The preferred method of management of the airway is by the patient with minimal assistance from the physician. The clinician can monitor the flow of air into the airway and observe

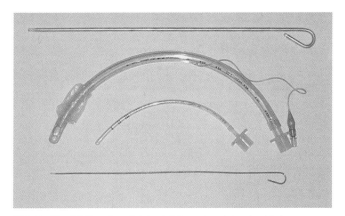
Figure 7 Adult and pediatric stylets and endotracheal tubes.

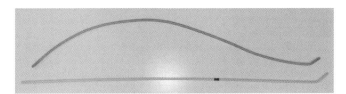
Figure 8 Semi-rigid gum-elastic bougies.

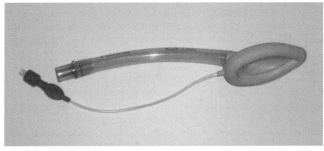
Figure 9 Laryngeal mask airway.

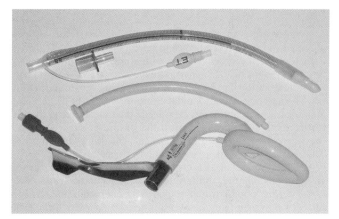
Figure 10 Intubating laryngeal mask airway (LMA). LMA-specific endotracheal tube (top), stylet (middle), and intubating LMA with intubating handle (bottom).

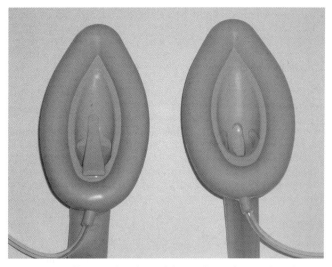
Figure 11 Pharyngeal orifices of the intubating laryngeal mask airway (LMA) (left) and regular LMA (right).

any difficulty in ventilation. Unfortunately, this is not always possible.

Once any of the aforementioned airway adjuncts have been unsuccessfully attempted and the patient has an unprotected airway and cannot be ventilated, a surgical approach to the airway is indicated.

Needle Cricothyroidotomy

This is a rapid, effective, and safe method of gaining access directly into the airway through the cricothyroid membrane. The advantages of this procedure are that it is relatively easy to use and requires minimal equipment. It bypasses obstructions at the level of the cords and allows for direct air entry into the tracheobronchial tree.

The disadvantages are that even a large-caliber needle is insufficient to adequately ventilate the patient for more than a few minutes. This method of airway control is designed to provide some oxygenation for a patient with inability to ventilate until a more formal surgical airway can be obtained.

Unfortunately, even though high-flow oxygen can be delivered through a 14-gauge or larger needle, there is minimal ability to exhale. Carbon monoxide levels rise and the ability to deliver oxygen to the alveoli is compromised.

Procedure

A syringe with a 14-gauge needle is obtained. A Y-connector is obtained and oxygen is attached to one branch of the Y. The other branch of the Y can be occluded with a finger to allow oxygen to flow into the trachea. The chest is then observed to rise with inspiration. Expiration can be effected by removing the occluding finger. The larynx is palpated and the inferior border of the larynx is identified. The cricothyroid cartilage is then identified as the first cartilaginous structure inferior to the larynx. The space between the larynx and the cricothyroid is the cricothyroid membrane. This is palpated with a finger and the needle attached to the syringe is advanced at a 45-degree angle through the skin, the cricothyroid membrane, and into the lumen of the trachea. As soon as the needle "pops" through the cricothyroid membrane, the barrel of the syringe should be aspirated. Air should flow easily into the syringe. The needle should then be withdrawn from the sheath and the cannulae secured in place. The oxygen line is then connected with the Y-connector to the barrel of the cannulae. Oxygen can then be delivered through the tubing directly into the trachea. By removing one's finger from one branch of the Y-connector, carbon dioxide can be vented from the endobronchial tree. Oxygen should be delivered at a high flow rate of 10–12 liters per minute.

Cricothyroidotomy

A formal cricothyroidotomy has considerable advantages over a needle cricothyroidotomy. A large cannula can be introduced through the cricothyroid membrane and adequate ventilation can then occur. The advantages are similar to the needle cricothyroidotomy in that the anatomy is easy to identify and the procedure is relatively easy to perform. The disadvantages are that this otomy is too superior in the neck to be long-term airway. For this reason, a cricothyroidotomy is to be used as a temporary measure until a tracheostomy can be performed in a controlled setting in the operating room.

Procedure

The larynx is identified in the midline and the cricothyroid ring is also identified. The diamond shaped cricothyroid membrane is palpated between both of these structures. It is essential to stay in the midline, as the midline is avascular. As the operator moves laterally, there is an opportunity to encounter the anterior jugular veins and the major vessels and nerves in the neck. The medial strap muscles are also just lateral to the midline. In the emergent situation, it is preferable to make a vertical incision directly over the cricothyroid membrane. The incision should be 1–2 cm in length. It is taken down through the skin and subcutaneous tissue and the platysma. As soon as the platysma is entered, a finger is introduced and the cricothyroid membrane is identified digitally. An incision is made with the scalpel through the cricothyroid membrane and into the trachea. The handle of the scalpel is then used to be introduced into the wound and turned through 90 degrees. This provides a generous otomy directly into the trachea. This scalpel handle technique is useful since there is a blood vessel at each lateral aspect of the cricothyroid membrane and it is preferable to perform a blunt dissection of the cricothyroid membrane. A tracheostomy tube is then introduced directly through the cricothyroid membrane into the trachea.

If the anatomy is distorted or if there is significant injury with a hematoma to this area, it is wise to pass a red rubber tube through the cricothyroid membrane into the trachea. The tracheostomy tube can then be advanced over the red rubber catheter. This will avoid creating a false passage or creating trauma to the trachea itself. Once the tracheostomy tube is in the trachea, the patient is then ventilated via the tracheostomy tube.

Emergency Surgical Tracheostomy

This procedure should be reserved for life-threatening situations. It is preferable to use any of the aforementioned airway adjuncts to gain control of the airway and adequately oxygenate the patient prior to performing an emergency tracheostomy. If there is adequate oxygenation, a transverse incision one finger-breadth above the suprasternal notch should be used. If, however, there is an emergency life-threatening procedure when time is of the essence, then a vertical incision should be made.

Procedure

The trachea is identified and controlled with one hand. An incision is made and carried down through the skin and platysma. Once the platysma is opened, it is essential that all dissection be performed in the midline. This will avoid the anterior jugular veins and the medial strap muscles. A dissection should be carried down to the trachea under direct vision. It is preferable to use a blunt clamp for dissection and then using the tip of the finger to identify the tracheal rings. If the isthmus of the thyroid is palpated on the surface of the trachea, it should be retracted cephalad and the trachea then identified. The membrane between the tracheal ring should be opened transversely for a distance of approximately 1 cm. A trapdoor can be created by placing a vertical incision at the lateral aspects of the wound and creating a flap in the trachea. A 2.0 Prolene suture should be placed through the trapdoor and left as a long retractor. The lumen of the trachea should be identified and a red rubber catheter introduced to ensure that there is no false passage. This is particularly important if there is an injury to the trachea and there is blood or mucosal hemorrhage in the trachea. The tracheostomy tube is then introduced into the tracheostomy and the cannulae removed. Ventilation should then occur. The tracheostomy tube should then be secured in place and the Prolene suture should be brought out through the wound and left in situ. This technique is extremely useful in event there is dislodgement of the tracheostomy tube. Traction on the suture opens the trapdoor and easily identifies the trachea. A new tube is then placed into the otomy in the trachea. This technique avoids difficulty in reintubation and the creation of false passages.

Management of Airway When Neck Is Lacerated

Lacerations to the anterior and lateral neck may involve the airway. It is essential to obtain a history as to how the laceration occurred. Whether this was a knife wound or an impaled object from a motor vehicle crash or a fall has different implications. An impaling object has the ability to create an injury to the cervical spine and spinal cord, and therefore, the neck has to be treated as if there was a potential injury to the spinal column. This requires stabilization of the neck.

In the event of a knife laceration in an assault, it is highly unlikely that there would be injury to the bony elements of the spinal cord and therefore, spinal cord injury is not a major factor.

The wound should be inspected for obvious pulsatile or nonpulsatile hemorrhage. Digital pressure should be applied to pulsatile arterial hemorrhage to control the hemorrhage. If the bleeding is nonpulsatile dark venous blood, it is important to remember that major venous injuries can precipitate air embolism by sucking air into the deep venous system and into the heart. This results in air embolism into the main pulmonary artery. An air lock is then created and pulmonary perfusion is significantly compromised. An air lock can also be created in the right ventricle with loss of function of the heart as an effective pump.

There are major nerves in association with the vascular structures in the neck, and therefore, blindly placing clamps into the wound should be avoided. Hemorrhage control should be either under direct vision or by a noncrushing clamp.

The wound should be palpated for pneumo crepitus. Air in the wound is a harbinger of an injury to the airway or the esophagus. Both of these structures would need to be identified and any injury dealt with in the operating room. The airway should be controlled either with an endotracheal tube or with a surgical airway. Once the airway is adequately controlled and the patient is effectively ventilated, then the patient should be transferred to the operating room for definitive control of hemorrhage and an evaluation of the aerodigestive tree either externally or with endoscopy in the operating room. The appropriate repair should then be carried out.

SUMMARY

Management of the airway in the trauma patient continues to be the most important life-saving event in the management of the severely injured and dying patient. It is essential that all surgeons are aware of the noninvasive and invasive methods of managing the airway. Identifying those patients who will not be able to be managed by conventional airway techniques such as endotracheal or nasotracheal intubation is critical. It is very important to determine when to proceed to a surgical airway and to be aware of the landmarks and potential pitfalls of obtaining an emergent surgical airway. Mastering all of these techniques and procedures will facilitate the emergent management of the severely injured patient's airway.

REFERENCES

1. American College of Surgeons: *Advanced Trauma Life Support® for Doctors Student Manual*, 6 ed. Chicago, American College of Surgeons Committee on Trauma, 2002.
2. Vesalius A: *de Humani Corporis Fabrica Libris Septum*. Basel, Oporinus, 1543.
3. University of Virginia Health System: Airway Management: Assessing the Patient, April 2004. Available at http://www.healthsystem.virginia.edu/Internet/Anesthesiology-Elective/airway/Assessment.cfm.
4. Shoemaker WC, et al: *Textbook of Critical Care*, 4 ed. Philadelphia, Saunders, 2000.
5. Mallampati SR, et al: A clinical sign to predict difficult tracheal intubation: a prospective study. *Can J Anaesth* 32:429, 1985.
6. Sellick B: Cricoid pressure to control regurgitation of stomach contents during induction of anesthesia. *Lancet* 2:404, 1961.
7. Mallampati SR: Recognition of the difficult airway. In Benumof JL, editor: *Airway Management: Principles and Practice*. St. Louis, MO, Mosby-Yearbook, Inc., 1996.
8. Benumof JL: Management of the difficult airway: with specific emphasis on awake tracheal intubation. *Anesthesiology* 75:1087, 1991.
9. Dunham CM, Barraco RD, et al: Guidelines for emergency tracheal intubation immediately after traumatic injury. *J Trauma* 55:162, 2003.
10. Parks SN: Initial assessment. In Matox KL, Feliciano DV, Moore EE, editors: *Trauma*, 5 ed. New York, McGraw-Hill, 2004, Chapter 10.
11. University of Virginia Health System: How to Intubate, April 2004. Available at http://www.healthsystem.virginia.edu/internet/anesthesiology-elective/airway/intubation.cfm.
12. Salem MR, Baraka A: Confirmation of tracheal intubation. In Benumof JL, editor: *Airway Management: Principles and Practice*. St. Louis, MO, Mosby-Yearbook, Inc., 1996, Chapter 27.
13. Wissler RN: The esophageal tracheal Combitube. *Anesth Rev* 20:147, 1993.
14. Smith CE, DeJoy SJ: New equipment and techniques for airway management in trauma. *Curr Opin Anaesthiol* 14(2):197, 2001.
15. Blostein PA, Koestner AJ, Hoak S: Failed rapid sequence intubation in trauma patients; esophageal tracheal Combitube is a useful adjunct. *J Trauma* 44:534, 1998.
16. Reynolds SF, Heffner J: Airway management of the critically ill patient: rapid sequence intubation. *Chest* 127:1397, 2005.
17. Viersen V: Rapid sequence induction for trauma, December 2005. Available at http://beta.trauma.org/traumawiki.
18. Perry JJ, Lee J, Wells G: Are intubation conditions using rocuronium equivalent to those using succinylcholine? *Acad Emerg Med* 9:813, 2002.
19. Schwartz DE, Mattay MA, Cohen NH: Death and other complications of airway management in critically ill adults. *Anesthesiology* 82:367, 1995.
20. Brain AI: The laryngeal mask—a new concept in airway management. *Br J Anaesth* 55:801, 1983.
21. Danne PD, Hunter M, MacKillop ADF: Airway control. In Matox KL, Feliciano DV, Moore EE, editors: *Trauma*, 5 ed. New York, McGraw-Hill, 2004, Chapter 11.

RESUSCITATION FLUIDS

Martin Schreiber, Brandon Tieu, Laszlo Kiraly, and Michael Englehart

The practice of giving intravenous fluids or medication has been used since the 1600s. Slow progress was made after William Harvey provided a modern description of the circulatory system in 1638. William O'Shaughnessy theorized that patients suffering from volume loss secondary to cholera would benefit from restoration of blood to its natural specific gravity. This became the first concept of contemporary intravenous fluid therapy. Thomas Latta was credited with actually applying O'Shaughnessy's theory and treating victims of cholera in 1832. Later in the century, Sydney Ringer described a physiologic solution with a focus on electrolyte concentrations in his animal models. Despite these early trials, application of these concepts was criticized and largely forgotten until the 20th century. The advent of modern surgery renewed interest in resuscitation as therapy to maintain intravascular volume.

World War I provided tremendous experience with resuscitation of hemorrhagic shock. Cannon's work eloquently described the natural history and presentation of shock with primary accounts of battlefield victims. His work suggested that a delay in surgical control of bleeding was accompanied by a large increase in mortality. Furthermore, he indicated that aggressive resuscitation without surgical control could worsen hemorrhagic shock. He also indicated that resuscitation with saline could worsen existing acidosis. In subsequent decades, however, much of his work was forgotten or ignored. Then in World War II and the Korean War, practice shifted to resuscitation with plasma and blood. Blalock supported this based on his dog studies, suggesting that crystalloid fluids were rapidly lost from the intravascular space. In 1963, Shires showed that shock is accompanied by a shift of interstitial fluid into the vasculature. This discovery brought renewed interest in salt solution therapy. Subsequent decades have been characterized by further optimization in aggressive resuscitation. Specific gains have been made in the realm of intensive care, monitoring, intravenous access, and endpoints of resuscitation. Despite these advances, many controversies and questions remain. Choice of fluid has been largely unchanged and unexamined. The study of the mechanism of shock at a cellular and molecular level has yet to reveal any applicable treatments. More importantly, the complications of modern resuscitation are commonly seen in trauma intensive care units. Before discussing details on fluids, it is important to understand hemorrhage and the physiologic response.

CLASSES OF SHOCK

Shock is inadequate tissue perfusion. The humoral sympathetic response to shock causes vasoconstriction in the clinical appearance of the patient. These findings were observed by Cannon when he correlated the volume of blood loss with the patient's clinical signs, symptoms, and blood pressure. His findings have since been validated with repeated observational studies in humans, as well as experimental studies in animals. The classes of shock are now well defined, and provide a quick means of assessing a patient's blood loss and the level of resuscitation required (Table 1).

AUTORESUSCITATION

The goal of the body's compensatory mechanisms during shock is to preserve perfusion to vital organs. Bickell's 1994 study of delayed fluid resuscitation for hypotensive patients with penetrating torso injuries demonstrated that, in the absence of resuscitation, blood pressure spontaneously increased prior to operative intervention. This finding validates observations made by Cannon, and has further been supported by subsequent data, which demonstrated that during hypotensive resuscitation blood pressure spontaneously rises toward normal in the absence of fluid therapy. Numerous mechanisms exist to account for these findings, specifically vasoconstriction, a reduction in capillary hydrostatic pressure, and hormonal responses. The sum of these responses is reflected in the phases of shock, which in turn help dictate the resuscitation strategy.

Vasoconstriction and Reduction of Capillary Hydrostatic Pressure

Peripheral and splanchnic vasoconstriction help to redirect blood flow away from muscle, skin, bowel, kidneys, and other nonvital organs. This is accomplished through the release of epinephrine, norepinephrine, and vasopressin. By increasing the peripheral vascular resistance, and effectively reducing the circulating volume through which the blood must pass, the mean arterial pressure is increased. Initially, during compensated shock, only the precapillary sphincter is constricted, reducing the capillary hydrostatic pressure and increasing the peripheral resistance. As the shock worsens, both the precapillary and postcapillary sphincters are constricted, leading to anaerobic metabolism, which results in excess lactate and acidosis. As the severity of shock increases, the postcapillary sphincter relaxes secondary to hydrogen ion buildup, releasing the metabolic byproducts into the circulation. The result is reperfusion injury. This is common when the system decompensates, and the patient shows signs of florid shock and global hypoperfusion.

The subsequent decrease in capillary hydrostatic pressure reduces the volume of plasma lost from the vasculature into the interstitial space, and increases return of interstitial fluid into the vascular space. This is an additional method of increasing venous return to the heart. Given the large capacitance of the venous system, larger volumes of circulating blood are stored within the veins compared to the arteries. According to the Frank-Starling laws of cardiac performance, the cardiac output is directly proportional to the venous return to the heart (preload) (Figure 1). As venous return decreases, so does cardiac output, and thereby arterial pressure to perfuse vital organs.

Hormonal Response

In response to hypotension, numerous hormonal pathways are initiated to restore circulating plasma volume. Vasopressin plays a major role in peripheral vasoconstriction. Additionally, it acts to increase free water absorption in the collecting ducts of the kidneys. In response to lower pressures at the afferent arteriole within the kidney, renin is released, triggering the renin/angiotensin/aldosterone cascade. The effect is to increase the absorption of sodium, which in turn increases water absorption. Additionally, angiotensin-II acts as a potent peripheral vasoconstrictor. Finally, cortisol acts to increase extracellular osmolarity and increased lymphatic flow.

The reduction of capillary hydrostatic pressure and the hormonal response increase venous return during the first 1–2 hours following injury, but this may be inconsequential in the setting of severe hemorrhage. Cessation or slowing of ongoing hemorrhage also

Table 1: Classes of Shock

	Class I	Class II	Class III	Class IV
Blood loss (ml)	<750	750–1500	1500–2000	>2000
Blood loss (% blood volume)	<15%	15%–30%	30%–40%	>40%
Urine output (ml/hr)	>30	20–30	5–15	Negligible
Mental status	Slight anxiety	Mild anxiety	Anxious, confused	Confused, lethargic
Skin	Warm	Cool, pale	Cool, pale	Cold, cyanotic, mottled
Thirst	Normal	Normal	Greater than normal	Much greater than normal
Fluid replacement	Crystalloid	Crystalloid	Crystalloid and blood	Crystalloid and blood

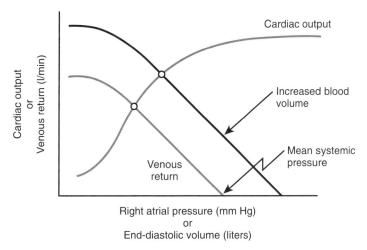

Figure 1 The effect of increased right atrial pressure on cardiac output. Increases in right atrial pressure are accomplished through either an increase in circulating blood volume, or a decrease in venous compliance. Cardiac output increases linearly in response to increased right atrial pressure. *(Adapted from Berne RM, Levy MN: Cardiovascular Physiology, 3rd ed. St. Louis, MO, Mosby, 1977.)*

contributes to a spontaneous rise in blood pressure by limiting ongoing fluid losses. The remainder of the response is carried out through vasoconstriction and the redistribution of blood flow, accounting for the majority of increased venous return. If prolonged, this can have a damaging, and sometimes irreversible effect upon the tissues supplied by the splanchnic circulation. This will result in ischemia and potential reperfusion injury.

Phases of Shock

Combined, the aforementioned physiologic effects produce the classic signs and symptoms exhibited by patients in hypovolemic shock. The progression from compensated to uncompensated shock gives rise to the physical findings of the systemic insult (Figure 2). Initially, compensated shock affects the periphery, manifesting the symptoms of cool extremities, cyanosis, mottling of the skin, and decreased capillary reperfusion (blanching). As the severity of shock progresses, vasoconstriction affects the torso, producing oliguria as the main clinical sign. Finally, in severe classes of shock, perfusion of the heart and brain are affected, producing cardiac dysrhythmias and a

reduced level of consciousness. Over the hours following injury, these mechanisms are in constant flux, in efforts to restore homeostasis to the injured system.

Lower cardiac output, variable tachycardia, oliguria, and decreased capillary pressure define the initial phase following hemorrhagic shock. The interstitial space is contracted in efforts to preserve circulating plasma volume. This occurs typically in the prehospital phase and extends into the early portions of the patient's initial resuscitation. During this period active replacement of blood loss is achieved through either crystalloid infusion or blood transfusion to restore circulating blood volume. The second phase is marked by extravascular fluid sequestration. This often occurs following surgical intervention and massive resuscitation. The intracellular and interstitial spaces expand as resuscitation continues, and blood pressure typically stabilizes. Crystalloids are given to maintain plasma volume based upon the patient's observed hemodynamic status. The third and final stage is marked by diuresis and mobilization of fluids with an increase in blood pressure. This response occurs only after appropriate volume resuscitation, surgical correction of the cause of the hemorrhage, and resolution of organ failure with return to a more homeostatic state.

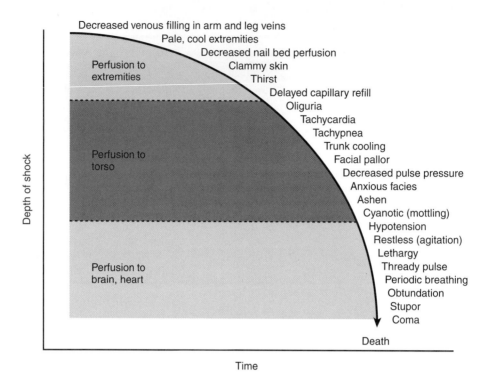

Figure 2 Signs and symptoms of shock.

HYPOTENSIVE RESUSCITATION

Traditional resuscitation strategies have been directed toward restoring normal intravascular fluid volumes and arterial blood pressures to maintain perfusion to vital organs. Since the early 1990s, this approach has been re-examined. The strategy of hypotensive resuscitation dictates delivery of limited volumes of intravenous fluids to sustain blood pressures lower than normal. In delayed resuscitation, fluids are withheld until control of the hemorrhage has been established. Tissue injury from regional hypoperfusion is a risk of these strategies. It depends on both length of time and severity of hypoperfusion. A single accurate method to assess regional hypoperfusion has not been established. Rapid resuscitation can exacerbate bleeding by dislodging fragile clots, decreasing blood viscosity, and creating compartment syndromes of the cranial vault, abdomen, and extremities. It also exacerbates the "lethal triad" of hypothermia, acidosis, and coagulopathy.

In a swine aortotomy model, Sondeen noted the average mean arterial pressure at which rebleeding occurred following uncontrolled hemorrhagic shock and spontaneous clotting was 64 mm Hg. This was independent of time of resuscitation. In addition, crystalloid solutions reduce the oxygen carrying capacity of the blood by dilution. The optimal volume of intravenous fluid administered is a balance between improving tissue perfusion and increasing blood loss by raising systolic blood pressure. Cannon stated that early control of hemorrhage was paramount and attempts at fluid resuscitation prior to this would result in increased bleeding and mortality. This concept has been evaluated in both animal and human studies. Previous animal studies used controlled hemorrhage models where hemostasis was achieved early allowing rapid restoration to a normovolemic state. Unfortunately, in the clinical setting the bleeding source may not be immediately known or immediate control is not possible. Using an aortotomy model in immature swine, Bickell and colleagues showed unfavorable outcomes in those swine resuscitated with lactated Ringer's or hypertonic saline/dextran compared with no fluid.

In a prospective randomized study, Bickell compared immediate and delayed fluid resuscitation in hypotensive patients (systolic blood pressure [SBP] <90 mm Hg) with penetrating injuries to the torso. There was a statistically significant difference in survival between the two groups, 62% versus 70% ($p=0.04$), suggesting delayed resuscitation improved outcomes in penetrating injuries to the torso. The study was criticized for its predominantly young, male patient population, and its urban setting with short transfer times. Subsequent subgroup analysis showed survival benefits only in patients with cardiac injuries and no difference in survival when deaths were divided into preoperative, intraoperative, and postoperative time periods. Dutton compared fluid resuscitation to SBP 70 mm Hg versus SBP of greater than 100 mm Hg in actively hemorrhaging patients. Resuscitation to a lower SBP did not affect overall mortality. Both blunt and penetrating trauma patients were included in this study.

Further randomized controlled trials are needed before a hypotensive resuscitation strategy can be defined. Currently, patients suffering from blunt injuries should be managed with traditional strategies. Although the ideal target blood pressure remains elusive, in penetrating injuries an SBP of 80–90 mm Hg may be adequate. A significant association exists between prehospital hypotension (SBP <90) and worse outcomes in severe traumatic brain injury (TBI). Attempts to maintain SBP above 90 may decrease adverse outcomes in head-injured patients, although no class I evidence is available to corroborate this.

The current literature on hypotensive resuscitation cannot be extrapolated to all trauma patients but it emphasizes the importance of rapid diagnosis and treatment. Early identification of bleeding sources and control of hemorrhage will lead to more rapid replacement of intravascular volume and decreased morbidity and mortality.

Choice of Fluids

The use of crystalloids versus colloids has been an ongoing debate for decades. In the Vietnam War, isotonic crystalloids were used when laboratory work from the 1960s by Shires and others showed larger volume resuscitation with isotonic crystalloids resulted in the best survival. They also noted that extracellular fluid redistributed into both intravascular and intracellular spaces during shock, and rapid correction of this extracellular deficit required an infusion of a 3:1 ratio of crystalloid fluid to blood loss. Figure 3 shows the influence of fluids on the extracellular fluid compartments. Using this resuscitation strategy, the rate of mortality and acute renal failure decreased but a new entity of shock lung, now better known as acute respiratory distress syndrome (ARDS), was discovered. In reviewing studies comparing crystalloids and colloids with respect to pleural effusions and pulmonary dysfunction, two trials reported no differences. Two other series showed more pulmonary complications among patients resuscitated with colloid. When mortality was used as an endpoint, the use of crystalloids in trauma patients was associated with increased survival.

There are advantages and disadvantages to the use of both crystalloids and colloids. Crystalloids replace interstitial as well as intravascular fluid loss, do not cause allergic reactions, and are inexpensive. Possible disadvantages include limited intravascular expansion and tissue edema, which can impair gas exchange in the lungs and diminish bowel perfusion. Colloids have a longer intravascular half-life, which may improve organ perfusion and may cause less tissue edema. This may be a short-term effect as the interstitial oncotic pressure increases

from diffusion of the colloid over time. Also, the choice of colloid may affect blood loss. Other possible disadvantages include increased incidence of allergic reactions, impaired blood cross matching due to dextrans, altered platelet function (dextrans, hetastarches), hyperchloremic acidosis due to high chloride content (hetastarch), and greater expense. A meta-analysis of clinical studies comparing crystalloids and colloids for fluid resuscitation failed to show any evidence of improved outcome with the use of colloids. In summary, there is no clear basis to give colloid products over crystalloid solutions for fluid resuscitation.

Crystalloid Solutions

The choice of lactated Ringer's (LR) and normal saline (NS) appears to be less controversial. Both are hypo-oncotic, balanced salt solutions (Table 2). It is well known that large volumes of NS resuscitation can lead to hyperchloremic metabolic acidosis. While large volumes of LR infused rapidly can increase lactate levels, this is not associated with acidosis. Koustova et al. have shown that LR influences neutrophil function by increasing production of reactive oxygen species and affects leukocyte gene expression, but Watters et al. showed that NS and LR have equivalent effects on alveolar neutrophils in a swine model of hemorrhagic shock. Healy et al. showed, in a rat model of

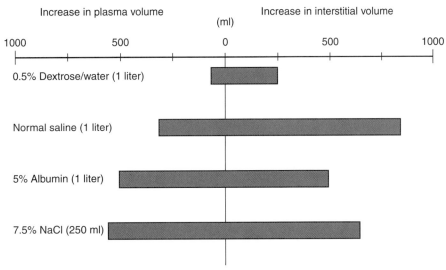

Figure 3 The influence of colloid and crystalloid fluids on the volume of the extracellular fluid compartments. *(Data from Imm A, Carlson RW: Fluid resuscitation in circulatory shock.* Crit Care Clin *9:313, 1993.)*

Table 2: Composition of Balanced Salt Solutions (meq/l)

Solutions	Glucose (g/l)	Na⁺	Cl⁻	NCO₃⁻	K⁺	Ca²⁺	Mg²⁺	HPO₄⁻	NH₄⁺
Extracellular fluid	1000	140	102	27	4.2	5	3	3	0.3
5% dextrose and water	50								
0.21% sodium chloride (0.25 NS)		34	34						
0.45% sodium chloride (0.5 NS)		77	77						
0.9% sodium chloride (NS)		154	154						
3% sodium chloride (HS)		513	513						
7.5% sodium chloride (HS)		1283	1283						
Lactated Ringer's solution		130	109	28ᵃ	4	2.7			

ᵃPresent in solution as lactate, but is metabolized to bicarbonate.

HS, Hypertonic saline; *NS,* normal saline.

massive hemorrhage and resuscitation, animals were significantly more acidotic (pH 7.14 ± 0.06 vs. 7.39 ± 0.04) and had a significantly worse survival (50% vs. 100%) when resuscitated with NS compared to LR. NS has been theoretically preferred when giving blood because of the concern that the calcium in LR could exceed the chelating capabilities of the citrate, resulting in clots that may enter the microcirculation. However, Lorenzo et al. showed that when fluid is given rapidly, LR does not increase clots, and at present there is no evidence that this is a clinically significant issue. In theory, NS is favored over LR for the treatment of severe head injuries due to its higher sodium content, which would reduce intracerebral swelling. Despite this concern, there is no literature supporting the use of NS over LR in this setting.

Ringer's ethyl pyruvate solution (REPS) is a calcium- and potassium-containing balanced salt solution. Ethyl pyruvate is derived from pyruvate, which is unstable in aqueous solutions, and acts as a potent reactive species of oxygen scavenger (e.g., H_2O_2, O_2, OH). It has been evaluated in several preclinical studies using animal models of mesenteric ischemia/reperfusion injury, hemorrhagic shock, and acute endotoxemia. In comparison to LR, REPS has been shown to improve survival and decrease expression of proinflammatory mediators. However, a recent study using a swine hemorrhagic shock model showed no short-term hemodynamic or tissue energetic advantage to using REPS as a resuscitation fluid when compared to LR. Further investigations are needed to evaluate the potential benefits of using REPS in hemorrhagic shock.

Hypertonic Saline

Hypertonic saline (HS) has osmotic properties that result in influx of fluid into the intravascular space. Because only small volumes are needed to achieve its desired effects, there has been significant interest in its use in the military and civilian settings. It is capable of rapidly expanding the intravascular volume and enhancing microcirculation by selective arteriolar vasodilatation. This occurs without causing swelling of red blood cells or the endothelium. Unfortunately, this improved microcirculation could also lead to increased bleeding. Adding dextran and hetastarch to HS can prolong its intravascular effects due to increased oncotic pressure. The volume of hypertonic saline solution that can be given is limited by the potential development of hypernatremia and intravascular volume overload. In a swine model of uncontrolled hemorrhagic shock, a single 250-ml bolus of 3% hypertonic saline plus 6% dextran produced an adequate and sustained rise in mean arterial pressure (MAP) and StO_2. More importantly, the increase in MAP was not associated with increased secondary bleeding. A meta-analysis by Wade et al. of both HS and HS with dextran (HSD) in the treatment of hypotension from traumatic injury suggests that HS is no different than isotonic crystalloids, but HSD did show a trend toward decreased mortality. In head trauma patients, its ability to draw fluid from the extravascular space can limit cerebral edema, lower intracranial pressure, and improve cerebral perfusion. Subgroup analysis in the previous study by Wade showed the greatest benefit with HSD to be in shock patients with concomitant severe closed head injuries. A recent prospective randomized study from Australia testing HS for field resuscitation in hypotensive and TBI patients failed to show any benefit in neurological outcome at 6 months when compared to LR. HS and HSD have also demonstrated a diminished inflammatory response, specifically neutrophil cytotoxicity, in animal models of hemorrhagic shock, ischemia/reperfusion, and sepsis.

Artificial Oxygen-Carrying Blood Substitutes

Although both crystalloids and colloids can replace intravascular volume, neither product restores the oxygen-carrying capacity of the lost red blood cells. Artificial hemoglobin products have the potential to improve oxygen-carrying capacity without the storage, availability, immune suppression, transfusion reaction, compatibility, or disease transmission problems associated with standard transfusions. Unfortunately, these products also fail to restore coagulation components, and hemostasis can be hindered with the loss of cellular elements that lower the viscosity of circulating blood. The use of a large volume of artificial oxygen-carrying solutions in severe hemorrhage has not been adequately studied.

Hemoglobin-based oxygen carriers have been derived from human blood, bovine blood, and recombinant DNA technology dating back to 1933. Carrier solutions need to be stroma-free polymerized or cross-linked hemoglobin tetramers with oxygen-carrying capabilities that remain within the intravascular space for a prolonged period of time. Early hemoglobin substitutes had a greater oxygen affinity because of the loss of 2,3 diphosphoglycerate (2,3 DPG). However, with pyridoxylation of the hemoglobin tetramer this problem was addressed. Hemoglobin-based oxygen carriers can also cause vasoconstriction. This occurs because tetrameric hemoglobin binds the nitric oxide in the vascular wall and results in unopposed vasoconstriction. Because of this phenomenon, blood pressures can be higher than expected for the level of intravascular volume replacement in hemorrhagic shock patients. Initial studies of these products in humans have been disappointing. A phase III trial of diaspirin cross-linked hemoglobin was prematurely stopped due to an unexpectedly high mortality in the treatment group (46 vs. 17%). Polyheme®, glutaraldehyde-polymerized pyridoxylated human hemoglobin, has proven to be safe and effective in phase I and II trials and is currently being studied in a multicenter phase III prehospital trial.

Perfluorocarbons are chemically and biologically inert liquids that dissolve large amounts of gas. They require dispersion in plasma-like aqueous fluids such as albumin or in physiologic electrolyte solutions to be an adequate oxygen-carrying substitute. They have a lower oxygen-delivering capacity than normal blood and require an FiO_2 of greater than 70% to carry physiologically useful concentration of oxygen. The long-term biological effects of absorption, distribution, metabolism, and excretion, and the effects on the reticular endothelial system (RES) require further evaluation. Concern about toxicity to the RES and high FiO_2 requirements may limit their use in severe hemorrhage.

Blood Transfusions

The use of blood transfusions in resuscitation has been an ongoing debate since its initial use in World War I and in World War II, when it became the standard of care. There was an increase in early survival, but many casualties later died of acute renal failure. It is generally accepted that a patient in shock who fails to respond adequately to 2 liters of crystalloid is in need of blood transfusions. It is clear in unstable patients with active bleeding and hemorrhagic shock that blood should be given immediately. When larger volumes of crystalloid and red blood cells are given, fresh frozen plasma, platelets, or cryoprecipitate may also be needed to reverse the associated dilutional coagulopathy. One must also consider the inherent risks of blood transfusion, such as transfusion reactions, transfusion-related acute lung injury, infection, and immunosuppression. It has been observed that blood transfusions contain proinflammatory mediators that both prime and activate neutrophils. This has been proposed as a key mechanism in the development of multiple organ failure. Stored red blood cells also undergo substantial shape changes and impaired deformability by the second week of storage. This decreased deformity can lead to microvascular obstruction, and has been found to be associated with the development of splanchnic ischemia. Malone et al. reported that trauma patients who underwent blood transfusions within the first 24 hours of admission, independent of shock severity, were almost three times more likely to die than those who did not receive transfusions.

Early clinical studies concluded that hemoglobin (HgB) levels of 10 g/dl were optimal for shock resuscitation; however, recent consensus panels have suggested that a lower concentration is adequate. A prospective randomized trial showed that ICU patients who received blood transfusion for HgB less than 7.0 g/dl and were maintained at HgB 7.0–9.0 g/dl did as well and possibly better than patients who were liberally transfused for a HgB level less than 10 g/dl and maintained at 10–12 g/dl. All these patients were without ongoing bleeding, acute myocardial infarction, or unstable angina. Subgroup analysis looking at the safety of a restricted red blood cell transfusion strategy in trauma patients showed there was no statistically significant difference in mortality, multiple organ dysfunction, or length of stay, when compared to those managed with the liberal transfusion strategy. Randomized, controlled investigations need to be conducted to provide evidence to help dictate the use of blood in critically ill trauma patients.

COMPLICATIONS OF RESUSCITATION

The focus in resuscitation has shifted to large-volume fluid resuscitation in acutely injured patients. With severe hemorrhagic shock and uncontrolled hemorrhage, interventions can commonly cause iatrogenic complications. Continued large volume crystalloid resuscitation in the setting of ongoing bleeding inevitably leads to acidosis, hypothermia, and coagulopathy. Individually, each of these conditions can worsen the other (Figure 4).

Hypothermia

The definition of hypothermia is a core body temperature of less than 35° C. The internal core temperature is a net result of heat production and heat loss. Heat loss or production can be a result of

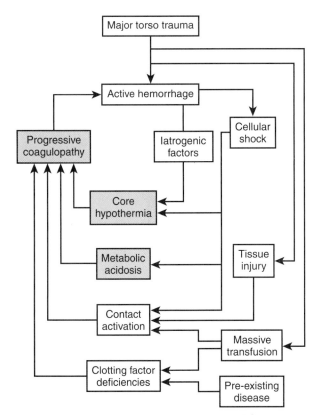

Figure 4 The lethal triad. (*Adapted from Moore EE: Staged laparotomy for the hypothermia, acidosis, coagulopathy syndrome. Am J Surg 172:405–410, 1996, with permission of publisher.*)

evaporation, radiation, conduction, or convection. Heat production largely occurs as a result of cellular metabolism while heat loss occurs through the skin and respiratory system. Acutely injured trauma patients have numerous sources of potential heat loss. Exposure in the field can cause the patient to be hypothermic on admission. Further exposure per ATLS protocols causes further losses. Operations involving exposure of body cavities cause significant losses through evaporative and conductive means. Trauma procedures involving large laparotomies or thoracotomies are especially threatening. In terms of resuscitation, intravenous fluids present the highest potential for heat loss. This can be quantified by the following equation:

$$Heat = mass \times specific\ heat \times (T_{body} - T_{fluid})$$

Given a specific heat of water of 4.19 kJ/kg/degree, 1 liter of 25° C crystalloid infused in a normothermic patient would result in a heat loss of 50.3 kJ. This heat loss exceeds the heat that can be returned to the patient by conventional methods in 1 hour. Given these findings, massive heat loss can occur in the setting of large-scale resuscitation.

The incidence of hypothermia in trauma patients during resuscitation has been described to be as high as 66%. Although Gregory et al. found that only 12% of patients arriving in the ED were hypothermic, 46% were hypothermic on arrival to the operating room (OR), and 57% were hypothermic when leaving the OR. This suggests that the majority of heat loss occurs in the resuscitation bay.

Hypothermia is commonly classified by severity. Mild hypothermia is a core temperature of 32°–35° C, and is characterized by tachypnea, tachycardia, hyperventilation, shivering, and impaired judgment. Increased urine output secondary to a "cold diuresis" has also been described. This is thought to be secondary to peripheral vasoconstriction, causing a temporary increase in the central intravascular volume. In moderate hypothermia, defined as 28°–32° C, heart rate and cardiac output are reduced. Decreased mental status and hyporeflexia are observed as well as decreased renal blood flow. Cardiac rhythm manifestations include atrial fibrillation and bradycardia. Severe hypothermia, that is, temperatures less than 28° C, can lead to pulmonary edema, oliguria, coma, hypotension, ventricular fibrillation, and asystole.

Hypothermia in the trauma patient is a poor prognostic indicator and it has been shown to be independently predictive of mortality. The mortality of victims of accidental exposure with moderate hypothermia has been documented to be 21%. However, trauma victims studied with similar core temperatures (<32° C) have 100% mortality. This difference has several explanations. Trauma patients do have similar losses secondary to exposure; however, they also have further losses secondary to hemorrhage and exposed body cavities. Beyond this, the decreased oxygen consumption secondary to blood loss and shock cause decreased heat production. Given these mechanisms, the mortality documented may be more a manifestation of the severity of injury rather than isolated hypothermia.

Because of the strong association of hypothermia to mortality and the other elements of the "lethal triad," rewarming and prevention of ongoing heat loss should be a priority of resuscitation (Table 3). The first step is to obtain an accurate core temperature. Esophageal or bladder temperatures have been shown to be more reliable than rectal or axillary measurements. Given the high rate of heat loss with infusion of room temperature fluids, all resuscitation solutions should be warmed. Operating room temperatures should be elevated to minimize losses due to conduction and radiation. Once the secondary evaluation is complete, the patient should be covered. A Bair Hugger or similar device can be used to actively warm the patient. For profound hypothermia, active internal rewarming can be used. This is done either with lavage of a body cavity (peritoneal or thoracic) or by intravascular rewarming. Options for intravascular rewarming include veno-venous rewarming, arteriovenous rewarming, or cardiopulmonary bypass. Continuous arteriovenous rewarming (Figure 5) has been shown to decrease early mortality in critically injured hypothermic trauma patients.

Table 3: Approximate Rate of Heat Transfer with Available Rewarming Methods

Rewarming Technique	Rate of Heat Transfer
Airway rewarming	33.5–50.3
Overhead radiant warmer	71.2
Heating blankets	83.8
Convective warmers	62.8–108.9
Body cavity lavage	150.8
Continuous arteriovenous rewarming	385.5–582.4
Cardiopulmonary bypass	2974.9

Source: Adapted from Gentilello LM: Practical approaches to hypothermia. In Maull KI, Cleveland HC, Feliciano DV, Rice CL, Trunkey DD, Wolferth CC, editors: *Advances in Trauma and Critical Care*, vol. 9. St. Louis, MO, Mosby, 1994, pp. 39–79, with permission.

Coagulopathy

Hemorrhage is a major cause of early trauma deaths. Coagulopathies in trauma patients are common during major resuscitations. The mechanisms are thought to be related to hypothermia, metabolic disturbances, dilution, and disseminated intravascular coagulation. Most of these mechanisms can be traced in some way to resuscitation.

Dilution is a major cause of coagulopathy in resuscitated trauma patients. Intravascular fluid containing coagulation factors is lost and replaced with solutions lacking these products. The actual amount of coagulopathy is not easily predictable as the plasma shifts are quite complex. Coagulation factors are continually produced and sequestered in the post trauma setting. Dilutional coagulopathy is not thought to play a significant role until approximately one blood volume of replacement fluids is infused into a patient. Therefore, giving prophylactic products without data or evidence of bleeding is generally not recommended. However, there is increasing evidence that the early administration of coagulation factors is indicated.

Hypothermia has a profound effect on coagulation activity. Reed and Rohrer in different experiments showed that hypothermia resulted in prolonged partial thromboplastin time (PTT) and prothrombin time (PT) independent of the actual level of enzymes. Gubler et al. showed that the effect of a dilutional coagulopathy is additive to this hypothermic effect (Figure 6). In addition to these enzyme effects, fibrinolysis is thought to be enhanced by hypothermia. Animal studies have suggested that platelets are sequestered by the spleen in the setting of hypothermia. Platelet adhesion is also decreased in hypothermic patients. A recent in vitro study suggests that platelet effects cause the majority of hypothermic coagulopathy at temperatures above 33° C. In this trial, enzymatic dysfunction did not have a significant effect until the temperature was below 33° C. Studies have shown that acidotic and hypothermic patients with adequate blood, plasma, and platelet replacement still develop clinically significant bleeding.

Logically, one could conclude that this coagulopathy would result in more hemorrhage and poor outcomes. This has been substantiated in clinical reviews. A recent review of trauma patients revealed that 24.4% were coagulopathic on admission. Nonsurvivors had a coagulopathy rate of 46 versus 10.9% for survivors.

As with any disease, treatment of coagulopathy begins with recognizing the problem. Any trauma patient with evidence of significant tissue injury or ongoing bleeding should be screened with an (INR), PTT, platelet count, and fibrinogen level. In the setting of active traumatic bleeding, the platelet count should be kept above 50,000/mcl, the INR is less than 2, the fibrinogen greater than 100 mg/dl, and the PTT less than 1.5 times normal. Again, close monitoring of these parameters is recommended as empiric therapy often yields unpredictable

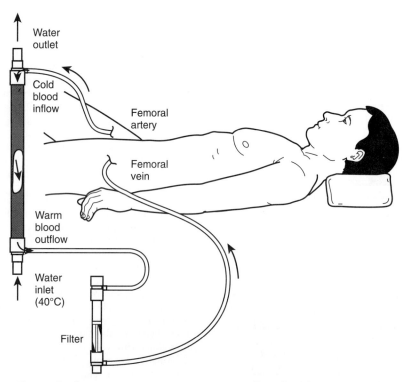

Figure 5 Continuous arteriovenous rewarming. *(From Gentilello LM, Jurkovich GJ, Stark MS, Hassantash SA, O'Keefe GE: Continuous arteriovenous rewarming: rapid reversal of hypothermia in critically ill patients. J Trauma 32(3):316–327, 1992, with permission.)*

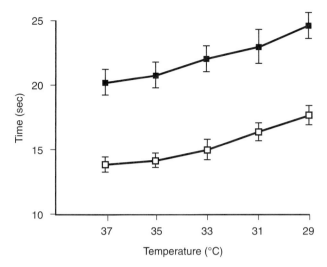

Figure 6   The effect of hypothermia and dilution on prothrombin time. Filled squares, diluted specimens; open squares, nondiluted specimens. *(From Gubler KD, Gentilello LM, Hassantash SA, Maier RV: The impact of hypothermia on dilutional coagulopathy. J Trauma 36(6):847–851, 1994.)*

results. In the absence of laboratory results, empiric therapy with platelets that contains plasma may be started.

Coagulopathy is also specifically linked to head trauma. The release of thromboplastin from injured brain tissue can cause severe consumptive coagulopathy leading to disseminated intravascular coagulopathy. More extensive coagulation monitoring is indicated in the setting of head trauma. There are reports and ongoing studies on the use of recombinant-activated factor VIIa in the setting of massive resuscitation and transfusion. This approach has not been widely accepted, but is likely effective in immediately reversing coagulopathy in the setting of continued bleeding.

Acidosis

Metabolic acidosis is commonly seen in trauma patients with hemorrhagic shock. This is postulated to occur secondary to tissue hypoperfusion in the setting of decreased cardiac output and oxygen-carrying capacity. This cascade of events eventually leads to anaerobic metabolism with the production of lactate. Massive resuscitation with crystalloid solutions has been associated with the development of a worsening metabolic acidosis. Following the Stewart model of acid base equilibrium, the administration of solutions with supraphysiologic levels of chloride relative to sodium results in a decreased strong ion difference (SID). $(Na + K + Ca + Mg - Cl - lactate)$. This decreased SID causes further dissociation of $H+$ from H_2O to maintain charge neutrality, and therefore a decreased pH.

Although the presence of a hyperchloremic acidosis has not been associated with increased mortality, there are many potential hazards of profound acidosis. Acidosis has a depressant effect on the myocardium and increases ventricular dysrhythmias. The sympathetic-adrenal axis is stimulated in the setting of acidosis. However, the myocardium has decreased responsiveness to circulating catecholamines. The prolonged acidotic state also increases respiratory drive, increases intracranial pressures in head-injured patients, and worsens coagulopathy. A more common danger exists in misinterpreting a hyperchloremic acidosis for continued hypoperfusion and shock leading to unnecessary therapies.

In order to avoid hyperchloremic acidosis, fluids with supraphysiologic concentrations of chloride should be avoided. LR contains a more physiologic concentration of chloride (109 meq/l) compared to normal saline (154 meq/l). Several clinical series and

animal studies document profound acidosis in the setting of large volume normal saline administration. Although less probable, this acidosis can be seen with LR, as its SID is less than physiologic. Careful monitoring of electrolytes with measurement of the anion gap can aid in guiding therapy. A normal or narrowed anion gap should be seen in the setting of an isolated hyperchloremic metabolic acidosis, as opposed to an elevated gap in lactic acidosis. Transitioning to fluids with less chloride (LR or Plasmalyte) or no chloride (Na acetate) can resolve the hyperchloremic acidosis.

The mechanism of coagulopathy in acidotic patients is a matter of active investigation. In vitro experiments have shown a decrease in the activity of factor VIIa-tissue factor and factor Xa-Va complexes. In vivo animal experiments have shown that acidosis independently decreases fibrinogen and platelet counts, increases PTT, and increases clinical bleeding time. In a study of patients undergoing massive transfusion, pH less than 7.10 independently predicted coagulopathy.

Compartment Syndromes

Tissue edema is a frequent result of large volume resuscitation in the setting of shock. In most cases, this edema has little immediately obvious harmful effects. However, in restricted body compartments, the resulting increase in pressure can lead to ischemia and subsequent tissue necrosis. The three affected areas are the extremities, abdomen, and cranial vault.

Extremity compartment syndrome most often results as a result of traumatic injury with or without an associated fracture. Although infrequent, compartment syndromes have been described in the absence of injury in the setting of large volume resuscitation. This entity has been labeled secondary extremity compartment syndrome. This process likely results from reperfusion after a period of severe shock. The subsequent release of inflammatory mediators results in a capillary leak phenomenon. When this is combined with large volumes of blood and fluids, the edema can overwhelm the fascial compartments leading to limb or muscle ischemia. As with any compartment syndrome, early recognition, diagnosis, and treatment are paramount for limb salvage.

The abdominal compartment syndrome (ACS) has been described over the past century, but was clearly recognized and defined in the early 1990s. It is defined as organ dysfunction secondary to intraabdominal hypertension. ACS was originally described in patients with abdominal operations or abdominal trauma. Since that time, ACS has been further classified as primary ACS, occurring from an insult to the intra-abdominal contents, and secondary ACS, occurring as a result of shock and massive resuscitation. Secondary ACS is theorized to occur by several mechanisms. As more intravenous fluid is given, more interstitial edema develops. Plasma proteins are also further diluted potentially diminishing intravascular oncotic pressure. The edema that forms increases intra-abdominal pressure and decreases splanchnic venous return. This process eventually causes decreased central venous return prompting further administration of fluids. This forms another vicious cycle of resuscitation.

Several studies have investigated the risk factors and mortality of secondary ACS. All studies indicate that severe shock and massive resuscitation are predisposing factors. Reviewed case series report a resuscitation volume averaging from 16–38 liters of crystalloid and 13–29 units of blood. Balogh et al. concluded that trauma patients undergoing supranormal resuscitation ($DO_2 > 600$) had received significantly more crystalloid and had a significantly higher rate of abdominal compartment syndrome (16% vs. 8%). The supranormal arm received an average of 13 liters of LR versus 7 liters in the standard resuscitation group. Patients suffering from secondary ACS had mortality rates ranging from 38% to 67%. This suggests that ACS may be prevented with judicious use of fluids and avoiding unnecessary volume overload.

Bladder pressures should be monitored in patients showing clinical signs of ACS or patients in shock who are receiving large resuscitations. A tense abdomen in the setting of low urine output, high airway pressures, and hypotension are diagnostic of ACS. Maxwell's series observed that nonsurvivors of secondary ACS had a time to OR of 25 hours versus 3 hours for survivors. This indicates that secondary ACS can happen very early in resuscitation. Furthermore, prompt diagnosis and treatment may be beneficial for survival.

Elevated intracranial pressure is a frequent result of traumatic brain injury and subsequent intracranial hemorrhage. The total volume of the intracranial vault is approximately 1600 cc. This is generally divided into 80% cerebral tissue, 10% blood, and 10% cerebral spinal fluid. Cerebral edema results from direct injury and a capillary leak phenomenon similar to the other compartment syndromes. Resuscitation with too much intravenous fluid can worsen this process. Given the composition of the vault contents, medical management offers limited treatment once pathologic intracranial hypertension develops. More invasive methods such as ventriculostomy or craniectomy should be used in a timely fashion when medical therapy fails.

SUMMARY

The resuscitation of trauma victims continues to evolve. Despite years of accumulated evidence, debate still rages over crystalloid and colloid solutions, hypotensive resuscitation, blood transfusions, and novel fluid therapy. Similarly, the goals of resuscitation are still controversial and the search for the perfect endpoint is ongoing. The focus in resuscitation should be to restore intravascular volume to provide protective physiology to the critically injured patient. Complications of resuscitation can be minimized with careful monitoring and respecting intravenous resuscitation as a potentially harmful medication rather than simply fluid.

SUGGESTED READINGS

Alderson P, Schierhout G, Roberts I, et al: Colloids versus crystalloids for fluid resuscitation in critically ill patients. *Cochrane Database Syst Rev* 2: CD000567, 2000.
Balogh Z, et al: Supranormal trauma resuscitation causes more cases of abdominal compartment syndrome. *Arch Surg* 138(6):637, 2003.

Bickell WH, et al: Immediate versus delayed fluid resuscitation for hypotensive patients with penetrating torso injuries. *N Engl J Med* 331:1105–1109, 1994.
Cannon WB, et al: The preventative treatment on wound shock. *JAMA* 70:618–621, 1918.
Cooper DJ, Myles PS, McDermott FT, et al: Prehospital hypertonic saline resuscitation of patients with hypotension and severe traumatic brain injury: a randomized controlled trial. *JAMA* 291(11):1350–1357, 2004.
Dutton MD, et al: Hypotensive resuscitation during active hemorrhage: impact on in-hospital mortality. *J Trauma* 52(6):1141–1146, 2002.
Gregory JS, et al: Incidence and timing of hypothermia in trauma patients undergoing operations. *J Trauma* 31(6):795–798, 1991.
Gubler KD, et al: The impact of hypothermia on dilutional coagulopathy. *J Trauma* 36(6):847–851, 1994.
Hebert PC, Wells G, Blajchman MA, et al: A multicenter, randomized, controlled clinical trial of transfusion requirements in critical care, *N Engl J Med* 340:409–417, 1999.
Jurkovich GJ, et al: Hypothermia in trauma victims: an ominous predictor of survival. *J Trauma* 27(9):1019–1024, 1987.
Malone DL, Dunne J, Tracy JK, et al: Blood transfusion, independent of shock severity, is associated with worse outcome in trauma. *J Trauma* 54: 898–905, 2003.
Martini WZ, et al: Independent contributions of hypothermia and acidosis to coagulopathy in swine. *J Trauma* 58(5):1002–1009, 2005.
McIntyre L, Hebert PC, Wells G, et al: Is a restrictive transfusion strategy safe for resuscitated and critically ill trauma patients? *J Trauma* 57(3): 563–568, 2004.
Reed RD, et al: Hypothermia and blood coagulation: dissociation between enzyme activity and clotting factor levels. *Circ Shock* 32(2):141–152, 1990.
Rohrer MJ, Natale AM: Effect of hypothermia on the coagulation cascade. *Crit Care Med* 20(10):1402–1405, 1992.
Schreiber MA, Aoki N, Scott BG, Beck JR: Determinants of mortality in patients with severe blunt head injury. *Arch Surg* 137(3):285–290, 2002.
Todd SR, Malinoski D, Schreiber MA: Lactated Ringer's is superior to normal saline in uncontrolled hemorrhagic shock. *J Trauma* 61(1): 57–64, discussion 64-5, 2006.
Watters JM, Brundage JM, Todd SR, et al: Resuscitation with lactated Ringer's does not increase inflammatory response in a Swine model of uncontrolled hemorrhagic shock. *Shock* 22(3):283–287, 2004.
Watters JM, Tieu BH, Differding JA, Muller PJ, Schreiber MA: A single bolus of 3% hypertonic saline with 6% dextran provides optimal resuscitation after uncontrolled hemorrhagic shock. *J Trauma* 61(1):75–81, 2006.
Wolberg AS, et al: A systematic evaluation of the effect of temperature on coagulation enzyme activity and platelet function. *J Trauma* 56(6): 1221–1228, 2004.

EMERGENCY DEPARTMENT THORACOTOMY

Juan A. Asensio, Patrizio Petrone, Luis Manuel García-Núñez, Dan L. Deckelbaum, Dominic Duran, Donald Robinson, Kenneth D. Stahl, Michael F. Ksycki, Francisco A. Ruiz Zelaya, Alexander D. Vara, John S. Weston, Allan Capin, and Carl Schulman

Emergency department thoracotomy (EDT) remains a formidable tool within the trauma surgeon's armamentarium. Since its introduction during the 1960s, the use of this procedure has ranged from sparing to liberal.[1] At many urban trauma centers, this procedure has found a niche as part of the resuscitative process.[1] Because of improvements in emergency medical services systems (EMS), many critically injured patients now arrive in extremis prompting trauma surgeons to perform this procedure to attempt saving their lives. This technically complex procedure should only be performed by surgeons familiar with the management of penetrating cardiothoracic injuries.

Indications for the use of EDT appearing in the literature range from vague to quite specific.[1] It has been used in a variety of settings including penetrating and blunt thoracic and/or thoracoabdominal injuries, cardiac and exsanguinating abdominal vascular injuries.[1-4] It has also been used rarely in exsanguinating peripheral vascular injuries arriving in cardiopulmonary arrest and also in pediatric trauma. Many studies in the literature have also reported its use in patients presenting in cardiopulmonary arrest secondary to blunt trauma.

HISTORIC PERSPECTIVE

In 1874, Schift[5] was first to promote the concept of open cardiac massage. Rehn[6] in 1896 reported the first successful repair of a cardiac injury, a stab wound of the right ventricle. In 1897, Duval[7] described the median sternotomy incision widely used today. Igelsbrud[5] in 1901 was the first to report successful resuscitation of a patient, sustaining a post-traumatic cardiac arrest patient with a thoracotomy and open cardiac massage. Spangaro[8] in 1906 described the left anterolateral thoracotomy widely used today for resuscitation as an intercostocondral thoracotomy.

Zolls[5] in 1956 was the first to introduce the concept of external defibrillation, and Kouwenhoven[5] in 1960 described closed cardiopulmonary resuscitation. Beall[9] et al. in 1961 was the first to propose that patients experiencing cessation of cardiac action should undergo immediate resuscitative thoracotomy and cardiac massage, whether in the ED, operating room (OR), or recovery ward, and was first to attempt this procedure. Similarly, in 1966, he advocated the use of immediate cardiorrhaphy in the emergency room and setting up an instrument tray; he was also the first to successfully perform this procedure.[10]

OBJECTIVES

Objectives of the EDT procedure include the following:

- Resuscitation of agonal patients with penetrating cardiothoracic injuries (Figure 1A and B)
- Evacuation of pericardial blood and clot to relieve cardiac tamponade
- Control of thoracic hemorrhage
- Perform open cardiac massage, which can produce up to 60% of the normal ejection fraction (EF)
- Repair of cardiac injuries
- Cross-clamp the pulmonary hilum to control pulmonary vessel hemorrhage
- Cross-clamp the descending thoracic aorta (Figures 2 and 3)
- Cross-clamp the pulmonary hilum and aspirate both the right and left ventricles to prevent and/or treat pulmonary embolism

PHYSIOLOGY

Some of the physiologic effects of thoracic aortic cross-clamping include positive and negative effects, while others are unknown.

Positive Effects

- Preservation and redistribution of remaining blood volume to improve coronary/carotid arterial perfusion

- Reduction of subdiaphragmatic blood loss
- Increases left ventricular stroke work index (LVSWI)
- Increases myocardial contractility

Negative Effects

- Decreases blood flow to abdominal viscera to approximately 10% of normal
- Decreases renal perfusion to approximately 10% of normal
- Decreases blood flow to the spinal cord to approximately 10%
- Induces anaerobic metabolism
- Induces hypoxia/lactic acidosis
- Imposes a tremendous afterload onto the left ventricle
- Unknown factors
- Length of safe cross-clamp time
- Incidence of reperfusion injury

INDICATIONS

Indications for EDT can be subdivided into three categories: accepted, selective, and rare.[1–4]

Accepted Indications

Emergency department thoracotomy is best applied to patients sustaining penetrating cardiac injuries who arrive in trauma centers after a short scene and transport time with witnessed or objectively measured physiological parameters (signs of life), pupillary reactivity, spontaneous ventilation even if agonal, presence of a carotid pulse, measurable or palpable blood pressure, extremity movement, and cardiac electrical activity.

Selective Indications

Emergency department thoracotomy should be performed selectively in patients sustaining penetrating noncardiac thoracic injuries due to its very low survival rate. Because it is difficult to ascertain whether injuries are noncardiac thoracic versus cardiac this procedure may be employed to establish a diagnosis.

EDT should be performed selectively in patients sustaining exsanguinating abdominal vascular injuries due to its very low survival

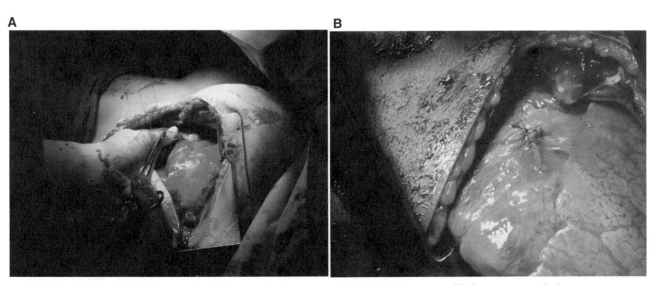

A   **B**

Figure 1 **(A)** Suturing a stab wound to the heart, after emergency department thoracotomy. **(B)** Same patient with the suture completed *(arrow)*.

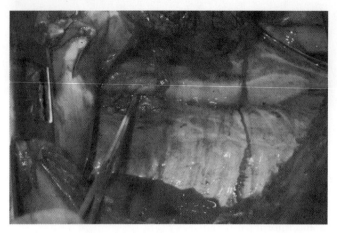

Figure 2   The descendent aorta when entering the aortic hiatus. The aorta was dissected prior to being clamped. Note the esophagus superiorly.

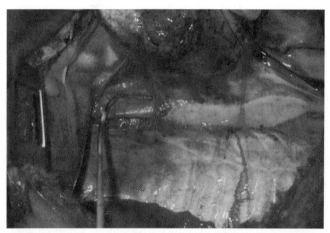

Figure 3   Aortic cross-clamp in place. Note the size of the left hemithorax cavity, which can hold the entire patient's volemia during exsanguinated injuries.

rate. Meticulous selection of patients should be exercised. This procedure should be used as an adjunct to definitive repair of abdominal vascular injuries.

Rare Indications

Emergency department thoracotomy should be performed rarely in patients sustaining cardiopulmonary arrest secondary to blunt trauma due to its very low survival rate and poor neurological outcomes. Extreme caution should be exercised in selecting patients for this procedure. It should be strictly limited to those who arrive with vital signs at the trauma center and experience a witnessed cardiopulmonary arrest. Most authors would caution against this indication.

TECHNIQUES FOR CARDIAC INJURY REPAIR

Incisions

There are two main incisions that are used in the management of penetrating cardiac injuries. Trauma surgeons should be aware that injuries caused by missiles can be unpredictable in their trajectory

and that a missile injury that penetrates a hemithoracic cavity may not remain confined in the original area of entrance and may produce injury to the contralateral cavity. This will require the trauma surgeon to access the contralateral hemithoracic cavity.[67,68,70,74,77]

Median sternotomy described by Duval[37] is the incision of choice for patients admitted with penetrating precordial injuries that arrive with some degree of hemodynamic instability and may either undergo preoperative investigation with FAST and/or chest x-ray. It is also the incision of choice or those that are thought to harbor occult cardiac injuries. The left anterolateral thoracotomy is the incision of choice in the management of patients who arrive in extremis. This incision is used in the ED for resuscitative purposes.[67,68,70,74,77]

The left anterolateral thoracotomy described by Spangaro[41] can also be extended across the sternum as bilateral anterolateral thoracotomies, if it is determined during the resuscitative period that the patient's injury extends into the right hemithoracic cavity (Table 1). Extension into bilateral anterolateral thoracotomies is also is the incision of choice for patients that are hemodynamically unstable after incurring mediastinal traversing injuries. This incision allows full exposure of the anterior mediastinum and pericardium as well as both hemithoracic cavities. It is important to note that upon transection of the sternum both internal mammary arteries are also transected and must be ligated after restoration of perfusion pressure. Uncontrolled, they can serve as a significant source of blood loss. This is a frequent pitfall during the institution of damage control; as trauma surgeons may forget to ligate these vessels prompting return to the operating room for a patient that can ill afford it. For patients that sustain thoracoabdominal injuries, the left anterolateral thoracotomy is also the incision of choice if patients deteriorate in the OR while undergoing a laparotomy.[67,68,70,74,77]

Adjunct Maneuvers

Trauma surgeons must possess several maneuvers in their armamentarium to deal with penetrating cardiothoracic injuries. The first adjunct maneuver dealing with these injuries was described by Sauerbuch[42] in 1907, as quoted by Brantigan. This maneuver entailed controlling blood flow to the heart by compression of the base. This maneuver is difficult to perform via a left anterolateral thoracotomy, has been abandoned, and is only mentioned because of historical interest only.

Total inflow occlusion to the heart is a complex maneuver that entails cross-clamping both the superior (SVC) and inferior vena cava (IVC) in their intrapericardial location to arrest total blood flow to the heart. Crafoord-DeBakey cross-clamps are employed, resulting in the immediate emptying of the heart. The trauma surgeon must recognize that cross-clamping the inferior vena cava intrapericardially at the space of Gibbons can be quite treacherous, as it is often fused with the posterior aspect of the pericardium. Inexperienced trauma surgeons will often force the cross-clamp in an attempt to rapidly achieve total occlusion leading to an iatrogenic injury of the intrapericardial IVC. Similarly, circumferentially dissecting this delicate vessel can also lead to iatrogenic injury. The clamp must be placed carefully and sometimes at an angle so as to totally occlude the intrapericardial IVC.[70,77]

Total inflow occlusion of the heart is indicated for the management of injuries in the lateral-most aspect of the right atrium and/or the superior or inferior atriocaval junction. Total inflow occlusion will lead to immediate emptying of the heart and allow the injury to be visualized and thus repaired. Frequently this procedure results in cardiopulmonary arrest, as tolerance by the injured, acidotic, hypothermic and ischemic heart is very limited. The safe period for this maneuver is unknown, although a 1–3 minute range is often quoted in the literature as the period of time after which clamps must be released. As the clamps are released, venous return fills the right-sided cardiac chambers and forward cardiac pumping motion will begin. More often than

Table 1: Algorithm for Emergency Department Thoracotomy

Operator	Well-trained surgeon
Initial assessment and resuscitation	Endotracheal intubation Immediate venous access Rapid infusion
Position	Supine with left arm elevated
Incision	Left anterolateral incision Fifth intercostal space from left sternocostal junction to latissimus dorsi m.
Procedure	Incision as above Sharp transection of intercostal m. Open pleura Place a Finnochietto retractor Open cardiac massage Elevate left lung medially Locate and dissect descending aorta Cross clamp aorta by Crafoord-Debakey clamp
If cardiac injury (bluish and tense pericardium)	Open pericardium longitudinally with preserving phrenic n. Evacuate blood clot Repair cardiac injury (mattress sutures of Halsted with Prolene 2/0)
If active bleeding at pulmonary hilum	Cross-clamp pulmonary hilum with Crafoord-Debakey clamp
If pulmonary parenchymal laceration	Clamp with Duval clamp
If associated injury in contralateral thoracic cavity	Extend incision to the contralateral side Transect sternum sharply Convert to bilateral anterolateral thoracotomy
If air embolism is suspected (air in coronary v)	Aspirate left ventricle
Miscellaneous	Ligate internal mammary a. Systemic or intraventricular epinephrine administration Internal defibrillation 10–50 joules Temporary pacemaker
Immediately transport to operating room after successful resuscitation	

not, the heart will fibrillate requiring immediate direct defibrillation along with pharmacologic manipulation. This may be unsuccessful, particularly if a period of 3 minutes has been exceeded. Restoration of a normal sinus rhythm is often impossible.[70,77]

Cross-clamping of the pulmonary hilum is another valuable maneuver indicated for the management of associated pulmonary injuries, particularly those that have hilar central hematomas and/or active bleeding. This maneuver arrests bleeding from the lung and prevents air emboli from reaching the systemic circulation. However, one of its negative effects is responsible for significantly increasing the afterload of the right ventricle, as half of the pulmonary circulation is no longer available for perfusion. We recommend sequential de-clamping of the hilum to be carried out as expediently as possible along with a direct approach by stapled pulmonary tractotomy[70,74] for identification and control of hemorrhaging intraparenchymal pulmonary vessels. This will promptly unload the right ventricle. In the presence of acidosis, hypothermia, and ischemia, the right ventricle may not be able to tolerate this maneuver leading to fibrillation and arrest.[70,74]

Grabowski[1] recently described a maneuver to facilitate exposure of posterior cardiac wounds by placing a Satinsky clamp at the right ventricular angle, which is formed at the acute anteroinferior margin of the right ventricle as it reflects on the right diaphragm. Grabowski[1] recommends that the clamp only grasp a small portion of the right ventricle. He recommends this maneuver for elevating the heart out of the pericardium to repair posterior injuries. We have no experience with this maneuver and cannot recommend it. We strongly feel that if used inappropriately, it will lead to the development of significant cardiac dysrhythmias.[70,74]

Maneuvers such as venting either the right or left ventricle postcardiorrhaphy are recommended to provide an avenue of egress for air emboli trapped in these chambers. This is usually accomplished by placing 16-gauge intravenous catheters. Theoretically, air should eject out of the repair chambers, thus preventing air emboli. Although the authors have used this maneuver successfully, little has been written in the literature describing its outcome.[70,74]

At times a trauma surgeon will need to elevate the heart out of the pericardium in order to repair certain injuries. Rapid and injudicious manipulation of the heart will often result in complex dysrhythmias that might include ventricular fibrillation and even cardiopulmonary arrest. Occasionally, given the degree of exsanguinating hemorrhage the heart must be extracted rapidly from pericardium in order to perform cardiorrhaphy. The trauma surgeon must communicate with the anesthesiologists whenever this maneuver is performed. If hemorrhage can be digitally controlled, gradual elevation of the heart by placing multiple laparotomy packs will allow better tolerance of this maneuver while decreasing the chances for the development of dysrhythmias.[70,74]

Recently described mechanical stabilizer systems to the heart have been utilized in the performance of conventional coronary artery bypass grafts (CABGs), which have traditionally used cardiopulmonary bypass to allow cardiac surgeons to operate on a motionless heart arrested by means of cardioplegic solutions. The deleterious systemic inflammatory effects of circulating blood through the extracorporeal circuit of the cardiopulmonary pump have prompted the development of mechanical stabilizer systems to allow off pump coronary artery bypass grafting (OPCABG) to be performed by cardiothoracic surgeons.

Waterworth[11] recently reported the first case in which the Octopus IV Mechanical Cardiac Stabilizer was used on a 20-year-old patient who sustained a 2-cm stab wound in the right ventricular outflow tract approximately 1 cm below the pulmonary valve. According to the author, this area was difficult to suture without causing further tearing due to tachycardia sustained by the patient and the fragile nature of this area. After control of hemorrhage by direct pressure, the Octopus IV Mechanical Cardiac Stabilizer was placed, which provided for immobility to this area of the heart and thus facilitated repair. In this case report, the author describes the use of this device, suggesting that cardiac stabilization devices with adjustable suction foot blades may be used to control hemorrhage in addition to facilitating repair, particularly in areas difficult or dangerous to handle manually. The recommended positioning parallel to the direction of the wound and approximating the foot plates may result in closure of the wound, providing a clear field for repair. This case report by Waterworth[11] appears to be the first and only case reported in the literature utilizing a mechanical cardiac stabilizer in the management of a penetrating cardiac injury. Whether stabilizers will be routinely used in the management of penetrating cardiac injuries in the future remains to be seen.

Repair of Atrial Injuries

Atrial injuries can usually be controlled by placement of a Satinsky partial occlusion vascular clamp. Control of the wound will allow the trauma surgeon to perform cardiorrhaphy. We recommend utilizing 2-0 or 3-0 polypropylene monofilament sutures on an MH needle in a running or interrupted fashion. It is important to visualize both sides of the atrial injury, particularly those caused by missiles. Missile injuries can usually cause a significant amount of tissue destruction, which might require meticulous debridement prior to closure. Similarly, a portion of the atria may be resected and cardiorrhaphy performed utilizing a running suture of 2-0 or 3-0 polypropylene monofilament suture. The trauma surgeon must be aware that the atria have fairly thin walls and demand gentleness during cardiorrhaphy, as they can easily tear and enlarge the original injury. The use of bioprosthetic materials in the form of Teflon pledgets is not recommended for management of these injuries.[70,74]

Repair of Ventricular Injuries

Ventricular injuries usually cause significant hemorrhage. They should be occluded digitally while simultaneously repaired by either simple interrupted or horizontal mattress sutures of Halsted. Ventricular cardiorrhaphy can also be accomplished with a running monofilament suture of 2-0 polypropylene on an MH needle. Performing cardiorrhaphy for ventricular for stab wounds is usually less challenging than for gunshot wounds. Missile injuries often produce some degree of blast effect that causes myocardial fibers to retract. Frequently, missile injuries that have been successfully sutured and controlled enlarge, as the damaged myocardium retracts and becomes more friable. Frequently, these injuries require multiple sutures to control significant hemorrhage. In the presence of this scenario, bioprosthetic materials such as Teflon strips and/or pledgets are often needed to buttress the suture line. This is usually performed by fashioning a Teflon strip that may measure anywhere from 1 to 5 cm (Figure 4A and B). This strip is held by two straight Crile clamps held by an assistant. Simultaneously, the trauma surgeon may then place double-armed 2-0 polypropylene monofilament sutures on an MH needle, first through the strip, and then through both sides of the injury. A second strip is then held in a similar fashion so that the trauma surgeon then places both needles thru the second Teflon strip. The sutures are then gently tied against the Teflon strip and/or pledget, which will buttress and reinforce the suture line. This maneuver must be repeated until total control of ventricular hemorrhage is achieved. The authors have recently used commercially made fibrin sealants to seal complex ventricular injuries.[70,74]

Coronary Artery Injuries

The repair of ventricular injuries adjacent to coronary arteries can be very challenging. Injudicious and/or inappropriate placement of sutures during cardiorrhaphy may narrow and/or occlude a

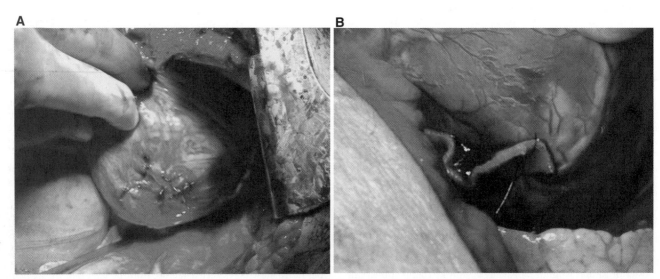

Figure 4 **(A)** Patient sustained a cardiac apex penetrating injury. **(B)** Same patient with Teflon patches used to reinforce the sutures.

coronary artery or one of its branches. Therefore, it is recommended that sutures be placed underneath the bed of the coronary artery. Coronary arteries are usually divided into three segments: proximal, middle, and distal. Injuries to the proximal segment of a coronary artery will usually require cardiopulmonary bypass for repair, although this is infrequently necessary. Injuries of the middle segment of the coronary artery may also require cardiopulmonary bypass, or if ligated in desperation, may result in immediate myocardial infarction at the operating table. These patients may benefit from the institution of intra-aortic balloon counterpulsation followed by aortocoronary bypass. Lacerations of the distal segment of the coronary artery particularly in the distal-most third of the vessel are managed by ligation.[70,74]

Use of Bioprosthetic and Autogenous Materials

Trauma surgeons are familiar with the use of Teflon pledgets and/or strips to buttress suture lines on friable myocardial tissue. Mattox[18] provided the first reference in the literature alluding to the use of this material. The authors strongly believe in the necessity to buttress complex suture lines and use Teflon when indicated. However, no studies have been performed to determine if the use of Teflon increases tensile strength of the repair. The use of autogenous materials such as the pericardium to bolster suture lines is also well known. A small flap is developed and excised from the pericardium to be used in a manner similar to use of Teflon pledgets. Inexperienced trauma surgeons will often suture the pericardium to a ventricular injury causing the chamber to be fixated, which leads to dysrhythmias. This is mentioned, as it is a pitfall that should be avoided at all costs.[70,74]

Complex and Combined Injuries

As trauma surgeons and trauma centers continue to develop greater expertise in the management of penetrating cardiac injuries, and patients are subjected to greater degrees of violence in urban arenas of warfare, a significant number of patients arrive harboring multiple associated injuries in addition to their penetrating cardiac injuries. Complex and combined cardiac injuries can be defined as a penetrating cardiac injury plus associated neck, thoracic, thoracic-vascular, abdominal, abdominal vascular, or peripheral vascular injuries. These injuries are quite challenging to manage. Priority should be given early to the injury causing the greatest blood loss or threatening the patient's life.[70,74]

Wall and Mattox described 60 patients with complex cardiac injuries, which they defined as those beyond lacerations of the myocardium. These injuries were defined as those with concomitant coronary artery injuries, cardiac valvular injuries, intracardiac fistulas, and other unusual injuries. In this series, the authors described 39 coronary artery injuries; 2 valvular injuries; and 14 intracardiac fistulas including ventriculoseptal defects, atrioseptal defects (ASD), and another 10 injuries that they considered unusual ranging from ventricular false aneurysms to coronary sinus injuries and two patients who developed missile emboli to the heart. These types of injuries can also be considered complex and combined injuries.

RESULTS

The literature abounds with retrospective series describing the use of EDT. Great difficulties, however, exist in evaluating the results of these series. Close scrutiny reveals several flaws; most series have been retrospective reviews, many from institutions that employ this technique infrequently. Furthermore, many institutions report many overlapping studies that encompass the experience of many years.

Whereas many series have selected physiologic parameters as predictors of outcome, none have statistically validated their predictive values. Invariably, these series omit data pertaining to the physiologic status of the patient upon initial presentation. To our knowledge, there is only one prospective study in the literature.[67] As a result, there are still many questions to be answered.[25]

Which patients should be subjected to this procedure?
Are there any prospectively validated physiologic predictors of outcomes that can safely and accurately identify patients who will benefit from the procedure and also safely exclude those who will not?
What are the true survival rates of this procedure?
Of the surviving patients, how many survive with severe neurologic impairment or remain in a persistent vegetative state?
How can we ensure that individuals performing this procedure are qualified?

Well-known physiologic factors predictive of poor outcome include prehospital and ED absence of vital signs, fixed and dilated pupils, absence of cardiac rhythm and motion in the extremities, and agonal breathing. Similarly, the absence of a palpable pulse in the presence of cardiopulmonary arrest is also predictive of poor outcome. These factors have been validated by Asensio and colleagues,[12,13] who tracked cases in the field, during transport, and upon arrival in the ED in two prospective studies dealing with penetrating cardiac injuries. Interestingly enough, many of these physiologic predictors of outcome, as well as any data describing the physiologic condition of the patient prior to EDT, are often absent in many studies.[1,2,25]

Previous work by Buckman et al.[17] and Asensio and colleagues[12,13] applied and validated the cardiovascular respiratory score (CVRS) of the trauma score (TS). The cardiovascular respiratory component of the trauma score reflects individual elements of blood pressure, respiratory rate, respiratory effort and capillary refill. The highest possible CVRS is 11, which denotes a systolic blood pressure of greater than 90 mm Hg, respiratory rates that fluctuate between 10 and 24/min along with a normal respiratory effort and capillary refill. The lowest possible CVRS score is zero, and reflects an absence of blood pressure, no palpable carotid pulse along with an absence of breathing, respiratory effort, and capillary refill. This score has been statistically validated and applied to the only three perspective cardiac injury series reported in the literature.

Asensio and colleagues,[2] in the only prospective study on the use of EDT reported in the literature, analyzed parameters measuring the physiologic condition of patients incurring cardiopulmonary arrest in the field, during transport, and upon arrival at the trauma center. The CVRS, injury mechanism, and anatomic site of injury along with restoration of blood pressure were tracked prospectively with the objectives of identifying a set of parameters that would reliably predict mortality and exclude patients from EDT. This 2-year prospective study had a single inclusion criterion—cardiopulmonary arrest secondary to traumatic injury—as well as a single intervention, EDT for resuscitation. The main outcome of this study was survival at 1 hour and survival to discharge.

A total of 215 patients who sustained cardiopulmonary arrest were studied prospectively. Of this total, 167 (78%) sustained penetrating injuries, including 142 (66%) gunshot wounds, 21 (10%) stab wounds, and 4 (2%) shotgun wounds. In addition, there were 48 (22%) who sustained blunt injuries. The mean revised trauma score (RTS) was 0.6, the mean injury severity score (ISS) was 42, and the mean CVRS was 1, denoting a severely injured and physiologically compromised patient population. The mean duration of cardiopulmonary resuscitation (CPR) prior to arrival at the trauma center was 12 minutes.

A total of 162 patients (75%) succumbed in the ED. Fifty-three patients (25%) survived up to 1 hour, after successful ED resuscitation with some restoration of vital signs so that they could be transported immediately to the OR. Of the 215 patients, only 6 (3%) survived, all of whom sustained cardiac injuries. None of the 48 patients who were

Table 2: Emergency Department Thoracotomy

Lead Author	Year	Type of Study	Survivors/Total EDT	Neurologic Impairment (n)	Survivors/Penetrating Trauma	Survivors/Blunt Trauma
Mattox[26]	1974	R	11/106	0	8/87	3/19
McDonald[27]	1978	R	3/28	0	3/26	0/2
Moore[28]	1979	R	12/146	4	11/98	1/48
Baker[29]	1980	R	32/168	2	31/108	1/60
Hamar[30]	1981	R	5/64	0	—	—
Ivatury[31]	1981	R	8/22	1	8/22	—
Flynn[32]	1982	R	4/33	0	4/13	0/20
Bodai[33]	1982	R	0/38	0	—	0/38
Rohman[34]	1983	R	24/91	0	24/91	—
Vij[35]	1983	R	5/63	1	5/57	0/6
Cogbill[36]	1983	R	16/400	4	15/205	1/195
Shimazu[37]	1983	R	6/267	2	4/50	4/217
Danne[38]	1984	R	10/89	1	10/60	0/29
Tavares[39]	1984	R	21/37	0	21/37	—
Washington[40]	1984	R	6/23	0	6/23	0
Washington[41]	1985	R	8/55	0	8/55	—
Brantigan[42]	1985	R	6/32	1	6/32	
Feliciano[43]	1986	R	28/335	1	25/280	3/53
Roberge[44]	1986	R	7/44	0	7/44	—
Schwab[45]	1986	R	14/51	0	14/36	0/15
Moreno[46]	1986	R	4/69	0	4/69	—
Ordog[47]	1987	R	6/80	1	5/64	2/16
Demetriades[48]	1987	R	5/73	0	5/73	—
Baxter[49]	1988	R	29/632	0	22/313	7/319
Clevenger[50]	1988	R	3/72	0	3/41	0/31
Hoyt[51]	1989	R	33/113	0	33/74	0/39
Mandal[52]	1989	R	7/23	0	—	0
Esposito[53]	1991	R	2/112	1	1/24	1/88
Ivatury[54]	1991	R	16/163	0	16/134	0/29
Lewis[55]	1991	R	8/45	0	8/32	0/13
Durham[56]	1992	R	32/389	0	32/318	0/69
Lorenz[57]	1992	R	41/424	4	37/231	3/193
Blake[58]	1992	R	5/22	0	5/22	—
Bond[59]	1992	R	2/28	0	2/11	0/17
Millham[60]	1993	R	13/290	4	13/290	—
Mazzorana[61]	1994	R	10/273	0	10/252	0/21
Velmahos[62]	1995	R	43/855	0	42/679	1/176
Jahangiri[63]	1996	R	1/16	0	1/4	0/12
Brown[64]	1996	R	4/160	0	4/149	0/11
Bleetman[65]	1996	R	8/25	0	8/24	0/1
Branncy[66]	1998	R	41/868	7	33/483	8/385
Asensio[67]	1998	P	6/215	0	6/167	0/48

EDT, Emergency department thoracotomy; *P*, prospective; *R*, retrospective.
From Working Group, Ad Hoc Subcommittee on Outcomes, American College of Surgeons, Committee on Trauma: Practice management guidelines for emergency department thoracotomy. *J Am Coll Surg* 193(3):303–309, 2001.

injured due to blunt trauma survived. Upon comparing patients succumbing in the ED with those who survived at least 1 hour, all physiologic parameters were predictive of outcome ($p<0.001$). When all patients who survived 1 hour were compared with overall survivors, none of the physiologic parameters predicted outcome. Duration of CPR ($p=0.04$), penetrating mechanism of injury ($p<0.001$), and exsanguination ($p<0.006$) were predictors of outcome. The CVRS showed a trend toward the prediction of survival ($p=0.07$). When all nonsurvivors were compared with survivors, restoration of blood pressure was a strong predictor of outcome ($p<0.001$).

The authors concluded from these data that physiologic parameters plus the CVRS score were predictive of survival for patients undergoing EDT. On the basis of these criteria, the authors estimated that 75% of these patients could be safely excluded from this procedure at a cost savings of over $500,000 at their institution, and recommended that EDT should be limited to patients sustaining penetrating cardiac injuries and should not be applied to patients sustaining cardiopulmonary arrest secondary to blunt trauma.

Precisely because of the lack of uniformity in the reporting process in many of the reports in the literature, Asensio and colleagues[25] in the working group of the Ad Hoc Subcommittee on Outcomes of the American College of Surgeons Committee on Trauma closely scrutinized the literature to generate practice management guidelines for EDT.

In an extensive literature search, studies were classified into three classes. Class I comprises prospective randomized controlled trials and remains the gold standard of all clinical trials. In this category, the studies found were generally poorly designed, had inadequate numbers, or suffered from methodological inadequacies, rendering them clinically nonsignificant. In this group, no prospective randomized controlled trials were found. Studies in class II included clinical studies in which data were collected prospectively, as well as retrospective analyses based on clearly reliable data. Included here are observational, cohort, prevalence, and case-controlled studies. The authors found 29 studies that qualified for class II, three of which were prospective. Finally, for class III—defined as retrospectively collected data including clinical series, databases or registries, case reviews, case reports, and expert opinion—the authors located 63 studies.[25]

Analysis was conducted by stratifying the series into series dealing with EDT, series reporting neurologic outcomes of patients subjected to EDT, series dealing exclusively with penetrating cardiac injuries, and series dealing with pediatric patients. In the 42 series[25–67] dealing with EDT (Table 2), there were 7035 EDTs and 551 survivors, for a

survival rate of 7.83%. When data were stratified according to mechanism of injury, there were 4482 thoracotomies for penetrating injuries; of these, 500 patients survived, yielding a survival rate of 11.16%. There were 2193 thoracotomies performed for blunt injuries; only 35 patients survived, for a survival rate of 1.60%.[25–67]

Of the 14 series reporting neurologic outcomes and their results,[27,28,30,34–37,41,42,46,52,56,59,65] a total of 4520 patients were subjected to EDT with 226 survivors, yielding a 5% survival rate. Of these 226 survivors, 34 (15%) survived with neurologic impairment. In the series dealing exclusively with EDTs performed to repair penetrating cardiac injuries (Table 3), in a total of 1165 EDTs, 363 patients survived, yielding a survival rate of 31.1%. Only four series were found that dealt exclusively with pediatric patients (Table 4). There were 142 EDTs performed. Of 57 thoracotomies performed for penetrating injuries, 7 patients survived, yielding a survival rate of 12.2%. Eighty-five thoracotomies were performed for blunt injuries; 2 patients survived, for a survival rate of 2.3%.

Although EDT does not lend itself to be studied with prospective randomized control trials, the authors have produced the following recommendations:

1. Emergency department thoracotomy should be performed rarely in patients sustaining cardiopulmonary arrest secondary to blunt trauma because of its very low survival rate and poor neurologic outcomes. It should be limited to those who arrive with vital signs at the trauma center and experience a witnessed cardiopulmonary arrest.[25]
2. Emergency department thoracotomy is best applied to patients sustaining penetrating cardiac injuries who arrive at trauma

Table 3: Emergency Department Thoracotomy for Cardiac Injuries

Lead Author	Year	Type of Study	Survivors/Total EDT	Survivors/Penetrating Trauma
Boyd[68]	1965	R	0/0	17/25
Beall[69]	1966	R	3/16	42/197
Sauer[70]	1967	R	12/0	12/13
Sugg[71]	1968	R	0/0	63/459
Yao[72]	1968	R	0/0	61/80
Steichen[73]	1971	R	7/21	35/58
Beall[74]	1971	R	29/52	42/66
Borja[75]	1971	R	0/0	24/145
Carrasquilla[76]	1972	R	8/30	20/245
Beall[77]	1972	R	0/0	67/269
Bolanowski[78]	1973	R	0/0	33/44
Trinkle[79]	1974	R	0/0	38/45
Mattox[80]	1974	R	25/37	31/62
Harvey[81]	1975	R	0/0	22/28
Symbas[82]	1976	R	0/0	50/98
Beach[83]	1976	R	0/4	26/34
Asfaw[84]	1977	R	0/0	277/323
Sherman[85]	1978	R	32/41	37/92
Trinkle[86]	1978	R	0/0	89/100
Evans[87]	1979	R	0/4	29/46
Breaux[87]	1979	R	39/44	78/197
Mandal[89]	1979	R	/38	26/55
Gervin[90]	1982	R	4/21	4/21
Demetriades[91]	1983	R	2/16	40/125
Demetriades[92]	1984	R	1/11	45

Continued

Table 3: Emergency Department Thoracotomy for Cardiac Injuries—cont'd

Lead Author	Year	Type of Study	Survivors/Total EDT	Survivors/Penetrating Trauma
Tavares[93]	1984	R	21/37	64
Feliciano[94]	1984	R	5/15	3/2
Mattox[95]	1985	R	50/119	204
Demertiades[96]	1986	R	1/18	70
Moreno[97]	1986	R	4/69	100
Ivatury[98]	1987	R	28/91	—
Jebara[99]	1989	R	4/17	—
Attar[100]	1991	R	21/55	—
Knott-Craig[101]	1992	R	5/13	—
Buchman[102]	1992	R	1/2	23
Benyan[103]	1992	R	1/13	—
Macho[104]	1993	R	12/24	—
Mitchell[105]	1993	R	7/47	—
Kaplan[106]	1993	R	2/23	
Henderson[107]	1994	R	6/122	215
Coimbra[108]	1995	R	0/20	
Arreola-Risa[109]	1995	R	11/40	
Karmy-Jones[110]	1997	R	3/6	16
Rhee[111]	1998	R	15/58	41/96
Asensio[112]	1998	P	6/37	6/37
Asensio[113]	1998	P	10/71	10/71

Note: There were no survivors of blunt trauma.
EDT, Emergency department thoracotomy; *P,* prospective; *R,* retrospective.
From Working Group, Ad Hoc Subcommittee on Outcomes, American College of Surgeons, Committee on Trauma: Practice management guidelines for emergency department thoracotomy. *J Am Coll Surg* 193(3): 303–309, 2001.

Table 4: Emergency Department Thoracotomy in Children

Lead Author	Year	Type of Study	Survivors/Total EDT	Survivors, Penetrating Trauma	Survivors, Blunt Trauma
Beaver[114]	1987	R	0/17	0/2	0/15
Powell[115]	1988	R	5/19	4/11	1/8
Rothenberg[116]	1989	R	3/83	2/36	1/47
Sheikh[117]	1993	R	1/23	1/8	0/15

EDT, Emergency department thoracotomy; *P,* prospective; *R,* retrospective.
From Working Group, Ad Hoc Subcommittee on Outcomes, American College of Surgeons, Committee on Trauma: Practice management guidelines for emergency department thoracotomy. *J Am Coll Surg* 193(3):303–309, 2001.

centers after a short scene and transport time with witnessed or objectively measured physiologic parameters (signs of life) such as pupillary response, spontaneous ventilation, presence of carotid pulse, measurable or palpable blood pressure, extremity movement, or cardiac electrical activity.[25]

3. Emergency department thoracotomy should be performed in patients sustaining penetrating noncardiac thoracic injuries, but these patients generally experience a low survival rate. Because it is difficult to ascertain whether the injuries are noncardiac thoracic versus cardiac, EDT can be used to establish a diagnosis.[25]

4. Emergency department thoracotomy should be performed in patients sustaining exsanguinating abdominal vascular injuries, but these patients generally experience a low survival rate. Judicious selection of patients should be exercised. This procedure should be used as an adjunct to definitive repair of the abdominal vascular injury.[25]

5. For the pediatric population, guidelines 1–4 are applicable.[25]

In conclusion, EDT remains a very powerful tool in the trauma surgeons' armamentarium. It should be employed wisely with strict indications, and should only be performed by trauma surgeons and surgeons properly trained. Only by judicious scientific inquiry can we push the envelope, save lives, and advance science.[1–4,25]

REFERENCES

1. Asensio JA, Tsai KJ: Emergency department thoracotomy. In Demetriades D, Asensio JA, editors: *Trauma Management.* Georgetown, TX, Landes Bioscience, 2000, pp. 271–279.
2. Asensio JA, Hanpeter D, Demetriades D: The futility of liberal utilization of emergency department thoracotomy. A prospective study. *Proceedings*

of the American Association for the Surgery of Trauma 58th Annual Meeting, September 1998, Baltimore, p. 210.

3. Asensio JA, Hanpeter D, Gomez H, et al: Exsanguination. In Shoemaker W, Greenvik A, Ayres SM, et al., editors: *Textbook of Critical Care*, 4 ed. Philadelphia, Saunders, 2000, pp. 37–47.

4. Asensio JA, Hanpeter D, Gomez H, et al: Thoracic injuries. In Shoemaker W, Greenvik A, Ayres SM, et al., editors: *Textbook of Critical Care*, 4 ed. Philadelphia, Saunders, 2000, pp. 337–348.

5. Biffl WL, Moore EE, Harken AH: Emergency department thoracotomy. In Mattox KL, Feliciano DV, Moore EE, editors: *Trauma*, 4 ed. New York, McGraw-Hill, 2000, 245–259.

6. Rehn L: Ueber Penetrerende Herzwunden und Herznaht. *Arch Klin Chir* 55:315, 1897. As quoted in Beck CS: Wounds of the heart: the technic of suture. *Arch Surg* 13:205–227, 1926.

7. Duval P: Le incision median thoraco-laparotomy. *Bull Mem Soc Chir Paris* 33:15, 1907. As quoted in Ballana C: Bradshaw lecture. The surgery of the heart. *Lancet* CXCVIII:73–79, 1920.

8. Spangaro S: Sulla tecnica da seguire negli interventi chirurgici per ferite del cuore e su di un nuovo processo di toracotomia. *Clin Chir Milan* 14:227, 1906. As quoted in Beck CS: Wounds of the heart: the technic of suture. *Arch Surg* 13:205–227, 1926.

9. Beall AC, Oschner JL, Morris GC, et al: Penetrating wounds of the heart. *J Trauma* 1:195–207, 1961.

10. Beall AC, Dietrich EB, Crawford HW: Surgical management of penetrating cardiac injuries. *Am J Surg* 112:686, 1966.

11. Waterworth PD, Musleh G, Greenhalgh D, Tsang A: Innovative use of Octopus IV stabilizer in cardiac truma. *Ann Thoracic Surgery* 80:1008–1010, 2005.

12. Asensio JA, Murray J, Demetriades D, et al: Penetrating cardiac injuries: a prospective study of variables predicting outcomes. *J Am Coll Surg* 186(1):24–34, 1998.

13. Asensio JA, Berne JD, Demetriades D, et al: One hundred five penetrating cardiac injuries. A 2-year prospective evaluation. *J Trauma* 44(6):1073–1082, 1998.

14. Asensio JA, Forno W, Gambaro E, et al: Penetrating cardiac injuries: a complex challenge. *Ann Chir Gynecol* 89(2):155–166, 2000.

15. Asensio JA, Hanpeter D, Gomez H, et al: Thoracic injuries. In Shoemaker W, Greenvik A, Ayres SM, et al, editors: *Textbook of Critical Care*, 4th ed. Philadelphia, Saunders, 2000, pp. 337–348.

16. Asensio JA, Stewart BM, Murray J, et al: Penetrating cardiac injuries. *Surg Clin North Am* 76(4):685–724, 1996.

17. Buckman RF, Badellino MM, Mauro LH, et al: Penetrating cardiac wounds: prospective study of factors influencing initial resuscitation. *J Trauma* 34(5):717–727, 1993.

18. Mattox KL, Espada R, Beall AC, et al: Performing thoracotomy in the emergency center. *J Am Coll Emerg Phys* 3:13–17, 1974.

19. Beall AC, Morris GC, Cooley DA: Temporary cardiopulmonary bypass in the management of penetrating wounds of the heart. *Surgery* 52:330–337, 1962.

20. Boyd TF, Strieder JW: Immediate surgery for traumatic heart disease. *J Thorac Cardiovasc Surg* 50:305–315, 1965.

21. Sugg WL, Rea WJ, Ecker RR, et al: Penetrating wounds of the heart: an analysis of 459 cases. *J Thorac Cardiovasc Surg* 56:531–545, 1968.

22. Beall AC, Gasior RM, Bricker DL: Gunshot wounds of the heart: changing patterns of surgical management. *Ann Thorac Surg* 11:523–531, 1971.

23. Steichen FM, Dargan EL, Efron G: A graded approach to the management of penetrating wounds to the heart. *Arch Surg* 103:574–580, 1971.

24. Mattox KL, Beall AC, Jordan GL, et al: Cardiorraphy in the emergency center. *J Thorac Cardiovasc Surg* 68:886–895, 1974.

25. Asensio JA, Wall M, Minei J, et al: Working Group, Ad Hoc Subcommittee on Outcomes, American College of Surgeons Committee on Trauma: Practice management guidelines for emergency department thoracotomy. *J Am Coll Surg* 193(3):303–309, 2001.

26. Mattox KL, Espada R, Beall AC: Performing thoracotomy in the emergency center. *J Am Coll Emerg Physician* 3:13–17, 1974.

27. McDonald JR, McDowell RM: Emergency department thoracotomies in a community hospital. *J Am Coll Emerg Physician* 7:423–428, 1978.

28. Moore EE, Moore JB, Galloway AC, et al: Postinjury thoracotomy in the emergency department: a critical evaluation. *Surgery* 86:590–598, 1979.

29. Baker CC, Caronna JJ, Trunkey DD: Neurologic outcome after emergency room thoracotomy for trauma. *Am J Surg* 139:677–681, 1980.

30. Hamar TJ. Oreskovich MR, Copass MK, et al: Role of emergency thoracotomy in the resuscitation of moribund trauma victims. 100 consecutive cases. *Am J Surg* 142:96–99, 1981.

31. Ivatury RR, Shah PM, Ito K, et al: Emergency room thoracotomy for the resuscitation of patients with "fatal" penetrating injuries of the heart. *Ann Thorac Surg* 32:377–385, 1981.

32. Flynn TC, Ward RE, Miller PW: Emergency department thoracotomy. *Ann Emerg Med* 11:45–48, 1982.

33. Bodai BI, Smith JP, Blaisdell FW: The role of emergency thoracotomy in blunt trauma. *J Trauma* 22:487–491, 1982.

34. Rohman M, Ivatury RR, Steichen FM, et al: Emergency room thoracotomy for penetrating cardiac injuries. *J Trauma* 23:570–576, 1983.

35. Vij D, Simoni E, Smith RF, et al: Resuscitative thoracotomy for patients with traumatic injury. *Surgery* 94:554–561, 1983.

36. Cogbill TH, Moore EE, Millikan JS, et al: Rationale for selective application of emergency department thoracotomy in trauma. *J Trauma* 23:453–460, 1983.

37. Shimazu S, Shatney CH: Outcome of trauma patients with no vital signs on hospital admission. *J Trauma* 23:213–216, 1983.

38. Danne PO, Finelli F, Champion HR: Emergency bay thoracotomy. *J Trauma* 24:796–802, 1984.

39. Tavares S, Hankins JR, Moulton AL, et al: Management of penetrating cardiac injuries: the role of emergency thoracotomy. *Ann Thorac Surg* 38:183–187, 1984.

40. Washington B, Wilson RF, Steiger Z: Emergency thoracotomies for penetrating trauma. *Curr Probl Surg* 14–17, 1984.

41. Washington B, Wilson RF, Steiger Z, et al: Emergency thoracotomy: a four-year review. *Ann Thorac Surg* 40:188–191, 1985.

42. Brantigan MW, Tietz G: Emergency thoracotomy in an urban community hospital: initial cardiac rhythm as a new predictor of survival. *Am J Emerg Med* 3:311–315, 1985.

43. Feliciano DV, Bitondo CG, Cruse PA, et al: Liberal use of emergency center thoracotomy. *Am J Surg* 152:654–659, 1986.

44. Roberge RJ, Ivatury RR, Stahl W, et al: Emergency department thoracotomy for penetrating injuries: predictive value of patient classification. *Am J Emerg Med* 4:129–135, 1986.

45. Schwab WC, Adcock OT, Max MH: Emergency department thoracotomy (EDT): a 26-month experience using an "agonal" protocol. *Am Surg* 52:20–29, 1986.

46. Moreno C, Moore EE, Majure JA, et al: Pericardial tamponade: a critical determinant for survival following penetrating cardiac wounds. *Trauma* 26:821–825, 1986.

47. Ordog GJ: Emergency department thoracotomy for traumatic cardiac arrest. *J Emerg Med* 5:217–223, 1987.

48. Demetriades D, Rabinowitz B, Sofianos C: Emergency room thoracotomy for stab wounds to the chest and neck. *J Trauma* 27:483–485, 1987.

49. Baxter TB, Moore EE, Moore JB, et al: Emergency department thoracotomy following injury: critical determinants for patient salvage. *World J Surg* 12:671–675, 1988.

50. Clevenger FW, Yarbrough DR, Reines HD: Resuscitative thoracotomy: the effect of field time on outcome. *J Trauma* 28:441–445, 1988.

51. Hoyt DB, Shackford SR, Davis JW, et al: Thoracotomy during trauma resuscitations-an appraisal by board-certified general surgeons. *J Trauma* 29:1318–1321, 1989.

52. Mandal AK, Oparah SS: Unusually low mortality of penetrating wounds of the chest-twelve years' experience. *J Thorac Cardiovasc Surg* 97:119–125, 1989.

53. Esposito TJ, Jurkovich GJ, Rice CL, et al: Reappraisal of emergency room thoracotomy in a changing environment. *J Trauma* 31:881–887, 1991.

54. Ivatury RR, Kazigo J, Rohman M, et al: "Directed" emergency room thoracotomy: a prognostic prerequisite for survival. *J Trauma* 31:1076–1082, 1991.

55. Lewis G, Knottenbelt JD: Should emergency room thoracotomy be reserved for cases of cardiac tamponade? *Br J Accid Surg* 22:5–6, 1991.

56. Durham LA, Richardson RJ, Wall MJ Jr, et al: Emergency center thoracotomy: impact of prehospital resuscitation. *J Trauma* 32:775–779, 1992.

57. Lorenz PH, Steinmetz B, Lieberman J, et al: Emergency thoracotomy: survival correlates with physiologic status. *J Trauma* 32:780–783, 1992.

58. Blake DP, Gisbert VL, Ney AL, et al: Survival after emergency 5 department versus operating room thoracotomy for penetrating cardiac injuries. *Am Surg* 58:329–333, 1992.

59. Bond M, Vanek VW, Bourguet CC: Emergency room resuscitative thoracotomy: When is it indicated? *J Trauma* 33:714–721, 1992.

60. Millham FH, Grindlinger GA: Survival determinants in patients undergoing emergency room thoracotomy for penetrating chest injury. *J Trauma* 34:332–336, 1993.

61. Mazzorana V, Smith RS, Morabito DJ, et al: Limited utility of emergency department thoracotomy. *Am Surg* 60:516–521, 1994.

62. Velmahos GC, Degiannis E, Souter I, et al: Outcome of a strict policy on emergency department thoracotomies. *Arch Surg* 130:774–777, 1995.

63. Jahangiri M, Hyde J, Griffin S, et al: Emergency thoracotomy for thoracic trauma in the accident and emergency department: indications and outcome. *Ann R Coll Surg Engl* 78:121–124, 1996.

64. Brown SE, Gomez GA, Jacobson LE, et al: Penetrating chest trauma: should indications for emergency room thoracotomy be limited? *Am Surg* 62:530–534, 1996.

65. Bleetman A, Kasem H, Crawford R: Review of emergency thoracotomy for chest injuries in patients attending a UK accident and emergency department. *Injury* 27:119–122, 1996.

66. Branncy SW, Moore EE, Feldhaus KM, et al: Critical analysis of two decades of experience with post injury emergency department thoracotomy in a regional trauma center. *J Trauma* 4:87–94, 1998.

67. Asensio JA, Hanpeter D, Demetriades D, et al: The futility of the liberal utilization of emergency department thoracotomy. A prospective study. *Proceedings of the American Association for the Surgery of Trauma 58th Annual Meeting*, September 1998, Baltimore, Maryland, p. 210.

68. Boyd TF, Strieder JW: Immediate surgery for traumatic heart disease. *J Thorac Cardiovasc Surg* 50:305–315, 1965.

69. Beall AC, Dietrich EB, Crawford HW, et al: Surgical management of penetrating cardiac injuries. *Am J Surg* 112:686–691, 1966.

70. Sauer PE, Murdock CE: Immediate surgery for cardiac and great vessel wounds. *Arch Surg* 95:7–11, 1967.

71. Sugg WL, Rea WJ, Ecker RR, et al: Penetrating wounds of the heart. *J Thorac Cardiovasc Surg* 56:530–545, 1968.

72. Yao ST, Vanecko RM, Printen K, Shoemaker WC: Penetrating wounds of the heart: a review of 80 cases. *Ann Surg* 168:67–78, 1968.

73. Steichen FM, Dargan EL, Efron G, et al: A graded approach to the management of penetrating wounds of the heart. *Arch Surg* 103:574–580, 1971.

74. Beall AC, Gasior RM, Briker DL: Gunshot wounds of the heart. *Ann Thorac Surg* 11:523–531, 1971.

75. Borja AR, Ransdell HT: Treatment of penetrating gunshot wounds of the chest. *Am J Surg* 122:81–84, 1971.

76. Carrasquilla C, Wilson RF, Walt AJ, et al: Gunshot wounds of the heart. *Ann Thorac Surg* 13:208–213, 1972.

77. Beall AC, Patrick TD, Ikles JE, et al: Penetrating wounds of the heart: changing patterns of surgical management. *J Trauma* 12:468–473, 1972.

78. Bolanowski PS, Swaminathan AP, Neville WE: Aggressive surgical management of penetrating cardiac injuries. *J Thorac Cardiovasc Surg* 66:52–57, 1973.

79. Trinkle JK, Marcos J, Grover FL, et al: Management of the wounded heart. *Ann Thorac Surg* 17:231–236, 1974.

80. Mattox KL, Beall AC, Jordan GL, et al: Cardiorrhaphy in the emergency center. *J Thorac Cardiovasc Surg* 68:886–895, 1974.

81. Harvey JC, Pacifico AD: Primary operative management method of choice for stab wounds to the heart. *South Med J* 68:149–152, 1975.

82. Symbas PN, Harlaftis N, Waldo WJ: Penetrating cardiac wounds: a comparison of different therapeutic methods. *Ann Surg* 183:377–381, 1976.

83. Beach PM, Bognolo D, Hutchinson JE: Penetrating cardiac trauma. Experience with thirty-four patients in a hospital without cardiopulmonary bypass capability. *Am J Surg* 131:411–415, 1976.

84. Asfaw I, Arbulu A: Penetrating wounds of the pericardium and heart. *Surg Clin North Am* 57:37–49, 1977.

85. Sherman M, Saini UK, Yardoz MD, et al: Management of penetrating heart wounds. *Am J Surg* 135:553–558, 1978.

86. Trinkle JK, Toon RS, Franz JL, et al: Affairs of the wounded heart: penetrating cardiac wounds. *J Trauma* 19:467–472, 1978.

87. Evans J, Gray LA, Payner A, et al: Principles for the management of penetrating cardiac wounds. *Ann Surg* 189:777–784, 1979.

88. Breaux EP, Dupont JB, Albert HM, et al: Cardiac tamponade following penetrating mediastinal injuries: improved survival with early pericardiocentesis. *J Trauma* 19:461–466, 1979.

89. Mandal AK, Awariefe SO, Oparah SS: Experience in the management of 50 consecutive penetrating wounds of the heart. *Br J Surg* 66:565–568, 1979.

90. Gervin AS, Fischer RP: The importance of prompt transport in salvage of patients with penetrating heart wounds. *J Trauma* 22:443–448, 1982.

91. Demetriades D, Vander Veen BW: Penetrating injuries of the heart: experience over two years in South Africa. *J Trauma* 23:1034–1041, 1983.

92. Demetriades D: Cardiac penetrating injuries: personal experience of 45 cases. *Br J Surg* 71:95–97, 1984.

93. Tavares S, Hankins JR, Moulton AL, et al: Management of penetrating cardiac injuries: The role of emergency thoracotomy. *Ann Thorac Surg* 38:183–187, 1984.

94. Feliciano DV, Bitondo CG, Mattox KL, et al: Civilian trauma in the 1980's. A 1-year experience with 456 vascular and cardiac injuries. *Ann Surg* 199:717–724, 1984.

95. Mattox KL, Limacher MG, Feliciano DV, et al: Cardiac evaluation following heart injury. *J Trauma* 25:758–765, 1985.

96. Demetriades D: Cardiac wounds. Experience with 70 patients. *Ann Surg* 203:315–317, 1986.

97. Moreno C, Moore EE, Majure JA, et al: Pericardial tamponade: a critical determinant for survival following penetrating cardiac wounds. *J Trauma* 26:821–825, 1986.

98. Ivatury RR, Rohman M, Steichen FM, et al: Penetrating cardiac injuries: Twenty-year experience. *Am Surg* 53:310–317, 1987.

99. Jebara VA, Saade B: Penetrating wounds to the heart: a wartime experience. *Ann Thorac Surg* 47:250–253, 1989.

100. Attar S, Suter CM, Hankins JR, et al: Penetrating cardiac injuries. *Ann Thorac Surg* 51:711–716, 1991.

101. Knott-Craig CJ, Dalron RP, Rossouw GJ, et al: Penetrating cardiac trauma: management strategy based on 129 surgical emergencies over 2 years. *Ann Thorac Surg* 53:1006–1009, 1992.

102. Buchman TG, Phillips J, Menker JB: Recognition, resuscitation and management of patients with penetrating cardiac injuries. *Surg Gynecol Obstet* 174:205–210, 1992.

103. Benyan AKZ, Al-A'Ragy HH: The pattern of penetrating cardiac trauma in Basrah province: personal experience with seventy-two cases in a hospital without cardiopulmonary by-pass facility. *Int Surg* 7:111–113, 1992.

104. Macho JR, Markinson RE, Schecter WP: Cardiac stapling in the management of penetrating injuries of the heart: rapid control of hemorrhage and decreased risk of personal contamination. *J Trauma* 34:711–716, 1993.

105. Mirchell ME, Muakkassa FF, Pool GV, et al: Surgical approach of choice for penetrating cardiac wounds. *J Trauma* 34:17–20, 1993.

106. Kaplan AJ, Norcross ED, Crawford FA: Predictors of mortality in penetrating cardiac injuries. *Am Surg* 9:338–342, 1993.

107. Henderson VJ, Smith SR, Fry WR, et al: Cardiac injuries: analysis of an unselected series of 251 cases. *J Trauma* 36:341–348, 1994.

108. Coimbra R, Pinto MCC, Razuk A, et al: Penetrating cardiac wounds: predictive value of trauma indices and the necessity of terminology standardization. *Am Surg* 61:448–452, 1995.

109. Arreola-Risa C, Rhee P, Boyle EM, et al: Factors influencing outcome in stab wounds of the heart. *Am J Surg* 169:553–556, 1995.

110. Karmy-Jones R, Van Wijngaarden MH, Talwar MK, et al: Penetrating cardiac injuries. *Injury* 28:57–61, 1997.

111. Rhee PM, Foy H, Kaufman C, et al: Penetrating cardiac injuries: a population-based study. *J Trauma* 45:366–370, 1998.

112. Asensio JA, Murray J, Demetriades D, et al: Penetrating cardiac injuries: prospective one-year preliminary report: an analysis of variables predicting outcome. *J Am Coll Surg* 186:24–33, 1998.

113. Asensio JA, Berne JD, Demetriades D, et al: One hundred and five penetrating cardiac injuries. A two-year prospective evaluation. *J Trauma* 44:1073–1083, 1998.

114. Beaver B, Colombani P, Buck J: Efficacy of emergency room thoracotomy in pediatric trauma. *J Pediatr Surg* 22:19–23, 1987.

115. Powell R, Gill E, Jurkovich G: Resuscitative thoracotomy in children and adolescents. *Am Surg* 54:188, 1988.

116. Rothenberg S, Moore E, Moore FA, et al: Emergency department thoracotomy in children: a critical analysis. *J Trauma* 29:1322–1325, 1989.

117. Sheikh A, Culbertson C: Emergency department thoracotomy in children: rationale for selective application. *J Trauma* 34:323, 1993.

The Role of Focused Assessment with Sonography for Trauma: Indications, Limitations, and Controversies

Michael Dunham,   Mark McKenney, and   David Shatz

Focused Assessment with Sonography for Trauma (FAST) has rapidly taken root in modern trauma care. FAST is an integral part of trauma algorithms, and is an important adjunct to the Advanced Trauma Life Support (ATLS) primary and secondary surveys. In 1997, the American Board of Surgery required the addition of ultrasonography into Accreditation Council for Graduate Medical Education (ACGME)–approved surgical training programs. The American College of Surgeons (ACS) has also incorporated FAST into the ATLS course and has sponsored multiple ultrasound training seminars.

The primary objective of FAST is the early identification of hemoperitoneum, hemopericardium, and hemothorax. With the advantage of providing an immediate, accurate, portable, noninvasive assessment of trauma patients, FAST has virtually replaced diagnostic peritoneal lavage (DPL) as a first-line tool in the evaluation of patients with thoracoabdominal trauma and has modified the use of computed tomography (CT).

FORMATION OF AN ULTRASOUND IMAGE

Proper visualization and accurate interpretation of an ultrasound image requires a basic understanding of ultrasound components, principles, physics, and terminology. The basic components of an ultrasound machine are listed in Table 1 and include the transmitter to send electrical signals to the transducer, the transducer to interconvert electrical energy and acoustic energy using the piezoelectric effect, the receiver to convert electrical signals into an image, and the monitor to display the image. An optional printer provides a hardcopy image.

There are three essential principles of ultrasonography (Table 2): the piezoelectric effect, pulse-echo principle, and acoustic impedance. Within the transducer, piezoelectric crystals expand and contract to interconvert electrical and mechanical energy, a process known as the piezoelectric effect. When an ultrasound wave contacts tissue, some of the signal is reflected and some is transmitted into tissue. The reflected waves bounce back and contact the crystals within the transducer, generating electrical impulses comparable to the strength of the returning wave. This is known as the pulse–echo principle. Acoustic impedance is the density of tissue multiplied by the speed of sound in tissue. The strength of the returning echo depends on the difference in density between the two structures imaged. Structures of different acoustic impedance (e.g., bile and gallstones) are relatively easy to distinguish from one another, whereas those of similar acoustic impedance (e.g., spleen and kidney) are more difficult to distinguish.[1]

The basic physics of ultrasonography are important for good image formation, and terminology used for ultrasonography is listed in Table 3. Ultrasound waves are high-frequency (>20 kHz) mechanical radiant energy transmitted through a medium. The frequency (number of cycles/second) of medical diagnostic ultrasound is 2.5–10 MHz. As frequency increases, resolution improves, but penetration to deeper tissue decreases. Generally, the highest frequency transducer that produces the best resolution of the target organ is chosen (3.5 MHz for FAST). Common clinical applications of different ultrasound frequencies are listed in Table 4.

Propagation speed (determined by density and stiffness of the medium) is greater in solids than in liquids, and greater in liquids than in gases. Ultrasonic waves travel poorly through gases and therefore the lungs, bowel, and organs underlying areas of subcutaneous emphysema are poorly visualized. Air-filled organs can be visualized when surrounded by liquid, which provides an acoustic window, allowing the passage of the ultrasound waves. Bone appears black on ultrasound because it attenuates sound waves strongly.

The amplitude, or height of a wave, is a measure of its intensity. As ultrasound waves travel through tissue, the amplitude is diminished or attenuated. Lower-frequency waves (3.5 MHz) have greater amplitude and are attenuated less, allowing for greater penetration. Conversely, high-frequency waves (7.5 MHz) are chosen for high resolution of superficial structures, but are unsuitable for deeper structures due to higher attenuation.

Ultrasound waves are attenuated by absorption, scattering, and reflection. Absorption is the conversion of sound waves to heat and scattering is the redirection of waves as they meet an irregular boundary. Reflection is the return of the wave to the transducer. The reflected waves form the image displayed on the monitor. Artifacts in ultrasound imaging, or errors in imaging, are features of the image that do not have precise correspondence to the image being scanned (e.g., shadowing of gallstones).

The degree of amplification or amplitude of returning waves can be adjusted by the gain setting. Increasing the gain will make the displayed image brighter, and conversely, decreasing the gain will make a bright image darker. Ultrasound waves are attenuated as they travel through tissue resulting in fewer and fewer waves penetrating to deep structures. Therefore, fewer ultrasound waves are reflected from deep organs and returned to the transducer. Time-gain compensation (TGC) will increase the amplitude of returning waves from deeper structures, which allows adequate visualization of deeper or thicker organs. TGC allows liver, for example, to appear uniform. Without TGC, the deeper liver parenchyma would appear darker as distance from the transducer increases.

The echogenicity of a structure is defined as the degree to which tissue echoes ultrasonic waves (generally reflected in ultrasound images as the degree of brightness). Tissues that reflect waves strongly will appear bright and are hyperechoic. Tissues that conduct ultrasound waves well are hypoechoic and are darker, while anechoic tissues conduct waves very well and appear black because essentially no waves are reflected back to the transducer. Isoechoic tissue transmits ultrasound similar to that of surrounding tissues, and is displayed with similar intensity (Table 5).[1]

TECHNIQUE

The patient's identifying information is first entered to annotate the hardcopy ultrasound images. With the patient in the supine position, a liberal amount of ultrasound transmission gel is applied to the subxiphoid, left and right upper quadrants, and suprapubic

Table 1: Components of Ultrasound Machine

Component	Description
Transmitter	Sends electrical signals to transducer
Transducer	Interconverts electrical energy and acoustic energy by piezoelectric effect
Receiver	Converts electrical signals into image
Monitor	Displays image
Printer	Records hard copy of image (optional)

Table 2: Essential Principles of Ultrasound

Principle	Explanation
Piezoelectric effect	Piezoelectric crystals expand and contract to interconvert electrical and mechanical energy.
Pulse-echo principle	When an ultrasound wave contacts tissue, some of the signal is reflected and some is transmitted into tissue. These waves are then reflected to crystals within the transducer, generating electrical impulse comparable to the strength of the returning wave.
Acoustic impedance	Acoustic impedance is the density of tissue X speed of sound in tissue. The strength of the returning echo depends on the difference in density between the two structures imaged: structures of different acoustic impedance (e.g., bile and gallstones) are relatively easy to distinguish from one another, whereas those of similar acoustic impedance (e.g., spleen and kidney) are more difficult to distinguish.

Table 3: Ultrasound Terminology

Term	Definition
Ultrasound	High-frequency (>20 kHz) mechanical radiant energy transmitted through a medium
Frequency	Number of cycles per second (medical diagnostic ultrasound: 2.5–10 MHz)
Propagation speed	Speed at which wave travels through soft tissue (1540 m/sec)
Amplitude	Strength or height of wave
Attenuation	Decrease in amplitude and intensity of wave as it travels through medium
Absorption	Conversion of sound waves into heat
Scattering	Redirection of wave as it strikes rough or small boundary
Reflection	Return of wave toward transducer
Artifact	Error in imaging
Gain	Amplitude of returning waves based on tissue depth

Table 4: Clinical Applications of Selected Transducer Frequencies

Frequency	Application
2.5–3.5 MHz	General abdominal
5 MHz	Transvaginal, pediatric abdominal, testicular
7.5 MHz	Vascular, soft tissue, thyroid

Table 5: Terminology Used in Interpretation of Ultrasound Images

Term	Definition
Echogenicity	Degree to which tissue echoes ultrasonic waves (generally reflected in ultrasound image as degree of brightness)
Anechoic	No internal echoes, appearing dark or black
Isoechoic	Having appearance similar to that of surrounding tissue
Hypoechoic	Less echoic (darker) than surrounding tissue
Hyperechoic	More echoic (brighter) than surrounding tissue

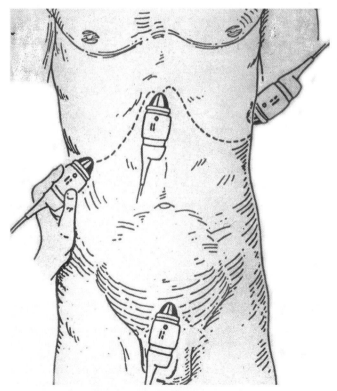

Figure 1 Transducer positions for focused assessment with sonography for trauma (FAST): 1, pericardial; 2, right upper quadrant; 3, left upper quadrant; and 4, pelvis.

areas. Using four transducer positions as shown in Figure 1, the pericardium and five dependent abdominal regions are examined for free fluid:

- Right subdiaphragmatic space
- Hepatorenal interface (Morrison's pouch)
- Left subdiaphragmatic space
- Splenorenal interface
- Pelvis

Although Morrison's pouch was shown by Rozycki and colleagues[2] to be the most sensitive for free intra-abdominal fluid, all five regions of the abdomen should be examined to maximize sensitivity of the test. Each area should be evaluated in two planes (longitudinal and transverse) with confirmation of positive regions using two views.

The FAST exam begins with the examination of the pericardial area. The gain is adjusted until the blood within the heart appears anechoic (black). Proper gain will ensure that any hemoperitoneum will appear anechoic. Correct superior/inferior and left/right orientation should be checked by noting the position of the visible indicator on the hand-held transducer.

A 3.5-MHz convex transducer is oriented for sagittal sections and positioned in the subxiphoid area directing the transducer superiorly. Often, mild pressure on the transducer below the xiphoid toward the pericardial sac is required to visualize the heart. If this is unsuccessful, a left, parasternal, 4th or 5th intercostal view will be required. Obesity, rib/sternal fracture, subcutaneous emphysema, and a narrow subcostal angle may necessitate the parasternal view, and/or make this part of the examination indeterminate. Hemoperi-

cardium is detected by an anechoic band between the heart and the pericardial/diaphragmatic interface, as seen in Figure 2.

The right upper quadrant is then visualized by placing the transducer in the right mid to posterior axillary line, 11th intercostal space, in both longitudinal and transverse planes to visualize the right subdiaphragmatic and hepatorenal interface. An anechoic band between the liver and kidney as shown in Figure 3 identifies the presence of a minimal amount of blood, and a moderate hemoperitoneum is shown in Figure 4.

The left upper quadrant is examined by directing the transducer between the 10th and 11th ribs in the posterior axillary line. The right sub-diaphragmatic and splenorenal spaces are examined in two planes for free fluid, detected again by an anechoic band separating the two organs. A normal view of the hyperechoic left kidney/spleen interface is shown in Figure 5 and a positive left upper quadrant view is shown in Figure 6.

Finally, the transducer is placed transversely just above the symphysis pubis and directed inferiorly looking for a coronal view of the bladder. This is ideally done before bladder catheterization to allow for a distended bladder, which optimizes ultrasound transmission and detection of free fluid posterior to the bladder in the rectovesical/uterine space. If a catheter has previously been placed, saline can be injected into the bladder through the catheter, or the catheter can simply be clamped and the pelvic view obtained after passive filling. Free intra-abdominal fluid is best detected on longitudinal plane in the rectovesical or rectouterine space by an anechoic band between the bladder and uterus or rectum as shown in Figure 7.

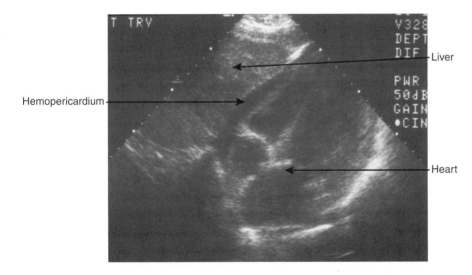

Figure 2 Positive pericardial view showing anechoic hemopericardium between liver and heart.

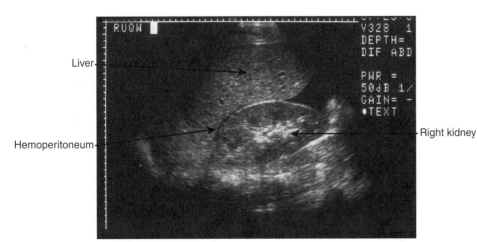

Figure 3 Sagittal view of right upper quadrant showing minimal hemoperitoneum between the right kidney and liver.

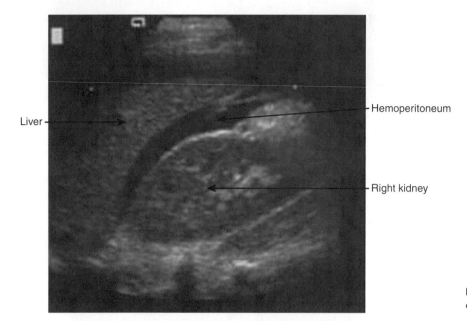

Liver

Hemoperitoneum

Right kidney

Figure 4 Sagittal view of right upper quadrant with moderate hemoperitoneum.

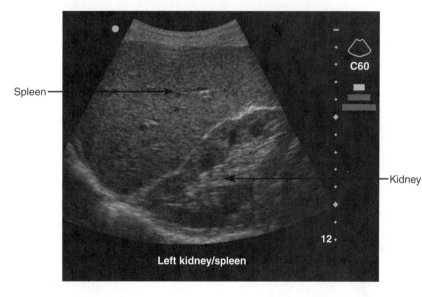

Spleen

Kidney

Left kidney/spleen

Figure 5 Normal sagittal view of left upper quadrant showing the hyperechoic left kidney/spleen interface.

TROUBLESHOOTING

Difficulties in image formation are often solved with the simple techniques and strategy changes found in Table 6. A common solution to improve visualization is to apply a liberal amount of gel and reapply whenever the image quality is poor. An image that is too dark or too bright may require an adjustment in the gain. Poor visualization of deeper structures may also require a lower-frequency (2.5-MHz) transducer or an increase in time-gain compensation of the far field. A 2.5-MHz transducer may be necessary for the obese trauma patient. A 5-MHz transducer may increase the resolution of FAST in pediatric trauma patients, and a 7.5-MHz transducer is optimal for superficial structures (vascular, soft tissue). Subcutaneous emphysema poses a significant problem for ultrasound waves and alternate sites such as the parasternal position may be necessary for adequate visualization.

One may become disoriented during a FAST exam, and ultrasonographers should remember to reestablish surface anatomy landmarks, confirm transducer orientation (superior/inferior, left/right), and identify obvious internal landmarks (e.g., liver, kidney, spleen). Difficulties visualizing the pericardial sac can be avoided by gentle pressure directing the transducer cephalad under the xiphoid process. Alternatively, moving to the left parasternal view between the 4th or 5th intercostal spaces can be helpful. Transducer movement should be slow with light pressure, watching for the motion of heart contraction. The right or left upper quadrant may be better visualized by moving up or down an intercostal space, moving posteriorly, or during end inspiration. In cooperative patients, requesting an end inspiration breath-hold may be helpful, especially if the shadow of a rib is obscuring a desired view. Oro/nasogastric tube decompression of the stomach may improve visualization of the left upper quadrant. Perhaps the most important maneuver to examine the splenorenal interface and left subdiaphragmatic space is to move the transducer posteriorly, flat on the stretcher, and then point the transducer anterior between the 9th or 10th interspace. The pelvic views should be done with a full bladder.

INDICATIONS

FAST should be performed on all trauma patients who require evaluation of the chest and abdomen and cannot be cleared by physical exam. It should not delay a patient with penetrating abdominal trauma and hypotension or peritonitis from surgical exploration. In the case of penetrating thoracoabdominal trauma, FAST is valuable in early identification of pericardial tamponade or hemoperitoneum.

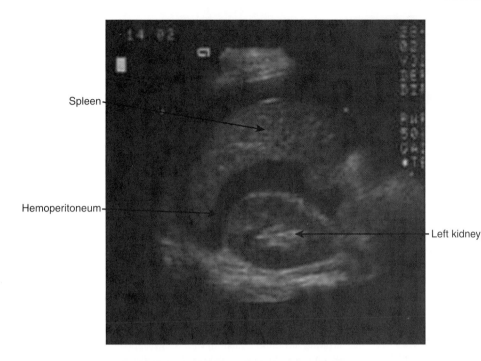

Figure 6 Sagittal view of left upper quadrant showing anechoic hemoperitoneum between left kidney and spleen.

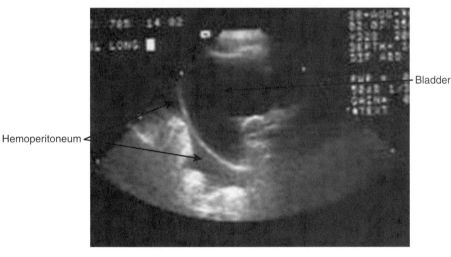

Figure 7 Positive longitudinal view of pelvis for hemoperitoneum posterior to bladder.

This early application of FAST can direct operative intervention toward the body cavity most likely injured.

FAST is indicated in the evaluation of the unstable, multitrauma patient with an unidentified cause of hypotension. In this scenario, CT is contraindicated and FAST provides a rapid screening test without moving the patient from the resuscitation area. A positive exam is most helpful in this situation and Rozycki et al.[3] reported 100% sensitivity and specificity (8 of 8 patients) for intra-abdominal injury in patients with a positive FAST and hypotension. McKenney et al.,[4] in a prospective evaluation of an ultrasound scoring system, reported similar results. In this series, 10 of 10 patients with initial hypotension (systolic blood pressure <90), and 32 of 36 patients with subsequent hemodynamic deterioration and a significant hemoperitoneum on FAST had a therapeutic laparotomy. Farahmand et al.,[5] in a study of 128 hypotensive patients suffering blunt abdominal trauma found FAST to be indispensable. The sensitivity of FAST for all injuries was 85%, for surgical injuries 97%, and 100% for fatal injuries. The authors found that FAST was able to virtually exclude surgical injury and detect surgical injury in 64% of positive studies. These studies strongly suggest that the combination of hemoperitoneum and hypotension mandate urgent laparotomy. A negative exam in the multi-injured, hypotensive patient should prompt further aggressive diagnostic and therapeutic evaluation.

The portable and noninvasive nature of ultrasound permits repeat FAST evaluations. A secondary ultrasound is most important in patients without obvious blood loss, a negative primary FAST, and continued hemodynamic instability despite ongoing resuscitation. Secondary FAST may also be performed on patients where CT is unavailable or delayed. Recently, Blackbourne and colleagues[6] prospectively evaluated 547 patients undergoing both a primary and secondary FAST exam (within 30 minutes to 24 hours of initial exam). Excluding patients with hemoperitoneum and hypotension (who went directly to the operating room), the secondary FAST exam increased the sensitivity of detecting intra-abdominal free fluid.

To summarize, all trauma patients at risk for thoracoabdominal injury who cannot be cleared by physical examination should have an initial FAST. In unstable, multitrauma patients, with blunt mechanisms, FAST should be used to rule out hemoperitoneum. FAST may also be helpful in directing operative strategy to the correct body cavity in patients with penetrating thoracoabdominal trauma. A secondary FAST should be performed on hemodynamically unstable patients with an initial negative FAST and ongoing instability despite adequate resuscitation.

Table 6: Troubleshooting

Problem	Solution
Image too dark	Increase gain, apply more gel
Image too bright	Decrease gain
Poor penetration of waves	Use lower-frequency transducer, increase gain, subcutaneous emphysema (use alternate site), apply more gel
Poor image	Adjust gain, higher frequency transducer, subcutaneous emphysema (use alternate site), inadequate gel, begin with light pressure, slow movements
Disorientation	Confirm correct surface anatomy, orient transducer position, find known landmark (e.g., liver, kidney)
Obesity	Use lower frequency transducer
Infants	Use higher frequency transducer
Pericardial	Gentle pressure beneath the xiphoid directing cephalad, use alternate left parasternal window, and with slow movements look for motion of heart
Right upper quadrant	Move up or down a rib space, move posterior, deep inspiration
Left upper quadrant	Place transducer as far posteriorly as possible (on bed) and direct anteriorly, insert an oro/nasogastric tube to decompress stomach gas, deep inspiration
Bladder	Ensure full bladder, clamp catheter or fill bladder with saline

ACCURACY

The accuracy of FAST is dependent on the examiner's technique, experience, and the volume of fluid within the abdominal cavity. Other factors such as massive hemothorax, subcutaneous emphysema, and mechanism of injury (penetrating vs. blunt) impact the accuracy of the examination. FAST accuracy also depends upon the exam to which it is compared. CT, DPL, course in hospital, and/or operative or postmortem findings have been used to calculate the accuracy of FAST.

Overall, FAST has proven to be an accurate, reliable, screening test for blunt trauma patients. Several large published series have reported sensitivity greater than 80% and specificity greater than 90%.[3,7] Dolich and coworkers[7] in a series of 2576 FAST studies reported a sensitivity of 86%, specificity of 98%, and an accuracy of 97%, with positive and negative predictive values of 87%, and 98%, respectively.

In a series of 1540 patients evaluated by FAST, Rozycki and colleagues[3] reported a sensitivity of 83.3% and a specificity of 99.7%. Hypotension coupled with a positive FAST produced a 100% sensitivity and specificity for therapeutic operative intervention. In the same study, FAST was used to evaluate for hemopericardium in 313 patients with a sensitivity of 100% and specificity of 99.3%. This was followed by a multicenter study by Rozycki et al.[8] examining 261 patients at risk for penetrating cardiac injury. They found a sensitivity, specificity, and accuracy of 100%, 96.9%, and 97.3%, respectively, for pericardial FAST.

While FAST for penetrating trauma to the pericardium has proven reliable, FAST for penetrating trauma to the abdomen has not been shown to be sensitive in detecting intra-abdominal injury. FAST for penetrating abdominal trauma is helpful only if it is positive; this group of patients should have immediate laparotomy. A negative FAST in

penetrating abdominal injury is not helpful. It does, however, have excellent specificity and positive predictive value. Soffer et al.[9] prospectively evaluated 177 stable patients with penetrating torso trauma and no clinical signs mandating operative exploration. They found FAST to have 48% sensitivity, 98% specificity, a negative predictive value (NPV) of 82%, a positive predictive value (PPV) of 92%, and an accuracy of 85%. The most common injury missed by FAST was hollow viscus injury. Interestingly, FAST altered the management in only three patients (1.7%) suggesting that it is not an accurate diagnostic tool. Similarly, Udobi and colleagues[10] also reported the inadequacy of FAST to detect intra-abdominal injury in penetrating trauma. This prospective study included 75 stable patients, evaluated by FAST, without obvious indication for laparotomy. They reported sensitivity, specificity, NPV, and PPV of 46%, 94%, 60%, and 90%, respectively, for this patient population. In 72 patients without clear indication for laparotomy, Boulanger et al.[11] reported similar results with FAST having a sensitivity, specificity, PPV, and NPV of 67%, 98%, 92%, and 89%, respectively. These investigators all conclude that a positive exam strongly suggests the need for laparotomy, and a negative exam requires additional diagnostic evaluation.

In summary, FAST is an accurate screening tool for blunt trauma and penetrating pericardial trauma. The presence of hypotension and positive FAST indicates the need for operative exploration for both blunt and penetrating trauma. The sensitivity of FAST for penetrating intra-abdominal injuries is low, and additional clinical and diagnostic evaluation is required for negative examinations.

LEARNING CURVE AND TRAINING

The learning curve associated with FAST has been studied, and guidelines have been established for training and credentialing. In 1997, the World Consensus Conference on Ultrasound, consisting of an international expert panel of surgeons, radiologists, and emergency physicians, recommended the following training requirements: (1) 1-day training course consisting of a 4-hour didactic component followed by a 4-hour practical component, and (2) 200 supervised examinations.[12] Alternative competency requirements exist consisting of a 1-day course followed by 50 supervised examinations.

The nature of FAST is a focused exam and not a comprehensive examination of the contents of the entire thoracic and abdominal cavities. FAST is designed to answer a specific clinical question: Is there free fluid within the pericardium or abdomen? FAST training and evaluation should be structured and evaluated based on a nonradiologist clinician's ability to detect the presence of free fluid. Identification of specific injuries to the various intra-abdominal and intra-thoracic organs is beyond the scope of FAST.

Based on studies evaluating training and learning curves for nonradiologist clinicians, several conclusions and recommendations can be made. First, nonradiologist clinicians can learn and become competent with FAST techniques. McKenney et al.,[13] in a prospective study comparing FAST accuracy of radiologists versus surgeons with limited training, found equal accuracy in interpreting FAST between both groups (99% vs. 99%). Thomas and colleagues[14] determined that the overall accuracy of trainees following a 1-day FAST course was 98%, with a sensitivity of 81%, and a specificity of 91%. Multiple other investigators have shown that surgeons can achieve accuracy of over 90%, which compares favorably to radiologist performed FAST.[3,7]

Second, to the beginner, sensitivity is initially poor, but with experience, and after 25–100 examinations, the learning curve flattens and minimal improvement is seen beyond 100 examinations. This is controversial, however. McCarter and colleagues[15] and Smith and colleagues[16] have reported no identifiable learning curve among novice ultrasonographers and have suggested that 25 examinations are adequate. Other studies do show that sensitivity improves over the first 100 exams. Shackford and coworkers[17] at the University of Vermont challenged the recommendation of more than 50 proctored examinations. In a prospective study, they observed a steep learning curve with a decrease in error rate from 17% after the first 5 examinations, to 5%

after 10 examinations. Notably, this steep curve was observed among a selected group of patients with a high risk of hemoperitoneum (21.2%). Jang et al.[18] found that 10 FAST examinations performed by emergency medicine residents was insufficient experience to ensure high sensitivity. After 20 examinations their sensitivity was 74%, but residents having 31 or more completed cases observed a rise in sensitivity to 95%.

Third, at least the first 25–100 examinations should be proctored and/or have gold standard confirmation. The number of proctored examinations is controversial and depends upon the individuals' own accuracy rate and the frequency of true positive exams in the patient population.

Fourth, total number of exams is not the only important factor in acquiring this skill. It is important to include an adequate number of positive examinations during the training period. In large series by Dolich et al.[7] and Rozycki and associates,[3] the positive FAST rate is between 9% and 13%, and therefore, it may take 100 FAST examinations to be exposed to sufficient true positives to accurately recognize the varying degrees of a positive exam. In addition, with liberal application of FAST to all trauma patients, true negative rates will be high, possibly falsely elevating the sensitivity of the exam. It has been noted by several investigators that error rates increase with an increasing prevalence of hemoperitoneum.[19] Peritoneal dialysis models for FAST training have been used to increase the experience in identifying positive studies. Gracias and colleagues[20] found that sensitivity increased from 45% to 87% after training using peritoneal dialysis patients as a model.

In conclusion, despite considerable controversy, it appears that a formal didactic session and between 30 and 100 proctored examinations of severely injured patients are adequate for a clinician to become competent with FAST.

FLUID VOLUME AND SCORING SYSTEMS

The differential diagnosis for free fluid within the abdomen found on FAST includes blood, urine, ascites, and bowel contents. Free fluid within the peritoneum has been shown to collect in the dependent regions of the abdomen: the right upper quadrant (Morrison's pouch), left upper quadrant (perisplenic), and in the pelvis. The minimal volume of intra-abdominal fluid reliably detected by FAST is usually more than 500 ml, ranging from 250 to 620 ml.[19] Abrams and colleagues[21] have shown that 5 degrees of Trendelenburg positioning increases the sensitivity of FAST. In patients requiring DPL, Branney and colleagues[22] found that a minimum of 619 ml was required for most examiners to detect free fluid within Morrison's pouch. Sensitivity of detecting 1000 ml of intra-abdominal fluid in this study was 97%.

Early experience with FAST taught clinicians that patients with large volumes of hemoperitoneum were most likely to require laparotomy. Two scoring systems were developed to identify which patients were most likely to require operative exploration. Huang and colleagues[23] gave 1 point for each of the five areas of the abdomen positive for blood, and an additional point for free-floating intestine. Two points were given for a fluid depth of greater than 2 mm in the hepatorenal or splenorenal space. They found that 96% of patients with 3 or more points required laparotomy; however, 38% of patients with a score less than 3 still required laparotomy. The sensitivity and specificity for hemoperitoneum greater than 1 liter at laparotomy was 84% and 71%, respectively.

McKenney and colleagues[4] developed a second scoring system and prospectively evaluated its performance. Using this system, the ultrasound score was defined as the depth in centimeters of the deepest pocket of fluid collection, plus the number of additional spaces where fluid was seen. They found that 85% of patients with a score greater or equal to 3, and only 15% of patients with a score less than 3 required laparotomy. In addition, this score was found to be more accurate than systolic blood pressure and base deficit in identifying patients in need of operative exploration. The sensitivity, specificity, and accuracy of this scoring system was 83%, 87%, and 85%, respectively.

To review, more than 500 ml of intra-abdominal fluid are reliably detected by FAST. Scoring and quantifying hemoperitoneum has been shown to be predictive in evaluating the need for laparotomy. A McKenney score higher than 3 predicts the need for laparotomy in the majority of cases. This may be more accurate than blood pressure and base deficit. Each patient should be evaluated individually however, with the understanding that a negative FAST does not exclude intra-abdominal injury.

ALGORITHM: BLUNT ABDOMINAL TRAUMA

All patients suspected of sustaining blunt abdominal trauma who cannot be cleared by physical examination should have an initial FAST exam. A positive FAST and hemodynamic instability should have immediate exploration in the operating room. Patients with a positive FAST and stable vital signs should proceed to CT to further define the source of free fluid because the majority hemodynamically stable patients with solid organ injuries characterized on CT are managed nonoperatively.

A negative FAST exam and instability should prompt further clinical and diagnostic evaluation (e.g., chest x-ray, diagnostic peritoneal lavage, anteroposterior pelvis x-ray, long-bone x-rays) to identify other potential sites of blood loss and a secondary FAST in 30 minutes. A negative FAST, stable vital signs, and risk factors for intra-abdominal injury should be followed up with CT or a secondary FAST if CT is unavailable. Risk factors for intra-abdominal injury include: spinal, pelvic, and rib fractures, hematuria, hypotension, abdominal tenderness, persistent base deficit, significant distracting injuries, head injury, and intoxication. Patients with these risk factors should have abdominal and pelvic CT. Ballard et al.[24] found a high incidence of missed intra-abdominal injuries in patients evaluated by FAST with pelvic fractures. There were 13 of 70 false-negative FAST exams in patients with pelvic fractures leading to four therapeutic laparotomies and nine patients with solid organ injuries managed nonoperatively.

Patients with blunt abdominal trauma and an equivocal FAST are followed by CT in stable patients, or a secondary FAST or DPL if CT is unavailable. Unstable patients with an equivocal FAST are resuscitated and evaluated with routine trauma diagnostic evaluation (chest x-ray, anteroposterior pelvis x-ray, long-bone x-rays) and DPL or secondary FAST. If the DPL or secondary FAST remains equivocal, the patient should have immediate laparotomy. The algorithm for blunt abdominal trauma is presented in Figure 8.

ALGORITHM: PENETRATING THORACOABDOMINAL TRAUMA

In patients with penetrating thoracoabdominal trauma, the accuracy of FAST in detecting hemopericardium is excellent, while the sensitivity of FAST in identifying intra-abdominal injury is poor. This is reflected in the FAST algorithm in Figure 9. Patients with penetrating thoracoabdominal trauma should have initial FAST to identify hemopericardium, hemothorax, or hemoperitoneum. FAST positive for hemopericardium warrants immediate median sternotomy and a hemothorax is managed with tube thorocostomy. In the presence of hemothorax, Rozycki et al.[8] have reported false-positive and -negative results for pericardial FAST. The hemothorax may obscure identification of intrapericardial blood, or a perforation of the pericardium may allow blood from the heart to enter the thoracic cavity.

Hemoperitoneum detected by FAST in penetrating trauma is followed by prompt laparotomy. Patients with a negative pericardial FAST are managed according to routine trauma protocols and equivocal FAST of the pericardium suggests the need for pericardial window. A negative FAST of the abdomen in penetrating trauma is not helpful, and should be followed by other diagnostic or operative evaluation.

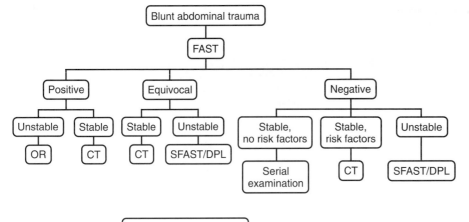

Figure 8 Algorithm for blunt abdominal trauma. *CT*, Computed tomography; *DPL*, diagnostic peritoneal lavage; *FAST*, focused assessment with sonography for trauma; *OR*, operating room; *SFAST*, secondary FAST. Risk factors include pelvic fracture, rib fracture, spine fracture, hematuria, transient hypotension, abdominal tenderness, head injury, intoxication, and persistent base deficit.

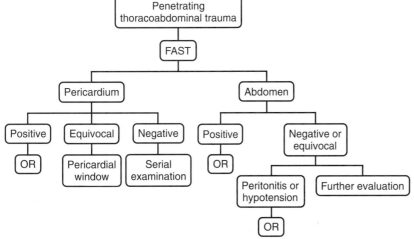

Figure 9 Algorithm for penetrating thoracoabdominal trauma. *FAST*, Focused assessment with sonography for trauma; *OR*, operating room.

EXTENSIONS TO FAST

Hemothorax

Evaluation for hemothorax is an extension of the right and left upper quadrant regions of FAST. The 3.5-MHz transducer is slowly moved cephalad until the hyperechoic diaphragm is identified. The supradiaphragmatic region is examined for anechoic fluid surrounding a hypoechoic "floating lung." There are obvious advantages to ultrasound diagnosis of hemothorax. As a part of FAST, detection of hemothorax is rapid and management decisions are expedited. Sisley et al.[25] compared the accuracy of ultrasonography and chest radiography in the detection of traumatic hemothorax. Three hundred sixty patients were examined with a sensitivity of 97.4% and specificity of 99.7%, versus 92.5% sensitivity and 99.7% specificity for chest x-ray. They also reported a significantly faster performance time for ultrasound compared to chest x-ray.

Pneumothorax

FAST has been extended by some investigators to include evaluation for pneumothorax. This has been termed extended FAST (eFAST) or FAST +2. Again, similar to detection of hemothorax, ultrasound diagnosis for pneumothorax is a rapid, noninvasive, and accurate test. Dulchavsky et al.[26] evaluated the performance of ultrasound in detecting pneumothorax in 382 trauma patients. Ultrasound identified 37 of 39 pneumothoraces (sensitivity 95%), with 2 pneumothoraces missed due to subcutaneous emphysema, and a true-negative rate of 100%. In a similar investigation, a group of emergency physicians[27] examined 176 patients for pneumothorax using ultrasound and compared their findings to

CT. Using CT as the gold standard they found that ultrasound outperformed chest radiography in the detection of pneumothorax (sensitivity 98% vs. 76%). These groups have concluded that ultrasound is a rapid and accurate modality for pneumothorax recognition, but still recommend routine chest x-ray for trauma patient evaluation.

The technique for ultrasound detection of pneumothorax requires a higher-frequency transducer (4.0–7.5 MHz) than for conventional FAST. The unaffected hemithorax is examined first, in the third to fourth intercostal space, midaxillary line. The transducer is moved slowly medially and laterally between the ribs in transverse and sagittal orientations. The normal examination will identify the acoustic shadow of the ribs and the pleura, visualized by a hyperechoic line between and below the ribs. The lung pleura is then examined for "pleural sliding" and "comet-tail" artifact. Pleural sliding occurs with apposition of visceral and parietal pleura seen as hyperechoic lines during the to-and-fro movement of respiration. A pneumothorax separates the visceral and parietal pleura and does not allow transmission of ultrasound waves. Visualization of the visceral pleura is lost and pleural sliding is not seen. The comet tail sign or artifact appears as a dense tapering trail of echoes just distal to a strongly reflecting structure. This reverberation type of artifact occurs when there is a marked difference in acoustic impedance between an object and its surrounding tissue. In the normal lung, ultrasound waves are strongly reflected by the lung and a tapering hyperechoic band (the comet tail artifact) is observed deep to the visceral pleura. This artifact is lost when a pneumothorax is present.

Sternal Fracture

Using a 7.5-MHz transducer, sternal fractures can be diagnosed with accuracy comparable to lateral sternal x-ray. Mahlfeld et al.[28] described the use of ultrasound in 11 patients suspected of sustaining a sternal fracture. In all 11 cases the fracture was detected by ultrasound and confirmed by lateral x-ray. Advantages to ultrasound diagnosis include its speed and apparent accuracy. Subcutaneous emphysema secondary to pneumothorax occasionally prevents adequate assessment of the sternum. Sternal fracture is rarely, if ever, life threatening and routine screening for this fracture is unlikely to become a part of the FAST protocol. However, it is important to recognize the degree of force required to fracture the sternum and the potential for associated thoracic and mediastinal injuries.

Ultrasound diagnosis of sternal fracture requires a liberal coat of transmission gel and a 7.5-MHz transducer. With the patient supine, the transducer is advanced slowly over the sternum in both transverse and longitudinal orientations. A fracture is diagnosed by observing a hypoechoic area over the sternum together with a hematoma, a disruption of the cortical bone, or a step in the bony outline.

Summarizing, extending the use of ultrasound for the diagnosis of hemothorax, pneumothorax, and sternal fracture has advantages for traumatically injured patients. Studies have confirmed ultrasound to provide rapid and accurate diagnosis and may direct early management decisions. Ultrasonography should not, however, replace routine chest radiography in the diagnostic evaluation of trauma patients and it is uncertain if screening for pneumothorax and sternal fracture should become part of routine FAST protocols.

FAST FOR PEDIATRIC TRAUMA

FAST performed by surgeons for the pediatric trauma population is a valuable screening modality. The technique for FAST in children is identical to that of adults, except a 5-MHz transducer may be substituted to improve resolution for imaging infants and young children. Like adults, FAST for children is rapid, portable, noninvasive, repeatable, and may be performed in the resuscitation area by surgeons.

The accuracy of FAST for pediatric blunt trauma patients is comparable to the adult blunt trauma population. In a prospective study, Thourani and colleagues[29] followed 196 pediatric trauma patients and found FAST to be 80% sensitive and 100% specific. In this study, FAST was positive in 5.3%, confirming the low frequency of hemoperitoneum in the pediatric trauma population. Four patients required immediate laparotomy after FAST and there were two false negatives confirmed on delayed CT; neither of these patients required laparotomy. All three patients with positive FAST and hypotension required therapeutic operative intervention. Five of five hemodynamically stable patients with positive FAST had splenic lacerations confirmed by CT and managed nonoperatively. These authors also found that the surgeon-sonographers were capable of performing FAST with adequate accuracy and the 3.5-MHz probe produced acceptable images. They concluded that FAST provides a rapid, accurate screening tool for pediatric trauma patients and provides efficient assessment of the abdomen allowing prioritization of injuries.

Soudack et al.[30] retrospectively reviewed 313 pediatric trauma patients evaluated by FAST. They reported 39 positive FAST exams with three false negatives and two false positives, with an overall sensitivity of 92.5%, specificity of 97.2%, and accuracy of 95.5%. They concluded that FAST was an effective screening tool. Coley et al.[31] in a report of 32 pediatric patients reported a sensitivity of only 55%; however, this study only included hemodynamically stable patients. Holmes et al.[32] studied FAST in 224 hemodynamically stable and unstable pediatric trauma patients. They report a sensitivity and specificity of 82% and 95%, respectively, for all patients. Seven of seven patients with positive FAST and hypotension had confirmed intra-abdominal injury at laparotomy. In total, 18 patients with positive FAST were taken to the operating room and only one patient had a nontherapeutic laparotomy. Fifteen patients in this study had a negative FAST and were determined to have intra-abdominal injury, six with intraperitoneal fluid and nine without intraperitoneal fluid. Two of these false negative exams included gastrointestinal tract injuries. They concluded that FAST is a rapid, accurate screening test and provides crucial information for the management of the hypotensive pediatric trauma patient. They also emphasize the need for CT in hemodynamically stable children with a positive FAST and in children where intra-abdominal injury cannot be ruled out by physical exam.

Ultrasound scoring systems have also been applied to the pediatric trauma population. Using the McKenney score, Ong et al.[33] retrospectively reviewed 193 pediatric trauma patients who had FAST. Thirty-seven patients had an initial positive FAST exam, with 22 patients scoring less than 3 and 15 patients scoring greater than or equal to 3. Of the 15 patients with a score greater than or equal to 3, eight required therapeutic laparotomy compared to only 1 of 22 in the group scoring less than 3. Interestingly, this patient had a jejunal perforation and mesenteric bleeding. One nontherapeutic laparotomy was performed in each group. The sensitivity, specificity, and accuracy for predicting therapeutic laparotomy using the McKenney score in this study was 89%, 75%, and 78%, respectively.

In summary, FAST performed by surgeons has been shown to be a rapid, accurate screening modality in pediatric blunt trauma patients. The finding of hypotension and a positive FAST in children strongly suggests immediate operative intervention. An ultrasound scoring system may be beneficial in predicting which patients with a positive FAST require laparotomy.

FAST FOR REPRODUCTIVE-AGE FEMALES

In reproductive-age female trauma patients, free fluid within the abdomen and pelvis detected by FAST suggests intra-abdominal injury until proven otherwise. Physiologic free fluid on transabdominal ultrasound has been estimated to range from 5–21 ml.[34] Ormsby et al.[34] reviewed 328 pregnant and 1804 reproductive-age women who presented with blunt abdominal trauma and were evaluated with FAST. Overall, they found that free fluid in the abdomen alone or abdomen and pelvis was strongly correlated with intra-abdominal injury compared to those with a negative FAST. In patients with free fluid in the abdomen alone, 57 of 70 (81.4%) nonpregnant and 4 of 9 (44%) pregnant patients had intra-abdominal injury. Of those with free fluid in the abdomen and pelvis, 67 of 74 (91%) nonpregnant and 7 of 10 (70%) pregnant patients had intra-abdominal injuries. Notably, 17 of 43 (40%) nonpregnant and 3 of 10 (30%) pregnant patients with free fluid isolated to the pelvis suffered intra-abdominal injury and the authors cautioned that isolated free fluid not be considered physiological in trauma patients. They also emphasized the need for a full bladder to visualize the pelvis adequately. In this study, 67 of 1804 (3.7%) nonpregnant patients, and 9 of 299 (3%) pregnant patients had a false-negative FAST, suggesting very good sensitivity of FAST in this patient population. Six of nine pregnant patients with intra-abdominal injury and a negative FAST had placental abruption. This underscores the need for obstetrical consultation and fetal monitoring in this unique trauma population. FAST in pregnant patients may have a lower sensitivity for detecting intra-abdominal injury. Richards et al.[35] reported FAST results from 328 pregnant patients. Twenty-three pregnant patients were FAST positive with a sensitivity, specificity, and accuracy of 61%, 94%, and 92%, respectively. Bochicchio and colleagues[36] have also suggested the FAST protocol should include routine screening in reproductive-age females for pregnancy. They confirmed pregnancy in 126 of 132 patients who reported that they were pregnant on admission, and diagnosed 8 incidental pregnancies using FAST alone.

The use of FAST in pregnant trauma patients should not alter trauma management algorithms. This group of patients must be managed aggressively together with obstetrical consultation and fetal monitoring. Free fluid on FAST indicates intra-abdominal injury until proven otherwise and must not be considered physiologic. Hypotensive pregnant patients with a positive FAST require laparotomy. Sensitivity of FAST in the pregnant population may be less than in nonpregnant patients, indicating a need for close surgical and obstetrical follow-up and/or further imaging such as CT or MRI.

LIMITATIONS OF FAST

Ultrasonography is a highly operator-dependent diagnostic modality that requires an understanding of ultrasound technology and experience in image formation and interpretation. Many studies have shown that surgeons are capable of learning and performing FAST with accuracy comparable to radiologists. Although FAST is feasible for almost all trauma patients, occasionally abrasions, lacerations, burns, or subcutaneous emphysema may make FAST difficult to complete. These problems can usually be overcome by alterations in technique and experience.

The primary goal of FAST is to identify hemopericardium, hemothorax, and hemoperitoneum, and is not a detailed evaluation of the heart, lungs, and solid organs of the abdomen. FAST protocols do not evaluate for injury to solid organ parenchyma, the gastrointestinal tract, the diaphragm, or retroperitoneal structures. Therefore, the major limitation of FAST is the detection of injuries that do not produce significant free intracavitary fluid. Intestinal injuries are a major limitation for FAST; the sensitivity of ultrasound in detecting intestinal injuries is poor. In a 15-year retrospective review of 1239 patients, Yoshii et al.[37] found that the overall sensitivity, specificity, and accuracy of ultrasound was 95%, 95%, and 95%, respectively. Individual organ injuries were identified with sensitivities of 92%, 90%, 92%, 71%, and 35% for the liver, spleen, kidneys, pancreas, and intestine, respectively. These authors concluded that ultrasound is a reliable method of diagnosing solid organ injuries, but insensitive for detecting intestinal injury.

Another limitation of FAST is the sensitivity of the exam for detecting free-intra-abdominal fluid in penetrating trauma patients and hemodynamically stable blunt trauma patients. Within these areas FAST does not perform as well. Sensitivities range from 46%–67% for penetrating trauma patients and 30%–80% for stable blunt trauma patients. These patients must proceed with further diagnostic evaluation.

The limitations of FAST include its highly operator dependant nature, occasional patient related obstacles, injuries causing minimal free body cavity fluid, and moderate to poor sensitivity in penetrating trauma and in hemodynamically stable blunt trauma patients.

CONTROVERSIES

Controversial issues surrounding FAST include whether nonradiologist clinicians can or should use ultrasonography. This question has been answered by large studies. Surgeon-performed FAST has been validated and shown to be a rapid, accurate, and useful screening modality.[3,7] Training requirements have been established by an international consensus conference,[12] and prospective studies have shown accuracy comparable to our radiology colleagues.[13] What constitutes an adequate number of examinations or volume of experience depends on a number of factors. Total number of exams, proctored evaluations, and number of positive studies all impact the learning curve of surgeon-performed FAST. As previously stated, it appears that 25–100 proctored studies evaluating multitrauma patients provides an adequate learning experience.

DPL has been essentially replaced by FAST. Although there has not been a randomized prospective trial comparing DPL to FAST, there remains little doubt that FAST is faster, less invasive, and carries less risk for procedure related morbidity. In a prospective study comparing FAST to DPL, Lentz et al.[38] examined 54 patients with FAST and subsequently DPL. They found that FAST compared favorably with sensitivity of 87%, specificity of 100%, and accuracy of 96% for detecting free intraperitoneal fluid. Previously, the sensitivity of DPL (>95%) had led to a high rate of negative laparotomy. With the advent of CT and FAST, the rate of negative laparotomy has decreased, but DPL is still a useful tool in the evaluation of FAST-negative, unstable patients with an undetermined source of hypotension (see Figure 8).

As the reliability, accuracy, cost-effectiveness, and training of surgeon-performed FAST have been established, some have questioned whether FAST can replace CT in certain patient populations. Certainly, hemodynamically unstable patients should not have CT, and FAST is an important tool in the evaluation of this group. The known risk factors for intra-abdominal injury in FAST-negative patients are rib, pelvic, and spinal fractures; brief hypotension; hematuria; intoxication; persistent base deficit; head injury; distracting injury; and abdominal tenderness. These patients should have CT to further evaluate the abdomen and pelvis. Ballard et al.[24] found FAST to be only 24% sensitive in detecting free abdominal fluid in patients with pelvic fractures. Four of the 13 false-negative patients in this group required operative intervention and the remaining 9 patients were successfully managed nonoperatively. In this study, FAST was compared to CT for patients with spinal injuries, but the data were insufficient for any recommendations. Other conditions that preclude detection of intra-abdominal injury by physical examination include intoxication, head injury, distracting injuries, and a persistent base deficit. Patients in this group commonly require CT, leaving a group of patients that can be reliably followed by clinical exam. Rose et al.[39] reported a study randomizing patients to receive either FAST or control (no FAST) to determine whether routine ultrasonography affected use of CT. A total of 104 patients were analyzed in each group, but the study was concluded early because an interim review recognized that FAST was becoming standard practice. Nevertheless, 52% of the control group and 36% of the FAST group received CT. The FAST group had sensitivity, specificity, and accuracy of 80%, 98%, and 96%, respectively. In the FAST group, three patients with a negative FAST and no CT had an intra-abdominal injury. Two of these three patients ultimately required therapeutic laparotomy. There were no missed injuries among patients receiving CT. Routine indications for CT after FAST included known risk factors for intra-abdominal injury, but this was not required per protocol. This trial did show a decrease in the use of CT with routine FAST, but the sample size was too small to make any firm conclusions. In the Netherlands, Bakker et al.[40] employed FAST as the primary screening tool in 1149 blunt abdominal trauma patients. Abdominal CT was employed in 7% resulting in delayed diagnosis of injury in 1.7% of patients without significant additional morbidity. Current practice suggests routine CT following FAST for stable patients with risk factors for intra-abdominal injury and where the abdominal examination is unreliable (see Figure 8).

The use of FAST in penetrating abdominal trauma is controversial. As mentioned previously, the sensitivity of FAST is 46%–67%[9–11] in detecting penetrating intra-abdominal injury. However, the reliability of a positive FAST is excellent, having a positive predictive value of 90%–92%, and specificity of 94%–98%.[9–11] Early application of FAST can also direct operative intervention toward the body cavity most likely injured resulting from single or multiple penetrating injuries. It must be emphasized, however, that a negative FAST does not rule out a significant intra-abdominal injury in penetrating trauma, and FAST must not delay operative intervention in patients with hypotension or peritonitis (see Figure 9). Decision making for operative intervention in penetrating abdominal trauma relies on clinical findings and FAST infrequently alters management. However, for penetrating injury to the pericardium, FAST has been shown to be over 96% sensitive, specific, and accurate.[8]

The presence of unstable pelvic fractures and free fluid on FAST is another area of controversy. Free fluid in this setting may be secondary to transperitoneal decompression of pelvic retroperitoneal blood or to concomitant intra-abdominal injuries. However, the rate of intra-abdominal injury and pelvic fracture in this patient population has been reported to be 67%. Ruchholtz et al.[41] reviewed 80 patients with AO/SICOT classification type B or type C pelvic ring fractures and FAST. Thirty-one patients had positive FAST, and 49 patients had negative FAST. Thirty of 31 patients with positive FAST had intra-abdominal or urogenital organ injury requiring surgical repair (2 patients with extraperitoneal bladder rupture in this group would probably have been managed nonoperatively in the United States). Twelve of 15 patients who presented with unstable pelvic ring fracture, hypotension, and positive FAST required therapeutic laparotomy. In the group of 49 patients with negative FAST, 3 required initial laparotomy (1 for perianal disruption, 1 for extraperitoneal disruption). An additional 3 patients required delayed laparotomy, 1 patient required splenectomy for ongoing bleeding, 1 patient developed abdominal compartment syndrome, and 1 patient had a delayed diagnosis and repair of the diaphragm. Although the sensitivity for detecting abdominal lesions with FAST in patients with type-B or -C pelvic ring fractures was 75% in this study, the positive predictive value of finding a relevant intra-abdominal/urogenital lesion was 97%. There was only positive FAST, due to transperitoneal blood from a pelvic fracture, which led to a non-therapeutic laparotomy. These authors report that positive FAST, in the setting of unstable type-B and -C pelvic fractures, strongly correlates with significant intra-abdominal/urogenital lesions requiring early laparotomy.

SUMMARY

Surgeon-performed FAST is an accurate, rapid, portable, cost-effective, noninvasive, and repeatable screening tool for trauma patients. FAST has replaced DPL as a primary screening modality for trauma patients. All trauma patients with risk factors for thoracoabdominal injury who cannot be cleared by physical examination should have an initial FAST exam. Stable trauma patients with no risk factors for intra-abdominal injury and a reliable examination may be cleared by FAST and serial examination. In unstable, multitrauma patients with blunt mechanisms, FAST should be used to rule out hemoperitoneum. A secondary FAST should be performed on hemodynamically unstable patients with an initial negative FAST. FAST is a sensitive and specific screening tool for blunt trauma and penetrating pericardial trauma. The presence of hypotension and a positive FAST indicates the need for operative exploration for both blunt and penetrating trauma. The sensitivity of FAST for penetrating intra-abdominal injuries is poor and additional diagnostic evaluation is required for negative examinations. A formal didactic session and between 30 and 100 proctored examinations of severely injured patients appears to be adequate to be competent with FAST. Scoring and quantifying hemoperitoneum has been shown to be predictive in evaluating the need for laparotomy. FAST is accurate in the detection of hemothorax, pneumothorax, and sternal fracture is an adjunct to chest radiography. FAST performed by surgeons in pediatric patients is a valid screening modality. Hypotension and a positive FAST in children, pregnant patients and patients with unstable pelvic fractures strongly suggests immediate operative intervention. Positive FAST in pregnant trauma patients and patients with pelvic fractures have a high incidence of intra-abdominal injury. Despite the limitations of surgeon-performed FAST, which include its highly operator-dependent nature, occasional patient-related obstacles, injuries causing minimal free body-cavity fluid, and moderate to poor sensitivity in penetrating trauma and in hemodynamically stable blunt trauma patients, FAST has been widely adopted by surgeons and trauma centers worldwide and is a valuable tool in modern trauma care.

REFERENCES

1. Rozycki GS, et al: Early detection of hemoperitoneum by ultrasound examination of the right upper quadrant: a multicenter study. *J Trauma* 5:878, 998.
2. Rozycki GS, et al: Surgeon-performed ultrasound in trauma and surgical critical care. In Moore EE, Feliciano DV, Mattox KL, editors: *Trauma*, 5 ed. New York, McGraw-Hill, pp. 311–328.
3. Rozycki GS, et al: Surgeon-performed ultrasound for the assessment of truncal injuries: lessons learned from 1540 patients. *Ann Surg* 228:557, 1998.
4. McKenney KL, et al: Hemoperitoneum score helps determine need for therapeutic laparotomy. *J Trauma* 50:650, 2001.
5. Farahmand N, et al: Hypotensive patients with blunt abdominal trauma: performance of screening US. *Radiology* 235:436, 2005.
6. Blackbourne LH, et al: Secondary ultrasound examination increases the sensitivity of the FAST exam in blunt trauma. *J Trauma* 57:934, 2004.
7. Dolich MO, et al: 2,576 Ultrasounds for blunt abdominal trauma. *J Trauma* 50:108, 2001.
8. Rozycki GS, et al: The role of ultrasound in patients with possible penetrating cardiac wounds: a prospective multicenter study. *J Trauma* 46:543, 1999.
9. Soffer D, et al: A prospective evaluation of ultrasonography for the diagnosis of penetrating torso injury. *J Trauma* 56:953, 2004.
10. Udobi KF, et al: Role of ultrasonography in penetrating abdominal trauma: a prospective clinical study. *J Trauma* 50:475, 2001.
11. Boulanger BR, et al: The routine use of sonography in penetrating torso injury is beneficial. *J Trauma* 51:320, 2001.
12. Scalea TM, et al: Focused assessment with sonography for trauma (FAST): results from an international consensus conference. *J Trauma* 46:466, 1999.
13. McKenney MG, et al: Can surgeons evaluate emergency ultrasound scans for blunt abdominal trauma? *J Trauma* 44:649, 1998.
14. Thomas B, et al: Ultrasound evaluation of blunt abdominal trauma: program implementation, initial experience, and learning curve. *J Trauma* 42:384, 1997.
15. McCarter FD, et al: Institutional and individual learning curves for ocused abdominal ultrasound for trauma: cumulative sum analysis. *Ann Surg* 231:689, 2000.
16. Smith RS, et al: Institutional learning curve of surgeon-performed trauma ultrasound. *Arch Surg* 133:530, 1998.
17. Shackford SR, et al: Focused abdominal sonogram for trauma: the learning curve of nonradiologist clinicians in detecting hemoperitoneum. *J Trauma* 46:553, 1999.
18. Jang T, et al: Residents should not independently perform focused abdominal sonography for trauma after 10 training examinations. *J Ultrasound Med* 23:793, 2004.
19. Rose JS: Ultrasound in abdominal trauma. *Emerg Med Clin North Am* 22:581, 2004.
20. Gracias VH, et al: The role of positive examinations in training for the Focused Assessment Sonogram in Trauma (FAST) examination. *Am Surg* 68:1008, 2002.
21. Abrams BJ, et al: Ultrasound for the detection of intraperitoneal fluid: the role of Trendelenberg positioning. *Am J Emerg Med* 17:117, 1999.
22. Branney SW, et al: Quantitative sensitivity of ultrasound in detecting free intraperitoneal fluid. *J Trauma* 39:375, 1995.
23. Huang M, et al: Ultrasonography for the evaluation of hemoperitoneum during resuscitation: a simple scoring system. *J Trauma* 36:173, 1994.
24. Ballard RB, et al: An algorithm to reduce the incidence of false-negative FAST examinations in patients at high risk for occult injury. *J Am Coll Surg* 189:145, 1999.
25. Sisley AC, et al: Rapid detection of traumatic effusion using surgeon-performed ultrasonography. *J Trauma* 44:291, 1998.
26. Dulchavsky SA, et al: Prospective evaluation of thoracic ultrasound in the detection of pneumothorax. *J Trauma* 50:201, 2001.
27. Blaivas M, et al: A prospective comparison of supine chest radiography and bedside ultrasound for the diagnosis of traumatic pneumothorax. *Acad Emerg Med* 12:844, 2005.
28. Mahlfeld A, et al: Ultrasound diagnosis of sternal fractures. *Zentrabl Chir* 126:62, 2001.
29. Thourani VH, et al: Validation of surgeon-performed emergency abdominal ultrasonography in pediatric trauma patients. *J Pediatr Surg* 33:322, 1998.
30. Soudack M, et al: Experience with Focused Abdominal Sonography for Trauma (FAST) in 313 pediatric patients. *J Clin Ultrasound* 32:53, 2004.
31. Coley BD, et al: Focused Abdominal Sonography for Trauma (FAST) in children with blunt abdominal trauma. *J Trauma* 48:902, 2000.
32. Holmes JF, et al: Emergency department ultrasonography in the evaluation of hypotensive and normotensive children with blunt abdominal trauma. *J Pediatr Surg* 36:968, 2001.
33. Ong AW, et al: Predicting the need for laparotomy in pediatric trauma patients on the basis of the ultrasound score. *J Trauma* 54:503, 2003.
34. Ormsby EL, et al: Pelvic free fluid: clinical importance for reproductive age women with blunt abdominal trauma. *Ultrasound Obstet Gynecol* 26:271, 2005.
35. Richards JR, et al: Blunt abdominal injury in the pregnant patient: detection with ultrasound. *Radiology* 233:463, 2004.
36. Bochicchio GV, et al: Surgeon-performed focused assessment with sonography for trauma as an early screening tool for pregnancy after trauma. *J Trauma* 52:1125, 2002.
37. Yoshii H, et al: Usefulness and limitations of ultrasonography in the initial evaluation of blunt abdominal trauma. *J Trauma* 45:45, 1998.
38. Lentz KA, et al: Evaluating blunt abdominal trauma: role for ultrasonography. *J Ultrasound Med* 15:447, 1996.
39. Rose JS, et al: Does the presence of ultrasound really affect computed tomographic scan use? A prospective randomized trial of ultrasound in trauma. *J Trauma* 51:545, 2001.
40. Bakker J, et al: Sonography as the primary screening method in evaluating blunt abdominal trauma. *J Clin Ultrasound* 33:155, 2005.
41. Ruchholtz S, et al: Free abdominal fluid on ultrasound in unstable pelvic ring fracture: is laparotomy always necessary? *J Trauma* 57:278, 2004.

THE USE OF COMPUTED TOMOGRAPHY IN INITIAL TRAUMA EVALUATION

L. Ola Sjoholm and **Steven Ross**

In the 1970s, computed axial tomography (CT) revolutionized the evaluation and management of brain injury. Since then, advances in technology leading to increased speed and resolution have similarly changed the assessment of other injuries. Following the primary and secondary survey and initial plain radiographic evaluation, CT is often essential in the work-up of hemodynamically stable victims of blunt trauma. With the introduction of multidetector arrays, CT now may replace invasive catheter angiography and/or magnetic resonance imaging in certain circumstances.

HISTORY

Computerized axial tomography was developed in the late 1960s and early 1970s, independently, by Hounsfield and Cormack. CT was first clinically applied in trauma situations in the mid-1970s. Initially, it was only possible to image the head and brain. After a period in which CAT scanners were not common, by the mid-1980s these devices were available in hospitals throughout the United States. This availability, as well as advances in CT technology, spurred the development of new applications and techniques.

Computed tomography is performed by passing rotating fan beams of x-rays through the patient in an axial plane. In the early scanners, the x-ray tube rotated around the patient to obtain a single image or "slice." The table then moved for the next slice. This process was quite time consuming. In modern scanners, the tube rotates continuously while the table is in motion, yielding a spiral or helical scan. The more recent scanners also have multiple rows of detectors that can obtain as many as 64 slices simultaneously. This makes it possible to scan the entire body from head to pelvis in only a few minutes.

The continuous data from the spiral scanning are stored in computer memory, which allows the data to be manipulated in various ways. If, for example, the chest and abdomen have been scanned, detailed reconstructions of images of the thoracic and lumbar spine can be obtained without exposing the patient to additional radiation. The computer can also generate three-dimensional (3D) rotating images, which can be useful in the interpretation of CT angiography and complex fractures.

Similar to plain radiographs, there are four basic densities on a CT image. Air is black; fat is dark gray; soft tissue is light gray; and bone/calcium and contrast agents are white. The x-ray absorption of a specific tissue can be measured in Hounsfield units (HU). The density of water is zero. Blood measures 40–70 HU. Urine, ascites, and bowel content measure close to water, 0–30 HU. Various "windows" for bone, brain, lung, abdomen, and so on, are used to best display tissues of various densities.

COMPUTED TOMOGRAPHY OF HEAD/BRAIN (CRANIUM)

Computed tomography of the head is indicated in patients with clinical evidence of traumatic brain injury, including loss of consciousness, amnesia, depressed level of consciousness, a mental state that is difficult to evaluate due to recreational or therapeutic drug administration, hemotympanum or cerebrospinal fluid leak, suspected skull fracture, severe headache, persistent nausea and vomiting, or post-traumatic seizures.

Scanning protocols may vary slightly from institution to institution. In adults the scan is usually performed with 5-mm cuts from the skull base to the vertex. In infants, the scan is commonly performed with finer cuts starting at the second cervical vertebra.

The study is performed without contrast. Acute hemorrhage appears white on the scan (Figure 1) except in very anemic patients, where it may appear isodense with brain. Active intracranial bleeding may also appear as gray swirls within the white clot, indicating hyperacute hemorrhage.

Computed tomography is very sensitive for intracranial hemorrhage, edema, and mass effect. As CT technology has advanced, detection of smaller lesions has become possible, leading to controversy regarding the significance of these lesions, and the indications for CT in mild head injury.[1] CT of the brain may be normal and not correlate well with the clinical picture in patients with diffuse axonal injury.

Computed tomography of the head may also detect fractures of the upper facial bones and orbits; however, dedicated CT of the face is required to provide adequate resolution to plan operative intervention. High-resolution CT of the base of the skull may be required to evaluate basilar skull fractures.

COMPUTED TOMOGRAPHY OF FACE AND ORBITS

Computed tomography is the best method to study facial fractures. Patients with clinical suspicion of fractures due to facial swelling, deformities, visual changes, or bony tenderness or instability on examination should undergo CT of the facial bones, concomitant with head scan (if necessary). If facial fractures or fluid in the sinuses are seen on CT of head, a formal CT of the face should be performed, as the resolution of head CT is insufficient.

Axial images are obtained using 3-mm slices from below the mandible to just above the frontal sinuses. The mandible may be excluded if no suspicion of injury is present. In a spiral CT scanner, coronal views can be reconstructed from the initial data. With multidetector CT scanners, 3D reconstructions (Figure 2) can be generated that are of value to the maxillofacial surgeon in planning reconstruction, and particularly in complex fractures.

COMPUTED TOMOGRAPHY OF SPINE

The cervical spine needs to be evaluated radiographically in victims of blunt trauma who present with cervical spine tenderness, acute neurologic deficit, or significant brain injury; or who cannot be adequately evaluated due to distracting injury, intoxication, or therapy (particularly those who are intubated and sedated). Debate continues regarding some of the "softer" indications for such imaging.[2] The mainstay of cervical spine imaging has been plain radiography for decades, with CT if the plain films are incomplete or inadequate, or the anatomy of injury requires delineation. Improvements in technology and technique have led some to advocate CT as the primary

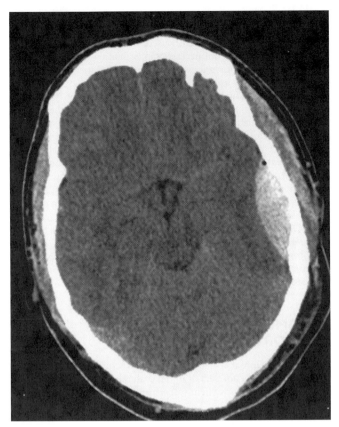

Figure 1 Computed tomography scan demonstrating a classic lenticular-shaped, acute epidural hematoma.

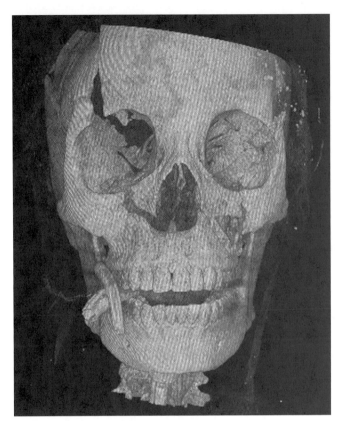

Figure 2 Three-dimensional reconstruction of the facial bones demonstrating multiple fractures, including a right-sided depressed skull fracture and bilateral orbital fractures.

imaging modality for the cervical spine.[3] The scan is done with 2.5–3-mm cuts from the skull base through the first thoracic vertebrae. In addition to the axial views, sagittal and coronal reconstructions are performed.

Computed tomography of the cervical spine has a sensitivity of 95%–100% and a specificity of 98%–100% for detecting cervical spine injury.[4] Indications for imaging the thoracic and lumbar spine are similar to those for the cervical spine. Patients with spine tenderness, deformity, distracting injuries, neurologic deficit, or spine fractures at other levels, or who cannot be properly evaluated due to depressed mental status (with appropriate mechanism of injury) should have anteroposterior and lateral x-ray views of their thoracic and lumbar spine. If the plain films are inadequate or if the patient has an impressive clinical exam with normal plain radiographs, the area of concern should be further evaluated with CT. If the chest and abdomen have been scanned, detailed images of the spine can be reconstructed from that data. Images with a 2.5-mm slice thickness, including two normal vertebral bodies above and below the injury, should be obtained with sagittal and coronal reconstruction.

COMPUTED TOMOGRAPHY OF NECK AND GREAT VESSELS

Patients with clinical signs of blunt neck injury, including laryngeal tenderness, subcutaneous emphysema, hemoptysis, hoarseness, hematomas, or significant contusions of the neck related to seat restraints should undergo CT of the soft tissues to evaluate the aerodigestive tract. CT is the study of choice to detect and define injuries of the larynx. Patients with cervical spine fractures (especially with transverse foramen involvement), severe facial fractures, basal skull fracture involving the carotid foramen, expanding hematoma in the neck, or with neurologic status not explained by traumatic brain in-

jury, are at risk for cervical vascular injury. Although four-vessel cerebral angiography is considered the gold standard for diagnosis of blunt cerebrovascular injury, CT angiography has shown promising results in some series, and is a rapid approach to identification of carotid or vertebral artery injuries in this setting.[5] For stable patients who have suffered penetrating neck trauma, CT-angiogram may be used to identify vascular, aerodigestive, and bony injuries, and may be useful to guide invasive studies and surgery.[6]

The study is carried out on multidetector scanner, with administration of 75–150 ml (1.5–2 ml/kg) of contrast material delivered at a rate of 3–5 ml/sec. When necessary, 3D images are reconstructed for interpretation and surgical planning.

COMPUTED TOMOGRAPHY OF CHEST

Computed tomography of the chest is performed routinely following blunt trauma in many institutions, whenever an abdominal scan is obtained. Chest CT is specifically indicated when the initial chest radiography or mechanism of injury suggests likelihood of blunt thoracovascular injury. CT angiography has replaced traditional angiography as the initial study of choice for blunt aortic injury (Figure 3), and may completely eliminate the need for arteriogram for both operative and "nonoperative" management.[7] Chest CT is also more sensitive for pneumothorax, hemothorax, pneumomediastinum, parenchymal lung injury, and bony thoracic injury, than plain chest radiography.

In hemodynamically stable transmediastinal gunshot wounds, a CT scan of the chest may be useful for initial screening to determine if further work-up or interventions are required.[8]

The chest is typically scanned in 2.5–3-mm slices with a contrast load of 150 ml (1.5–2 ml) given at a rate of 3–5 ml/sec. A delay of 20 seconds is used in order to optimize great artery opacification during the scan.

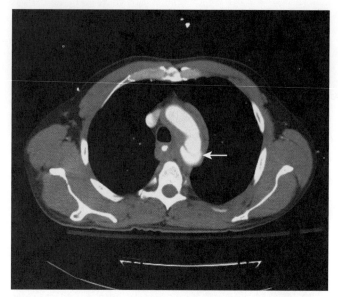

Figure 3 Axial image in the arterial phase of a patient suffering from blunt chest trauma demonstrating large mediastinal hematoma thoracic aortic intimal disruption near the ligamentum arteriosum *(white arrow)*.

COMPUTED TOMOGRAPHY OF ABDOMEN AND PELVIS

Computed tomography has become the study of choice for evaluating the abdomen in hemodynamically stable blunt trauma victims. It is sensitive to the presence and extent of injuries of solid organs (e.g., liver, spleen, and kidneys), but is less sensitive in detecting injuries of the diaphragm, pancreas, and the gastrointestinal tract. Indirect findings, such as free fluid without solid viscus injury, or mesenteric streaking, are important when suspicion of these injuries exists.

The scan is performed in 5-mm slices from the lower chest through the perineum. In the trauma setting, there is no place for CT of the abdomen without concomitant pelvic CT. Intravenous contrast is used to enhance the solid organs and to detect active bleeding. A "blush" suggests active arterial bleed when seen in the area of a pelvic fracture, or in a solid organ injury, even in a stable patient (Figure 4). This find-

ing should prompt an invasive approach to care, including interventional angiography and embolization and/or surgery.

Oral contrast is also frequently used, although many studies have demonstrated that it is not necessary in evaluating the gastrointestinal tract for injury. Radiologist preference and patient compliance should determine its use.[9]

In penetrating trauma, CT of the abdomen and pelvis may be useful in evaluating asymptomatic patients with stab wounds of the back or flank. In these situations, the triple-contrast technique yields sensitivity of 97%–100% and specificity of 96%–98% for retroperitoneal or abdominal visceral injury and peritoneal penetration. It may also be of value in identifying tangential gunshot wounds, at low risk for intra-abdominal or retroperitoneal injury. In institutions where nonoperative management of gunshot wounds of the liver is an option, CT of the abdomen of stable patients with suspicion of such injuries is a requirement.[10,11]

A CT cystogram can be performed in patients at risk for bladder injury. This has a diagnostic accuracy approaching 100%. Bladder distention is achieved by instilling at least 350 ml of diluted contrast solution via a Foley catheter under gravity. Postdrainage images are unnecessary.[12]

COMPUTED TOMOGRAPHY OF ORTHOPEDIC INJURIES

Other than for initial evaluation of pelvic fractures, CT study of orthopedic injuries is not part of initial evaluation. In otherwise stable patients, it may be convenient to perform them concomitantly with other studies.

Computed tomography of the acetabulum is indicated after hip dislocation to detect intra-articular bone fragments or acetabular fractures and for presurgical evaluation of unstable fractures. It is also useful in the evaluation of shoulder/scapular injury, tibial plateau fractures, and complex fractures of the ankle involving the articular surfaces and talus/calcaneal fractures.

REFERENCES

1. Stiell IG, Clement CM, et al: Comparison of the Canadian CT Head Rule and the New Orleans Criteria in the patients with minor head injury. *JAMA* 294:1551–1553, 2005.
2. Griffen MM, Frykberg ER, et al: Radiographic clearance of blunt cervical spine injury: plain radiograph or computed tomography scan. *J Trauma* 55:222–226, 2003.
3. Sanchez B, Waxman K, et al: Cervical spine clearance in blunt trauma evaluation of a computed tomography-based protocol. *J Trauma* 59(1):179–183, 2005.
4. Hoffman JR, Mower WR, et al: Validity of a set of clinical criteria to rule out injury to the cervical spine in the patients with blunt trauma. National Emergency X-Radiology Utilization Study Group. *N Engl J Med* 343(2):94–99, 2001.
5. Miller PR, Fabian TC, et al: Prospective screening for blunt cerebrovascular injuries: analysis of diagnostic modalities and outcomes. *Ann Surg* 236(3):386–393, 2002.
6. Munera F, Soto JA, et al: Penetrating neck injuries: helical CT angiography for initial evaluation. *Radiology* 224(2):366–372, 2002
7. Fabian TC, Davis KA, et al: Prospective study of blunt aortic injury: helical scan is diagnostic and antihypertensive therapy reduces rupture. *Ann Surg* 227(5):666–676, 1998.
8. Stassen NA, Lukan JK, et al: Reevaluation of diagnostic procedures for transmediastinal gunshot wounds. *J Trauma* 53(4):635–638, 2002.
9. Stuhlfant JN, Soto JA, et al: Blunt abdominal trauma: performance of CT without oral contrast material. *Radiology* 233(3):689–694, 2004.
10. Shanmuganathan K, Mirvis SE, et al: Penetrating torso trauma: triple contrast helical CT in peritoneal violation and organ injury—a prospective in 200 patients. *Radiology* 231(2):775–784, 2004.
11. Demetriades D, Gomez H, et al: Gunshot injuries to the liver: the role of selective nonoperative management. *J Am Coll Surg* 188(4):343–348, 1999.
12. Deck AJ, Shaves S, et al: Current experience with computed tomographic cystography and blunt trauma. *World J Surg* 25(12):1592–1596, 2001.

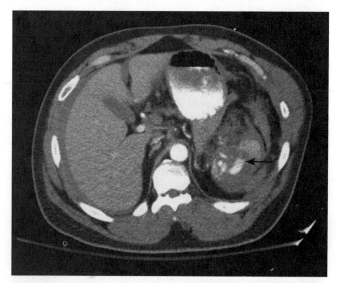

Figure 4 Abdominal computed tomography demonstrating a splenic injury with extravasation of contrast ("blush") *(black arrow)*.

INTERVENTIONAL RADIOLOGY: DIAGNOSTICS AND THERAPEUTICS

George Maish   and   Timothy Fabian

Radiology has always been an important component of a Level I trauma center. This relationship has increased over the last two decades such that it is almost impossible to conceive of caring for a trauma patient without the ability to perform trauma imaging. Interventional radiology techniques, including angiography, angioembolization, and stent placement, have evolved from infrequently used adjuncts in the care of trauma patients into pivotal adjuncts in the nonoperative management of solid organ injury and hemorrhage associated with pelvic trauma. Historically, these techniques have only been available in a dedicated angiographic suite that was physically separate from the resuscitation area and operating room. This required that patients were hemodynamically normal so that they could tolerate the transportation to the angiographic suite. In addition, commitment to availability 24 hours a day from angiographic technologists and staff was necessary to ensure that these techniques would be available. This distinction among resuscitation area, operating room, and angiographic suite has been gradually dissolving over the past decade. Many centers have built angiographic suites into or next to their emergency department so that the risk of transportation has been decreased. In addition, the development of better radiolucent operating room tables and portable fluoroscopy machines with digital subtraction capabilities has enabled some interventional radiology techniques to be performed in the operating room. Several institutions have built endovascular suites in their operating room suites for the performance of endovascular techniques by vascular surgeons. This ever increasing fusion of resuscitation area, operating room, and angiographic suite has made interventional radiology techniques available to more trauma patients than ever before.

While the angiography suite has been undergoing an evolution over the past decade, the practitioner who is capable of performing these techniques has been changing as well. Historically, endovascular techniques were the exclusive domain of the interventional radiologist. This has changed. Endovascular techniques are now completely incorporated into the training of vascular surgeons, with many vascular surgeons offering both endovascular and traditional vascular techniques for the management of peripheral vascular disease, aortic aneurysms, and aortic dissections. In addition, interventional cardiologists are placing carotid stents for the management of carotid stenosis. Due to difficulty in obtaining interventional radiology coverage 24 hours a day, 7 days a week, some trauma surgeons have obtained additional training in endovascular techniques so that trauma patients have access to these less invasive techniques.

While interventional radiology techniques have become more accessible for the trauma patients, developments in the technology of computed tomography (CT) scanners, particularly the development of the multidetector CT scanner, have allowed for the development of CT angiography for diagnosis. CT angiography is beginning to challenge conventional angiography as a gold standard in the diagnosis of some injuries. However, for now, angiography remains the gold standard for the diagnosis of most vascular injuries.

In order to make the angiographic suite available to the trauma patient, it is important that the patient is either hemodynamically normal or accompanied by a physician and a nurse to make sure that the patient is being appropriately resuscitated. Good communication between the interventional radiology staff and the trauma team is essential to ensure safe care of the severely injured trauma patient.

INDICATIONS

The indication for using interventional radiology techniques in the care of trauma patient depends on the technique being used and the medical condition of the trauma patient. It is not appropriate to transport a hemodynamically abnormal patient to the angiographic suite for a diagnostic arteriogram. The arteriogram should either be performed in the operating room or delayed until the patient is resuscitated. Alternatively, patients with severe pelvic trauma should undergo relatively prompt arteriography and possible embolization to try to achieve hemostasis. These patients may be hemodynamically abnormal but the interventional radiology techniques are part of their resuscitation. In other injuries, interventional radiology techniques may be used to provide definitive therapy for hemorrhage. The development of intravascular covered stents has allowed for the management of certain injuries, including arterial disruption and arteriovenous fistulas, to move from the operating room to the angiographic suite. Venous injuries including lacerations, thrombosis, and compression can be managed by the placement of uncovered intravascular stents. The decision to use interventional radiology techniques and the timing of these techniques requires that the trauma surgeon understands the indications and limitations of these techniques.

BLUNT CEREBROVASCULAR INJURY

Over the past decade, there has been an increased awareness of blunt cerebrovascular injury (BCVI), which includes carotid artery injuries (CAI) and vertebral artery injuries (VAI). Several studies have identified an incidence of 1.5%–2% for BCVI among blunt trauma victims. Historically, blunt carotid artery injuries had been diagnosed by onset of neurologic symptoms. The outcomes for this injury were poor. Blunt carotid injuries had an associated mortality rate of 31% and a stroke rate of 43%. Blunt carotid injuries have been shown to have worse outcomes compared to penetrating carotid injuries. Seventy-eight percent of patients with penetrating carotid injuries have been found to be independent with locomotion at the time of discharge compared to 37% of those with blunt carotid injuries. Blunt carotid injuries also have a worse outcome compared to the overall blunt trauma population. Fifty-five percent of blunt trauma patients are able to be fully independent at the time of discharge compared to 33% of patients with blunt carotid injury. VAI occurs in 0.53% of blunt trauma patients, and has an associated stroke rate of 25%. Screening protocols using four-vessel angiography have been used to successfully identify these injuries prior to the development of neurologic symptoms. The institution of early treatment with anticoagulation or antiplatelet therapy in VAI has been shown to decrease the stroke rate from 14% to 0%. When anticoagulation or antiplatelet therapy is used in the management of blunt carotid injuries, the stroke rate decreases from 60% to less than 10%. It is clear that there is significant morbidity and mortality when BCVI is missed. However, they occur relatively infrequently, such that it is not practical to screen all blunt trauma patients.

Several screening triggers have been suggested in the literature including cervical spine fracture, neurologic findings not explained by radiographic findings, Horner's syndrome, LeFort II or III facial fractures, skull base fractures involving the foramen lacerum, and neck soft tissue injury. A good screening test should be relatively inexpensive, have a low morbidity rate, and a high sensitivity rate. It should find all the true positive results with some false positives and no false negatives. In a comparison of magnetic resonance angiography (MRA), computed tomographic angiography (CTA), and four-vessel cerebral angiography between 2000 and 2002, the sensitivity of MRA and CTA for BCVI was 47%–53%. These rates are too low for a test to be an effective screening modality. Four-vessel cerebral angiography has been identified as the gold standard for the diagnosis of BCVI. However, its cost and major complication rate of 1%–3% in large series make it a less than ideal screening test. The development of the multidetector CT scanner has increased the resolution of the CT scanner. Two recent studies demonstrated that CTA performed on multidetector CT scanners has dramatically improved ability to diagnose these injuries. A head-to-head comparison of CTA with multidetector CT scanners and four-vessel cerebral angiography has yet to be done. As a result, four-vessel cerebral angiography remains the gold standard for diagnosis and screening of these injuries. It will be important to continue to monitor improvements in CTA, MRA, and possibly even ultrasound technologies for less invasive, cheaper, and safer screening modalities for BCVI.

Blunt cerebrovascular injuries have been effectively managed by anticoagulation or antiplatelet therapy in patients with contraindications to anticoagulation. With the development of endovascular technologies including balloons, coils, and stents, there have been several single-institution, small series that have demonstrated good efficacy in the treatment of traumatic pseudoaneurysms of the carotid artery with good short-term follow-up. However, one large series with 46 patients over an 8-year period demonstrated a 21% complication rate and 45% occlusion rate for patients treated with endovascular stents. Patients who had received antithrombotic agents alone only had a 5% occlusion rate. This study concluded that antithrombotic therapy was the recommended therapy for blunt carotid injuries, and that the role of stents remains undefined. The indications for the use of endovascular techniques in the management of BCVI remain unclear and their long-term results are unproven. Clearly, further study of these techniques is warranted.

BRACHIOCEPHALIC TRAUMA

The use of diagnostic angiography in penetrating neck injuries is based on which zone of the neck is involved. Penetrating injuries to zone 1 of the neck are usually evaluated with angiography of the carotid and subclavian arteries, if the patient is hemodynamically normal. Penetrating injuries to zone 2 of the neck can be managed by unilateral or bilateral neck exploration. If the patient is hemodynamically normal, evaluation of the injury with four-vessel cerebral angiography, esophagoscopy or soluble-contrast esophagography, and bronchoscopy can be performed. Some authors have reported using a multidetector CT scan of the neck with CT angiography (CTA) to evaluate these injuries. At this time, CTA has not been directly compared with four-vessel cerebral angiography and future studies will determine whether CTA can replace four-vessel cerebral angiography. Penetrating injuries to zone 3 of the neck are usually evaluated with four-vessel cerebral angiography because of the difficulty in achieving adequate surgical exposure of either the internal carotid artery or the vertebral artery at this level. Endovascular techniques including coil embolization and endovascular stents have been used successfully to manage vascular injuries in this area of the neck.

Angioembolization has also been successfully used to control hemorrhage associated with blunt and penetrating facial injuries. Attempting to obtain hemostasis of these injuries operatively can be very difficult. As a result, arteriography with angioembolization has become the first-line treatment for many of these injuries.

There have been several case and short series reports regarding the use of endovascular stents to repair blunt and penetrating injuries to the subclavian, axillary, and brachial arteries. All of them have demonstrated excellent success in acutely managing these injuries and few complications in short-term follow-up. The long-term success of these devices remains unknown.

THORACIC INJURY

Blunt aortic injury (BAI) may be caused by either rapid horizontal or vertical deceleration. Rapid horizontal deceleration usually results in an injury to the aorta at the isthmus, just distal to the origin of the left subclavian artery. The injury may be a dissection or transection of the aorta which can lead to hemorrhage, pseudoaneurysm formation, or thrombosis. Seventy to 90% of patients with traumatic injury to the thoracic aorta die at the scene. An additional 30% of these remaining patients die in the hospital prior to undergoing definitive surgical treatment. Surgical repair has been associated with mortality rates between 5%–25% and spinal cord infarction rates as high as 13%. It remains important to promptly diagnose this injury so that the patient can be appropriately managed. BAI may be suggested on routine chest radiograph. Findings such as a widened superior mediastinum, an indistinct aortic knob, or widening of the paratracheal stripe are all suggestive of a BAI. However, the specificity of these findings is only about 5%–10%. A CT scan of the chest may be performed to further delineate the aorta. The absence of a mediastinal hematoma on a helical CT scan of the chest has been shown to have a negative predictive value of 97%–99%. The evolution of the multi-detector CT scanner over the last 5 years has allowed for the development of CT angiography (CTA), which appears to have high sensitivity and specificity according to preliminary reports. Some institutions have begun using CTA as their diagnostic test of choice for BAI. At this time, aortography remains the gold standard for diagnosis of BAI, but it will most likely be replaced by CTA if its sensitivity and specificity are as high as early studies suggest. Alternatively, patients with evidence of blunt aortic injury could undergo transesophageal echocardiography to evaluate the aorta. The decision to obtain aortography or transesophageal echocardiography depends on which of these modalities is more readily available to the trauma team and the preference of the surgeon performing the repair of the aorta.

The management of BAI has been changing over the last several years. If the patient is hemodynamically normal, the patient is admitted to the ICU and conservatively managed until the associated injuries are resolved. Conservative management includes the use of beta-blockers and vasodilators to prevent tachycardia and hypertension. Several studies have demonstrated a decreased rate of in-hospital mortality and paraplegia with delayed repair of BAI. Endovascular stents have been used to repair BAI in both the emergent and delayed settings. The reported cases have all demonstrated few acute complications and 30-day mortality rates below 15%. While these results are encouraging, long-term results are unknown. One long-term study on endovascular repair of aortic aneurysms demonstrated a 65% endoleak rate, 35% graft migration, and 78% graft deformation. In fairness, this study involved some of the first generation of endovascular stents, and hopefully, the results for newer generation of stents will be better. Figure 1 demonstrates a traumatic pseudoaneurysm of the descending aorta. Figure 2 demonstrates the completion aortogram after placement of an endovascular stent. The first commercially available endovascular stents for the thoracic aorta only became available in the United States in 2005. There is currently a prospective analysis of the use of these grafts in the management of BAI being conducted by the American Association for the Surgery of Trauma (AAST). The ultimate success of these devices will be based on their long-term performance. It is important to remember that the average age of a trauma patient is much lower than that of patients undergoing aortic aneurysm or dissection repair. These grafts may need to last 40–60 years when placed in a young trauma patient. These results are simply unknown at this time.

Angiography can be useful in the evaluation of victims of both penetrating and blunt trauma. Patients who have suffered transmediastinal penetrating injuries should undergo aortography as part of their evaluation. CTA using multidetector CT scanners is still being evaluated, but it will most likely replace conventional catheter aortography as the screening test of choice.

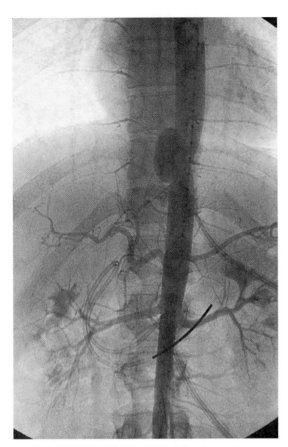

Figure 1   Traumatic pseudoaneurysm of the descending aorta.

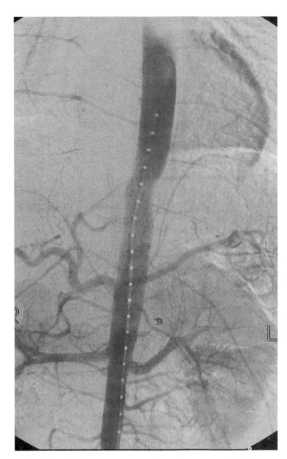

Figure 2   Completion aortogram after placement of endovascular stent.

ABDOMINAL TRAUMA

The two most commonly injured abdominal organs in blunt trauma are the liver and spleen. If patients are hemodynamically abnormal and have evidence of abdominal injury, either by a positive diagnostic peritoneal lavage (DPL) or a positive focused abdominal sonogram for trauma (FAST), the patient is taken to the operating room for surgical exploration. If the victim of blunt trauma is hemodynamically normal, they are evaluated with a contrast-enhanced CT scan of the abdomen. If the patient is hemodynamically normal, has a Glasgow coma score (GCS) of 15, does not have a distracting injury, and is not impaired by alcohol or illicit drugs, the patient's abdomen can be evaluated by clinical examination. The development of the CT scanner has allowed for the nonoperative diagnosis of injuries to the spleen and liver and the development of scoring systems for these injuries. During the late 1980s and early 1990s, several large studies demonstrated that hemodynamically normal patients with blunt injuries to the spleen and liver could be successfully managed nonoperatively with success rates of 70%–85%. This is now the routine practice for the management of blunt injury to the liver and spleen in hemodynamically normal patients.

At the same time that nonoperative management of blunt splenic injuries was developing, there were some case reports of using angioembolization to manage hemorrhage from blunt splenic injury. As a result, some groups of trauma surgeons began routinely performing arteriography on all blunt splenic injuries that qualified for nonoperative management. Any evidence of active hemorrhage or pseudoaneurysm formation was managed with angioembolization. This included proximal splenic artery embolization with coils or large gelfoam and more selective embolization of arterial branches with smaller coils or gelfoam. This strategy increased the success rate of nonoperative management of blunt splenic injuries to 93%–97%. Other groups looked for more selective criteria for using angioembolization in the nonoperative management of blunt splenic injuries. Several studies demonstrated that evidence of

active contrast extravasation or pseudoaneurysm formation on contrast-enhanced CT scan was predictive of failure of nonoperative management. Angioembolization was used as an adjunct in patients with evidence of active contrast extravasation or pseudoaneurysm to achieve nonoperative management success rates similar to those achieved with the routine use of arteriography on all splenic injuries. As a result, most institutions have incorporated angioembolization into their nonoperative management algorithms for splenic injuries in a selective fashion, usually based on findings on CT scan. There is a low complication rate for angioembolization of the spleen, which includes total splenic infarction, splenic abscess formation and complications, related to the arterial access for the procedure. This complication rate is lower when selective angioembolization of branch vessels of the splenic artery is performed rather than occlusion of the main splenic artery. In addition, angioembolization is not technically feasible in every patient. However, despite these few limitations and complications, angioembolization has clearly established itself as a useful adjunct to the nonoperative management of blunt splenic injuries. It is now possible to manage 70%–75% of all blunt splenic injuries nonoperatively with success rates over 90%.

The role of angioembolization in the management of blunt hepatic trauma has developed over the last 25 years as well. Initially, angioembolization was reported as being useful in the management of hemobilia after blunt hepatic trauma and iatrogenic injury. These case reports and small series demonstrated that angioembolization of the liver could be used to successfully manage hemobilia. The operative management of hepatic trauma, whether the mechanism is blunt or penetrating, has evolved over last 15 years as well. Historically, the operative mortality for grade IV and grade V liver injuries has been reported as between 50% and 80%. About 10 years ago, the concept of damage control laparotomy was developed to try and avoid the "triad of death": hypothermia, acidosis, and coagulopathy. This concept revolves around minimizing the length of the initial laparotomy in severely injured patients so that they arrive at the ICU for further resuscitation as soon as possible. This technique involves packing liver injuries rather than performing extensive operative maneuvers to gain hemostasis, repairing vascular injuries, and resecting bowel injuries, but leaving the bowel in discontinuity and temporary abdominal closure. This operative strategy has been reported to lower the operative mortality rate of grades IV and V liver injuries to 25%–40%. Angioembolization has been successfully used as an adjunct to damage control laparotomy to further decrease mortality and achieve hemostasis. Today, most authors would recommend a damage control laparotomy with packing of the injured liver for severe (AAST grade IV and V) hepatic trauma with angioembolization as an adjunct to further achieve hemostasis rather than extensive operative attempts to gain hemostasis. Angioembolization is also used as an adjunct to the nonoperative management of blunt hepatic injuries. Those patients who are seen to have active contrast extravasation from a liver injury on CT scan can undergo angioembolization to control their hemorrhage. This approach has improved the success rate of nonoperative management of blunt hepatic trauma to over 85%. The complications of hepatic embolization include hepatic necrosis, hepatic abscess, and bile leaks. If the patient has an intact portal vein with hepatopetal flow, the risk of hepatic necrosis is markedly reduced. For victims of both penetrating and blunt hepatic trauma, angioembolization can be a very useful adjunct to control the hemorrhage associated with significant liver trauma regardless of whether the patient is managed operatively or nonoperatively.

Angioembolization and endovascular stents have also been used in the management of renal trauma. Blunt renal injuries with evidence of active contrast extravasation on CT scan have been managed with arteriography and embolization of associated renal artery branches to achieve hemostasis. Endovascular stents have been used to manage both blunt and penetrating injuries to the renal arteries. The kidney is very sensitive to warm ischemia and that restoration of blood flow to the kidney needs to occur within the first 4–6 hours after injury. Due to time spent in transportation from the scene, resuscitation and evaluation in the trauma room and possibly CT scan, it is often 2–3 hours after injury that the diagnosis of a renal artery injury is made. As a result, the operative kidney salvage rate for exploration of the renal artery has been reported to be 5%–10%. This rate is so low that some authors do not recommend attempting to revascularize a unilateral blunt renal artery occlusion. There have been several small series and case reports of using endovascular stents in blunt renal artery injuries, which suggest that the kidney salvage rate for this approach may be as high as 25%. It is important to remember that all of the patients in these studies were hemodynamically normal and did not require operative exploration for associated injuries. Figure 3 demonstrates a blunt dissection of the left renal artery after a motor vehicle collision. Figure 4 is a CT scan after placement of 17 mm × 6 mm renal artery stent with restoration of perfusion to the left kidney. Further study of the use of endovascular stents in the management of both blunt and penetrating renal artery injuries is clearly warranted.

Angioembolization has also been used to successfully manage retroperitoneal hematomas with evidence of active extravasation and is the treatment of choice for these injuries due to the complexity of attemptng to control these injuries operatively.

PELVIC TRAUMA

Angioembolization has become part of the first-line treatment for pelvic hemorrhage associated with severe blunt pelvic fractures such as open-book or wind-swept pelvic fractures. An external binder such as the T-pod or an external fixator is placed to restore the conformation of the pelvis to allow for tamponade of pelvic venous bleeding. If the patient responds to resuscitation and does not have an indication for operative exploration, angioembolization is then used to control any arterial bleeding. Arterial hemorrhage is identified in approximately 10%–20% of these patients with significant pelvic trauma. Subselective transcatheter embolization can be performed with either gelfoam frag-

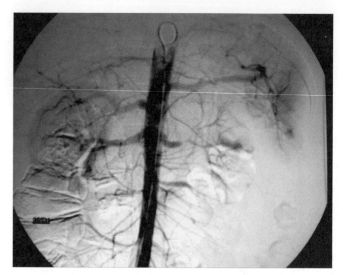

Figure 3 Dissection of the left renal artery and pseudoaneurysm of the splenic artery.

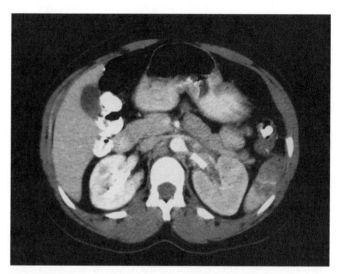

Figure 4 Computed tomography scan after placement of 17 mm × 6 mm renal stent with restoration of perfusion to the left kidney.

ments, which dissolve over 1–3 weeks, or metallic coils, which are essentially permanent. Usually, attempts are made to occlude the bleeding artery as distally as possible. However, in the setting of massive pelvic hemorrhage, it is sometimes necessary to occlude one or both internal iliac arteries with gelfoam to achieve hemostasis. Vertical shear pelvic fractures are associated with injury to the superior gluteal artery that can be diagnosed and managed by angioembolization of the superior gluteal artery. In addition to angioembolization for control of arterial hemorrhage associated with severe pelvic trauma there have been a few case reports of the use of endovascular stents to treat iliac vein injuries associated with blunt pelvic trauma. There have been case reports of using endovascular stents to repair penetrating injuries to the iliac artery and vein with good initial results.

EXTREMITY TRAUMA

Arteriography of the extremity, whether intraoperative or in the interventional radiology suite, can be used to evaluate the injured extremity. In penetrating trauma patients who have "hard" signs of vascular injury, which includes expanding hematoma, pulse discrepancy, and pulsatile bleeding, usually surgical exploration is all that is performed. However, for patients with multiple penetrating wounds to the same extremity, it may be desirable to perform arteriography to more precisely locate the injury. In blunt trauma patients with posterior knee dislocations, floating knees (distal femur fracture with tibial plateau fracture), supracondylar knee fractures and tibial plateau fractures, there is an increased incidence of blunt popliteal injury. If there is a pulse discrepancy in an extremity with one of these injuries, arteriography is usually performed prior to or at the time of operative exploration to confirm the diagnosis of blunt popliteal injury. This assumes that obtaining the arteriogram will not significantly delay appropriate treatment of the vascular injury. Duplex scanning is increasing in specificity and sensitivity for these injuries but the gold standard remains arteriography. Development of the multidetector CT scanner and resultant ability to perform CTA may ultimately replace traditional catheter arteriography.

MANAGEMENT OF LATE COMPLICATIONS

Abscess formation can occur after many of the injuries associated with blunt trauma. Intra-abdominal abscesses can occur after blunt or penetrating abdominal trauma, especially when there has been an associated injury to the bowel. If technically possible, these abscesses are often best managed by the placement of a percutaneous drain. These are usually placed under ultrasonography or CT guidance. The infected material should be sent for Gram stain and culture to allow for appropriate antibiotic therapy. The catheter is left in place until drainage stops, and there is evidence of resolution of the abscess cavity on CT scan or other radiographic test. Percutaneous catheters are usually not able to drain hematomas completely because of the viscosity of the hematoma. Bilomas and bile leaks can complicate hepatic trauma. Bilomas can be treated by percutaneous drainage and bile leaks are managed by endoscopically placed biliary stents. Occasionally, a bile leak will need to be managed by percutaneous transhepatic cholangiography and catheter placement.

Suggested Readings

Andrassy J, et al: Stent versus open surgery for acute and chronic traumatic injury of the thoracic aorta: a single-center experience. *J Trauma* 60:765, 2006.

Asensio JA, et al: Approach to the management of complex hepatic injuries. *J Trauma* 48:66, 2000.

Biffl WL, et al: The unrecognized epidemic of blunt carotid arterial injuries—early diagnosis improves neurologic outcome. *Ann Surg* 228:462, 1998.

Biffl WL, et al: The devastating potential of blunt vertebral artery injuries. *Ann Surg* 231:672, 2000.

Castelli P, et al: Endovascular repair of traumatic injuries of the subclavian and axillary arteries. *Injury* 36:778, 2005.

Cooney R, et al: Limitations of splenic angioembolization in treating blunt splenic injury. *J Trauma* 59:926, 2005.

Davis KA, et al: Improved success in nonoperative management of blunt splenic injuries: embolization of splenic artery pseudoaneurysms. *J Trauma* 44:1008, 1998.

Dent D, et al: Blunt splenic injuries-high nonoperative management rate can be achieved with selective embolization. *J Trauma* 56:1063, 2004.

Fabian TC, et al: Blunt carotid injury—importance of early diagnosis and anticoagulant therapy. *Ann Surg* 223:513, 1996.

Haan JM, et al: Splenic embolization revisited: a multicenter review. *J Trauma* 56:542, 2004.

Johnson JW, et al: Hepatic angiography in patients undergoing damage control laparotomy. *J Trauma* 52:1102, 2002.

Leurs LJ, et al: Endovascular treatment of thoracic aortic diseases: combined experience from the EUROSTAR and United Kingdom thoracic endograft registries. *J Vasc Surg* 40:670, 2004.

Martin MJ, et al: Functional outcome after blunt and penetrating carotid artery injuries—analysis of the national trauma data bank. *J Trauma* 59:860, 2005.

Miller PR, et al: Blunt cerebrovascular injuries—diagnosis and treatment. *J Trauma* 51:279, 2001.

Miller PR, et al: Prospective screening for blunt cerebrovascular injuries—analysis of diagnostic modalities and outcomes. *Ann Surg* 226:386, 2002.

Pacini D, et al: Traumatic rupture of the thoracic aorta—ten years of delayed management. *J Thorac Cardiovasc Surg* 129:880, 2005.

Shapiro M, et al: The role of repeat angiography in the management of pelvic fractures. *J Trauma* 58:227, 2005.

Wahl WL, et al: The need for early angiographic embolization in blunt liver injuries. *J Trauma* 52:1097, 2002.

Wheatley GH III, et al: Midterm outcome in 158 consecutive Gore TAG thoracic endoprostheses: single center experience. *Ann Thorac Surg* 81:1570, 2006.

Wong YC, et al: Mortality after successful transcatheter arterial embolization in patients with unstable pelvic fractures: rate of blood transfusion as a predictive factor. *J Trauma* 49:71, 2000.

ENDPOINTS OF RESUSCITATION

Michael Englehart,   Brandon Tieu, and   Martin Schreiber

The optimal endpoint of resuscitation has been debated since the early 20th century when Cannon espoused his controversial viewpoints concerning limited volume resuscitation, and it continues to be a topic of tremendous discussion and study. The ideal endpoint should be readily obtainable and easily interpretable. The goal is to provide adequate oxygen delivery (DO_2) and therefore tissue perfusion without producing the complications of over-resuscitation. This is accomplished primarily by increasing cardiac output via increases in preload (volume loading) or vasoactive drugs. Multiple diagnostic measurements have been used to determine both optimal cardiac performance and adequate tissue perfusion. While no single value can be used exclusively, various measurements do allow uniformity in comparing adequacy of resuscitation. The values provide the ability over time to determine whether a patient is being properly resuscitated. These can be categorized into hemodynamic parameters, metabolic parameters, and regional perfusion endpoints.

HEMODYNAMIC PARAMETERS

Vital Signs and Clinical Endpoints

Shock has been defined in a multitude of ways, but can best be described as a lack of adequate tissue perfusion, and thereby an impairment of oxygen delivery and removal of waste products. The six basic advanced trauma life support (ATLS) physiologic parameters that have been used to identify shock are heart rate, respiratory rate, blood pressure, urine output, level of consciousness, and pulse pressure. Urine output and level of consciousness are direct measurements of tissue perfusion, and are defined by the classes of shock. Renal blood flow correlates with arterial pressure, but can be subject to significant autoregulation during periods of hypoperfusion. Level of consciousness is less reliable when influenced by intoxication, central nervous system injury, and medication. Heart rate and respiratory rate can be notoriously misleading (Table 1). Anxiety, pain, and stress secondary to the emotional impact of trauma can falsely elevate these physiologic parameters. This can confuse the picture and mask the underlying severity of shock. The diagnosis of shock is best made by observing the body's main compensatory mechanism: redistribution of blood flow.

Due to austere conditions and inability to measure blood pressure, combat medics in Operation Iraqi Freedom and Operation Enduring Freedom have been trained to resuscitate patients until they are conscious, or when consciousness cannot be assessed, until they have a palpable radial pulse. During World War I, Cannon stated that 75 mm Hg is the critical systolic blood pressure to maintain. For patients with traumatic brain injury, many have advocated avoiding hypotension to ensure adequate cerebral perfusion pressure. The presence of hypotension is predictive of a bad outcome after head injury. Additionally, patients with previous hypertension may display symptoms of organ hypoperfusion despite a "normal" mean arterial pressure (MAP). Due to complex interactions of the patients' pre-existing disease states and the severity of the injury, there is unfortunately no clear "goal" MAP to determine adequate resuscitation.

Invasive Monitoring

Oxygen delivery is a function of hemoglobin concentration, oxygen saturation, and cardiac output. Hemoglobin concentration and high oxygen concentration are relatively easy to manipulate and monitor, but cardiac output can be more problematic. Adequate cardiac performance is largely a function of preload. Multiple methods have been devised to best estimate the patient's volume status indirectly by evaluating the venous return to the heart. With the introduction of central venous and pulmonary artery catheters, central venous and pulmonary capillary wedge pressures have been used as better measurements of volume status. While these measurements serve as guides in determining the accuracy and trend of the resuscitation, absolute values should be interpreted with caution. Valvular or global cardiac dysfunction, as well as restrictive pulmonary disease can dramatically alter these measurements.

Newer pulmonary artery catheters (volumetric or oximetric catheters) have the capability for dynamic measurement of additional hemodynamic parameters that were previously unobtainable. Cardiac output can be continuously monitored, and cardiac performance can be evaluated using calculations of ventricular power and end diastolic volume index. A recent study has demonstrated that the

right-ventricular, end diastolic volume index (RVEDVI) is a more sensitive measurement of preload than central venous pressure or wedge pressure, particularly in the mechanically ventilated patient. Cheatham et al. demonstrated that cardiac index correlated better with RVEDVI than with pulmonary artery wedge pressure at up to very high levels of positive, end expiratory pressure. In a comparison of RVEDVI with splanchnic perfusion in trauma patients, both Miller et al. and Chang et al. found that supranormal resuscitation to a RVEDVI of greater than 120 ml/m^2 during shock was associated with better outcomes.

Despite the advances in pulmonary artery catheters (PACs), their effectiveness has been in question since the mid-1990s. Connors et al. published an observational study suggesting that PACs were associated with increased mortality and increased utilization of resources. Despite the study's limitations, critically ill patients who had a PAC placed had a higher 30-, 60-, and 180-day mortality, increased hospital cost, and longer ICU stays. A recent meta-analysis of 13 randomized controlled trials evaluating PACs showed that the use of PACs did not improve survival or decrease length of stay in hospital. It did not show an increased mortality in the patients with a PAC. The meta-analysis included 5051 patients and is a combination of surgical and medical ICU patients. The results suggest that PACs should not be used routinely in surgical ICU patients unless effective therapies can be found that improve outcomes when used in conjunction with this diagnostic tool.

Less invasive techniques for measuring cardiac performance have been developed. Thoracic electrical bioimpedance measures the resistance of the chest to low voltage currents. It is inversely related to thoracic fluid content, thereby allowing calculation of cardiac output. Several studies have proven that this method correlates well with thermodilution measurements of cardiac output. However, a meta-analysis demonstrated clinical utility in trend analysis but not accuracy for diagnostic interpretation. There can also be significant imprecision with tachycardia or with pathologic fluid collections such as pleural effusions. Transesophageal echocardiography can assess preload and peak velocity measurements as well as continuous cardiac output monitoring. It has been validated with thermodilution techniques. In animal models of hemorrhagic shock, it has accurately reflected the magnitude of change on cardiac output. Pulse contour–derived CO measurement (PCCO) can also continuously measure cardiac output and it correlates with thermodilution. PCCO requires placement of an arterial catheter and a central venous catheter on opposite sides of the diaphragm. It may be a more accurate indicator of cardiac preload than central venous or wedge pressure. Unfortunately, rapid changes in hemodynamic status, including changes in blood pressure and systemic vascular resistance, can alter the monitoring, and recalibration is necessary.

Many have attempted to define the oxygen consumption/delivery endpoint itself, but with no clear results. The Fick equation states that DO_2 and VO_2 are functions of cardiac performance (CI),

Table 1: Relationship of Degree of Shock to Pulse Rate (106 Cases)

Pulse Rate	Degrees of Shock			
	None (n=13)	Slight (n=24)	Moderate (n=34)	Severe (n=35)
Minimum	70	88	80	60
Maximum	140	150	160	144
Average	103 + 7.2	111 + 3.4	113 + 3.6	116 + 3.3

Notes: These data were gathered in the North African–Mediterranean Theater during World War II. There was minimal variability observed between groups despite significant differences in the severity of shock. Slight shock = 80% of normal blood volume; moderate shock = 70% of normal blood volume; severe shock = 55% of normal blood volume.
Source: Office of the Surgeon General, The Board for the Study of the Severely Wounded: *The Physiologic Effect of Wounds*, 1952.

hemoglobin (Hb), and arterial and venous oxygen saturations (SaO$_2$ and SvO$_2$, respectively):

$$DO_2 = CI \times 13.4 \times Hb \times SaO_2$$

$$VO_2 = CI \times 13.4 \times Hb \times (SaO_2 - SvO_2)$$

Unfortunately, DO$_2$ and VO$_2$ are both derived from cardiac output, and the stable plateau described in Figure 1 is virtually impossible to obtain. Goal-directed therapy, aimed at ensuring CI greater than 4.5 l/min/m^2, DO$_2$ index greater than 600 ml/min/m^2, and VO$_2$ index greater than 170 ml/min/m^2, has been advocated by Shoemaker and others, showing reduced morbidity and mortality in critically ill patients. However, Gattinoni in a multicenter randomized controlled trial, and Heyland in a meta-analysis, have shown that no such benefit exists. Furthermore, a prospective, randomized controlled trial by Velmahos comparing conventional versus supranormal endpoints demonstrated that despite all efforts, only 70% of patients were able to reach these endpoints. They concluded that regardless of the resuscitation strategy, the ability of the patient to achieve "optimal hemodynamic values" significantly affected outcome. Looking at O$_2$ delivery alone, McKinley et al. found that there was no difference in outcome between groups resuscitated to an O$_2$ delivery goal of 600 ml/min/m^2 versus 500 ml/min/m^2.

Resuscitation to supranormal endpoints has been associated with numerous complications. Shoemaker's protocol included volume loading with crystalloids and blood, and enhancement of cardiac output with dobutamine. Improvements in blood pressure and cardiac performance by vasoactive drugs can be negated by reduced tissue perfusion, and can often result in tissue ischemia. Hayes et al. found in medical and surgical critically ill patients that the use of dobutamine to augment O$_2$ delivery may actually increase mortality. Over-resuscitation with crystalloid solutions can lead to the development of compartment syndromes, coagulopathy, and congestive heart failure in patients with cardiac disease.

METABOLIC PARAMETERS

Lactate

Measurable metabolic endpoints allow the clinician to effectively assess the microcirculation. Accumulation of lactate occurs under anaerobic conditions, and therefore, is a marker of inadequate microcirculatory oxygen delivery. Thus, lactate levels can provide a measure of the extent of shock. While elevated levels indicate worsening degrees of shock,

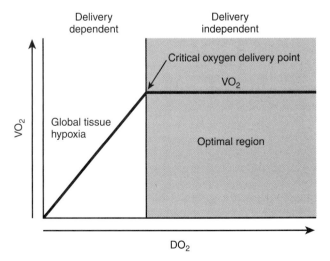

Figure 1   Relationship between oxygen delivery (DO$_2$) and oxygen extraction (VO$_2$).   *(From Bilkovski RN, et al: Targeted resuscitation strategies after injury. Curr Opin Crit Care 10:529–538, 2004, with permission.)*

there is no clear cutoff value for when resuscitation is "satisfactory" and adequate oxygen delivery to the tissues is present. Manikas et al. found that initial and peak lactate levels, along with duration of hyperlactatemia, correlated with the development of multiple organ dysfunction syndrome after trauma. Lactate clearance over time is more predictive of mortality than isolated values. Serial lactate levels in trauma patients have been associated with 0%–10% mortality if cleared (lactate level <2 mmol/l) within 24 hours, 25% mortality if cleared by 24–48 hours, and 80%–86% mortality if cleared beyond 48 hours.

Base Deficit

Base deficit has been advocated as a useful clinical marker for assessing reduced tissue perfusion and as a convenient marker of elevated lactate levels. It is defined as the amount of base (millimoles) required to raise 1 liter of whole blood to a normal pH. Davis first classified the base deficit according to severity: mild (2–5 mmol/l), moderate (6–14 mmol/l), or severe (>15 mmol/l). The severity of the deficit directly correlated with the volume of crystalloid and blood replaced within the first 24 hours. It has been shown that serum bicarbonate levels, which may be more readily available, correlate well with base deficits, but they are affected by the patient's ventilatory status. Similar to lactate, the absolute base deficit can estimate the severity of shock, but no single value can be used as an endpoint. Persistently high or worsening base deficits may be an indicator of complications such as abdominal compartment syndrome or ongoing hemorrhage. Greater severity of base deficit does predict diminished oxygen consumption, increased risk of multiple organ dysfunction syndrome, and greater mortality. However, base deficit secondary to hyperchloremic acidosis is not associated with increased mortality or complications as demonstrated by Brill et al. (Table 2). The inaccurate interpretation of an elevated base deficit that is truly related to hyperchloremic acidosis may result in unnecessary interventions such as ongoing fluid resuscitation, blood transfusion, or even operative interventions. As with lactate, the trend of the base deficit over time is more useful in predicting outcomes.

REGIONAL PERFUSION ENDPOINTS

A multitude of devices that directly measure the tissue microcirculation have been developed. These include gastric tonometry, sublingual capnography, and near-infrared spectroscopy (NIRS). Gastric tonometry monitors the gastric intramucosal pH (pHi), by measuring the level of tissue pCO$_2$. pHi decreases as splanchnic perfusion decreases. For this test to be accurate, gastric feedings need to be withheld and gastric acid secretion needs to be suppressed. Unfortunately, it correlates poorly with lactate and base deficit, and has a prolonged calibration time. It has been suggested in studies that a lower pHi correlates with the development of multiorgan dysfunction syndrome and increased mortality. Sublingual capnography uses the premise that global tissue hypoperfusion causes systemic hypercarbia. It has been proven to correlate with lactate levels, as well as the severity of shock, and has been used as a predictor of mortality. Finally, NIRS can be used to determine tissue oxygen saturation (StO$_2$) (Figure 2). The NIRS technology allows the simultaneous measurement of tissue pO$_2$, pCO$_2$, and pH. In animal models of hemorrhagic shock, StO$_2$ closely correlated with measured oxygen delivery, and was a superior measurement of shock compared to lactate, base excess, or SvO$_2$. McKinley et al. found that StO$_2$ correlated with oxygen delivery, base deficit, and lactate levels in severely injured trauma patients. NIRS can also monitor mitochondrial function by monitoring the redox state of cytochrome aa3, which reflects mitochondrial oxygen consumption. Under normal conditions, tissue oxyhemoglobin levels (HbO$_2$) and cytochrome aa3 levels are tightly coupled. Cairns et al. noted that in a study of 24 severely injured trauma patients, 9 patients who developed multiorgan failure (MOF) had HbO$_2$ and cytochrome aa3 decoupling. Only 2 of 16 patients who did not develop MOF had decoupling. Many of these

Table 2: Hyperchloremic Group vs. Combined High and Mixed Anion Gap Group

	Hyperchloremic Group	Combined Group	p Value
Number of patients	37	38	
Mean age	53.9 ± 19.8	54.8 ± 22.9	0.85
Male sex (%)	54	60	0.71
APACHE II	12.2 ± 6.01	15 ± 7.5	0.10
Mean days SICU	7.8 ± 6.9	10.4 ± 9.9	0.19
Mean estimated blood loss (ml)	1088 ± 1835	1343 ± 1930	0.61
Mean resuscitation (ml)	5598 ± 3950	6500 ± 5227	0.41
Mean lactate (mg/dl)	1.5 ± 0.29	3.9 ± 2.2	<0.001
Mean blood density	5.3 ± 2.5	7.8 ± 5.4	0.01
Deaths	4	13	0.03

Note: Mortality is significantly reduced in surgical intensive care unit patients when acidosis is secondary to hyperchloremic acidosis as opposed to lactic acidosis.
APACHE II, Acute Physiology and Chronic Health Evaluation II; *SICU,* surgical intensive care unit.
Source: Brill SA, et al: Base deficit does not predict mortality when secondary to hyperchloremic acidosis. *Shock* 17(6):459–462, 2002.

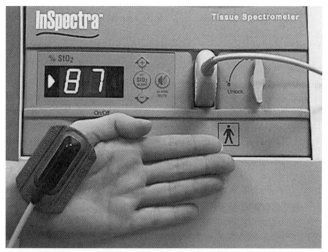

Figure 2 Near-infrared spectroscopy measuring tissue oxygen saturation (StO₂). InSpectra™ Tissue Spectrometer with thenar shield in place. Shield may also be used on the deltoid muscles.

devices have failed to gain widespread use and have not been standardized.

SUMMARY

In conclusion, the goals of resuscitation should be to optimize preload, cardiac performance, blood pressure, oxygen delivery, and end-organ perfusion. Unfortunately, no single hemodynamic value or laboratory test will be universally helpful. The best method is to incorporate and optimize each of these endpoints. Given that shock remains a clinical diagnosis, the assessment of resuscitation is best made at the bedside, relying on an accurate assessment of the physical signs and symptoms.

SUGGESTED READINGS

Abramson MD, et al: Lactate clearance and survival following injury. *J Trauma* 35(4):584–589, 1993.
Bishop MH, et al: Prospective, randomized trial of survivor values of cardiac index, oxygen delivery, and oxygen consumption as resuscitation endpoints in severe trauma. *J Trauma* 38(5):780–787, 1998.

Boyd O, Grounds R, Bennett ED: A randomized clinical trial of the effect of deliberate perioperative increase of oxygen delivery on mortality in high-risk surgical patients. *JAMA* 270(22):2699–2707, 1993.
Brain Trauma Foundation, American Association of Neurological Surgeons, Joint Section on Neurotrauma and Critical Care: Hypotension. *J Neurotrauma* 17(6–7):591–595, 2000.
Brill SA, et al: Base deficit does not predict mortality when secondary to hyperchloremic acidosis. *Shock* 17(6):459–462, 2002.
Chang MC, et al: Gastric tonometry supplements information provided by systemic indicators of oxygen transport. *J Trauma* 37:488–494, 1994.
Cheatham ML, et al: Right ventricular end-diastolic volume index as a predictor of preload status in patients on positive end-expiratory pressure. *Crit Care Med* 26:1801–1806, 1998.
Connors AF Jr, et al: The effectiveness of right heart catheterization in the initial care of critically ill patients. SUPPORT Investigators. *JAMA* 276(11): 889–897, 1996.
Davis JW, et al: Base deficit as a guide to volume resuscitation. *J Trauma* 28:1464–1467, 1988.
DeFigueiredo LF, et al: Cardiac output determination during experimental hemorrhage and resuscitation using a transesophageal Doppler monitor. *Artif Organs* 28:338–342, 2004.
Gattinoni L, et al: A trial of goal-oriented hemodynamic therapy in critically ill patients. *N Engl J Med* 333(16):1025–1032, 1995.
Hussain FA, et al: Serum lactate and base deficit as predictors of mortality and morbidity. *Am J Surg* 185:485–491, 2003.
Ivatury RR, et al: A prospective randomized study of end points of resuscitation after major trauma: global oxygen transport indices versus organ-specific gastric mucosal pH. *J Am Coll Surg* 183:145–154, 1996.
Kincaid EH, et al: Elevated arterial base deficit in trauma patients: a marker of impaired oxygen utilization. *J Am Coll Surg* 187(4):384–392, 1998.
Miller PR, Meredith JW, Chang MC: Randomized, prospective comparison of increased preload versus inotropes in the resuscitation of trauma patients: effects on cardiopulmonary function and visceral perfusion. *J Trauma* 44:107–113, 1998.
Shah MR, et al: Impact of the pulmonary artery catheter in critically ill patients: meta-analysis of randomized clinical trials. *JAMA* 294(13): 1664–1670, 2005.
Schreiber MA, et al: Determinants of mortality in patients with severe blunt head injury. *Arch Surg* 137(3):285–290, 2002.
Shoemaker WC, et al: Prospective trial of supranormal values of survivors as therapeutic goals in high-risk surgical patients. *Chest* 94:1176–1186, 1988.
Velmahos GC, et al: Endpoints of resuscitation of critically injured patients: normal or supranormal? A prospective randomized trial. *Ann Surg* 232(3):409–418, 2000.
Weil MH, et al: Sublingual capnometry: a new noninvasive measurement for diagnosis and quantitation of severity of circulatory shock. *Crit Care Med* 27:1225–1229, 1999.

HEAD AND CENTRAL NERVOUS SYSTEM INJURIES

TRAUMATIC BRAIN INJURY: PATHOPHYSIOLOGY, CLINICAL DIAGNOSIS, AND PREHOSPITAL AND EMERGENCY CENTER CARE

Alex B. Valadka   and   **Mark J. Dannenbaum**

Death. Long-lasting or even permanent loss of function. Those are the burdens borne by many traumatic brain injury (TBI) patients and their families. Even some patients who initially appeared to have injuries that were mild according to clinical or radiographic criteria can suffer permanent injury.

Emergency craniotomies and insertion of intracranial monitors are the most high-profile aspects of management of TBI patients. However, the vulnerability of the injured brain to even mild and transient metabolic derangements underscores the major impact that systemic parameters can have on influencing outcome from TBI. Thus, non-neurosurgeons can influence management in ways that are just as important, and in some cases perhaps more so, than the interventions performed by neurosurgeons.

This chapter will discuss a few principles of the underlying pathophysiology, initial assessment, and prehospital and emergency center management of TBI patients. The following chapter addresses topics relevant to the acute hospital admission. This discussion is weighted toward patients with severe TBI, but many of the basic principles apply to patients with mild or moderate TBI as well.

INCIDENCE

It is frequently stated that in multiply injured patients, the head is the most commonly injured part of the body. Outcome from polytrauma is more dependent on the extent of brain injury than on injury to other organ systems. Perhaps a third of the entire cost of trauma, including medical and rehabilitative care, lost income to the patient, and lost productivity to society, is attributable to brain injury.

According to data reported by the Centers for Disease Control and Prevention in the 1990s, 1.5 million Americans sustain a TBI every year. Of this number, hospitalization and ultimate survival occur in approximately 230,000 patients, but 50,000 will die. Long-term disability will occur in 80,000-90,000 patients annually. It has been estimated that more than 5 million men, women, and children in the United States are living with a permanent TBI-related disability.[1]

Motor vehicle crashes are the most common cause of TBI that produces hospitalization, whereas violence is the major cause of TBI-related deaths. Falls predominate as the leading cause of TBI in elderly patients. In 1990, gunshot wounds to the head overtook falls as the most common cause of TBI-related death in the United States.

The TBI death rate in the United States is approximately 20 per 100,000 population. In all age groups, the mortality rate is higher in males than in females. The incidence of TBI-related mortality peaks in the late teens and early twenties, subsequently decreasing during the next few decades until taking off exponentially at about retirement age.

MECHANISM OF INJURY

Although an epidural, subdural, or intraparenchymal hematoma may have a dramatic appearance on a computed tomography (CT) scan, the clinician must remember that these lesions are distinct from the cerebral parenchymal injury that is the true cause of long-term neurologic deficits. TBI is best thought of as a diffuse disturbance of cerebral function, not as a blood clot or contusion. This diffuse disturbance may occur in parallel with, but may also be independent of, those processes that lead to the development of traumatic mass lesions.

Subdural Hematoma

Classically, a subdural hematoma (SDH) (Figure 1) has been said to develop after tearing of a bridging vein, that is, a vein passing directly from the cortex to the overlying dura. The mechanical forces of the trauma can cause tearing of these veins. More recent evidence indicates that at least some of these hematomas actually form from splitting of inner and outer layers of the dura, that is, they may actually be "intradural hematomas." Finally, some SDHs are caused by direct bleeding into the subdural space from parenchymal contusions or hematomas or from injured cortical arteries or veins.

Epidural Hematoma

Epidural hematomas (EDHs) classically arise after a blow to the side of the head results in a fracture of the thin temporal bone immediately overlying the middle meningeal artery. The patient may briefly lose consciousness after the initial impact, but he or she quickly awakens; thus, the brain injury was mild. Unfortunately, the fracturing of the skull lacerated the middle meningeal artery. Continued

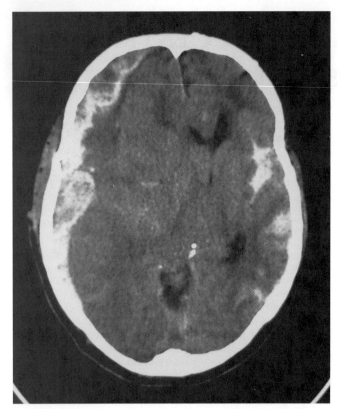

Figure 1 Large acute subdural hematoma (SDH) with midline shift. Subarachnoid hemorrhage is evident contralateral to the SDH.

bleeding from this source produces an enlarging EDH, the presence of which may be signaled by such symptoms as severe and worsening headache, vomiting, and decreasing level of consciousness. The period between awakening from the initial concussion and subsequent lapsing into a coma has historically been described as a "lucid interval." Importantly, loss of consciousness does not always occur after the skull is fractured, and many patients with large EDHs are awake until they begin to lapse into a terminal coma. It must also be mentioned that many EDHs are not associated with meningeal arterial bleeding. In these cases, perhaps the source of the hematoma is oozing from the overlying edges of fractured bone.

Referring again to the classic scenarios, patients with EDHs are said to fare better than patients with similarly sized SDHs. Why should this be so? The answer is that a "pure" EDH essentially represents a skull fracture with no direct parenchymal injury to the brain. On the other hand, the rotational forces that are said to be an important cause of SDHs via tearing of bridging veins may also cause widespread axonal injury, as discussed later. Thus, SDH is said to be associated with a greater burden of parenchymal injury, which explains the worse outcomes. Of course, this explanation refers only to the extreme ends of the spectrum of the pathophysiology of EDHs and SDHs. Many patients with EDHs will do poorly, while SDH patients often recover well from their injuries. Nevertheless, this explanation is a useful way to conceptualize the interactions between mass lesions and diffuse injury.

Subarachnoid Hemorrhage

The most common post-traumatic intracerebral hemorrhage is not a mass lesion, but rather diffuse subarachnoid hemorrhage (SAH) (see Figure 1). Several retrospective series report that SAH after TBI is independently associated with worse outcomes, but the mechanism that might explain such an association is unclear. In the acute setting,

SAH does not seem to have much effect on patient management, which is driven instead by more immediately pressing concerns.

Parenchymal Lesions

Contusions occur commonly after TBI, especially at the base of the frontal lobes and at the anterior edges of the temporal lobes. The brain in these regions is said to continue moving over or into the skull base after the head suddenly stops moving after a violent blow or rapid rotational movement. Fortunately, most such contusions remain small and surgically insignificant. Emergency surgery may be required, however, for larger lesions or for smaller ones that subsequently enlarge.

Unlike contusions, in which extravasated blood mixes freely with brain tissue, parenchymal hematomas consist of solid blood clots within the brain itself. They occur less commonly than contusions. They tend to be more variable in their distribution.

Ischemia

Diffuse injury may be of several types. Ischemia is a common form of diffuse injury. In some cases, mass effect from a traumatic hematoma may cause elevated intracranial pressure (ICP) and local compression of underlying tissue that can lead, respectively, to global and local reduction of cerebral blood flow (CBF). However, post-traumatic cerebral ischemia may also occur when no mass lesion is present, especially very early after injury. Although the CT scans in these cases may be relatively unimpressive, these patients may be quite vulnerable to the effects of such secondary insults as hypotension or hypoxia. Over the subsequent hours and days, CBF usually increases, but the damage from early ischemia may have already been done long before the increase in CBF (Figure 2). Some centers have used xenon CT or perfusion CT to measure CBF and identify ischemia immediately after injury.

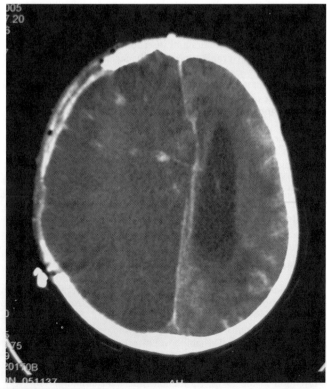

Figure 2 Infarction of an entire cerebral hemisphere is evident on the left side of this computed tomography scan.

Diffuse Axonal Injury

Another common type of diffuse injury is diffuse axonal injury (DAI). Although the axonal disconnection that characterizes DAI is commonly thought to occur at the time of injury, such immediate loss of axonal continuity probably occurs only when an injury produces severe cerebral parenchymal disruption. Instead, it appears more likely that the rotational and mechanical forces that are operant during the traumatic event produce a focal impairment of axoplasmic flow, which, in turn, culminates in axonal disconnection several hours after injury.[2] This slight delay creates hope that a therapeutic window may exist for the administration of a yet-to-be-developed treatment that would prevent loss of axonal integrity and function.

Of course, axonal pathology cannot be visualized on a CT scan. However, DAI frequently occurs in conjunction with small scattered parenchymal hemorrhages commonly described as "shear injuries," probably because they have been postulated to occur as tissues at different depths of the brain undergo rotation at different velocities. The interface between these regions is said to undergo shearing, resulting in the small punctuate hemorrhages. Regardless of whether this explanation is true, the presence of scattered small hemorrhages may serve as a clue that DAI may be present.

Cellular and Molecular Factors

At the cellular level, the abnormalities caused by TBI are numerous and complex. Release of glutamate and other excitatory neurotransmitters may lead to excessive neuronal depolarization and intracellular calcium influx, with activation of proteases and other processes that lead to cell death. Inadequate blood flow can cause a conversion from aerobic to anaerobic metabolism. The lactic acid that is produced lowers local tissue pH, and the consequent acidosis contributes to tissue injury and death. Trauma-induced apoptosis may promote further cell death. These and other biochemical and cellular processes take place against the backdrop of an individual patient's genetic makeup; the presence of specific alleles for various genes may make an individual more or less susceptible to the damaging effects of various pathophysiologic processes.

CLINICAL DIAGNOSIS

Clinical Examination

Ideally, the severity of TBI is determined and classified according to a patient's neurologic examination. The size and appearance of a mass lesion as seen on imaging studies are not as important as the effect that the lesion may be having on a patient's neurologic function and level of alertness.

The single most important question in the evaluation of a potentially head-injured patient is whether he or she obeys simple one-step commands. A simple definition of coma is that a person will not do such things as hold up two fingers or stick out the tongue when asked to do so. Failure to obey commands is widely used as an indicator of the presence of severe TBI. Other simple but important observations are the type of movement exhibited by the patient (localization of noxious stimuli, withdrawal, flexion, extension, etc.); whether the right and left sides are symmetrical; the type of speech; the presence or absence of eye opening; and pupillary size, reactivity to light, and bilateral symmetry.

Because the nerve fibers that mediate pupillary constriction lie on the surface of the third cranial nerve, compression of this nerve by herniating brain tissue that is being displaced by a large mass lesion may cause inactivation of the pupilloconstricting fibers. The resulting pupil appears large and unable to constrict in response to bright light. This physical finding in a comatose TBI patient suggests that an immediate CT scan is needed to identify a large acute hematoma. However, fixed and dilated pupils may also be caused by brainstem ischemia or by direct ocular trauma.

Many scales have been developed for the assessment of consciousness or neurologic status after injury, but by far the most widely used is the Glasgow Coma Scale (GCS)[3] (Table 1). In conjunction with such information as the status of pupillary reactivity and the tempo or rate of change of a patient's neurologic condition, the GCS is an extremely useful tool for assessing a patient's baseline condition and subsequent progress.

INITIAL CLINICAL INTERVENTIONS: PREHOSPITAL AND EMERGENCY CENTER CARE

The basic principles of TBI care, which have remained unchanged for decades, are maintenance of normal homeostasis and prevention and prompt treatment of secondary insults. The acutely traumatized brain is much more vulnerable than the uninjured brain to even mild deviations from normal, such as transient episodes of hypotension or hypoxia.[4] Some evidence suggests that events like febrile episodes, seizures, and hyperglycemia may also worsen outcome. Brief insults are usually tolerated well by the normal brain, but they may have a profound detrimental effect on the injured brain.

The basics of TBI care revolve around the ABCs: airway, breathing, and circulation. Although some of the specifics of management of these parameters differ between the prehospital setting and the intensive care unit (ICU), it is important to view management of the ABCs as a continuum with goals that remain constant throughout the acute phase of a patient's illness. Because of this continuity, the following discussion of the ABCs begins with the prehospital setting but then moves into ICU considerations as well.

Airway

In terms of control of the airway, prehospital endotracheal intubation should be considered in patients with severe TBI or with other problems that may impair movement of air or protection of the airway from aspiration. Recent retrospective reports in the trauma literature associate worse outcomes with prehospital intubation of severe TBI patients. One possible explanation of these findings may be the difficulty of performing successful endotracheal intubation in the prehospital setting, especially if prehospital providers do so only infrequently.

Breathing

In terms of breathing, standard recommendations advocate the lowest FiO_2 capable of maintaining adequate oxygenation. Although the minimum acceptable PaO_2 based on the oxygen-hemoglobin dissociation curve is 60 mm Hg, most practitioners

Table 1: Glasgow Coma Scale

Score	Motor	Verbal	Eye Opening
6	Obeys commands	—	—
5	Localizes stimulus	Oriented	—
4	Withdraws from stimulus	Confused	Spontaneously
3	Flexes arm	Words/phrases	To voice
2	Extends arm	Sounds	To pain
1	No response	No response	Remains closed

target a minimum of 80-100 mm Hg in TBI patients in order to create a bit of a cushion.

Hyperventilation is no longer recommended as a prophylactic measure to prevent intracranial hypertension.[5] Hyperventilation is known to cause constriction of the cerebral vasculature, and the resultant decrease in cerebral blood volume can acutely lower ICP. However, the constriction of cerebral arteries may cause CBF to drop to critical levels. Also, within 24 hours of initiation of hyperventilation, the cerebral arteries probably dilate back to their original diameter.[6] Subsequent attempts to allow the $PaCO_2$ to increase can cause the arteries to dilate even further, possibly raising ICP.

Most clinicians aim for the low-normal range of $PaCO_2$, targeting a value of approximately 35 mm Hg. Keeping the $PaCO_2$ toward the lower end of the normal range may optimize the ability of the cerebral vasculature to autoregulate.

Hyperventilation should be reserved for acute deterioration accompanied by signs of a mass lesion, such as raised ICP with asymmetrical pupils or asymmetrical motor exam. In such cases, the assumption is that the patient will need emergency surgery to treat the lesion. Hyperventilation and other measures, like administration of mannitol, are intended only to buy a few minutes to obtain an emergency CT scan prior to going to surgery. If the scan reveals that no surgical lesion is present, attempts should be made to manage the elevated ICP without hyperventilation by using some of the steps explained in the next chapter.

Circulation

The "C" in ABCs stands for circulation. For brain-injured patients, this can be thought of as management of blood pressure and intravenous fluids.

In years past, common practice was to dehydrate patients "to prevent the brain from swelling." In the 1990s, the pendulum swung the other way as TBI patients were aggressively managed with intravenous fluids and pressors in order to artificially elevate their blood pressure. However, subsequent studies showed that patients treated with aggressive elevation of blood pressure through fluids and pressors did not have improved neurologic outcomes and, in fact, had a five-fold higher likelihood of developing acute respiratory distress syndrome.[7]

Current management strategies call for maintenance of a normal blood pressure, with aggressive elevation of blood pressure reserved for those patients in whom clinical or physiologic monitoring suggests a need for such therapy, such as to treat cerebral hypoxia or to reverse neurologic deterioration.

Direct monitoring of brain tissue oxygen tension ($PbtO_2$) is now possible via small intraparenchymal catheters. Although some clinicians treat low $PbtO_2$ by increasing the FiO_2, we prefer to treat low brain tissue PO_2 by raising blood pressure in order to optimize perfusion of the affected tissue. Ischemic thresholds of brain tissue are difficult to identify with precision. A $PbtO_2$ below 15-20 mm Hg is generally regarded as low, whereas values below 8-10 mm Hg may suggest that further evaluation and/or intervention might be appropriate.

IMAGING MODALITIES: WHAT, WHEN, AND WHY

Computed Tomography Scanning

After initial assessment and stabilization of a TBI patient, the next order of business is the procurement of imaging studies. The most important radiologic study for the evaluation of acute TBI is a CT scan. This imaging modality is excellent for revealing acute hemorrhage, cerebral edema, and mass effect, which are the features of greatest interest during the initial assessment. Bone settings can also detect calvarial and skull base fractures. Another advantage is that CT scanning is a quick procedure that is widely available, at least in the United States. To overcome difficulties with prehospital intubation and the frequent use of sedation in these patients, Marshall et al.[8] devised a TBI classification scheme based on CT scan findings (Table 2).

Magnetic Resonance Imaging

Magnetic resonance imaging (MRI) has limited application in the acute setting for several reasons. Obtaining a study requires a fair amount of time, access to the patient is limited during the study, and ferromagnetic monitoring and resuscitative equipment must be removed before the patient can enter the magnet. After patients have been stabilized, MRI may reveal the presence of subtle parenchymal injuries that may shed light on the unexplained failure of some patients to improve.

Angiography

Angiography continues to have an ambiguous role in the initial evaluation of the brain-injured patient. Prior to the development of CT scanning in the 1970s, neurosurgeons were limited to pneumoencephalography or angiography for detecting midline shift or other types of mass effect. Skull radiography could also indicate displacement of the calcified pineal gland.

Since the advent of CT scanning, cerebral angiography has usually been reserved for cases in which a high index of suspicion for intracranial vascular injury exists, such as pseudoaneurysm formation or arterial dissection. However, the optimal treatment of any such findings is unclear. Most acutely brain-injured patients should not receive heparin or warfarin, yet interventional radiologic procedures often require that the patient be anticoagulated. Similarly, critically low cerebral blood flow is present in a sizeable percentage of severe TBI patients. The wisdom of occluding a major artery in a patient who may already be ischemic is questionable.

Continuing advances in CT angiography may soon make this technology comparable to conventional angiography for detecting vascular injury. Thus, angiography will probably continue its historical trend of declining use in the acute assessment of TBI patients.

Table 2: Marshall CT Classification Scheme

Category	Definition
Diffuse injury I (no visible pathology)	No intracranial pathology visible on CT scan
Diffuse injury II	Cisterns present with midline shift 0-5 mm and/or: Lesion densities present No high- or mixed-density lesion >25 cc
Diffuse injury III (swelling)	Cisterns compressed or absent with midline shift 0-5 mm; no high- or mixed-density lesion >25 cc
Diffuse injury IV (shift)	Midline shift >5 mm, no high- or mixed-density lesion >25 cc
Evacuated mass lesion	Any lesion surgically evacuated
Nonevacuated mass lesion	High- or mixed-density lesion >25 cc, not surgically evacuated

CT, Computed tomography.

INJURY GRADING

Glasgow Coma Scale

Many different schemes have been proposed for the grading and classification of brain injury. As discussed previously, the best known is the GCS. Introduction of this scale reinforced the need for an accurate neurologic examination as part of the assessment and classification of brain-injured patients. This point is as fundamental today as when the GCS was initially described. Because this scale made possible a more objective assessment of patients, interobserver and intercenter variability could be reduced, thus enabling the creation of multicenter and even multinational studies.

However, accurate determination of the GCS score is often difficult in patients who are intoxicated with alcohol or other drugs or in patients with injuries that cause such extensive periorbital edema that the eyes are swollen shut, making assessment of eye opening impossible. Other factors that complicate the determination of the GCS score reflect changes in prehospital and emergency department practices since the initial description of the GCS over a generation ago. Nowadays, many patients are endotracheally intubated in the prehospital setting, and paralytics and sedatives are often administered before an accurate and thorough neurologic assessment is performed. These problems have led to the creation of other assessment tools, such as those based on CT findings.[8] Another way of getting around the problem of an inaccurate neurologic examination might be the use of serum markers to identify trauma patients who are likely to have serious central nervous system injury, analogous to the manner in which serum levels of cardiac enzymes are used in the diagnosis of acute myocardial injury.[9] This is an area of rapidly growing interest.

Common practice classifies brain injury as mild, moderate, or severe based on the GCS score. Mild TBI is traditionally equated with a GCS score of 13-15, whereas moderate TBI refers to a GCS score of 9-12. Some authorities, however, consider a score of 13 to be more indicative of moderate injury. Severe TBI refers to patients with a GCS score of 8 or less.

It is worth emphasizing that this widely used scheme of classifying TBI is based on functional, not anatomic, criteria. This approach contrasts with that used in much of the general trauma literature, in which anatomic criteria are used as the primary means of classifying injuries.

Marshall Computed Tomography Scale

Marshall and colleagues developed a CT-based classification scheme using data from the Traumatic Coma Data Bank (see Table 2). This system, commonly referred to as the Marshall scale or the TCDB scale, classifies CT scans according to such factors as midline shift and compression of cerebrospinal fluid cisterns. Although this scale is useful in certain circumstances, it should not be considered a substitute for an accurate neurologic examination.

Abbreviated Injury Scale

The Abbreviated Injury Scale (Table 3) for the head assigns a score of 1 for minor scalp injuries such as abrasions, contusions, and lacerations.[10] Longer and deeper lacerations receive a score of 2, whereas scalp injuries accompanied by significant blood loss or characterized by total scalp loss are scored as 3. Cranial nerve injuries are coded as 2.

Injuries to major cerebral vessels are generally coded as 3 or 4 for thrombosis or traumatic aneurysm formation, or as 4 or 5 for laceration.

Scores for fractures of the skull and skull base range from 2 for simple fractures of the vault, to 3 for skull base fractures or

Table 3: Abbreviated Injury Scale for Head Injury

Score	Injury Severity	Head Injury Examples
1	Minor	Minor scalp injuries
2	Moderate	More severe scalp injuries Cranial nerve injuries Simple calvarial fractures LOC <1 hour Post-traumatic amnesia
3	Serious	Worst scalp injuries Cerebral vascular injuries Skull base fractures Comminuted calvarial fractures Small parenchymal contusions Traumatic subarachnoid hemorrhage LOC 1–6 hours
4	Severe	Worse cerebral vascular injuries Worst skull fractures Hematomas LOC 6–24 hours
5	Critical	Worst cerebral vascular injuries Larger hematomas LOC >24 hours
6	Lethal	Massive destruction Crush injuries

LOC, Loss of consciousness.

comminuted vault fractures, to 4 for the most complex open fractures with exposed brain tissue or for significantly depressed closed fractures.

Scoring for brain parenchymal injuries ranges from 3 to 5. Small single or multiple contusions receive a score of 3, as does SAH, edema, or infarction directly related to trauma. Hematomas are scored as 4 or 5, depending on their size.

Massive destruction or crush injuries are scored as a 6.

The duration of loss of consciousness and presence of associated neurologic deficits may be used to score injury severity if such scores exceed those based on anatomical injuries. Such scores range from 2 to 5.

The American Association for the Surgery of Trauma organ injury scale does not address brain injuries.

Mild and Moderate Traumatic Brain Injury

This chapter and the following one focus on patients with severe TBI. Those with moderate brain injury, who are commonly described as patients with a GCS score of 9–12, often have significant intracranial pathology and yet still obey commands. Their management is similar to that of severe TBI patients in the sense that careful observation and prevention of secondary insults are of paramount importance. However, intracranial monitors may not be needed in many of these patients, and they may not require the same intensity of care for the same amount of time as severe TBI patients.

The vast majority of patients seeking medical attention after a brain injury have mild TBI. They are often diagnosed as having had a concussion. Importantly, the diagnosis of mild TBI (or concussion) does not require that a patient lose consciousness. Some data indicate that the majority of patients with mild TBI never lose consciousness, but they may complain of a variety of symptoms like headache, post-traumatic amnesia, difficulty concentrating, ringing in the ears, unsteadiness of gait, and so on.

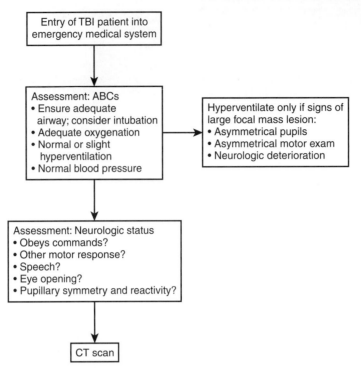

Figure 3 Basic initial assessment and management of traumatic brain injury patients.

Unlike the situation with severe TBI, the major concern with mild TBI is not whether a patient will live or die or whether a patient will become vegetative or severely disabled. Almost all these patients survive. Instead, the major morbidity relates to disturbances of memory, cognition, attention, emotional stability, and related areas. The lack of "hard" evidence of neurologic impairment leads many physicians to downplay the significance of these symptoms. However, these patients often go on to lose their jobs, drop out of school, divorce their spouses, or go through other major upheavals in their lives. Eventually, most of them recover, but such a process may take months. Reassurance of the patient and family may be all that is needed, and in fact, may be all that can be offered. Counseling and formal testing may be appropriate if objective documentation of injury is needed or if a physician suspects malingering or symptom magnification for secondary gain.

CONCLUSIONS AND ALGORITHM

Figure 3 summarizes the priorities in assessment and initial management of TBI patients. Accurate neurologic assessment and careful attention to the ABCs are of paramount importance. These goals continue to be emphasized while patients are transported to a hospital, resuscitated, and taken to a CT scanner.

REFERENCES

1. Centers for Disease Control and Prevention: Traumatic Brain Injury in the United States: A Report to Congress. Available at http://www.cdc.gov/doc.do/id/0900f3ec8001012b.
2. Stone JR, Okonkwo DO, Dialo AO, et al: Impaired axonal transport and altered axolemmal permeability occur in distinct populations of damaged axons following traumatic brain injury. *Exp Neurol* 190:59-69, 2004.
3. Teasdale G, Jennett B: Assessment of coma and impaired consciousness. A practical scale. *Lancet* 2(7872):81-84, 1974.
4. Miller JD, Sweet RC, Narayan R, Becker DP: Early insults to the injured brain. *JAMA* 240:439-442, 1978.
5. Muizelaar JP, Marmarou A, Ward JD, et al: Adverse effects of prolonged hyperventilation in patients with severe head injury: a randomized clinical trial. *J Neurosurg* 75:731-739, 1991.
6. Muizelaar JP, van der Poel HG, Li ZC, et al: Pial arteriolar vessel diameter and CO_2 reactivity during prolonged hyperventilation in the rabbit. *J Neurosurg* 69:923-927, 1988.
7. Robertson CS, Valadka AB, Hannay HJ, et al: Prevention of secondary ischemic insults after severe head injury. *Crit Care Med* 27:2086-2095, 1999.
8. Marshall LK, Marshall SB, Klauber MR, et al: A new classification of head injury based on computerized tomography. *J Neurosurg* 75:S14-S20, 1991.
9. Wang KK, Ottens AK, Liu MC, et al: Proteomic identification of biomarkers of traumatic brain injury. *Expert Rev Proteomics* 2:603-614, 2005.
10. Association for the Advancement of Automotive Medicine: *The Abbreviated Injury Scale.* 1990 rev., update 1998. Barrington, IL, Association for the Advancement of Automotive Medicine, 1998, 2001.

Traumatic Brain Injury: Imaging, Operative and Nonoperative Care, and Complications

Alex B. Valadka   and   Mark J. Dannenbaum

The previous chapter described pathophysiology and initial management of traumatic brain injury (TBI) patients. This chapter provides an overview of selected aspects of surgical management, nonoperative care, complications, and outcome.

SURGICAL MANAGEMENT

The strength and rigidity of the skull, its covering by the highly vascular scalp, and the need to do something with the overlying hair all combine to make it harder to get to the brain than to most other organs. Consequently, the surgeon must prepare carefully prior to any craniotomy, especially an emergency. Disaster can occur if the original positioning and exposure prove to be inadequate to deal with the known pathology, much less with the unexpected contingencies that seem to arise all too frequently during emergency craniotomies. If additional exposure should suddenly become necessary in the middle of a case, the price that might need to be paid to gain this additional access may include considerable blood loss, brain swelling, or other complications.

Positioning

Most traumatic lesions can be accessed by positioning the patient supine, with the head turned to the contralateral side (i.e., to the right for a left-sided craniotomy). A large roll of sheets or other support placed parasagittally under the ipsilateral shoulder blade and upper chest can also facilitate rotation of the head. Rigid fixation of the head via pins is not needed for most trauma craniotomies. Instead, the hospital's usual doughnuts, foam head holders, or other devices are typically used. In most trauma cases, the goal is to have the midline of the head more or less parallel to the floor.

In patients with rigid cervical collars, this goal may be achieved by varying the positioning described previously so that the patient is placed in the lateral position. Putting a patient into such a position requires more work from all members of the surgical team, but an experienced crew should be able to secure a patient in this position quickly.

The seemingly infinite variety of anatomical lesions that may be found in head-injured patients makes it necessary for the surgeon to know how to gain access to all parts of the brain and skull. Treatment of occipital, posterior temporal and parietal, and posterior fossa pathology may require that the patient be positioned prone. Injuries to the anterior midline skull base, such as depressed frontal sinus fractures, are usually operated on with the head neutral and the neck slightly extended. A detailed discussion of the variety of positionings and approaches that are used in neurosurgery is beyond the scope of this book. The essential message is that flexibility and familiarity with different surgical approaches are key parts of the management of head and brain injury.

Bone Flap

Another general principle of surgery for TBI is to create a large bone flap. This principle is especially true for an acute subdural hematoma (SDH). The blood in these lesions often layers out over much of the cerebral hemisphere. Trying to remove a clot from far under the edges of a small bony opening is often frustrating for the surgeon and may be dangerous for the patient. Furthermore, the intradural bleeding that often accompanies SDHs may arise almost anywhere: from draining veins that enter the superior sagittal sinus near the midline, from the floor of the anterior or middle cranial fossa, from inferior or medial to the frontal pole, or from the transverse sinus, to name just a few common areas. A large bone flap is the best way to ensure that as many potential bleeding sites as possible have been made accessible.

Most trauma incisions begin at the posterior root of the zygoma, just anterior to the tragus. They then curve posteriorly, above and behind the ear. In trauma cases, this posterior extension should extend as far as possible. The incision then curves medially and superiorly. It is wise to take the skin incision to the midline to permit access to the superior sagittal sinus in the event that troublesome bleeding arises from the midline.

Although the scalp flap extends near or to the midline, it is wise to keep the medial edge of the bone flap several centimeters off the midline. Attempts to remove bone on or near the midline may produce brisk epidural bleeding from arachnoid granulations or severe dural bleeding from dural venous lakes. Such bleeding is usually controllable with gentle pressure, but these maneuvers delay and distract attention from the goal of rapid evacuation of the SDH. Similarly, recurrence of this bleeding may go unnoticed while the surgeon is preoccupied with evacuation of the clot. If brisk bleeding originates from underneath the medial edge of the craniotomy opening, the best treatment may be tamponade with absorbable hemostatic agents and placement of numerous closely spaced dural tack-up sutures.

The size of the opening needed to evacuate an epidural hematoma (EDH) may often be smaller than that for a SDH because the tight adherence of the dura to the overlying skull constrains the spread of these lesions. For this reason, EDHs often appear to be "short and fat" on computed tomography (CT) scans, but SDHs often spread out and appear to be "long and thin" because of the absence of barriers to their spread over the surface of the hemisphere. Care must still be taken, however, not to make the bony opening too small when attempting evacuation of an EDH.

Intraparenchymal lesions like hematomas and contusions are often amenable to evacuation via smaller openings. In fact, even large lesions can be evacuated through very small openings in the cerebral cortex. Careful retraction of the cortical edges is made easier because of the cavity that is left behind as the clot is removed.

Brain Swelling

Rapid brain swelling is a major concern after evacuation of an acute SDH. The speed with which this phenomenon occurs suggests that defective autoregulation may play an important role. A popular current practice is simply to leave the native dura open (but loosely cover the brain with a dural graft) and not replace the bone flap. Some neurosurgeons strongly advocate this practice, and it does seem to be effective in lowering intracranial pressure (ICP), but its effects on outcome remain unclear. Publications going back several decades report that a persistent vegetative state was commonly seen in survivors.[1] Other concerns are that decompressive craniectomies may be performed too frequently or for poor or inadequate indications. Often, the bony opening that is left behind is too small, causing the swollen brain to strangulate and die, with the resulting edema tracking back intracranially and further aggravating intracranial hypertension.

Although the surgeon sometimes has no choice but to leave the bone flap off, a better strategy is to undertake several steps to minimize the likelihood of being placed in such a situation. Instead of a wide dural opening, slits may be made in the dura in the four different quadrants of the exposure, and the clot carefully aspirated through these slits. Slow, controlled evacuation of the hematoma may prevent sudden massive brain swelling more than immediate removal of the entire clot. If it appears that most of the hematoma has been removed, and if there is no evidence of ongoing intradural bleeding, the slits can be closed quickly if the brain begins to swell. However, if continued intradural bleeding persists, a wider dural opening must be created by connecting two or more of the slits in order to identify and control the source of the bleeding. Such a maneuver must be performed as rapidly as possible so that dural closure can be achieved before the brain begins to swell.

Implicit in the previous discussion is the need to close the dura before brain swelling makes this impossible. As mentioned previously, this goal may seem antiquated in light of the current popularity of simply not replacing the bone flap. However, the authors have rarely encountered problems using this strategy, even when a retractor had to be used to gently depress swelling brain while the dural edges were forcibly pulled together with forceps so that they could be sutured together. This experience is consistent with laboratory data suggesting that decompressive craniectomy may actually promote cerebral edema.[2]

Epidural Hematomas

Surgery for EDHs is usually more straightforward. Occasionally, the surgeon may feel the need to make a small opening in the dura to verify that no subdural blood is present. It is common to see a thin layer of subdural blood when this maneuver is carried out, but this can usually be irrigated away without too much difficulty. Another common problem in the epidural space is persistent bleeding, either from dural veins or the dural venous sinuses or from underneath the bony edges of the craniotomy. If epidural venous bleeding cannot be stopped with cautery, gentle pressure with any of the various commercially available neurosurgical hemostatic agents is usually effective. In most cases, leaving these bioabsorbable materials in place is better than attempting to remove them. Of note, bleeding from the middle meningeal artery is not encountered as frequently as some books suggest, but when seen, it is usually possible to cauterize the bleeding artery directly.

Intraparenchymal Lesions

Evacuation of intraparenchymal hematomas and contusions can often be performed via a small corticectomy. Fortunately, as soon as one of these lesions is evacuated, the brain becomes much more relaxed. The main difficulties in these cases are ensuring complete lesion evacuation and verifying hemostasis. These goals may be difficult if the hematoma cavity is large. Occasionally, for large contusions or hematomas, a second corticectomy may facilitate lesion evacuation and hemostasis of parts of the lesion that would be inaccessible via the original cortical opening.

Intracranial Pressure Monitoring

The question of whether these patients require postoperative ICP monitoring is often difficult to answer. In general, if a patient is not expected to "wake up" after surgery, that is, not expected to obey commands and/or to have a Glasgow Coma Scale score greater than 8, insertion of a monitor should be strongly considered. Ventriculostomies are preferred because they permit therapeutic drainage of cerebrospinal fluid (CSF) in the event that ICP becomes elevated.

Insertion of these devices during the initial craniotomy is usually possible, but some surgeons prefer to wait until the craniotomy has been closed and then insert the ventriculostomy in the operating room (OR) or in the intensive care unit (ICU). If the ventricles cannot be cannulated, a parenchymal monitor may be used.

Coagulopathy

If patients appear to be coagulopathic, the blood bank should be given early notification that platelets and fresh frozen plasma are urgently needed in the OR. Severe diffuse oozing may require the use of recombinant factor VIIa. Laboratory studies can be used during surgery to track the effects of these interventions on coagulation studies and platelet counts, but an easier way to gauge the status of hemostasis is simply to check whether blood that trickles down into the dependent parts of the surgical field is able to form a solid clot.

Summary

In summary, the surgeon can often avoid trouble by thinking ahead about possible setbacks and their avoidance. Planning the exposure to permit adequate clot evacuation is crucial. Elevating the head of the bed slightly may minimize venous bleeding. Major bleeding should be anticipated if depressed fractures overlying major dural venous sinuses are elevated. A controlled dural opening during evacuation of an acute SDH may be helpful for minimizing massive brain swelling.

NONOPERATIVE MANAGEMENT

Location of Care

The complexity of TBI management and the tremendous impact of TBI on long-term outcome suggest that brain-injured patients should initially be admitted to an ICU with physicians and nurses experienced in the care of TBI patients. This specialized experience in TBI may be more important than expertise only in general trauma or critical care. During the first few days after injury, TBI patients may require blood pressure monitoring, frequent checking of hemoglobin concentrations, complex ventilator management, and other interventions that are standard for patients without a brain injury, but in addition to these basic measures, careful assessment and management of the brain injury and integration of systemic management practices with brain-specific therapies must also occur. Although many general ICUs or trauma ICUs are not comfortable with the nuances of TBI management, most neurosurgical ICUs are quite capable of managing patients with major systemic illnesses.

If a TBI patient improves or remains neurologically stable for a few days, he or she can then be transferred to another ICU, to an intermediate care unit, or to a regular care ward. This approach differs from the commonly advocated view that patients should initially be admitted to a standard trauma unit instead of to a neurosurgical ICU. In many standard surgical ICUs, however, management is based on a patient's systemic parameters, which may not necessarily be optimal for the brain injury. In the real world, these discrepancies are handled differently at each institution according to whatever arrangements have been made among the different parties who care for these patients.

Secondary Insults

The prehospital emphasis on prevention and early treatment of secondary cerebral insults continues during the ICU management of these patients and, in fact, forms the foundation of their management. Special attention should be paid to basic metabolic and physiologic parameters, including blood pressure, oxygenation, hemoglobin concentration, and serum sodium concentration. Surgery for associated injuries that do not absolutely require immediate treatment, such as facial fractures, hand or foot injuries, and even most long-bone fractures, is best deferred while the injured brain is still vulnerable to possible intraoperative metabolic disturbances.

Ventilator Weaning and Tracheostomy

Attempts at weaning and eventual extubation are dictated by the patient's clinical course. Many intensivists advocate very early tracheostomy in these patients. However, if patients appear to be recovering consciousness, there is usually little harm in gradually decreasing the intermittent mandatory ventilation rate. In most TBI patients, the indication for continued intubation is the brain injury, not a primary pulmonary problem. Thus, the decision to extubate is based primarily on improvement in mental status. Even if a patient is clearly not going to wake up soon, continued intubation may be necessary because of the potential risk of aggravating intracranial hypertension if a tracheostomy is performed while the patient is still having frequent or continual elevations of ICP.

Sedation

In many ICUs, there exists an automatic reflex among practitioners to sedate patients heavily and to administer pharmacologic paralytics, often via simultaneous intravenous infusions of multiple drugs. Few people seem to ask why the patient receives such extensive medication. If a TBI patient's ICP is not elevated and if he or she is not thrashing about, there is probably little need for heavy sedation beyond reasonable doses of analgesics on an as-needed basis. This philosophy permits accurate assessment of neurologic status and also facilitates more rapid weaning from the ventilator. Partly for this reason, we are less eager than some other institutions to perform immediate tracheostomies on these patients, preferring instead to allow them the opportunity to recover to the point of extubation if they demonstrate early progress toward that goal.

Cerebral Monitoring

Monitoring of cerebral physiologic function can provide important information that may be used to titrate treatment toward the goal of preventing and promptly treating secondary insults.

ICP monitoring has been widely available for decades. Whenever possible, a ventriculostomy catheter is preferred because of its relatively low cost, its ability to act as a therapeutic tool by draining CSF, and the ability to re-zero the monitor as needed. The development of antibiotic-impregnated catheters seems to have lowered the risk of ventriculostomy infection.[3]

Additional cerebral monitoring devices are commercially available. Jugular venous oxygen saturation may be tracked continuously via oximetric catheters inserted in a retrograde manner up the jugular vein and into the jugular bulb. A decrease in the oxygen saturation of the blood in the jugular bulb signals an increase in cerebral oxygen extraction because of ischemia or other causes.

Intraparenchymal monitors of the oxygen tension of the brain ($PbtO_2$) have generated considerable interest because of the usually good relationship between $PbtO_2$ and cerebral blood flow (CBF). Importantly, interpretation of these data requires knowledge of whether the catheter is measuring normal brain or whether it lies near contused or injured brain. Such positioning dictates whether the catheter is acting like a monitor of global metabolism or a gauge of the regional metabolism of the brain around the probe. Large areas with significantly abnormal regional metabolism may get lost in the background and not be detected if only a global monitor is used.

Our preference has been to use local monitors like $PbtO_2$ catheters to target brain tissue around contused or otherwise injured areas.[4]

Other monitors provide methods of tracking CBF, performing cerebral microdialysis, following brain electroencephalographic activity, and measuring other physiologic parameters. These can all provide valuable information that supplements careful neurologic assessments and CT scans. It will be difficult to conduct prospective, randomized, controlled trials to demonstrate the utility—or lack thereof—of these devices. However, judicious use of these monitoring techniques and careful interpretation of the data gathered can facilitate targeted patient management.

Nutrition

Nutrition should be started as soon as possible, usually via the enteral route. If feedings via this route cannot be initiated despite several days of trying, consideration should be given to parenteral nutrition. The increasing attention being paid to the association between poor outcomes and elevated glucose levels suggests that protocols for frequent monitoring and, if needed, treatment of serum glucose concentration should be considered. Dextrose is omitted from intravenous fluids for the same reason.

Fluids and Electrolytes

Other basic principles include maintenance of a normal intravascular volume to avoid either dehydration or fluid overload. We aim for a serum sodium in the normal range and do not deliberately drive the sodium to supranormal levels. However, we have become more concerned that hyponatremia may contribute to cerebral edema and increased ICP. Thus, we have become more liberal about treating serum sodium values in the 120s or even low 130s with hypertonic saline to establish a more desirable osmotic gradient between the brain and the vasculature.

Physical, Occupational, and Speech Therapy

Early involvement of physical therapy and occupational therapy can be quite helpful to preserve range of motion of extremities and, later during a patient's recovery, to expedite sitting up and even ambulation. Speech therapy may also be helpful for some patients.

Fever

Hyperthermia is receiving more scrutiny as a contributor to adverse outcomes in patients with neurologic injuries. Continuous intravascular cooling devices might be considered in patients who remain febrile despite antipyretics, external cooling, and treatment of known sources of fever.

Deep Venous Thrombosis

Prevention of deep venous thrombosis (DVT) is important in comatose patients who may be bedridden for a prolonged period. Application of sequential compression devices immediately upon patient arrival in the ICU has been effective in our unit. We have not generally used pharmacologic prophylaxis immediately after injury for fear of aggravating potential coagulopathy and possibly contributing to delayed or recurrent intracranial hemorrhage. Occasionally, however, we have added low-molecular-weight heparin (LMWH) in patients who seemed to be at especially high risk. We have also used LMWH to treat DVT when it occurs. We do not routinely place prophylactic inferior vena cava (IVC) filters. Instead, we have generally reserved IVC filters in TBI patients for cases of documented DVT. We are more aggressive with patients who are paralyzed as a result of a spinal cord injury.

Transfusion Thresholds

Transfusion thresholds continue to be a controversial area. Historically, neurosurgeons have advocated that hemoglobin levels be maintained at approximately 10 mg/dl in patients with TBI or aneurysmal subarachnoid hemorrhage. Although the O_2-carrying capacity of blood is decreased at this subnormal value, the nonlinear relationship between O_2-carrying capacity and viscosity causes the viscosity to be reduced much more than the O_2-carrying capacity at this hemoglobin level. Thus, the improvement in flow from the lower viscosity was felt to more than offset the reduction in O_2-carrying capacity. Several studies, however, have demonstrated that blood transfusion increases the risk of mortality and that patients fare better with a "permissive" transfusion strategy of not administering blood until the hemoglobin decreases as low as 7 mg/dl. On the other hand, some data suggest that patients with myocardial ischemia do better when hemoglobin is maintained at 10 mg/dl rather than 7 mg/dl. Debate rages about whether these findings apply to patients with TBI, stroke, and other neurologic diseases. At the present time, we favor the traditional approach of targeting a hemoglobin level of approximately 10 mg/dl.

Treatment of Intracranial Hypertension

Many algorithms exist for the treatment of elevated ICP (Figure 1). These generally begin with safe, noninvasive interventions. If ICP continues to be elevated, progressively more aggressive treatments are applied. The variety of the algorithms that are available reflects the differences with which various centers embrace the individual treatments that make up those algorithms. Of note, use of steroids to treat TBI is not recommended.

Computed Tomography Scanning

Repeat CT scanning should be considered if there is any suspicion that elevated ICP readings may be caused by a delayed or recurrent hematoma, by hydrocephalus or ventriculostomy malfunction, by a large infarction, and so on (Figure 2).

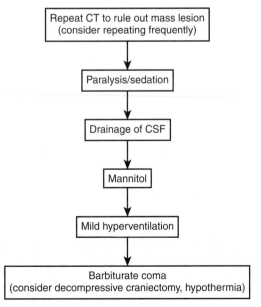

Figure 1 Basic algorithm for the management of elevated intracranial pressure.

Sedation and Paralysis

Sedation and analgesics may help to lower ICP, supplemented if needed by neuromuscular blockade.

Cerebrospinal Fluid Drainage

Persistently elevated ICP may respond to CSF drainage if a ventriculostomy has been inserted. The older practice of routinely changing a ventriculostomy catheter every 5–7 days to prevent infection does not seem to be justified by more recent studies,[5] and some centers have reported leaving catheters in place for 2 weeks or even longer without an increase in infection rates. The subsequent development of antibiotic-coated ventriculostomy catheters seems to have had a considerable impact on lowering the incidence of ventriculostomy-related infections.[6]

Osmotic Diuretics

Administration of mannitol is often a useful step. Mannitol has an osmotic effect that pulls fluid from the brain into the vascular compartment. It also decreases blood viscosity, which enables cerebral arteries to constrict (and thereby lower intracerebral blood volume) without decreasing CBF because the decrease in viscosity facilitates adequate flow through the narrower artery.[7] Hypertonic saline is receiving a great deal of interest as a possible surrogate or supplement to mannitol. Its use has become especially widespread among pediatric intensivists. Although preliminary reports are encouraging, more solid data are still pending about the optimal method of administration and about relative indications, contraindications, and adverse events.

Hyperventilation

Continued elevations of ICP may respond to judicious use of mild hyperventilation. Whenever possible, we attempt to use monitors of cerebral oxygenation to make sure that cerebral ischemia does not result from hyperventilation that is more aggressive than the brain can tolerate.

Barbiturate Coma

Persistent intracranial hypertension may respond to pentobarbital-induced coma.[8] This treatment is effective at lowering ICP, but hypotension is a major problem. Prior to administering barbiturates, we usually insert a pulmonary artery catheter to ensure that intravascular volume is adequate. Likewise, we have pressors ready for immediate infusion if the blood pressure begins to decrease.

Decompressive Craniectomy

Intracranial hypertension that persists despite initiation of the treatments listed in Figure 1 is a serious problem. Decompressive craniectomy, in which a large part of the skull is temporarily removed so that the injured brain has room to swell, is currently a popular intervention. It seems clear that a large craniectomy can lower ICP, but uncertainty remains about whether it improves patient outcomes. It is possible that many of these operations are performed prematurely and/or with inadequate removal of bone (Figure 3). The complications of decompressive craniectomy can also be troubling, including development of contralateral subdural fluid collections and herniation of brain through the craniectomy defect (Figure 4).

Hypothermia

Another potential treatment is hypothermia. The results of the National Acute Brain Injury Study: Hypothermia demonstrated lack of effect when this treatment was applied indiscriminately to all patients.[9] However, like decompressive craniectomy or any other intervention, it is likely that a specific subpopulation of TBI patients can benefit. The difficulty for investigators and clinicians lies in identifying patients for whom an intervention has the most optimal benefit:risk ratio.

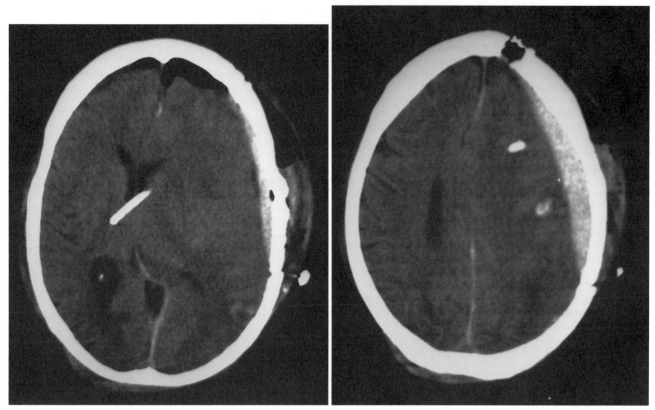

Figure 2 Postoperative computed tomography (CT) scans from a patient who had undergone evacuation of an acute subdural hematoma. Intracranial pressure readings remained elevated after surgery. CT scan revealed postoperative epidural hematoma, for which the patient had to be taken back to surgery.

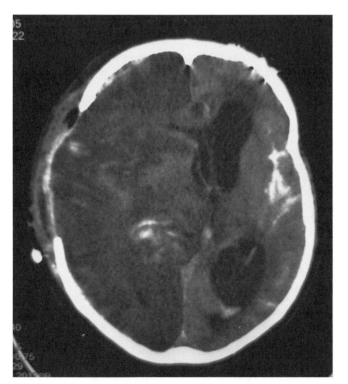

Figure 3 Postoperative computed tomography (CT) scan from the patient whose initial CT scan is shown in Figure 1 of the previous chapter. The bone flap was not replaced, but the size of the craniectomy was too small to prevent subsequent midline shift.

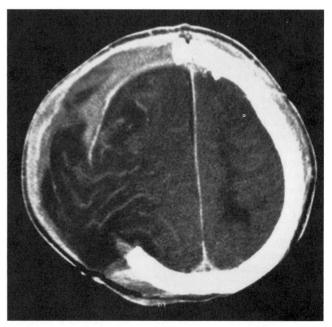

Figure 4 Massive herniation of necrotic brain through a craniectomy defect.

Individualization of Treatment

Although most algorithms recommend that patients be treated according to the same sequence of interventions, patients are in fact unique. Ideally, treatments would be applied not according to an algorithm that forces all patients into the same pathway, but rather according to a patient's particular metabolic picture. In terms of treating elevated ICP, patients with considerable amounts of cerebral edema might benefit most from osmotic diuretics, those with obstructed CSF flow may need a ventriculostomy, and those with elevated CBF might benefit from mild hyperventilation performed early in their course.

It is highly likely that each of these ICP-lowering treatments represents the optimal intervention for a certain type of patient. Our weakness lies in our inability to identify which treatment represents the best intervention for a given patient at that particular time in a patient's course. Part of this weakness is explained by the fact that clinical trials in severe TBI have generally enrolled all severe TBI patients, regardless of their pathophysiologic picture. A treatment that may be beneficial in only certain types of patients might not be proven "effective" in a clinical trial because of the background noise from all the other patients who do not benefit. Targeted trials are more difficult to perform, but there appears to be a great need for the type of information that they can provide.

Failure of Intracranial Pressure Prophylaxis

Another important lesson that has been learned over and over again is that treatments for elevated ICP cannot be applied proactively. Doing so is not beneficial and, in fact, may cause harm in many cases. Our natural inclination as clinicians is to try to prevent ICP from rising by aggressively instituting treatments known to lower ICP; we worry that waiting until ICP rises may subject patients to the risk of harm. However, over the years, prophylactic use of hyperventilation, barbiturate coma, pharmacologic paralysis, hypothermia, or blood pressure elevation has been shown in class I or class II studies to have no benefit and, in many cases, to have significant risks. Thus, the best we can do at this time is to monitor patients carefully, to focus on the ABCs (airway, breathing, and circulation) and on prevention of secondary insults, and to intervene promptly when ICP elevation or another adverse event occurs.

Guidelines

Various guidelines for the management of brain-injured patients have enjoyed widespread circulation. Properly constructed, guidelines summarize a review of the literature with a weighting of that literature based on the quality of the design and execution of the reviewed studies. Methodologically solid studies are given a higher classification than trials that are poorly conceived or carried out. The resulting recommendations are weighted accordingly.

Not surprisingly, most clinical decisions have little in the way of randomized, prospective, controlled trials to support them. At the same time, such well-constructed trials are usually designed to answer a specific question in a specific population, and with specified outcome measures. Generalizability of findings to a larger population is often problematic.

These limitations of guidelines suggest that it is unwise to follow their recommendations blindly. Instead, a much more reasoned approach is to integrate evidence-based guidelines with a particular physician's judgment and experience, with a particular patient's situation, and with the particular aspects of the environment in which care is being delivered. This approach should avoid unthinking adherence to guidelines while, at the same time, ensuring that they receive serious and appropriate consideration.

Failure of Clinical Trials

Millions of dollars and countless hours of effort have been poured into clinical trials to test drugs and other treatments that were designed to improve outcome after TBI. These have all failed. Analysis of these trials and recommendations for improving the design of future trials have become dynamic fields of inquiry, but such considerations are beyond the scope of this chapter. The lesson learned from these failures is that, for the time being, we must continue to focus on the basics of patient care instead of placing unjustified optimism in the development of a single pharmacologic "cure" for TBI.

MORBIDITY AND COMPLICATIONS

Traumatic brain-injured patients are prone to the same complications as any other trauma patients. These include infections of the respiratory tract, urinary tract, and other body systems, as well as infections of therapeutic devices like central and peripheral venous catheters and arterial lines. Deep venous thrombosis, decubitus ulcers, myocardial infarction, and loss of lean body mass are just a few of the many other adverse events that may develop during a critically ill patient's prolonged stay in an ICU.

For the most part, these complications are managed just as they would be in a patient without a brain injury. A common temptation is to blame unusual developments on the brain injury by ascribing them to a "central process." However, that must be a diagnosis of exclusion that is appropriate only after a thorough work-up has eliminated more likely sources.

Some complications are unique to the brain-injured patient. Elevated ICP and its management have already been discussed. Excessive and inappropriate sedation not only impairs accurate neurologic assessment of a patient, but may also unnecessarily subject a patient to the risks of sedation and of a lengthened stay in the ICU.

Prophylaxis against seizures is currently recommended for the first week after injury. After that time, anticonvulsants may be discontinued in patients who have not had a seizure. If seizures occur in a patient who is already receiving anticonvulsants, serum levels of the drug should be checked. Options include administering a bolus and increasing the maintenance dose of the drug, or adding a second agent. The optimal duration of seizure treatment in these patients remains unclear, but certainly treatment is reasonable for at least several months and probably longer.

Rebleeding or delayed intracranial bleeding can be catastrophic (see Figure 2). Some of these events may be caused by suboptimal surgical technique in which inadequate time was spent ensuring that hemostasis was present. Often, however, patients may have a pre-existing history of liver disease, and the trauma itself can predispose to a coagulopathic state. Aggressive use of fresh frozen plasma and sometimes platelets may help achieve hemostasis in patients with persistent diffuse oozing. Recent reports describing the successful use of recombinant factor VIIa in such cases have generated considerable interest.

MORTALITY

Many studies in the trauma literature report outcomes in terms of patient mortality at hospital discharge. This choice of outcome measure is often driven by the data contained in a hospital's trauma registry. Such an endpoint is an understandable choice for reports about chest and abdominal injuries, from which patients tend to either recover reasonably well or die soon after admission from their initial injuries or from subsequent complications.

Unfortunately, mortality rate at hospital discharge is a poor outcome measure for TBI. Survival is not considered to be a good outcome if a patient will remain in a persistent vegetative state. Most TBI studies have considered death, persistent vegetative state, or severe disability to be a poor outcome, whereas good recovery or moderate disability has been viewed as a good outcome. These outcome categories are based on the Glasgow Outcome Scale (GOS) (Table 1). In addition or instead of the GOS, some studies use more detailed instruments to assess outcome, especially if data are sought about less obvious measures, such as neuropsychological function.

The timing of outcome assessment is important. A patient who begins to recover quickly may have a high level of function upon discharge from the acute care hospital, which may take place just a week or two after injury. Another patient who is transferred early to a long-term care facility or to a rehabilitation hospital may have a low level of function upon leaving the acute care hospital. Yet at 6 months after injury, both these patients may have comparable levels of function if the second patient makes gradual progress. Recovery from brain injury may continue for several years. For practical reasons, most TBI studies collect outcome data at 6 months.

Some recent studies report quite good outcomes after TBI, with mortality rates of approximately 20% or lower. However, many of these studies did not enroll patients with a Glasgow Coma Scale score of 3, with fixed and dilated pupils, or with other findings to suggest that they were unlikely to have a good recovery. The Traumatic Coma Data Bank, which enrolled all patients who presented to four academic centers, included 753 patients. Approximate outcomes were as follows: 27% good recovery, 16% moderate disability, 16% severe disability, 5% persistent vegetative state, and 36% mortality.[10] Current experience suggests that these percentages remain valid today. However, these data were collected in the 1980s. Because of subsequent advances in emergency medical services systems and in neurocritical care, it might be interesting to collect such data again to see if these advances have resulted in a noticeable improvement in outcomes.

Penetrating Brain Injury

Most penetrating brain injuries are caused by gunshot wounds to the head. The vast majority of these result in death before the patient ever reaches the hospital, and most studies indicate that the majority of patients who reach the hospital alive proceed to die. On the other hand, among survivors, there is a reasonable likelihood of reaching a good outcome.

Some authors recommend that heroic measures not be instituted in patients with a GCS score of 3 or 4, and perhaps for a score of 5 as well. Others, however, report that good outcomes can occasionally be attained by patients whose initial neurologic examination was quite poor. Thus, they advocate uniformly aggressive resuscitation and stabilization of these patients. The extent of surgical intervention that is necessary varies from extensive craniotomy and reconstruction to simple debridement that can be accomplished at the bedside.

It is important to remember that the possibility of organ donation represents the only good thing that can come from many of these often tragic cases.

CONCLUSIONS AND ALGORITHM

Figure 5 lists some basic principles and goals in the management of TBI patients. As always, the main goal remains the avoidance of secondary insults. The best monitor is a reliable neurologic examination repeated at regular intervals. Patients who do not obey commands may require monitoring of ICP and other parameters to facilitate prompt detection of adverse metabolic events. Generic algorithms are available for the treatment of intracranial hypertension (see Figure 1). Patient-specific interventions may supplement or replace these algorithms if monitoring data suggest the existence of particular pathophysiologic patterns in given patients.

Table 1: Glasgow Outcome Scale

Score	Category	Description
5	Good recovery (GR)	Able to live and work independently despite minor disabilities.
4	Moderate disability (MD)	Able to live independently despite disabilities. Can use public transportation, work with assistance/supervision, and so on.
3	Severe disability (SD)	Conscious but dependent on others for self-care. Often institutionalized.
2	Persistent vegetative state (PVS)	Not conscious, but may appear "awake."
1	Death (D)	Self-explanatory.

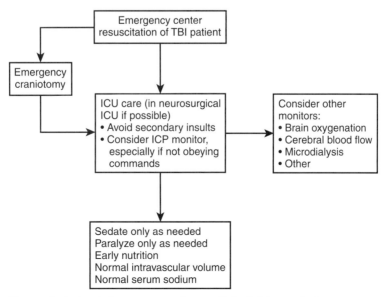

Figure 5 In-hospital management of traumatic brain injury patients.

REFERENCES

1. Cooper PR, Rovit RL, Ransohoff J: Hemicraniectomy in the treatment of acute subdural hematoma: a re-appraisal. *Surg Neurol* 5:25–28, 1976.
2. Cooper PR, Hagler H, Clark WK, Barnett P: Enhancement of experimental cerebral edema after decompressive craniectomy: implications for the management of severe head injuries. *Neurosurgery* 4:296–300, 1979.
3. Zabramski JM, Whiting D, Darouiche RO, et al: Efficacy of antimicrobial-impregnated external ventricular drain catheters: a prospective, randomized, controlled trial. *J Neurosurg* 98:725–730, 2003.
4. Gopinath SP, Valadka AB, Uzura M, Robertson CS: Comparison of jugular venous oxygen saturation and brain tissue PO_2 as monitors of cerebral ischemia after head injury. *Crit Care Med* 27:2337–2345, 1999.
5. Holloway KL, Barnes T, Choi S, et al: Ventriculostomy infections: the effect of monitoring duration and catheter exchange in 584 patients. *J Neurosurg* 85:419–424, 1996.
6. Muizelaar JP, Wei EP, Kontos HA, Becker DP: Mannitol causes compensatory cerebral vasoconstriction and vasodilation in response to blood viscosity changes. *J Neurosurg* 59:822–828, 1983.
7. Eisenberg HM, Frankowski RF, Contant CF, et al: High-dose barbiturate control of elevated intracranial pressure in patients with severe head injury. *J Neurosurg* 69:15–23, 1988.
8. Clifton GL, Miller ER, Choi SC, et al: Lack of effect of induction of hypothermia after acute brain injury. *N Engl J Med* 344:556-563, 2001.
9. Marshall LF, Gautille T, Klauber MR, et al: The outcome of severe closed head injury. *J Neurosurg* 75:S28–S36, 1991.

SPINE: SPINAL CORD INJURY, BLUNT AND PENETRATING, NEUROGENIC AND SPINAL SHOCK

Vartan S. Tashjian, Nestor R. Gonzalez,
and Larry T. Khoo

In the acute setting, spinal cord injury (SCI) represents a complex management issue, with optimal patient care depending on the smooth execution of diagnostic and therapeutic interventions, involving several different disciplines within the medical field. These include emergency medical system (EMS) personnel, emergency department (ED) staff, radiologists, orthopedic and neurological surgeons, intensivists, and physiotherapists. Of these, the immediate interventions employed within hours of injury often dictate the overall prognosis, and provide the patient with the best opportunity to improve long-term functional outcome. For this reason, adequate spinal immobilization, prompt diagnosis, and early consultation of the appropriate surgical service are measures that every ED physician should strive to incorporate into the evaluation each individual trauma patient. This chapter focuses on the epidemiology, classification, and management of SCI, as well as the complications that are typically encountered in both the acute and chronic spine-injured patient. It is through a healthy understanding of the diagnostic and therapeutic guidelines and recommendations that the morbidity and mortality associated with SCI can continue to trend downward, as it has consistently over the past 30 years.

INCIDENCE

Spinal cord injury as a whole most often afflicts young men between the ages of 16 and 30. The mean age is 29.7 years, and there is an 82% male gender bias, likely reflecting the greater tendency of young males to engage in risk-related activities.[1-3] Injury most often occurs in the warmer summer months, especially during the weekend, with 53% of all SCI occurring between Friday and Sunday.[4] With regard to specific etiologies of SCI, results often vary from one trauma center to the next, based largely on the socioeconomic setting of the respective institution. Vehicle trauma is common to both rural and urban healthcare centers as the leading cause of SCI. Prevention programs, including mandatory seatbelt laws, coupled with evolving innovations in automobile safety have served to drastically reduce the overall proportion of SCI attributable to motor vehicle accidents in recent years. In one 10-year period between 1980 and 1990, the overall proportion of SCI caused by vehicle trauma decreased from 47.2% to 38.1%.[2] In rural centers, falls account for the second highest cause of SCI. Whereas in urban centers, violence has rivaled vehicle trauma as the leading cause of SCI. Specifically, gunshot wounds (GSW) from handguns represents approximately 90% of all SCI resulting from violence in urban centers, with an over-representation of minorities in these specific cases. Sports-related injuries continue to play a significant role in the overall incidence of SCI, regardless of the socioeconomic setting. In a study focusing on sports-related SCI out of the University of Alabama, Birmingham, the following sports contributed most to SCI in descending order: diving/surfing, football, winter sports, gymnastics, wrestling, and horseback riding.[5] With the ever-increasing geriatric population, and youth violence on the rise, it is likely that falls and penetrating SCI will represent an increasing proportion of total SCI cases in years to come.

SCI represents a major economic burden on the healthcare industry for a variety of reasons. At the core of the problem is the fact that SCI patients not only represent an acute management challenge, with the average first year postinjury costs ranging from $123,000 to $417,000 depending on the neurologic level of injury, but they also represent a chronic financial burden, when long-term direct and indirect costs are factored in.[2,6] Whereas direct costs are absorbed as a direct result of the injury, including rehospitalizations, nursing home care, durable equipment, and attendant care, indirect costs are more esoteric, and include loss of future wages, fringe benefits, and productivity. While it is indeed a triumph of modern medicine and critical care that greater than 95% of SCI patients survive their initial hospitalization, with an overall lifespan now approaching that of the average citizen, these factors have only further contributed to the escalating direct and indirect costs associated with the life-long care for SCI patients.[1,2] The young average age of SCI patients at the onset of injury contributes further to the economic impact of SCI, with the estimated lifetime direct and indirect costs in excess of $2.5 million for high cervical injury patients (injury between C1 and C4).[2]

MECHANISM OF INJURY

First described by Denis,[7] the three-column model of spinal anatomy divides the spine into three distinct longitudinally-oriented anatomical columns (Figure 1). The anterior column includes the anterior longitudinal ligament (ALL), the anterior half of the vertebral body, and the intervertebral disc. The middle column consists of the posterior half of the vertebral body/intervertebral disc and posterior longitudinal ligament (PLL). Finally, the posterior column represents all bony/ligamentous elements posterior to the PLL (pedicles, lamina, spinous process, ligamentum flavum, and the interspinous ligament). By definition, SCI resulting in disruption of at least two of these three columns is considered an unstable injury. This somewhat simplistic representation of spinal anatomy serves to provide a mental framework for appreciating spine biomechanics and the potential injuries that may result from various blunt and penetrating forces to the spinal column.

Biomechanics of the Spine

Prior to delving into potential mechanisms of SCI, a healthy understanding of the biomechanics of the spine is imperative. As is frequently the case, there is often a certain degree of discrepancy between the actual level of deforming injury to the spine, and the resultant radiographic findings and neurologic deficits associated with the injury. Multiple mechanisms are often simultaneously involved in producing SCI. In their simplest forms, the four types of injurious forces that may be imparted to the intact spinal column are (1) flexion and extension (deflexion) injuries, (2) vertical compression and longitudinal distraction trauma, (3) rotational injuries, and (4) injuries with combined mechanisms.[1,6]

Regarding flexion-extension injuries, the spinal cord is often damaged by compression, transverse/longitudinal shear, torsion, and rotational forces. These injuries typically involve the cervical spine, and often result in disk protrusion, and/or interspinous/anterior column/posterior column ligamentous tears. When an associated disk protrusion and/or subluxation is present, there is a high incidence of concomitant local cord damage with mainly central cord necrosis and hemorrhage seen. In children under the age of 8, extreme hyperflexion injuries are often associated with complete cord transection, secondary to the physiologic high cervical ligamentous laxity normally found in the pediatric population.[8–10]

Hyperextension (retroflexion) injuries most often result in damage to the spinal cord at the C5–C6 level, as extension is maximal at this specific level from a biomechanical perspective. These injuries are often associated with bony dislocation, ventral fracture-dislocation, avulsion of articular processes, disruption/displacement of the intervertebral disks, and disruption of the anterior longitudinal ligament/posterior longitudinal ligament, all of which result in significant compromise of the anteroposterior diameter of the spinal canal and subsequent central cord lesions.[9]

Compression and longitudinal distraction injuries are most often seen in the setting of vertical stress to the spinal column secondary to the falls on the head, buttocks, or neck. They also often occur with an acute increase in axial load forces during a motor vehicle accident (MVA). Radiographically, these injuries are typically characterized by vertebral body flattening, end-plate fractures, and acute disk herniations. Often, there is associated retropulsion of bony fragments/disk material into the spinal canal, and varying degrees of resultant cord

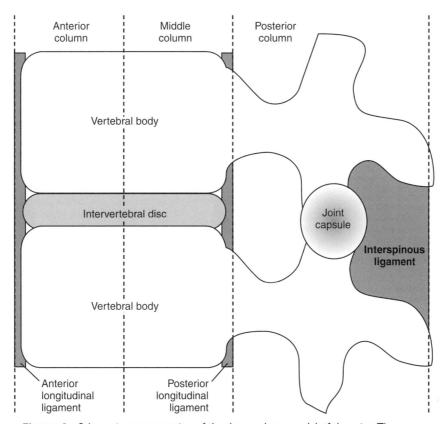

Figure 1   Schematic representation of the three-column model of the spine. The anterior column consists of the anterior longitudinal ligament (ALL) and the anterior half of the vertebral body/intervertebral disc complex. The middle column is composed of the posterior half of the vertebral body/intervertebral disc complex and the posterior longitudinal ligament (PLL). The posterior column includes the intact vertebral arch and associated ligamentous structures.

compression. When the mechanism of injury involves a fall, the majority of these injuries occur at the thoracolumbar junction, the most mobile segment of the spinal column. Conversely, the lower cervical spine is more often involved in cases where a vertical axial load is imparted the spinal column.

Similar to compression/longitudinal distraction injuries, rotational injuries of the spine most often involve the thoracolumbar junction and upper lumbar spine. By definition, they may involve all parts of the vertebral body, including the pedicles, articulating facets, and ligamentous complex. These injuries often result in unilateral or bilateral dislocation, or stable/unstable fracture dislocation due to interlocking of the vertebral bodies and distraction of the intervertebral disks.[9,11]

Mechanism of Injury

Spinal cord trauma is a broad term describing an injurious event that results in disruption of the functional and/or anatomic integrity of the spinal cord at a particular level(s). Although isolated lumbar spine injuries represent a significant proportion of SCI, the majority of debilitating SCI involve trauma to the cervical and thoracic spine. It is for this reason that the focus of this discussion will be injury of the spine from the cervical spine down to the thoracolumbar junction. With respect to the general mechanism of injury, all SCI can be categorized in one of three subgroups: (1) direct (penetrating) SCI, (2) indirect (blunt) SCI, or (3) combined direct/indirect SCI. Depending on the underlying mechanism of injury involved, the pathogenesis of SCI can be further subclassified. Primary traumatic lesions are due to direct mechanical disruption of the cord parenchyma, typically occurring at the time of the original injury. Secondary traumatic (reactive) lesions do not develop directly from the injurious stimulus, but instead evolve as a consequence of injury-related factors, including the development of edema, ischemia, improper immobilization with secondary mechanical injury, and other biochemical disorders. Finally, common to both primary and secondary traumatic lesions is the potential for delayed neurologic sequelae, including scar formation, secondary degeneration, or regenerative phenomena.[9]

Penetrating Spinal Cord Injury

Historically, the management of penetrating spinal cord injury (PSI) was a task relegated mainly to military physicians, as the majority of these injuries occurred in the setting of active combat. Unfortunately, the emergence of violence as a leading cause of SCI in many urban centers over the past 20 years, has served to underscore the importance of emergency room physician familiarity with the acute management of these injuries in civilian practice. In general, PSI can be classified as either gunshot wound–related (GSW-PSI) or lacerating (non-GSW) PSI. Both types of PSI most commonly involve the thoracic spine, and seldom involve more than one vertebral segment.[12] Depending on the series, 52%–57% of all PSI results in complete neurological deficit (no sacral motor/sensory sparing), although lacerating PSI often results in incomplete neurologic injury.[13–15] Although by definition, PSI implies direct dural/parenchymal disruption, in some cases the pathogenesis of PSI resembles that of a concussive model. This has been demonstrated in numerous military-based studies in which normal-appearing dura was encountered at the time of laminectomy in numerous cases.[16–19]

Blunt Spinal Cord Injury

In clinical practice, closed injuries of the spine are typically the most frequent type of SCI encountered. They often occur in the setting of MVA, industrial accidents, falls, and sport-related activities. In these cases, underlying injury to the spinal cord may occur in the

presence/absence of concomitant soft tissue injuries, including fracture dislocation and subluxation of the spine. Biomechanics and mechanism of injury play a central role in the type and extent of spinal cord injury incurred. A thorough understanding of the potential types of mechanical forces distributed throughout the spine at the time of injury is paramount in order to be able to anticipate the evolution of secondary reactive lesions following the initial insult. In general, closed SCI can be distilled down into two broad categories. The first involves indirect cord injury arising from blunt trauma without space-occupying or penetrating lesions within the spinal canal. This type of injury is frequently observed in cases where the mechanism of injury involves longitudinal shearing/distraction, flexion, rotation, rotation-flexion, and/or posteroanterior acceleration.[9] The second type of closed SCI involves direct cord injury secondary to blunt or penetrating forces resulting in canal compromise from a variety of space-occupying lesions. These include bony/ligamentous damage, fracture dislocation, or subluxation. It is important to note that SCI is rarely confined to the anatomic point of impact. In approximately 15% of SCI cases, lesions are observed at multiple levels due to both primary and secondary traumatic changes.[20]

SEVERITY/GRADING OF SPINAL CORD INJURIES

The neurologic level of injury (NLI) is a specific term that refers to the most caudal spinal cord level at which normal motor/sensory function persists following SCI. Although some degree of correlation often exists between the anatomic and neurologic level of injury, this relationship is not always consistent. Several factors including the spinal segment involved, and the underlying mechanism of injury, contribute to the ultimate NLI, once secondary traumatic lesions have manifested. Overall, according to the American Spine Injury Association (ASIA) database, approximately 53% of SCI patients are tetraplegic, 46% are paraplegic, and the remaining 1% experience complete recovery by the time they are discharged from the hospital. The classification of SCI can be further categorized as complete or incomplete injury, referring to the absence/presence of sacral motor/sensory sparing, respectively. The most common neurologic category is incomplete tetraplegia (31.2%), followed by complete paraplegia (26%), complete tetraplegia (21.9%), and incomplete paraplegia (20%).[1,2]

Neurological and Functional Outcome Scales

Numerous classification schemes have been devised to describe patients with SCI over the years. Generally speaking, two types of assessment scales exist, neurological examination scales and functional outcome scales. It is now generally accepted that the most meaningful description of SCI in the acute setting occurs when a neurological assessment tool is applied in conjunction with a functional outcome assessment scheme, in order to provide perspective on the significance of any neurological recovery on the day-to-day life of SCI patients. The first standardized neurological assessment scale for SCI was proposed by Frankel and associates in 1969.[21] In this scheme, a five-grade scale (A to E) is employed to discriminate SCI patients on the basis of differing degrees of motor/sensory function preserved after their injury. Frankel grade A patients are those with complete motor and sensory lesions. Grade B patients have sensory only functions below the level of injury. Grade C patients have some degree of motor and sensory function below the level of injury, but their retained/recovered motor function is useless. Grade D patients have useful, but abnormal, motor function below the level of injury. And grade E patients are fortunate enough to experience complete motor/sensory recovery prior to discharge from the hospital. The main deficiencies involving the Frankel scale proved to be the difficulty involved in discerning grade C from grade D patients, as well as the relatively poor interobserver reliability with practical application of the scale. Despite these shortcomings, the Frankel scale provided an important classification framework from which several contemporary classification schemes have been derived. In fact, the ASIA impairment scale, largely regarded as the most studied and useful of the SCI neurological classification schemes, is essentially a permutation of the original Frankel scale, in which objective parameters are provided to better assess the significance of retained motor function between grade C and grade D patients.[22]

Analogous to the Frankel scale as a neurologic examination tool in SCI is the Functional Independence Measure (FIM) as a functional outcome scale. The FIM is an 18-item, seven-level scale designed to assess the severity of patient disability, estimate the burden of care, and to prognosticate on medical rehabilitation and overall functional outcome. Specifically, the FIM complements neurological assessment by providing scores for activities of grooming, bathing, eating, dressing the upper body, dressing the lower body, and toileting.[22]

Concomitant assessment of both the neurological and functional deficits in acute SCI is imperative in assessing the impact of injury on the patient as a whole. Additionally, linkage of these independent scales allows clinicians to specifically evaluate whether therapeutic interventions resulting in improvement of the gross neurological assessment score also result in enhanced functional recovery for the patient. It is on the basis of functional outcome that the overall significance of various therapeutic interventions can be truly assessed. Omission of such functional outcome assessment in the National Acute Spinal Cord Injury Study (NASCIS) I and II clinical trials assessing the benefit of acute

methylprednisolone (MP) therapy in acute SCI patients is often cited as a critical shortcoming of the design study, rendering the interpretation of improved neurological outcome scores essentially impossible. A recent meta-analysis of the current literature regarding classification schemes for SCI prompted the Section on Disorders of the Spine and Peripheral Nerves of the American Association of Neurological Surgeons (AANS) and the Congress of Neurological Surgeons (CNS) to recommend the ASIA standards for neurological and functional classification of SCI as the preferred neurological examination for clinicians involved in the evaluation and management of acute SCI.[22] This recommendation was based largely on the finding that the ASIA scale provided the greatest discrimination in grouping subjects with SCI into mixed-injured categories, with a relatively high degree of interobserver reliability. Similar to the other SCI classification schemes, the ASIA scale has undergone several revisions since its inception in 1984. Currently, the scale now consists of several components, including the ASIA impairment scale, the ASIA motor index score, the ASIA sensory score, and the FIM (Figure 2).

Spinal Cord Syndromes

Several spinal cord syndromes have been described in the setting of acute SCI. Central cord syndrome typically occurs with a cervical region injury leading to greater weakness in the upper limbs than

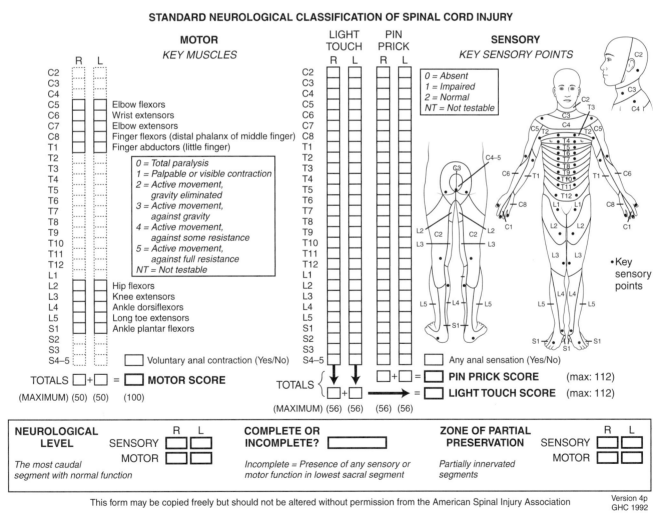

Figure 2 The American Spinal Injury Association (ASIA) Impairment Scale, and ASIA neurological classification scheme for spinal cord injury (SCI). The Impairment Scale is a permutation of the original Frankel Scale for SCI. The actual ASIA classification scheme includes the ASIA Impairment Scale and ASIA motor/sensory indices, as well as the Functional Independence Measure (FIM), which is not pictured. *(The American Spinal Cord Injury Association [ASIA] and The International Medical Society of Paraplegia [IMSOP].)*

the lower limbs, associated with sacral sparing. Brown-Sequard syndrome is classically seen in the setting of penetrating SCI resulting in a hemisection lesion of the cord. It is typically associated with a relatively greater ipsilateral proprioceptive and motor loss, with contralateral loss of sensitivity to pain and temperature below the NLI. Conversely, anterior cord syndrome is associated with a lesion causing variable loss of motor function and sensitivity to pain and temperature, while posterior tracts including proprioception are spared. Conus medullaris syndrome is associated with injury to the sacral cord and lumbar nerve roots, leading to areflexic bladder, bowel, and lower extremity, while sacral segments may occasionally demonstrate preserved reflexes. Finally, cauda equine syndrome is due to injury involving the lumbosacral nerve roots within the spinal canal, resulting in areflexic bladder, bowel, and lower extremities. Similar to the various brainstem vascular syndromes (e.g., Wallenberg's syndrome), spinal cord syndromes often do not present with the classic textbook constellation of signs/symptoms. However, as is the case with brainstem vascular syndromes, an understanding of the various spinal cord syndromes serves to provide a rough neuroanatomical framework regarding the complex structural organization intrinsic to the spinal cord.

DIAGNOSIS

The organization of the central nervous system provides the physician with the opportunity to localize traumatic lesions to the spinal cord with a relatively high degree of accuracy, based on careful neurologic examination alone. However, adequate presurgical care, as well as optimal surgical planning, are both heavily dependent upon accurate imaging of the spine. For decades, plain roentgenograms of the spine have been an invaluable localization tool in SCI for several reasons. First, unlike other more sophisticated imaging modalities, the technology and resources required are not typically a limiting factor. Second, the portability of x-ray technology and the relative ease of acquisition provide the physician the opportunity to rapidly attain important anatomic information, even under the most hectic conditions. Lastly, plain films of the spine can provide a whole host of information regarding underlying SCI, including the presence/absence of fractures, subluxation/dislocation, and spinal canal patency (Figure 3). Although soft tissue structures are not well-visualized with standard x-ray technology, malalignment/angulation of the spine detected on a plain film may hint to underlying acute ligamentous or disk injury.

Within the past 10–15 years, the increased availability of computerized tomography (CT) in most trauma centers has served to revolutionize the diagnosis of SCI in the acute setting. In many centers, CT has supplanted plain x-ray as the acute imaging modality of choice for the evaluation of the spine in trauma patients, due largely to the improved accessibility of this technology. CT is superior to plain x-ray in many respects. It provides an outstanding view of the osseous structures, unparalleled by any other imaging modality. Additionally, the recent advent of three-dimensional reconstruction software now provides the added benefit of viewing the relevant anatomy in the axial, coronal, and sagittal planes (Figure 4). For these reasons, CT is generally considered to be able to detect vertebral fractures with greater sensitivity/specificity than plain x-ray alone. Although far inferior to magnetic resonance imaging (MRI) technology with regard to the associated soft-tissue anatomy, CT can provide some resolution of soft tissue, including the presence of paraspinous hematoma, which further raises the likelihood of underlying unstable ligamentous injury. Combined with myelography, CT technology can provide a view of intracanal anatomy that approaches MRI specificity in diagnosing space-occupying lesions of the spinal canal. Unfortunately, the technical burden and logistics involved with myelography on polytrauma patients has limited its applications for assessment of the acute spine-injured patient.

Since its inception as a medically applicable imaging modality by Raymond Damadian in 1971, MRI technology has continuously

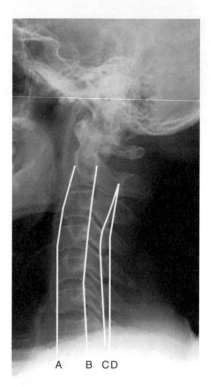

Figure 3 Lateral radiograph of the nonpathologic cervical spine, demonstrating normal alignment of **(A)** the anterior vertebral bodies, **(B)** the posterior vertebral bodies, **(C)** the laminar-facet line, and **(D)** the spino-laminar line.

evolved into the diagnostic tool that it is today. This evolution in technology has been mirrored by a concomitant increase in its availability. Although inferior to CT technology in terms of resolution of bony architecture, MRI undoubtedly provides the most information regarding injury to soft tissue structures, particularly the spinal cord itself. In particular, T2 sequencing provides valuable information regarding the actual NLI, once secondary traumatic lesions, such as cord edema, have manifested (Figure 5). Most importantly, active mechanical compression of the spinal cord and direct spinal cord parenchymal injury can be directly ascertained by MRI, thus guiding the overall time table for surgical decompression/stabilization.

MANAGEMENT OF ACUTE SPINAL CORD INJURY

The optimal management of acute SCI represents a daunting task, requiring a well-executed multidisciplinary effort in order to provide patients with the greatest chance for meaningful neurological recovery. In the broadest sense, the management of acute SCI can be fractionated into several important phases, beginning with care rendered by emergency medical service (EMS) personnel in the field, and culminating with intensive spinal cord rehabilitation following the acute hospitalization. In between, careful orchestration of patient care between emergency department (ED) personnel, radiologists, surgeons, intensivists, and physiotherapists, all play an equally important role in the overall prognosis and outcome of SCI patients. In general, the phases of management in SCI include (1) prehospital care, (2) acute ED evaluation/care, (3) postacute care, and (4) posthospital care/rehabilitation. Certain aspects of care rendered during a particular phase of treatment may overlap with subsequent phases of management. For instance, pharmacotherapy initiated during acute evaluation in the ED often continues into the postacute phase

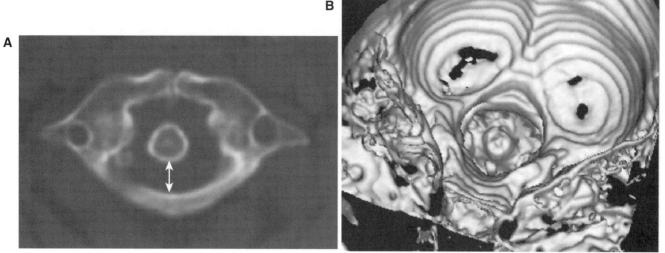

Figure 4 An example of post-traumatic atlantoaxial subluxation in a 35-year-old patient with Down syndrome. **(A)** Note the generous atlanto-dens interval, as well as the marked reduction in the anteroposterior canal diameter *(double-headed arrow)* appreciated more readily on the three-dimensional reconstruction **(B).**

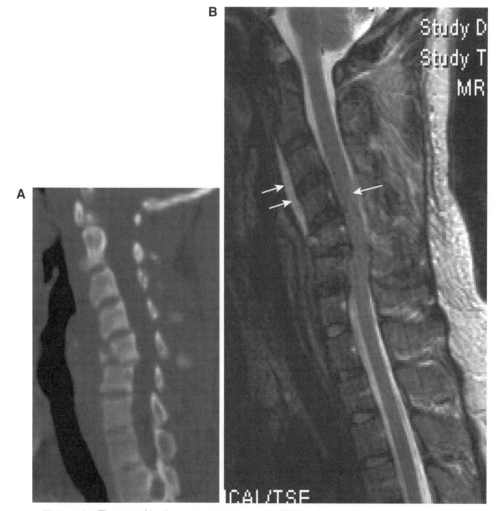

Figure 5 The use of both computed tomography (CT) and magnetic resonance imaging (MRI) technology to evaluate spinal cord injury can provide complementary pieces of information. **(A)** Whereas CT provides a superb view of the C5 anterior teardrop fracture and focal kyphotic deformity present in this specific example, **(B)** MRI technology provides a greater resolution of the associated spinal cord edema *(single arrow)* and prevertebral hematoma *(double arrow)*.

of care. Additionally, certain treatment options, such as surgery, may be offered at different points of care (e.g., acute vs. subacute surgical intervention).

Prehospital Care

The main tenet of prehospital care of SCI has remained rapid and effective spinal immobilization, in order to prevent further neurological deterioration secondary to pathological motion of the unstable spine. It is estimated that approximately 3%–25% of SCIs occur after the initial traumatic insult, either during transport, or early in the course of management.[22] For this reason, it is recommended that complete spine immobilization utilizing a rigid cervical-spine collar with supportive blocks on a rigid backboard with straps, be performed on all trauma patients in which the underlying mechanism of injury suggests potential underlying SCI. The judicious use of spine immobilizers must be tempered with their rapid discontinuation once definitive evaluation and treatment has been rendered, given concern over immobilization device-associated morbidity. Specifically, elevated intracranial pressure (ICP), development of pressure sores, significant patient discomfort/distress, falls, and increased risk of aspiration have all been associated with spinal immobilization devices.[23,24] Once a patient is safely extricated and immobilized, timely transport to a regional medical center capable of evaluating and treating acute SCI is paramount.

Acute Emergency Department Evaluation/Management

Once the patient has made it to the ED, the onus then falls on the evaluating physician to expeditiously perform the patient work-up. Early in the evaluation of a trauma patient, an important responsibility of the ED physician is to ensure that appropriate spine precautions have been implemented in the field, and to closely adhere to these precautions during the primary and secondary surveys. Care must be taken to adequately palpate the spinal column in its entirety, to assess for potential bony separation malalignment, and/or associated soft-tissue swelling/injury. A thorough neurological examination and physical palpation should be performed in conjunction with the primary survey, and any overt neurological deficit should prompt early consultation of the appropriate surgical service (neurosurgery or orthopedic surgery), if available. Next, rapid acquisition of the appropriate radiographic studies should be obtained, as well as interpreted by the staff radiologist. Any radiographic structural abnormality potentially representing acute spinal injury should further prompt surgical consultation. If neurosurgery or orthopedic surgery services are not available at a given institution, then transfer of the patient to the closest ED with appropriate surgical coverage is warranted at the earliest sign of neurological impairment or radiographic abnormality. Transfer should be delayed only in cases where the patient is hemodynamically unstable, requiring additional resuscitation prior to transport.

Depending on the institution, evaluation of acute SCI lies within the realm of either neurological or orthopedic surgery. In many regards, the most important aspect of the surgeon's involvement actually begins in the setting of the ED. It is the surgeon's responsibility to rapidly process several diverse pieces of information including the neurological examination findings, radiographic findings, and the presence of other detracting injuries, in order to arrive at the major branch point in the early management of the spine-injured patient: acute surgical intervention versus conservative management with the potential for delayed surgical intervention. The decision to intervene surgically is typically made on a case-by-case basis, as each case represents a unique set of circumstances to consider and diagnostic/therapeutic obstacles to overcome. Generally speaking, the decision to operate in the acute setting is heavily influenced by the specific type of injury radiographically present, the patient's neurological exam findings, and the overall stability of the patient vis-a-vis other potentially immediately life-threatening traumatic injuries. Polytrauma in the SCI patient is common, with the following injuries occurring with decreasing frequency: fractures of the trunk (17.2%), long-bone fractures (13.9%), head and facial trauma (13.8%), pneumothorax and chest injury (8.8%), and abdominal injury (8.6%).[1] In these cases, surgery should be delayed until the patient is first adequately resuscitated, including treatment of immediately life-threatening injuries, maintenance of adequate blood pressure parameters, and the employment of cervical traction and corticosteroid therapy if deemed appropriate.

Surgical Intervention

Regarding surgical intervention in SCI, the Section on Disorders of the Spine and Peripheral Nerves of the AANS and CNS recently undertook the herculean task of reviewing the pertinent literature in order to provide recommendations on surgical management of various types of cervical spine injury. The surgical options advanced in this section are a reflection of their recommendations, albeit in a more condensed format.

Traumatic atlanto-occipital (C1-occipital) dislocation injuries may be best treated with internal fixation and arthrodesis utilizing any variety of craniocervical fusion techniques. Although traction and external immobilization have been used to successfully treat a subset of these injuries, transient or permanent neurological worsening, or delayed instability, have been observed more often in these cases than in cases with surgical stabilization. Occipital condyle fractures may be most optimally treated with external cervical immobilization. Management of isolated fractures of the atlas (C1) is typically dictated by the specific atlas fracture present. It is recommended that all isolated atlas fractures with preservation of the transverse ligament be treated with immobilization alone. Whereas isolated atlas fractures occurring in the context of transverse ligament disruption may be treated with either external cervical immobilization alone, or with surgical fixation. The rule of Spence states that in the setting of atlas fractures, when the sum of the displacement of the lateral masses of C1 on C2 exceeds 8 mm on plain open-mouth x-ray, the likelihood of underlying transverse ligament disruption is especially high, and may require an MRI for further assessment. Management of fractures of the axis (C2) similarly depends on the type of fracture present. Type I (tip of dens), type II (base of dens), and type III (involvement of dens with extension into the body of C2) odontoid fractures may all be initially managed conservatively with external immobilization (Figure 6). However, surgical fixation should be entertained in cases of type II/III odontoid fractures where the dens is displaced greater than 5 mm, there is comminution of the dens fracture (type IIA), or where fracture alignment is difficult to maintain with external immobilization alone. Additionally, initial surgical fixation should be considered in patients over age 50, with type II odontoid fractures, given the relatively high rate of non-union in this subset of patients. Hangman's fractures of C2 (traumatic spondylolisthesis of the axis) may also be managed with external immobilization in most cases, although it is important to balance these considerations with the morbidities associated with HALO vest use. Surgical stabilization should be considered in cases of severe C2–C3 angulation, disruption of the C2–C3 disk space, or inability to maintain alignment with external immobilization. Isolated fractures of the axis body should be treated with external immobilization alone. The management of combination fractures

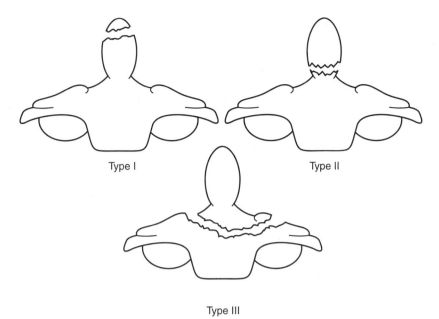

Figure 6 Schematic representation of odontoid fracture types. Type I fractures involve the tip of the dens. Type II fractures involve the base of the dens. Type III fractures involve the base of the dens with extension into the vertebral body of C2.

of the atlas and axis should be based primarily on the specific characteristics of the underlying axis fracture. The majority of C1–C2 combination fractures may be treated with external immobilization, with the exception of C1-type II odontoid combination fractures with an atlanto-dens interval of 5 mm or more, and C1-Hangman's combination fracture with C2–C3 angulation of 11 degrees or more. The surgical technique employed must be modified to accommodate for any loss of integrity of the ring of the atlas.

Management of subaxial cervical facet dislocation and fracture/dislocation injuries may be treated with either closed or open reduction, followed by rigid external immobilization, anterior arthrodesis with plate fixation, or posterior arthrodesis with plate, rod, or interlaminar clamp fixation.

Thoracolumbar Fractures

The three-column model of spine anatomy is particularly helpful in evaluating injuries to the thoracic and lumbar spine. In general, there are four main types of blunt injury that can be imparted to the thoracolumbar spine: (1) compression fractures, (2) burst fractures, (3) flexion distractions, and (4) fracture dislocations. Compression fractures are characterized by intact middle/posterior columns, with compression and loss of height of the anterior column. Conversely, burst fractures typically involve both the anterior and middle columns, and are most often generated by pure axial load injuries. They most commonly occur between T10 and L2, and, by definition, are associated with retropulsion of bone/ligament complex into the spinal canal, often resulting in significant cord compression (Figure 7). Flexion distraction injuries typically involve horizontal fractures that can extend exclusively through bone (type I), through bone and ligament (type II), and through the disk, facet capsule, and the interspinous ligament (type III). These injuries may be missed by conventional axial CT, due to the horizontal orientation of the fractures. Fracture dislocations are typically caused by shear forces, are highly unstable injuries, and are often associated with significant canal compromise (Figure 8).

Optimal Timing of Surgical Intervention in Spinal Cord Injuries

The role of surgical decompression in acute SCI remains a topic of considerable debate. Whereas experimental data involving early surgical decompression in animal models has consistently demonstrated enhanced neurological recovery, these results have proven difficult to extrapolate back to actual SCI patients, mainly due to the lack of clinical trials needed to demonstrate definitive and unequivocal benefit of acute surgical decompression in SCI.[25–27] The majority of studies on surgical decompression in the literature represent retrospective case series with historical controls. Generally speaking, most studies comparing decompressive surgery with conservative management actually fail to definitively demonstrate improved outcome with surgery. Interestingly, in a recent meta-analysis by La Rosa et al.,[28] early surgical decompression performed within 24 hours of injury resulted in statistically significant neurological improvement when compared to both delayed surgical intervention (more than 24 hours postinjury) and conservative management, particularly in patients with initial incomplete injury. Despite the lack of irrefutable supportive evidence, early surgical decompression remains the recommended treatment option in patients with acute cord compression.

Surgery in Penetrating Spinal Cord Injuries

Similar to early surgical intervention for blunt (nonpenetrating) SCI, the value of early surgical intervention in PSI remains debatable. Retrospective analyses of PSI typically do not demonstrate any improved outcome with early surgical intervention. Additionally, the rate of complication tends to be higher in PSI patients that have been treated with laminectomy in the acute setting.[12] For this reason, early surgical intervention in the setting of acute PSI is only recommended as a treatment option in cases associated with progressive neurological deterioration. However, open wounds or wounds with suspicion of CSF leakage may require surgical debridement/exploration and dural repair.

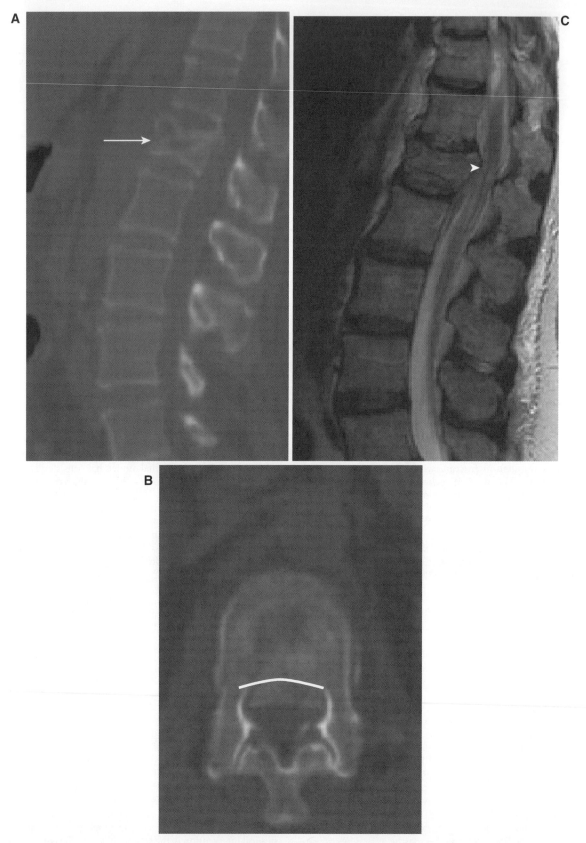

Figure 7 **(A)** Sagittal computed tomography reconstruction demonstrating an L1 burst fracture *(arrow)*, with marked canal compromise secondary to retropulsion of bony elements noted on the axial views **(B).** The white line represents the normal posterior boundary of the vertebral body. Magnetic resonance imaging scan **(C)** demonstrates significant compression of the conus medullaris secondary to the retropulsed fragments *(arrowhead).*

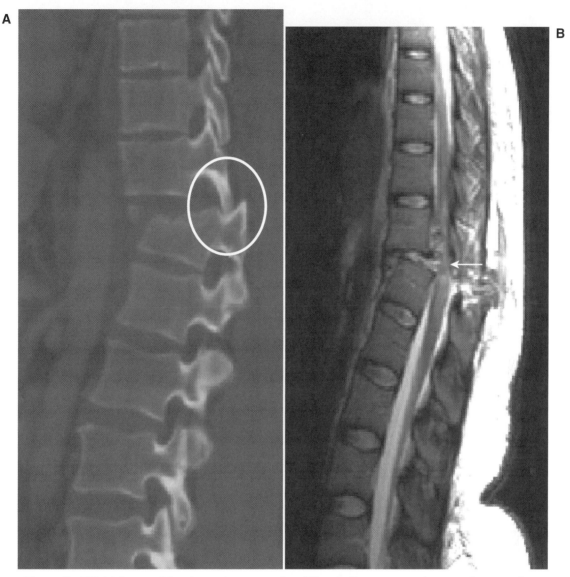

Figure 8 T12–L1 fracture dislocation as demonstrated on **(A)** sagittally reconstructed computed tomography, with complete facet dislocation *(circle)*, and on magnetic resonance imaging **(B),** with significant compression of and T2 signal changes within the conus *(arrow)*.

Nonoperative Acute Interventions

Concomitant with the assessment for potential acute surgical intervention, several other interventions may be implemented during the acute phase of SCI, while the patient is still in the ED. These include closed reduction of C-spine dislocation injuries, pharmacotherapeutic intervention, and correction/prevention of hypotension. Awake patients with isolated cervical fracture dislocation injuries should undergo early closed reduction with cranio-cervical traction, in order to restore the anatomical alignment of the spine. The overall rates of transient and permanent neurological complication associated with closed reduction are 2%–4% and 1%, respectively.[22] If the patient is alert and can be examined, then the risk of reduction/traction without a prior MRI is low. Therefore, external cervical reduction should be performed as soon as possible, after the diagnosis has been made radiographically. Prereduction MRI examination is recommended only in cases when the patient cannot be examined during the reduction. The presence of a significant disc herniation under these conditions represents a relative indication for open ventral decompression prior to reduction. Additionally, MRI is recommended for patients who fail

initial attempts at closed reduction. An algorithm for the clearance of the cervical spine in a trauma patient is presented in Figure 9.

Pharmacotherapy and Spinal Cord Injury

Unlike the case of closed reduction for cervical dislocation injuries, the role of pharmacotherapy in the treatment of acute SCI has been less definitive. Of the various agents available for treatment of acute SCI, methylprednisolone (MP) has, by far, been the most extensively studied. After initial enthusiasm over the potential benefit of early corticosteroid (MP) therapy in acute SCI, recent studies and intense scrutiny of the study parameters and data interpretation employed in the original NASCIS clinical trials have served to weaken the argument that MP therapy is associated with a meaningful improvement in functional outcome of SCI patients. The main criticisms of the NASCIS trials have been related to the determination of optimal timing of therapy, the method of motor assessment, and the apparent lack of correlation between motor recovery scores and functional outcome measures. These shortcomings, coupled with the inability to

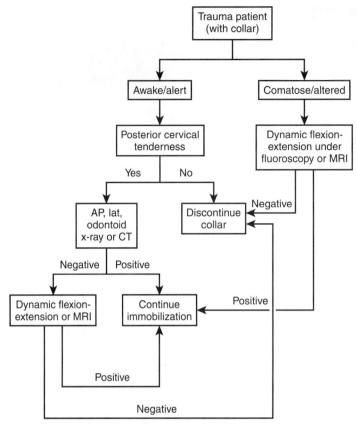

Figure 9 Algorithm for the clearance of the cervical spine in a trauma patient.

demonstrate any clear therapeutic benefit of MP therapy on outcome of SCI in several independent studies, have prompted the AANS and CNS to recommend MP therapy as a treatment option only, which should only be undertaken with the knowledge that evidence suggesting harmful side effects is more consistent than any suggestion of clinical benefit.[22] Harmful side effects of MP therapy include pneumonia, sepsis, hyperglycemia, gastrointestinal ulcers/bleeding, and avascular necrosis of the femoral head, all of which have been observed to occur at significantly higher rates in NASCIS II/III protocol MP-treated SCI patients.[29–31] GM-1 ganglioside has similarly been implicated in enhancement of neurological recovery in acute SCI. However, available medical evidence does not support such a benefit, and thus, the administration of GM-1 ganglioside in the setting of acute SCI is recommended only as a potential treatment option at this time. Nimodipine, naloxone, and tirilazad mesylate have also been implicated as potential neuroprotectants following SCI, and are currently the focus of ongoing clinical trials.[30,32–34]

Institution of Blood Pressure Parameters

Yet another intervention that should be implemented in acute SCI patients relatively early in their course is the maintenance of adequate blood pressure parameters. Hypotension is commonly encountered in the setting of acute SCI, and is often due to associated traumatic injuries with resultant hypovolemia, and/or spinal/neurogenic shock. Whatever the underlying mechanism at play, hypotension should be avoided in the setting of acute SCI, due to the potential for cord hypoperfusion, ischemia, and exacerbation of secondary traumatic lesions. Due to associated ethical concerns, only retrospective (class III) evidence is available in the literature on neurological outcome in SCI patients with hypotensive episodes early in their hospital course.

Based on the available data, the prevailing recommendation by the AANS and CNS is to avoid systolic blood pressure less than 90 mm Hg in acute spine-injured patients, with the goal of maintaining mean arterial pressure (MAP) greater than 85 mm Hg for the first seven days postinjury. This often entails placement of a central venous catheter, and use of intravenous pressor agents.

Subacute Management of SCI

Following initial resuscitation and acute surgical intervention, SCI patients then enter the subacute phase of their initial hospitalization. Review of the literature suggests that severe SCI patients are susceptible to life-threatening cardiovascular instability and respiratory insufficiency in the first 7–14 days postinjury.[22] This is particularly true for severe cervical SCI patients. For this reason, it is strongly recommended that patients with severe cervical level SCI be managed in an intensive care unit (ICU) setting, and that cardiac, hemodynamic, and respiratory monitoring devices be employed in their care to detect any cardiopulmonary dysfunction. Even in otherwise stable patients, maintenance of MAP parameters with continuous infusion of pressor agents often necessitates ICU nursing care. While in the ICU, as well as afterward on the wards, SCI patients benefit from prompt evaluation by physical and occupational therapy (PT/OT) services, and early participation in associated rehabilitation activities. Care should be taken to prevent the development of pressure ulcers and extremity contractures, as these factors negatively impact neurological recovery potential, as well as outcome in general. Once the patient has been transferred out of the ICU setting, priority should be placed on timely transfer to a qualified rehabilitation center, in order to provide SCI patients with the greatest opportunity to regain neurological function and improve their overall functional outcome.

MORBIDITY AND COMPLICATIONS MANAGEMENT IN SPINAL CORD INJURY

In discussing the various complications associated with SCI, it is helpful to classify these events by their typical timeline to presentation following the initial injury. Acute complications tend to occur within the first hours to weeks following acute SCI, often occurring during the acute hospitalization. These complications include hemodynamic instability, cardiopulmonary events, pneumonia, urinary tract infection (UTI), sepsis, and thromboembolic phenomena. Conversely, chronic complications tend to occur weeks to years following the initial insult, and include respiratory, genitourinary, psychiatric, thromboembolic, musculoskeletal, gastrointestinal, infectious, and skin care issues. Many of the complications encountered during the acute management of SCI, including pulmonary, genitourinary, and thromboembolism, require the employment of aggressive preventive/prophylactic measures in order to reduce risk of occurrence in the chronic setting.

Neurogenic Shock

Of the potential complications commonly encountered in the context of acute SCI, those implicated in development of hemodynamic compromise are associated with a significant proportion of morbidity and mortality in the early management of these patients. Neurogenic shock is classically associated with the triad of hypotension, bradycardia, and core hypothermia, in the setting of acute SCI with the NLI localized to T6 and above. The loss of thoracic sympathetic outflow produces a state of unopposed predominant vagotonia, with resultant end-organ effects including decreased peripheral vascular resistance, impaired thermoregulation, and bradycardia. The diminished vascular tone, in combination with diminished cardiac output (CO) secondary to bradycardia, often results in profound hypotension that may be refractory to crystalloid/colloid resuscitation. Untreated, systemic hypotension can contribute to cord ischemia, facilitating the progression and severity of secondary traumatic lesions. It is this premise that has underscored the rationale of maintaining MAP goals in the acute SCI patient. Typically this is achieved through fluid/colloid resuscitation, the use of pressor agents, or a combination of the two.[35–37] Pressors with intrinsic β1-agonist chronotropic activity, including dobutamine and dopamine, are of particular usefulness, as they address both the vasomotor and cardiogenic aspects of neurogenic shock. Persistent bradycardia may be treated with intermittent atropine, with the knowledge that atropine may exacerbate pulmonary dysfunction by thickening secretions. In general, sympathetic tone begins to return in 3–7 days.[35] However, during this period of time, the SCI patient is at greatest risk for developing a cardiopulmonary complication, and thus continued ICU monitoring of these patients during the first 1–2 weeks postinjury is strongly recommended.[22]

Spinal Shock

Unlike neurogenic shock, spinal shock is a state of transient physiologic reflex depression of cord function below the level of injury, with an associated loss of all sensory/motor functions. Hypertension due to an initial release of catecholamines may be encountered, typically followed by profound hypotension. Flaccid paralysis, including of the bowel and bladder, is the hallmark feature of spinal shock. In many instances, sustained priapism is also observed. These findings typically last from hours to days following the injury, until the reflex arc below the level of injury resumes function. The bulbocavernosus reflex refers to anal sphincter contraction in response to squeezing the glans penis or tugging on the Foley catheter. The reflex involves the S1, S2, and S3 nerve roots and is a spinal cord-mediated reflex arc.

Following spinal cord trauma, the presence or absence of this reflex carries prognostic significance. Specifically, in cases of cervical or thoracic cord injury, absence of this reflex documents continuation of spinal shock, or spinal injury at the level of the reflex arc itself. The period of spinal shock usually resolves within 48 hours and return of bulbocavernosus reflex signals termination of spinal shock. Complete absence of distal motor or sensory function or perirectal sensation, together with recovery of the bulbocavernosus reflex, indicates a complete cord injury, and in such cases it is highly unlikely that significant neurologic function will ever return. Therefore, if no motor or sensory recovery below the level of injury is present, the patient has a complete SCI and no further distal recovery of motor function can be expected. On the other hand, any spared motor or sensory function below the level of injury is considered an incomplete injury. In the acute setting, the type of shock present may be difficult to discern given the presence of other detracting injuries. Therefore, invasive monitoring of pulmonary artery pressures may be necessary to differentiate among neurogenic, hypovolemic, and cardiogenic shock.

Pulmonary Complications

Pulmonary complications represent a significant source of morbidity and mortality in SCI patients, in both the acute as well as the chronic setting. Injury to the cervical and midthoracic cord often results in underlying respiratory dysfunction, which, in turn, increases susceptibility to pulmonary infections. SCI above C4 often compromises phrenic nerve function, resulting in subsequent diaphragmatic dysfunction. The majority of patients with a high cervical injury thus require prolonged mechanical ventilation, often necessitating tracheostomy to avoid laryngotracheal malacia associated with prolonged intubation. Injury at lower cervical and upper thoracic levels can impair innervation to accessory muscles of respiration, including the intercostal muscles, resulting in a progressive loss of vital capacity, tidal volume, and negative inspiratory pressure. This serves to effectively reduce lung volume, create ventilation-perfusion mismatches with intrapulmonary shunting, and decrease the arterial oxygen saturation.[37] Loss of the ability to produce an adequate cough and the normal sigh mechanism, leads to the accumulation of uncleared secretions, and plugging/collapsing of the terminal pulmonary segments. This serves to promote an optimal intra-alveolar environment for the development of repetitive, and in many cases fatal, pneumonias. The excessive use of analgesia and sedatives can further depress respiratory function. In order to decrease the risk of pulmonary complications, it is imperative that an aggressive pulmonary toilet regimen be immediately instituted, consisting of aerosol treatments, chest physiotherapy, intermittent positive pressure breathing (IPPB), and frequent suction in mechanically ventilated patients. Bronchoscopy has been a valuable tool for retrieval of tenacious mucus plugs in chronically debilitated patients. Additionally, early mobilization, if possible, also serves to improve overall pulmonary function.

Thromboembolism

Thromboembolic phenomena, including deep venous thrombosis (DVT) and pulmonary embolism (PE), represent a significant, and potentially fatal, complication in the SCI patient population. DeVivo and colleagues[38] have documented a 500-fold increased risk of dying from a PE in the first month following SCI when compared against both age- and gender-matched controls. Although the risk of DVT and PE appears to decline proportionately with time from injury, SCI patients, especially those with complete injury, are perpetually at an elevated risk for thromboembolism due to immobility. For this reason, prophylaxis for at least 3 months following injury has been advanced as a standard of care in SCI patients.[22] A variety of methods have been used to achieve this end, including the use of low-molecular-weight heparins, caval filters, rotating beds, adjusted-dose heparin, low-dose warfarin, pressure stockings, pneumatic compression stockings, and electrical stimulation.[35,36] Of these, low-dose heparin, in combination with pneumatic compression stockings, represents the prophylactic regimen of choice in most centers, despite the lack of any direct evidence of synergy. Use of a prophylactic regimen has been observed to reduce the risk of DVT in SCI from 27.3%–10.3%.[35] In the event of a documented DVT or PE, a 4–6 month duration of full anticoagulation is warranted. Caval filters are recommended for SCI patients who experience refractory thromboembolic events despite anticoagulation, and in patients in whom anticoagulation is contraindicated (e.g., recent or impending surgery). The diagnosis of DVT can be accomplished with duplex Doppler ultrasound with a sensitivity of approximately 90%.[22] More invasive diagnostic techniques such as venography should be reserved for cases in which the index of suspicion for DVT remains high, despite a negative Doppler study. Similarly, invasive diagnostic modalities for PE such as transfemoral pulmonary angiogram should be reserved only for cases where suspicion of PE remains high, despite a negative ventilation-perfusion or spiral pulmonary CT angiogram study.

Genitourinary Complications

Urinary complications due to elevated bladder pressure, infections, and bladder/renal calculi, remain a significant source of morbidity in SCI patients. Alteration of detrusor motor function and bladder sensation, along with compromised sphincter activity, all play a role in incomplete bladder emptying, which, in turn, leads to elevated bladder pressures and secondary genitourinary insult. Chronically elevated bladder pressures can lead to the serious sequelae of hydroureteronephrosis and vesicoureteral reflux. Additionally, urinary stasis increases the risk of UTI, as well as urosepsis, the leading cause of morbidity in SCI. In order to limit these complications, a strict bladder regimen is recommended. The use of indwelling bladder catheters should be limited to the ICU course. Should urinary retention/incontinence prove to be an issue, intermittent clean catheterization every 4–6 hours should be employed, with the goal of maintenance of bladder volume under 500 ml at all times. Prophylactic antibiotics are not recommended. However, any indication of possible UTI should be diagnosed and treated promptly.

Gastrointestinal Complications

In the acute setting, SCI patients are at risk of developing stress ulcers of the upper gastrointestinal tract, likely related to gastric capillary bed ischemia, resulting in a diminished resistance of the gastric-enteric mucosa to the normal digestive secretions of the stomach. The utilization of high-dose MP therapy in the treatment of acute SCI also places these patients at higher risk of developing stress ulcers. In recent years, the incidence of bleeding gastric ulcers has gradually decreased in the SCI population, thought to be due, in large part, to the implementation of stress ulcer prophylaxis with histamine receptor type 2 (H2)-blockers, sucralfate, or proton-pump inhibitors (PPI). With neurological injury, institution of a bowel care regimen is of importance given the likelihood of associated adynamic ileus. A healthy bowel regimen often includes a combination of stool softeners, high-fiber diet, digital stimulation, suppositories, enemas, and manual disimpaction.

Skin Care

In the setting of neurological injury, the development of pressure ulcers is a significant source of discomfort, and represents yet another potential route of infection. The sacral prominence, femoral greater trochanters, ischial tuberosities, and heels are particularly vulnerable to ulcer formation. The incidence of pressure necrosis

requiring surgical debridement within 2 years of SCI is approximately 4%.[36] Prevention is paramount, and typically involves early patient mobilization, air mattresses, limited use of braces/orthotics, and aggressive skin inspection and wound care.

Post-Traumatic Syringomyelia

Typically occurring on a more chronic timetable, post-traumatic syringomyelia (PTS) has been encountered with increasing frequency in SCI over the past 20 years, likely due to a combination of factors including increased life expectancy in SCI patients, as well as the emergence of MRI technology as a highly sensitive diagnostic tool. By definition, PTS is a central cavitation of the spinal cord, typically occurring months to years after the initial injury. Although presenting symptoms vary based on the location and severity of the syrinx, persistent local or radicular pain, motor weakness, spasticity, dissociated sensory loss, autonomic dysreflexia, sphincter loss, sexual dysfunction, Horner's syndrome, and respiratory dysfunction have all been described. Extension of cervical syrinx cavities into the medulla, termed syringobulbia, has also been described, and typically manifests with corticobulbar dysfunction. Although the exact pathognomic mechanism involved in syrinx formation has not been definitively elucidated, the prevailing hypothesis favors a progression of post-traumatic cystic myelopathy. Alteration in spinal subarachnoid cerebral spinal fluid (CSF) flow dynamics secondary to post-traumatic arachnoiditis may also play a role. The incidence of PTS ranges from 1.1% to greater than 50%, with the duration of time of injury to diagnosis of syrinx ranging from 2 months to 33 years.[39] Development of symptomatic syringomyelia is a poor prognostic sign. Although several surgical procedures have been employed in the treatment of PTS, including placement of cysto-peritoneal and cysto-pleural shunts, the overall success of these interventions is generally poor.

MORTALITY

Despite significant advances made in first responder management of SCI, approximately 10%–20% of acute SCI patients do not survive to reach hospitalization, and another 3% of patients die during their acute hospitalization.[3,6,14,38,40] For those patients who survive the acute hospitalization, the major cause of death is pneumonia and other respiratory complications, followed by heart disease, subsequent trauma, and septicemia. The leading causes of death among incomplete paraplegics are cancer and suicide. Suicide is also the leading cause of death in complete paraplegics, followed by heart disease. In general, the suicide rate is higher among the SCI population under the age of 25 years. In terms of life expectancy, individuals aged 20 years at the time of their injury have life expectancies of approximately 33 years as tetraplegics, 39 years as low tetraplegics, and 44 years as paraplegics.

CONCLUSION

Thanks in large part to marked improvements made in the first-responder and ED management of acute SCI, overall morbidity and mortality in this patient population have substantially decreased over the past 30 years. Similarly, the implementation of aggressive prophylactic/preventative measures against many of the common complications of SCI, including thromboembolism, urinary tract infections, pulmonary infections, and pressure ulcers, have served to further improve the quality of life for these patients. With the average life span of SCI patients approaching that of the general public, the economic burden associated with lifelong treatment of these patients will undoubtedly continue to increase in the years to come. Timely diagnosis, in conjunction with the application of appropriate treatment guidelines/recommendations in the acute setting, provides patients with the best opportunity to improve functional neurological outcome. Whereas certain interventions, including spinal immobilization, closed reduction of cervical dislocation injuries, and maintenance of blood pressure parameters, have gained universal acceptance in the management of SCI, others, including the role of MP therapy and acute surgical decompression, are more widely debated and open for interpretation.

REFERENCES

1. Zigler JE, et al: Epidemiology of spinal cord injury: a perspective on the problem. In Levine AM, et al, editors: *Spine Trauma*. Philadelphia, W.B. Saunders, 1998, pp. 2–15.
2. Garland DE, et al: Epidemiology and costs of spine trauma. In Capen DA, Haye W, editors: *Comprehensive Management of Spine Trauma*. St. Louis, MO, Mosby, 1998, pp. 1–5.
3. Devivo MJ, et al: Prevalence of spinal cord injury. *Arch Neurol* 37: 707–708, 1980.
4. Stover SL, et al: *Spinal Cord Injury: The Facts and Figures*. Birmingham, University of Alabama, 1986.
5. Harvey C, et al: New estimates of traumatic SCI prevalence: a survey-based approach. *Paraplegia* 28:537–544, 1990.
6. Kurtzke JF: Epidemiology of spinal cord injury. *Exp Neurol* 48:163–236, 1975.
7. Denis F: The three column spine and its significance in the classification of acute thoracolumbar spinal injuries. *Spine* 8:817–831, 1983.
8. Papadasiliou V: Traumatic subluxation of the cervical spine during childhood. *Orthop Clin North Am* 9:945–954, 1978.
9. Jellinger K: Pathology of spinal cord trauma. In Errico TJ, Bauer RD, Waugh T, editors: *Spinal Trauma*. Philadelphia, Lippincott, 1991, pp. 455–495.
10. Gilles FH, et al: Infantile atlantoocipital instability. *Am J Dis Child* 133: 30–37, 1979.
11. Adams JH, et al: *Greenfield's Neuropathology: Disease of the Spine and Spinal Cord*, 4th ed. London, Edward Arnold and Company, 1984, pp. 779–812.
12. Simpson RK, et al: Penetrating spinal injuries. In Pitts LH, Wagner FC, editors: *Craniospinal Trauma*. New York, Thieme Medical Publishers, 1990, pp. 197–212.
13. Stauffer ES, et al: Gunshot wounds of the spine: effects of laminectomy. *J Bone Joint Surg* 61:389–392, 1979.
14. Yashon D, et al: Prognosis and management of spinal cord and cauda equina bullet injuries in sixty-five civilians. *J Neurosurg* 32:163–170, 1970.
15. Karim NO, et al: Spontaneous migration of a bullet in the spinal subarachnoid space causing delayed radicular symptoms. *Neurosurgery* 18:97–100, 1986.
16. Six E, et al: Gunshot wounds to the spinal cord. *South Med J* 72:699–702, 1979.
17. Meirowsky AM: Penetrating spinal cord injuries. In Coates JB, Heaton LD, Meirowsky AM, editors: *Neurological Surgery of Trauma*. Washington, DC, Office of the Surgeon General, 1965, pp. 257–344.
18. Haynes WG: Acute war wounds of the spinal cord. *Am J Surg* 72:424–433, 1946.
19. Frazier CH: Stab and gunshot wounds to the spine. In Frazier CH, editor: *Surgery of the Spine and Spinal Cord*. New York, D. Appleton, 1918, pp. 457–497.
20. McCormick WF: Trauma. In Rosenberg RN, editor: *The Clinical Neurosciences: Neuropathology*. New York, Churchill Livingstone, 1983, p. 241.
21. Frankel HL, Hancock DO, Hyslop G, et al: The value of postural reduction in the initial management of closed injuries of the spine with paraplegia and tetraplegia. *Paraplegia* 7:179–192, 1969.
22. Guidelines for management of acute cervical spine injury. *Neurosurg Suppl* 50(3), 2002.
23. Linares HA, et al: Association between pressure sores and immobilization in the immediate post-injury period. *Orthopedics* 10:571–573, 1987.
24. Davies G, et al: The effect of a rigid collar on intracranial pressure. *Injury* 27:647–649, 1996.
25. Tarlov IM: Spinal cord compression studies III. *Arch Neurol Psychiatry* 71:588–597, 1954.
26. Tarlov IM, et al: Spinal cord compression studies II. Time limits for recovery after acute compression in dogs. *Arch Neurol Psychiatry* 71:271–290, 1954.
27. Brodkey JS, et al: Reversible spinal cord trauma in cats. Additive effects of direct pressure and ischemia. *J Neurosurg* 37:591–593, 1972.
28. La Rosa G, et al: Does early decompression improve neurological outcome of spinal cord injured patients? Appraisal of the literature using a meta-analytical approach. *Nature* 42(9):503–512, 2004.
29. Wing PC, et al: Risk of avascular necrosis following short-term megadose methylprednisolone treatment. *Spinal Cord* 36:633–636, 1998.
30. Bracken MB, et al: Effects of timing of methylprednisolone or naloxone administration on the recovery of segmental and long-tract neurological function in NASCIS 2. *J Neurosurg* 79:500–507, 1993.
31. Hurlbert RJ: Methylprednisolone for acute spinal cord injury: an inappropriate standard of care. *J Neurosurg* 93(Suppl 1):1–7, 2000.
32. Bracken MB: National Acute Spinal Cord Injury Study of methylprednisolone or naloxone. *Neurosurgery* 28:628–629, 1991.
33. Bracken MB, et al: A randomized, controlled trial of methylprednisolone, or naloxone in the treatment of acute spinal cord injury: results of the Second National Acute Spinal Injury Study (NASCIS-2). *N Engl J Med* 322:1405–1411, 1990.
34. Bracken MB, et al: Methlyprenisolone or tirilazad mesylate administration after acute spinal cord injury: 1-year follow-up results of the Third National Acute Spinal Cord Injury Randomized Controlled Trial. *J Neurosurg* 89:699–706, 1998.
35. Schaffery C: Medical complications. In Benzel EC, editor: *Spine Surgery: Technique, Complication Avoidance, and Management*. New York, Elsevier, 2005, pp. 2027–2032.
36. Rimoldi RL, et al: Immediate post-operative care. In Levine AM, et al, editors: *Spine Trauma*. Philadelphia, W.B. Saunders, 1998, pp. 562–566.
37. Ruben BH: Cardiopulmonary management of spinal cord injury. In Greenberg J, editor: *Handbook of Head and Spine Trauma*. New York, Marcel Dekker, 1993, pp. 497–502.
38. DeVivo MJ, et al: Cause of death for patients with spinal cord injury. *Arch Intern Med* 149:1761–1766, 1989.
39. Madsen III PW, et al: Post-traumatic syringomyelia. In Levine AM, et al, editors: *Spine Trauma*. Philadelphia, W.B. Saunders, 1998, pp. 608–629.
40. Bracken MS, et al: Incidence of traumatic spinal cord injury in the United States, 1970–1971. *Am J Epidemiol* 113:615–622, 1981.

MAXILLOFACIAL AND OCULAR INJURIES

MAXILLOFACIAL INJURIES

Guy J. Cappuccino, Samuel T. Rhee, and Mark S. Granick

While facial injuries may be dramatic in appearance, they are infrequently life threatening, and often not the most critical injuries the patient has sustained. Developing a systematic approach to the examination of patients with multiple wounds and prioritizing treatment is of paramount importance.

When craniofacial injuries occur in the setting of multiple injuries, the Advanced Trauma Life Support® guidelines should be followed beginning with a primary survey. The primary survey is called "the ABCs" because it stabilizes airway, breathing, and circulation. The application of these fundamental principles as they apply to facial trauma deserves special attention.

AIRWAY AND BREATHING

Early death as a result of airway obstruction most often occurs in the setting of multiple mandibular fractures or the combination of nasal, maxillary, and mandibular fractures. Since the tongue is suspended in the mouth by the mandible, fracture can cause the tongue to fall unsupported into the posterior oropharynx causing airway obstruction. In addition, surrounding tissue edema and hematoma can significantly narrow the airway. Fractured or avulsed teeth, broken dentures, blood, vomitus, or foreign bodies can also cause obstruction and need to be evacuated. If the patient exhibits signs of impending respiratory obstruction, including stridor, cyanosis, or drooling, or is unable to protect the airway with an effective gag reflex, endotracheal intubation or a surgical airway is indicated. Nasotracheal and nasogastric intubation may be contraindicated with midface instability due to the risk of passing the tube through the fractured cranial base into the brain. Early tracheostomy or cricothyroidotomy should be considered for the setting of pan-facial fractures, profuse nasal bleeding, severe soft-tissue edema surrounding the airway, comatose patients requiring intermaxillary fixation, severe facial burns, high spinal cord injuries, and concerns about difficult reintubation or prolonged intubation.

All trauma patients should be considered to have cervical spine instability and kept in a cervical collar until it can be cleared by physical or radiographic examination.

CIRCULATION AND CONTROL OF HEMORRHAGE

The head and neck receive 20% of the cardiac output; however, hemorrhage from facial wounds alone rarely cause systemic shock. Veins of the head and neck have no valves, and this can increase venous bleeding.

Despite this, most bleeding can be controlled with pressure, whether by direct digital pressure or packing. Instruments should not be inserted into wounds in attempts to stem arterial bleeders. The parotid duct, facial nerve, and other delicate structures are at risk of injury. The risk of airway obstruction from hemorrhage is the most serious concern.

Epistaxis

Nasopharyngeal bleeding can usually be controlled by direct pinch pressure on the nose. Thirty minutes of direct pressure without release is often sufficient. If this fails to control the hemorrhage, nasal packing should be performed. Anterior nasal bleeding can be treated by direct external pressure or cautery of the bleeding vessel. If the bleeding cannot be controlled by these measures, packing is indicated. Ribbon gauze impregnated with petroleum jelly works well for this purpose. Bayonet forceps and a nasal speculum are used to approximate the accordion-folded layers of the gauze, which should extend as far back into the nose as possible. Each layer should be pressed down firmly before the next layer is inserted. Posterior epistaxis requires posterior packing, which is accomplished by passing a catheter through one or both nares, through the nasopharynx, and out the mouth. A gauze pack then is secured to the end of the catheter and positioned in the posterior nasopharynx by pulling back on the catheter until the pack is seated in the posterior choana, sealing the posterior nasal passage, and applying pressure to the site of the posterior bleeding. Various balloon systems are effective for managing posterior bleeding and are less complicated than the packing procedure. If nasal packs or balloon systems are not available, a Foley catheter (10 to 14 French) with a 30-ml balloon may be used. The catheter is inserted through the bleeding nostril and visualized in the oropharynx before inflation of the balloon. The balloon then is inflated with approximately 10 ml of saline, and the catheter is withdrawn gently through the nostril, pulling the balloon up and forward. The balloon should seat in the posterior nasal cavity and will tamponade a posterior bleed. With traction maintained on the catheter, the anterior nasal cavity is then packed as previously described. Traction is maintained by placing an umbilical clamp or suture across the catheters outside the nostrils, with padding in between to prevent pressure necrosis of the columella.

Scalp Lacerations

The scalp is richly vascularized and thus lacerations can cause profuse bleeding. A surgical stapler can be used to quickly control this bleeding in an emergent situation. Both edges of the laceration should be stapled, parallel to the wound edge. This will provide hemostasis on a temporary basis until a formal repair can be performed.

Tongue Lacerations

Deep tongue lacerations may cause injury to the lingual artery. Control of this bleeding can be performed by suture ligation of the damaged lingual artery. After a bite block is placed in the mouth, a towel clip or a large suture is used to retract the tongue forward. The bleeding vessel then can be ligated and a formal repair of the tongue can be performed at this time if more serious injuries have already been addressed.

Hemorrhage from LeFort Fractures

In the case of severely displaced LeFort fractures, hemorrhage can be controlled by manually reducing the fracture. This is performed by grasping the maxillary arch of the hard palate and realigning the displaced segments.

HISTORY AND PHYSICAL EXAM

Once all life-threatening injuries have been addressed, a short history should be conducted. The acronym AMPLE can serve as a preliminary assessment: allergies (A), medications (M), past medical history (P), last meal (L), and events of the injury (E). A more involved history pertaining to maxillofacial trauma should investigate the mechanism of injury. This can be useful since certain force vectors produce predictable fracture patterns. Ask patients about any dental or orthodontic history, including the nature of their occlusion prior to injury (e.g., overbite, cross-bite). Ask about any prior facial injuries or surgery. In addition, old photographs of the patient can prove useful in reconstructive efforts.

The physical examination should proceed in a systematic and orderly fashion. Examination from superior or inferior is an acceptable pattern. No specific approach is preferred as long as the examiner is consistent. The face should be evaluated for symmetry and obvious deformity. All bony surfaces should be palpated to assess for step off, crepitus, or point tenderness. When examining the mandible and maxilla, broken or missing teeth should be noted, as well as jaw excursion. Normal excursion is 5–6 cm measured from the incisal edges of the incisors. Normal lateral movement of the mandible is 1 cm in relation to the maxilla. The patient's occlusion should be documented. When evaluating soft tissue, any contusions, abrasions, or lacerations should be noted. An examination for occult injuries should be performed, including within the ear canal, nares, and oral cavity. A complete sensory and motor exam should also be conducted. Cranial nerves 2–12 are easily tested (Table 1).[1]

RADIOGRAPHS

Computed tomography (CT) scans and Panorex films are the studies of choice in facial injuries. CT scans have generally replaced plain films in the diagnosis of facial fractures. Both axial and coronal sections, obtained with 1–2-mm cuts, help determine the location and displacement of facial fractures. Three-dimensional reconstructions can aid in visualization with panfacial fractures and bone loss. A

Table 1: Testing Cranial Nerve Function

Cranial Nerve	Test of Function
(II) Optic	Visual acuity
(III) Occulomotor	Evaluation of extraocular eye movements
(IV) Trochlear	
(VI) Abducens	
(V) Trigeminal	Test motor function by asking the person to clench his or her teeth while you palpate the masseter and temporal muscle for firmness. Test all three divisions of the trigeminal for intact sensation.
(VII) Facial	Test the facial nerve by asking the person to shut eyes, smile, and frown noting function and asymmetry.
(VIII) Vestibulocochlear	Test the cochlear portion of this cranial nerve by evaluating hearing acuity.
(IX) Glossopharyngeal	Test by checking for an intact gag reflex.
(X) Vagus	Look for symmetrical elevation of the soft palate.
(XI) Spinal accessory nerve	Have patient shrug shoulders against resistance.
(XII) Hypoglossal	Ask the person to stick out the tongue. Note symmetry, atrophy, and involuntary movements.

Panorex film is the study of choice for finding fractures of the body, ramus, angle, and condylar regions of the mandible. In lieu of a Panorex, a maxillofacial CT with cuts through the mandible can be obtained.

SOFT TISSUE INJURIES

General Considerations

The initial evaluation of most facial injuries frequently takes place in a busy emergency department or trauma bay. While this may be an acceptable location for diagnosis, it rarely provides a suitable environment for repair of facial trauma. Before beginning any reconstructive effort, an adequate light source, assistants, and all requisite supplies should be present. Extensive soft tissue injuries are optimally repaired in the operating room.

Local Anesthesia

Local anesthesia is the preferred modality for repair of most soft tissue injuries. While general anesthesia is required for major injuries, it is best avoided if possible since trauma patients may bear significant risks for aspiration, either due to intoxication or gastric contents. Local anesthesia can be combined with intravenous sedation to increase patient comfort and cooperation. Depending upon the choice of anesthetic, the effects of local anesthesia can last up to 7 hours (Table 2). When combined with epinephrine, the duration of anesthesia is extended and more importantly, the resultant vasoconstrictive effect

Table 2: Local Anesthetics Used in the Face

Drug	Plain Solution		Epinephrine Solution	
	Maximum Dose	Duration (Minutes)	Maximum Dose	Duration (Minutes)
Lidocaine (Xylocaine)	5 mg/kg	30–120	7 mg/kg	120–360
Bupivacaine (Marcaine)	2.5 mg/kg	120–240	3 mg/kg	180–420

provides increased hemostasis in the operative field. Onset of action is from 2 to 5 minutes for all drugs; however, waiting 7 minutes provides maximal effects.[2]

Cocaine (5% solution) is the topical anesthetic of choice for nasal mucous membranes. It can be introduced on cotton pledgets or gauze soaked with the solution.

Antibiotics

The use of antibiotics depends on the location and mechanism of the facial injury. Most soft tissue injuries of the face can be prophylaxed with a first-generation cephalosporin or aminoglycoside in the case of penicillin allergic patients. In the case of animal or human bites, gram negative and anaerobic organism coverage should be provided. Wounds with intraoral involvement should also cover these organisms. Duration of treatment should be determined based upon the extent of injury, contamination, and immune status of the patient[3] (Table 3).

Abrasions

Abrasions should be cleaned with a mild soap solution. If debris is embedded in the dermis, the skin should be anesthetized and scrubbed using a surgical scrub brush to remove the foreign material and prevent traumatic tattooing. The wound should ideally be cleaned within 12–24 hours. The wound should be kept moist, to facilitate epithelialization, and a sterile dressing placed.

Foreign Bodies

Foreign bodies larger than those that cause traumatic tattooing should be removed from facial wounds to prevent cellulitis and abscess formation. Metal fragments from bullets can be left if removal requires extended dissection since most bullets are relatively aseptic when they penetrate skin.

Treatment of Lacerations—General Concepts

Given the rich vascular supply to the face, wounds usually can be safely closed up to 24 hours following injury. Basic principles that apply to all facial lacerations include debridement of devitalized tissue or jagged wound edges, irrigation, and closure of the wound in layers. Conservative trimming should be performed to create healthy, perpendicular skin edges that are conducive to healing with minimal scarring. Suturing should be done in layers. The deepest layers should be closed with interrupted, buried, absorbable sutures. This will serve to minimize dead space, and help approximate and relieve tension on skin edges. Epidermis should be closed using a fine 5-0 or 6-0 suture. Interrupted sutures allow removal of select stitches for drainage of purulence or hematoma; however, a simple running suture can provide equally good results and save time. The wound should then be kept covered with sterile adhesive strips or antibiotic ointment for 48 hours to allow for epithelialization. Nonabsorbable epidermal sutures should be removed 4–7 days after placement. Areas with thin skin such as the eyelid should have sutures removed by day 4.

Lip Lacerations

Repair of lip lacerations should be done with reference to anatomic landmarks, carefully aligning the edges of the vermilion border and the wet–dry margin. The first suture should be placed at the vermilion border with the remainder of the wound closed in layers. Muscle should be repaired with a braided absorbable suture. The vermilion and mucosa can be repaired with an absorbable chromic gut suture. Finally, skin is closed with a nylon or fine fast-absorbing gut suture.

Nasal Lacerations

Nasal lacerations can be simple, involving skin only, or complex, which involve a combination of the mucosal lining, cartilaginous framework, and skin. Repair should be performed in layers. Cartilage

Table 3: Tetanus Prophylaxis

Immunization Status	Tetanus Toxoid (0.50 ml)	Tetanus Immunoglobulin
Unknown status or no history of immunization	Immediate dose plus two more at monthly intervals	One dose 250 IU
Last immunization greater than 5 years ago	One dose	
Contaminated wounds with immunization greater than 2 years ago	One dose	One dose 500 IU

Source: Immunization Practices Advisory Committee: Diphtheria, tetanus, and pertussis: guidelines for vaccine prophylaxis and other preventive measures. *MMWR Morb Mort Wkly Rep* 34:426, 1985.

should be repaired with interrupted 4-0 or 5-0 absorbable monofilament or chromic gut sutures. Mucosa is generally repaired in a similar fashion with 4-0 or 5-0 chromic gut suture. Skin can be closed with a fine nylon (5-0 or 6-0) or fast-absorbing gut suture. Nasal septal hematomas can occur after blunt or penetrating trauma and deserve special attention, since failure to drain the hematoma can cause pressure necrosis of the nasal septum. A septal hematoma can be drained within 24 hours of injury with a large-bore needle and syringe or a small scalpel incision followed by intranasal packing with petroleum gauze.

Ear Lacerations

Ear trauma ranges from simple lacerations to complete amputations. Primary repair is paramount since secondary repair is more difficult and often yields significantly less favorable results. The ear has abundant cutaneous blood supply. Lacerations which involve cartilage do not always require repair of the cartilage. If approximation of skin edges or perichondrium brings the severed edges of the cartilage into adequate apposition, then repair of the cartilage is not required. Skin should be repaired with 5-0 or 6-0 nylon or fast-absorbing gut. If the cartilaginous damage is extensive, or the edges are considerably irregular, primary repair of the cartilage should be performed with 4-0 or 5-0 chromic gut or absorbable monofilament sutures in simple interrupted fashion. Following repair, contoured bolsters can be fashioned from petroleum gauze with antibiotic ointment and placed postauricularly and within the conchal bowl of the ear for support. This can be held in place with a gauze head wrap dressing. Avulsion injuries of the ear can be closed primarily if the defect is small enough or may necessitate composite grafting or local flap creation for reconstruction. Total ear avulsion or amputation should be referred for consideration of microsurgical replantation. Care of the amputated part includes placing it in a moist gauze wrap in a sealed container or bag. The container then is placed in an ice water bath. The amputated part should never be placed directly on ice, as this can cause a cold burn.

Orbital Soft Tissue Injuries

Blunt or penetrating trauma to the globe can cause bleeding into the anterior chamber of the eye, which is called hyphema. Any injury involving the periorbital area warrants a basic eye exam for visual acuity and extraocular muscle patency. Frequently, an ophthalmology consultation is indicated. However, in mild cases of hyphema, no treatment is required and the blood is absorbed within a few days. Bed rest, eye patching, and sedation to minimize activity and reduce the likelihood of recurrent bleeding, may be prescribed for hyphema. In severe cases, surgical intervention to evacuate the hematoma is necessary.

Eyelid lacerations warrant special consideration due to their complex anatomy and relationship with the eye. Before repair is attempted, underlying injury to the globe must be ruled out. Removal of all foreign bodies should be performed by avoiding further injury in the removal process. Irrigation can be performed with a syringe and an 18-gauge intravenous catheter. Debridement should be kept to a minimum. Blood clot around the globe must be evacuated with caution, as it may be adherent to the richly vascular iris, which also can resemble clot. While attempting eyelid repair, remember to keep the globe lubricated. Lidocaine jelly and a corneal protector can provide adequate anesthesia for an awake patient. Eyelid lacerations can be divided into two categories: superficial, involving skin only, and deep. Superficial lacerations are then subdivided into those that are parallel to the lid margin and those that are perpendicular to it. Lacerations that run parallel require only a few simple interrupted sutures of 6-0 nylon. Smaller lacerations may not require any suturing or may heal well with a topical dermal adhesive such as cyanoacrylate glue. Conjunctival repair can be performed with 6-0 plain gut suture; small lacerations may not require any suturing. Lacerations which run perpendicular tend to spread and require suturing to close.

Deep lacerations which involve subcutaneous musculature or transect the lid margin generally require special attention. Realignment of the lid margin must be precise. A 6-0 silk suture on a nontraumatic ophthalmic needle is passed into the tarsus through a meibomian gland on one side of the wound, across the wound margin, and exited through a meibomian gland orifice on the opposing side. Tension can be held on this suture while two more sutures are placed, one at the anterior margin and the other at the posterior margin of the meibomian gland. These sutures are then retracted superiorly to align the edges of the laceration inferior to the lid margin. The pretarsal and muscle layers are repaired first with a fine absorbable suture and then the skin is closed with a fine nonabsorbable monofilament suture.

Lacrimal System Injuries

Any injury near the medial canthus should raise suspicion for a lacrimal duct injury. Disruption of the lacrimal duct can lead to epiphora, or tear overflow as a result of outflow obstruction. This is often seen as a late complication of naso-orbito-ethmoid (NOE) fractures. In cases of incomplete division of the duct, the surrounding tissues can be repaired which in most cases is enough to restore patency of the ductal system. More severe injuries require a dacryocystorhinostomy (DCR), which is a procedure in which the duct is cannulated and sutured around a silastic tube. DCR is most often a secondary reconstructive procedure, performed months after the injury if symptoms dictate its use.

Parotid Duct Injuries

The parotid, or Stensen's, duct arises from deep within the parotid gland and emerges from the superior third of the gland at its anterior border. From there it courses below the zygomatic arch, into the buccal space, through the buccinator muscle, and enters the oral cavity in the buccal mucosa, opposite the upper second molar. Its course can be visualized by the middle third of a line drawn from the tragus of the ear to the midportion of the upper lip. Since the parotid duct is more superficial than the facial nerve, it is more susceptible to injury trauma. Disruption of Stensen's duct can result in a parotid fistula or sialocele if left unrepaired. If injury is suspected, the ostium of the duct can be cannulated with a small-gauge silastic tube. A 22-gauge intravenous catheter can be used for this purpose. Once catheterized, the disrupted ends of the duct can be sutured around the tube with fine absorbable suture material on an atraumatic needle. The end of the tube should be anchored in place in the mouth with nonabsorbable sutures and left in place for approximately 1–2 weeks. Persistent fluid accumulation can be treated with percutaneous drainage or re-insertion of the tube.

Facial Nerve Injuries

The 7th cranial nerve exits the skull from the stylomastoid foramen and enters the parotid gland at its deep surface. Adjacent to the parotid duct, the nerve divides into two major branches, the temporofacial branch and the cervicofacial branch. The nerve courses more superficially as it passes across the surface of the masseter muscle to its terminal branches, which have intercommunications. The major branches of the facial nerve lie deep to the muscles of facial expression and are thus well protected from trauma. Nerve injury anterior to a line perpendicular to the lateral canthus does not necessitate repair. Injury distal to this arborization allows maintenance of cross-innervation to the musculature. Injury to the larger, more proximal branches warrants repair of the nerve with loupe or microscopic magnification.

Intraoral Injuries

Intraoral injuries should be treated with copious irrigation and debridement of devitalized tissues. Then the mucosa should be loosely approximated using absorbable sutures such as 4-0 chromic gut. The patient should be encouraged to rinse the mouth with half-strength peroxide, or oral chlorhexidine solution to reduce bacterial load.

FACIAL FRACTURES

General Principles

A CT scan is the preferred modality for diagnosing facial fractures. Three-millimeter cuts in the coronal, sagittal, and axial planes with three-dimensional reconstruction are usually adequate for diagnosis. Facial fractures are classified as either open or closed, and by anatomic location. Anatomically, fractures are divided into upper, middle, and lower third fractures. The upper third of the face consists of the frontal bones and the orbits. Orbital fractures are subdivided into orbital rim fractures and internal orbital fractures. The middle third of the face contains the zygoma, maxilla, and nasal bones. The lower third is represented by the mandible.

Facial fractures tend to occur in reproducible patterns due to weaker areas that fracture first despite the location of impact. Some common patterns are the zygomaticomaxillary complex (ZMC) fractures, Le Fort fractures, NOE fractures, orbital blowout fractures, and frontobasilar fractures. Knowledge of these patterns can help in the identification of their component fractures and extent of injury which helps in preoperative planning. Primary treatment consisting of open reduction and internal fixation of facial fractures yield the best cosmetic and functional results. This may be delayed, however, for up to a week to allow coordination of a multidisciplinary approach. Open reduction and internal fixation is the treatment of choice allowing anatomical reduction of fractures, stable internal fixation, and early jaw mobilization. Reestablishment of the effective occlusion is of prime importance when addressing fractures that involve the occlusal plane. Most often this involves placing the patient in intermaxillary fixation.

Frontal Sinus/Frontobasilar Fractures

Frontal sinus fractures often result from forceful blunt trauma to the forehead, commonly from a steering wheel when involved in a motor vehicle collision. The frontal bone is comprised of a thicker outer (anterior) table and relatively thinner inner (posterior) table. Just deep to the posterior table are the meninges; any displaced fracture of the posterior table should raise suspicion of dural injury and warrants neurosurgical consultation. Clinical signs of anterior table fracture include forehead depression and malleability upon palpation. Signs of dural involvement include cerebrospinal fluid rhinorrhea and pneumocephaly. Extensive fractures of the frontal sinus can cause disruption of the nasofrontal drainage system. Obstruction of the nasofrontal ducts can cause late post-traumatic complications such as recurrent suppurative sinusitis or mucopyelocele formation. Acute obstruction of the nasofrontal ducts is generally treated by obliteration of the frontal sinus. This process consists of removing the mucosal lining of the sinus, obliteration of the nasofrontal duct and sinus with graft material, and reconstruction of the anterior table. Cranialization of the sinus, where the posterior table

is completely removed and the brain is allowed to expand into the sinus, is reserved for severely comminuted or displaced posterior table fractures.[10,11]

Naso-Orbital-Ethmoid Fractures

Naso-orbital-ethmoid fractures consist of injury to the frontal processes of the maxilla and nasal bones; these can be some of the most difficult facial fractures to manage. The frontal process of the maxilla contains the attachment of the medial canthal tendon (MCT), which shapes the medial palpebral fissure and supports the globe. Disruption of the medial canthal tendon in NOE fractures results in traumatic telecanthus. These injuries are of significant clinical importance because of all facial fractures they have the great potential for subsequent deformity. Signs of NOE fractures include telecanthus (intercanthal distance greater than 30–35 mm), rounded medial palpebral fissures, a flattened nasal dorsum, and a mobile medial canthus on physical examination. Mobility of the frontal process of the maxilla on direct finger pressure over the medial canthal tendon is a reliable sign of NOE fracture. The Manson test consists of palpating the frontal process with one hand while applying lateral pressure with an instrument inserted into the nostril and advanced to a position medial to the frontal process.[5] NOE fractures are classified by the extent of the fracture and the involvement of the MCT attachment. Type 1 NOE fractures contain a single, central segment fracture. Type 2 NOE fractures contain a comminuted central fragment not involving the attachment of the medial canthal tendon. Type 3 NOE fractures involve a comminuted fracture disrupting the attachment of the medial canthal tendon.[6] Treatment is generally open reduction and fixation of fragments with miniplates, screws, and/or interfragmentary wiring.[10,11]

Orbital Fractures

The bony framework of the orbit can be divided into the rim and internal orbit. The anterior orbit is comprised of thick bone, the middle third is relatively thin bone and posteriorly the bone becomes thick again. The weakest areas of the orbit are the floor and medial wall. Orbital fractures are described as pure or impure. A pure orbital fracture involves only the inner orbit while an impure fracture also involves the rim. An orbital blowout fracture refers to a pure fracture of the orbital floor and medial wall where orbital contents herniate into the maxillary and ethmoid sinuses. This can cause entrapment of adjacent medial and inferior rectus muscles. These are generally the result of a low energy impact. Impure fractures involving the rim are often the result of high energy impact. Signs of orbital fractures include subconjunctival and palpebral hematoma, paresthesias in the infraorbital nerve distribution, and diplopia. Diplopia and abnormal extraocular movements may indicate entrapment. If entrapment is suspected, a forced duction test should be performed. This is done by instilling topical anesthetic into the conjunctival sac. Forceps are used to grasp the inferior rectus muscle approximately 7 mm from the limbus. The globe is then rotated in all directions to assess resistance to motion which would indicate entrapment. Enophthalmos is another complication of orbital fractures and can become clinically apparent with an increase in orbital volume of 5%.[7] Correction of these defects requires reconstruction of the orbital floor and medial wall with titanium mesh, synthetic orbital plate constructs, or bone grafting.

Superior orbital fissure syndrome consists of abnormal extraocular movements, forehead and brow paresthesias, and pupillary dilation. This results from injury or compression of cranial nerves III, IV, ophthalmic division of V, and VI as they pass between the greater and lesser wings of the sphenoid bone, which comprises the superior orbital fissure.[10,11]

Orbital fractures have a significant incidence of associated ocular injures including vitreous hemorrhage, hyphema, damage to optic nerve, and globe laceration. A thorough eye exam is indicated in the presence of such fractures. If the optic nerve is involved, it is termed orbital apex syndrome.

Zygoma Fractures

Due to the prominent and superficial position of the zygoma, it is frequently fractured. With the exception of an isolated zygomatic arch fracture, all fractures of the zygoma include fractures of the adjacent orbital bones. This pattern is called a zygomaticomaxillary complex (ZMC) fracture. The zygoma has four bony attachments to the skull at the frontal, maxillary, temporal, and sphenoid bones. Thus, ZMC fractures should be referred to as "tetrapod" fractures, and not "tripod" fractures, by which they are commonly known. Most ZMC fractures are posteroinferiorly displaced due to the pull of attached muscles including the masseter, zygomaticus, and temporalis.

Clinical signs and symptoms of a ZMC fracture include periorbital ecchymosis/edema, painful and limited jaw motion, inferior displacement of lateral palpebral fissure, anesthesia in the distribution of the infraorbital nerve, palpable step-off deformity of inferior orbital rim and zygomatico-frontal region, and enophthalmos with laterally displaced ZMC fractures. Nondisplaced zygomatic fractures can be treated nonoperatively with observation. Displaced fractures, or fractures causing functional impairment, require reduction and fixation. Late complications of untreated ZMC fractures include malunion, enophthalmos, ectropion, diplopia, and permanent dysesthesia of the infraorbital nerve.[10,11]

Maxillary LeFort Fractures

Fractures of the maxilla generally involve multiple midface structures. In 1901, Rene LeFort described reproducible patterns of fracture propagation in midface trauma. He concluded that predictable patterns of fractures follow certain injuries. Three predominant types were described.[8] A LeFort I fracture (horizontal fracture) is a fracture separating the maxillary alveolus from the upper midface. A LeFort II fracture (pyramidal fracture) separates a pyramid shaped fragment containing the maxillary alveolus, nasal bones, and inferior medial orbit from the remainder of the face. A LeFort III fracture (transverse fracture or craniofacial disjunction) separates the midface at the level of the upper zygoma, orbital floor, and naso-ethmoid region from the remaining upper facial skeleton. Most LeFort III fractures are combinations of LeFort I, II, and III fractures with a high degree of comminution. Physical findings include midfacial edema, profuse epistaxis, malocclusion, and palpable bony defects, depending on the fracture type. The most significant physical findings on exam are the mobility of the maxilla in relation to the remainder of the facial skeleton. The level at which the mobility occurs dictates the type of LeFort fracture. Isolated maxilla movement with intact upper facial structures point toward a LeFort I fracture. Mobility at the nasofrontal region upon manipulation of the palate indicates a LeFort II. Movement at the zygomaticofrontal sutures with manipulation of the palate is consistent with LeFort III fractures. A small percentage of LeFort fractures are not mobile and are classified as incomplete. One must rely on CT findings in this scenario. Ten percent of LeFort fractures include palatal fracture.[9] Displacement of LeFort fractures is in the posteroinferior vector as a consequence of pull from the pterygoid musculature. Often the patient will appear to have a sunken and elongated midface with an open bite deformity.

Emergency management of LeFort fractures is required only with airway compromise and massive hemorrhage. Manual anterior distraction of the maxilla can be attempted in the event of oropharyngeal obstruction which precludes endotracheal intubation. If this maneuver fails, emergency cricothyroidotomy should be performed. Reducing a badly displaced LeFort fracture can help to tamponade hemorrhage in conjunction with packing. Definitive surgical treatment can be delayed up to 7 days to allow time for stabilization of the patient. The goal of surgery is to restore proper anatomic relationships. In particular, attempt to normalize the integrity of the support bolsters of the facial skeleton, the midfacial height and projection, and dental occlusion.[10,11]

Nasal Fractures

Nasal fractures are the most common facial fractures encountered in facial trauma, and often go undiagnosed. Isolated nasal bone fractures are uncommon, and more often are seen in combination with septal disruption. Nasal fractures can be displaced posteriorly or laterally. Nasal bone fractures are easily seen on CT scans, but can be diagnosed by visual inspection and palpation. Pain, crepitus, and mobility of the nasal pyramid upon palpation are common physical findings. Epistaxis is often present. Visual inspection of the septum is paramount to rule out a septal hematoma.

Closed reduction of displaced nasal pyramid and septal fractures can be performed in the acute care setting. Adequate closed reduction usually leads to minimally noticeable subsequent deformity which can be addressed by rhinoplasty if needed 6 months to a year after injury. The procedure for acute closed reduction involves local anesthesia and IV sedation if available. The upper lateral cartilages, the base, the columella, and the infraorbital foramen are infiltrated with local anesthetic. If available, 4% cocaine soaked pledgets are placed intranasally. Using the thumb and index finger, the laterally displaced nasal bone fractures are reduced medially. Medially displaced nasal bone fractures can be reduced with a scalpel handle placed within the nares and pressed laterally against the displaced structures. Septal deviation is best reduced with an Asch or Walsham forceps. Steri-strips should be placed across the dorsum of the nose and a moldable thermoplast nasal splint is applied for 1 week.[10,11]

Mandibular Fractures

Mandibular fractures are the second most common facial fractures seen in trauma. Signs and symptoms include malocclusion, anesthesia in the distribution of the inferior alveolar nerve, preauricular pain, and limited or painful jaw excursion. A Panorex film is the study of choice; however, a CT scan can provide useful information as well. Physical exam should include palpation for pain and step-off as well as an intraoral exam to inspect for lacerations and possible open fractures. Mandibular fractures are classified by anatomic location, symphysis, alveolar, body, angle, ramus, coronoid, or condyle. Due to the ring shaped configuration of the mandible, a fracture will also have a contralateral (indirect) fracture. Fractures can be classified as open or closed, displaced or nondisplaced. Restoration of occlusion is the primary goal of treatment. Treatment options range from intermaxillary fixation with wires and arch bars for closed, minimally displaced fractures to open reduction and internal plating for more severe fractures.[10,11]

REFERENCES

1. Seidel H, Bass J, Dains J, Benedict GW: *Mosby's Guide to Physical Examination*, 4th ed. St. Louis, MO, Mosby, 1999.
2. Brown D: *Atlas of Regional Anesthesia*, 2nd ed. Philadelphia, W.B. Saunders, 1999.
3. Brook I, Frazier EH: Aerobic and anaerobic bacteriology of wounds and cutaneous abscesses. *Arch Surg* 125:1445, 1990.
4. Immunization Practices Advisory Committee: Diphtheria, tetanus, and pertussis: guidelines for vaccine prophylaxis and other preventive measures. *MMWR Morb Mort Wkly Rep* 34:426, 1985.

5. Paskert JP, Manson PN: The bimanual examination for assessing instability in naso-orbitoethmoidal injuries. Plast Reconstr Surg 83:165, 1989.

6. Gruss JS: Naso-ethmoid-orbital fractures: classification and role of primary bone grafting. Plast Reconstr Surg 75:303, 1985.

7. Saunders CJ, Whetzel TP, Stokes RB, et al: Transantral endoscopic orbital floor exploration: a cadaver and clinical study. Plast Reconstr Surg 100:575, 1997.

8. Manson PN: Some thoughts on the classification and treatment of LeFort fractures. Ann Plast Surg 17(5):356, 1986.

9. Manson P, Glassman D, Vander Kolk C, Petty P: Rigid stabilization of sagittal fractures of the maxilla and palate. Plast Reconstr Surg 85:711–716, 1990.

10. Moore E, Feliciano D, Mattox K: Trauma, 5th ed. New York, McGraw-Hill, 2004.

11. Aston S, Beasley R, Thorne C: Grabb and Smith's Plastic Surgery. Philadelphia, Lippincott-Raven, 1997.

TRAUMA TO THE EYE AND ORBIT

Mario A. Meallet

Trauma and emergency physicians are frequently confronted with evaluating and managing severe eye injuries, most of which will require immediate consultation and referral to an ophthalmologist. We hope to describe the types of ocular emergencies that can be managed by the emergency and trauma physician, and clearly illustrate the techniques employed.

When facial fractures are limited to the orbital bones, an ophthalmology evaluation is sufficient to develop a management plan. In more extensive fractures involving the nasopharynx, skull, maxilla, and mandible, a more collaborative approach with the aid of plastic surgery, ophthalmology, head and neck, and oral-maxillofacial surgery may be needed. The decision for appropriate triage is made within the emergency department and we hope to provide useful guidelines to aid in decision making.

Direct injury to the eye requires the immediate involvement of eye care providers. Severely injured patients are often unable to cooperate with extensive ocular examination, and management decisions will be based on objective eye findings. In obvious open globe injuries, the emergency physician and the trauma surgeon can aid in obtaining a clear history of the injury and making the prompt decision for radiologic evaluation. Where an intraocular foreign body is suspected, or a thorough history cannot be elicited, an immediate orbital computed tomography (CT) should be obtained. A fox shield should be placed over the eye for protection and the remainder of the evaluation and management should be deferred to an ophthalmologist. In particular, the emergency medical physician should defer performing a slit-lamp examination and absolutely avoid measurement of intraocular pressure. The patient should also be asked to avoid maneuvers that may cause intraocular hemorrhage, such as coughing or Valsalva, and be urged to rest quietly until the wound has been repaired (Figure 1).[1,2]

When an open globe is not clearly obvious, a full ocular examination is carried out in a methodical and rational fashion, beginning with gross external inspection and visual acuity measurement in each eye, independently. Optic nerve function is assessed by testing for a relative afferent pupillary defect and, if appropriate, intraocular pressure is measured and a careful slit-lamp examination is performed. Dilated fundus exam can only be performed by trained personnel and can be left to the ophthalmologist. If the combination of clinical findings and ancillary testing is not clearly indicative of an open globe injury, but the suspicion remains high, then formal exploration under anesthesia is recommended. Photodocumentation is recommended whenever feasible.[1] Prompt management by the initial emergency and trauma surgeons can have a profound impact on the ultimate visual function of these patients, and familiarity with the various types of urgent eye injuries will promote a system of ideal triage (Figure 2).

INCIDENCE

Ocular trauma in the United States occurs at an estimated rate of 2 million eye injuries per year (7 per 1000 population). Data gathered by McGwin et al.[3,4] from national ambulatory care surveys and hospital discharge records reveal that most eye injuries in the United States are treated in emergency departments (50.7%), followed by private physicians' offices (38.7%), and outpatient (8.1%) and inpatient (2.5%) facilities. Demographic analysis of the highest-risk groups reveals that eye injury rates are highest among males in their 20s, with no clear difference among ethnic groups.

The rate of eye injury begins to climb later in childhood, with peak incidence in the third decade, followed by a slow decline. A second peak occurs with very advanced age.[4,5] This bimodal incidence in younger and older adults, as well as higher rates in males, is a reflection of the types of high-risk activities younger males engage in and the propensity for injuries and falls seen in older adults. These trends apply to injuries in these groups in general.

The setting in which an injury occurs has a marked impact on the severity and the prognosis for visual recovery. A study on the rate of eye injuries in the workplace reported that open globe injuries were the most common (46%), followed by injury to the surrounding ocular adnexal structures (20%), orbital fractures (11%), and traumatic hyphemas (11%).[4,6] Interestingly, the vast majority (approximately 90%) of eye injuries occur in settings where protective eyewear can have a major impact (e.g., workplace, sports activities). In fact, in many of these settings, eyewear is mandated but is not being worn at the time of injury. Thus, it is estimated that up to 90% of eye injuries could be prevented if protective eyewear were worn in these settings.

Of the small number of motor vehicle–related eye injuries (estimated at 1.8% of all eye injuries in the United States), very few present as open globe injuries. The mandated use of seatbelts has resulted in a twofold decrease in the number of eye injuries. Curiously, this has been offset by a twofold increase in eye injuries in accidents where airbags have been deployed. The most frequent injury mechanism related to MVA is impact with the windshield, followed by the airbag, steering wheel, and flying glass.[7] However, these statistics must be viewed in the context of the decreased number of fatalities with the advent of airbag and seatbelt use.

Overall, only a small percentage (2.3%) of eye injuries encountered in the emergency setting present as lacerations and punctures (Table 1 and Figure 3). The most common causes of eye injuries in this setting are foreign bodies (44.6%) and blunt trauma (33.0%) (Table 2 and Figure 4).[4] In the subgroup of patients with blunt trauma, many of these represent ruptures of the sclera that may not be clearly obvious to the examiner. In these cases, the examiner must rely on the key clinical findings associated with occult scleral rupture, as outlined in the section on diagnosis. Werner et al.[5] reported on these occult scleral ruptures and found that they can represent up to 25% of all potential ruptured

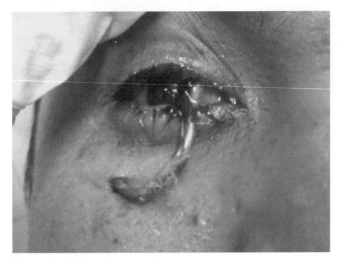

Figure 1   Nail-gun injury to the eye.

Table 1: Post-Traumatic Eye Findings in Emergency Setting

Type of Eye Injury	%
Contusion/abrasion	44.6
Foreign body	30.8
Conjunctivitis	10.2
Hemorrhage	9.9
Laceration	1.8
Puncture	0.5

Adapted from McGwin G Jr., Owsley C: Incidence of emergency department-treated eye injury in the United States. *Arch Ophthalmol* 123:662–666, 2005.

globes that present to physicians. Of these suspected cases of occult rupture, roughly one-third were actually found to have eye ruptures at the time of surgical exploration.

There is a significant association of orbital fractures found in patients presenting with head trauma. In a large study of 4426 U.S. Army soldiers with facial and orbital fractures, orbital floor fractures were found in 26%. Within this group, there was also a 30% incidence of injury to the globe and a 70% incidence of concomitant bodily injury.[8] Fractures of the orbital floor and medial wall make up the majority of fractures, with the lateral wall being the third most likely site of fracture and a smaller number of fractures occurring in the orbital roof (Figure 5).[9] The floor is most susceptible just medial to the infraorbital groove, whereas the medial wall is most likely to rupture at the lamina papyracea, a paper-thin bony septum.[10]

MECHANISM OF INJURY

The mechanisms of injury to the eye and surrounding structures are largely associated with foreign bodies, blunt trauma, and thermal and chemical burns. Machinery, motor vehicle, and firearms are among the less common causes (see Table 2 and Figure 4).[4] There is often appreciable overlap, and the physician must consider the impact of these mechanisms in combination and treat each injury individually. For example, a ruptured globe from blunt trauma may require a short course of systemic steroids for traumatic optic neuropathy if an afferent

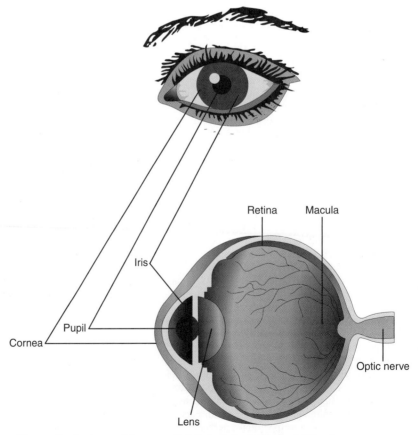

Figure 2   Anatomy of the eye.   *(Artistic rendering by Narina Sokolova.)*

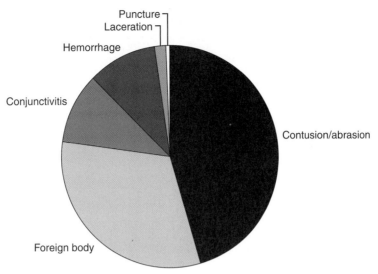

Figure 3 Post-traumatic eye findings in the emergency setting. See Table 1. *(Data from McGwin G Jr, Owsley C: Incidence of emergency department–treated eye injury in the United States. Arch Ophthalmol 123: 662–666, 2005.)*

Table 2: Key Mechanisms of Eye Injury in Emergency Setting

Mechanism of Eye Injury	%
Foreign body	44.6
Blunt trauma	33.0
Fire/burn	12.0
Machinery	3.1
Motor vehicle accident	2.3
Fall	1.8
Firearm	< 1.0

Adapted from McGwin G Jr, Owsley C: Incidence of emergency department-treated eye injury in the United States. *Arch Ophthalmol* 123:662–666, 2005.

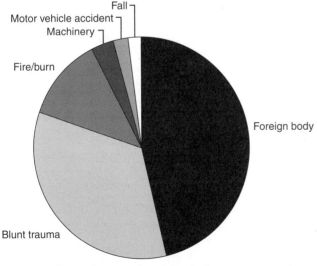

Figure 4 Key mechanisms of eye injury in the emergency setting. See Table 2. *(Data from McGwin G Jr, Owsley C: Incidence of emergency department–treated eye injury in the United States. Arch Ophthalmol 123:662–666, 2005.)*

pupillary defect is noted. Blunt force on an eye can also be described as coup–contrecoup, or compressive force in a manner similar to brain injury. Examples of coup injuries are corneal abrasions, subconjunctival hemorrhages, choroidal hemorrhages, and retinal necrosis. The best example of a contrecoup injury is commotio retinae, with anterior forces being transmitted to the retina and causing shearing of the retinal layers.[11] Compression of the globe usually causes scleral rupture. These open globe injuries are described below.

Orbital fractures can be caused by blunt forces with an increase of intraorbital pressure resulting in blowout fractures of the medial wall and floor, or caused by direct injury to the bones of the face resulting in fracture of any of the four walls. Because the lateral wall and roof are the most resistant to fracture, injury of these bones is an indicator of significant force to the face and eyes and concomitant injury to the globe should be carefully evaluated. Foreign body penetration of the orbit can involve the eye directly or any of the surrounding structures.

Chemical and thermal injuries to the eyelids and adnexa must be evaluated long term, well beyond the healing period for the superficial tissues. Burns to the eyelids and skin lead to scarring and contraction of the eyelids, which place these patients at risk for eyelid retraction and exposure damage to the cornea and ocular surface. Thus, long-term follow-up is important in this patient group, particularly if they are in a critical care setting. They must be treated with aggressive lubrication to the eyes until they demonstrate an ability to blink voluntarily and protect the eye. It is urged that all ICU and trauma wards have written eye care protocols for the management of these patients.

Open globe injuries are classically divided into penetrating and non-penetrating injuries. The latter group is caused by blunt trauma that causes a forceful compression of the eye and results in the physical rupture of the eye wall. The location of the rupture is typically in the areas where the eye wall is the thinnest, namely the corneo–scleral junction (the limbus), at the muscle insertion sites, and at the posterior attachment of the optic nerve. Ruptures posterior to the limbus may be difficult to identify and the clinician must be familiar with the signs of occult rupture, which are described in the section on diagnosis.

When the mechanism of injury involves penetration of the globe, the site of entry is usually visible and the decision for surgical intervention is straightforward. The three variables to consider when an entry wound is identified are whether the penetrating object has

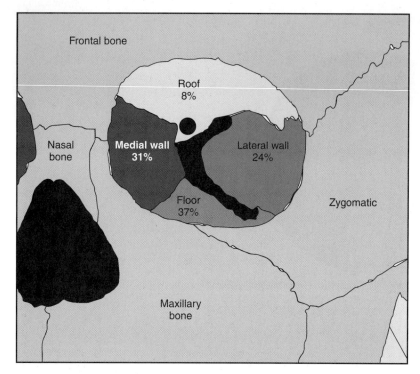

Figure 5 Diagram of orbital bones with incidence of orbital fractures. *(Original image obtained from Yanoff M, Duker JS: Ophthalmology, 2nd ed. St. Louis, Mosby, 2004, figure 83-1. Data from Shere JL, Boole JR, Holtel MR, Amoroso PJ: An analysis of 3599 midfacial and 1141 orbital blowout fractures among 4426 United States Army Soldiers, 1980–2000. Otolaryngol Head Neck Surg 130:164–170, 2004.)*

exited the eye, whether a foreign body is within the eye, or whether it has passed through the entire eye (perforation), in which case a posterior exit wound should be suspected and the foreign body may be located within the orbit.

If there is evidence of an intraocular or intraorbital foreign body, the type of material may also have implications in toxicity to the eye and the risk of infection to the orbit and the eye (Table 3). When the history of the type of injury is unclear, an orbital CT should be requested immediately and a shield placed over the eye. Even if the foreign body is easily accessible and protruding from the eye or surrounding structures, the emergency or trauma surgeon should make no attempt to remove the object. A shield should be carefully placed over the eye and no manipulation at-

tempted. The extent of injury can be assessed at the time of surgical repair.

DIAGNOSIS

Orbital Trauma

The key clinical features that aid in the decision for urgent management in cases of orbital trauma involve (1) significant limitation of ocular motility, (2) the presence of an afferent pupillary defect, (3) the presence of proptosis (abnormal anterior bulging of the eye),

Table 3: Manifestations of Intraocular Metal Toxicity

Type of Metal	Cornea	Iris	Lens	Vitreous	Retina	Signs/Symptoms
Iron (siderosis)	Rust-colored corneal stromal staining	Anisocoria/ heterochromia	Flower-shaped cataract	Brownish opacities	Diffuse retinal pigmentation	Night blindness, visual field loss
Copper (<85%) (chronic chalcosis)	Fleischer ring	Greenish discoloration	Sunflower cataract	Brownish-red opacities	Metallic flecks on vessels and macula	Progressive vision and field loss
Copper (>85%) (acute chalcosis)	Severe inflammation	Greenish discoloration	Sunflower cataract	Diffuse vitritis	Metallic flecks on vessels	Fulminant inflammation/ loss of eye
Gold	—	—	Anterior capsule deposits	—	—	—
Aluminum/zinc	Minimal inflammation	—	—	—	—	—

Based on data from Yanoff M, Duker JS: *Ophthalmology*, 2nd ed. St. Louis, Mosby, 2004.

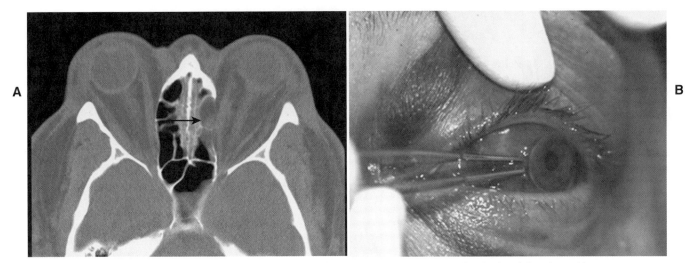

Figure 6 Young male after blunt trauma to left eye. **(A)** Patient had limited ocular motility when looking left and possible entrapment on orbital CT *(arrow)*. **(B)** Forced duction testing revealed full abduction, and entrapment was ruled out.

and (4) the presence of enophthalmos (abnormal posterior displacement of the eye). Any of these features requires an immediate orbital CT scan, ophthalmologic evaluation and consideration of surgical intervention. In a study by Lee et al.[10] on the role of CT in orbital trauma, of those patients who suffered visual loss secondary to orbital trauma, the causes in order of decreasing frequency were retrobulbar hemorrhage, optic nerve thickening presumably secondary to edema, intraorbital emphysema, optic nerve impingement, retinal detachment, and ruptured globe. In addition to assessing the findings described previously the clinician should palpate the orbital rim for fractures (step-offs) and assess for hypoesthesia just below the eye in the distribution of the infraorbital nerve, and note the presence of hypoglobus (inferior displacement of the eye). Presence of hypoesthesia is indicative of a blowout fracture involving the infraorbital canal and nerve, but it has no urgent significance in itself.

Evaluation of ocular motility involves assessing for limitation of eye movement and eliciting symptoms consistent with decreased motility. The patient will often complain of double vision that disappears with the occlusion of one eye. Defining the orientation of the diplopia (horizontal, vertical, or oblique) can also help focus the exam. During the acute inflammatory period, ocular motility is often affected due to orbital congestion or muscle contusion, and supplementary tests can help distinguish between muscle palsy and muscle restriction or entrapment. Forced duction testing, where the eye is physically displaced using forceps to grasp the eye, can help discern the presence of mechanical restriction. A drop of anesthetic is placed on the eye and the patient is asked to look in the direction of the limited movement. The eye is then physically displaced in that direction to assess for a "tethering" effect (Figure 6). If significant resistance is encountered, entrapment must be suspected and an orbital CT should be obtained immediately. Clinical signs of entrapment supported by radiologic evidence require immediate surgical intervention to prevent muscle ischemia and necrosis.

The finding of post-traumatic proptosis requires immediate measurement of eye pressures to assess for retrobulbar hemorrhage. Proptosis and elevated intraocular pressures are indicative of an orbital compartment syndrome and an axial and coronal orbital CT should be obtained immediately (Figure 7). The findings on further examination are resistance to retropulsion, diffuse subconjunctival hemorrhage, tight eyelids and orbit, vision loss, an afferent pupillary defect, and decreased color vision. Medical therapy should be initiated immediately with pressure-lowering agents as described in the management section in this chapter, and intraocular pressure should be measured frequently to ensure the efficacy of the medical therapy. If the pressures are very high (>30) or if there is no response to

medical therapy, a lateral canthotomy and cantholysis should be performed (described in the management section). This can be performed prior to obtaining an orbital CT if pressures are significantly elevated and there is evidence of an afferent pupillary defect.[12]

The presence of an afferent pupillary defect should prompt an immediate orbital CT to rule-out the presence of bone fragments or a foreign body within the orbit impinging on the optic nerve. With evidence of this type of compression, immediate surgery must be performed to relieve the pressure on the nerve. In the absence of impingement on the optic nerve and absence of obvious lesions of the anterior visual pathway, an afferent pupillary defect is highly suggestive of traumatic optic neuropathy and a 3-day course of intravenous steroids should be instituted.[10]

There is a wide variety of imaging modalities that can be used to visualize the orbit and surrounding bony architecture. The standard head CT consisting of 4-mm sections that is obtained in the emergency setting is often inadequate to assess orbital trauma. The subtle findings of trauma to the orbit, eye and visual pathway require evaluation with 2-mm axial and coronal sections extending from the eyelids to the optic chiasm. However, signs on the routine head CT that are suggestive of orbital fracture include opacification of the paranasal sinuses, periorbital subcutaneous emphysema and surrounding soft tissue edema. Presence of these features should prompt the attainment of a full orbital series.[10] The key features of a variety of important CT findings are highlighted in Figures 8, 9, and 10.

Ocular Trauma

The most crucial aspect in evaluating direct trauma to the eye is in determining the presence of an open globe injury. With penetrating injuries, the site of rupture is usually obvious at examination and darkly pigmented uveal structures (iris and choroid) can be seen protruding through the wound (Figure 11). This can usually be seen at the bedside with the use of a penlight. With a reliable history that the penetrating object was removed from the eye intact, radiologic studies can be deferred. Given a history of a foreign body entering the eye, an orbital CT consisting of 2-mm axial and coronal sections should be obtained immediately. In this scenario, MRI is contraindicated as it may cause movement of a metallic object. The eye should be covered with a shield immediately and the remainder of the exam performed by an ophthalmologist, possibly under general anesthesia at the time of surgical repair.[1,2] The diagnosis of a ruptured globe should not be made by CT alone, although the status of the eye can

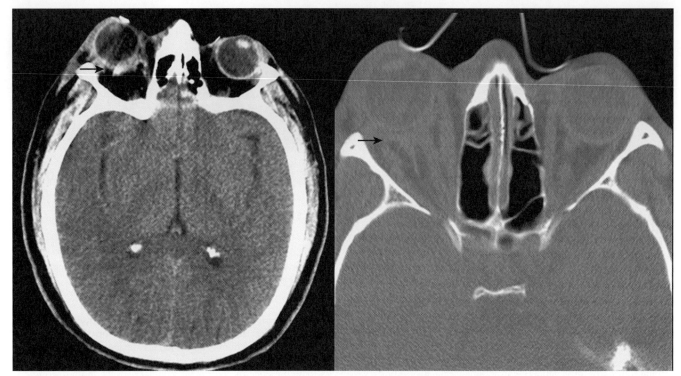

Figure 7   Male victim of blunt trauma to the right eye with significant proptosis and radiodensity posterior to the right eye on computed tomography scan (retrobulbar hemorrhage indicated by *arrows*). His intraocular pressure was measured to be 40 and was rapidly lowered to 20 with a lateral canthotomy and cantholysis.

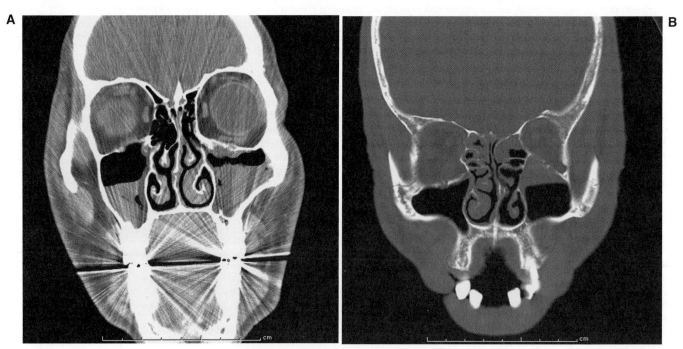

Figure 8   Bilateral orbital fractures. **(A)** Note air fluid levels in maxillary sinuses and soft tissue prolapse of the left orbit. **(B)** Left orbital fracture with orbital fat prolapse.

often be assessed based on its appearance on CT scan (Figure 12). There is a proven decrease in the rate of infection with prompt diagnosis and repair.[13] The risk of post-traumatic sympathetic ophthalmia must be considered in all ruptured globes. This condition, in which the injured "inciting" eye stimulates the formation of antibodies that can then attack the noninjured "sympathizing" eye and cause

a severe sight-threatening inflammation in the healthy eye, is estimated to be as high as 1 in 500 following an open globe injury.

The most likely areas of rupture from blunt trauma to the eye are the sites where the eye wall is thinnest, namely at the corneal-scleral junction (the limbus), at the rectus muscle insertions, and at the attachment of the optic nerve to the eye (Figure 13). However, the

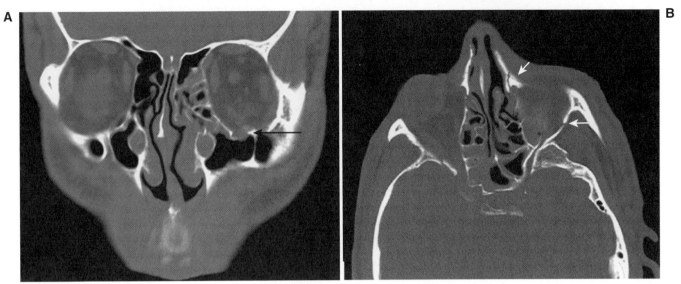

Figure 9   Left orbital fracture with muscle entrapment. **(A)** The radio-opaque muscle can be seen protruding into the "trapdoor" of the fracture *(arrow)*. **(B)** Fracture of nasal bone and lateral orbital wall *(arrows)*. The eye was intact in this case.

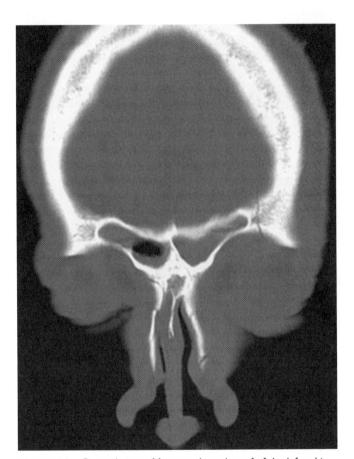

Figure 10   Coronal view of fracture through roof of the left orbit.

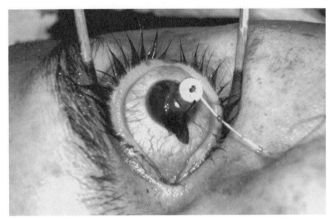

Figure 11   Patient with stun-gun probe injury to left eye. Note dark uveal tissue protruding from the cornea. This patient's eye was immediately covered with a cup and he was sent to the eye clinic for further management.

sclera may rupture posterior to the limbus in a manner that is not clearly obvious by standard slit-lamp examination. In these difficult cases, the examiner must rely on the cardinal features of occult scleral rupture to determine the need for surgical exploration of the eye. Werner et al.[5] studied 49 eyes with suspected scleral rupture and found that the factors most indicative of true rupture, as determined by surgical exploration, were visual acuity worse than 20/400, lower intraocular pressure in the traumatized eye, the presence of hyphema, an afferent pupillary defect, and vitreous hemorrhage. In using these criteria, 17 of 49 patients were found to have true ruptures at surgical exploration. The presence of hemorrhagic chemosis and a peaked pupil has also been found to be sensitive in determining the presence of occult scleral rupture. These data are similar to those of Kylstra et al.[14] The clinical finding of vitreous hemorrhage can only be confirmed by the trained ophthalmologist, often requiring ultrasound exam. This finding is important in the development of proliferative vitreoretinopathy, a fibrous proliferation within the vitreous that causes traction on the retina and predisposes to complicated retinal detachment, as established by Cleary and Ryan.[15] When taken in combination, these findings are very useful in guiding the decision for exploration and repair of a suspected scleral rupture. Figures 14 and 15 illustrate three of these key findings. Their sensitivities and specificities are summarized in Table 4.

Two particularly important subgroups of open eye injuries are those involving intraocular foreign bodies (IOFB) and the infected open eye. The presence of a foreign body places the patient at greater

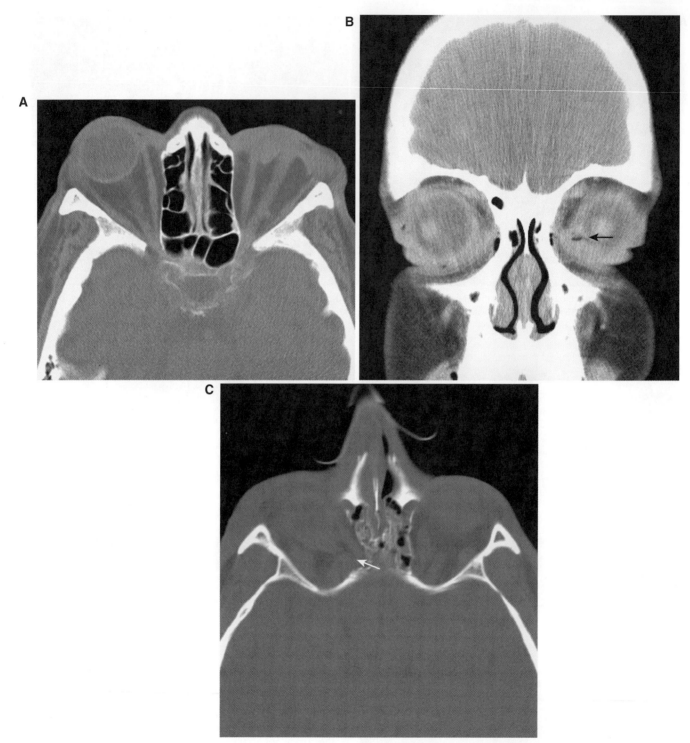

Figure 12 Three examples of globe injuries on computed tomography scan. **(A)** Flattened left eye. **(B)** Scleral rupture of left eye. **(C)** Optic nerve avulsion of right eye.

risk of infection and toxicity, and often requires emergent vitreoretinal surgery to salvage the eye. The materials can range from metals to wood and other organic objects. Orbital CT is very sensitive in detecting metallic foreign bodies (Figure 16); however, ultrasound examination should be performed on all eyes with suspected IOFB. With an obvious corneal laceration and a history of a small solid projectile to the eye, the anterior chamber angle must be carefully inspected with gonioscopic techniques.

If there is evidence of wound contamination at the time of examination (e.g., injury with plant matter), the concern for infection becomes very acute and must be managed aggressively. Post-traumatic endophthalmitis has been reported to occur in approximately 4%–8% of open globe injuries and in up to 30% of injuries in a rural setting.[16–19] The classic finding of hypopyon in an infected eye is not commonly seen in the context of a ruptured globe, as the anterior segment is often distorted and obscured by blood. The role of the trauma and emergency

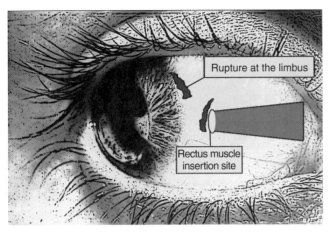

Figure 13 The most likely areas of rupture from blunt trauma to the eye. *(Artistic rendering by Narina Sokolova.)*

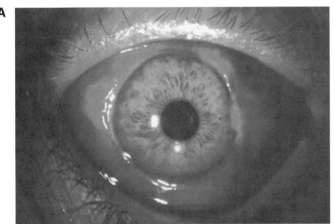

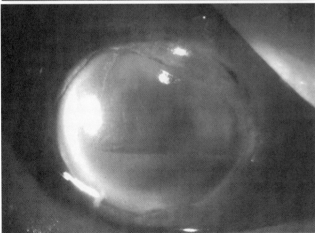

Figure 14 **(A)** Hemorrhagic chemosis. Note that the conjunctiva is elevated and boggy, not flat as seen with subconjunctival hemorrhage, a benign condition. **(B)** Hyphema of 45% elevation. These are both indicators of occult scleral rupture.

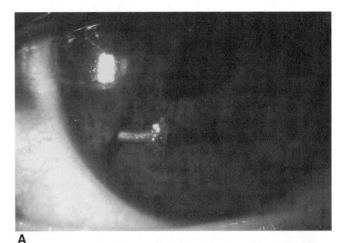

A

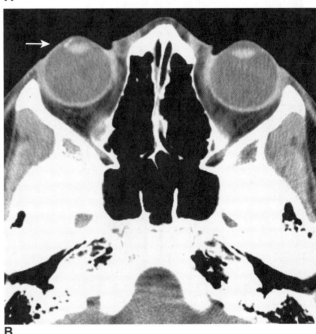

B

Figure 15 Patient with pencil lead penetration into globe (note the "peaked" pupil). Orbital CT reveals that foreign body does not extend beyond the anterior chamber *(arrow)*.

physician in this setting is as with all other open globes, to obtain in immediate ophthalmology consult and obtain an urgent orbital CT. Further management requires the expertise of eye care providers.

One of the most useful modalities in evaluating globe rupture is the ultrasound. Marked lid swelling and patient discomfort often make evaluating ocular trauma very difficult, and the examiner must take the utmost care not to further disturb the open eye. Skilled use of the

Table 4: Sensitivity and Specificity of Specific Signs in Detecting Eye Rupture

Finding	Sensitivity (%)	Specificity (%)
Vision worse than 20/400	88	47
Intraocular pressure nontraumatized eye > intraocular pressure traumatized eye	71	61
Hyphema	69	55
Afferent pupillary defect	80	56
Vitreous hemorrhage	93	38

Adapted from Werner MS, Dana MR, Viana MA, Shapiro M: Predictors of occult scleral rupture. *Ophthalmology* 101:1941-1944, 1994.

A

B

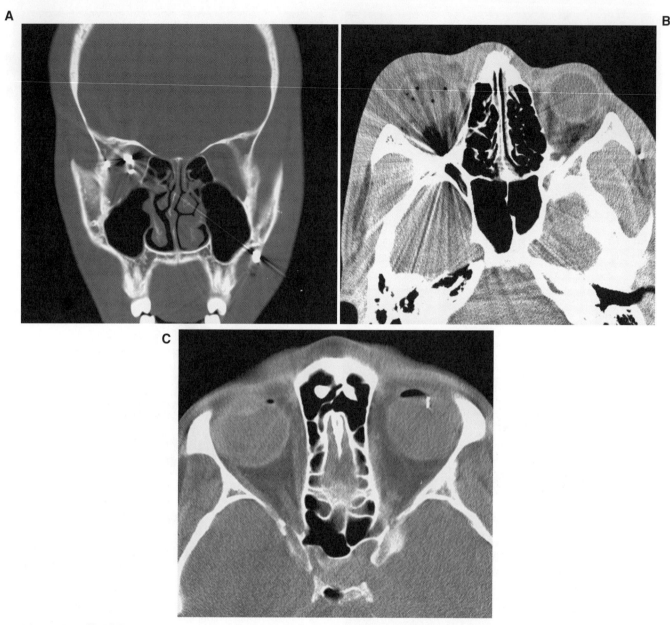

C

Figure 16 **(A, B)** Shotgun pellets in right eye. **(C)** Metallic foreign body and air in anterior chamber of left eye.

ultrasound can yield sufficient information on the status of the intra-ocular contents and on the presence of intraocular foreign bodies. The eye can be examined from the cornea to the optic nerve, through closed eyelids with virtually no pressure exerted on the globe. In the presence of hyphema or vitreous hemorrhage, the posterior pole of the eye may be difficult to view, in which case an ultrasound exam may allow thorough evaluation. Posterior scleral rupture usually presents with marked hemorrhagic chemosis and vitreous hemorrhage (Figure 17). These cases are typically occult with no external signs of rupture and normal intraocular pressure. A clue to the trajectory and ultimate location of an intraocular foreign body is the presence of a hemorrhagic tract as seen on ultrasound. By following this tract, the foreign body and its path of destruction can be tracked and defined (Figure 18). Ultrasound examination should be performed on all forms of intraocular foreign bodies, even if the foreign body has been previously localized on orbital CT (Figure 19). Ultrasound has the advantage of more precisely localizing the position of a foreign body, in assessing the intraocular contents, and in detecting foreign bodies that are not readily visible on CT scan, such as wood, glass, and plastic. Moreover, with a foreign body

that is adjacent to the scleral wall, ultrasound is able to determine whether it lies just inside or outside of the globe.[20]

Chemical and thermal burns are often associated with open eye injuries or can occur in isolation. The mainstay of treatment is copious irrigation and treatment with topical steroids and antibiotics. However, in the presence of an open globe, repair of the rupture is of primary importance and should then be followed by management of the chemical and thermal injury. The pH of the ocular surface should be tested with litmus paper and irrigation initiated promptly with a Morgan lens. Between each liter of irrigation, the pH should be reassessed and irrigation continued until the pH becomes neutral. The upper and lower fornices should be swept with a cotton swab for crystallized particles if the pH does not neutralize and lid eversion may be required to remove the particles.[12]

Acids and bases have very distinct effects on the ocular surface. Acids tend to cause denaturation and precipitation of proteins within the cornea and sclera, and a proteinaceous barrier is formed that prevents the further penetration of acids into the deeper layers. Acidic compounds rarely penetrate into the anterior chamber to cause

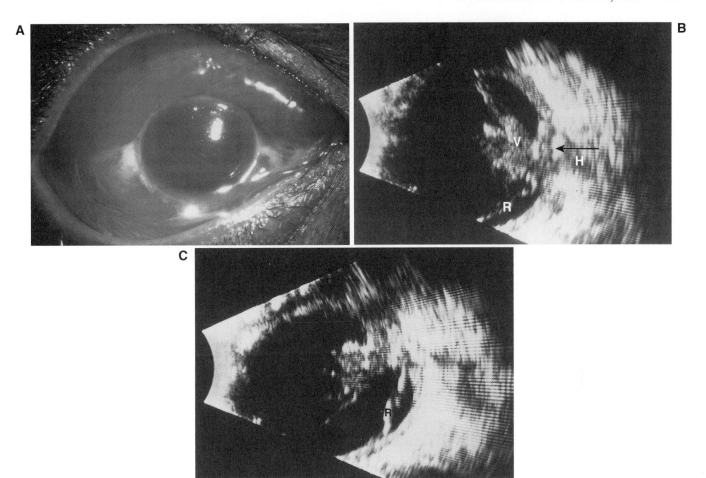

Figure 17   Scleral rupture following blunt trauma. **(A)** External photograph showing anterior chamber hyphema and hemorrhagic chemosis. **(B)** Longitudinal B-scan displays vitreous hemorrhage (V), incarceration of vitreous into scleral rupture *(arrow)*, and inferior RD (R). **(C)** Transverse B-scan view through area of scleral rupture shows vitreous incarcerated into scleral wound and RD (R). *H*, Orbital hemorrhage.   *(Courtesy Byrne SF, Green RL: Ultrasound of the Eye and Orbit, 2nd ed. St. Louis, Mosby, 2002.)*

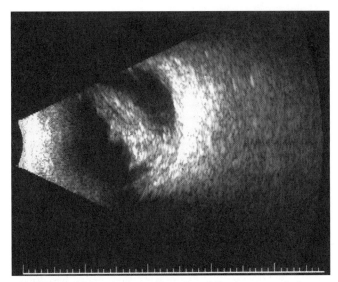

Figure 18   Hemorrhagic tract in patient following removal of stun-gun probe from the eye (see Figure 11).

further damage. On the other hand, bases have the capacity to saponify the superficial lipophilic layers of the cornea and readily penetrate the deeper tissues, frequently causing damage to the intraocular structures and leading to glaucoma and cataract.[21] The eye can appear unusually quiet and the severity of the burn is overlooked. The rule of thumb in these cases is that the quieter the appearance after a chemical burn, the worse the prognosis. This is due to the fact that the vasculature of the ocular surface has been obliterated and the eye will be deceptively blanched in appearance. Over time, the ocular surface becomes inflamed and scarred (Figure 20). These cases require extensive ocular surface reconstruction, glaucoma surgery and transplantation of the cornea to regain visual function. Aggressive irrigation within the first few minutes and hours has the most profound impact on the final outcome. Treatment with topical antibiotics and steroids in the first few days is of paramount importance. This is often initiated in the emergency/trauma setting and can be done well before the patient is seen by an eye care provider.

ANATOMIC LOCATION OF INJURY AND INJURY GRADING—OCULAR TRAUMA CLASSIFICATION GROUP

In 1996, the Ocular Trauma Classification Group established a classification of ocular trauma to standardize the definitions for physicians and researchers. One of the goals of this process was to promote the use

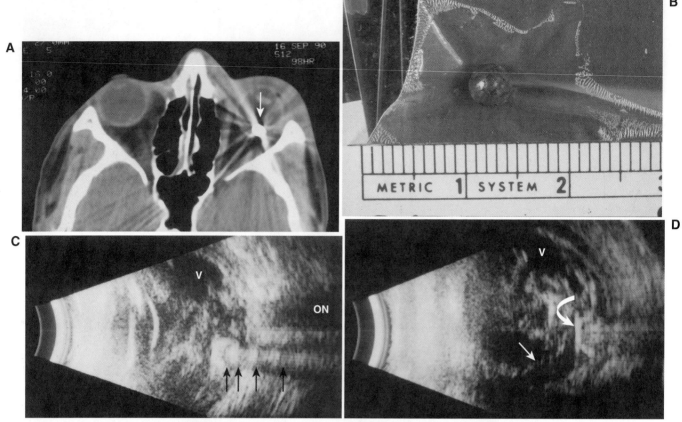

Figure 19   Intraocular subretinal BB (gunshot). **(A)** Axial computed tomography scan shows spherical foreign body *(straight white arrow)* in vicinity of posterior ocular wall. **(B)** Spherical BB removed from eye in A. **(C)** Axial B-scan view at high gain shows dense vitreous hemorrhage (V) and large, echo-dense signal from BB. Note the characteristic chain of multiple signals (comet tail artifact) produced by BB *(small black arrows)*. **(D)** Transverse B-scan at reduced gain shows RD *(straight white arrow)* and underlying BB *(curved white arrow)*.   *(Courtesy Byrne SF, Green RL:* Ultrasound of the Eye and Orbit, *2nd ed. St. Louis, Mosby, 2002.)*

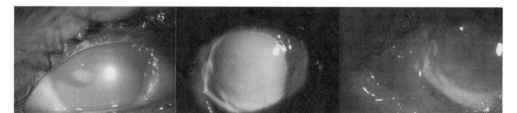

Figure 20   Patient with severe alkali burn. Note the white and quiet nature of the eye. The patient has a total corneal epithelial defect as seen with fluorescein stain and cobalt blue light. Despite aggressive management, the patient has a total burn of the ocular surface with extensive inflammation and obliteration of the fornices.

of trauma specific terminology in describing eye injuries. This classification applies to both closed and open globe injuries (Table 5).[22] Pieramici et al.[23] studied the prognostic significance of this system for classifying mechanical injuries of the eye. The four specific variables in the classification system include (1) the mechanism of injury, (2) the visual acuity in the injured eye at initial examination, (3) the presence or absence of an afferent pupillary defect in the injured eye, and (4) the location of the eye-wall opening. These variables were chosen because they have been shown to be prognostic of visual outcome, and they can be assessed clinically on initial examination or during the initial surgical procedure. The location of the eye-wall opening and the presence of an

afferent pupillary defect had the strongest prognostic value. The key recommendations for the trauma and emergency physician are to assess for visual acuity and the presence of an afferent pupillary defect. However, as previously mentioned, with an obvious rupture, the trauma surgeons and emergency physicians are urged to cover the eye with a fox shield and allow the trained ophthalmologist to perform the remainder of the exam. With a keen understanding of the findings of closed and open globe injuries, the trauma surgeons and emergency physicians should be able to appropriately categorize these eye injuries and aid the eye care provider in making effective medical and surgical management decisions.

Table 5: New Standard Classification of Ocular Trauma Terminology

Term	Definition
Eye wall	Sclera and cornea
Closed-globe injury	Eye wall does not have full-thickness corneal wound
Open-globe injury	Eye wall has full-thickness corneal wound
Rupture	Full-thickness eye wall wound caused by a blunt object; impact results in momentary increase of intraocular pressure and an inside-out injury mechanism
Laceration	Full-thickness wound of eye wall, usually caused by a sharp object; wound occurs at impact site by outside-in mechanism
Penetrating injury	Single laceration of eye wall, usually caused by sharp object
Intraocular foreign body	Retained foreign object(s) causing entrance laceration(s)
Perforating injury	Two full-thickness lacerations (entrance plus exit) of eye wall, usually caused by sharp object or missile

Source: Ryan S: *Retina*, 4th ed., vol. 3. St. Louis, Mosby, 2004, table 140-1, p. 2380.

MEDICAL AND SURGICAL MANAGEMENT

Trauma to the Orbit

Conservative medical management of orbital fractures consists of broad spectrum oral antibiotics and nasal decongestants, particularly with CT evidence of disease of the paranasal sinuses or evidence of foreign body penetration into the orbit. If the patient has no complaints of diplopia and very little restriction of ocular motility, surgical intervention is not indicated and the patient can be observed weekly. The findings that require immediate repair (within 24 hours) are the white-eyed blowout fracture (normal appearing eye with marked restriction of motility) and fractures with evidence of entrapment clinically and on CT that are associated with nonresolving bradycardia, heart block, nausea, vomiting, or syncope (the oculo-cardiac reflex). Fractures of the orbital roof, fractures associated with CSF rhinorrhea and orbital fractures associated with intracranial hemorrhage require neurosurgical evaluation, and often are repaired collaboratively by neurosurgery and ophthalmology.[12]

Retrobulbar hemorrhage is diagnosed by the presence of significant proptosis and elevated intraocular pressure in the presence of a tight orbit (very tense eyelids) and evidence of retrobulbar bleeding on orbital CT. If the clinical suspicion is high, a lateral canthotomy and cantholysis can be performed primarily and the orbital CT can be obtained afterward. Performing a lateral canthotomy and cantholysis requires application of local anesthetic and the use of toothed forceps and straight scissors. The lateral orbital rim is palpated and the tissue extending from the lateral canthal angle to the orbital rim is cut in a vertical fashion, splitting the upper and lower connection of the eyelids. The lower lid is grasped with the forcep and tension is placed on the canthal tendon. The tendon can be identified by strumming with scissors and the tendon is cut as close to the orbital rim as possible (Figure 21). The same approach is taken to locating and incising the upper canthal tendon. Many physicians take a step-wise approach to performing this procedure by cutting the lower canthal tendon and re-measuring the intraocular pressure. If the pressure normalizes by this step alone, cutting the upper canthal tendon can be deferred. Intraocular pressure lowering agents consisting of intravenous or oral carbonic anhydrase inhibitors, topical beta-blockers, and hyperosmotic agents should be initiated.[12] On completion of this procedure, there is often a release of blood from the retrobulbar space and the eye becomes even more proptotic. However, the result should be the lowering of intraocular pressure and re-establishment of normal blood flow to the eye.

The treatable causes of an afferent pupillary defect in cases of trauma include orbital compartment syndrome, mechanical optic nerve compression (by a bone fragment or foreign body), or traumatic optic neuropathy. Central retinal artery occlusion, optic nerve avulsion, and damage to the nerve within the optic canal (fracture or compression within the canal) are less amenable to medical or surgical intervention. Traumatic optic neuropathy (TON) is the diagnosis of exclusion once the other causes have been ruled-out. If TON is suspected, the recommended treatment involves intravenous Solu-Medrol, 5.4 mg/kg every 6 hours over 3 days in 12 divided doses.[12] No oral steroid taper is necessary with this regimen. This treatment has been extrapolated from the results of the spinal cord treatment trial, which showed limited benefit for recovery of function in patients who sustained spinal cord injuries when treated with systemic steroids.[24,25] Studies published in the ophthalmic literature do not conclusively show a benefit of systemic steroids in treating traumatic optic neuropathy, but this approach is widely accepted.[26] Because of the questionable benefit and significant side-effect profile, this treatment is used with the utmost caution in young children, the elderly, patients with brittle diabetes, and patients predisposed to infection.

An additional consideration in patients with orbital trauma is the presence of lacerations to the eyelids and surrounding soft tissues. Emergency physicians and trauma surgeons are capable of suturing the majority of these lacerations. Exceptions include lacerations involving the eyelid margin and the lacrimal drainage system (punctum and canaliculus) associated with ptosis (droopy eyelid) and with exposed orbital fat. Repair of these injuries must often be done in the operating room and are often associated with trauma to the eye. Consider tetanus prophylaxis and systemic antibiotics if contamination is suspected (e.g., animal bite). Fast-absorbing suture should be used for the deep aspect of the wound, and slow-absorbing suture for the superficial aspect (e.g., 6-0 Vicryl), particularly if removal after 7–10 days proves to be difficult (e.g., children or patients where follow-up may be questionable).

The immediate medical and surgical management of injury to the eye will be directed by the eye care provider. The initial examination by the emergency physicians and trauma surgeons should lead to the rapid decision to obtain an urgent eye consult and to obtain the necessary ancillary tests. Data that will be important to the anesthesiologist are the overall hemodynamic and electrolyte status, pulmonary and neurologic status, and time since last food intake. Also important to the anesthesiologist is to avoid the administration of succinylcholine in the operating room if a ruptured globe is suspected. Depolarizing paralytic agents cause constriction of the extraocular muscles which may result in the expulsion of the intraocular contents. The repair of lacerations to the eye wall are performed by an ophthalmologist and consists of careful reapproximation of the

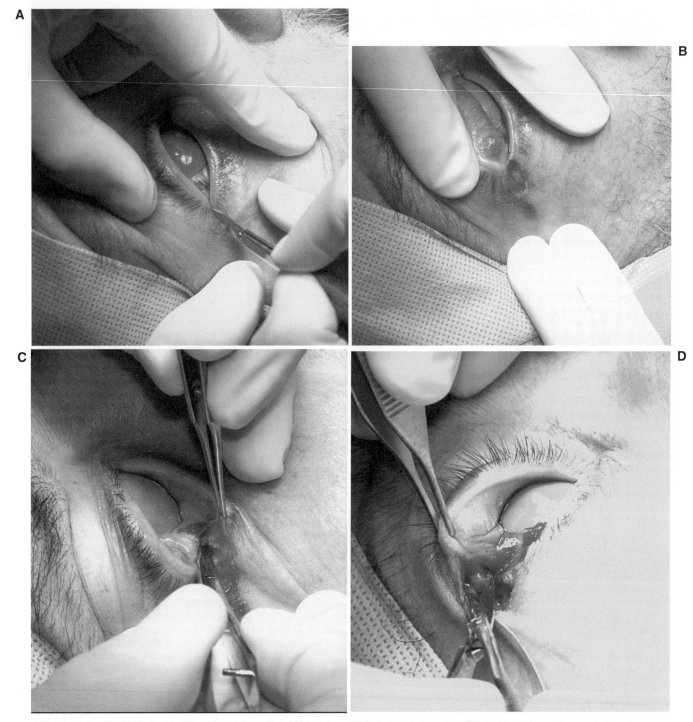

Figure 21   **(A, B)** Vertical incision of lateral canthus. **(C)** Incision of inferior canthal tendon. **(D)** Incision of superior canthal tendon.

eye wall in a manner that minimizes the degree of postoperative astigmatism and distortion of the globe and will allow further vitreo-retinal surgery if indicated (Figure 22).

CONCLUSIONS AND ALGORITHM

Although the advanced management of eye injuries requires the experience and training of an ophthalmologist, emergency physicians and trauma surgeons often make the most important decisions in the care of these patients. Below are concise summaries of these key

concepts described in this chapter for quick reference. By using this step-wise approach, the critical factors of trauma to the orbit and eye can be documented, and rapid decisions for further management can be made.

The key components of a thorough orbital and ocular exam in the trauma setting are as follows:

1. The initial examination involves the assessment of visual acuity and the presence of an afferent pupillary defect (APD). The presence of an APD (even if visual acuity is not severely affected) is a reflection of optic nerve compromise. The potentially treatable

A

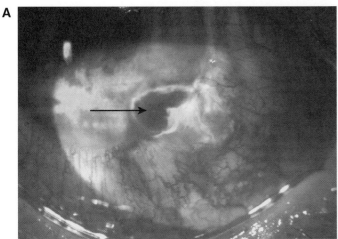

B

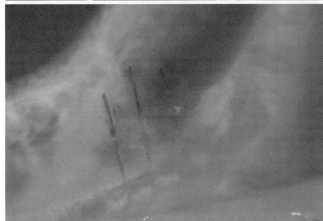

Figure 22 Patient shot with "blank" bullet and suspected plastic shell injury to left eye. Fluorescein stain shows evidence of leak of aqueous at the limbus *(arrow)* with wound extending onto cornea. No extension onto sclera was found on surgical exploration and wound was easily closed with three 10-0 nylon sutures.

causes are retrobulbar hemorrhage with elevated intraocular pressures (orbital compartment syndrome), mechanical compression by a bone fragment or foreign body within the orbit, and traumatic optic neuropathy (nerve contusion). The first two can be diagnosed within the emergency room by the trauma specialist, while the third cause is a diagnosis of exclusion with very few findings on imaging studies. The decision to obtain an orbital CT with 2 mm axial and coronal sections is straightforward in these cases. If the clinical suspicion for orbital compartment syndrome is high (significant proptosis and elevated intraocular pressure), a lateral canthotomy and cantholysis can be performed prior to obtaining imaging studies and is relatively easy to repair once the condition has been treated. Other causes of an APD that must be ruled out are central retinal artery occlusion, ischemic optic neuropathy and retinal detachment. These entities are diagnosed only with full examination of the eye.

2. The next step of the examination is to assess for an open globe injury. If rupture or perforation is seen, further examination should be deferred, and the eye should be covered with a shield. An ophthalmologic consult should be obtained immediately and the patient should be started on systemic antibiotics. The patient should be advised to avoid coughing and Valsalva-type maneuvers. Assess for signs of occult rupture: lower intraocular pressure, hyphema, APD, vitreous hemorrhage, hemorrhagic chemosis, and peaked pupil. If

rupture is not evident and intraocular pressures are normal, further ocular examination can be safely performed by the trauma physician or the ophthalmologist. Traumatic hyphema is managed with topical steroids and topical atropine 1% for 5 days. The highest rate of re-bleeding in cases of traumatic hyphema occurs in the first 5 days and the patient must be seen daily during this time. Intraocular pressure must be monitored closely and the patient is kept on low dose topical steroids until the hyphema resolves.

3. Evaluation of ocular motility is performed by asking the patient to look in the four main directions of gaze (up, down, left, right) and the eyes are observed for any limitation of movement. The patient should also be asked about double vision either when looking straight or in either direction (the double vision disappears if one eye is covered). If limitation is observed, forced duction testing can be done after placing a drop of topical anesthetic on the eye and asking the patient to look in the same direction of limitation. The physician then attempts to move the eye in the same direction with a forcep. With moderate suspicion of limitation, an immediate orbital CT should be obtained to rule out entrapment of the muscle or orbital fat. Ominous signs of entrapment include bradycardia, nausea, vomiting and syncope. Also, the quiet appearing eye with significant limitation of movement (the white-eyed blowout) is concerning in children. Oral antibiotics and nasal decongestants are recommended if there is significant disease of the paranasal sinuses (mucosal thickening) on orbital CT.[12]

4. History and presentation consistent with an intraocular foreign body (IOFB) requires an immediate orbital CT scan consisting of 2-mm axial and coronal sections. An IOFB on CT should prompt an immediate ocular ultrasound to better localize the foreign body and to assess the extent of intraocular injury. Wood, glass, and organic foreign body is better visualized on ultrasound than orbital CT (i.e., the absence of an obvious IOFB on CT scan does not rule out wood, glass, or organic matter). The ultrasound must be performed by experienced personnel as this must be done with the utmost care so as not to further disrupt the open eye. An immediate eye consult must be obtained and the patient should be started on systemic antibiotics and must remain NPO for anticipated surgery.

5. Evidence of chemical burn requires the measurement of the pH of the ocular surface and initiation of irrigation if an abnormal pH is detected. The physician must be aware that a white, quiet eye following a chemical burn is an ominous sign and must be managed urgently. Continuous irrigation with lactated Ringer's or balanced saline solution is initiated and continued until the repeat pH is normal. Thermal burns must be assessed for direct burn to the eye and managed with antibiotics and lubrication as needed. Burns involving only the eyelids must be monitored until the skin is healed, as contracture may occur and the eye can become exposed. In this setting, lubrication is the mainstay of treatment.

6. The presence of enophthalmos (posterior displacement of the eye) is an indicator of a large fracture of the orbital walls and will require early surgical repair. With a fracture involving more than 50% of the floor, it is assumed that enophthalmos will develop and these patients are scheduled for surgery within 1–2 weeks of injury. The other signs of orbital fracture should be thoroughly assessed (hypoesthesia of the cheek below the eye, bony "step-off" of the orbital rim, and limitation of eye movements).

The points described in this chapter will serve as useful guidelines in assessing the majority of eye trauma cases that present in the emergency room or to trauma surgeons. Additional considerations in the trauma setting involve that of nonaccidental trauma in children (shaken-baby syndrome), Horner's syndrome associated with intracranial and neck injury, aneurysmal compressions affecting the cranial nerves to the eye, and the occasional case of carotid-cavernous fistula that can occur in relation to trauma. Although saving the sight of a severely injured patient may seem of secondary concern in the acute setting, it becomes of primary importance once the patient has recovered and is trying to regain normal activity and function.

REFERENCES

1. Harlan JB Jr, Pieramici DJ: Evaluation of patients with ocular trauma. *Ophthalmol Clin North Am* 15:153–161, 2002.
2. Runyan TE: Ophthalmic considerations in the severely injured patient. *Surg Clin North Am* 62:301–308, 1982.
3. McGwin G Jr, Xie A, Owsley C: Rate of eye injury in the United States. *Arch Ophthalmol* 123:970–976, 2005.
4. McGwin G Jr, Owsley C: Incidence of emergency department-treated eye injury in the United States. *Arch Ophthalmol* 123:662–666, 2005.
5. Werner MS, Dana MR, Viana MA, Shapiro M: Predictors of occult scleral rupture. *Ophthalmology* 101:1941–1944, 1994.
6. Baker RS, Wilson RM, Flowers CW Jr, et al: A population-based survey of hospitalized work-related ocular injury: diagnoses, cause of injury, resource utilization, and hospitalization outcome. *Ophthalmic Epidemiol* 6:159–169, 1999.
7. McGwin G Jr, Owsley C: Risk factors for motor vehicle collision-related eye injuries. *Arch Ophthalmol* 123:89–95, 2005.
8. Shere JL, Boole JR, Holtel MR, Amoroso PJ: An analysis of 3599 midfacial and 1141 orbital blowout fractures among 4426 United States Army Soldiers, 1980–2000. *Otolaryngol Head Neck Surg* 130:164–170, 2004.
9. Yanoff M, Duker JS: Ophthalmology, 2nd ed. St. Louis, Mosby, 2004.
10. Lee HJ, Jilani M, Frohman L, Baker S: CT of orbital trauma. *Emerg Radiol* 10:168–172, 2004.
11. Tasman W, Jaeger EA, editors: *Duane's Clinical Ophthalmology.* Philadelphia, Lippincott Williams & Wilkins, 2004.
12. Kanitkar KD, Makar M, editors: *The Wills Eye Manual,* 4th ed. Philadelphia, Lippincott Williams & Wilkins, 2004.
13. Essex RW, Yi Q, Charles PG, Allen PJ: Post-traumatic endophthalmitis. *Ophthalmology* 111:2015–2022, 2004.
14. Kylstra JA, Lamkin JC, Runyan DK: Clinical predictors of scleral rupture after blunt ocular trauma. *Am J Ophthalmol* 115:530–535, 1993.
15. Cleary PE, Ryan SJ: Mechanisms in traction retinal detachment. *Dev Ophthalmol* 2:328–333, 1981.
16. Boldt HC, Pulido JS, Blodi CF, et al: Rural endophthalmitis. *Ophthalmology* 96:1722–1726, 1989.
17. Lieb DF, Scott IU, Flynn HW Jr, et al: Open globe injuries with positive intraocular cultures: factors influencing final visual acuity outcomes. *Ophthalmology* 110:1560–1566, 2003.
18. Thompson JT, Parver LM, Enger CL, et al: Infectious endophthalmitis after penetrating injuries with retained intraocular foreign bodies. *Ophthalmology* 100:1468–1474, 1993.
19. Thompson WS, Rubsamen PE, Flynn HW, et al: Endophthalmitis after penetrating trauma: risk factors and visual acuity outcomes. *Ophthalmology* 102:1696–1701, 1995.
20. Frazier Byrne S, Green RL: *Ultrasound of the Eye and Orbit,* 2nd ed. St. Louis, Mosby, 2002.
21. American Academy of Ophthalmology: Basic *Clinical Science Course. Vol. 8: External Disease and Cornea.* San Francisco, American Academy of Ophthalmology, 2005.
22. Ryan SJ, editor: *Retina,* 4th ed., vol. 3. Philadelphia, Elsevier/Mosby, 2006.
23. Pieramici DJ, Sternberg P Jr, Aaberg TM Sr, et al: A system for classifying mechanical injuries of the eye (globe). The Ocular Trauma Classification Group. *Am J Ophthalmol* 123:820–831, 1997.
24. Bracken MB, Shepard MJ, Collins WF Jr, et al: Methylprednisolone or naloxone treatment after acute spinal cord injury: 1-year follow-up data. Results of the second National Acute Spinal Cord Injury Study. *J Neurosurg* 76:23–31, 1992.
25. Bracken MB, Shepard MJ, Holford TR, et al: Methylprednisolone or tirilazad mesylate administration after acute spinal cord injury: 1-year follow-up. Results of the third National Acute Spinal Cord Injury randomized controlled trial. *J Neurosurg* 89:699–706, 1998.
26. Steinsapir KD, Goldberg RA: Traumatic optic neuropathy. *Surv Ophthalmol* 38:487–518, 1994.

Penetrating Neck Injuries: Diagnosis and Selective Management

Leonard J. Weireter   and   L. D. Britt

The neck has been a source of tremendous interest in the trauma surgical literature for several hundred years. Its anatomic compactness places vital anatomic structures in close proximity to each other making the patient prone to multisystem injuries as the result of a single traumatic event. The debate about the proper treatment of neck trauma has persisted since the 16th century when Ambroise Paré reportedly attended to a victim of a laceration to the common carotid artery and internal jugular vein sustained in a duel. While Paré's patient survived, he was rendered hemiplegic and aphasic. Complications still highlight discussions today regarding the appropriateness of aggressive surgical management of penetrating cervical injuries.

ANATOMY OF THE NECK

The neck contains a number of important structures all in close proximity. The carotid artery and the internal jugular vein are juxtaposed immediately deep to the sternocleidomastoid muscle. The pharynx and its junction with the esophagus at the level of the cricopharyngeus musculature are immediately deep to the larynx and the trachea. The thyroid gland and the associated parathyroids are located in the anterior neck overlying the upper trachea. The thoracic duct is well protected as it traverses the neck and enters the jugular-subclavian system in the left neck deep to the sternocleidomastoid muscle. The cervical vertebra and the spinal cord are the most posterior structures except for the long cervical musculature.

The neck is conventionally divided into a series of triangles.[1] Most surgical discussions center on the anatomy of the anterior triangles which encompass the area between the sternocleidomastoid muscles. Functionally, the neck is divided into three zones (Figure 1). The boundaries for zone 1 include the cricoid cartilage (superiorly), the thoracic inlet (interiorly), and the sternocleidomastoid (laterally). Its surgical significance is the fact that this zone encompasses the major cervicothoracic vasculature, along with components of the aero-digestive tract. Zone III is the horizontal region of the neck cephalad to the angle of the mandible which superior border is the base of skull. It is important to note that the internal carotid artery which is cephalad to the angle of the mandible is not readily accessible surgically, necessitating special maneuvers to achieve vascular control (e.g., surgical dislocation of the mandible). However, zone II (the area between the cricoid cartilage and the angle of the mandible), is readily accessible with the most direct surgical approach being achieved with an incision along the anterior border of the sternocleidomastoid muscle (Figure 2).

INITIAL EVALUATION

The initial evaluation of the patient suffering neck injury should be dictated by the Advanced Trauma Life Support® guidelines. Such guidelines provide a management framework to expeditiously identify life-threatening injuries and appropriately prioritize treatment. Presentations which warrant urgent surgical intervention, usually referred to as "hard signs" (Table 1) of neck injury, include subcutaneous emphysema, expanding and/or pulsatile hematoma, or brisk bleeding from the wound. All are overt findings suggestive of a major vascular or aero-digestive tract injury. Diagnostic studies are not essential for these presentations. Optimal airway management is always the first priority.

Without the "hard signs" of injury and, consequently, a need for immediate surgical intervention, a more selective or expectant approach can be initiated. The armamentarium of this selective approach include esophagoscopy, esophagography, laryngoscopy/tracheoscopy, arteriography, or Doppler ultrasonography. Although subtle findings (so-called "soft signs"—see Table 1) such as difficulty speaking or change in voice tone could prompt such a selective evaluation, the major controversy centers around whether patients with zone II injury and no "hard findings" should undergo selective management or just observation (expectant management).

A detailed neurologic examination is required for all cervical injuries. Penetrating wounds should never be explored locally. This maneuver should only be done in the operating theater as part of a formal neck exploration. In order to limit patient gagging and coughing, insertion of nasogastric tubes or nasal tracheal suctioning should be withheld, if possible, until the induction of anesthesia in the operating theater.

AERO-DIGESTIVE INJURY

Simultaneous injuries of the airway and digestive tract are not uncommon due to the close proximity of the trachea and esophagus in the neck. According to Asensio and associates,[2] aero-digestive tract injuries are seen in 10% of penetrating injuries. As highlighted previously, optimal airway management is the top priority.

In a patient who requires urgent airway management, the translaryngeal endotracheal approach is still the best option, particularly

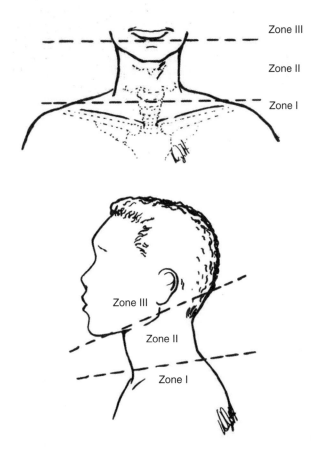

Figure 1   Zones of the neck for injury stratification.   *(Drawing by Doris Holloman.)*

when it is performed by skilled practitioners.[3] The role of the surgical airway should always be considered when approaching any patient who might have a difficult airway for conventional management. However, someone who is an expert with airway management should make an attempt at rapid translaryngeal endotracheal intubation. The surgical airway of choice in a true emergency setting is a cricothyroidotomy. A tracheostomy should only be considered in the adult when there is an urgent need for an airway in a patient who you suspect might have

a partial laryngo-tracheal separation. Even in that setting, an attempt should be made, if possible, by an airway expert to perform a careful translaryngeal endotracheal intubation (Figure 3).

After achieving airway control, and if a selective management approach is chosen, the available modalities include flexible fiber-optic laryngoscopy, flexible esophagoscopy, flexible bronchoscopy and contrast esophagography. Using a water-soluble contrast agent and multiple views of the esophagus, extravasation can be safely excluded. The 85% sensitivity and specificity of this study can be increased to near 100% by the addition of esophagoscopy.[6] With increased experience with flexible fiber-optic scopes and enhanced technology, dependence on the use of contrast studies has lessened. Visualization of the proximal 3–5 cm of the cervical esophagus immediately inferior to the cricopharyngeal constrictor is critical for this area can be easily missed during scope insertion and withdrawal. This area has to be specifically inspected.

While direct laryngoscopy should be used to determine if there is a laryngeal injury, fiber-optic bronchoscopy is used for detection of a tracheal or bronchial injury. Alternatively, computed tomography (CT) scan of the neck may identify injuries that require further investigation or operative intervention.

If a tracheal injury is found, it should be repaired by interrupted absorbable suture reapproximating the lacerated trachea after appropriate debridement of devitalized tissue. An accompanying tracheostomy is often not needed unless there is a complex injury.

For suspected laryngeal injuries, fiber-optic endoscopy is the diagnostic procedure of choice and can be combined with surgical exploration depending on the preference of the evaluating team and the suspicion for more severe injury. Laryngeal injury, including the thyroid cartilage, vocal cords, and the arytenoid processes, may require specialized reconstruction. The grading system (Table 2) advocated by Bent et al.[5] details their retrospective experience over an 18-year period with laryngeal injuries. The emphasis is on securing an adequate airway and addressing all associated life-threatening injuries. With laryngeal injuries, airway control is best obtained by performing a tracheostomy. Treatment delay in laryngeal injuries beyond 48 hours can lead to inferior results. However, the delay often reflects the fact that the patient is severely injured and is unable to undergo definitive management. Mucosal coaptation and fracture reduction should be performed at the time of initial exploration.

Injury to the cervical esophagus can be difficult to diagnose and result in the development of a fulminant mediastinitis. Weigelt and associates[6] reported only 7 of 10 injured patients with signs or symptoms of the esophageal injury. The authors noted that there is a false-negative rate of approximately 20% for either

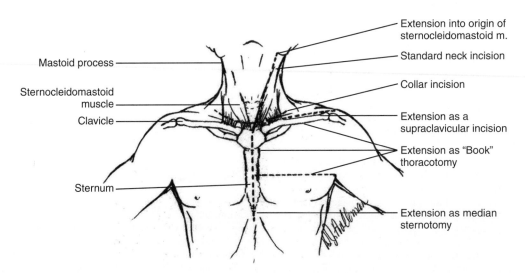

Figure 2   Incisions for operative exposure of penetrating neck injuries.   *(Drawing by Doris Holloman.)*

Table 1: Signs of Penetrating Neck Injury

Hard Signs	Soft Signs
Active bleeding	Dysphagia
Expanding or pulsatile hematoma	Voice change
Subcutaneous emphysema or air bubbling from wound	Hemoptysis
	Wide mediastinum

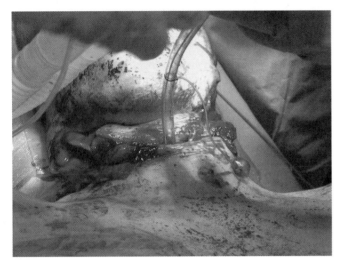

Figure 3 Neck wound sustained during an altercation. Note that the airway is established by direct intubation of the lacerated trachea through the wound. Maintaining the patient in the sitting position until intubation is accomplished facilitates airway exposure and minimizes the risk of drowning in secretions.

Table 2: Laryngeal Injury Classification

Group 1	Minor endolaryngeal hematoma or laceration without detectable fracture
Group 2	Edema, hematoma, minor mucosal disruption without exposed cartilage, nondisplaced fractures noted on computed tomography scan
Group 3	Massive edema, mucosal tears, exposed cartilage, cord immobility, displaced fractures
Group 4	Same as group 3 with more than two fracture lines or massive trauma to laryngeal mucosa
Group 5	Complete laryngotracheal separation

Source: Bent JP, Silver JR, Porubsky ES: Acute laryngeal trauma: a review of 77 patients. *Otolaryngol Head Neck Surg* 109:441–449, 1993.

endoscopy or esophagography. When the two procedures were combined in evaluation, the false-negative rate decreased to 0%. Armstrong et al.[7] reported a retrospective series of 23 patients with penetrating cervical esophageal injury. Contrast esophograms were only 62% sensitive, while rigid esophagoscopy was 100% sensitive. With advanced fiber-optic technology and greater operative experience, flexible endoscopy has essentially supplanted rigid esophagoscopy.

Most esophageal injuries require the basic surgical principles. Minimal debridement precedes primary closure, which should be done in two layers. An inner absorbable is followed by an outer

nonabsorbable suture layer. For concomitant tracheal and esophageal wounds, interposition of viable endogenous tissues, such as muscle flaps, is essential. Complications of treatment, such as esophageal stenosis, tracheo-esophageal fistula, and infection are frequent.

Injury to the pharynx, often subtle, requires simple primary repair and drainage.

SOFT TISSUE INJURY

Care of the soft tissue follows the same principles of debridement of devitalized skin. Although primary closure can be done, constructing a flap or free tissue graft may be required in order to provide adequate soft tissue coverage, especially in large, open wounds. Penetrating wounds to the thyroid are best controlled by suture ligature although lobectomy may be warranted depending on the degree of hemorrhage, devascularization, and tissue destruction. Identified injuries to major nerves of the neck or brachial plexus should be tagged for future repair.

THORACIC DUCT INJURY

Injury at the base of the left neck risks laceration of the thoracic duct. Soft tissue injury and bleeding make identifying this injury difficult. Therefore, the classic chylous drainage may not be readily apparent at the time of initial surgical exploration.

VASCULAR INJURY IN THE NECK

In the early 20th century during U.S. military campaigns, major vascular injuries of the neck had very poor outcomes. A 30% neurologic deficit rate was reported after World War I when carotid injuries were treated by ligation.[8] It was not until the 1950s and the military experience in Korea with vascular repair that carotid injury repairs became popular. The superior results were quickly appreciated, and a more aggressive management approach focusing on diagnosis and repair of vascular injuries was established.[9] The first civilian report of carotid injuries appeared in 1956 when Fogelman and Stewart[10] concluded that operative intervention was necessary and that mortality increased the longer surgery was delayed. This report was the basis for mandatory exploration of the neck as the standard of care for the next two decades.

Reports challenging the mandatory exploration for penetrating central neck injuries began being widely published in the mid-70s. Sheely and colleagues[11] reported a series of 632 cases of penetrating neck injuries that still supported mandatory exploration but acknowledged that selected patients might be observed safely, provided they are treated by experienced personnel. Contrary opinion was presented by Saletta et al.,[12] who reported a series of 246 patients that underwent mandatory neck exploration. While the negative exploration rate was high at 63%, morbidity was low and there was no mortality. Although they had negative clinical evaluations, 13 patients had findings at exploration of major injury. Mandatory exploration was thought to be justified. Concurring with this logic, Bishara et al.[13] reported a series where 53% of the patients underwent mandatory exploration and had normal operative findings. However, 23% of the patients had injuries that were not suspected on preoperative clinical evaluation. These were most often isolated venous injuries or isolated pharyngoesophageal injuries. Surgical exploration for a zone II injury was felt to be safe and appropriate. Nevertheless, the high negative exploration rates noted with mandatory neck exploration prompted several institutions to question this approach. Elerding[14] and coworkers reported a series with a 56% negative exploration rate on the basis of a mandatory exploration policy. All the patients with injuries were noted to have clinical signs suggestive of injury preoperatively. Selective exploration was felt to be a legitimate option in the evaluation and management of these patients.

Jurkovich et al.[15] reported that the diagnostic yield of combined angiographic and fluorographic studies of the vascular and aerodigestive anatomy was 23%. Only 9% of patients benefited from such studies. Using the zone of injury to determine the management approach, Jurkovich advocated aggressive use of angiography, chest radiographs and esophagography for zone I injury and angiography for zone III. It was emphasized that zone II injuries could be safely observed, if the patients were asymptomatic. Additional support for a more selective approach to the management of these injuries was published by Obeid and associates[16] who, in a retrospective review, concluded that mandatory exploration should be supplanted by a selective management policy. The rationale behind this support was predicated on several findings, including the fact that missed injuries still occurred with mandatory explorations and that there was morbidity associated with negative exploration and considerable number of hospital days. Obeid et al.[16] felt that patients with "hard signs" of injury needed operative intervention, while those patients with negative physical examinations could be observed. Patients with equivocal findings on physical examination or with changing findings needed ancillary diagnostic studies to determine whether any clinically significant injuries exist. Additional support for a selective exploration policy was published by Belinke et al.[17] In this study, 44 patients were treated with a selective exploration policy, based on physical findings. Twenty-two patients underwent immediate exploration with a negative exploration rate of 23%. In the group of patients observed, there were no delayed operations or complications. If all the patients had been subject to immediate exploration, the negative exploration rate would have been 60%, prompting the authors to advocate a selective approach to penetrating zone II injuries.

Metzdorff and colleagues,[18] who also endorsed a selective management theme, reported 83 patients with a 56% negative exploration rate. When clinical signs of injury were noted preoperatively, an injury was found in 82% of the patients. If the preoperative physical examination was negative, there were no injuries found in 80% of the patients.

In 1987, Meyer and associates[19] reported a prospective trial of 120 patients with penetrating neck wounds. Seven patients underwent emergency exploration for hemorrhage. The remaining patients underwent arteriography, upper aero-digestive endoscopy, and esophagography plus surgical exploration. Five patients were found to have six major vascular injuries that were not expected preoperatively. The authors concluded that selective management missed too many major vascular injuries and that mandatory exploration was a more prudent approach.

Wood and colleagues[20] advocated selective management based on presenting physical findings. Equivocal findings required diagnostic studies to clarify the need for surgical exploration. In a similar argument, Narrod and Moore[21] confirmed the safety and efficacy of selective management of these patients. Mansour et al.[22] endorsed selective nonoperative management when it was determined that only one patient in a cohort of 119 patients required a delayed operation for an occult injury.

Beitsch et al.[23] reported a retrospective review of penetrating wounds to the neck. A negative physical examination ruled out 99% of the vascular injuries. Seventy-one angiograms were performed. Only one patient required operative repair. In the light of a normal physical examination, mandatory exploration and the role of angiographic evaluation were questioned.

Scalfani and colleagues[24] reported on a study of proximity angiograms, and noted that physical examination had a sensitivity of 61% and a specificity of 80%. The authors argued that not incorporating proximity angiography in the evaluation of penetrating neck injuries was premature. However, Menawat et al.[25] reported that in a series of 110 patients with penetrating neck injuries, only one patient had an injury not predicted by physical examination findings. Nine arterial

injuries were treated nonoperatively without sequelae. Atteberry and coworkers[26] reported on a prospective study of 66 patients which highlighted that in the absence of definitive or "hard signs" of vascular injury, these patients could be safely watched. Sekharan et al.[27] reported a missed injury rate of 0.7% with physical examination alone. Also, Jarvik et al.[28] reported that physical examination was sensitive and specific enough for detecting clinically significant vascular injuries. Physical examination had a sensitivity of 93.7%. Azuaje and associates'[29] series of penetrating neck injuries demonstrated a sensitivity and negative predictive value of 100% for physical examination in detecting surgically significant vascular injuries. When considering injuries detected by angiography, physical examination showed a sensitivity of 93% and a negative predictive value of 97%. No patient in this series with a negative physical examination required a vascular repair, regardless of the zone of injury.

Referring specifically to zone III wounds, Ferguson et al.[30] reports a series of 72 patients with penetrating wounds. The absence of "hard signs" reliably excluded surgically significant injuries. Sixty percent of the patients with "hard signs" of injury were explored. Only one patient in this group had no identifiable injury. The remainder of the patients with "hard signs" of injury underwent emergent angiography with endovascular angiographic treatment. The authors recommended that zone III injuries with "hard signs" of vascular injury should undergo angiography, as they may be amenable to endovascular intervention.

A variety of complementary diagnostic modalities have been proposed as adjuncts to the evaluation of penetrating neck injuries. Ginzburg et al.[31] demonstrated, in a prospective double-blind evaluation of angiography and duplex scanning in stable patients with zone I, II, or III penetrating wounds, that duplex scans had 100% sensitivity and 85% specificity.

Newer imaging modalities have emerged. Munera and colleagues[32] prospectively studied 60 patients, and reported that helical CT had a sensitivity of 90%, a specificity of 100%, a positive predictive value of 100%, and a negative predictive value of 98%. The authors concluded that helical CT was an excellent diagnostic study in the evaluation of neck injuries. Also, Mazolewski et al.[33] performed a prospective evaluation of 14 stable patients with penetrating zone II injuries. All patients underwent thorough physical examination, infusion CT scan, and operative exploration. Three of the 14 patients had five injuries. Those patients had a high probability for injury based on the CT scan findings. Although a small sample size, results indicated that the CT scan had a sensitivity of 100%, specificity of 91%, positive predictive value of 75%, and negative predictive value of 100%. The authors felt that the CT scan should play a pivotal role in the evaluation of neck injuries. Gracias and coworkers[34] conducted a retrospective series of 23 patients evaluated by CT scan for penetrating neck trauma that spanned all three zones. All the patients lacked "hard signs" of vascular or aero-digestive injury. Thirteen patients had the trajectory of injury remote from important structures identified and no further evaluation carried out. There were no adverse events. Gonzalez et al.[35] reported on a prospective study of computed tomography in patients with zone II penetrating wounds without "hard signs" of injury necessitating immediate exploration. The authors concluded that CT added little to the information obtained by physical examination with zone II injuries.

Hollingsworth et al.[36] conducted a meta-analysis of computed tomographic angiography (CTA) for detection of carotid and vertebral lesions of either atherosclerotic or traumatic origin. It was concluded that there were insufficient high-quality data to comment on the sensitivity or specificity of CTA for trauma.

Woo and colleagues[37] studied patients with zone II penetrating wounds who underwent CTA as a diagnostic test. They reported that with increase utilization of CTA and enhanced staff experience, there was an associated decrease in the number of negative neck explorations. The authors highlighted that with this imaging, wound tracts could be visualized. This could assist in determining if other diagnostic studies would be needed. For example, the CT could show that the injury tract was away from any major structure thus obviating any further investigation. Alternatively, an injury may be demonstrated and surgical exploration or conventional angiography for endovascular intervention could be performed. Finally, an indeterminate study may prompt other investigations depending on the finding in question.

Angiography has been advocated for zone I injuries at the base of the neck because injury in the thoracic outlet would be difficult to diagnose and control. Eddy et al.[38] conducted a multi-institutional retrospective study surveying patients over a 10-year period. A total of 138 patients were studied and 28 arterial injuries were found. However, the group concluded that in the presence of a normal physical examination and a normal chest radiograph, angiographic study may not be needed.

Gasparri and associates[39] confirmed this finding after conducting a retrospective review of 100 patients. All patients with "hard signs" of vascular injury were taken for expeditious surgical exploration. Eighty-one patients without "hard signs" of injury underwent angiography, and 11 occult injuries were discovered. When a normal physical examination and a normal chest radiograph are combined, they have a sensitivity of 100%, a specificity of 80%, a positive predictive value of 40%, and a negative predictive value of 100%. The group concluded that proximity alone does not mandate angiography.

A prospective trial by Demetriades et al.[40] evaluating the role of physical examination in penetrating neck wounds demonstrated that the lack of hard clinical signs of vascular or aero-digestive injury had a negative predictive value of 100% and reliably excluded all such wounds needing operative repair. The algorithm used by this group specifically looked for physical examination information regarding vascular and aero-digestive injury. Asymptomatic patients were observed safely.

Our own approach is outlined in the algorithm in Figure 4. Patients presenting with "hard signs" of vascular or aero-digestive injury go immediately to the operating room for neck exploration. The surgical approach is at the discretion of the attending surgeon. Patients without "hard signs" are observed. Recently, we have

incorporated helical CT to evaluate such patients. If the wound tract is obviously away from major structures of concern, no specific therapy is initiated. Our results do not support that CT has offered a substantial advantage over astute physical examination at this time.

What is clear is that a policy of mandatory surgical exploration of the neck for penetrating zone II wounds will result in a high negative exploration rate. Routine use of ancillary diagnostic procedures (selective approach) will result in a large expenditure of time and effort and appears to offer no advantage over expectant management only. The presence of "hard signs" of vascular and/or aero-digestive injuries requires surgical exploration. Less overt signs of vascular or aero-digestive injury can be evaluated at the discretion of the surgical team. Astute physical examination directed at signs of vascular injury will detect the overwhelming majority of patients needing surgical exploration and repair. The role of CT or CT angiography is evolving but appears to offer little benefit compared with thorough physical examination.

TREATMENT OF CAROTID ARTERY INJURIES

The surgical approach to the cervical vasculature is predicated on the zone of injury. Zone II injuries are best approached via an incision along the anterior border of the sternocleidomastoid muscle with the head turned to the opposite side. Placement of a towel roll under the patient's shoulders is very helpful. Dissection along this line will encounter the common facial vein, which can be sacrificed, and will allow complete visualization of the common carotid artery, the carotid bulb, the proximal internal carotid and the external carotid arteries, and the internal jugular vein. Carotid arterial injuries are best treated by surgical repair. The use of a vein patch taken from adjacent facial vein or Gortex™ is an alternative to direct suture repair. Shunts are not routinely used in these circumstances. When to repair versus ligate is complicated by the poor ability to discriminate between severe ischemia and evolving infarction. Patients with fixed neurologic deficits do poorly with revascularization. Injuries distal in the common carotid may require special maneuvers to gain access for repair. Disarticulation of the temporomandibular joint allowing forward displacement of the mandible will allow access to the internal carotid cephalad to the angle of the mandible. The skull base is not surgically accessible and may require interventional techniques to control. Injuries to the proximal internal carotid not amenable to repair may benefit from ligation of the proximal external carotid and utilization of it as a conduit for restoration of internal carotid flow. Pro-grade flow in the carotid at the time of surgical exploration is a good indication for repair. In the absence of pro-grade flow ligation may be preferable. Ligation of the injured carotid should be reserved only for those patients with devastating neurologic injuries. Liekweg and Greenfield's[41] review of the literature demonstrated less morbidity and mortality in the revascularization group compared to the ligation group. Unger et al.[42] and Brown et al.[43] in separate reports confirm this recommendation for revascularization over ligation.

Lacerations of the internal jugular are best treated by lateral venography although ligation is a reasonable alternative especially when dealing with injuries than near completely transect the vein or will result in narrowing greater than 50% of the luminal diameter. Injuries that extend proximally into the thoracic outlet are amenable to surgical exposure by extending the anterior sternocleidomastoid incision as a median sternotomy or a thoracic trapdoor incision. This allows in continuity access to the aortic arch and the take off of the carotid and subclavian vessels if needed. Likewise the supraclavicular fossa can be explored by an extension of the anterior neck incision laterally. This may facilitate exposure of the subclavian vessels or vertebral take-off if necessary.

An extended collar incision, as used for thyroid or parathyroid procedures, can be used for bilateral neck explorations. Transcervical

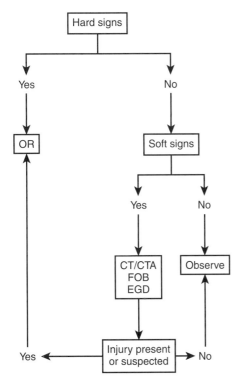

Figure 4 Algorithm for evaluation of penetrating neck wounds.

gunshot wounds with the potential for bilateral vascular injury might be better approached through this incision as bilateral control is easy to obtain from one position. This incision may need to be moved cephalad in the neck to facilitate exposure on occasions.

The role of endovascular therapy for penetrating cervical wounds involving the subclavian, carotid and vertebral vessels is evolving. Experience gained in the treatment of atherosclerotic diseases will, undoubtedly, spill over into injury care but currently there is insufficient experience to broadly endorse its application. Also, the use of endoluminal stents requires lifelong patient follow-up.

CONCLUSION

Penetrating neck wounds still present serious challenges in diagnosis and management. Astute physical examination with attention to the overt findings of vascular and aero-digestive injury "hard signs" appears to be the most efficient approach to evaluation of penetrating neck injuries. Surgical therapy is usually straightforward although endovascular approaches are evolving. In the absence of the "hard signs" of injury, careful observation with or without additional diagnostic studies can be a very successful strategy.

REFERENCES

1. Basmajian JV, editor: *Grant's Method of Anatomy,* 9th ed. Philadelphia, Williams and Wilkins, 1975.
2. Asensio JA, Valenziano CP, Falcone RE, et al: Management of penetrating neck injuries: the controversy surrounding zone II injuries. *Surg Clin North Am* 71:267–296, 1991.
3. Mandavia DP, Qualls S, Rokos I: Emergency airway management in penetrating neck injury. *Ann Emerg Med* 35(3):221–225, 2000.
4. Shearer VA, Giesecke AH: Airway management for patients with penetrating neck trauma: a retrospective study. *Anesth Analg* 77:1135–1138, 1993.
5. Bent JP, Silver JR, Porubsky ES: Acute laryngeal trauma: a review of 77 patients. *Otolaryngol Head Neck Surg* 109:441–449, 1993.
6. Weigelt JA, Thal ER, Snyder WH, et al: Diagnosis of penetrating cervical esophageal injuries. *Am J Surg* 154:619, 1987.
7. Armstrong WB, Detar TR, Stanley RB: Diagnosis and management of external penetrating cervical esophageal injuries. *Ann Otol Rhino Laryngol* 103(11):863–871, 1994.
8. Makins GH: Injuries to the blood vessels. In: *Official History of the Great War Medical Services. Surgery of the War.* London, 1922, pp. 170–296.
9. Hughes CW: Acute vascular trauma in Korean war casualties: an analysis of 180 cases. *Surg Gynecol Obstet* 99:91–100, 1954.
10. Fogelman MJ, Stewart RD: Penetrating wounds of the neck. *Am J Surg* 91:581–596, 1956.
11. Sheely CH 2nd, Mattox KL, Reul GJ Jr, et al: Current concepts in the management of penetrating neck trauma. *J Trauma* 15(10):895–900, 1975.
12. Saletta JD, Lowe RJ, Lim LT, et al: Penetrating trauma of the neck. *J Trauma* 16(7):579–587, 1976.
13. Bishara RA, Pasch AR, Douglas DD, et al: The necessity of mandatory exploration of penetrating zone II. *Neck Inj Surg* 100(4):655–660, 1986.
14. Elerding SC, Manart FD, Moore EE: A reappraisal of penetrating neck injury management. *J Trauma* 20(8):695–697, 1980.
15. Jurkovich GJ, Zingarelli W, Wallace J, et al: Penetrating neck trauma: diagnostic studies in the asymptomatic patient. *J Trauma* 25(9):819–822, 1985.
16. Obeid FN, Haddad GS, Horst HM, et al: A critical reappraisal of a mandatory exploration policy for penetrating wounds of the neck. *Surg Gynecol Obstet* 160(6):517–522, 1985.
17. Belinke SA, Russell JC, Dasilva J, et al: Management of penetrating neck injuries. *J Trauma* 23(3):235–237, 1983.
18. Metzdorff MT, Lowe DK: Operation or observation for penetrating neck wounds? A retrospective analysis. *Am J Surg* 147(5):646–649, 1984.
19. Meyer JP, Barnett JA, Schuler JJ, et al: Mandatory versus selective exploration for penetrating neck trauma: a prospective assessment. *Arch Surg* 122(5):592–597, 1987.
20. Wood J, Fabian TC, Mangiante EC: Penetrating neck injuries: recommendations for selective management. *J Trauma* 29(5):602–605, 1989.
21. Narrod JA, Moore EE: Selective management of penetrating neck injuries: a prospective study. *Arch Surg* 119(5):5748, 1984.
22. Mansour MA, Moore EE, Moore FA, et al: Validating the selective management of penetrating neck wounds. *Am J Surg* 162(6):517–520, 1991.
23. Beitsch P, Weigelt JA, Flynn E: Physical examination and arteriography in patients with penetrating zone II neck wounds. *Arch Surg* 129(6):577–581, 1994.
24. Scalfani SJ, Cavaliere G, Atwew N, et al: The role of angiography in penetrating neck trauma. *J Trauma* 31(4):557–562, 1991.
25. Menawat SS, Dennis JW, Laneve LM: Are arteriograms necessary in penetrating zone II neck injuries? *J Vasc Surg* 16(3):397–400, 1992.
26. Atteberry LR, Dennis JW, Menawat SS, et al: Physical examination alone is safe and accurate for the evaluation of penetrating zone II neck trauma. *J Am Coll Surg* 179(6):657–662, 1994.
27. Sekharan J, Dennis W, Veldenz C, et al: Continued experience with physical examination alone for the evaluation and management of penetrating zone 2 neck injuries: results of 145 cases. *J Vasc Surg* 32(3):483–489, 2000.
28. Jarvik JG, Philips GR 3rd, Schwab CW, et al: Penetrating neck trauma: sensitivity of clinical examination and cost effectiveness of angiography. *Am J Neuroradiol* 16(4):647–654, 1995.
29. Azuaje RE, Jacobson LE, Glover J, et al: Reliability of physical examination as a predictor of vascular injury after penetrating neck injury. *Am Surg* 69(9):804–807, 2003.
30. Ferguson E, Dennis JW, Frykberg ER: Redefining the role of arterial imaging in the management of penetrating zone 3 neck injuries. *Vascular* 13(3):158–163, 2005.
31. Ginzburg E, Montalvo B, LeBlanc S, et al: The use of duplex ultrasonography in penetrating neck trauma. *Arch Surg* 131(7):691–693, 1996.
32. Munera F, Soto JA, Palacio D, et al: Diagnosis of arterial injuries caused by penetrating trauma to the neck: comparison of helical CT angiography and conventional angiography. *Radiology* 216(2):356–362, 2000.
33. Mazolewski PJ, Curry JD, Browder T, et al: Computer tomographic scanning can be used for surgical decision making in zone II penetrating neck injuries. *J Trauma* 51(2):315–319, 2001.
34. Gracias VH, Reilly PM, Philpot J, et al: Computed tomography in the evaluation of penetrating neck trauma. *Arch Surg* 136:1231–1235, 2001.
35. Gonzalez RP, Falimirski M, Holevar MR, et al: Penetrating zone II neck injury: does dynamic computed tomographic scan contribute to the diagnostic sensitivity of physical examination for surgically significant lesions? A prospective blind study. *J Trauma* 54(1):61–64, 2003.
36. Hollingworth W, Nathens AB, Kanne JP, et al: The diagnostic accuracy of computed tomographic angiography for traumatic or atherosclerotic lesions of the carotid and vertebral arteries: a systematic review. *Eur J Radiol* 48(1):88–102, 2003.
37. Woo K, Magner DP, Wilson MT, et al: CT angiography in penetrating neck trauma reduces the need for operative neck exploration. *Am Surg* 71(9):754–758, 2005.
38. Eddy VA: Is routine arteriography mandatory for penetrating injury to zone I of the neck? Penetrating Injury Study Group. *J Trauma* 48(2):208–213, 2000.
39. Gasparri MG, Lorelli DR, Kralovich KA, et al: Physical examination plus chest radiography in penetrating peri-clavicular trauma: the appropriate trigger for angiography. *J Trauma* 49(6):1029–1033, 2000.
40. Demetriades D, Theodorou D, Cornwell E, et al: Evaluation of penetrating injuries of the neck: prospective study of 223 patients. *World J Surg* 21:41–48, 1997.
41. Liekweg WG, Greenfield LJ: Management of penetrating carotid arterial injury. *Ann Surg* 188:587, 1978.
42. Unger SW, Tucker W, et al: Carotid arterial trauma. *Surgery* 87:477, 1980.
43. Brown JM, Graham JM, Feliciano DV: Carotid artery injury. *Am J Surg* 144:748, 1982.

CAROTID, VERTEBRAL ARTERY, AND JUGULAR VENOUS INJURIES

Vincent L. Rowe, Patrizio Petrone,
Luis Manuel García-Núñez, and Juan A. Asensio

CAROTID ARTERY INJURIES

Over the centuries, management of carotid artery injuries has been reported. The first report of successful management of a carotid artery injury by ligation was by Ambroise Paré[1] in 1552, who ligated both the common carotid artery and the jugular vein. The patient survived but he developed an aphasia and hemiplegia. Fleming[2] reported a successful outcome after ligating an injured common carotid artery. Ligation continued to be used routinely in the surgical management of carotid artery injuries and was associated with high rates of hemiplegia and death. The Korean conflict marked the beginning of primary repair of arterial injuries, and carotid repair was attempted with success. Subsequently, these reconstructive techniques were applied to civilian carotid arterial injuries.

Incidence

Cervical vessels are involved in 25% of head and neck trauma, and carotid artery injury constitutes 5%[3] of all arterial injuries. Penetrating injury is the leading mechanism of injury, with gunshot wounds accounting for half of them, while blunt trauma comprises less than 10%,[4] most of them due to motor vehicle crashes. Mortality still has been very high, ranging between 10% and 30%, with an incidence of permanent neurologic deficit of 40%.[5]

Mechanism of Injury

Carotid artery injuries usually result from high-velocity missiles or direct impacts to the head. While high-velocity missiles may injure directly or by concussive forces, or cause secondary injury by bone fragments, low-velocity missile injuries are confined to the missile tract. Blunt injuries may result from direct impacts to the vessel causing disruption of the wall or as a result of bony fragments from associated injuries.[6] Motor vehicle crashes account for the majority of blunt neck injuries. Drivers and passengers on motorcycles, bicycles, jet skis, and snowboards can also sustain blunt neck injuries from direct impact.[7]

In order to provide a guideline in the management of penetrating neck injuries, the wounds to the neck have been grouped into three separate zones: zone I, injuries from the clavicle to the cricoid cartilage; zone II, injuries between the cricoid and angle of mandible; and zone III, injuries above the angle of mandible and the base of the skull.[8]

Of the three zones of the neck, zone II is the easier to expose via an incision parallel to the anterior border of the sternocleidomastoid muscle. Zone I often requires a median sternotomy for the more proximal portions of the common carotid artery. In zone III, the internal carotid artery is approached by extending the sternocleidomastoid incision to the ear into the postauricular space.

Diagnosis

Physical examination of patients with traumatic neck injuries is of paramount importance. The importance is confirmed by the fact that vascular injuries of the neck are associated with mortality rates up to 30% and are present in approximately 25% of all neck injuries. Signs such as expanding hematoma of the anterior or posterior triangle of the neck, audible cervical bruit, palpable thrill, abrasions on the neck secondary to seatbelts, and neurological deficits, are highly suggestive of a vascular injury of the neck. Additional findings include ipsilateral Horner's syndrome, active bleeding from oropharyngeal wounds, cranial nerves IX to XII deficits, and a diminished pulse in the ipsilateral superficial temporal artery.

Color-flow duplex (CFD) has emerged a valuable and accurate tool in the assessment of traumatic vascular injuries. Numerous studies have documented the accuracy CFD in the diagnosis of cervical vascular trauma, especially in zone II injuries to the neck.[9–15] When performed by a trained technologist and interpreted by a practitioner familiar with the nuances of flow disturbances, CFD correlates with contrast angiography in over 90% of zone II carotid injuries. Color-flow duplex has the advantage of being noninvasive and does not require contrast agents, thus making in-hospital follow-up examinations safe. Unfortunately, due to the adjacent bony structures, CFD is not useful in diagnosis of zone I and III injuries. Also, because the accuracy of CFD is so highly dependent on the personnel performing and interpreting the study and the availability of the personnel is variable after hours, use of CFD is limited even in trauma centers with Level 1 distinction. As usage of emergency-room ultrasound imaging increases in the secondary assessment of intracavitary trauma patients, extension of the scanning to include the neck may become commonplace. Color-flow capability of the ultrasound machine and appropriate training for acute care practitioners would be required.

With advances in the speed of acquisition and the enhanced software allowing elaborate reconstructive views, computerized tomography angiography (CTA) has become more commonly used as a diagnostic modality in traumatic neck injuries. With many patients already being evaluated with CT scans of the cervical spine, chest, and abdomen, CTA has the advantage of not requiring additional transport of the critically injured patient. This is especially the case in head-injured patients where a CT scan of the head is crucial to evaluate the existence of concurrent intracranial hematomas, parenchymal brain injury, or cerebral edema; here CTA of the neck to screen for extracranial and intracranial major vascular trauma is efficacious. In comparing CTA to CFD, Mutze and associates[16] demonstrated that CTA was more sensitive in detecting blunt carotid injuries and recommended contrast material-enhanced studies to avoid the morbidity of a missed cervical vascular injury. Unfortunately, CTA requires the use of nephrotoxic contrast agents to adequately delineate the vascular anatomy, which, when combined with the contrast load required for scanning of the chest and abdomen, increases the possibility of renal toxicity in the hemodynamically compromised trauma patient.

Magnetic resonance arteriography (MRA) is a viable imaging tool to evaluate the extracranial and intracranial vasculature; however, application to trauma patients is not widely accepted. MRA shares the advantage of CTA in that other areas can be imaged simultaneously and in being noninvasive, but unlike CTA, MRA uses a nonnephrotoxic contrast agent. Miller and colleagues[17] prospectively screened selected patients for blunt cerebrovascular injuries and compared the diagnostic modalities, CTA, and MRA, and contrast angiography (CA) in 143 trauma patients. Compared to CA, MRA and CTA had sensitivities of 50% and 47%, respectively, for carotid artery injuries. Similar results were demonstrated for blunt vertebral artery screening with MRA and CTA having respective sensitivities of 47% and 53%. Based on their findings, these authors cautioned against routine use of these modalities for screening of cervical vascular injuries. Compounding this report is the fact that MRA is not easily accessible in the majority of hospitals, and the presence of metallic orthopedic instrumentation limits widespread usage for trauma patients.

Contrast angiography still remains the gold standard with which all other diagnostic modalities are compared. This is especially true in zones I and III vascular injuries where accurate definition of the vascular pathology is essential to planning operative approaches. With the advent of endovascular surgery, CA has the distinct advantage of being the only diagnostic modality where treatment of the vascular abnormality can be rendered immediately after the diagnosis is established.

Treatment

Surgical reconstruction remains the mainstay therapy for carotid arterial injuries. Ligation, a treatment option of the past, is only reserved for cases of extensive injury or life-threatening exsanguination. In patients with signs of extensive pulsatile hemorrhage, expanding hematomas with or without airway compromise, immediate surgical exploration is recommended. Neurological evaluation should always be document prior to surgical intervention. Despite having a dense neurological deficit preoperatively, surgical repair is still recommended. Weaver and associates[18] demonstrated that regardless of the initial neurological deficit, mortality and final neurological status improved after surgical arterial repair. Since this report, subsequent studies documented similar success with surgical repair.[19,20]

Despite the success of operative intervention, nonoperative management of carotid injuries is justified in certain clinical scenarios. For example, in patients diagnosed with a carotid artery occlusion, a significant neurological deficit, and a large cerebral infarct on the ipsilateral side, observation is the preferred treatment of choice due to the poor prognosis in this subgroup of patients. Similarly, in patients with carotid artery occlusion and a normal neurological examination, observation and anticoagulation therapy for a period of at least 3 months is recommended to avoid any propagation of existent thrombus.

Likewise, patients diagnosed with "minimal" vascular injuries based on CFD or CA do not require as aggressive surgical approach. Minimal injuries can be described as nonobstructive or adherent intimal flaps and pseudoaneurysms less than 5 mm in size. Initial work by Stain and coworkers[21] documented the safety of observation in 24 nonocclusive arterial injuries. Patients in this study were managed nonoperatively and subsequently studied arteriographically at 1–12 weeks after injury. Resolution, improvement, or stabilization of the injury occurred in 21 injuries (87%). Progression was noted in three, and only one required repair. There were no cases of acute thrombosis or distal embolization. Later, Frykberg et al.[22] documented a similar report with data extending to 10 years with comparable excellent results, thus confirming the wisdom of this approach.

In patients undergoing open surgical repair, basic surgical principles and techniques for the management of arterial injuries must be followed. In preparation for the procedure, availability of vascular clamps and instrumentation, as well as intraluminal shunts should be confirmed. The operative field should include not only the area of injury, but also the ipsilateral chest wall, an area up throughout zone III of the neck, and a thigh for a vein graft harvest site. In general, zone I injuries require exposure through a median sternotomy and

zone II via an incision along the anterior border of the sternocleidomastoid muscle. Zone III injuries of the neck are more difficult to expose and to gain adequate exposure of the distal internal carotid artery, anterior subluxation or osteotomy of the mandible is required.

Once proximal and distal vascular control is established, injured vessels are debrided to macroscopically normal arterial wall. Fogarty catheters should be passed selectively and gently, both proximal and distal to the arterial injury, to remove any intraluminal thrombus. It is extremely important not to overinflate the balloon, lest the endothelial lining be damaged and arterial spasm or thrombosis result. Both proximal and distal arterial lumens are flushed with heparinized saline solution. Systemic heparinization, if not contraindicated, is of benefit to decrease the risk of thrombus formation or clot propagation. Placement of an intraluminal shunt is a helpful adjunct to maintain antegrade flow to the ipsilateral cerebral cortex and is strongly recommended particularly for proximal internal carotid artery or carotid bulb injuries. In this scenario, standard indications for the selective use of shunting in elective carotid artery surgery should not apply. Proximal common carotid injuries may be repaired without distal shunting because the external carotid artery provides adequate collateral flow. The type of repair is dictated by the extent of arterial damage. Repair of injured vessels can be accomplished by lateral suture patch angioplasty, end-to-end anastomosis, interposition graft, or, when adjacent soft injury is extensive, a bypass graft. If possible, an all-autogenous arterial repair with a vein graft is recommended. However, prosthetic grafts, such as expanded polytetrafluoroethylene (ePTFE), can be used with excellent outcomes, especially in the common carotid artery reconstructions.

Monofilament 5-0 or 6-0 sutures are suitable for most peripheral vascular repairs, and all completed repairs should be tension free and covered by viable soft tissue. We consider intraoperative completion arteriography or duplex scanning to be mandatory to document technical perfection of the vascular reconstruction, visualize arterial runoff, and detect persistent missed distal thrombi. Intra-arterial vasodilators such as papaverine or tolazoline may be helpful, particularly in the pediatric age group, in reversing severe spasm in the distal arterial tree or the repaired arterial segment.

The use of endovascular therapy to treat traumatic arterial injuries has gained popularity in the management of traumatic arterial injuries. Endovascular management has the advantage of being able to treat the vascular abnormality at the time of diagnosis, if contrast angiography is the diagnostic modality being used. In addition, catheter-based treatment can access lesions that would be either difficult to surgically expose (i.e., zone III injuries) or lesions that would require extensive operative incisions (i.e., lower zone I injuries). The disadvantages to endovascular treatment are the requirement for contrast material, and the lingering possibility for surgical exploration for concomitant injuries or to evacuate extensive hematomas.

Traditionally used for treatment of small arteriovenous fistulae and short-segment dissections, covered and uncovered stents are being used for more significant arterial lesions. Joo and associates[23] reported successful management of 10 traumatic carotid arterial injuries. The lesions involved both the intracranial and extracranial carotid artery with the all arterial pathology consisting of arteriovenous fistulae or pseudoaneurysms. The authors did comment that long-term follow-up was not available in their study group; a concern with the application of this newest vascular technology. Regardless, as technology continues to advance, endovascular treatment of cervical arterial lesions should be considered, especially in high-risk patients with multiple concomitant injuries. As more operating room suites transform into high resolution fluoroscopic units and surgeons become more adept in endovascular treatment modalities, expeditious diagnosis and management of traumatic cervical vascular injuries should be expected in the future.

VERTEBRAL ARTERY INJURIES

The vertebral artery is the first branch of the subclavian artery. It is located in the posterior triangle of the neck, and is divided into four parts. The first part begins at the subclavian artery and ends at the foramina in the transverse process of the sixth cervical vertebra. The second portion includes its travel as it continues within the bony vertebral foramina. The last two parts, the third and the fourth, are beyond the first cervical vertebra.[24]

In 1853, Maissoneuve reported a first successful outcome after ligating a vertebral artery injury.[25] This report documenting 42 cases of extracranial vertebral artery injuries was the largest description at that time. Rich[26] reported only three cases in the military literature from World War I through the Vietnam conflict, and at the same time only 12 civilian cases were reported.

Vertebral artery injuries are uncommon, and historically many of them have gone unrecognized. In recent years the diagnosis and management of these injuries have undergone some major changes because of newer diagnostic and therapeutic procedures. However, the majority of vertebral artery injuries are not life threatening.

Incidence

The incidence reported in the literature of vertebral injuries in penetrating neck trauma varies from 1.0%–7.4%, depending on the mechanism (gunshot or stab wounds). In 1967, Stein[27] reported 200 consecutive penetrating neck injuries with only two patients (1.0%) with vertebral artery injuries. In a prospective study[28] of 223 penetrating neck injury patients evaluated with routine four-vessel angiography, there were 13 cases (7.4%) with vertebral injuries reported.

The incidence in blunt trauma is very low, and is usually associated with cervical spine fractures.

Mechanism of Injury

The most common mechanism is a gunshot wound, followed by stab wound and other penetrating neck trauma. Blunt trauma includes mechanisms such as closed head injury, ligamentous cervical spine injury, bony disruptions, and direct impacts to the neck.[29–32] Other situations in which arterial vertebral injuries can be seen are during internal jugular catheterization, angiographic procedures, cervical spine internal fixation, and diskectomy.[33]

Associated Injuries

Gunshot wounds to the vertebral artery are often associated with major injuries to other vessels, the aero-digestive tract, the cervical spine, and nerves. Stab wounds are often associated with brachial plexus and internal jugular vein injuries, along with injuries to the esophagus, and occasionally a hemothorax.[34] Injuries to the vertebral injuries due to blunt mechanisms should be suspected in patients with facet joint dislocation or transverse foramen fracture, and closed head injuries.[29] According to Asensio, associated vascular injuries occur in a range from 13 to 19%, and arteriovenous fistulas between the vertebral artery and the two paired vertebral veins occur with a frequency of 11%. Similarly, associated pharyngo-esophageal injuries occur with a frequency of 11%–22%.[35]

Diagnosis

Presentation of patients with vertebral artery trauma is highly variable. In patients presenting after penetrating vertebral artery trauma, the "hard signs" of a vascular injury (expanding hematoma, cervical bruit, pulsatile hemorrhage) were only present in 50% of patients and only 30% presented with "soft signs" (history of bleeding, proximity wound, neurological abnormality).[36] In fact, close to 20% of patients with vertebral artery trauma present with no overt clinical signs. As opposed to carotid arterial trauma where occlusion of a single vessel can lead to permanent neurological alterations, single occlusion of one vertebral artery often remains clinically silent. However, if bilateral vertebral artery occlusions occur, neurological symptoms would manifest.

Color-flow duplex has a limited role as a reliable diagnostic tool. Unlike the carotid artery where a long segment of artery can be evaluated in both longitudinal and transverse planes, because of the course within the cervical spine, only the most proximal segment of the vertebral artery can be visualized in a very short longitudinal plane. Therefore, outside of documenting an occlusion, CFD can only provide information about abnormal flow patterns suggestive of pathology more distal in the vessel.

Because of the difficulty in physical examination and CFD in diagnosing vertebral arterial injuries, CTA and MRA will be the diagnostic modalities that identify the majority of abnormalities. Both imaging techniques allow visualization of all segments of the vertebral artery without obstructed shadowing from the cervical spine, thus becoming one of the main screening tools for vertebral artery trauma. Contrast angiography remains the gold for imaging the vertebral artery. Because of the ability to endovascularly treat the revealed lesion at the time of diagnosis, contrast angiography may be the preferred imaging selection.

Treatment

Contrary to the treatment of carotid artery injuries, which are managed operatively, the majority of vertebral artery injuries either do not require treatment or are treated with angiographic embolization. The only indication for operative management is for patients with active hemorrhage or those that have failed angiographic treatment methods. Also, because of the anatomical relationship with both vertebral arteries, vertebral artery occlusion is infrequently accompanied by a major neurological event. Regardless, angiographic evaluation should still be undertaken to treat underlying arteriovenous fistulae and to confirm occlusion.

Anatomy of the vertebral artery can be divided into four segments. The first portion of the vertebral artery (V-1) begins where the vertebral artery originates from the subclavian artery and extends to the sixth cervical vertebrae transverse process foramen. This area of the artery is the most accessible for surgical exposure. After positioning the patient with the head angled away from the affected side, exposure to the vertebral artery can be through an incision along the sternocleidomastoid muscle (SCMM) or a transverse supraclavicular approach (the authors' preference). Note, however, that the incision along the SCMM does allow continuation of the incision superiorly or inferiorly to provide additional exposure. After mobilizing and retracting the SCMM laterally, and retracting the carotid sheath medially, the anterior scalene muscle with the overlying phrenic nerve is encountered. With careful medial retraction of the anterior scalene muscle and the phrenic nerve, the vertebral vein is visualized. The vertebral artery is directly posterior. To gain additional exposure, the omohyoid and the clavicular head of the SCMM may be divided.

The second portion (V-2), or the interosseous portion, extends from the transverse foramina of C-6 to C-2. Exposure of this segment of the vertebral artery requires dissection through the transverse foramina to expose the vertebral canal. Through the same exposure discussed previously, the longus coli muscle is encountered in the deep posterior aspect of the neck. Once this muscle is swept off of the underlying bony structure with a periosteal elevator, the anterior tubercle of the transverse process and the vertebral bodies are visualized. Bone rongeurs are used to remove the anterior rim of the vertebral foramen to expose the vertebral artery.[36,37] Moderate bleeding may be anticipated during this part of the dissection. Additional anterior rims may be excised for increased exposure. The vertebral artery may be safely ligated at this point. Care should be taken not to blindly place surgical clips for arterial occlusion because cervical nerve roots lie directly posterior to the artery and may be injured.

The third part of the vertebral artery (V-3) courses from where the vertebral artery exits the foramina of C-2 and extends to the foramen magnum at the base of the skull. A posterior auricular approach is required to expose this segment of the artery. The fourth part of the vertebral artery (V-4) starts at the foramen magnum and ends where both vertebral arteries join to form the basilar artery. The fourth segment of the vertebral artery can only be exposed with a craniotomy. Exposure of this segment of vertebral artery is most challenging to both the trauma and vascular surgeon, and assistance from a neurosurgeon is often required.

The preferred method for management of vertebral artery injuries is angiographically. Lesions ranging from aneurysms, arteriovenous fistulae, and pseudoaneurysms can all be treated with an array of detachable balloons, stents, coils, liquid tissue adhesives, and other hemostatic agents. Numerous authors have documented successful endovascular management of traumatic vertebral artery injuries. With the continued improvement of endovascular technology, the scope of traumatic lesions will certainly increase.

JUGULAR VENOUS INJURIES

Jugular venous injuries are caused almost exclusively by penetrating neck trauma. The low-pressure venous system usually tamponades or occludes without a major hemorrhage or hematoma. Most isolated jugular venous injuries go unrecognized, and the true incidence of traumatic jugular injuries is unknown. In one of the first retrospective studies of venous injuries,[38] jugular venous injuries constituted 3.5% of all injuries. These injuries are often diagnosed during exploration following an arterial injury.

When the patient is in shock, any venous injury should be managed by ligation. An injury to the internal jugular vein should be repaired by a lateral venorrhaphy.[7] If repair is difficult or the patient is critically unstable, ligation is the option of choice. The external jugular vein can be ligated without adverse sequelae. Air emboli can result from venous injuries. Van Ieperen[39] reported 11 patients who died due to air emboli after penetrating neck injuries.

REFERENCES

1. Watson WL, Silverstone SM: Ligature of common carotid artery in cancer of the head and neck. *Ann Surg* 109:1, 1939.
2. Fleming D: Case of rupture of the carotid artery: the wounds of several of its branches successfully treated by tying the common trunk of the carotid itself. *Med Circ J* 3:2, 1812.
3. Ward RE: Injury to the cervical cerebral vessels. In Blaisdell FW, Trunkey DD, editors: *Trauma Management.* Vol. III, *Cervicothoracic Trauma.* New York, Thieme, 1986, pp. 262–268.
4. Martin RF, Eldrup-Jorgensen J, Clark DE, et al: Blunt trauma to the carotid arteries. *J Vasc Surg* 14:789–795, 1991.
5. Weaver FA, Yellin AE, Wagner WH, et al: The role of arterial reconstruction in penetrating carotid injuries. *Arch Surg* 123:1106–1111, 1988.
6. Kumar SR, Weaver FA, Yellin AE: Cervical vascular injuries: carotid and jugular venous injuries. *Surg Clin North Am* 81:1331–1344, 2001.
7. Britt LD: Neck injuries: evaluation and management. In Moore EE, Feliciano DV, Mattox KL, editors: *Trauma,* 5th ed. New York, McGraw-Hill, 2004, pp. 445–458.
8. Saletta JD, Lowe RJ, Lim LT: Penetrating trauma of the neck. *J Trauma* 16:579–587, 1976.
9. Kuzniec S, Kauffman P, Molnar LJ, et al: Diagnosis of limbs and neck arterial trauma using duplex ultrasonography. *Cardiovasc Surg* 6:358–366, 1998.
10. Guinzburg E, Montalvo B, LeBlang S, et al: The use of duplex ultrasonography in penetrating neck trauma. *Arch Surg* 131:691–693, 1996.
11. Fry WR, Dort JA, Smith RS, et al: Duplex scanning replaces arteriography and operative exploration in the diagnosis of potential cervical vascular injury. *Am J Surg* 168:693–695, 1994.
12. Cogbill TH, Moore EE, Meissner M, et al: The spectrum of blunt injury to the carotid artery: a multicenter perspective. *J Trauma* 37:473–479, 1994.
13. Bynoe RP, Miles WS, Bell RM, et al: Noninvasive diagnosis of vascular trauma by duplex ultrasonography. *J Vasc Surg* 14:346–352, 1991.
14. Meissner M, Paun M, Johansen K: Duplex scanning for arterial trauma. *Am J Surg* 161:552–555, 1991.
15. Greenwold D, Sessions EG, Haynes JL, et al: Duplex ultrasonography in vascular trauma. *J Vasc Tech* 15:79–82, 1991.
16. Mutze S, Rademacher G, Matthes G, et al: Blunt cerebrovascular injury in patients with blunt multiple trauma: diagnostic accuracy of duplex Doppler US and early CT angiography. *Radiology* 237:884–892, 2005.
17. Miller PR, Fabian CT, Croce MA, et al: Prospective screening for blunt cerebrovascular injuries: analysis of diagnostic modalities and outcome. *Ann Surg* 236:386–393, 2002.
18. Weaver FA, Yellin AE, Wagner WH, et al: The role of arterial reconstruction in penetrating carotid injuries. *Arch Surg* 123:1106–1111, 1988.
19. Brown MF, Graham JM, Feliciano DV, et al: Carotid artery injuries. *Am J Surg* 144:748–753, 1982.
20. Kuehne JP, Weaver FA, Papanicolaou G, et al: Penetrating trauma of the internal carotid artery. *Arch Surg* 131:942–947, 1996.
21. Stain SC, Yellin AE, Weaver FA, et al: Selective management of nonocclusive arterial injuries. *Arch Surg* 124:1136–1140, 1989.
22. Frykberg ER, Vines FS, Alexander RH: The natural history of clinically occult arterial injuries: a prospective evaluation. *J Trauma* 29:577–583, 1989.
23. Joo JY, Ahn JY, Chung YS, et al: Therapeutic endovascular treatments for traumatic carotid artery injuries. *J Trauma* 58:1159–1166, 2005.
24. Blickenstaff KL, Weaver FA, Yellin AE, et al: Trends in the management of traumatic vertebral artery injury. *Am J Surg* 158:101–106, 1989.
25. Matas R: Traumatisms and traumatic aneurysms of the vertebral artery and their surgical treatment, with the report of a cured case. *Ann Surg* 18:477–521, 1893.
26. Rich N: *Vascular Trauma.* Philadelphia, W.B. Saunders, 1978.
27. Stein A, Seaward P: Penetrating wounds of the neck. *J Trauma* 7:238–247, 1967.
28. Demetriades D, Theodorou D, Cornwell E, et al: Evaluation of penetrating injuries of the neck: prospective study of 223 patients. *World J Surg* 21:41–48, 1997.
29. Biffl W, Moore E, Elliot J, et al: The devastating potential of blunt vertebral artery injuries. *Ann Surg* 231:672–681, 2000.
30. Dragon R, Saranchak H, Laskin P, et al: Blunt injuries to the carotid and vertebral arteries. *Am J Surg* 141:497–500, 1981.
31. Hayes P, Gerlock AJ Jr, Cobb CA: Cervical spine trauma: a case of vertebral artery injury. *J Trauma* 20:904–905, 1980.
32. Knoop M, Kroger JC, Schulz K, et al: Diagnosis and management of an intraoperative vertebral artery injury. *Chirurg* 70:789–794, 1999.
33. Wright N, Lauryssen C: Vertebral artery injury in C1-2 transarticular screw fixation: results of a survey of the AANS/CNS section on disorders of the spine and peripheral nerves. *J Neurosurg* 88:634–640, 1998.
34. Roberts LH, Demetriades D: Vertebral artery injuries. *Surg Clin North Am* 81:1345–1356, 2001.
35. Asensio JA, Valenziano CP, Falcone RE, et al: Management of penetrating neck injuries: the controversy surrounding zone II injuries. *Surg Clin North Am* 71:267–296, 1991.
36. Demetriades D, Theodorou D, Asensio JA: Management options in vertebral artery injuries. *Br J Surg* 83:83–86, 1996.
37. Henry A: *Extensile Exposure,* 2nd ed. Edinburgh, Churchill, Livingstone, 1973.
38. Gaspar MR, Treiman RL: The management of injuries to major veins. *Am J Surg* 100:171–175, 1960.
39. Van Ieperen L: Venous air embolism as a cause of death: a method of investigation. *South Afr Med* 63:442–443, 1983.

BLUNT CEREBROVASCULAR INJURIES

C. Clay Cothren and Ernest E. Moore

Over the past decade, a wealth of studies has provided the scientific rationale to promote the early screening and treatment of blunt cerebrovascular injuries (BCVI). Initially, BCVI were thought to have unavoidable, devastating neurologic outcomes, but several reports suggested anticoagulation improves neurologic outcome in patients suffering ischemic neurologic events.[1,2] If untreated, carotid artery injuries (CAIs) have a stroke rate up to 50% depending on injury grade, with increasing stroke rates correlating with increasing grades of injury; vertebral artery injuries (VAIs) have a stroke rate of 20%–25%.[3] Screening protocols, based on patient injury patterns and mechanism of injury, have been instituted to identify these injuries in asymptomatic patients and to initiate treatment, prior to neurologic sequelae. Current studies suggest early antithrombotic therapy in patients with BCVI reduces stroke rate and prevents neurologic morbidity. [3–8]

SIGNS AND SYMPTOMS

Blunt cerebrovascular injuries were first reported over 30 years ago, in patients who presented with stroke following injury.[9] The patient's symptom of cerebral ischemia or the distribution of their symptoms usually indicates the underlying cerebrovascular lesion (Figure 1). Carotid artery injuries generally result in contralateral sensorimotor deficits, which to the general practitioner is classically defined as a stroke. Aphasia occurs when the dominant hemisphere is involved, while nondominant hemisphere strokes may result in hemineglect. Vertebral artery injuries typically manifest as more vague symptomatology, namely ataxia, dizziness, vomiting, facial or body analgesia, or visual field defects. Symptoms of carotid-cavernous fistulae include orbital pain, exophthalmos, chemosis, and conjunctival hyperemia.

Although some patients may present with symptoms of BCVI-related ischemia within an hour of injury, the majority exhibit a latent period. This asymptomatic phase has been inferred based upon the time to onset of symptoms in patients with defined injuries who did not receive antithrombotic therapy. This timeframe appears to range from hours up to 14 years, but t he majority seems to develop symptoms within 10–72 hours.[1,3,4,10] The goal, then, is diagnosing BCVI during this "silent period" prior to the onset stroke. After all, the theory is that if you diagnose these injuries during the asymptomatic period you can effectively treat the patient to prevent stroke. Screening for BCVI during the asymptomatic period was initially suggested in the mid-1990s after the recognition that specific patterns of injuries were associated with BCVI. Although optimal screening criteria have yet to be defined, current screening algorithms include patients considered at high risk based on their injury pattern.

MECHANISM AND PATTERNS OF INJURY

Crissey and Bernstein originally postulated three fundamental mechanisms of injury resulting in BCVI.[9] The first is a direct blow to the neck. This mechanism is often seen with patients in motor vehicle collisions with inappropriately fitting seatbelts who end up with a seatbelt sign across the neck; it can also be seen in mountain bikers with a direct blow to the neck after falling during riding. The second proposed mechanism is hyperextension with contralateral rotation of the head. This is the most common mechanism causing CAI with the hyperextension resulting in a stretching of the carotid artery over the lateral articular processes of C1–C3 (Figure 2). VAI may also be due to a hyperextension-stretch injury due to the tethering of the vertebral artery within the lateral masses of the cervical spine. The third mechanism of injury is a direct laceration of the artery by adjacent fractures involving the sphenoid or petrous bones. Although originally described as the mechanism in association with CAI, this may also be the cause of VAI. With a fracture of any of the bony elements comprising the vertebral foramen, also termed the foramen transversarium, it is not surprising that the vertebral artery could be directly injured. Regardless of the type of injury mechanism, there is intimal disruption of the carotid or vertebral artery. This intimal tear becomes a nidus for platelet aggregation that may lead to emboli or vessel occlusion, and subsequent stroke.

Although the mechanism of injury is important for determining patients at high risk for BCVI, the patient's associated injuries are also critical to determine which asymptomatic patients undergo screening for BCVI. Aggressive screening for BCVI was initially suggested after recognition that specific patterns of injuries were associative. Current screening algorithms include patients with signs or symptoms, as well as those considered at high risk by injury pattern (Table 1). BCVI screening protocols have remained relatively unchanged over the past decade since their institution, aside from refinements in patients with cervical spine fractures. Initially, screening protocols included all patients with cervical spine fractures to rule out BCVI. However, there were a significant number of patients with isolated cervical spine fractures that could be managed by the local orthopedic surgeons without referral to Level I trauma facilities; therefore, we questioned the need to evaluate every patient with a cervical spine fracture.[11] In our population, excluding patients who underwent screening for associated injuries or other injury patterns, only patients with three patterns of spine fracture were identified as having a BCVI, barring other symptoms of neurologic compromise: cervical spine subluxation, fractures involving the transverse foramen, and upper cervical spine fracture of C1–C3 (Figure 3). Therefore, only this subpopulation of patients with cervical spine fractures undergoes screening for BCVI.

DIAGNOSTIC IMAGING

Using defined screening protocols, high-risk patients undergo imaging to identify BCVI. Historically, four-vessel arteriography has been the gold standard to diagnose BCVI. Undoubtedly, many clinicians question the need for subjecting patients to angiography. Angiography is labor intensive, costly, and not without risks; and, if not available at smaller hospitals, requires emergent transfer of a patient for definitive evaluation. Currently, CTA remains an unproven diagnostic modality for this injury. In particular, injuries that may be missed by such noninvasive studies are typically grade I and II injuries; however, pseudoaneurysms and occlusions have also been misdiagnosed.[12,13] The risk of angiography in our screened trauma population is 0.1%, while the stroke risk of an undiagnosed grade I CAI is 8% and VAI is 6%.[3,4] Recent preliminary studies report improved imaging and visualization of injuries with multislice CT scanners (16 or more slices). These promising

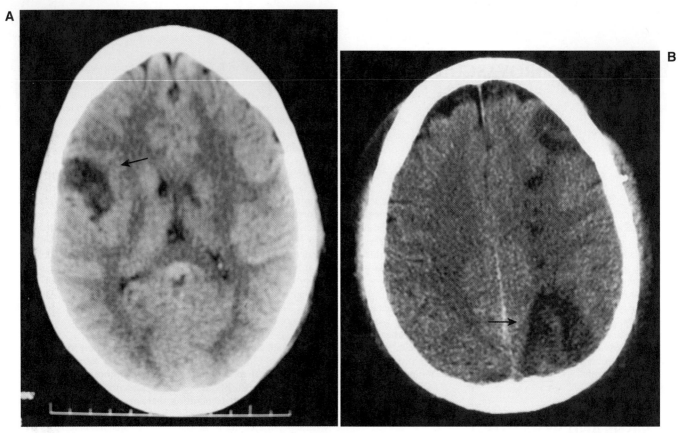

Figure 1   Computed tomography scan imaging of blunt cerebrovascular injury–related strokes from a carotid artery injury **(A)** and a vertebral artery injury **(B)**.

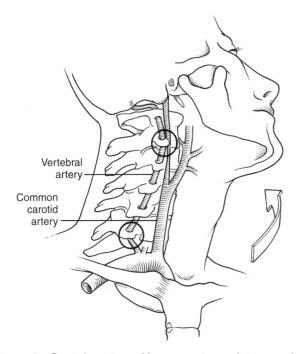

Figure 2   Cervical rotation and hyperextension result in a stretch injury of the carotid and vertebral vasculature.   *(Adapted from Biffl WL, Moore EE, Elliot JP, et al: Blunt cerebrovascular injuries. Curr Prob Surg 36:505, 1999.)*

Table 1: Denver Screening Criteria for Blunt Cerebrovascular Injuries

Signs/Symptoms of BCVI

Arterial hemorrhage
Cervical bruit in patient <50 years of age
Expanding cervical hematoma
Focal neurologic deficit
Neurologic exam incongruous with head CT scan findings
Stroke on secondary CT scan

Risk Factors for BCVI

High-energy transfer mechanism with:
LeForte II or III fracture
Cervical-spine fracture patterns: subluxation, fractures extending into transverse foramen, fractures of C1–C3
Basilar skull fracture with carotid canal involvement
Diffuse axonal injury with Glasgow Coma Scale <6
Near hanging with anoxic brain injury

BCVI, Blunt cerebrovascular injury; CT, computed tomography.
Courtesy of Denver Health Medical Center.

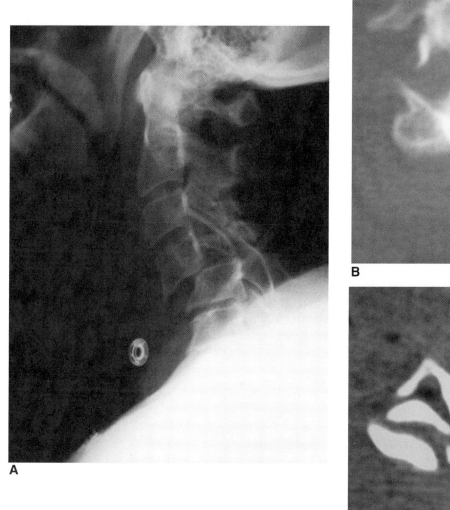

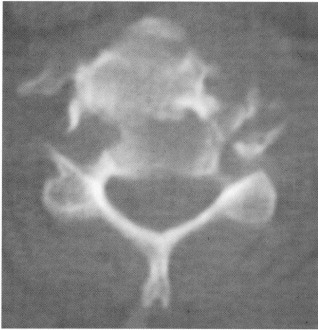

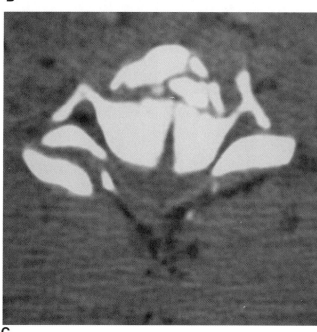

Figure 3 Cervical spine fracture patterns associated with blunt cerebrovascular injury: subluxation **(A)**, transverse foramen involvement **(B)**, and C1–C3 fractures **(C)**.

advances in technology, which would allow noninvasive evaluation of patients, will clearly facilitate the screening process.

All patients with indications for screening, and no contraindications to antithrombotic therapy, undergo imaging as soon as possible. Patients with documented BCVI undergo repeat imaging 7–10 days after their initial diagnostic study. The importance of routine follow-up imaging is particularly salient in patients with grade I and II injuries; over half of grade I injuries completely heal, allowing cessation of antithrombotic therapy.[3] While only 8% of grade II injuries heal, over 40% progress to grade III injuries despite therapy; in patients with CAI, this increase in injury grade

also correlates with an increase in stroke risk. Patients with carotid or vertebral artery occlusions are not as important for reimaging, as over 80% display no change on follow-up imaging.

INJURY GRADING SCALE

The identification of disparate outcomes associated with varied luminal irregularities comprising BCVI (dissection, occlusion, transection, and pseudoaneurysms) prompted us to propose a grading scale.[10] An injury grading scale was developed to provide not only an accurate description of the injury, but also to define stroke risk by injury grade (Figure 4 and Table 2). Untreated injuries have an overall stroke rate of approximately 20%; CAIs have increasing stroke rate by increasing grade, while VAIs tend to have a more consistent stroke rate of approximately 20% for all grades of injury (Table 3).

INCIDENCE OF BLUNT CEREBROVASCULAR INJURIES

Originally thought to be a rare injury, BCVIs are currently diagnosed in 1% of all blunt trauma patients. Previously, BCVI-related strokes were likely attributed to a patient's primary head injury, rather than as a sequelae of cervical arterial injury with subsequent embolic stroke. Therefore, BCVIs were felt to be rare with an incidence less than 0.1% in all trauma patients, and with blunt

CAI accounting for less than 3% of all traumatic carotid injuries. Once the patient's neurologic changes were ascribed to a vascular source, and appropriate imaging was instituted to identify the injured artery, the incidence of BCVI identified tripled. In the first multicenter review of BCVI, performed by the Western Trauma Association, only 49 patients with carotid artery injuries were identified at 11 medical institutions over a 6-year period. With the recognition of BCVI as a specific injury causing significant morbidity and stroke-related mortality, was the associated silent period. With the advent of injury screening in asymptomatic high-risk patients, there has been a relative epidemic of BCVI diagnosed. Currently, in centers with a comprehensive screening approach, the screening yield is over 30% in high-risk populations. In our most recent Denver Health Medical Center institutional review over an 8½–year period, 0.1% of blunt injury patients presented with neurologic symptoms and 4% underwent screening angiography, with a 34% screening yield for diagnosing

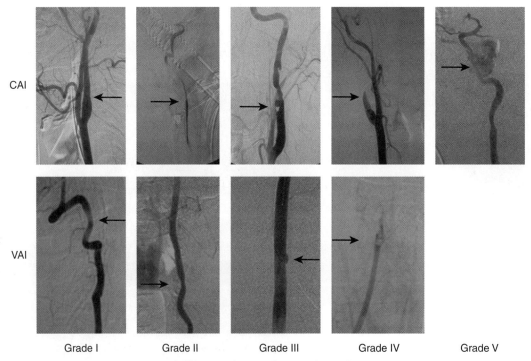

Figure 4   Representative images of blunt cerebrovascular injury by grade.

Table 2: Denver Grading Scale for Blunt Cerebrovascular Injuries

Grade I	Irregularity of vessel wall or dissection/ intramural hematoma with less than 25% luminal stenosis
Grade II	Intraluminal thrombus or raised intimal flap is visualized, or dissection/intramural hematoma with 25% or more luminal narrowing
Grade III	Pseudoaneurysm
Grade IV	Vessel occlusion
Grade V	Vessel transection

Courtesy of Denver Health Medical Center.

Table 3: Stroke Rate by Blunt Cerebrovascular Injury Grade

	Grade of Injury	Stroke Rate (%)
Carotid arterial injury	I	3
	II	14
	III	26
	IV	50
	V	100
Vertebral arterial injury	I	6
	II	38
	III	27
	IV	28
	V	100

BCVI and an overall incidence of 1.5% in all blunt trauma victims.

ANTITHROMBOTIC TREATMENT

Following the recognition that BCVI were responsible for patients' adverse neurologic events, treatment modalities were debated. If the injury occurs in a surgically accessible area of the carotid artery, particularly the common carotid artery, operative management is warranted (Figure 5). The vast majority of BCVI lesions, however, occur in surgically challenging or inaccessible areas of the blood vessels, either high within the carotid canal at the base of the skull or within the foramen transversarium (Figure 6). Such a location makes the standard vascular repair approaches including reconstruction or thrombectomy difficult if not impossible. Heparin was initially the treatment of choice for BCVI, with the assumption that this promoted clot stabilization if present and clot resolution through intrinsic fibrinolytic mechanisms, and prevented further thrombosis. Treatment with anticoagulation was shown to improve neurologic outcome in patients sustaining BCVI-related ischemic neurologic events (INEs).[2,6] Initial reports, including a multicenter study by the Western Trauma Association,[1] indicated that patients who were treated with anticoagulation had an improved outcome compared to those who were either not treated or had a contraindication to anticoagulation due to associated head injuries. In these studies, up to 45% of patients achieved good neurologic status, and anticoagulation therapy was independently associated with survival and improvement in neurologic outcome.

Subsequently, intravenous heparin was thought to be the treatment of choice for those asymptomatic patients with blunt injuries.[3,6] Initially, standard heparinization protocols were used, but due to a moderate incidence of bleeding in multisystem trauma patients the protocol was modified (Figure 7).[7,10] Currently, anticoagulation with systemic heparin is initiated using a continuous infusion of heparin at 15 U/kg/hr, without a loading dose; heparin drips are titrated to achieve a partial thromboplastin time (PTT) in 40–50 seconds. With this adjustment in the BCVI heparin protocol, less than 1% of patients have had bleeding complications necessitating transfusion in our experience.[4] For patients with a contraindication to heparin, antiplatelet agents (aspirin 325 mg/day and clopidogrel 75 mg/day) have been administered. Antithrombotic therapy is not started in patients with closed head injury or intraparenchymal hemorrhage without input from the neurosurgery service. Antithrombotic therapy in patients with significant solid organ injuries or a complex pelvic fracture with associated retroperitoneal hematoma is typically not started until 24–48 hours of physiologic stability without transfusion have passed.

Currently there is controversy regarding the ideal antithrombotic therapy for any type of arterial disease—anticoagulation versus antiplatelet agents. A retrospective study by Chimowitz et al.[17] indicated that warfarin is superior in patients with vertebrobasilar occlusive disease, while a more recent prospective double-blind comparison by the same authors[18] demonstrated that aspirin is the therapy of choice for patients with symptomatic intracranial atherosclerotic arterial stenosis, due to equivalent stroke prevention rates as warfarin, but decreased hemorrhagic complications. A recent review of vertebrobasilar disease supported the use of antiplatelet agents in patients with arterial stenosis but warfarin in patients with severe, flow-limiting lesions or dissections.[19] Which therapeutic agent is used, and whether the choice of antithrombotic should be determined by the patient's injury grade, must continue to be evaluated in prospective studies.

Most importantly, patients who are diagnosed with BCVI early and are treated with antithrombotics almost universally avoid INE.[4,8,12] The Memphis group showed a reduction in stroke rate for CAI from 64% in untreated patients to 6.8% in patients treated with antithrombotics (either anticoagulation or antiplatelet agents), and for VAI a reduction from 54% to 2.6% in treated patients.[12] Our group's most recent evaluation demonstrated a stroke rate of 0.5% in 187 patients with BCVI treated with antithrombotics, while untreated patients had an overall stroke rate of 21%.[8] Although the optimal regimen remains unanswered, there appears to be equivalence between the two therapies (anticoagulation and antiplatelet agents) with regard to stroke rate.[3,4,8,12]

Following initiation of antithrombotics, treatment is empirically continued for 6 months. Our current protocol is to transition the patient to warfarin if the initial antithrombotic therapy was heparin, with a goal INR of 2.0. If the patient was started on antiplatelet agents, these are continued after hospital discharge. Although complete healing of grade I injuries on repeat imaging at 7–10 days has been documented in more than half of affected patients, the vast majority of grades II, III, and IV injuries persist. Comprehensive long-term follow-up beyond the acute hospitalization has not been reported in the literature, as is true in most trauma population studies. Therefore, whether these injuries heal or persist at 3–6 months is unknown.

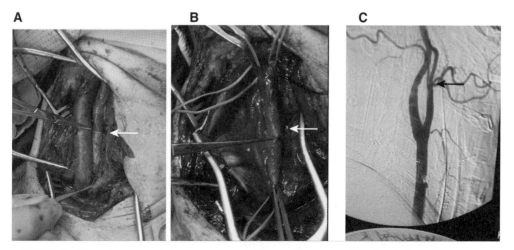

Figure 5 Operative approach to a common carotid pseudoaneurysm following angiographic **(A)** diagnosis; identification of the injury **(B)** is followed by primary end to end repair **(C)**.

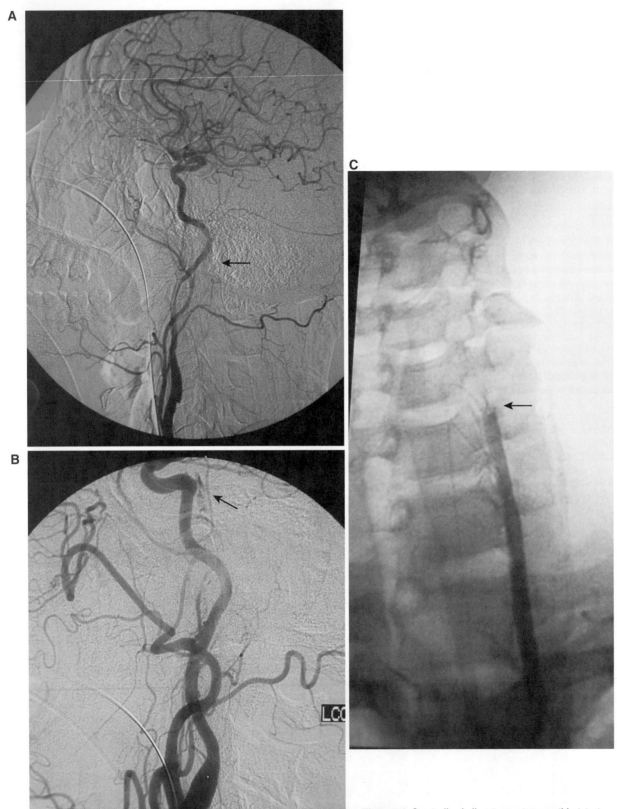

Figure 6 Surgically challenging or inaccessible injuries include carotid arterial injury at the base of the skull (**A** and **B**) and vertebral arterial injury within the transverse foramen (**C**).

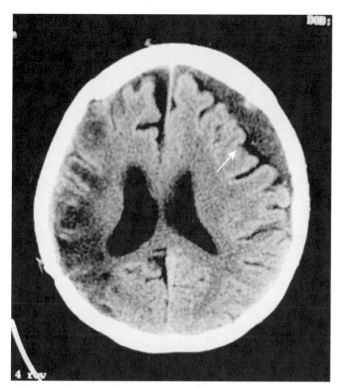

Figure 7 Intracranial bleeding complications associated with heparinization of a patient for blunt cerebrovascular injury.

ROLE OF ENDOVASCULAR STENTS

Over the past decade, there has been an explosion in the use of percutaneous transluminal arterial interventions for both traumatic injuries and atherosclerotic lesions. Although the role of carotid stents for atherosclerotic disease is being explored with randomized, well-controlled trials, the indication for percutaneous intervention for traumatic injuries is less well defined. Carotid stents have been used in patients with blunt injury with persistent pseudoaneurysms, due to the concern for subsequent embolization or rupture. In theory, the uncovered carotid stent acts as a filter to trap any thrombus within the pseudoaneurysm, thereby preventing embolization and stroke. The stent may also decrease flow into the pseudoaneurysm by increasing laminar flow within the stented portion of the carotid lumen itself. Decreasing flow into the aneurysmal sac may then reduce any egress of blood from the sac, which in turn may reduce turbulence within the lumen. There are anecdotal reports of carotid pseudoaneurysm rupture, particularly in the petrous portion of the canal leading to epistaxis. However, aside from limited cases, few other reports of late events are evident in the literature. With so little long-term data, it is difficult to confidently state either the true healing rate of these injuries or the risk of rupture or delayed embolic stroke.

Several isolated case reports have advocated the use of percutaneous angioplasty and stenting of carotid injuries. Not surprisingly, these case reports represent a diverse range of pathologies, symptoms, mechanisms of injury, and time to diagnosis. Although the majority appears to have patency of the stented carotid artery documented in follow-up radiographic evaluation, several cases of carotid artery occlusion following stent placement have been reported. Our most recent evaluation indicates a prohibitive stroke and carotid occlusion rate associated with carotid stents placed in acutely injured vessels.[20] During the 8½–year study period, 140 patients sustained blunt carotid injury, of whom 46 (33%) had a carotid artery pseudoaneurysm. Carotid stents were placed in 23

patients, while the remaining 23 patients were treated with antithrombotic therapy alone. In the group undergoing stent placement, three patients suffered stroke and one patient sustained a subclavian artery dissection. Carotid occlusion rate in this group was 45%. In patients treated solely with antithrombotics, including heparin or antiplatelet agents, there were no ischemic neurologic events and the occlusion rate on follow-up angiography was 5%. Additionally, long-term follow-up in patients with traumatic pseudoaneurysms who were treated with anticoagulation alone is needed. Further understanding and evaluation of the role of appropriate concurrent antithrombotic therapy, as well as evolving stent technology including smaller delivery systems and covered stents, may improve the outcome for postinjury intraluminal carotid stents. In the interim, however, our experience suggests carotid stenting should be performed in selective cases and antithrombotic therapy remains the cornerstone of treatment for post-traumatic pseudoaneurysms.

LONG-TERM FOLLOW-UP AND OUTCOME

Following initiation of antithrombotics, treatment is continued for 6 months empirically. Repeat evaluation of the patient's injury and a determination of antithrombotic therapy should be considered at 6 months. Although no long-term studies have been performed to date, we currently recommend multislice CTA for long-term follow-up. Patients with persistent injuries on repeat imaging are often treated with lifelong aspirin. Although, as is true for any long-term therapy, the risks of treatment should be discussed with the patient.

The morbidity and mortality of BCVI-related ischemic neurologic events are well documented. Historically, BCVI stroke-related permanent neurologic morbidity was greater than 80% with associated mortality rates of 40%. Modern series report lower rates of morbidity but mortality due to BCVI is significant, with CAI patients having a 13%–21% stroke-related mortality and patients with VAI-related strokes a 4%–18% mortality rate.[21] A less studied variable is the impact of neurologic morbidity on the need for prolonged acute patient care. Our recent evaluation points to a greater need for discharge and overall rate of discharge to rehabilitation services in patients suffering BCVI-related INE.[8] Such prolonged acute patient care increases costs to the patient, insurance companies, and ultimately to society. Performing a cost analysis of direct BCVI-related costs is difficult in these multisystem trauma patients; however, a cost analysis of patient life is even more problematic. In our series, overall mortality in patients sustaining CAI was 7% for those without neurologic event versus 32% for those with neurologic event; in patients with VAI, those without neurologic event had a mortality of 7% while those with a neurologic event had a mortality rate of 18%. The impact on mortality due to BCVI-related strokes appears independent of a patient's associated injuries, as the ISS was not significantly different between those with and without INE.

CONCLUSIONS

Diagnosis and treatment of BCVI has evolved over the past three decades. Originally thought to be a rare occurrence, BCVIs are now diagnosed in approximately 1% of blunt trauma patients. The recognition of a clinically silent period allows for screening for injuries based on mechanism of trauma and the patient's constellation of injuries. Currently, protocols exist for screening, hence limiting invasive procedures to those with the highest risk of injury (Figure 8). Comprehensive evaluation of patients has resulted in the early diagnosis of BCVI during the asymptomatic phase, thus allowing prompt initiation of treatment. Although the ideal regimen of antithrombotic therapy has yet to be determined, treatment with either antiplatelet agents or anticoagulation reduces the BCVI-related stroke rate. BCVI is a rare but

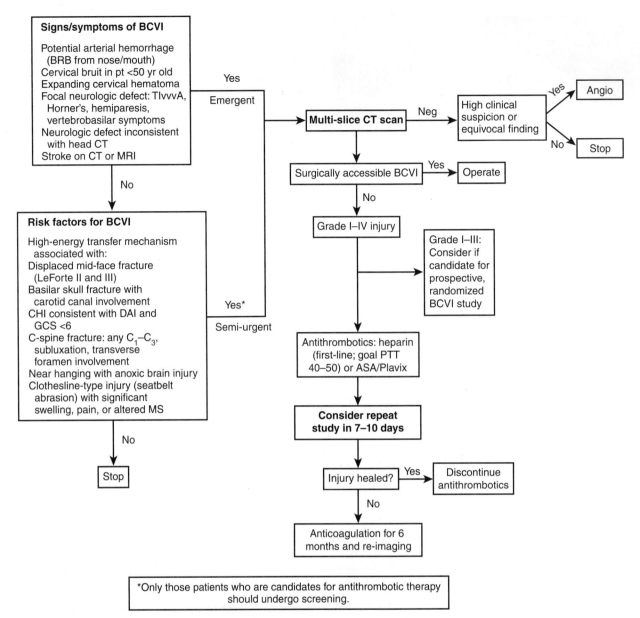

Figure 8 Denver Health Medical Center's current BCVI screening algorithm. *BCVI*, Blunt cerebrovascular injury; *BRB*, bright red blood; *CHI*, closed head injury; *CT*, computed tomography; *DAI*, diffuse axonal injury; *GCS*, Glasgow Coma Scale; *MRI*, magnetic resonance imaging; *MS*, mental status; *TIA*, transient ischemic attack. *(Courtesy of Denver Health Medical Center.)*

potentially devastating injury; appropriate screening in high-risk patients should be performed and prompt treatment initiated to prevent ischemic neurologic events.

REFERENCES

1. Cogbill TH, Moore EE, Meissner M, et al: The spectrum of blunt injury to the carotid artery: a multicenter perspective. *J Trauma* 37:473–479, 1994.
2. Davis JW, Holbrook TL, Hoyt DB, et al: Blunt carotid artery dissection: incidence, associated injuries, screening, and treatment. *J Trauma* 30:1514–1517, 1990.
3. Biffl WL, Ray CE Jr, Moore EE, et al: Treatment-related outcomes from blunt cerebrovascular injuries: importance of routine follow-up arteriography. *Ann Surg* 235:699–706, 2002.
4. Cothren CC, Moore EE, Biffl WL, et al: Anticoagulation is the gold standard therapy for blunt carotid injuries to reduce stroke rate. *Arch Surg* 139:540–545, 2004.
5. Miller PR, Fabian TC, Bee TK, et al: Blunt cerebrovascular injuries: diagnosis and treatment. *J Trauma* 51:279–285, 2001.
6. Fabian TC, Patton, JH, Croce MA: Blunt carotid injury. Importance of early diagnosis and anticoagulant therapy. *Ann Surg* 223:513–522, 1996.
7. Biffl WL, Moore EE, Ryu RK et al: The unrecognized epidemic of blunt carotid arterial injuries: early diagnosis improves neurologic outcome. *Ann Surg* 228:462–470, 1998.
8. Cothren CC, Moore EE, Ray CE, et al: Screening for blunt cerebrovascular injuries is cost effective. *Am J Surg* 190:845–849, 2005.
9. Crissey MM, Bernstein EF: Delayed presentation of carotid intimal tear following blunt craniocervical trauma. *Surgery* 75(4):543–549, 1974.
10. Biffl WL, Moore EE, Offner PJ, et al: Blunt carotid arterial injuries: implications of a new grading scale. *J Trauma* 47(5):845–853, 1999.
11. Cothren CC, Moore EE, Johnson JL, Ciesla DJ, Moore JB, Burch JM: Cervical spine fracture patterns mandating angiography to rule out blunt cerebrovascular injury. *Surgery* 141:76–82, 2007.
12. Miller PR, Fabian TC, Croce MA, et al: Prospective screening for blunt cerebrovascular injuries: analysis of diagnostic modalities and outcomes. *Ann Surg* 236:386–393, 2002.

13. Malhotra AK, Camacho M, Ivatury RR, et al: Computed tomographic angiography for the diagnosis of blunt carotid/vertebral artery injury: a note of caution. *Ann Surg* 246:632–641, 2007.
14. Biffl WL, Egglin T, Benedetto B, Gibbs F, Cioffi WG: Sixteen-slice computed togographic angiography is a reliable noninvasive screening test for clinically significant blunt cerebrovascular injuries. *J Truma* 60(4): 745–751, 2006.
15. Utter GH, Hollingworth W, Hallam DK, Jarvik JG, Jurkovich GJ: Sixteen-slice CT angiography in patients with suspected blunt carotid and vertebral artery injuries. *J Am Coll Surg* 203(6):838–848, 2006.
16. Eastman AL, Chason DP, Perez CL, McAnulty AL, Minei JP: Computed tomographic angiography for the diagnosis of blunt cervical vascular injury: is it ready for primetime? *J Trauma* 60(5):925–929, 2006.
17. Chimowitz MI, Kokkinos J, Strong J, et al: The Warfarin-Aspirin Symptomatic Intracranial Disease Study. *Neurology* 45(8):1488–1493, 1995.
18. Chimowitz MI, Lynn MJ, Howlett-Smith H, et al: Comparison of Warfarin and Aspirin for symptomatic intracranial arterial stenosis. *N Engl J Med* 352:1305–1316, 2005.
19. Savitz SI, Caplan LR: Vertebrobasilar disease. *N Engl J Med* 352: 2618–2626, 2005.
20. Cothren CC, Moore EE, Ray CE, et al: Carotid artery stents for blunt cerebrovascular injury: risks exceed benefits. *Arch Surg* 140:480–486, 2005.
21. Miller RS, Patton M, Graham RM, Hollins D: Outcomes of trauma patients who survive prolonged lengths of stay in the intensive care unit. *J Trauma* 48:229–234, 2000.

TRACHEAL, LARYNGEAL, AND OROPHARYNGEAL INJURIES

Luis G. Fernandez, Scott H. Norwood,
and John D. Berne

Structural mobility and elasticity are characteristics of the upper airway that make injury to these structures infrequent. Skeletal protection is also provided anteriorly by the mandible and sternum and posteriorly by the bony spinal column[1] (Figure 1). Upper airway injuries are identified in only 0.03% of patients admitted to major trauma centers. These injuries are frequently lethal, which explains their higher reported occurrence in autopsy series.[2,3] Penetrating mechanisms of injury are more common than blunt mechanisms of injury,[1,2,4] the true incidence of which is unknown.[1,5] Twenty-one percent of patients with upper airway injuries die within the first 2 hours after hospitalization.[6] The diagnosis is often delayed in patients without immediate life-threatening upper airway trauma.[6,7] Such delays often result in serious late complications.[8,9] Limited experience in nonoperative and operative management of airway injuries has led to a wide variety of recommendations that may be considered under various clinical scenarios. For unstable, immediate life-threatening upper airway injuries, rapid airway control by any available means is essential for patient survival. Most authors agree that tracheal intubation through an open wound that communicates with the tracheobronchial tree is appropriate.[1] Stable patients may benefit from bronchoscopic-guided tracheal intubation distal to the injury site, and blind endotracheal tube placement is almost always a poor choice for airway control.[10] Airway injuries are always challenging to even the most experienced surgeon since traditional approaches to airway control are often contraindicated.

ANATOMY OF UPPER AIRWAY

Oral Cavity

The oral cavity is designed for the articulation of speech and mastication. It also provides an alternate pathway (to the nasopharynx) for the upper airway system.

Boundaries

Anterior—lips
Posterior—anterior tonsillar pillars
Roof—hard and soft palate
Floor—mucosa overlying sublingual and submandibular glands
Walls—buccal mucosa

Contents

Alveolar processes and teeth
Anterior tongue to circumvallate papilla
Orifice of parotid gland (Stenson's duct) in buccal mucosa opposite upper second molars
Orifice of submandibular duct (Wharton's duct) in anterior floor of mouth
Orifices of sublingual glands

Pharynx

Surgical Anatomy

The pharynx consists of the following elements:

Nasopharynx: Extends from posterior choanae of the nose to the soft palate. It is related posteriorly to the base of the skull. The nasopharynx contains adenoid tissue and the orifices of the Eustachian tubes. This area is not accessible to direct inspection and must be examined by mirrors or optical instruments.

Oropharynx: Portion that is visible via the mouth. The oropharynx extends from the soft palate superiorly to the vallecula inferiorly. The posterior and lateral walls of the oropharynx are formed by the superior and middle pharyngeal constrictors.

Palatine tonsils: Lymphoid aggregates between the mucosal folds created by the palatoglossus and palatopharyngeus muscles. The palatine tonsils are covered by stratified squamous epithelium, which continues down into deep crypts. Tonsils vary widely in size and may be sessile or pedunculated.

Hypopharynx: Portion of the pharynx that lies inferior to the tip of the epiglottis. The posterior and lateral walls are formed by middle and inferior pharyngeal constrictors. The hypopharynx extends inferiorly to the cricopharyngeus muscle, where the pharynx empties into the cervical esophagus. Anteriorly, it extends from the vallecula and contains the epiglottis and the larynx. Lateral to the larynx are the pyriform sinuses, two mucosal pouches

A

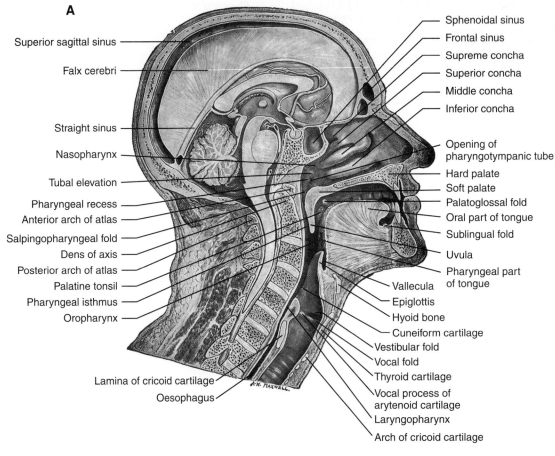

Superior sagittal sinus

Falx cerebri

Straight sinus

Nasopharynx

Tubal elevation

Pharyngeal recess

Anterior arch of atlas

Salpingopharyngeal fold

Dens of axis

Posterior arch of atlas

Palatine tonsil

Pharyngeal isthmus

Oropharynx

Lamina of cricoid cartilage

Oesophagus

Sphenoidal sinus

Frontal sinus

Supreme concha

Superior concha

Middle concha

Inferior concha

Opening of pharyngotympanic tube

Hard palate

Soft palate

Palatoglossal fold

Oral part of tongue

Sublingual fold

Uvula

Pharyngeal part of tongue

Vallecula

Epiglottis

Hyoid bone

Cuneiform cartilage

Vestibular fold

Vocal fold

Thyroid cartilage

Vocal process of arytenoid cartilage

Laryngopharynx

Arch of cricoid cartilage

B

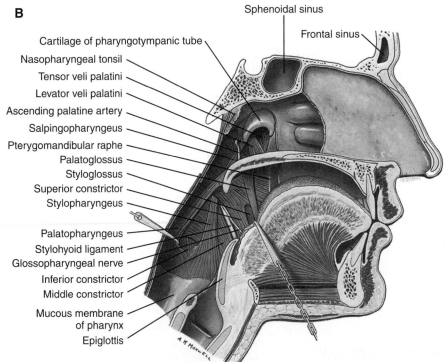

Sphenoidal sinus

Frontal sinus

Cartilage of pharyngotympanic tube

Nasopharyngeal tonsil

Tensor veli palatini

Levator veli palatini

Ascending palatine artery

Salpingopharyngeus

Pterygomandibular raphe

Palatoglossus

Styloglossus

Superior constrictor

Stylopharyngeus

Palatopharyngeus

Stylohyoid ligament

Glossopharyngeal nerve

Inferior constrictor

Middle constrictor

Mucous membrane of pharynx

Epiglottis

Figure 1   **(A)** Median sagittal section through the head and neck. **(B)** Median sagittal section of the head, showing a dissection of the interior of the pharynx, after the removal of the mucous membrane.   *(From Gray's Anatomy, 39th ed. St. Louis, Churchill Livingstone/Mosby, 2004, figures 35.1 and 35.3, with permission.)*

whose medial borders are the lateral walls of the larynx. The posterior aspect of the hypopharynx contains the posterior pharyngeal wall and postcricoid mucosa (Figures 2, 3, and 4).

PHARYNGEAL INJURY

Incidence

Isolated blunt pharyngeal injury is exceedingly rare. It is more often associated with concomitant cervical facial trauma. Penetrating pharyngeal injury occurs more commonly in the pediatric population from lacerations caused by intraoral foreign bodies.[11]

Mechanism of Injury

Pharyngeal trauma may occur from foreign body ingestion, blunt or penetrating trauma, or following laryngoscopy or other endoscopic procedures.[12–15]

Diagnosis

The initial clinical scenario varies. Patients with nonlethal injuries commonly present with dysphagia and odynophagia. Patients with more severe injuries may present with aphonia, dyspnea, hemoptysis, and severe acute respiratory failure that may rapidly lead to asphyxia if not treated.[16] Injuries to the esophagus and pharynx are difficult to diagnose and may be missed during the management of other immediate life-threatening injuries. Oral bleeding, drooling, and subcutaneous emphysema all suggest upper digestive tract or airway injury.[16] When possible, careful examination of the oropharynx and hypopharynx should be performed at the bedside.

Lateral views of the neck and cervical CT scan may identify soft tissue air (Figures 5 and 6). A nonionic contrast-enhanced esophagram

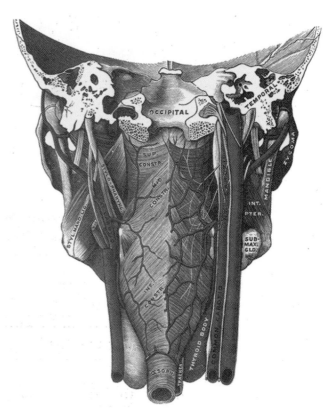

Figure 3 Muscles and blood supply of the pharynx. Muscles of the pharynx, viewed from behind, together with the associated vessels and nerves. *(Adapted from Gray H: Anatomy of the Human Body. Philadelphia, Lea & Febiger, 1918. Available at www.bartleby.com/107/.)*

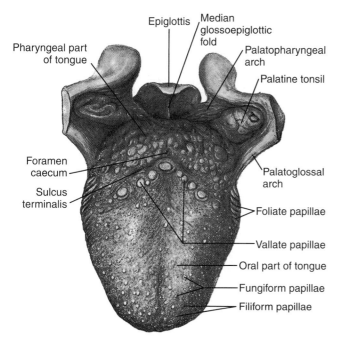

Figure 2 Contents of the oropharynx. *(From Gray's Anatomy, 39th ed. St. Louis, Churchill Livingstone/Mosby, 2004, figure 33.4, with permission.)*

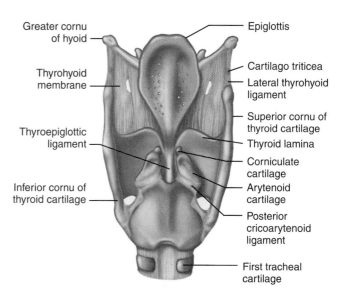

Figure 4 Posterior view of the laryngeal cartilages and ligaments. *(From Gray's Anatomy, 39th ed. St. Louis, Churchill Livingstone/Mosby, 2004, figure 36.3, with permission.)*

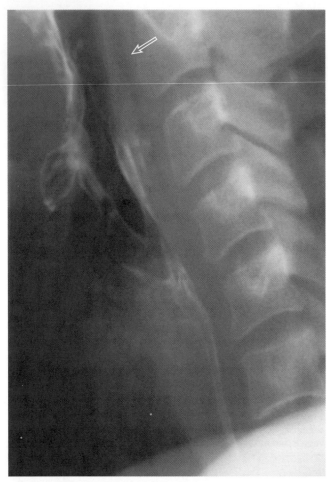

Figure 5   Retropharyngeal air *(black arrow)* as seen on a lateral cervical spine radiograph/esophagogram.

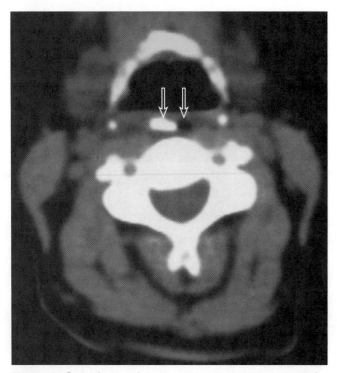

Figure 6   Retropharyngeal air as seen on a noncontrast computed tomography scan of the neck.

and/or esophagoscopy are indicated if injury is clinically suspected.[17] Contrast leak may be revealed on esophagram (see Figure 5).

LARYNX

Surgical Anatomy

The larynx is a functional "valve" separating the trachea from the upper aero-digestive tract. It is primarily an organ of communication (the voice box), but also serves as an important regulator of respiration. The larynx is necessary for effective coughing and for creating Valsalva maneuvers. The larynx also prevents aspiration during swallowing.

The larynx is composed of the following elements:

Skeleton (Figure 7)
Hyoid bone: Attaches to epiglottis and strap muscles.
Thyroid cartilage: Anterior attachment of vocal folds. Posterior articulation with cricoid cartilage.
Cricoid cartilage: Complete ring. Articulates with thyroid and arytenoid cartilages.
Arytenoids: Two cartilages that glide along the posterior cricoid and attach to posterior ends of vocal folds.
Divisions
Supraglottis: Usually covered with respiratory epithelium containing mucous glands.
Epiglottis: Leaf-shaped mucosal-covered cartilage, which projects over larynx.
Aryepiglottic folds: Extend from the lateral epiglottis to the arytenoids.
False vocal cords: Mucosal folds superior to the true glottis. Separated from true vocal folds by the ventricle.
Ventricle: Mucosal-lined sac, variable in size which separates the supraglottis from the glottis.
Glottis: The true vocal folds attach to the thyroid cartilage at the anterior commissure. The posterior commissure is mobile, as the vocal folds attach to the arytenoids. Motion of the arytenoids effects abduction or adduction of the larynx. The bulk of the vocal

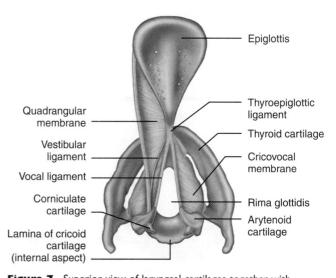

Figure 7   Superior view of laryngeal cartilages together with cricothyroid, quadrangular, and related ligaments and membranes. *(From Gray's Anatomy, 39th ed. St. Louis, Churchill Livingstone/Mosby, 2004, figure 36.7, with permission.)*

fold is made up of muscle covered by mucosa. The free edge is characterized by stratified squamous epithelium. The vocal folds abduct for inspiration and adduct for phonation, cough, and Valsalva. Subglottis: Below the vocal folds, extending to the inferior border of the cricoid cartilage.

Innervation—branches of the vagus nerve

Superior laryngeal nerve: Sensation of the glottis and supaglottis. Motor fibers to the cricothyroid muscle, which tenses the vocal folds. This nerve leaves the vagus high in the neck.

Recurrent laryngeal nerve: Sensation of the subglottis and motor fibers to intrinsic muscles of the larynx. This nerve branches from the vagus in the mediastinum, then turns back up into the neck. On the right, it travels inferior to the subclavian artery and on the left, the aorta.

Laryngeal Injury

Incidence

Laryngeal and cervical tracheal injuries account for less than 1% of trauma cases seen in most major trauma centers.[2,17] These injuries are rare compared to the total number of injuries that occur to the head and neck area. Experience in managing laryngeal trauma is limited because of these small numbers. External laryngeal trauma occurs in 1/30,000 emergency room visits.[18,19] The rare nature of laryngeal injuries is a consequence of multiple factors, including protection by the mandible and sternum, delayed or missed diagnoses of minor laryngeal injuries in major multitrauma victims, and patient mortality at the scene from airway loss and asphyxiation.[20]

Although rare, initial management of laryngeal injuries affects the immediate probability of patient survival and long-term quality of life. The larynx is a well-protected structure that is both anatomically and functionally complex. Blunt and penetrating laryngeal injuries may cause chronic problems with aspiration, phonation, and respiration.[20]

Mechanism of Injury

The mechanisms of laryngeal injury can be divided into blunt trauma (including crushing, clothesline, and strangulation injuries) and penetrating trauma. The degree and location of blunt laryngotracheal trauma are multifactorial. Sheely et al.[21] found that 88% of injuries occurred above the fourth tracheal ring. Penetrating injury can occur at any level of the cervical trachea.

Diagnosis

Adherence to the essential principles of initial assessment delineated in the *Advanced Trauma Life Support (ATLS)®* Manual is recommended. The ABCs (airway, breathing, circulation), concomitant resuscitation of the trauma victim, and a thorough secondary survey are essential for optimal management of airway injuries.[22] Early recognition of these injuries requires a high index of suspicion based on mechanism of injury and findings identified during cervical and chest examination. Clinical signs and symptoms may include stridor, acute respiratory distress, cervical tenderness, subcutaneous emphysema, and cervical hematoma when associated with major vascular injury.[23] Hemoptysis suggests that an intralaryngeal laceration may be present.[23] This is more common with penetrating injury, but also occurs from blunt laryngeal trauma with an associated laryngeal cartilage fracture.[23] Diagnostic procedures such as direct laryngoscopy, fiberoptic bronchoscopy, and cervical helical, contrast-enhanced multidetector (16 slices minimum) computed tomography (CT) with angiography are all beneficial if the patient's clinical condition permits performing these tests.[17,24] A sample algorithm for the evaluation of patients with laryngeal injuries is described (Figure 8).

TRACHEA

Surgical Anatomy

The trachea is a cartilaginous and membranous tube. It extends from the lower part of the larynx, at the level of the sixth cervical vertebra, to the upper border of the fifth thoracic vertebra. There it divides into the two main stem bronchi. The trachea is an ellipsoid cylinder that is flattened posteriorly. The average adult trachea measures about 11 cm in length with a diameter that varies from 2 to 2.5 cm. The pediatric trachea is smaller, more deeply placed, and more mobile. Half of the trachea lies within the neck and half is intrathoracic. The anterior two thirds of the trachea are composed of 18 to 22 "U"-shaped cartilages. The membranous posterior wall of the trachea is in apposition with the anterior wall of the esophagus. The bifurcation of the mainstem bronchi forms the carina at approximately the fourth to fifth thoracic vertebrae. The trachea is supplied with blood by the inferior thyroid arteries. Similarly named veins form the thyroid venous plexus. Tracheal innervation is derived from the vagus nerves, the recurrent laryngeal nerves, and from the sympathetic chain. The recurrent laryngeal nerve lies within the tracheoesophageal groove formed by the close proximity of the lateral aspects of the trachea and the esophagus (Figures 9, 10, and 11).

Tracheal Injury

Incidence

Disruption of the tracheobronchial tree is a rare occurrence and most surgeons' experience is limited. On average, one such case is seen per year in large trauma centers.[25] Bertelsen and Howitz[4] reviewed 1178 postmortem reports of trauma deaths and found 33 (2.8%) with tracheal and/or bronchial disruptions. Of these 33 cases, 27 were dead at the scene.[4]

Complete cervical transection is rarer still. The true incidence (and tracheobronchial injuries in general) is unknown.[26,27] There have been a number of case reports and small series described in the literature; however, the extant surgical experience remains limited.[26]

Knowledge of emergency airway management is essential. Loss of the airway in this clinical circumstance can rapidly lead to serious complications and/or the patient's demise.[17,28]

Mortality in those patients who do not have complete airway loss at the time of injury is due to the severity of associated injuries. Those patients who arrive alive to a trauma center with isolated tracheobronchial injuries, including complete transection, have a reasonable chance for survival if the trauma surgeon has mastered the skills required for managing a difficult airway.[29]

Beskin[30] reported the first successful repair of a complete cervical transection after blunt trauma in 1957. Hood and Sloan[31] in 1959 collected 18 cases of tracheobronchial injury in the world literature. Complete tracheal transection was "rarely found." In a more recent series, Eckert et al.[3] reported a total of 105 tracheobronchial injuries, of which 75 were from penetrating trauma and 30 from blunt trauma. Of these, only 24 patients survived the transfer from the scene of the accident to the trauma center. Of the 30 blunt trauma victims reported in this series, 18 were dead on arrival at the emergency department. The majority of those who arrived alive, regardless of the mechanism of injury, had no other associated injuries (15 of 24 [63%]), and the remainder had only one other associated injury, including esophageal injuries (9 of 24 [37%]).[3] In the same series, the most commonly injured segment of the tracheobronchial tree in survivors was the cervical trachea (37%). The total number of complete tracheal transections in Ecker and associates' series is unknown.

Kelly et al.[6] reviewed 106 patients with tracheobronchial injuries of which only 6 had a blunt mechanism of injury.[6] They concluded

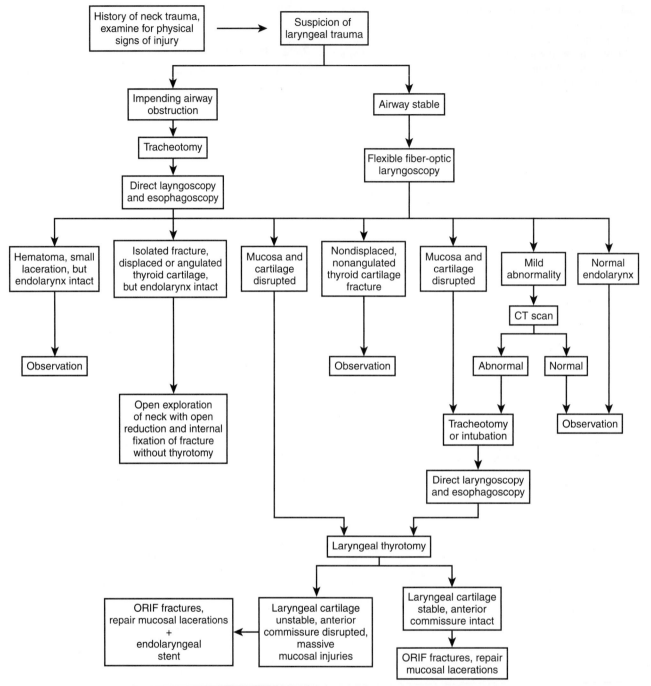

Figure 8 Algorithm for evaluating patient with suspected laryngeal injury. *CT,* Computed tomography; *ORIF,* open reduction with internal fixation. *(Adapted from Pancholi SS: Fractures, laryngeal. Department of Otolaryngology, Three Rivers Medical Center, Louisa, KY, November 3, 2005, http://www.emedicine.com/ent/images/ and http://www.emedicine.com/ent/topic488.htm.)*

that a surgeon must adopt a rapid, aggressive surgical approach to these patients in order to prevent lethal outcomes.[6]

Mechanism of Injury

Cervical trachea

Injuries to the cervical trachea may be caused by blunt or penetrating trauma. Penetrating injury is relatively straightforward. With the exception of shrapnel wounds, this consists of a traumatic defect created by the trajectory of the knife or bullet. Knife wounds more commonly occur in the cervical trachea, while gunshot wound injuries may occur at any point along the course of the tracheobronchial tree.[17–27]

In one review, blunt injury to the cervical tracheal was reported to occur in less than 1% of all 1248 blunt trauma patients admitted over the study period. In this anatomic region, blunt injuries to the larynx are the most frequent.[17] They usually result from motor vehicle accidents or sports injuries, and direct blows to this area (e.g., "clothesline injury").[17–27]

Intrathoracic tracheal injury

Injuries in this region are more commonly caused by blunt trauma, but may also result from penetrating injuries. In the former, the exact mechanism is unknown. Several theories have been advanced. This injury is often associated with sudden and forceful

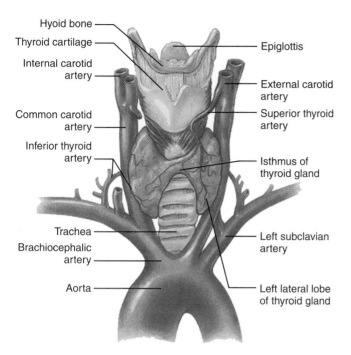

Figure 9 Anatomy of the larynx, cervical, and upper thoracic trachea. *(Copyright 2001 Benjamin Cummings, an imprint of Addison Wesley Longman, Inc.)*

compression of the thorax. It is postulated that a rapid anteroposterior compression of the trachea in combination with a closed glottis causes markedly increased tracheal intraluminal pressure. When shearing forces are added to the tracheobronchial tree between the relatively stationary cricoid cartilage and carina (encountered during rapid deceleration), bronchial rupture may occur. Intrathoracic tracheal disruption usually occurs at the junction of the membranous and cartilaginous trachea within 2 cm of the carina. Vertical lesions are rare. When they do occur, they are more commonly located posteriorly where the cartilage is less evident. Bronchial injuries more commonly involve the main bronchi. They tend to occur within 2.5 cm of the carina.[7–9,27]

Gunshot wounds are the most frequent penetrating injuries. The incidence of thoracic tracheobronchial injury increases with transmediastinal gunshot wounds. Injuries to the heart, great vessels, and esophagus are common in these cases, and are major contributors to morbidity and mortality.[27]

Diagnosis

A thorough physical examination and knowledge of the mechanism of injury are the first and most important steps in diagnosing a tracheobronchial injury. Clinical findings suggesting airway injury vary according to the mechanism of injury. Cicala et al.[32] reviewed nine patients following stab wounds. A laceration directly communicating with the airway was present in five cases. Subcutaneous emphysema was apparent on physical examination and on lateral cervical spine radiograph in three cases. Only one patient had no obvious clinical or radiographic findings to suggest an airway injury. This patient had a small puncture laceration of the cricotracheal membrane which was diagnosed by bronchoscopy. The majority of patients presenting with gunshot wounds to the trachea will show physical or radiographic finding that suggest airway injury on a plain radiograph of the neck or chest.[32] In the study by Cicala and colleagues,[32] two patients with gunshot wounds to the cervicothoracic trachea developed tension pneumothorax with massive air leak during resuscitation. Two others had fractures of the thyroid cartilage without any airway compromise. One was diagnosed by direct palpation on physical examination. The other patient was diagnosed by cervical CT scan. Hemoptysis, in addition to other findings, was noted in two of the gunshot wound victims.[32]

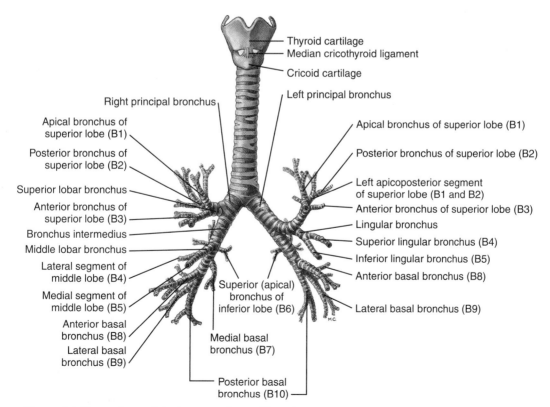

Figure 10 The cartilages of the larynx, trachea, and bronchi: anterior aspect. *(From Gray's Anatomy, 39th ed. St. Louis, Churchill Livingstone/Mosby, 2004, figure 63.12, with permission.)*

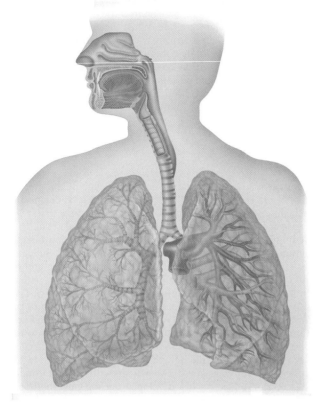

Figure 11   The respiratory tract. Those parts of the tract in the head and upper neck are shown in sagittal section, in the lower neck turned anteriorly and, in the remainder of the tract, from the anterior aspect. The right lung shows the bronchial tree in detail whereas the left lung shows the pulmonary vasculature.   *(From Gray's Anatomy, 39th ed. St. Louis, Churchill Livingstone/Mosby, 2004, figure 63.1, with permission.)*

Blunt trauma patients who survive to the emergency department may present with a wide spectrum of clinical signs and symptoms dependant on the severity and location of the injury to the cervical thoracic trachea. Blunt cervical tracheal injury may create severe respiratory compromise leading to rapid acute respiratory failure and asphyxia. Alternatively, patients with less severe injuries may present with stridor, hoarseness, hemoptysis, and subcutaneous emphysema.[24,32]

Plain radiographs of the neck and chest may be diagnostic. Subcutaneous emphysema in the neck and chest wall on plain radiographs or CT scan should prompt further evaluation if clinical suspicion favors a major airway injury.[1–6,10–12,32] Fiberoptic bronchoscopy is the first step in confirming a tracheal injury.[27,33] Indications for bronchoscopy include a large pneumomediastinum, persistent pneumothorax, or a large, persistent air leak after placement of a functional thoracostomy tube; persistent atelectasis; and expanding severe subcutaneous emphysema.[34] Bronchoscopy is the most accurate and reliable means to establish the diagnosis, determine the site and define the extent of the injury.[35] Debate remains as to whether rigid or flexible bronchoscopy is superior in this setting. Disadvantages of rigid bronchoscopy include the need for a general anesthetic and a stable cervical spine. Flexible bronchoscopy does not require a general anesthetic, and may be used in patients whose cervical spine may be injured. Fiber-optic bronchoscopy is not only diagnostic, but may also be useful in establishing an airway with bronchoscopically guided endotracheal tube placement.[36]

Preoperative assessment of the vocal cords in this setting is strongly recommended. Direct laryngoscopy may be necessary to evaluate the function of the vocal cords. The presence of a recurrent laryngeal nerve injury causing vocal cord paralysis may assist the operating surgeon in determining whether tracheostomy is needed regardless of the location or extent of airway injury.[37,38]

SURGICAL MANAGEMENT

Surgical management includes appropriate nonoperative observation (by a trauma surgeon) as well as operative intervention. Initial airway management must be approached with caution. Patients who are spontaneously breathing and maintaining adequate oxygenation and ventilation should not be intubated unless their clinical condition deteriorates. Patients intubated prior to arrival in the emergency department should undergo flexible bronchoscopy as soon as possible. Careful intubation over a bronchoscope, performed by an experienced bronchoscopist, is the optimal approach for those patients who require early airway control for clinical deterioration or for treatment of other life-threatening injuries. Intubation is ideally performed in the operating room where emergent cricothyroidotomy or tracheostomy can be performed if necessary. The trauma surgeon must be prepared to extend the tracheostomy incision to a median sternotomy if the distal trachea retracts into the mediastinum. Clinical deterioration may still occur as positive pressure ventilation is applied if the injury is distal to the tracheostomy. High-frequency ventilation or low tidal volume ventilation with additional tube thoracostomies may be necessary.

Nonoperative Management

Small iatrogenic injuries from endotracheal intubation or from minimal blunt force trauma can often be safely observed. Most injuries from high energy blunt force trauma and all penetrating injuries are not generally considered for nonoperative management.

Gomez-Caro et al.[39] recently reported the successful management of 17 patients with iatrogenic tracheobronchial injuries between 1993 and 2003. Many of these lesions were as large as 4 cm in length. The authors reported no complications or deaths directly caused by nonoperative management. Clinical and endoscopic follow-up in 14 of 17 patients was uneventful. Guidelines for nonoperative management include vital signs stability, no associated esophageal injury, no issues with mechanical ventilation or intubation (if necessary), no development of severe subcutaneous emphysema or mediastinal emphysema, and no signs of sepsis.[39] Additional requirements for nonoperative management have been published.[27] These include only small tracheobronchial lacerations, such as those with less than one-third of the circumference of the trachea, well-opposed edges, no significant tissue loss, no associated injuries, and no need for positive pressure ventilation. Intubation as well as tracheostomy should ideally be avoided. When necessary, endotracheal intubation with placement of the endotracheal tube balloon distal to the tear has been proposed by Marquette et al.[40] This technique has been successfully used on three occasions by one of the authors (SN). Nonoperative management includes administering prophylactic antibiotics and proton pump inhibitors, very close observation, and close bronchoscopic follow-up.[27] A sample algorithm is provided in Figure 12.

Operative Management

Patients diagnosed with a major tracheobronchial injury should always undergo surgery unless medical instability or severe associated injuries are significantly prohibitive.[41,42] In those situations, all efforts are made to support and stabilize the patient while maintaining adequate oxygenation and ventilation. High-frequency ventilation may be helpful. Permissive hypercapnia using very low tidal volumes (less than 5 ml/kg) has also been successfully used.[43]

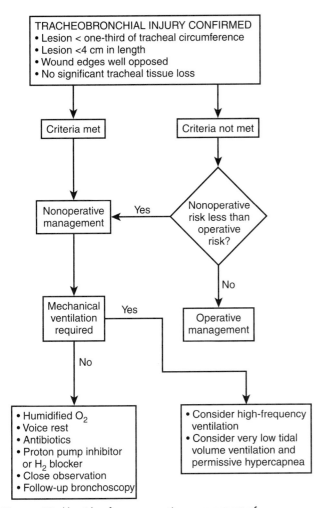

Figure 12 Algorithm for nonoperative management of tracheobronchial injuries.

The majority of patients are optimally managed with early surgery. The site of injury dictates the operative approach. These injuries are often challenging to even the most experienced surgeon, and appropriate consultation with an otolaryngologist for high cervical injuries or a thoracic surgeon for more distal intrathoracic injuries may be helpful.

Most cervical injuries are approached through a transverse collar incision. This incision can be extended cephalad along the anterior border of either sternocleidomastoid muscle, depending on the location of the primary and any associated injuries. Penetrating cervical injuries can often be approached directly, incorporating the wound into the incision. This may be necessary to achieve early airway control.

Blunt cervical tracheal injuries are also approached through a transverse collar incision just above the sternal notch. The chest should always be prepped for median sternotomy. An upper median sternotomy is immediately performed if the distal trachea retracts into the chest. Do not necessarily expect to find the trachea in its usual midline position. We have experienced one case where the distal trachea, upon entry into the chest, retracted 10 cm below the sternal notch and 10 cm to the left of midline.

Most blunt intrathoracic tracheobronchial injuries occur within 2–3 cm of the carina. A right posterolateral thoracotomy through the fourth or fifth intercostal space provides the best exposure unless the injury is on the left more than 2–3 cm distal to the carina. In this situation, a left posterolateral thoracotomy through the fifth intercostal space is preferred.

Prior consultation with the anesthesiologist is crucial. A variety of endotracheal tubes, connectors, and ventilator tubing should be available on the operative table prior to opening the chest. Intubation over a bronchoscope in the operating room is best for optimal tube placement. Double-lumen tubes are beneficial for providing single-lung ventilation. However, their larger size may cause further damage and hinder the operative repair. Positioning the patient for thoracotomy and opening the chest may cause rapid deterioration from hypoxemia and hypoventilation. Opening the chest quickly with direct intubation of a major bronchus through the operative field may be necessary. The surgeon may also be able to direct the orotracheal tube from the upper trachea into the uninjured bronchus to provide one lung ventilation. If the anatomy of the injury is not completely known, two ventilators should be available in the operating room so that bilateral single lung ventilation can be provided if needed. The Univent® endobronchial blocker may also be helpful if there is active bleeding from one of the mainstem or segmental bronchi. This device incorporates an endotracheal tube with a maneuverable device that can be directed into and occlude a mainstem bronchus, an intermediate trunk, or a lobar bronchus.[44]

Repair of the trachea and bronchi requires optimal debridement of all devitalized tissue and primary end-to-end anastomosis. Either permanent or absorbable monofilament sutures are preferred. The authors prefer a running monofilament absorbable suture. All knots are tied external to the lumen to reduce the risk of granuloma formation. Management "pearls" are provided in Table 1.

MORBIDITY

Early Complications

In the early postinjury period following tracheal or laryngeal injury, *loss of airway* represents the greatest immediate threat. The need for definitive airway control is dictated by clinical signs of respiratory insufficiency such as dyspnea, tachypnea, hypoxemia, or massive hemoptysis. When laryngeal injury is suspected, care should be taken when passing the tube through the area of injury as partial tears can be converted into complete tears. Tension pneumothorax and massive subcutaneous emphysema may lead to mechanical ventilatory failure from mechanical constraints limiting pulmonary expansion. Endotracheal intubation can be attempted with extreme caution. When advancing the tube past the vocal cords care should be taken if tracheal injury is present or suspected. Nasotracheal intubation with a no. 7 or smaller cuffed endotracheal tube over a flexible bronchoscope has been proposed as one option in the stable patient.[12,45] This should ideally be performed in the operating room or wherever conditions for performing an immediate surgical airway are optimal. Identification of the injury and strategically guided tube placement may be possible while minimizing iatrogenic trauma during intubation. This technique may be particularly useful in cases of near-complete or complete tracheal transection when suspected preopera-

Table 1: Management Pearls for Acute Laryngotracheal Trauma

Avoid searching for recurrent laryngeal nerves
Avoid tracheostomy through the repair
Conservation of viable trachea
Thorough evaluation of associated injuries
Flexion of neck postoperatively to reduce tension on tracheal repair
Proper airway management
Separation of tracheal and esophageal suture lines

Source: Mathisen DJ, Grillo H: Laryngotracheal trauma. *Ann Thorac Surg* 43(3):254–262, 1987.

tively to advance the tube into the distal tracheal segment.[45] This maneuver must be performed by an experienced bronchoscopist. Even in cases when complete tracheal transection has occurred, adequate ventilation and oxygenation may be achieved with intubation of only the proximal tracheal remnant provided that the paratracheal tissues of the neck and superior mediastinum are still intact. Caution should be taken in this setting at the time of operation or attempted surgical airway control when entering this space from a cervical incision; rapid ventilatory failure and cardiopulmonary collapse can occur when this air space is entered and this distal tracheal segment has not been secured with an airway.[26,46] The distal tracheal segment may retract back into the superior mediastinum and be difficult to access from a cervical incision. This may be prevented by performing a sternotomy prior to entering the pretracheal space when complete tracheal transection is suspected preoperatively.[26]

Tension pneumothorax can lead to rapid cardiopulmonary collapse if not quickly recognized and treated. While temporary improvement may be achieved, needle thoracostomy should be reserved for patients with impending cardiopulmonary collapse in the prehospital or emergency department setting. Immediate placement of one or more tube thoracostomies is the ideal treatment and may be lifesaving. Patients with tracheobronchial injuries may develop a large air leak following pleural space drainage. In addition to increasing the negative pressure suction applied to the pleural space, advanced ventilatory strategies may be required to improve gas exchange. Low tidal volume ventilation, high-frequency jet ventilation, and high-frequency oscillatory ventilation have all been used with success to reduce peak airway pressure, increase mean airway pressure, reduce air leak, and promote healing at the site of injury.[43,47,48]

Pneumomediastinum may occur following tracheobronchial injury. Although hemodynamic compromise has been reported from air under pressure in the mediastinum, this appears to be unusual.[35,49] Treatment is directed toward the underlying injury and resolution following injury repair, and recovery is the rule.

Subcutaneous emphysema can be massive, spreading to all areas of the body very quickly. Although treatment with multiple incisions or drains has been advocated,[50,51] the emphysema itself has no direct adverse sequelae and is usually self-limiting.

Massive bleeding into the airways suggests an associated major vascular injury. Initial treatment should be directed at identification and control of hemorrhage from this injury. Large volumes of bloodshed into the airway can lead to airway obstruction and profound hypoxemia from impaired gas exchange. Following definitive airway control the endotracheal cuff should be advanced beyond the site of bleeding into the airway if possible. Bronchoscopic lavage of retained blood and clots may be of further benefit in clearing retained hemorrhage and improving hypoxemia.

Associated injuries are common and account for a substantial portion of early morbidity. A high index of suspicion for these injuries is maintained throughout early evaluation. Patient management based on ATLS® guidelines will minimize associated morbidity.[52]

Late Complications

Late complications following tracheal injury are often related to the integrity of the area of injury or site of surgical repair.

The incidence of tracheobronchial stenosis following injury is 3.8%–9.3% following surgical repair.[41,53] Stenosis may also occur when nonoperative management of a tracheal or bronchial tear is attempted.[43] Initial measures to reduce inflammation include corticosteroid therapy and proton pump inhibitors or H2 blockers to reduce aspiration of acidic gastric contents. Steroid therapy is controversial. The risks of immunosuppression and compromised wound healing must be compared to the benefits of reduced scarring and stenosis.[54,55] Steroids may be beneficial during nonoperative management to reduce stenosis from hypertrophic granulation tissue, but there are currently no large studies to refute or support this therapy. Factors associated

with a higher incidence of tracheal stenosis include degree of tracheal injury and increased time to operative repair.[56] Others have not found increased stenosis rates when operative repair is delayed.[41,57] Timing of operative repair is determined by associated injuries and overall physiologic status. Surgical repair should proceed as soon as possible to reduce this potential complication. Good surgical technique can reduce postoperative tracheal stenosis. Complete debridement of devitalized tissue, wide mobilization to reduce anastomotic tension and possibly the use of absorbable sutures are principles that may reduce inflammation and enhance normal healing repair site. Vascularized pedicles of muscle, usually the sternocleidomastoid or the strap muscles, sewn as a buttress to the anastomotic site have been shown to reduce the rate of anastomotic dehiscence, leak, and subsequent fistula formation.[41] Tracheal stenosis is suspected when stridor, dyspnea, or air hunger develop following tracheal repair or injury.[54] Usually the history is one of worsening progression over several days to weeks. Voice changes may occur simultaneously. Other symptoms may include postobstructive atelectasis or pulmonary sepsis, particularly following bronchial or distal segment repairs.[57]

Flexible or rigid bronchoscopy provides an accurate diagnosis and an opportunity for simultaneous treatment. Modern multidetector CT scanners are also highly sensitive and specific for diagnosing tracheobronchial pathology.[58,59] Anatomic detail with three-dimensional reconstruction is very useful in planning operative or interventional repair. Treatment options include (1) endoscopic dilatation with steroid therapy[60]; (2) silicone, metal, or Teflon stent placement[61,62]; (3) Nd-Yag laser ablation of scar tissue[63]; or (4) open surgical repair. All of these treatments have been individually successful, and the therapeutic approach in any given patient must be individualized based on the extent of stenosis, severity of comorbid conditions and the experience and resources of each surgeon and facility. Many different open surgical techniques have been described but general principles should include resection and debridement of tracheal scar with tracheal mobilization and primary end-to-end anastomosis with absorbable suture.

Tracheoesophageal fistula may occur following a delay in diagnosis and/or treatment of esophageal and/or tracheal injuries. A high index of suspicion for esophageal or tracheal injury must be maintained whenever the other is identified, and thorough evaluation with bronchoscopy, esophagoscopy, or esophagography is usually required. Careful and thorough intraoperative evaluation at surgery is mandatory. Full mobilization of the cervical esophagus and intraluminal instillation of methylene blue have been advocated to avoid missing a subtle esophageal tear. Following identification of a late tracheoesophageal fistula, delayed repair is planned following medical stabilization, treatment of aspiration pneumonitis or pneumonia, and gastrostomy tube placement. Repair consists of wide esophageal and tracheal mobilization, debridement to healthy tissue, and primary end-to-end anastomosis. Transposition of a vascularized pedicle of muscle between the areas of repair to be dictated by the anatomic location of the fistula is mandatory to reduce anastomotic dehiscence and recurrent fistula formation.[41]

Voice changes such as dysphonia and laryngeal stenosis can occur following laryngeal injury when architectural relationships within the voice box are altered by healing. Poor outcomes are associated with injuries that create significant mucosal disruption, arytenoid dislocation, or exposed cartilage. One series reported an association between delays in operative repair beyond 24 hours and increased rates of airway stenosis ranging from 13%–31%.[64] Laryngeal stenting, particularly when one or both vocal cords are mobile, helps preserve the voice by normalizing the shape of the anterior commissure. Stents should be removed as soon as possible (usually 10–14 days) because of the risk of compromised mucosal perfusion with prolonged usage.[65]

Vocal cord paralysis from recurrent laryngeal nerve injury may be unilateral or bilateral following tracheal or laryngeal injuries. Cricotracheal separation carries a 60% risk of recurrent nerve injury, which is often bilateral.[55] Resolution of neurapraxia and nerve regeneration may occur up to 1 year following injury, resulting in resolution of vocal cord paralysis in some cases.

Laryngeal webs, granulomas, and hypertrophic granulation can develop several months following laryngeal trauma. Follow-up endoscopy with laser ablation can prevent chronic problems from these less serious complications.[64]

Other Potentially Life-Threatening Complications

Pharyngeal injuries can lead to serious complications particularly when the diagnosis is delayed. Retropharyngeal abscess is uncommon but potentially life threatening if upper airway obstruction or mediastinitis develops.[66] A short course of prophylactic antibiotics may reduce the risk of this complication. The diagnosis is usually apparent upon inspection of the oropharynx and palatine tonsils. Retropharyngeal air may be present on lateral cervical radiograph. If present, further evaluation should include cervical and mediastinal CT scan. Surgical drainage of the abscess and broad spectrum intravenous antibiotics are indicated. Surgical intensive care unit admission and possible intubation may be necessary in severe cases.[67]

Injury to the internal carotid artery should also be considered whenever an impalement injury of the posterior pharynx is diagnosed. Asymptomatic dissection of the internal carotid artery followed by arterial occlusion or embolization to the cerebral vasculature may develop over several hours to days resulting in severe neurologic deficits. Therefore, a high index of suspicion and screening with angiography should be performed when clinical presentation suggests this possibility.[67] CT angiography (CTA) has improved in recent years with the multidetector scanners. Experience suggests that CTA may be a good screening tool to identify these injuries.[68-70] Anticoagulation to prevent propagation and occlusion of the dissection is standard therapy, but experience with carotid stents is growing. Carotid stenting may be an alternative in selected cases. Surgical repair of the internal carotid artery is usually impossible due to the distal location of most lesions.[70]

■ MORTALITY

The mortality rate for tracheobronchial injuries in most modern series is less than 30%.[29,41,53,57] A large literature review pooled all patients with blunt tracheobronchial injury reported between 1873 and 1996 and found a 9% mortality rate since 1970 for patients who arrived alive at the hospital.[57] Left-sided injuries, high-speed deceleration, and crush mechanisms are associated with the poorest outcomes. Autopsy series suggest that 80% of patients with tracheobronchial injuries die at the scene.[57] Early mortality results from associated injuries and loss of airway.

Mortality from laryngeal injuries has been reported as high as 40% and is primarily attributable to asphyxiation from airway compromise. Penetrating laryngeal injuries appear to have a lower mortality (20%). Death from penetrating injuries is more attributable to associated injuries, particularly esophageal and major vascular injuries.[55]

Attributable mortality from pharyngeal injuries is difficult to determine since these injuries are rarely life threatening. Death is usually attributable to the internal carotid artery thrombosis, cervical infection, or mediastinitis. When present, the outcome for each of these complications is dependent on early diagnosis and treatment.[67]

REFERENCES

1. Roger SC, Kenneth AK, Alan, et al: Initial evaluation and management of upper airway injuries in trauma patients. *J Clin Anesth* 3:91–98, 1991.
2. Gussack GS, Jurkovich GJ, Luterman A: Laryngotracheal trauma: a protocol approach to a rare injury. *Laryngoscope* 96:660–665, 1986.
3. Ecker RR, Libertini RV, Rea WJ, et al: Injuries of the trachea and bronchi. *Ann Thorac Surg* 11:289–298, 1971.
4. Bertelson S, Howitz P: Injuries of the trachea and bronchi. *Thorax* 27:188–194, 1972.
5. Nahum AM: Immediate care of acute blunt laryngeal trauma. *J Trauma* 9:112–125, 1969.
6. Kelly JP, Webb WR, Moulder PV, et al: Management of airway trauma. I: Tracheobronchial injuries. *Ann Thorac Surg* 40(6):551–555, 1985.
7. Mahaffey DE, Creech O, Boren HG, et al: Traumatic rupture of the left-main bronchus successfully repaired eleven years after injury. *J Thorac Surg* 32:312–331, 1956.
8. Kirsh MM, Orringer MB, Behrendt DM, et al: Management of tracheobronchial disruption secondary to nonpenetrating trauma. *Ann Thorac Surg* 22(1):93–101, 1976.
9. Grillo HC: Surgery of the trachea. In Ravitch MM, editor: *Current Problems in Surgery.* Chicago, Year Book Medical Publishers, 1970, pp. 3–59.
10. Trone TH, Schaefer SD, Carder HM: Blunt and penetrating laryngeal trauma: a 13-year review. *Otolaryngol Head Neck Surg* 88(3):257–261, 1980.
11. Fitz-Hugh GS, Powell JB: Acute traumatic injuries of the oropharynx, laryngopharynx, and cervical trachea in children. *Otolaryngol Clin North Am* 3(2):375–393, 1970.
12. Demetriades D, Velmahos GG, Asensio JA: Cervical pharyngoesophageal and laryngotracheal injuries. *World J Surg* 25(8):1044–1048, 2001 (review).
13. Pereira W Jr, Kovnat DM, Snider GL: A prospective cooperative study of complications following flexible fiberoptic bronchoscopy. *Chest* 73(6):813–816, 1978.
14. Heater DW, Haskvitz L: Suspected pharyngoesophageal perforation after a difficult intubation: a case report. *AANA J* 73(3):185–187, 2005.
15. Carey WD: Indications, contraindications and complications of upper gastrointestinal endoscopy. In Sivak MV Jr, editor: *Gastroenterologic Endoscopy.* Philadelphia, W.B. Saunders, 1987, pp. 296–306.
16. Goudy SL, Miller FB, Bumpous JM: Neck crepitance: evaluation and management of suspected upper aerodigestive tract injury. *Laryngoscope* 112(5):791–795, 2002.
17. Fuhrman G, Steig F, Buerk C: Blunt laryngeal trauma: classification and management protocol. *J Trauma* 30:87–92, 1990.
18. Jewett BS, Shockley WW, Rutledge R: External laryngeal trauma analysis of 392 patients. *Arch Otolaryngol Head Neck Surg* 125(8):877–880, 1999.
19. Biller HF, Moscoso J, Sanders I: Laryngeal trauma. In Ballenger JJ, Snow JB, editors: *Otorhinolaryngology: Head and Neck Surgery,* 15th ed. Media, PA, Lippincott Williams & Wilkins, 1996, pp. 518–525.
20. Meislin HW, Iserson KH, Kabak KR, et al: Airway trauma. *Emerg Med Clin North Am* 1:295–312, 1983.
21. Sheely CH 2nd, Mattox KL, Beall AC Jr: Management of acute cervical tracheal trauma. *Am J Surg* 128(6):805–808, 1974.
22. American College of Surgeons: *Advanced Trauma Life Support for Doctors: Instructor Course Manual.* Chicago, American College of Surgeons, 1997.
23. Snow JB Jr: Diagnosis and therapy for acute laryngeal and tracheal trauma. *Otolaryngol Clin North Am* 17(1):101–106, 1984.
24. Schaefer S: Primary management of laryngeal trauma. *Ann Otorlaryngol* 91:399–402, 1982.
25. Major CP, Floresguerra CA, Messerschmidt WH, Lewis JV: Traumatic disruption of the cervical trachea. *J Tenn Med Assoc* 85(11):517–518, 1992.
26. Norwood SH, McAuley CE, Vallina VL, et al: Complete cervical tracheal transection from blunt trauma. *J Trauma* 51(3):568–571, 2001.
27. Riley RD, Miller PR, Meredith JW: Injury to the esophagus, trachea, and bronchus. In Moore EE, Feliciano DV, Mattox KL, editors: *Trauma,* 5th ed. New York, McGraw-Hill, pp. 544–550.
28. Lazar HL, Thomashow B, King TC: Complete transection of the intrathoracic trachea due to blunt trauma. *Ann Thorac Surg* 37(6):505–507, 1984.
29. Flynn AE, Thomas AN, Schecter WP: Acute tracheobronchial injury. *J Trauma* 29:1326, 1989.
30. Beskin CA: Rupture-separation of the cervical trachea following a closed chest injury. *J Thorac Surg* 34:392–394, 1957.
31. Hood RM, Sloan HE: Injuries to the trachea and major bronchi. *J Thorac Cardiovasc Surg* 38:458–480, 1959.
32. Cicala RS, Kudsk KA, Butts A, et al: Initial evaluation and management of upper airway injuries in trauma patients. *J Clin Anesth* 3:91–98, 1991.
33. Roberge RJ, Squyres NS, Demetropoulous S, et al: Tracheal transection following blunt trauma. *Ann Emerg Med* 17:47–52, 1988.
34. Spencer JA, Rogers CE, Westaby S: Clinico-radiological correlates in rupture of the major airways. *Clin Radiol* 43:371, 1991.
35. Hancock BJ, Wiseman NE: Tracheobronchial injuries in children. *J Pediatr Surg* 26:1316–1319, 1991.
36. Angood PB, Attia EL, Brown RA, Mulder DS: Extrinsic civilian trauma to the larynx and cervical trachea—important predictors of long-term morbidity. *J Trauma* 26:869, 1986.
37. Iwasaki M, Kaga K, Ogawa J, et al: Bronchoscopy findings and early treatment of patients with blunt tracheo-bronchial trauma. *J Cardiovasc Surg* 35:269, 1994.

38. Hara KS, Prakash UBS: Fiberoptic bronchoscopy in the evaluation of acute chest and upper airway trauma. *Chest* 96:627, 1989.

39. Gomez-Caro A, Diez FJM, Herrero PA, et al: Successful conservative management in iatrogenic tracheobronchial injury. *Ann Thorac Surg* 79: 1872–1878, 2005.

40. Marquette CH, Bocquillon N, Roumilhac D, et al: Conservative treatment of tracheal rupture. *J Thorac Cardiovasc Surg* 117:399–401, 1999.

41. Richardson JD: Outcome of tracheobronchial injuries: a long-term perspective. *J Trauma* 56:30–36, 2004.

42. Thompson EC, Porter JM, Fernandez LG: Penetrating neck trauma: an overview of management. *J Oral Maxillofac Surg* 60(8):918–923, 2002.

43. Self ML, Mangram A, Berne JD, et al: Nonoperative management of severe tracheobronchial injuries with positive end-expiratory pressure and low tidal volume ventilation. *J Trauma* 59:1072–1075, 2005.

44. Nishiumi N, Maitani F, Yamada S, et al: Chest radiography assessment of tracheobronchial disruption associated with blunt chest trauma. *J Trauma* 53:372–377, 2002.

45. Schoem SR, Choi SS, Zalzal GH: Pneumomediastinum and pneumothorax from blunt cervical trauma in children. *Laryngoscope* 107:351–356, 1997.

46. Bowley D, Plani F, Murillo D, et al: Intubated, ventilating patients with complete tracheal transection: a diagnostic challenge. *Ann R Coll Surg Engl* 85:245–247, 2003.

47. Naghibi K, Hashemi SL, Sajedi P: Anaesthetic management of tracheobronchial rupture following blunt chest trauma. *Acta Anaesthesiol Scand* 47(7):901–903, 2003.

48. Clark RH, Wiswell TE, Null DM: Tracheal and bronchial injury in high-frequency oscillatory ventilation compared with conventional positive pressure ventilation. *J Pediatr* 111(1):114–118, 1987.

49. Liistro G, Goncette L, Rodenstein DO: Tracheal laceration and tension pneumomediastinum of spontaneous favorable outcome. *Acta Clin Belg* 53:44–46, 1998.

50. Sherif HS, Ott DA: The use of subcutaneous drains to manage subcutaneous emphysema. *Tex Heart Inst J* 26:129–131, 1999.

51. Herlan DB, Landreneau RJ, Ferson PF: Massive spontaneous subcutaneous emphysema: acute management with infraclavicular "blow holes." *Chest* 102:503–505, 1992.

52. American College of Surgeons Committee on Trauma: *Advanced Trauma Life Support for Doctors,* 7th ed. Chicago, American College of Surgeons, 2004.

53. Balci AE, Erin N, Erin S, et al: Surgical treatment of post-traumatic tracheobronchial injuries: 14-year experience. *Eur J Cardiothorac Surg* 22: 984–989, 2002.

54. Healy GB: Subglottic stenosis: pediatric otolaryngology. *Otolaryngol Clin North Am* 22(3):599–605, 1989.

55. Atkins BZ, Abbate S, Fisher SR, et al: Current management of laryngotracheal trauma: case report and literature review. *J Trauma* 56:185–190, 2004.

56. Reece GP, Shatney CH: Blunt injuries of the cervical trachea: review of 51 patients. *South Med J* 81(12):1542–1548, 1988.

57. Kiser AC, O'Brien SM, Detterbeck FC: Blunt tracheobronchial injuries: treatment and outcomes. *Ann Thorac Surg* 71:2059–2065, 2001.

58. Lim KE, Liu YC, Hsu YY: Tracheal injury diagnosed with three dimensional imaging using multidetector row computed tomography. *Chang Gung Med J* 27:217–221, 2004.

59. Moriwaki Y, Sugiyama M, Matsuda G, et al: Usefulness of the 3-dimensionally reconstructed computed tomography imaging for diagnosis of the site of tracheal injury (3D-tracheography). *World J Surg* 29:102–105, 2005.

60. Clement P, Hans S, de Mones E, et al: Dilation for assisted ventilation-induced laryngotracheal stenosis. *Laryngoscope* 115:1595–1598, 2005.

61. Huang C: Use of the silicone t-tube to treat tracheal stenosis of tracheal injury. *Ann Thorac Cardiovasc Surg* 7:192–196, 2001.

62. Mandour M, Remacle M, Van de Heyning P, et al: Chronic subglottic and tracheal stenosis: endoscopic management vs. surgical reconstruction. *Eur Arch Otorhinolaryngol* 260:374–380, 2003.

63. Dowd NP, Clarkson K, Walsh MA, et al: Delayed bronchial stenosis after blunt chest trauma. *Anesth Analg* 82:1078–1081, 1996.

64. Thal ER, Nwariaku FE: Neck injuries. In Maull MI, Rodriguez A, Wiles CE III, editors: *Complications in Trauma and Critical Care.* Philadelphia, W.B. Saunders, 1996, pp. 270–272.

65. Leopold DA: Laryngeal trauma. *Arch Otolaryngol* 109:106–112, 1983.

66. Luqman, Z, Khan MAM, Nazir Z: Penetrating pharyngeal injuries in children: trivial trauma leading to devastating complications. *Pediatr Surg Int* 21:432–435, 2005.

67. Schoem SR, Choi SS, Zalzal GH, et al: Management of oropharyngeal trauma in children. *Arch Otolaryngol Head Neck Surg* 123:1267–1270, 1997.

68. Brietzke SE, Jones DT: Pediatric oropharyngeal trauma: what is the role of CT scan? *Int J Otorhinolaryngol* 69:669–679, 2005.

69. Berne JD, Norwood SH, McAuley CE, Villareal DH: Helical CT angiography: an excellent screening test for blunt cerebrovascular injuries. *J Trauma* 57:11–19, 2004.

70. Berne JD, Reuland KS, Norwood SH, et al: Sixteen-slice multi-detector computed tomographic angiography improves the accuracy of screening for blunt cerebrovascular injury. *J Trauma* 60:1204–1209, 2006.

THORACIC INJURIES

PERTINENT SURGICAL ANATOMY OF THE THORAX AND MEDIASTINUM

Paul Schipper, Mithran Sukumar, and John C. Mayberry

The thorax consists of the chest wall comprising the sternum, ribs, and thoracic vertebrae; the mediastinum containing the pericardium, heart, esophagus, trachea, great vessels, thoracic duct, and thymus; and the paired pleural cavities containing the lungs. This chapter will discuss the anatomy of these structures and spaces, as pertinent to trauma surgery and the surgical intensive care unit.

CHEST WALL

The muscular, tendinous, and bony structures of the chest serve several functions. The chest wall must be rigid enough to protect the thoracic viscera and serve as a fixation point against which the muscles of the upper extremity and abdomen can work yet flexible enough to expand and contract with vigorous respirations.

With gentle respirations, the chest wall is a cylinder with the diaphragm as its piston. With inspiration, the diaphragm contracts, its dome is flattened, and, like a piston, it descends in the chest. This motion increases the volume of the thorax, and actively expands the lungs by drawing in air through the trachea. The lungs are very elastic and tend to collapse without outward forces keeping them expanded. With exhalation, the diaphragm relaxes, the elasticity of the lungs causes lung volume to decrease, and air is expelled. Ultimately, the tendency of the lung to collapse is countered by the outward force/rigidity of the chest wall. With vigorous respirations, the intercostal muscles, scalenes, and other accessory muscles of respiration elevate the ribs and increase the thoracic volume much more than usual. With vigorous respirations, the chest wall and diaphragm act in concert like a bellows increasing thoracic volume and then relaxing and allowing the elasticity of the lung to decrease thoracic volume.

The bony structures of the chest wall include 12 ribs, 12 thoracic vertebrae, and the sternum. All ribs articulate posteriorly with the transverse processes and vertebral bodies of their respective thoracic vertebrae and the vertebral body directly superior (Figure 1). Ribs 1 through 7 are called true ribs because they articulate anteriorly directly with the sternum through their own costal cartilage. Ribs 8, 9, and 10 are called false ribs because they articulate anteriorly to the costal cartilage of the rib above. This creates a construct of stair-stepping costal cartilages, which ultimately articulates with the sternum and creates the costal arch or costal margin. Ribs 11 and 12 are called floating ribs because they do not articulate with any structure anteriorly (Figure 2). Rather, they attach to the abdominal wall musculature, primarily the internal oblique muscle.

Because ribs 1 through 10 are fixed anteriorly and posteriorly, they function much like a bucket handle (Figure 3A). When performing a tube thoracostomy, as you approach the sternum anteriorly and the transverse processes posteriorly, the size of the interspace becomes fixed and narrow. Laterally, away from these points of attachment, the ribs separate and the interspace opens. The widest portion of the interspaces can be found at the lateral apogee or "keystone" of the rib. Tube thoracostomies placed laterally will be easier to place through the interspace and more comfortable for the patient (Figure 3B). Also, when creating a thoracotomy, division of the intercostal muscles far anterior and posterior will create a larger working space without tearing the intercostal muscle or fracturing a rib with placement of the rib spreader. The skin need only be divided over the working space, not over the entire intercostal incision.

The sternum has three parts, the manubrium, the body, and the xiphoid process. The manubrium is thick and broad, articulating with the clavicle, first rib, and sharing the second rib articulation with the body of the sternum. The sternoclavicular articulation is the only bony articulation of the thorax to the shoulder girdle (see Figure 2). Understanding the angle of the clavicle, manubrium, and first rib is important in safe placement of central venous catheters into the subclavian vein. The subclavian vein and artery leave the arm and enter the thoracic inlet over the top of the first rib and under the clavicle. Once under the clavicle, a needle directed parallel to the clavicle and first rib will not enter the chest and cause a pneumothorax before finding the subclavian vein. A needle directed too steeply in its approach will quickly enter and exit the triangle where the subclavian vein is found, penetrate the intercostal space, and puncture the lung (Figure 4).

The second rib inserts into the sternomanubrial junction (angle of Louis). This can be easily palpated in most people as a horizontal ridge in the sternum or where the two planes that make up the sternum intersect (Figure 5). The interspace immediately below the angle of Louis is the second interspace. The angle of Louis serves as a landmark to rapidly locate the second rib and second interspace for placement of a catheter to decompress a tension pneumothorax or to place an anterior tube thoracostomy for an apical pneumothorax.

The first rib is short, broad, flat, and arches sharply from posterior to anterior (Figure 6). The second rib is longer than but very similar to the first rib (Figure 7). The first slip of the serratus anterior muscle attaches to the second rib approximately one-third of the arc from posterior to anterior—this slip also attaches to the inferior aspect of the first rib. Posterior to this attachment, the scalenus posterior attaches to the second rib.

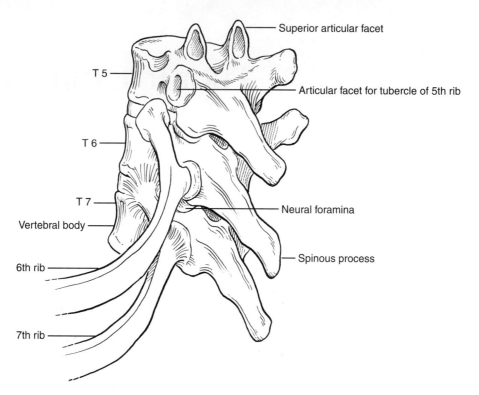

Figure 1   Costovertebral junction. Lateral view showing two left ribs and three vertebrae. Note that ribs articulate with transverse process and body of one vertebrae and body of vertebrae above.   *(Redrawn from* Grant's Atlas of Anatomy, *11th ed., Philadelphia, Lippincott Williams & Wilkins, 2005, figures 1.13–1.14, pp. 14–15.)*

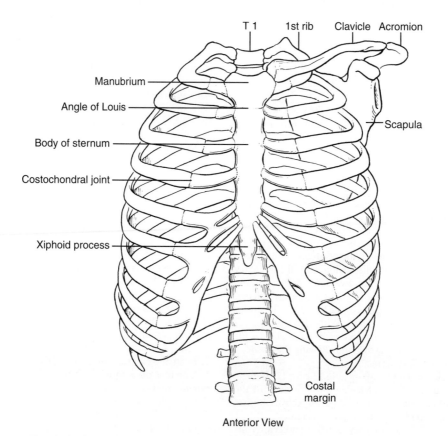

Anterior View

Figure 2   Bony chest wall. Anterior view.   *(Redrawn from* Grant's Atlas of Anatomy, *11th ed., Philadelphia, Lippincott Williams & Wilkins, 2004, figure 1.8, p. 9.)*

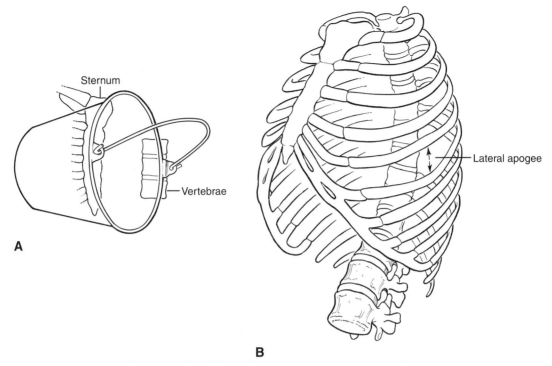

Figure 3 Bucket handle motion of ribs. Ribs are fixed anteriorly at the sternum and posteriorly at the vertebrae. The ribs will move like a "bucket handle." The widest space between the ribs will be at the lateral apogee or "keystone." *(Redrawn from Pearson FG, editor: Thoracic Surgery, 2nd ed. Philadelphia, Churchill Livingstone, 2002, figure 48-3, p. 1327.)*

When performing a thoracotomy, counting ribs can identify the correct interspace. Once the latissimus dorsi muscle has been divided and the serratus anterior muscle divided or swept anterior, the scapula is elevated. Thin fibrous attachments hold the undersurface of the scapula to the chest wall. A hand placed deep to the scapula, posterior near the spine, and apically can palpate ribs. The first rib is identified by its conspicuously broad and flat contour. Inferior to this, the second rib can be identified by the attachment of the scalenus posterior muscle. This muscle body is palpable by sweeping the finger from posterior to anterior along the second rib (Figure 8). Less distinct will be the third rib, which seems to "turn the corner" from the apex of the chest to the lateral chest wall (Figure 9). In a lateral decubitus position, the tip of the scapula overlies the sixth interspace. In a male, the nipple overlies the fourth interspace.

MUSCLES OF THE CHEST WALL

Integral to safe thoracentesis, placement of a tube thoracostomy, or a thoracotomy, is understanding the layers of the chest wall and the anatomy of the interspace.

The paired pectoralis major muscles cover the majority of the anterior chest wall. The pectoralis major muscle originates from the clavicle and anterior aspects of ribs 1 through 6 inserting on the proximal humerus. Its origin from the chest wall is broad and an anterior thoracotomy will divide or separate its fibers. Inferiorly, the rectus abdominus muscle inserts onto the costal cartilages of ribs 5 through 7 and the xiphoid process. Lateral to this, the muscle fibers of the external oblique insert onto ribs 5 through 12. The external oblique muscle interdigitates with the serratus anterior muscle as it inserts on ribs 1 through 8 (Figure 10). Most thoracotomies do not traverse the interspaces guarded by the rectus abdominus and external oblique. These muscles will be encountered with thoracoabdominal incisions crossing the costal margin.

Laterally and posteriorly, two musculo-fascial layers guard the ribs. The more superficial layer contains the latissimus dorsi muscle laterally. Posteriorly, at the ausculatory triangle, or posterior border of the latissimus dorsi, this layer becomes a thin but tough layer of fascia, which more posteriorly envelopes the trapezius muscle. The second musculo-fascial layer contains the serratus anterior muscle laterally, becoming a broader sheet of thin but tough fibrous tissue posteriorly and then becoming the rhomboid major muscle then the rhomboid minor muscle posteriorly and superiorly (Figure 11). A tube thoracostomy will traverse these muscle layers to reach the ribs and interspaces. Knowing where you are in these layers allows precious time to be saved in traversing them and getting to where you need to be to complete the procedure.

A typical tube thoracostomy is placed in the fifth interspace at the anterior axillary line. The muscle bodies traversed are thinner here. From superficial to deep, the surgeon will separate skin, subcutaneous fat, the latissimus dorsi/trapezius musculo-fascial layer, and then the serratus anterior musculo-fascial layer. At this depth, the shiny surface of the periosteum of the ribs and the oblique fibers of the external intercostal muscle can be seen. As discussed later, tube thoracostomies are performed over the superior aspect of the rib. It is much easier to locate the superior aspect of the rib when you do not have intervening layers of muscle and fascia.

A thoracotomy can be fashioned to divide or spare these muscles as needed in order to gain access to the rib cage. A full thoracotomy will divide the latissimus dorsi laterally and the trapezius posteriorly. The incision sweeps from horizontal across the lateral chest to vertical and parallel to the spine posteriorly (Figure 12). Deep to this layer, the serratus anterior can be swept anterior or divided. Posteriorly, the fascial layer coming off the serratus anterior is divided and then the rhomboid major and rhomboid minor muscles are divided. The innervation of the trapezius muscle and rhomboid muscles runs from medial to lateral. The more muscle body that is left medially, the more muscle function will be retained. Enough muscle needs to

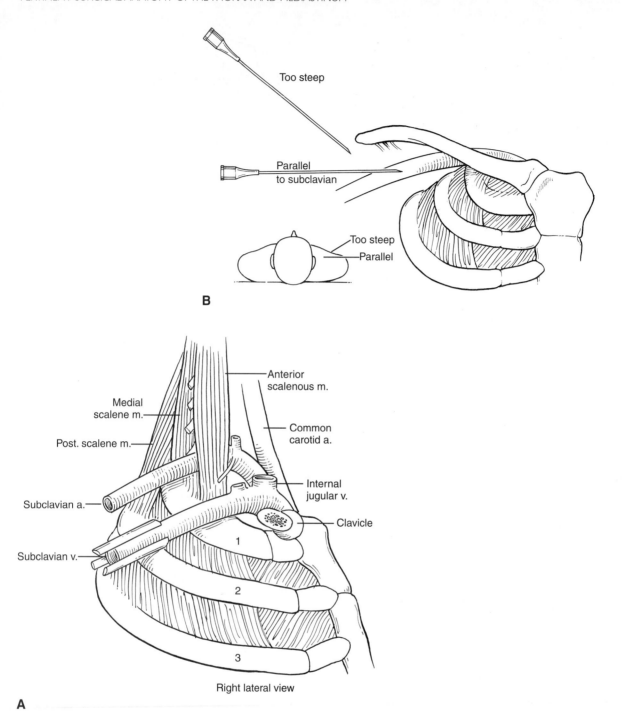

Figure 4 Central venous cannulation of subclavian vein. **(A)** The clavicle and rib cage form a triangle through which the subclavian vein courses. The vein runs roughly parallel to both the clavicle and the rib cage. **(B)** A needle, once passed under the clavicle, directed parallel to the rib cage and clavicle will have a far greater chance of finding the vein. A needle directed too steeply will enter and exit this triangle, penetrate the intercostal space, and puncture the lung. *(Redrawn from* Grant's Atlas of Anatomy, *11th ed., Philadelphia, Lippincott Williams & Wilkins, 2004, figures 1.8, 6.29, pp. 9, 379.)*

be left attached to the scapula to allow suture repair of the muscle, and the muscle should not be stripped from the scapula. The posterior and vertical aspect of this incision where the trapezius and rhomboids are divided is done to elevate the scapula off the chest wall, to access the interspaces underneath.

A thoracotomy can be extended anterior, dividing the pectoralis major muscle overlying the interspace of interest. The sternum can be split transversely, and a thoracotomy continued on the contralateral side. This is termed a "clam shell" thoracotomy. The left and right mammary artery will be found 1 cm lateral to and on either side of the sternum, deep to the ribs and intercostal muscles, but superficial to the pleura. These vessels can be cauterized if speed is needed, but are prone to spasm and late bleeding, and should be sought and ligated when possible.

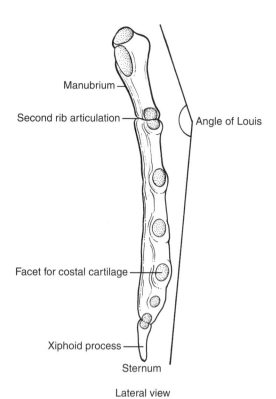

Lateral view

Figure 5 Sternum, lateral view. Angle of Louis can be palpated in the midline as a raised horizontal ridge or as the point where the plane of the manubrium and body intersect. The second rib articulates directly lateral to the angle of Louis. *(Redrawn from Gray's Anatomy, 39th ed., figure 57.5, p. 954.)*

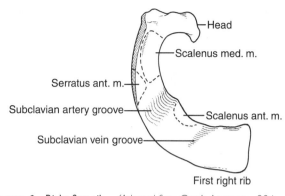

Figure 6 Right first rib. *(Adapted from Gray's Anatomy, 20th ed., plate 124.)*

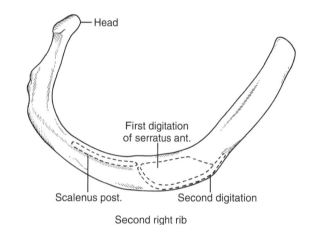

Figure 7 Right second rib. *(Adapted from Gray's Anatomy, 20th ed., plate 125.)*

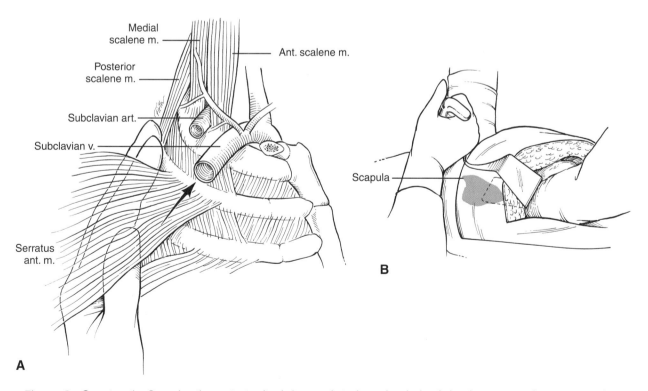

Figure 8 Counting ribs. Once the rib cage is visualized, the scapula is elevated, and a hand placed posterior and superior to palpate and count ribs. Note that the first rib is broad, short, and flat; the second rib has the insertion of the scalenus posterior; and the third rib "turns the corner" from apex to lateral chest wall.

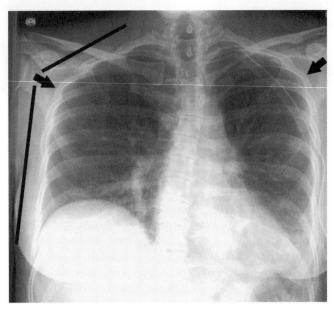

Figure 9 Third rib "turns the corner." Anteroposterior chest radiograph illustrating how the rib cage forms a loose box with the third rib at a corner. Arrows denote third rib.

INTERCOSTAL SPACE

Each intercostal space from superficial to deep, has two layers of muscle; an artery, a vein, and a nerve; and a diminutive inner layer of muscle. The external intercostal muscles run obliquely with fibers in the same orientation as the external oblique muscle of the abdomen (fingers in pockets). Deep are the internal intercostal muscles running in the opposite direction. The intercostal artery, vein, and nerve run along the inferior aspect of each rib, occasionally running underneath a ledge in the costal groove. To avoid injury to these three structures, tube thoracostomies and thoracotomies are directed over the superior aspect of each rib or through the middle of the interspace, but not the inferior aspect of the rib (Figure 13). The innermost intercostal muscles are located deep to the neurovascular bundle and run in the same direction as the internal intercostal muscles. While mentioned in anatomy texts, surgically, the innermost intercostal muscles do not need to be considered separately from the internal intercostal muscle (Figure 14). The intercostal arteries originate as segmental branches off the descending aorta. The intercostal space, including the underlying pleura, can be harvested as a posteriorly based pedicled muscle flap (Figure 15). This flap is useful for reinforcing bronchial or esophageal repairs.

The internal mammary artery originates from the subclavian arteries bilaterally, and descends on the inside of the chest wall, approximately 1 cm lateral to the sternum bilaterally (Figure 16).

PLEURAL SPACE

Normally the lung is coupled to the chest wall by the vacuum, which exists between the visceral and parietal pleura. With penetration of the chest wall air is allowed into the pleural space from the outside or more commonly, penetration of the lung allows air to escape from air spaces within the lung (alveoli, bronchioles, bronchi) into the pleural space. The coupling of the visceral and parietal pleura is broken and the potential space, which is the pleural space, becomes a real space. The elasticity of the lung causes it to collapse and a pneumothorax is formed. The pleural space extends superiorly to where it rises above the circumference of the first rib to inferiorly where the diaphragm inserts on the costal margin and the 12th rib. Lung may or may not be present between the diaphragm and ribs in the lower most recesses of the pleural space. Anterior to the pericardium and posterior to the sternum, the two pleural cavities can abut but rarely communicate.

DIAPHRAGM

The diaphragm is the movable dome-shaped partition between the thoracic and abdominal cavities. With full exhalation, the dome of the diaphragm can rise to the level of the fourth interspace anteriorly (nipple level). With full inhalation, the diaphragm flattens, bringing the thoracic cavity down to the level of the costal margin anteriorly and the 12th rib posteriorly. The muscle fibers of the diaphragm originate from the sternum, the ribs, and the vertebral column. All three groups insert on a tough, fibrinous central tendon. Fibers of the sternal portion are short, arising as small slips from the back of the xiphoid process. Laterally on either side of the xiphoid, fibers originate from the inner surface of the lower six costal cartilages (costal margin). Posteriorly, fibers originate from a thick band arching over the quadratus lumborum (lateral arcuate ligament) and the psoas major (medial arcuate ligament). The paired lateral arcuate ligaments extend from the tip and lower margin of the 12th ribs and arch over the quadratus lumborum muscle to the transverse processes of L1. The paired medial arcuate ligaments complete the journey, arching over the psoas major from the tip of the transverse process of the first lumbar vertebrae to the tendinous portion of each diaphragmatic crus (Figure 17).

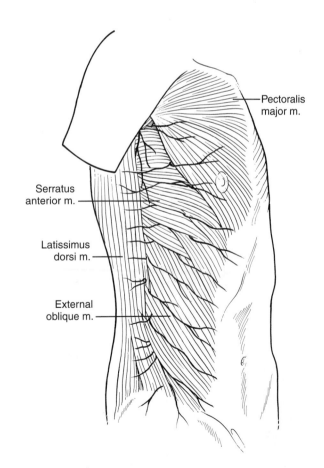

Pectoralis major m.

Serratus anterior m.

Latissimus dorsi m.

External oblique m.

Figure 10 Muscles of thorax: left lateral view. *(Adapted from Gray's Anatomy, 20th ed., plate 392.)*

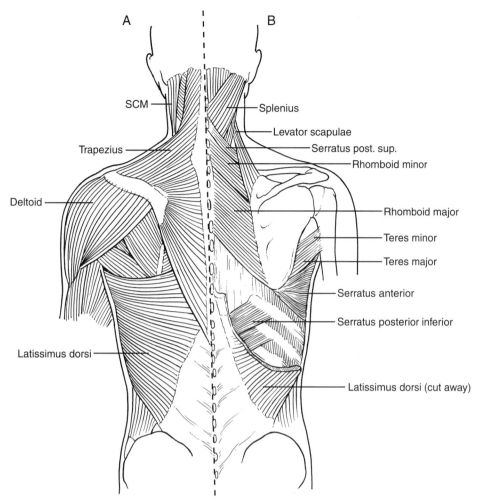

A   B

SCM

Splenius

Levator scapulae

Trapezius

Serratus post. sup.

Rhomboid minor

Deltoid

Rhomboid major

Teres minor

Teres major

Serratus anterior

Serratus posterior inferior

Latissimus dorsi

Latissimus dorsi (cut away)

Figure 11   Muscles of the thorax. **(A)** Superficial layer containing latissimus dorsi m. and trapezius m. **(B)** Deep layer containing serratus anterior m., rhomboid major m., and rhomboid minor m.   *(Redrawn from Grant's Atlas of Anatomy, 11th ed., Philadelphia, Lippincott Williams & Wilkins, 2004, figures 4.47, 4.48, 6.13, pp. 233, 234, 367.)*

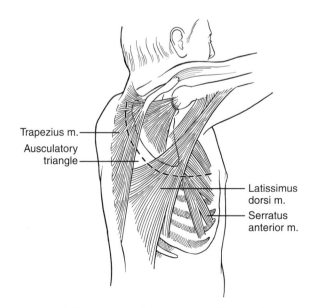

Trapezius m.

Ausculatory triangle

Latissimus dorsi m.

Serratus anterior m.

Figure 12   Full posterolateral thoracotomy.   *(Redrawn from Grant's Atlas of Anatomy, 11th ed., Philadelphia, Lippincott Williams & Wilkins, 2004, Figs. 4.47, 4.48, 6.13, pp. 233, 234, 367.)*

The posterior medial portion of the diaphragm is composed of two crura—an anatomic right crus originating from the upper three lumbar vertebral bodies and an anatomic left crus originating from the upper two lumbar vertebral bodies. Anterior to the aorta, the medial margins of the two crura form a poorly defined arch called the median arcuate ligament. Anterior to this arch, either the anatomic right crus (64%) or the anatomic left crus (2%) or both (34%) form the esophageal hiatus. While anatomists name the crura left or right by their origin from the left or right side of the vertebral bodies, surgeons name the crura left or right by their relationship to the esophagus. In the abdomen, visualization of the esophagus and division of the crus running to the left of the esophagus will expose the distal thoracic aorta above the level of the celiac artery and renal arteries. A clamp can be applied here to obtain vascular control. Alternatively, a retractor wrapped with a laparotomy pad can be used in this position to occlude the aorta by compressing it against the posteriorly located vertebral body (Figure 18).

The phrenic nerve and twigs from the lower intercostal nerves innervate the diaphragm. The phrenic nerve originates primarily from the C4 nerve root, but receives innervation from C3 and C5 (C3, C4, and C5 keep the body alive). In the neck, the phrenic nerve originates lateral to the scalenus anterior muscle and descends from lateral to medial on the superficial surface of this muscle, deep to the sternocleidomastoid muscle. It enters the thoracic inlet and is found on the medial aspect of the mediastinum just deep to the pleura

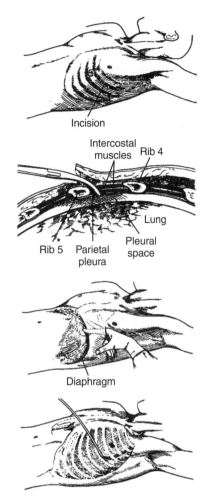

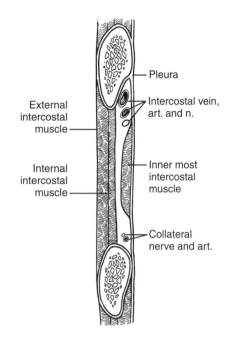

Figure 14 Intercostal space in cross-section. Note main intercostal bundle along the inferior aspect of the rib. The collateral nerve and artery, while present, are diminutive. *(Adapted from Crafts RC: A Textbook of Human Anatomy, 3rd ed., New York, John Wiley & Sons, 1985.)*

Figure 13 Technique for tube thoracostomy. Tubes placed emergently for trauma are placed along the anterior axillary line, fourth or fifth interspace. The intercostal space is entered on the superior aspect of the rib. Finger palpation confirms entrance into the pleural cavity and avoids inadvertent subscapular or intraabdominal placement of tubes as well as injury to adhesed lung. *(From Moore FA, Moore EE: Trauma resuscitation. In Wilmore DN, Brennan MF, Harken AH, et al., eds. Care of the Surgical Patient. New York, Scientific American, 1989.)*

and a third posteriorly. The posterior branch bifurcates into a branch directed toward the 12th rib and one toward the crus. Safe incisions in the diaphragm are fashioned to avoid cutting major branches of the phrenic nerve (Figure 19). A peripheral and circumferential incision will avoid all but distal twigs of the phrenic nerve. Radial incision can be placed but must be done with care to avoid major branches of the phrenic nerve.

Because the primary innervation of the diaphragm, the phrenic nerve, enters centrally and spreads centrifugally, the diaphragm can be transposed to higher or lower origins from the thoracic cage while maintaining its innervation. This is occasionally required in repair of a diaphragmatic rupture when surface area of the diaphragm is lost or the chest wall has lost its rigidity and can no longer subserve its cylinder function. Care should be taken to maintain a dome shape to the diaphragm. A diaphragm that is flattened at rest will pull the walls of the thorax closer together when contracting. With contraction, instead of increasing intrathoracic volume, the diaphragm will now decrease intrathoracic volume and become a muscle of expiration (Figure 20).

PERICARDIUM

The pericardial space is considerably smaller than the pleural space and a small increase in the volume of fluid in this space can have a dramatic impact on cardiac function. The parietal pericardium is a thick, fibrous sac with an inner serosal surface containing the heart, the proximal ascending aorta, the distal superior vena cava, the distal inferior vena cava, the pulmonary trunk and bifurcation, proximal left and right main pulmonary arteries, and a short segment of all four distal pulmonary veins. From this description, it can be visualized that all vessels flowing into and out of the heart have short segments contained in the pericardial sac (Figure 21). It is also these vascular structures, which fix the heart in the pericardial sac. If the

bilaterally. Superiorly, it is very anterior in the chest and vulnerable to injury, especially with a median sternotomy and dissection of the great vessels where it is often not readily visible in the wound, but very close to the dissection. On the left, it descends outside the pericardium, deep to the pleura, passing over the arch of the aorta, anterior to the hilum of the lung, and anterior to the inferior pulmonary ligament. As it nears the diaphragm, it is often invested in a veil of pericardial fat, hanging like a curtain between the pericardium and the diaphragm. The nerve reaches the diaphragm just lateral to the left border of the heart and in a plane slightly more anterior than the right phrenic nerve (see Figure 33). The right phrenic nerve descends along the right lateral border of the superior vena cava, passes anterior to the hilum of the lung, and anterior to the inferior pulmonary ligament. It is also invested in a veil of pericardial fat as it approaches the diaphragm. The right phrenic nerve enters the diaphragm just lateral to the inferior vena cava (see Figure 32).

Both left and right phrenic nerves immediately trifurcate into three muscular branches after entering the hemi-diaphragm. One is directed anterior-medially toward the sternum, one anterior-laterally,

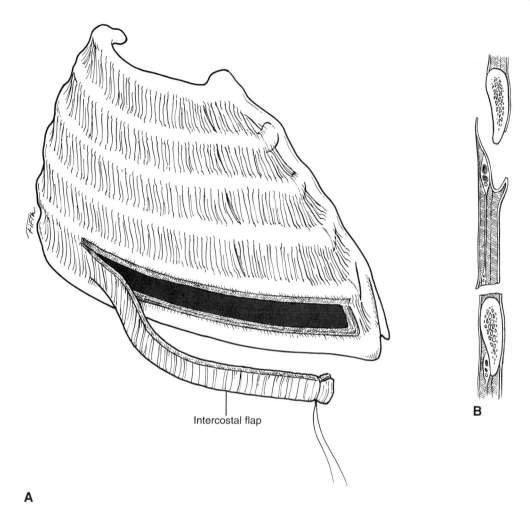

A

Figure 15 **(A)** Intercostal muscle flap. Based on intercostal artery with pedicle posterior.
(B) Transverse view of this flap.

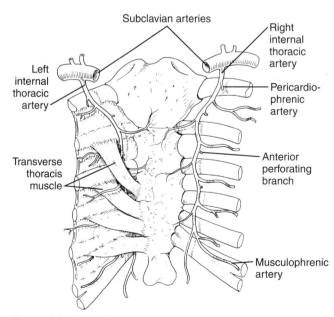

Figure 16 Internal mammary arteries as viewed from inside the chest. *(From Pearson FG, editor: Thoracic Surgery, 2nd ed. Philadelphia, Churchill Livingstone, 2002, figure 48-8, p. 1330.)*

heart is allowed to rotate, these structures will be twisted or kinked, impeding blood flow. Because they are the lowest pressure conduits, the superior vena cava and inferior vena cava are the most vulnerable to kinking and impedance of flow. With decreased blood flow into the heart, there is decreased blood flow out of the heart, and systemic blood pressure falls. This is the physiology of hypotension associated with tension pneumothorax and with cardiac herniation.

There are two sinuses behind the heart. The oblique pericardial sinus is a cul-de-sac behind the heart bounded by pericardial attachments to the inferior vena cava and the four pulmonary veins. Because of the oblique sinus, with a median sternotomy, a hand can be placed around the apex of the heart and the apex gently elevated into the wound. This allows visualization of the lateral and posterior walls of the left ventricle, including the vascular distribution of the diagonal, circumflex, and obtuse marginal coronary arteries. This maneuver is generally poorly tolerated without opening the right pericardium vertically, parallel to the phrenic nerve. This allows the right heart to fall into the right pleural space and maintain filling as the heart is lifted. In addition, severe Trendelenburg and an apically placed suction retraction device will aid exposure and improve hemodynamics. Internal defibrillating paddles should be open and ready prior to performing this maneuver, as ventricular fibrillation is not uncommon.

The transverse pericardial sinus allows a finger or clamp to be placed along the right side of the ascending aorta, behind the aorta and pulmonary trunk, and be visualized to the left of the pulmonary trunk and superior to the left superior pulmonary vein in the vicinity of the left atrial appendage (see Figure 21).

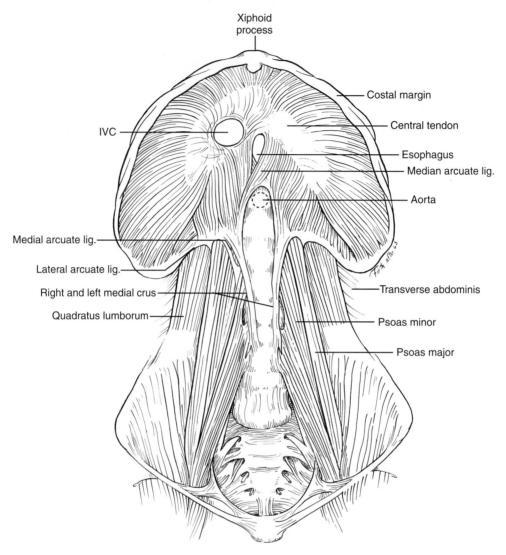

Figure 17 Diaphragm as viewed from the abdomen. The diaphragm originates bilaterally from the xiphoid process, costal margin, lateral arcuate ligament, and medial arcuate ligament, and inserts into the central tendon. The left and right crus originate from the lumbar vertebral bodies and insert into the central tendon. *(Adapted from Langley LL, Telford IR, Christensen JB: Dynamic Anatomy and Physiology, 5th ed., New York, McGraw-Hill, 1980.)*

The pericardium can be drained through a median sternotomy, left or right thoracotomy, subxiphoid approach, or laparotomy. From a left or right thoracotomy, an incision is made anterior or posterior to and parallel to the phrenic nerve. From the left chest the left ventricle and from the right chest the right atrium will be encountered in the pericardial space behind these incisions (Figure 22).

From a laparotomy, a modification of the subxiphoid approach can be used to enter the pericardium. Alternatively, the central portion of the diaphragm makes up the inferior fibrous parietal pericardial sac. An incision in the diaphragm in this location will enter the pericardial sac, visualizing the inferior wall of the heart.

Subxiphoid Space

The subxiphoid space is a favored access to the pericardium for diagnosis and treatment of pericardial effusions. Both the linea alba and the diaphragm attach to the xiphoid. The peritoneum on the diaphragm is continuous with the peritoneum on the deep surface of the posterior fasciae of the anterior abdominal wall. An incision from above the xiphoid process to 4 cm below will pass through skin, fat, and linea alba. Incising the linea alba will reveal the xiphoid superiorly and the peritoneum inferiorly. The diaphragmatic attachments to the xiphoid can be divided flush with the xiphoid and the xiphoid resected to the level of the sternal body/costal margin. A large vein is routinely encountered at the angle between the xiphoid, costal margin, and sternal body. Posterior retraction of the diaphragm and superior retraction of the sternum will reveal the pericardial reflection on the diaphragm. Incising the pericardium will enter the pericardial space. The acute margin of the right ventricle will be visible through this incision (Figure 23). Since this incision is at the corner where two perpendicular planes meet, fluid can be aspirated in two directions. First, straight posterior, parallel to the diaphragm, along the inferior border of the heart, and second, superior, parallel to the sternal body, anterior to the anterior surface of the heart (Figure 24).

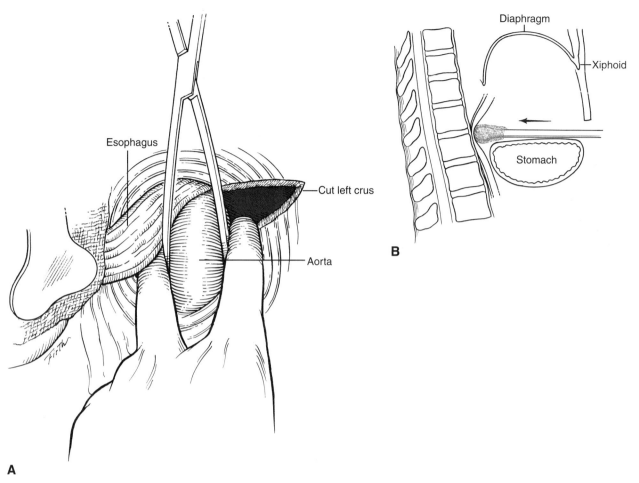

Figure 18 Cross-clamping of distal descending thoracic aorta from abdomen. **(A)** Left crus divided and thoracic aorta found deep. **(B)** Lateral view, aorta occluded by compression against vertebral body.

HEART

The heart occupies the central and left portion of the thorax and is the primary content of the middle mediastinum. It is bounded on all sides by the parietal pericardium. Outside this pericardium, it is bounded anteriorly by the sternum and posteriorly by the esophagus, vertebral column and descending aorta. On the right, mediastinal pleura and lung are present with the phrenic nerve running just anterior to the hilum of the lung. On the left, the same structures are present but the phrenic nerve runs more anteriorly. Extra care is required to protect this nerve when the heart is approached from the left.

Body Surface Markings for Heart

The surface projection of the superior border of the heart is a line joining a point 2 cm lateral to the sternum in the left second intercostal space to a point just to the right of the sternum in the same space. This marks the line of the main pulmonary arteries. The right border extends inferiorly to the sixth costal cartilage adjacent to the sternum. This is formed by the right atrium. The inferior border extends from the right sixth costal cartilage to the point of maximum cardiac impulse, which is usually in the left fifth intercostal space just medial to the mid-clavicular line. The right ventricle forms the inferior border. The left border extends superiorly to the second intercos-

tal space 2 cm lateral to the sternal edge. The left ventricle forms the left border (Figure 25).

External Features

The heart consists of four chambers divided by three grooves. The atrioventricular groove contains the coronary sinus, which is the largest vein of the heart and lies posteriorly opening into the right atrium. The interatrial groove is covered anteriorly by the ascending aorta and the main pulmonary artery. The interatrial groove is visible to the right of the heart as a fatty line between the superior vena cava and right superior pulmonary vein. The interventricular groove runs anteriorly toward the apex and contains the great cardiac vein. Posteriorly, it continues along the inferior surface of the heart toward the right margin and contains the middle cardiac vein. The heart has five surfaces, anterior, posterior, inferior, and a right and left. The anterior surface is formed primarily by the right ventricle and the right atrium, and is therefore at risk from any frontal injury. Two-thirds of the right atrium and ventricle face anteriorly. The posterior surface or the base of the heart is formed by the left and right atria. The two pulmonary veins on either side, inferior and superior, open into the left atrium at this posterior location. The superior and inferior vena cava open into the right atrium. The posterior surface of the heart is related to the sixth through the ninth thoracic vertebrae being separated from them

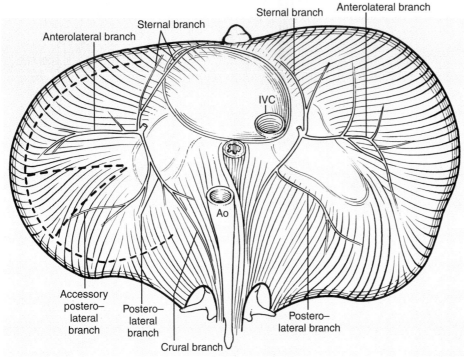

Superior view of diaphragm

Figure 19 Diaphragmatic incisions and branches of the phrenic nerve. Incisions are fashioned to avoid denervating large portions of the diaphragm. *(From Meredino KA, Johnson RS, Skinner HH, et al: The intradiaphragmatic distribution of the phrenic nerve with particular reference to the placement of diaphragmatic incisions and controlled segmental paralysis. Surgery 39:189, 1956.)*

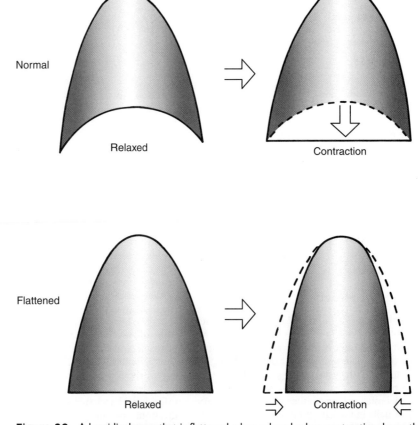

Figure 20 A hemidiaphragm that is flattened when relaxed, when contracting draws the rib cage in and causes expiration, not inspiration.

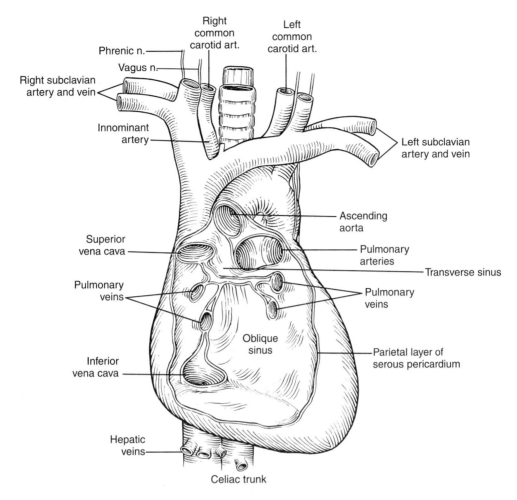

Figure 21   Pericardial sac, posterior and lateral aspects. Anterior pericardial sac has been removed. Heart has been removed.   *(Adapted from Grant's Atlas of Anatomy, 11th ed., Philadelphia, Lippincott Williams & Wilkins, 2004, figure 1.61, p. 55.)*

only by the pericardium, right pulmonary veins, esophagus, and aorta (from right to left). One-third of the right ventricle and two-thirds of the left ventricle form the inferior or diaphragmatic surface of the heart. This part of the heart is in contact with the central portion of the diaphragm. The right atrium and the right ventricle form the right surface of the heart. They are related to the pericardium, the right lung, and the right phrenic nerve just anterior to the hilum. The left ventricle and the left atrium form the left surface. They are related to the same structures as on the right but the phrenic nerve runs across the middle of the surface (Figure 26).

Coronary Arteries and Veins

Right and left coronary arteries arise from the ascending aorta. The right coronary artery supplies the right atrium, the right ventricle, the posterior one-third of the interventricular septum and the inferior portion of the septum. The left coronary artery supplies the left atrium, the left ventricle and the anterior two-thirds of the interventricular septum. Collateral circulation in the heart is minimal therefore occlusion of a coronary artery results in a specific area of myocardial infarction and dysfunction (Figure 27).

The named coronary arteries travel just under the epicardium, superficial to the myocardium. Lacerations close to a coronary

artery, but not including the artery, can be repaired with unpledgeted horizontal mattress sutures of Halsted. Alternatively, pledgeted horizontal mattress sutures may also be used, placed under the coronary bed, effectively repairing the myocardium but not occluding the coronary artery (Figure 28). Care should be taken in placing and tying the suture so as not to kink the coronary by incorporating too much myocardium. If the left anterior descending artery is the adjacent vessel being avoided, it is possible with this suture to occlude a major septal perforator diving deep to the vessel.

The venous system of the heart is centered on the coronary sinus, which receives the tributaries from the different areas of the heart and drains into the posterior aspect of the right atrium just superior to the tricuspid valve (see Figure 26B).

Conduction System

The sinoatrial node is the pacemaker of the heart and is located just to the right and anterior to the opening of the superior vena cava. The impulses are transmitted to the atrioventricular node through the wall of the atrium. The atrioventricular node is situated in the posteroinferior portion of the interatrial septum just superior to the opening of the coronary sinus. From here the impulses travel through the bundle of His (atrioventricular bundle) along the

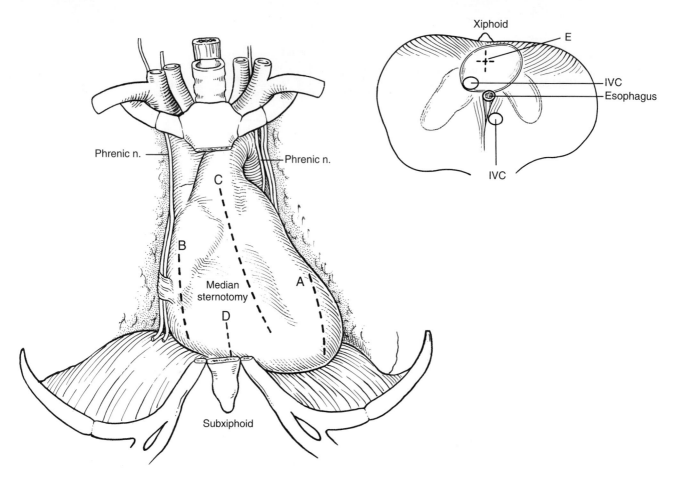

Figure 22 Approaches to a pericardial window. The pericardium can be opened from **(A)** left thoracotomy, **(B)** right thoracotomy, **(C)** median sternotomy, **(D)** subxiphoid, or **(E)** abdominal approach. *(Adapted from* Grant's Atlas of Anatomy, *11th ed., Philadelphia, Lippincott Williams & Wilkins, 2004, figure 1.49.)*

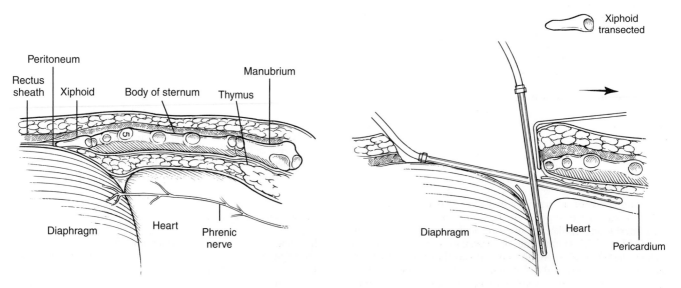

Figure 23 Subxiphoid space.

Figure 24 Subxiphoid pericardial window.

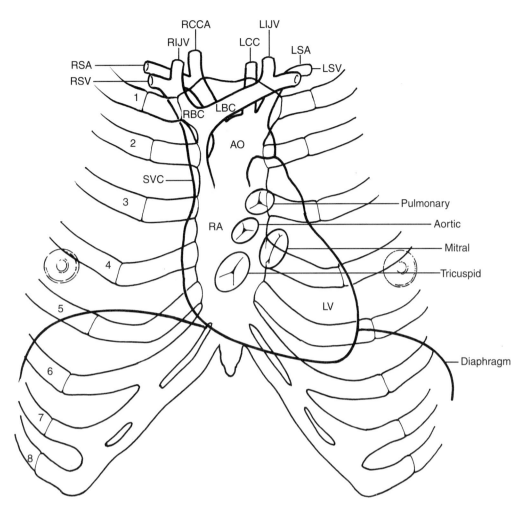

Figure 25 Surface projections of heart and lungs. *(Adapted from Gray's Anatomy, 20th ed., plates 1216, 1218.)*

posterosuperior edge of the muscular interventricular septum to the right and left bundle branches. These run through the interventricular septum to the papillary muscles in the left and right ventricle and then form a subendocardial network (Purkinje fibers) (Figure 29).

Internal Features of Heart Chambers

The right atrium has a smooth-walled posterior aspect onto which the vena cava and the coronary sinus open. Anteriorly, the wall is trabeculated muscle. Posteromedially is the interatrial septum with a depression called the fossa ovalis, which marks the previous foramen ovale or communication between the atria that existed in utero. Anteroinferiorly is the orifice of the tricuspid valve opening into the right ventricle.

The right ventricle is triangular in shape and muscular with an inflow area from the tricuspid valve and an outflow area, which is smooth leading to the pulmonary valve.

The ventricular wall gives rise to three (anterior, posterior, septal) conical projections of the papillary muscles. Tendinous structures arise from the apex of each of these to attach to cusps of the tricuspid valve. Injury to any portion of the valve apparatus can give rise to incompetence of the valve. Placed medially and obliquely is the interventricular septum separating the two ventricles.

The left atrium is quadrangular in shape and has smooth walls. The left atrial appendage projects to the left and is the only portion of the atrium that can be seen anteriorly. The openings of the veins lie posteriorly on the left and right. The interatrial septum lies to the right and slopes posteriorly making the left atrium lie behind the right atrium. The mitral valve orifice lies in the anteroinferior part of the atrium (Figure 30).

The left ventricle is muscular and has an inflow area from the mitral orifice and an outflow area to the aortic root. The ventricular wall gives rise to anterior and posterior papillary muscles that have chordae tendineae that attach to the anterior and posterior mitral valve leaflets (cusps). The anterior leaflet separates the inflow of the mitral valve orifice from the outflow of the aortic root. The aortic orifice is therefore positioned anterior to the mitral orifice. The interventricular septum is present to the right and anteriorly (see Figure 30).

ANATOMY OF PULMONARY ARTERY/ SWAN-GANZ CATHETER PLACEMENT

A pulmonary artery catheter is usually introduced via the subclavian or internal jugular vein but the femoral vein can also be used. The catheter passes through these veins into the superior or inferior vena cava and then into the right atrium. The flow of blood carries the tip through the tricuspid valve orifice into the right ventricle and then through the right ventricular outflow tract and the pulmonary valve into the main pulmonary artery. Due to the

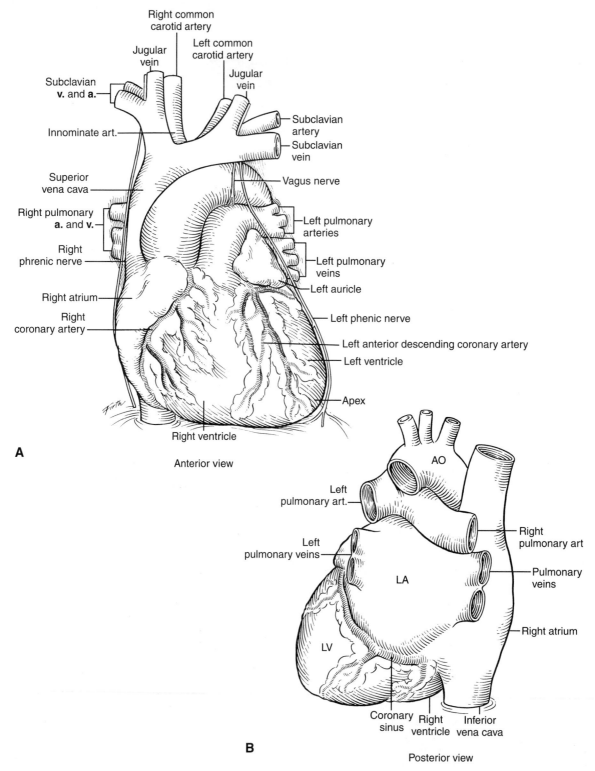

Figure 26 Heart. **(A)** Anterior. **(B)** Posterior. *(Adapted from Gray's Anatomy, 39th ed., plate 970, and figure 60.2.)*

orientation of the right main pulmonary artery to the pulmonary trunk the catheter tends to pass to the right preferentially and lodge in the distal pulmonary artery.

Occasionally the catheter may pass into the inferior vena cava or the coronary sinus while traversing the right atrium. Entry into the coronary sinus can be recognized by loss of right atrial tracing soon after it appears. Persistence of this tracing after considerable length of

the catheter has been introduced suggests coiling within the atrium or passage into the inferior vena cava.

Traditional instruction on pulmonary artery catheter placement includes orienting the coil of the catheter such that it enters the atrium from the SVC and is directed toward the tricuspid valve. The coil of the catheter is oriented on a coronal plane with the tricuspid valve perceived to be a hole in a sagittal plane (Figure 31A). The

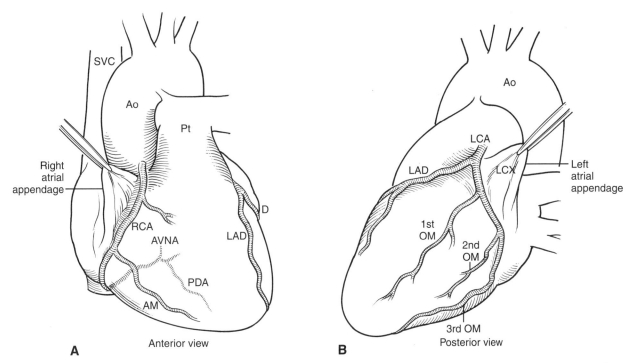

Figure 27 Coronary arteries. *LCA,* Left coronary artery; *LAD,* left anterior descending; *LCx,* left circumflex; *D,* diagonal branch of LAD; *OM,* obtuse marginal branch of LCx; *RCA,* right coronary artery; *AM,* acute marginal branch of right coronary artery; *PDA,* posterior descending coronary artery; *AVNA,* AV nodal artery.

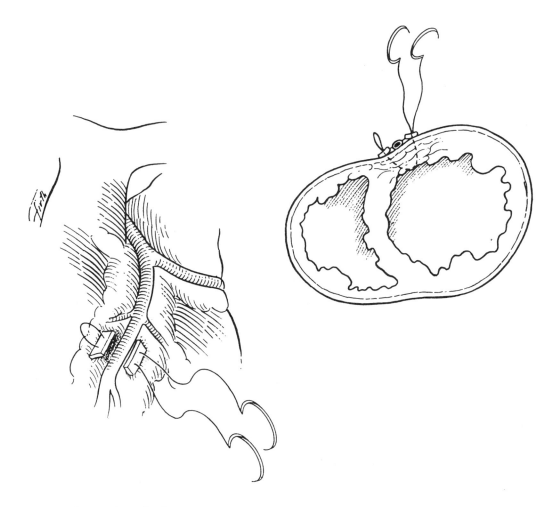

Figure 28 Repair of a cardiac laceration near a coronary artery.

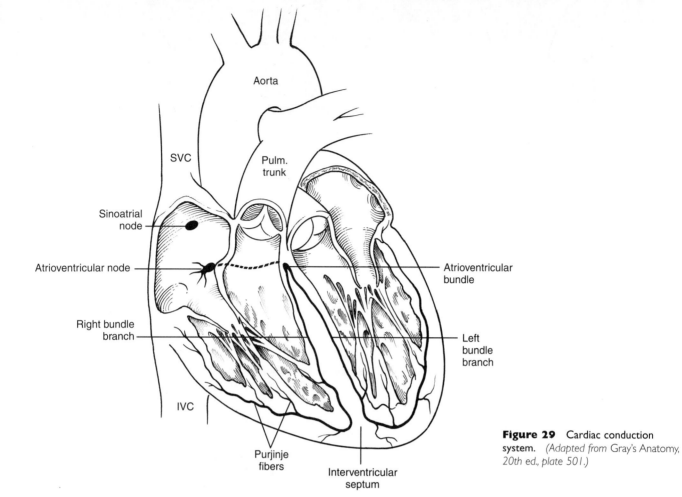

Figure 29 Cardiac conduction system. *(Adapted from Gray's Anatomy, 20th ed., plate 501.)*

Aorta

SVC

Pulm. trunk

Sinoatrial node

Atrioventricular node

Right bundle branch

IVC

Purjinje fibers

Interventricular septum

Atrioventricular bundle

Left bundle branch

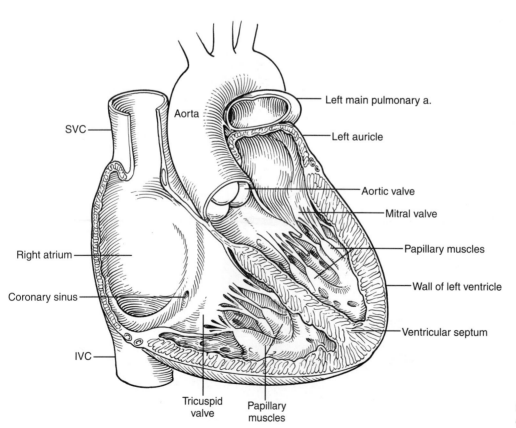

Figure 30 Left and right heart chamber anatomy. *(Adapted from Gray's Anatomy, 20th ed., plate 498.)*

SVC

Aorta

Left main pulmonary a.

Left auricle

Aortic valve

Mitral valve

Papillary muscles

Wall of left ventricle

Ventricular septum

Right atrium

Coronary sinus

IVC

Tricuspid valve

Papillary muscles

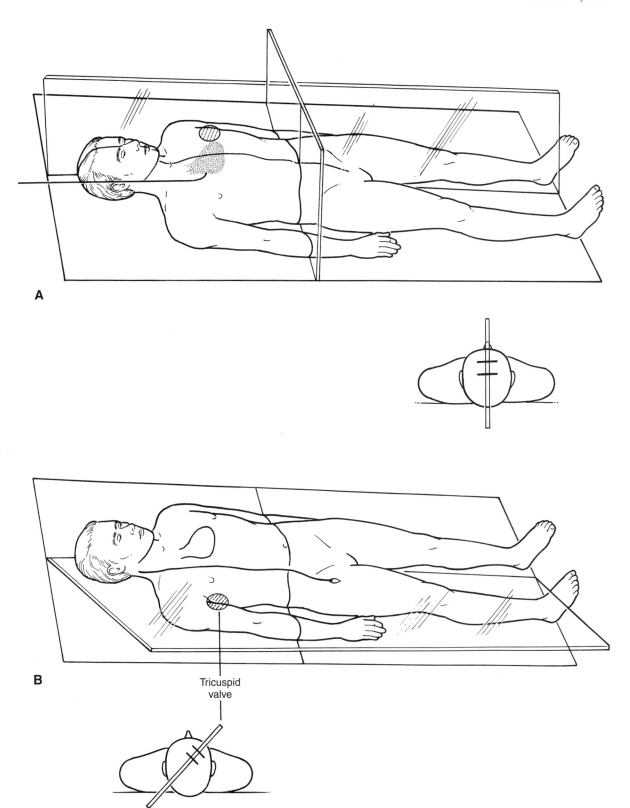

Figure 31 Placement of pulmonary artery catheter. **(A)** Traditional placement of coil is directed toward the wall to the patient's left on a coronal plane, perceiving the tricuspid valve as an opening on a sagittal plane. **(B)** Tricuspid valve is actually an opening on a plane 40–50 degrees off the sagittal plane, and correct orientation will direct the catheter 40–50 degrees more toward the ceiling.

tricuspid valve, however, truly exists on a plane rotated 40–50 degrees off the sagittal plane (Figure 31B). In a patient lying supine, blood flows from a right posterior position in the right atrium, through the tricuspid valve diagonally anterior and to the left. The coil of the catheter should therefore have its tip directed 40–50 degrees toward the ceiling rather than straight toward the left wall. The right ventricular outflow tract, however, is in the sagittal plane. Once the pressure tracing indicates the tip of the catheter is in the right ventricle, it should be rotated counterclockwise such that the coil is directed toward the left wall.

HILUM OF LUNG

The hilum of the lung is the point where the airway and pulmonary artery enter the lung and the pulmonary veins leave. It represents a fixed point where the relatively mobile lung is tethered to the mediastinum. The reflection of the visceral onto parietal pleura occurs at the hilum, adding additional support.

Much thoracic surgery is done through exposures retracting the lung anterior or posterior or looking directly at the anterior or posterior surface of the hilum. Bilaterally, the respective phrenic nerves run anterior to the hilum. On the right (Figure 32), the esophagus, vagus nerve, thoracic duct, and azygous veins are posterior. On the left (Figure 33), the descending aorta, esophagus, and vagus nerve are posterior.

Right Hilum

The inferior pulmonary ligament is a reflection of the visceral pleura of the medial aspect of the right lower lobe. This ligament attaches the lung to the mediastinum. Dividing this ligament will bring the right lower lobe into view for inspection or repair through a standard fifth interspace thoracotomy. The ligament should be divided as close to the lung as possible without injuring lung parenchyma to avoid injury to the underlying thoracic duct, esophagus, and vagus nerve. The superior most aspect of the inferior pulmonary ligament is the inferior pulmonary vein. This can be visualized as a reflection of the pericardium into the lung. A lymph node will often guard the inferior pulmonary vein at the top of this ligament.

At the superior aspect of the right hilum is the azygous vein coursing posterior to anterior to join the backside of the superior vena cava. Deep to the azygous vein the trachea bifurcates. Traveling under or medial to the azygous vein is anteriorly the right main stem bronchus and posteriorly the esophagus. The right main pulmonary artery enters the right chest underneath the superior vena cava just inferior to the azygous vein and anterior to the trachea and right mainstem bronchus. The right main pulmonary artery travels further than the left main pulmonary artery before reaching the pleural space and before branching. After entering the right chest, the pulmonary artery takes an abrupt turn inferior into the deepest part of the horizontal and oblique fissures. It gives off branches to the right upper lobe, right middle lobe, and right lower lobe, respectively. It should be remembered that the pulmonary artery branches distally into the lung like a deciduous tree. Larger vessels will be found close to the hilum and in the horizontal and oblique fissures. Progressively smaller vessels will be found as you approach the outer surface of the lung (Figure 34). The first branch of the right main pulmonary artery goes to the right upper lobe. This branch may come off the pulmonary artery very proximal and course under the superior vena cava separate from the main pulmonary artery. This branch is often located just anterior to the right upper lobe bronchus, and just inferior to the azygous vein as it arches over the hilum. In this

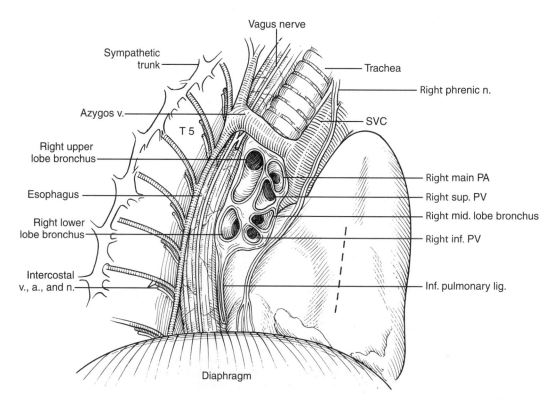

Figure 32 Hilum of right lung. Dotted line marks incision for pericardial window from right chest. *(Redrawn from Grant's Atlas of Anatomy, 11th ed., Philadelphia, Lippincott Williams & Wilkins, 2004, figure 1.43, p. 40.)*

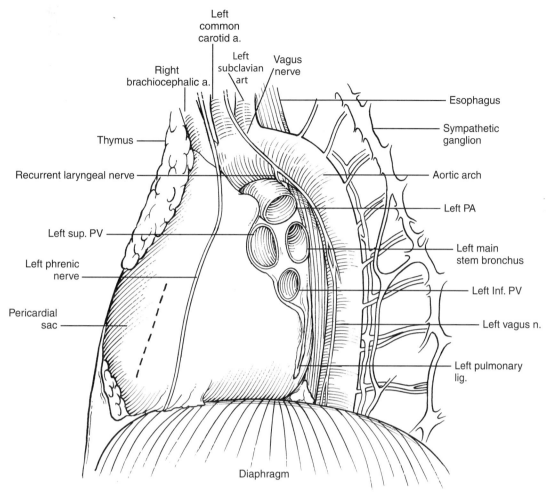

Left
common
carotid a.

Left
subclavian
art

Vagus
nerve

Right
brachiocephalic a.

Esophagus

Sympathetic
ganglion

Thymus

Recurrent laryngeal nerve

Aortic arch

Left PA

Left sup. PV

Left main
stem bronchus

Left phrenic
nerve

Left Inf. PV

Pericardial
sac

Left vagus n.

Left pulmonary
lig.

Diaphragm

Figure 33 Hilum of left lung. Dotted line marks incision for pericardial window. *(Adapted from Grant's Atlas of Anatomy, 11th ed., Philadelphia, Lippincott Williams & Wilkins, 2004, figure 1.44, p. 44.)*

location, it is very susceptible to iatrogenic traction injury by too vigorously pulling the lung inferior.

Proximal vascular control of the right pulmonary artery can be obtained as it courses under the superior vena cava either by encircling the vessel with a vessel loop, careful vascular clamping (Figure 35), or if needed, applying a nonselective clamp across the entire hilum (Figure 36). A nonselective clamp is sometimes referred to as "dirty" clamping because the immediate need is control of hemorrhage and structures other than the offending vessel may initially be included in the clamp.

From the right chest or a median sternotomy, the superior vena cava and inferior vena cava can be clamped. This is termed inflow occlusion and will cause cardiac standstill that can be tolerated no more than 3–5 minutes. In desperate circumstances, this allows time and visualization to obtain vascular control of a large hemorrhage such as from a main or branch pulmonary artery. Once the hemorrhage is contained, blood should be allowed to return to the heart before performing a definitive repair. Cardioversion will be necessary if the heart has fibrillated and should be anticipated.

The remaining vascular structure making up the hilum of the right lung is the superior pulmonary vein. This vein is seen anteriorly, sending a superior branch to the upper lobe, which crosses anterior to the pulmonary artery traveling in the horizontal fissure and variable branches to the right middle lobe.

The right mainstem bronchus can be visualized on the posterior superior right hilum. It bifurcates from the carina and travels underneath the azygous vein. While visualizing the bronchus from the posterior hilum, the delicate membranous airway is seen, with the bases of the arching bronchial cartilages visible and palpable on either side.

Left Hilum

As with the right lung, the left inferior lobe is tethered to the mediastinum by the left inferior pulmonary ligament. The superior most aspect of this ligament is the left inferior pulmonary vein, often with a lymph node in the ligament, just inferior to the vein. The superior aspect of the left hilum has the arch of the aorta crossing from the right to the left and from anterior to posterior. The superior most structure in the hilum proper is the left main pulmonary artery. The left main pulmonary artery is shorter than the right main pulmonary artery. Its first branch is to the left upper lobe and is often buried in the medial substance of the lung parenchyma. This branch is also vulnerable to injury during inferior retraction of the lung. The vagus nerve descends in the left chest anterior to the left subclavian artery, crossing the lateral surface of the arch of the aorta and diving anterior to the descending aorta to join and travel next to the more medially placed esophagus. The vagus

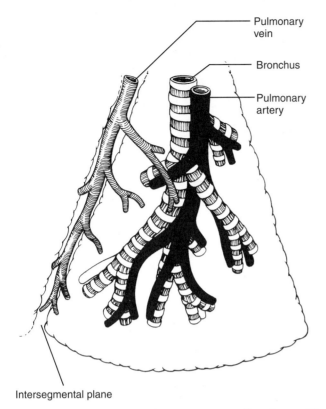

Figure 34   Generic bronchopulmonary segment.   *(From Pearson FG, editor: Thoracic Surgery, 2nd ed. Philadelphia, Churchill Livingstone, 2002, figure 20-1, p. 428.)*

nerve gives off the left recurrent laryngeal nerve just below the arch of the aorta. The left recurrent laryngeal nerve will dive around the ligamentum arteriosum and also join the esophagus, but travel superiorly in the tracheoesophageal groove back into the neck to innervate the larynx. The ligamentum arteriosum is the vestigial ductus arteriosus. It is fibrous, possibly calcified, and connects the top of the bifurcation of the pulmonary trunk to the arch of the aorta. It is visible in the left chest and emphasizes the proximity of

the bifurcation of the pulmonary trunk to the left hilum of the lung. Minimizing the use of electrocautery in this region and keeping dissections close to the pulmonary artery and away from the aorta and ligamentum arteriosum can avoid injury to the recurrent laryngeal nerve. Proximal control of the left pulmonary artery can be obtained by encircling the pulmonary artery, application of vascular clamps, or by hilar clamping. Because the left pulmonary artery is so short, it is sometimes necessary to incise the pericardium anterior to the left main pulmonary artery, taking care not to injure the phrenic nerve. The pulmonary trunk and intrapericardial course of the left main pulmonary artery can then be visualized and the left main pulmonary artery clamped. Immediate vascular collapse after placement of this clamp may mean blood flow to the right pulmonary artery was occluded as well and the clamp should be reapplied. The left atrial appendage will be present in this location. It is mobile and often an unwelcome companion. It is susceptible to injury, hemorrhage, and air embolism by clamping and retraction and should be treated with respect.

The left main pulmonary artery turns sharply after entering the chest and descends in the deepest part of the oblique fissure. Like the right superior pulmonary vein, the left superior pulmonary vein is only visible anteriorly. It can be seen inferior to the pulmonary artery as a fold of pericardium entering the lung. The left mainstem bronchus, while long, is hidden by the arch of the aorta and main pulmonary artery. It is often not visible at all without incising the reflection of the parietal and visceral pleura posteriorly and developing the plane between the membranous portion of the left mainstem bronchus and the esophagus.

The left hilum can also be nonselectively clamped to obtain vascular control (see Figure 36).

LUNG ANATOMY

The right lung has three lobes, the right upper, right middle, and right lower. The left lung has two lobes, the left upper and left lower. The lingula of the left upper lobe is analogous to the middle lobe on the right. Fissures of the lung are usually present, but variably complete. On the right, the horizontal fissure, usually incomplete, divides the right upper lobe from the right middle lobe. The horizontal fissure joins the oblique fissure posteriorly. The oblique fissure divides the right upper lobe from the superior segment of

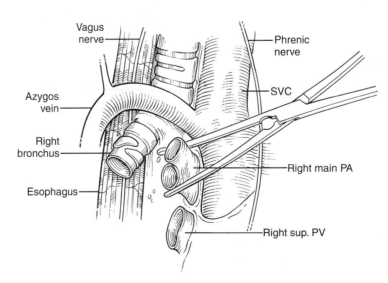

Figure 35   Clamping the right main pulmonary artery as it courses under the superior vena cava.

bifurcate toward the periphery. Pulmonary veins travel in the border zones between lung segments and along the walls of the horizontal and oblique fissures (see Figure 34).

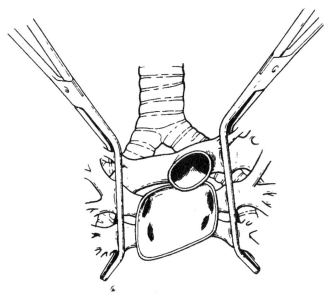

Figure 36 "Dirty" clamping of the left or right pulmonary hilum. *(From Pearson FG, editor: Thoracic Surgery, 2nd ed. Philadelphia, Churchill Livingstone, 2002, figure 68-3, p. 1837.)*

the right lower lobe and the right middle lobe from the right lower lobe. The right lower lobe rests on the diaphragm posteriorly. The right middle lobe will often rest on the diaphragm anteriorly and is mistaken for the right lower lobe in this position. On the left, the oblique fissure divides the left upper lobe from the left lower lobe. The left lower lobe rests on the diaphragm posteriorly. The lingula of the left upper lobe can extend down to the diaphragm anteriorly.

Figure 37 shows the lung segments. Pulmonary arteries and the airway will enter the middle of their respective lung segment and

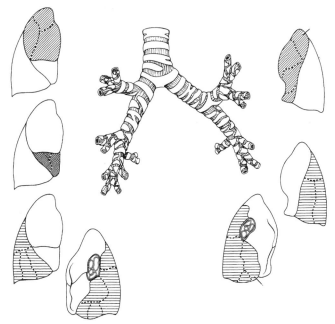

Figure 37 Segmental anatomy of the lung. *(From Pearson FG, editor: Thoracic Surgery, 2nd ed. Philadelphia, Churchill Livingstone, 2002, figure 20-2, p. 428.)*

AORTA, TRACHEA, ESOPHAGUS, AND THORACIC DUCT

Posterior to the heart, outside the pericardium, several tubular structures travel parallel to each other. They are the aorta, trachea, esophagus, and thoracic duct (Figure 38).

Aorta

The thoracic aorta originates from the fibrous trigone of the heart at the aortic valve. The coronary arteries originate immediately distal to the valve from the aortic sinuses of Valsalva. The left coronary artery commonly originates from the left sinus, which is located posteriorly and toward the pulmonary valve. The right coronary artery originates from the right sinus of Valsalva, which is anterior and to the right. The right coronary may be seen coursing from left to right across the anterior wall of the right ventricle from its origin at the aorta. The ascending aorta is short, ending in the aortic arch. The aorta arches mostly from anterior to posterior with some movement from the midline to the left to come to lie just to the left of the vertebral column in the left chest. The great vessels originate at the top of this arch. From proximal to distal and anterior to posterior, they are the right brachiocephalic artery, the left carotid artery, and the left subclavian artery. The right brachiocephalic artery will have the right vagus nerve crossing anteriorly with the right recurrent nerve branching posteriorly from the right vagus just after crossing this vessel. The right recurrent nerve travels to the right tracheoesophageal groove and then superiorly back into the neck. On the underside of the aortic arch, the ligamentum arteriosum attaches the aorta to the pulmonary trunk. The combination of the great vessels and ligamentum arteriosum fix the aortic arch in the chest. The descending thoracic aorta is relatively mobile. The aorta just distal to the left subclavian artery is in the transition zone between fixed and mobile and is a common site for aortic injury in acceleration/deceleration injuries. The descending thoracic aorta gives off segmental branches to the chest wall as intercostal arteries as well as braches to the esophagus, trachea, carina, and proximal bronchi. The aorta enters the abdomen through the aortic hiatus of the diaphragm from T11 to T12. Between T8 and L2, but usually near L2 is the origin of the artery of Adamkiewicz. This is a large segmental artery, most commonly left sided, which anastomosis with the anterior spinal artery and supplies up to 2/3 of spinal cord blood flow. Occluding the aorta proximal to this vessel may cause spinal cord ischemia.

TRACHEA

The trachea begins in the neck at the cricoid cartilage, enters the thorax anterior to the esophagus and posterior to the great vessels, including posterior to the arch and ascending aorta and the pulmonary arteries. Distally, near the carina, the arch of the aorta crosses to the left of the trachea. The trachea bifurcates into the right and left mainstem bronchi at the carina. The carina is at the level of the angle of Louis anteriorly and T4/T5 posteriorly. The average adult trachea is 11 cm in length and varies according to the height of the person. In a young person, hyperextension of the neck can bring 50% of the trachea out of the chest and into the neck. Conversely, in a kyphotic elderly patient, the cricoid cartilage can be at the level of the sternal notch. In the neck, the trachea is anterior and subcutaneous. As it enters the chest, it travels obliquely posterior to the posterior mediastinum. The shortest distance from a point to a line is a perpendicular from that line, intersecting

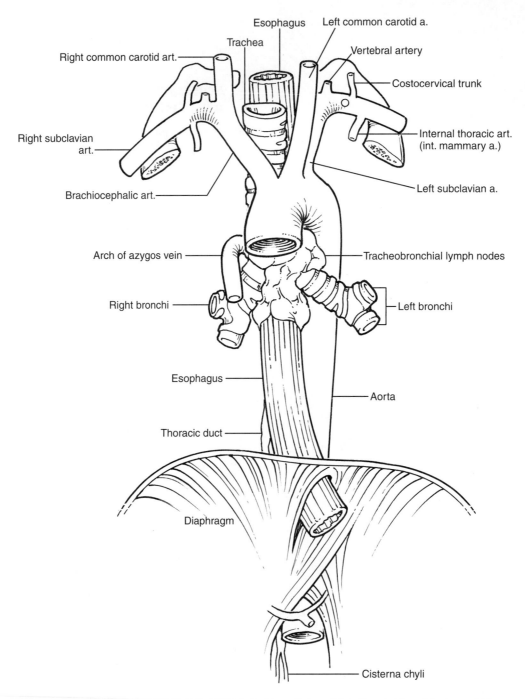

Figure 38 Aorta, trachea, esophagus, and thoracic duct. *(Adapted from Grant's Atlas of Anatomy, 11th ed., Philadelphia, Lippincott Williams & Wilkins, 2004, figure 1.78, p. 68.)*

the point. If the trachea is a line, obliquely posterior, the shortest distance from a point on the skin to the trachea will be in a trajectory slightly superior. Visualizing this relationship aids in tracheostomy and cricothyroidotomy incisions (Figure 39). The trachea is composed anteriorly of cartilaginous arches with fibrous tissue in between. The posterior wall of the trachea is membranous. The blood supply to the trachea is segmental, superiorly primarily from the inferior thyroidal arteries and inferiorly from the bronchial arteries. The subclavian artery, highest intercostal artery, internal thoracic arteries, and innominate artery also supply it. These vessels also supply the esophagus. The blood supply enters the trachea laterally at 3 and 9 o'clock.

ESOPHAGUS

The esophagus travels through the posterior mediastinum anterior to the vertebral bodies, to the right of the descending aorta, and to the left of the azygous vein (see Figure 38). Its blood supply is from segmental branches of the descending aorta, draining into intercostal veins. Above the level of the carina, the esophagus is posterior to the trachea and immediately abuts the membranous trachea. Above the level of the ligamentum arteriosum, the recurrent laryngeal nerve travels in the left tracheoesophageal groove. Above the level of the right brachiocephalic artery the right recurrent laryngeal nerve travels in the right tracheoesophageal groove. Below the carina, the

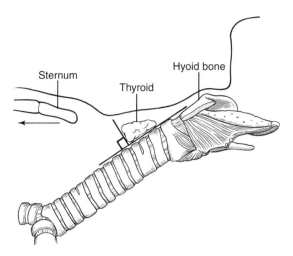

Figure 39 Trachea travels diagonally posterior as it leaves the neck and enters the chest. The shortest distance between a point and a line is perpendicular to that line through the point.

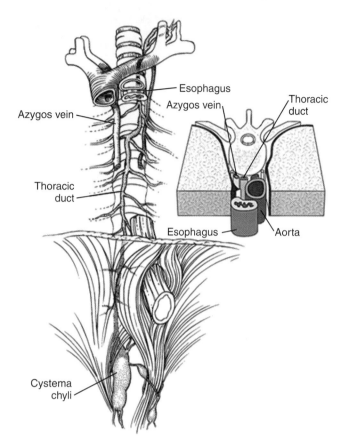

Figure 40 Thoracic duct. *(From Pearson FG, editor:* Thoracic Surgery, *2nd ed. Philadelphia, Churchill Livingstone, 2002, figure 20-7, p. 431.)*

esophagus directly abuts the posterior pericardium. To its left and right from superior to inferior are the superior pulmonary veins, the inferior pulmonary veins, and the inferior pulmonary ligaments. The esophagus enters the diaphragm through the esophageal hiatus at the level of T10 or T11. The area to the left and right of the esophagus at and below the inferior pulmonary ligament and before entering the diaphragm represents an anatomic weak spot. The wall of the esophagus is not buttressed by other firm mediastinal structures and is exposed to the negative pressure of the pleural space. It is for this reason that increased intraesophageal pressure causing a perforation of the esophagus most commonly occurs here (Boerhaave's syndrome).

THORACIC DUCT

The thoracic duct originates from the cisterna chyli (Figure 40). The cisterna chyli is located in the abdomen, at the level of the celiac axis, anterior to the vertebral body and to the right of the aorta. The thoracic duct travels superiorly, entering the thorax through the aortic hiatus of the diaphragm. It ascends in the posterior mediastinum between the aorta and the azygous vein. Above the arch of the aorta, it travels posterior to the esophagus, arches behind the internal jugular vein to join the venous system at the junction of the internal jugular vein and subclavian vein. The thoracic duct is thin walled and often invisible to the naked eye if not distended with lymph. Injury to the duct is visible as a pooling of lymph in the vicinity of the leak. Fat delivered to the small bowel will within 10–20 minutes turn this lymph milky white, enhancing visualization. Ligation of the thoracic duct is accomplished by ligating all fatty material and lymphatics bounded by four walls, consisting of the azygous vein, the parietal pleura, the esophagus, and the aorta below the level of the suspected leak.

SUGGESTED READINGS

Agur AMR: *Grant's Atlas of Anatomy*, 9th ed. Baltimore, Williams and Wilkins, 1991.

Christensen JB, Telford IR: *Synopsis of Gross Anatomy*, 5th ed. Philadelphia, J.B. Lippincott, 1988.

Collis JL, Kelly TD, Wiley AM: Anatomy of the crura of the diaphragm and the surgery of hiatus hernia. *Thorax* 9:175–189, 1954.

Collis JL: Surgical control of reflux in hiatus hernia. *Am J Surg* 115:465–471, 1968.

Graeber GM, Szwerc MF: Anatomy and physiology of the chest wall and sternum. In Pearson FG, editor: *Thoracic Surgery*, 2nd ed. Philadelphia, Churchill Livingstone, 2002, pp. 1325–1335.

Mathisen DJ, Grillo H: The trachea. In Baue A, et al., editors: *Glenn's Thoracic and Cardiovascular Surgery*, 6th ed., vol. I. Stamford, CT, Appleton & Lange, 1996, pp. 665–690.

Mehran RJ, Deslauriers J: Anatomy and physiology of the pleural space. In Pearson FG, editor: *Thoracic Surgery*, 2nd ed. Philadelphia, Churchill Livingstone, 2002, pp. 1133–1139.

Plestis KA, Fell SC: Anatomy, embryology, pathophysiology, and surgery of the phrenic nerve and diaphragm. In Pearson FG, editor: *Thoracic Surgery*, 2nd ed. Philadelphia, Churchill Livingstone, 2002, pp. 1499–1507.

Rice T: Anatomy of the lung. In Pearson FG, editor: *Thoracic Surgery*, 2nd ed. Philadelphia, Churchill Livingstone, 2002, pp. 427–441.

THORACIC WALL INJURIES: RIBS, STERNAL SCAPULAR FRACTURES, HEMOTHORACES, AND PNEUMOTHORACES

Alisa Savetamal   and   David H. Livingston

Although many chest injuries are potentially lethal, early man sustained and survived blunt and penetrating chest trauma. Examinations of Neanderthal skeletons have shown evidence of healed penetrating and blunt rib fractures. The Edwin Smith Papyrus, written circa 3000 BC, gave explicit instructions for the management of chest injuries including soft tissue and bony injuries.[1] In fact, 8 of the 43 cases discussed concerned chest injuries, suggesting that even at that time, chest injuries accounted for 20%–25% of all trauma.

Trauma to the chest wall and the underlying lung parenchyma either in isolation or as part of multisystem trauma remains exceedingly common and are a frequent source of trauma mortality and morbidity. Hemothoraces and pneumothoraces, while technically not injuries to the thoracic wall, occur commonly in conjunction with such injuries will be considered here as well. Flail chest and its accompanying pulmonary contusion are mentioned only briefly here and are more completely discussed on pages 269–277.

INCIDENCE

Thoracic injuries remain common and are directly attributable for 20%–25% of all trauma deaths; chest injuries are further associated with another 25% of trauma deaths. Chest injuries commonly accompany other injuries and contribute to organ failure in the multiply-injured patient. Rib fractures are among the most commonly encountered injuries. In a review of over 7000 patients seen in a Level I trauma center, 10% had rib fractures; of these, 94% had associated injuries, and 12% died. Half of patients with rib fractures required operation or intensive care unit (ICU) admission, one-third developed complications, and one-third ultimately required extended care in an outpatient facility.[2]

Pneumothorax is found in over 20% in patients arriving to a trauma center.[3] Hemothoraces are encountered with similar frequency. The incidence of both hemothoraces and pneumothoraces is underestimated by plain films, as these injuries are much better visualized by computed tomography (CT) of the chest than the traditional supine anteroposterior chest radiograph (AP CXR).

Fractures to the bony thorax other than the ribs most commonly occur in the clavicles, which constitute 5%–10% of all fractures. Fractures of the sternum and scapula are much less common (0.5%–4% and 0.8%–3%, respectively) and are more likely to occur in association with other injuries than clavicular fractures. Again, the more liberal use of chest CT has resulted in an increase in the identification of nondisplaced scapular and sternal fractures. Complete scapulothoracic dissociation is a rare but dramatic injury with severe associated neurovascular injury.

MECHANISM

Injuries of the chest wall may vary enormously in severity. In routine emergency room settings, chest trauma may be incurred as a result of a low energy impact, and be relatively minor. On the other hand, chest injuries sustained by patients treated in trauma centers following high-energy trauma from motor vehicle collisions (MVC) are typically severe and are often life-threatening. The most common causes of chest wall injuries and rib fractures in adults are MVC followed by falls and direct blows to the chest with blunt objects. It is important to recall that rib fractures in infants and younger children occur almost exclusively in the setting of child abuse. In older populations, falls and pedestrian in motor vehicle accidents become the predominant mechanism of injury.

Rib fractures are normally the hallmark of significant blunt chest trauma, and increasing numbers of rib fractures are related to increasing morbidity and mortality. The presence of more than three rib fractures in adults is a marker for associated solid visceral trauma and mortality, and thus has been used as a marker for trauma center transfer.[4] In hemodynamically stable patients, the presence of blunt chest trauma has also been shown to double the rate of intra-abdominal injuries detected by abdominal CT.[5] Rib fractures are less common in children due to the resilience of their bony chest wall. Thus, children may suffer major intrathoracic injury without rib fractures and the presence of any rib fracture in a child should be considered a marker for severe injury.[6] The presence of acute rib fractures in a young child whose mechanism of injury is unclear or the finding of rib fractures of varying ages should also serve as an indicator for potential child abuse.[7,8] Conversely, elderly patients with brittle bones will occasionally have little in the way of intrathoracic injury despite extensive rib fractures.[9]

The different mechanisms of injury provide somewhat different patterns of injury. Penetrating injury causes parenchymal lacerations with hemopneumothoraces. Blunt injury to the lung is most often due to displaced rib fractures, and can result in hemopneumothoraces or pulmonary contusions. Pneumothoraces after blunt trauma occur through (1) alveolar rupture with resultant air leak due to a sudden increase in intrathoracic pressure, (2) laceration of the lung due to displaced rib fractures, (3) tearing of the lung in a deceleration injury, and (4) direct crush injury from a blow to the chest.

DIAGNOSIS

Physical Examination

Expeditious inspection and palpation of the chest will provide much information regarding the patient's injuries (Figure 1). Auscultation and percussion tend to be less reliable due to the high ambient noise of the trauma ED. Hypotension, tachycardia, pallor, or cyanosis suggests shock. In the presence of a known or suspected thoracic injury, shock must be assumed to be from an intrathoracic source. Inspection of the chest itself should include assessment of use of the accessory muscles suggestive of airway obstruction, the symmetry of the chest wall, number and location of wounds, presence of open chest wounds, subcutaneous emphysema, and the presence of "flail" segments. While tracheal deviation in the neck is also frequently cited as a sign of tension pneumothorax, in reality it is rarely if ever seen, even in patients with gross mediastinal deviation on chest x-ray. Palpation can reveal mobile segments of chest wall and further allows appreciation of the symmetry of chest wall motion and of crepitance. Auscultation in trauma has a high specificity but very poor sensitivity, so focus should be placed only on the presence and symmetry of

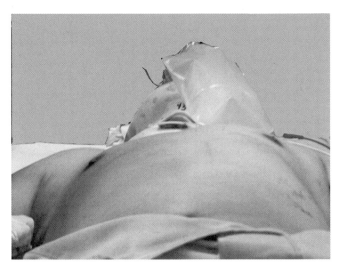

Figure 1   Physical examination of the chest in a driver of a motor vehicle discloses marked asymmetry of the right and left hemithoraces.

air entry. Heart sounds, such as the muffled heartbeat in Beck's triad or the "mediastinal crunch" of Hamman's sign, are also difficult to obtain clearly in the trauma bay. The absence or asymmetry of breath sounds, however, is very suggestive of significant pathology; in the unstable patient, this is an indication for intervention on clinical grounds and a contraindication for imaging studies. Thoracic percussion, even more than auscultation, is difficult to interpret in the trauma setting and is rarely useful.

Physical examination often, but not always, reveals the presence of a hemopneumothorax. It may be suspected in hemodynamically unstable patients by physical exam. In the patient with greatly diminished or absent breath sounds on the affected side, the diagnosis is quickly made on clinical grounds. In the noisy trauma bay, however, auscultation can unreliable even in the presence of a sizeable hemothorax or pneumothorax. In addition, breath sounds can be well-transmitted from the contralateral lung, further obscuring the results of auscultation. The finding of any subcutaneous emphysema following blunt trauma or at some distance from a penetrating wound is ample evidence of a pneumothorax that requires treatment. An open pneumothorax, of course, is readily appreciated on examination. Confirmation of the hemothorax or pneumothorax occurs with the placement of a chest tube with evacuation of blood and/or air.

Radiographic Studies

The supine AP CXR is the initial and sometimes most important study in the management of chest trauma. The trauma surgeon must be comfortable interpreting these films, which are often sub-optimal due to the patient's body habitus, supine position, the presence of a spine board, and the use of portable x-ray machines. Still, the portable AP CXR can diagnose or exclude a number of life-threatening injuries, and it must be obtained and reviewed before the patient is transported for any other imaging or procedures.

Interpretation of the CXR should begin with review of the lung parenchyma and pleura. Lung expansion, pulmonary infiltrates or contusions, the position of the endotracheal tube if present, and the presence of hemothoraces or pneumothoraces should be noted. The mediastinum should be evaluated for evidence of great vessel injury, which is suggested by mediastinal widening, blunting of the aortic knob, apical capping, or a medial displacement of the left mainstem bronchus or of the nasogastric tube. Diaphragmatic elevation or injury should also be noted. Finally, any fractures of the bony thorax—ribs, clavicles, and scapulae—should be sought. Alignment

of the thoracic vertebrae can be appreciated on CXR, but full imaging of the spine as well as specific radiographs of the bony thoracic structures should be deferred until the patient's airway, respiratory, and cardiovascular status has been stabilized.

Radiographic imaging is extremely useful in the diagnosis of a hemothorax or pneumothorax. Indeed, in a hemodynamically stable patient, the diagnosis is often made on the portable AP CXR obtained for the secondary survey. In the supine position the AP CXR will reveal hemothorax only when at least 200–300 ml of blood is present in the pleural space, and is suggested by an overall opacification or haziness compared to the contralateral hemithorax as the fluid will layer posteriorly (Figure 2). False "negative"–appearing CXR may occur in the setting of bilateral hemothoraces (no difference between the two sides) or when there is a simultaneous anterior pneumothorax (decreasing the relative density more similar to the other side). In the patient with penetrating chest trauma, the CXR is best taken with the patient upright which increases the sensitivity for both hemothoraces and pneumothoraces. Chest ultrasound may help to identify the presence of pleural fluid, but its sensitivity and specificity for this purpose have not been well-defined.

As routine truncal (chest, abdomen, and pelvis) CT scanning has become more prevalent, many patients with blunt trauma have been found to have significant anterior pneumothoraces not seen on plain CXR. The incidence of missed pneumothoraces on supine AP CXR has been estimated to be between 20%–35%. A patient with a relatively minor pneumothorax on CXR who nonetheless develops dyspnea and hypoxia may thus in fact have a significant pneumothorax that is better visualized by chest CT. In stable patients, CT scanning will reveal also pleural fluid collections and help to distinguish them from parenchymal injury such as pulmonary contusion.

The appropriate management of the patient with "CT-only" pneumothorax is a matter of some controversy (Figure 3). The reported

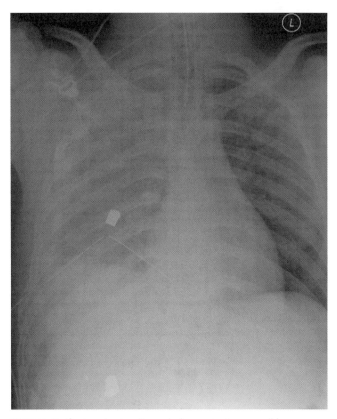

Figure 2   Supine chest radiograph demonstrating overall hazy appearance that is diagnostic of a right hemothorax (in this case incompletely drained by a tube thoracostomy). Note the difference between the right and left sides.

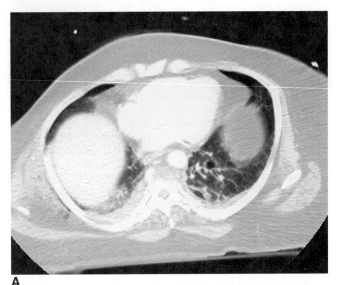

A

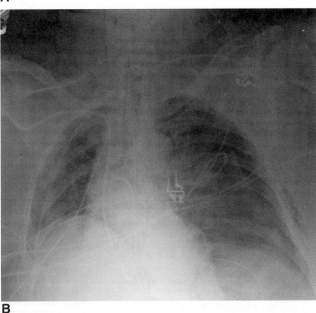

B

Figure 3   CT scan **(A)** demonstrating small bilateral "CT-only" pneumothoraces. Chest radiograph of the same patient **(B),** following mechanical ventilation. Note the large left pneumothorax, demonstrating the somewhat unpredictable outcome of these small pneumothoraces. The patient never developed a pneumothorax on the right. *CT,* Computed tomography.

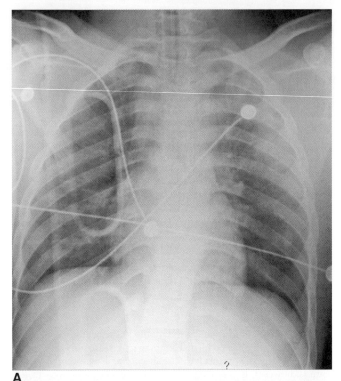

A

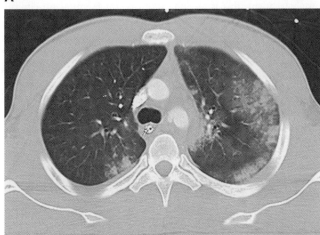

B

Figure 4   Chest radiograph of patient ejected from a motor vehicle at high rate of speed **(A).** The lung fields are essentially clear, although the mediastinal contour is abnormal. CT scan **(B)** of the same patient demonstrating significant pulmonary contusions, which helped explain the patient's clinical hypoxemia. In addition, an injury to the descending aorta is also visualized. *CT,* Computed tomography.

incidence of these pneumothoraces in blunt trauma patients is 2%–8%.[10,11] The available literature suggests that 20% of these patients will require tube thoracostomy. The decision to place a chest tube, however, should be dictated by the patient's overall status. Patients who are multiply injured, are in hemorrhagic shock, or have sustained a traumatic brain injury will not tolerate progression of even a small pneumothorax (see Figure 3). These patients would benefit from tube thoracostomy. In patients where the clinical picture appears stable, observation can be undertaken, with serial radiographs taken at 6 and 24 hours after diagnosis.

Computed tomography (CT) of the chest has become increasingly accepted in the early management of trauma. CT can reveal injuries not seen on initial CXR in about two-thirds of major trauma patients[12] and can lead to therapeutic changes in 5%–30%

of cases[13,14] (Figure 4). In addition, CT scanning may reveal additional findings that are only suggested by an abnormal CXR (Figure 5). There are a number of specific situations in which chest CT contributes significantly to trauma management. CT of the thoracic spine is the "gold-standard" imaging modality for assessing vertebral body as well as posterior element fractures, and is also helpful in imaging the spine at the cervicothoracic junction.[12,14,15] In patients with the nonspecific finding of a widened mediastinum on CXR, use of CT can help to limit the use of aortography to assess aortic injuries.[16–18] As CT technology improves

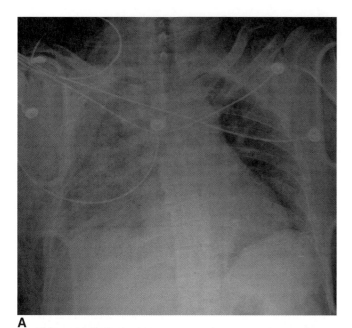

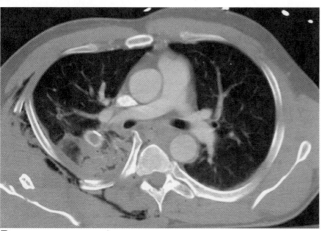

Figure 5 **(A)** The impact of CT scanning with more obvious severe chest trauma following a motor vehicle collision. Physical examination demonstrated no paradoxical motion in the upper right hemithorax. There are multiple (seven) rib fractures, a haziness over the entire right hemithorax and subcutaneous emphysema but no obvious pneumothorax. **(B)** CT scan of the same patient. A chest tube was inserted based on the marked subcutaneous emphysema present on physical exam that drained no air on insertion and minimal amount of blood. The haziness turned out to be only a modest pulmonary contusion with a minimal hemothorax. The scan revealed a total of 18 distinct rib fractures with considerably more displacement than was noted on the plain radiograph. The reason for the lack of paradoxical motion is explained by the posterior nature of the flail segments. In addition, a nondisplaced scapula fracture and six thoracic transverse process fractures were identified. *CT,* Computed tomography.

and as further studies become available, the role of CT in chest trauma will become better-defined.

Ultrasonography has become important in the assessment of intra-abdominal hemorrhage and pericardial fluid collections in the trauma patient. Recent reports also suggest that it might be useful to assess the pleural spaces for pneumothoraces and hemo-thoraces.[19–21] The pleural space is interrogated by placing the

ultrasound probe between the ribs and looking for the characteristic signs of pneumothorax.[19,22]

AAST-OIS GRADING

The American Association for the Surgery of Trauma-Organ Injury Scale (AAST-OIS) grading scales for chest wall and lung injury developed by Moore et al.[23] are listed in Tables 1 and 2.

MANAGEMENT OF SPECIFIC INJURIES TO CHEST WALL

Chest Wall Defects

Chest wall defects create open pneumothoraces and are potentially rapidly lethal. Large sucking chest wounds can allow rapid equilibration of pleural and atmospheric pressure, preventing lung inflation and alveolar ventilation and causing death by asphyxia. As a result, patients sustaining chest wall defects with significant tissue loss rarely survive long enough to be seen in the trauma bay. Patients who do come to medical attention are usually found to have penetrating injuries such as close shotgun blasts or impalements.

The field approach to the relatively small chest wall defect is placement of an occlusive dressing taped on three sides to allow gas to exit from, but not to enter, the thorax. Subsequent treatment consists of tube thoracostomy through clean nontraumatized skin, after which the primary wound may be temporarily closed or dressed with an occlusive dressing. Definitive wound closure is then performed in the operating room.

In large chest wall defects, the occlusive dressing is of no value. These patients must be endotracheally intubated with positive pressure ventilation. Operative management then focuses on control of

Table 1: Chest Wall Injury Scale

Grade	Injury Type	Description of Injury
I	Contusion	Any size
	Laceration	Skin and subcutaneous
	Fracture	<3 ribs, closed; nondisplaced clavicle, closed
II	Laceration	Skin, subcutaneous, and muscle
	Fracture	>3 adjacent ribs, closed
		Open or displaced clavicle
		Nondisplaced sternum, closed
		Scapular body, open or closed
III	Laceration	Full thickness, including pleural penetration
	Fracture	Open or displaced sternum
		Flail sternum
		Unilateral flail sternum (<3 ribs)
IV	Laceration	Avulsion of chest wall tissues with underlying rib fractures
	Fracture	Unilateral flail chest (>3 ribs)
V	Fracture	Bilateral flail chest (>3 ribs on both sides)

Adapted from Moore EE, Cogbill TH, Malangoni MA, et al: Organ injury scaling. *Surg Clin North Am* 75(2):293–303, 1995.

Table 2: Lung Injury Scale

Grade	Injury Type	Description of Injury
I	Contusion	Unilateral, <1 lobe
II	Contusion	Unilateral, 1 lobe
	Laceration	Simple pneumothorax
	Contusion	Unilateral, L1 lobe
III	Laceration	Persistent (>72 hours) air leak from distal airway
	Hematoma	Nonexpanding intraparenchymal
	Laceration	Major (segmental or lobar) air leak
IV	Hematoma	Expanding intraparenchymal
	Vascular	Primary branch intrapulmonary vessel disruption
V	Vascular	Hilar vessel disruption
VI	Vascular	Total uncontained transaction of pulmonary hilum

Adapted from Moore EE, Cogbill TH, Malangoni MA, et al: Organ injury scaling. *Surg Clin North Am* 75(2):293–303, 1995.

hemorrhage from the chest wall and from any associated injuries. Chest wall hemorrhage in these cases may be life-threatening and may mandate emergent thoracotomy. "Damage control" with packing may be the optimal initial management of these patients. The chest defect can be temporarily closed with skin or prosthetic material. The definitive closure of these defects, which may require tissue-transfer procedures, is best deferred until the patient is fully resuscitated, physiologically sound, and able to tolerate a lengthy operation.

Rib Fractures and Flail Chest

Rib fractures can result in chest wall pain, chest wall hemorrhage, and less commonly, chest wall instability. A flail chest is said to exist when three or more adjacent ribs are segmentally fractured. The resultant chest wall instability combined with underlying pulmonary contusion is responsible for the respiratory insufficiency that develops in patients after this injury. The pathophysiology and treatment of flail chest injuries are covered in greater detail on pages 269–277.

Failure to provide sufficient analgesia in the setting of chest wall injuries has been shown to result in hypoventilation, retained secretions, increased atelectasis and lobar collapse, pneumonia, and respiratory failure.[24] Persistence of pain may perpetuate the stress response to injury and may have a negative impact on post-traumatic immune function.[25] Poor pain control will hamper the ability of mechanically ventilated patients to be weaned and extubated. The pharmacological approach to pain management in chest injury has consisted of the use of narcotics with or without regional anesthesia. The addition of nonsteroidal anti-inflammatory drugs (NSAIDs) such as ketorolac have also proven effective in relieving pain from mild to moderate injuries.

Narcotics

Narcotics are the mainstay for pain control in the majority of trauma patients. Narcotic preparations can be given orally, intramuscularly, or intravenously. But whereas intramuscular administration has been the standard for decades, we strongly advise against this route of administration because it is both painful to the patient and results in unreliable absorption of the narcotic. With the exception of meperidine (Demerol) however, which narcotic chosen is far less important

than ensuring adequate dosing for pain control.[26] The amount of narcotic required for pain control may vary greatly depending upon previous or current narcotic use, age, and other factors that alter the patient's perception of pain.

The use of pain scales in combination with performance on incentive spirometry can be very effective in determining the adequacy of pain control.[27] Our current approach is to begin most awake patients on a patient-controlled analgesia (PCA) regimen using morphine or fentanyl. Later, patients are transitioned to long-acting narcotic preparations such as OxyContin or MS-contin with the use of oxycodone for breakthrough pain. The addition of an NSAID may reduce inflammation and augment the effect of the oral narcotics. It is also important to avoid narcotic induced constipation. This can result in severe abdominal pain, nausea, and vomiting in patients requiring long-term opioids.

Regional Anesthesia

Rib blocks can be accomplished using a mixture of 1%–2% lidocaine with 0.25% bupivacaine to decrease the pain of rib fractures. This simple technique involves the administration of 2–3 ml of the anesthetic mixture to the inferior rib margin several centimeters posterior to the site of the rib fracture. Optimal analgesia requires blocking at least one rib above and one rib below the fracture. The limitations of the technique are that the pain control is short-lived and that it can only be used for patients with mid or lower rib fractures. Last, in our experience the results vary widely and the risks of pneumothorax in patients without a chest tube are real.[28]

Epidural analgesia/anesthesia is the delivery mode that has been shown to have the greatest impact on pulmonary mechanics following moderate to severe chest trauma, especially in patients with bilateral injuries.[29] There are various combinations of local anesthetics and narcotics which have been employed. In our institution, the most common combination is fentanyl with bupivacaine. Combination therapy can be advantageous because it works via two different mechanisms of action. Opioids modulate presynaptic and postsynaptic nerve transmission in dorsal horn neurons by effects on their specific receptors. Local anesthetics work by blocking sodium channels. Thus, the analgesic effects of the two classes of drug are synergistic. Moreover, the potential for side effects is lessened in combination therapy because the doses of each drug used can be lower than the amount used if either were administered alone.

Epidural analgesia has significant practical problems including ileus, pruritus, and urinary retention as well as transient hypotension. The use of epidural analgesia requires that the spine be documented to be free of injury, which may be difficult to accomplish for several days in severely injured patients. Also, the concomitant use of low-molecular-weight heparin (LMWH) in patients with an epidural catheter has been implicated in the development of spinal epidural hematomas with resultant neurologic deficits. Last, epidural catheters can only be left in place safely for 7–10 days because of the possibility of epidural abscess formation. Thus, it is strongly recommended that epidural catheters not be placed in mechanically ventilated patients until they are ready to be weaned.

The data supporting the use of epidural analgesia is strong. Mackersie et al.[30] demonstrated that the use of epidural fentanyl was associated with significant improvements in pulmonary mechanics with 85% of the patients requiring no additional parenteral narcotics. Intravenous narcotics were associated with increases in $PaCO_2$ and decreases in PaO_2 that were not observed in the epidural group. In a randomized prospective trial, Bulger et al.[31] reported epidural analgesia was associated with half the number of ventilator days compared to patients in the opioid group. They also point out that the technique was limited in trauma patients due to the presence of exclusion criteria in over 50%. Despite these limitations the use of epidural analgesia, when feasible, is of considerable benefit to patients following severe chest injury, as it has been strongly associated with a decrease in the rate of nosocomial pneumonia and a shorter duration of mechanical ventilation.

Pneumothorax and Hemothorax

Rib fractures can also cause injury to the underlying lung parenchyma, with resultant hemothoraces or pneumothoraces, although these can also occur without evidence of rib fractures. The severity of pneumothorax ranges from clinically insignificant to life-threatening. Pneumothoraces can be categorized as simple, open, and tension. A simple pneumothorax is a collection of air arising from leakage of air from an injured lung into the pleural space. An open pneumothorax arises when air enters the thoracic cavity from an open chest wound, with equalization of pressure between the thorax and the atmosphere. A tension pneumothorax occurs from a "ball-and-valve" effect in which air enters but does not exit the thoracic cavity, causing intrapleural pressure to exceed atmospheric pressure. The resultant pressure can cause the heart and great vessels to shift away from the side of injury and result in progressive circulatory compromise (see Figure 3).

Hemothorax, the presence of blood in the pleural space, can arise from either thoracic or abdominal sources. Bleeding from thoracic sources can occur from injured lung parenchyma, lacerated intercostal or internal mammary arteries, or the heart and great vessels. Hemothorax from an abdominal source occurs in the setting of diaphragmatic injury with associated abdominal injury, most commonly the liver or spleen.

Treatment of pneumothorax depends upon the type. Small simple pneumothoraces can generally be observed, though larger ones require tube thoracostomy. If the patient is stable and a simple pneumothorax is suspected, a CXR is obtained before any intervention. This (1) confirms the diagnosis and prevents unnecessary chest tube placement, (2) helps to exclude unexpected pathology such as a diaphragmatic rupture, and (3) may demonstrate other findings (such as a large hemothorax or chest wall hematoma) that would affect the size or location of chest tube placement. Patients with small pneumothoraces who are stable from the hemodynamic and respiratory standpoints may be observed with serial radiographs. Supplemental oxygen may be administered to enhance reabsorption of the pneumothorax. Patients with larger pneumothoraces may be treated either with standard tube thoracostomy or in select patients a "pigtail" catheter.

Open and tension pneumothoraces require urgent treatment. The treatment of open pneumothoraces requires temporary closure of the defect, tube thoracostomy, and then definitive operative closure of the chest wall defect. Tension pneumothorax is treated with needle decompression followed by tube thoracostomy. If a tension pneumothorax is suspected and the patient manifests any respiratory distress or hemodynamic instability, decompression should be performed without awaiting radiologic imaging. Emergent chest decompression is performed by inserting a 14-gauge IV catheter in the second or third intercostal space (approximately two finger-breadths below the clavicle) in the midclavicular line. A large chest tube is then placed (see below).

The treatment goal for hemothoraces, as for pneumothoraces, is evacuation of the pleural space and re-expansion of the lung. This is accomplished initially through tube thoracostomy. Apposition of the visceral and parietal pleurae generally provides definitive control of hemorrhage, and thoracotomy is required in less than 10%–15% of all chest trauma patients. Patients may occasionally present to the trauma bay several hours after injury with a large amount of initial drainage from the chest tube. This usually represents the slow accumulation of blood rather than rapid active bleeding, particularly in the patient who remains hemodynamically stable. If the hemothorax cannot be adequately drained by one chest tube, another one may need to be placed. CXR should be obtained immediately after tube thoracostomy to demonstrate successful drainage of the pleural space and lung re-expansion. If residual blood in the pleural space is still suspected and the patient is stable, CT of the chest may help to resolve the issue. If an acute hemothorax cannot be adequately drained because the chest tube is clotted, operative drainage may be necessary as continued bleeding cannot be assessed (Figure 6). Operative treatment can be accomplished either through thoracotomy or, in selected stable patients, through video-assisted thoracoscopic surgery (VATS).

The chest tube output from any moderate- to large-sized acute hemothorax should be collected and auto-transfused. Collection systems should be readily available in the trauma emergency department (ED), as the largest amount of blood loss occurs immediately upon placement of the chest tube. Autotransfusion in our experience appears to diminish the coagulopathy and inflammatory response to injury in these patients.

For patients with hemopneumothoraces, admission to a monitored setting and observation are appropriate for patients who remain hemodynamically stable, have little or no further hemorrhage from the chest tube, demonstrate evacuation of the pleural space on CXR, and have no other emergent operative indications. Rapid active bleeding or persistent brisk bleeding suggests a significant lung injury. The need for emergent thoracotomy is strongly suggested when more than a liter of blood is immediately evacuated on placement of a chest tube. In patients in whom a lower initial volume is drained, continued chest tube output of 200 ml/hr for 4 hours is an indication for thoracotomy. Observation of patients in this latter group should include a repeat CXR to ensure that the slowing of chest tube output is not resulting from a clotted hemothorax.

Tube Thoracostomy: Technique and Management

Once the decision is made to place a chest tube, the patient should be positioned to allow easy access to the midaxillary line in the fifth or sixth intercostal space. This location is preferred because (1) it is usually safely above the diaphragm and (2) the chest wall musculature is thinnest in this area, thus facilitating the procedure. The chest should be cleansed with an antiseptic solution and anesthetized with 10 ml of 1% lidocaine in all layers of the chest wall down to the pleura. There should be no fear of entering the pleural space when inserting a tube thoracostomy! To provide longer analgesia and increase patient comfort following insertion we suggest mixing the lidocaine with an equal volume of 0.25% bupivacaine. Conscious sedation may be administered if the patient's hemodynamic and respiratory status permits. A 2-cm skin incision is made over the rib immediately below the interspace selected for tube insertion. Sharp dissection proceeds

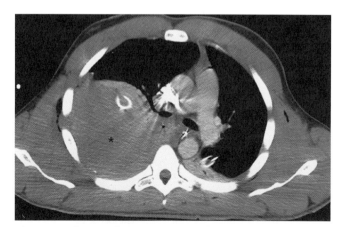

Figure 6 Computed tomography scan of patient in Figure 2. The large right retained hemothorax (*) is easily seen and can be easily differentiated from the lung parenchyma. The clotted hemothorax was successfully evacuated by video-assisted thoracoscopic surgery.

directly to the rib, and the pleural space is entered at its superior margin, care being taken to avoid the intercostal neurovascular bundle at the inferior border of the adjacent superior rib. While a clamp is commonly used to "pop" through the pleural space, we advocate continuing with the scalpel as it is both easier and less painful to the patient. Once the pleural space is entered, digital exploration will confirm entry into the thorax rather than the lung or abdominal cavity. The presence or absence of adhesions should be noted as well. Digital exploration is particularly important in the patient who may have a diaphragmatic rupture or who has a history of thoracic surgery or pulmonary infection. If no adhesions, diaphragmatic injury, or pulmonary pathology is encountered, the chest tube can be safely placed. The blind placement of chest tubes with trocars is ill-advised.

Chest tubes, like most medical devices, have markings to aid in placement. Unfortunately, in our experience these are too often ignored by residents placing the tube in the heat of battle, which results in tubes that may be poorly positioned. One of the most common mistakes is to insert the tube too far in to ensure that it will not "fall out." The tube will often bend at the last hole, which will prevent adequate drainage (see Figure 2). To prevent this type of malposition, the mark at the skin should be evaluated. If the tube is place in the midaxillary line at the fifth interspace, the mark at the skin level in most patients should be between 10 and 12. A tube placed deeper is likely to be kinked. In addition, once the tube is positioned it should be rotated 360 degrees before securing it in place. A tube that cannot be rotated freely is presumably kinked or otherwise malpositioned.

Once inserted, the chest tube is connected to suction with an underwater seal at a negative pressure of 20 cm of water. A chest radiograph should be obtained after tube placement to confirm placement, evacuation of air or fluid, and proper re-expansion of the lung. If intrapleural air or fluid remains, a second chest tube should be placed. Complete evacuation of the pleural space with full pulmonary re-expansion will help to decrease bleeding and air leaks, as well as the risk of a post-traumatic empyema. Early surgical intervention is indicated for retained blood in the pleural space.

Chest radiographs should be obtained daily to confirm resolution of the hemopneumothorax. It is not our practice to use prophylactic antibiotics with tube thoracostomies, although opinion in the literature is divided on this issue.[32,33] The chest tube can subsequently be removed when there is no air leak and when there is less than 100–150 ml of drainage over 24 hours. A prospective study has shown that a 6–8 hour trial of water seal decreases the incidence of recurrent pneumothorax when compared to chest tube removal with no water seal.[34]

Should a new air leak be discovered or the lung fails to re-expand, several potential causes should be investigated. The connections between chest tube, canisters, and wall suction should be inspected for leaks. The chest tube must be checked to ensure that the last hole has not migrated out of the chest wall. If the chest tube is noted to be "out" immediately after placement, it can be re-prepped and advanced a small distance; if detection is delayed, however, the chest tube should be removed and replaced at a different site. Placement of the tube into the major fissure may result in inadequate re-expansion, and parenchymal tube placement will result in continuing air leaks. These will also require removal and replacement. It is not uncommon for pleural space to become loculated or the chest tube occluded some time following injury and a tension pneumothorax is always a possibility in a patient on mechanical ventilation even in the presence of a chest tube.

Sternal Fractures

Sternal fractures are relatively uncommon and occur most often following blunt trauma. The usual mechanism of injury involves an unrestrained driver who strikes the sternum against the steering column of an automobile in a deceleration crash. A fall or other direct impact to the chest may also cause a sternal fracture. Most sternal fractures occur in the upper or mid-portion of the bone.[35] As with scapular fractures, the presence of a sternal fracture should be regarded as a marker of potential severe multiple trauma, including rib fractures (40%), long-bone fractures (25%), and head injuries (18%).

The fracture itself often needs no treatment acutely, and more than 95% of patients are treated nonoperatively. While a baseline EKG should be obtained, particularly in patients over 40 years of age, the need for continuous cardiac monitoring is determined by the associated injuries and the patient's cardiac status rather than by the presence of the sternal fracture itself. Most patients will be found to have a transient right ventricular dysfunction. The patient with an isolated sternal fracture and otherwise normal ED evaluation may be discharged.[36–38] Similar to rib fractures, the management of sternal fractures is symptomatic and consists of analgesic administration and the avoidance of motion. Occasionally, patients who have grossly displaced fractures or who have persistent pain due to nonunion may require operative reduction and internal fixation (ORIF). Sternal repair can be accomplished though various techniques utilizing wires or small plates.

Scapular Fractures

Fractures of the scapula are uncommon, occurring with an incidence of 1%–3% in blunt trauma.[39] Because of its location and structure, the scapula requires considerable direct force to fracture. As a result, associated injuries are common (80%–98%), and a patient with a scapular fracture should be considered to have sustained a severe chest trauma. Careful examination for thoracic, neurologic, vascular, and abdominal injuries, as well as other orthopedic injuries, should be undertaken. Findings on physical examination include local pain or tenderness, swelling, and crepitus. Although most scapular fractures will be seen on initial CXR, they may be obscured or overlooked. Many scapular fractures may have hitherto gone undetected, with increasing detection of nondisplaced fractures with the increasing use of modern CT technology[40] (see Figure 5). CT of the shoulder may be necessary to evaluate the fracture and to look for extension into the shoulder joint.

Management of scapular fractures in the vast majority of cases consists of analgesic administration and immobilization initially, followed by progressive physical therapy. Surgical intervention is rarely required and is undertaken primarily for those fractures that will likely cause significant disability. Minimally displaced fractures of the scapular body, neck, coracoid, acromion, and scapular spine are treated nonoperatively and typically result in healing with normal or near-normal function. Glenoid fracture-dislocations, unstable fractures of the neck, and significantly displaced fractures of the coracoid, acromion, and scapular spine, on the other hand, will require operative fixation for restoration of function. Other indications for operative treatment of scapular fractures include intra-articular fractures with step-off of greater than 5 mm or with instability, angulation of greater than 40 degrees of the glenoid neck, displacement of greater than 1–2 cm, or disruption of the superior suspensory complex of the shoulder.

Scapulothoracic Dissociation

Scapulothoracic dissociation results from severe blunt trauma with traction to the shoulder girdle causing the scapula, humerus, musculature of the shoulder, and neurovascular structures to be pulled away from the body. While this injury is relatively rare, it can be dramatic, involving not only the structures of the shoulder girdle, but also thoracic, craniocerebral, and spinal injuries. Damschen et al.,[41] in a review of 58 cases, reported complete brachial plexus injury in 81% of patients and partial injury in 13%; subclavian or axillary artery disruption was found in 88%. Because these patients almost universally have severe neurologic deficits in the affected limb, the likelihood of a good functional outcome is low. This should be borne in mind before extensive reconstruction to salvage an essentially de-functionalized limb is undertaken.

Clavicular Fractures

Clavicular fractures, unlike scapular or sternal fractures, often occur in isolation. They also occur in association with thoracic and extra-thoracic trauma. The clavicle is most commonly fractured in the middle third (80%) after a fall or lateral blow to the shoulder. Clinical findings include local tenderness, crepitus, and deformity. If the fracture is displaced, the shoulder may be found to be positioned inferiorly and medially. Most of these fractures are readily appreciated on AP CXR. The majority (85%) of mid-shaft clavicular fractures will heal without intervention, and initial management consists of immobilization with a figure-of-eight dressing or shoulder immobilizer.

Operative reduction and fixation of the clavicle is indicated in open fractures, displaced fractures with tenting of the overlying skin, and those associated with neurologic or vascular injury. Fractures with greater than 2 cm of shortening, widely displaced fragments with associated chest injuries, a floating shoulder (combined clavicular and scapular fractures), and nonunion are relative indications for operative intervention. Operative treatment consists of either intramedullary fixation or placement of fixation plates.

COMPLICATIONS OF HEMOPNEUMOTHORAX

Empyema

Empyema has been reported to have an incidence of 0%–18%.[33,42–44] At least some of the culture-negative "empyemas" in blunt trauma patients are probably sterile pleural collections that, being rich in inflammatory mediators, produce systemic effects clinically indistinguishable from true empyema collections.[45,46] The true empyema rate in major trauma patients is probably closer to 5%, although, with the increasing survival of severely injured patients, the incidence of this complication may be increasing. Risk factors for the development of empyema include an inadequately drained pleural collection, mechanism of injury, location and number of chest tubes, presence of pulmonary contusion, and pneumonia.

The clinical presentation of empyema includes unexplained fever, elevated white count, and respiratory failure. Most patients in whom an empyema is suspected are critically ill. AP CXR in this group may be of little or no help, and liberal use of CT scanning can more easily identify pathology that is not evident on plain films (Figure 7). Early use of CT can prevent the diagnostic delay that may result in the need for more extensive surgical procedures.

Treatment includes (1) drainage via chest tube or CT-guided catheter, (2) chest tube drainage with intrapleural fibrinolytic therapy, (3) VATS, or (4) thoracotomy and decortication. As the empyema progresses from an exudative effusion to a loculated effusion and then to an organized empyema, the pleural fluid becomes increasingly more viscous, and the intervention required becomes more invasive. Early diagnosis and treatment is thus important.

In those patients undergoing decortication, the initial postoperative CXR may look worse rather than better initially. The patient, however, will begin to improve even though the CXR does not. Vigorous pulmonary toilet, suctioning, and culture-specific antibiotics should be administered to all patients.

Pneumatocele

A post-traumatic cyst or pneumatocele can occur after chest trauma. This is usually an air collection within the lung that arises after airway disruption without connection to the pleural space. Most such lesions require no specific treatment and resolve after weaning from the ventilator. If the lesion is large, continues to enlarge, or becomes infected, CT-guided percutaneous drainage is an effective treatment.

Persistent Air Leaks and Bronchopleural Fistula

Air leaks are not uncommon after chest trauma, and typically resolve with tube thoracostomy. A large air leak, however, requires workup for a tracheobronchial injury. If such injury is excluded, then complete lung expansion is the cornerstone of therapy. Air leaks may persist for days or even weeks in patients requiring mechanical ventilation with high positive end-expiratory pressure (PEEP); only with weaning from the ventilator will air leaks begin to seal. Tracheostomy can, by decreasing the anatomic dead space, help

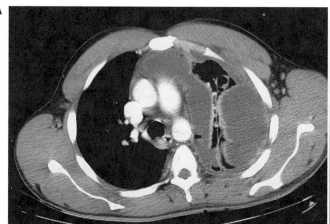
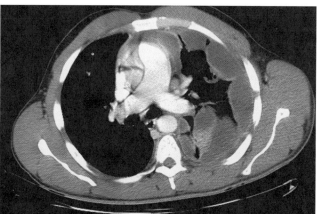

Figure 7 **(A, B)** Computed tomography scans of a loculated empyema of the chest in a patient 2 weeks following a gunshot wound to the chest and evacuation of a hemothorax. Note the enhancement around the collections. Patient was successfully treated with a thoracotomy and decortication.

to lower the peak airway pressures and thus at least slow the air leak. VATS can also help in those hemodynamically stable patients with prolonged air leaks.

Complications of Bony Injuries

Complications of bony injuries to the chest are most commonly related to pain. Sternal fractures in isolation or with only mild associated injury appear to have a relatively low incidence of post-injury sequelae; in one study, only 3% of patients at a 6-week follow-up had complaints requiring further intervention, including surgical intervention for a displaced fracture.[48] Twenty-one percent of patients in that same study reported pain at 6 weeks but required no further intervention.

Scapular fractures are rarely associated with nonunion, but can cause chronic pain. Pain and disability are particularly associated with the degree of glenoid angulation and displacement if the fracture is treated nonoperatively.[49]

Clavicular fractures, by contrast, do carry an incidence of nonunion, though that number is somewhat in dispute. Early studies of nonoperative treatment of clavicle fractures revealed a nonunion rate as low as 0.1%.[50] The nonunion rate has in more recent studies been reported to be much higher, with a rate of 15% for conservative treatment of displaced middle-third fractures.[51] Even with operative fixation, some nonunion occurs. An analysis of 8 studies and 14 case series of midshaft clavicle fractures revealed an overall nonunion rate of 4.2%. Nonoperative treatment resulted in a nonunion rate of 5.9%. When results for displaced fractures were identified, a nonunion rate of 4.8% was noted with IM fixation, while displaced fractures treated nonoperatively had a nonunion rate of 15.1%.[52]

Other long-term sequelae of clavicular fractures include pain, cosmetic deformity, or thoracic outlet compression. For these patients, ORIF can successfully manage severe symptoms.

Scapulothoracic dissociation, as would be expected, has significant long-term sequelae. A retrospective cohort study with a mean follow-up over 12 years revealed that patients with a complete brachial plexus avulsion had significant physical and mental impairments as measured by the standard SF-36 questionnaire.[53] Primary amputation of the affected limb, though a difficult decision, should be considered to avoid a defunctionalized limb where complete brachial avulsion has occurred.

CONCLUSIONS

Chest wall injuries and concomitant hemopneumothoraces are frequent following blunt and penetrating trauma and are significant cause of trauma mortality and morbidity. As the spectrum of thoracic injury is great and occurs in isolation as well as in part of multisystem trauma providers need to understand the pathophysiology and impact of these injuries on overall patient care. While most thoracic injuries may be managed nonoperatively, vigilance is required to detect those injuries that are potentially life threatening and require urgent intervention. More importantly, these injuries often drive ventilator usage and ICU length of stay and thus have a tremendous impact on overall trauma outcome.

REFERENCES

1. Breasted J: *The Edwin Smith Surgical Papyrus*. Chicago, University of Chicago Press, 1980.
2. Ziegler DW, Agarwal NN: The morbidity and mortality of rib fractures. *J Trauma* 37:975, 1994.
3. Di Bartolomeo S, Sanson G, Nardi G, et al: A population-based study on pneumothorax in severely traumatized patients. *J Trauma* 51:677, 2001.
4. Lee RB, Bass SM, Morris JA Jr, et al: Three or more rib fractures as an indicator for transfer to a Level I trauma center: a population-based study. *J Trauma* 30:689, 1990.
5. Livingston D, Lavery R, Passannante M, et al: Admission or observation is not necessary after a negative abdominal computed tomographic scan in patients with suspected blunt abdominal trauma: results of a prospective, multi-institutional trial. *J Trauma* 44:273, 1998.
6. Garcia VF, Gotschall CS, Eichelberger MR, et al: Rib fractures in children: a marker of severe trauma. *J Trauma* 30:695, 1990.
7. Bulloch B, Schubert CJ, Brophy PD, et al: Cause and clinical characteristics of rib fractures in infants. *Pediatrics* 105:E48, 2000.
8. Cadzow SP, Armstrong KL: Rib fractures in infants: red alert! The clinical features, investigations and child protection outcomes. *J Paediatr Child Health* 36:322, 2000.
9. Cameron P, Dziukas L, Hadj A, et al: Rib fractures in major trauma. *Aust N Z J Surg* 66:530, 1996.
10. Neff M, Monk JJ, Peters K, et al: Detection of occult pneumothoraces on abdominal computed tomographic scans in trauma patients. *J Trauma* 49:281, 2000.
11. Rhea J, Novelline R, Lawrason J, et al: The frequency and significance of thoracic injuries detected on abdominal CT scans of multiple trauma patients. *J Trauma* 29:502, 1989.
12. Gray L, Vandemark R, Hays M: Thoracic and lumbar spine trauma. *Neuroimaging Clin North Am* 11:421, 2001.
13. Guerrero-Lopez F, Vazquez-Mata G, Alcazar-Romero PP, et al: Evaluation of the utility of computed tomography in the initial assessment of the critical care patient with chest trauma. *Crit Care Med* 28:1370, 2000.
14. Grieser T, Buhne KH, Hauser H, et al: Significance of findings of chest x-rays and thoracic CT routinely performed at the emergency unit: 102 patients with multiple trauma. A prospective study. *Rofo Fortschr Geb Rontgenstr Neuen Bildgeb Verfahr* 173:44, 2001.
15. Jelly LM, Evans DR, Easty MJ, et al: Radiography versus spiral CT in the evaluation of cervicothoracic junction injuries in polytrauma patients who have undergone intubation. *Radiographics* 20:S251, 2000.
16. Parker MS, Matheson TL, Rao AV, et al: Making the transition: the role of helical CT in the evaluation of potentially acute thoracic aortic injuries. *Am J Roentgenol* 176:1267, 2001.
17. Downing SW, Sperling JS, Mirvis SE, et al: Experience with spiral computed tomography as the sole diagnostic method for traumatic aortic rupture. *Ann Thorac Surg* 72:495, 2001.
18. Pate JW, Gavant ML, Weiman DS, et al: Traumatic rupture of the aortic isthmus: program of selective management. *World J Surg* 23:59, 1999.
19. Dulchavsky SA, Schwarz KL, Kirkpatrick AW, et al: Prospective evaluation of thoracic ultrasound in the detection of pneumothorax. *J Trauma* 50:201, 2001.
20. Rozycki GS, Feliciano DV, Davis TP: Ultrasound as used in thoracoabdominal trauma. *Surg Clin North Am* 78:295, 1998.
21. Rozycki GS, Ballard RB, Feliciano DV, et al: Surgeon-performed ultrasound for the assessment of truncal injuries: lessons learned from 1540 patients. *Ann Surg* 228:557, 1998.
22. Lichtenstein D, Meziere G, Biderman P, et al: The "lung point": an ultrasound sign specific to pneumothorax. *Intensive Care Med* 26(10):1434–1440, 2000.
23. Moore EE, Cogbill TH, Malangoni MA, et al: Organ injury scaling. *Surg Clin North Am* 75(2):293–303, 1995.
24. Desai P: Pain management and pulmonary dysfunction. *Crit Care Clin* 15:151, 1999.
25. Yokoyama M, Itano Y, Mizobuchi S, et al: The effects of epidural block on the distribution of lymphocyte subsets and natural-killer cell activity in patients with and without pain. *Anesth Analg* 92:463, 2001.
26. Clark RF, Wei EM, Anderson PO: Meperidine: therapeutic use and toxicity. *J Emerg Med* 13:797, 1995.
27. Gallagher EJ, Liebman M, Bijur PE: Prospective validation of clinically important changes in pain severity measured on a visual analog scale. *Ann Emerg Med* 38:633, 2001.
28. Shanti CM, Carlin AM, Tyburski JG: Incidence of pneumothorax from intercostal nerve block for analgesia in rib fractures. *J Trauma* 51:536, 2001.
29. Mackersie RC, Karagianes TG, Hoyt DB, et al: Prospective evaluation of epidural and intravenous administration of fentanyl for pain control and restoration of ventilatory function following multiple rib fractures. *J Trauma* 31:443, 1991.
30. Mackersie RC, Shackford SR, Hoyt DB, et al: Continuous epidural fentanyl analgesia: ventilatory function improvement with routine use in treatment of blunt chest injury. *J Trauma* 27:1207, 1987.
31. Bulger EM, Edwards T, Klotz P, Jurkovich GJ: Epidural analgesia improves outcome after multiple rib fractures. *Surgery* 136:426, 2004.

32. Wilson R, Nichols R: The EAST Practice Management Guidelines for Prophylactic Antibiotic Use in Tube Thoracostomy for Traumatic Hemopneumothorax: a commentary. *J Trauma* 48:758, 2000.

33. Luchette F, Barrie P, Oswanski M, et al: Practice Management Guidelines for Prophylactic Antibiotic Use in Tube Thoracostomy for Traumatic Hemopneumothorax: the EAST Practice Management Guidelines Work Group. Eastern Association for Trauma. *J Trauma* 48: 753, 2000.

34. Martino K, Merrit S, Boyakye K, et al: Prospective randomized trial of thoracostomy removal algorithms. *J Trauma* 46:369, 1999.

35. Buckman R, Trooskin S, Flancbaum L, et al: The significance of stable patients with sternal fractures. *Surg Gynecol Obstet* 164:261, 1987.

36. Hills M, Delprado A, Deane S: Sternal fractures: associated injuries and management. *J Trauma* 35:55, 1993.

37. Jackson M, Walker W: Isolated sternal fracture: a benign injury? *Injury* 23:535, 1992.

38. Chiu W, D'Amelio L, Hammond J: Sternal fractures in blunt chest trauma: a practical algorithm for management. *Am J Emerg Med* 15: 252, 1997.

39. Thompson D, Flynn T, Miller P, et al: The significance of scapular fractures. *J Trauma* 25:974, 1985.

40. Haapamaki VV, Kiuru MJ, Koskinen SK: Multidetector CT in shoulder fractures. *Emerg Radiol* 11(2):89–94, 2004.

41. Damschen D, Cogbill T, Siegel M: Scapulothoracic dissociation caused by blunt trauma. *J Trauma* 42:537, 1997.

42. Aguilar M, Battistella F, Owings J, et al: Posttraumatic empyema. Risk factor analysis. *Arch Surg* 132:647, 1997.

43. Eddy AC, Luna GK, Copass M: Empyema thoracis in patients undergoing emergent closed tube thoracostomy for thoracic trauma. *Am J Surg* 157: 494, 1989.

44. Mandal A, Thadepalli H, Mandal A, et al: Posttraumatic empyema thoracis: a 24-year experience at a major trauma center. *J Trauma* 44:764, 1997.

45. Watkins J, Spain D, Richardson J, et al: Empyema and restrictive pleural processes after blunt trauma: an under-recognized cause of respiratory failure. *Am Surg* 66:210, 2000.

46. Adams JM, Hauser CJ, Livingston DH, et al: The immunomodulatory effects of damage control abdominal packing on local and systemic neutrophil activity. *J Trauma* 50:792, 2001.

47. Carrillo E, Schmacht D, Gable D, et al: Thoracoscopy in the management of posttraumatic persistent pneumothorax. *J Am Coll Surg* 186:636, 1998.

48. Velissaris T, Tang ATM, Patel A, et al: Traumatic sternal fracture: outcome following admission to a thoracic surgical unit. *Injury* 34:924–927, 2003.

49. Romero J, Schai P, Imhoff AB: Scapular neck fracture—the influence of permanent malalignment of the glenoid neck on clinical outcome. *Arch Orthop Trauma Surg* 121(6):313–316, 2001.

50. Neer CS: Nonunion of the clavicle. *JAMA* 172:1006–1011, 1960.

51. Hill JM, McGuire MH, Crosby LA: Closed treatment of displaced middle-third clavicular fractures of the clavicle gives poor results. *J Bone Joint Surg Br* 79-B(4):537–539, 1997.

52. Zlowodski M, Zelle BA, Cole PA, et al: Treatment of acute midshaft clavicle fractures: systematic review of 2144 fractures. *J Orthop Trauma* 19:504–507, 2005.

53. Zelle BA, Pape H-C, Gerich TG, et al: Functional outcome following scapulothoracic dissociation. *J Bone Joint Surg Am* 86:2–8, 2004.

DIAGNOSTIC AND THERAPEUTIC ROLES OF BRONCHOSCOPY AND VIDEO-ASSISTED THORACOSCOPY IN THE MANAGEMENT OF THORACIC TRAUMA

Ajai K. Malhotra, Michel B. Aboutanos, Rao Ivatury, and Therese M. Duane

Direct injury to the chest and pulmonary complications after any major trauma account for a significant proportion of trauma-related morbidity and mortality. In the past the role of thoracic endoscopy was limited to bronchoscopic diagnosis of major airway injury and assistance with pulmonary toilet. Major injuries to the tracheobronchial tree, significant hemorrhage within the chest, failure of nonoperative management of chest injuries, and major pulmonary complications invariably required thoracotomy with its high morbidity and mortality. Technical advances in fiber optics and videoscopic imaging have led to rapid advances in the field of minimally invasive surgery. In the thoracic region, this has led to the advent of video-assisted thoracoscopic surgery (VATS) and the broadening of the role of bronchoscopy, both in terms of diagnosis and therapy. These minimally invasive endoscopic techniques have significantly lower morbidity and mortality. The current chapter focuses on the evolving role of thoracic endoscopy (thoracoscopy and bronchoscopy) following chest trauma and major pulmonary complications after any trauma.

INCIDENCE

Thoracic trauma accounts for a significant burden of disease in terms of morbidity and mortality. Twenty percent of trauma-associated deaths involve chest injury, and chest trauma is second only to head and spinal cord injuries as a cause of death following trauma.[1] Death as a result of chest trauma in the acute setting is related to either airway injury, direct trauma to the heart, or massive bleeding in the chest cavity. In addition to the acute deaths that are a direct result of chest trauma, pulmonary complications following chest trauma or any trauma add to the mortality and morbidity attributable to the chest.[2]

Most chest trauma comprises of abrasions, rib fractures, and simple pneumothoraces that are easily diagnosed with chest x-rays and/or computed tomography (CT) and can be treated with simple measures—pulmonary toilet, pain management, and tube thoracostomy. The indications for open thoracotomy in the acute setting are principally major airway disruption and massive bleeding in the chest or airway. Approximately 1% of all trauma admissions require open thoracotomy in the acute setting.[3] Open thoracotomy in this setting is associated with a very high morbidity and mortality.[3] Bronchoscopic control of bleeding within the airway and stenting of major airway injury can offer a lower-risk alternative to open surgery in selected patients.[4,5] Similarly, VATS offers a lower-risk alternative for managing hemorrhage within the chest cavity.[6] In the nonacute setting, trauma patients with or without direct injury to the chest have a high incidence of pulmonary complications, including pneumonia, retained hemothorax, fibrothorax, empyema, and acute respiratory distress syndrome (ARDS), posing diagnostic and therapeutic challenges.[1,2] Thoracic endoscopy in this setting is playing an increasingly important role in early diagnosis and therapy for these complications, and possibly improving outcome.

DIAGNOSTIC AND THERAPEUTIC ROLES OF VATS IN CHEST TRAUMA

Indications and Patient Selection

The first diagnostic and therapeutic application of thoracoscopy for the management of thoracic pathologies such as pleural effusions, pleural adhesions, empyemas, and thoracic malignancy, was recorded by Jacobaeus at the University of Stockholm in 1922.[7] Thoracoscopy for the treatment of traumatic injuries was first described in 1946 by Branco for the management of hemothorax in penetrating chest injuries.[8] In the last decade, the advent of minimally invasive access to the thoracic cavity combined with video-assisted technology and selective lung ventilation has revolutionized the diagnosis and the treatment of thoracic injuries with improved use and outcomes.[9,10]

Patient selection is very important for the application of VATS in thoracoabdominal trauma. The current indications are both diagnostic and therapeutic and include mainly the evaluation of a structural injury (the diaphragm, the pericardium, lung parenchyma, the thoracic duct, etc.) or the drainage of a pleural collection and repair of any structural damage. Aside from the usual bleeding disorders, the main contraindications of VATS include an unstable patient, or a patient with underlying lung and cardiac pathologies that preclude the use of single lung ventilation. Table 1 lists the current indications and contraindications for the use of VATS.

Diaphragmatic Injuries

The incidence of blunt diaphragmatic injuries have been reported as low as 0.8% and as high as 7%.[11,12] Blunt trauma accounts for 10%–30% of traumatic diaphragmatic ruptures (TDR) in North American series from urban trauma centers.[13] The incidence of diaphragmatic injuries has been reported to be as high as 67% in penetrating thoracoabdominal trauma.[14]

Table 1: Indications and Contraindications of VATS in Trauma

Indications	Contraindications
Persistent pneumothorax	Hemodynamic instability

Retained collections
  Hemothorax
  Chylothorax
  Bilothorax
  Pleural effusion
	Poor lung and cardiac functions with inability to tolerate single lung ventilation (chronic obstructive pulmonary disease, heart failure)
	Contraindication to lateral decubitus position
	History of bleeding diatheses

Empyema	Massive hemothorax (>1.5 liters initially or 200 ml/hr over 3–4 hours)
Detection of intrathoracic organ injury (diaphragm, lung, thoracic duct, pericardium)	Obliterated pleural cavity (infection, pleuritis, previous surgery)
Intrathoracic foreign body	Suspected cardiac injury
Acute hemorrhage in stable patients	Indication for laparotomy

Diaphragmatic injuries are particularly difficult to diagnose with the use of radiographic imaging such as chest x-ray or CT and can be missed in up to 30% of patients.[14,15] Together with laparoscopy, thoracoscopy has become the diagnostic tool of choice for diaphragmatic injuries when compared with other nonoperative modalities.[16,17] Thoracoscopy is particularly useful when laparoscopy may not be optimal or feasible. It is useful for evaluation of right-sided diaphragmatic injuries and of posterior wounds from the posterior axillary line to the spine.[18] It is also useful for avoidance of abdominal procedures, particularly in patients with previous laparotomies and expected presence of extensive adhesions.

The therapeutic role of VATS in the treatment of diaphragmatic injuries is well documented.[14,19] In a report of 24 patients who underwent VATS for thoracic injuries, 9 of 10 patients were successfully diagnosed with diaphragmatic injuries. VATS was used for repair of the diaphragm in four patients.[19] Martinez et al.[14] evaluated 52 patients with penetrating thoracoabdominal trauma admitted to the General Hospital for Accidents in Guatemala City. VATS was used to diagnose 35 patients with diaphragmatic injuries. All 35 diaphragmatic injuries were successfully repaired thoracoscopically. Even though successful thoracoscopic repair of diaphragm injuries is reported as feasible, safe, and expeditious, currently no long-term outcome results are available.

In areas where other abdominal injuries are suspected, a laparoscopic or open surgical approach is preferable depending on the available surgical expertise. A combined thoracic and abdominal cavitary endoscopy can also be useful. Figure 1 shows the thoracoscopic evaluation of a right diaphragm injury from an impaled object in the chest of a patient evaluated in our trauma center. This was followed by the thoracoscopic repair of the diaphragm after the laparoscopic confirmation of a nonbleeding liver laceration, and no other associated abdominal injuries. In all cases where a diaphragm injury is found, an exploratory laparoscopy or laparotomy is mandatory to rule out associated intra-abdominal injuries.

Retained Thoracic Collection

The evacuation of a retained hemothorax is one of the main indications for VATS. Inadequate evacuation of blood from the pleural space and prolonged thoracostomy tube drainage put the patient at risk for developing empyema and fibrothorax with prolonged hospital stays and increasing costs.[9,20] The incidence of a retained hemothorax and empyema post–tube thoracostomy placement ranges from 4% to 20% and from 4% to 10%, respectively.[8,9,19,21–23] A prospective randomized study of 39 patients with thoracic trauma and retained hemothoraces from Parkland Memorial Hospital showed that early evacuation with VATS compared with conventional therapy of a secondary chest tube placement lead to a significantly shorter duration of tube drainage (2.5 days), shorter hospital stay (2.7 days), and reduced hospital costs ($6000).[9] These advantages of VATS were attributed to rapid and complete evacuation of the pleural space, optimal video-assisted positioning of the thoracostomy tubes, and identification and treatment of the sources of the bleeding and of other associated intrathoracic injuries.

It is important to note that these advantages rest on the early use (day 4–7 postinjury) of VATS for the evacuation of the hemothorax. In a study by Heniford et al.,[20] 19 of 25 patients (76%) with retained hemothorax were successfully treated with VATS. Failure of VATS correlated with time interval from injury to operation, and with the type of fluid collection (hemothorax vs. empyema). The mean time between admission and operation for the successful versus unsuccessful thoracoscopic drainage was 4.5 days and 14.5 days, respectively.[20]

The application of VATS for traumatic empyema is dependent on the phase of the empyema. For the acute/exudative empyema occurring between 1 and 5 days, VATS is uniformly effective. The success rate for the transitional/fibrinopurulent stage (day 6–14) is around 75%–85%, with a sharp drop to around 50% in the organized/chronic phase (>2 weeks).[24,25] The presence of a thick fibrin peel with

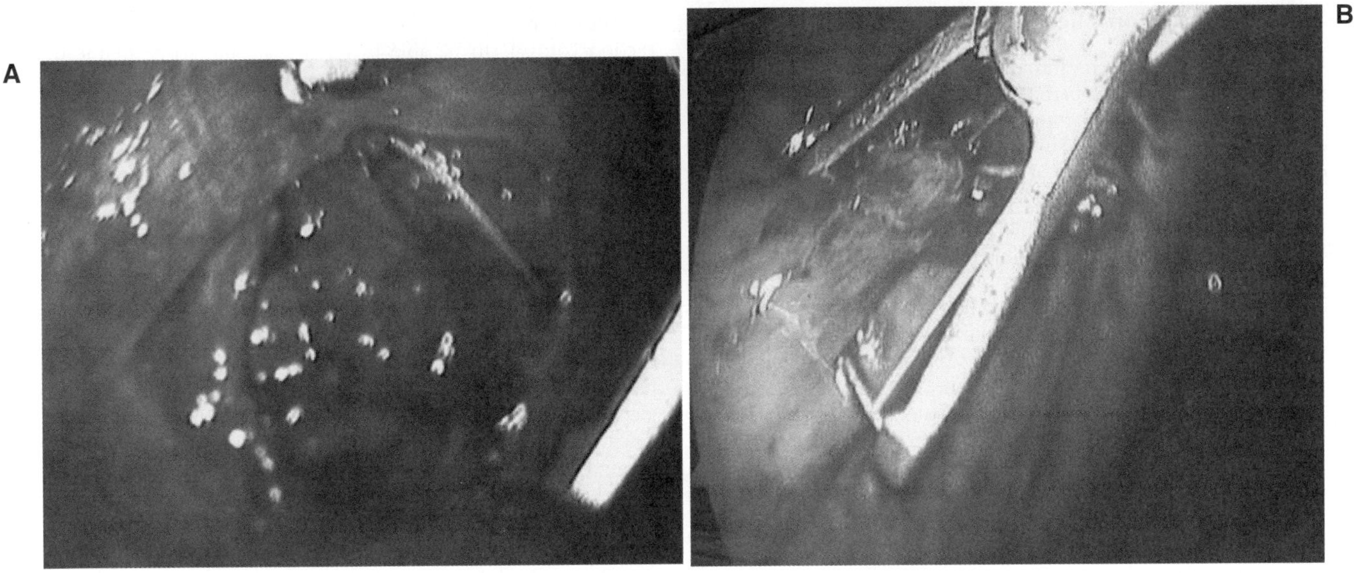

Figure 1 This 48-year-old construction worker was impaled with a 4×4 wooden object. **(A)** Large 5-cm, full-thickness diaphragm injury was noted with underlying liver laceration. **(B)** Diaphragm was repaired thoracoscopically.

entrapped lung requires mature surgical judgment for early conversion to open thoracotomy and avoidance of the risk of further pulmonary parenchymal injury or the creation of a bronchopleural fistula.

Persistent Hemorrhage

Video-assisted thoracoscopic surgery is also useful for patients with persistent but slow hemorrhage and no hemodynamic instability. Unstable patients with suspected thoracic bleed require open thoracotomy. Smith et al.[26] performed VATS on five hemodynamically stable patients for persistent hemorrhage from intercostal vessels. In three patients, the bleeding was successfully controlled with diathermy. Other techniques for hemorrhage control, including endoclips or argon beam coagulators, can be used.[15] Intracorporeal suture placement around the rib was used successfully in our center for control of a persistent intercostal bleed not amenable to endoclip placement. The success rate for the thoracoscopic control of a nonhemodynamically compromising hemorrhage is around 80% with a thoracotomy conversion rate of 15%–20%.[24,27]

Persistent Pneumothorax

The incidence of persistent air leak and lung re-expansion 72 hours post–thoracostomy tube placement ranges from 4% to 23%.[27,28] Conservative management with continuous pleural suction leads to prolonged chest tube drainage, prolonged hospital length of stay (LOS), and increased hospital costs.[28] VATS has been shown to be safe and effective in the treatment of persistent pneumothorax with decreased number of chest tube days, hospital LOS, and cost.[9,28,29] In our trauma center, endo-GIA staplers are routinely employed to staple off the affected lung parenchyma. Recently the use of a topical synthetic nonreactive surgical sealant (Coseal by Baxter, Freemont, CA) for the creation of an elastic watertight seal has also been reported.[17] Chemical pleurodesis or pleural scarification by electrocoagulation remains a viable option especially in recurrences post-VATS. Carillo et al.[28] reported the successful use of VATS in 10 of 11 patients with persistent pneumothorax post-traumatic injuries. The 11th patient was successfully treated with chemical pleurodesis. The inflammatory reaction that occurs with chemical pleurodesis, however, is often associated with increased pleural edema, drainage, and postoperative pain.[15] Prior to committing a patient to VATS, it is

important to aggressively evaluate the cause of the air leak and rule out a malfunctioning or a malpositioned chest tube, the presence of a foreign body, or a deeply penetrating rib fragment. The patient should be evaluated thoroughly with chest CT and bronchoscopy to evaluate the tracheobronchial tree, the distal parenchyma, and the pleural cavity.

Other Indications/Application

Other indications for use of VATS in chest trauma include diagnosis of bronchopleural fistulas, removal of retained foreign bodies, ligation of injured thoracic duct, drainage of chylothorax, and assessment of cardiac and mediastinal structure.[10,15] Although pericardioscopy for suspected penetrating cardiac injury has been reported as feasible and safe in the hemodynamically stable patient, it remains very controversial, with potential for iatrogenic life-threatening injuries.[30] In a stable patient, the gold standard approach for suspected cardiac injury remains the use of echocardiography or subxyphoid pericardial window followed by immediate sternotomy or left thoracotomy for evacuation of hemopericardium and repair of cardiac injury.

Surgical Approach

The operation is performed under general endotracheal intubation with a dual lumen endotracheal tube. The position of the tube is confirmed bronchoscopically. The patient is positioned in the lateral decubitus position and flexed at the hip to open the rib spaces. The initial port is 10 mm, placed at the site of the existing chest tube or in the midaxillary line in the fifth intercostal space. This port is used to introduce a camera with a 30- or 45-degree scope into the pleural cavity and to aid in the placement of additional 5-mm working ports. A maximum of two working ports are typically used, along with a 5-mm 30-degree scope to allow complete inspection of the lung and pleural spaces. Insufflation is not required, although it can be helpful when full lung collapse is not achieved. At the end of the procedure, chest tubes are placed under direct observation through existing port sites. The lung is then inflated under direct vision. Patient-controlled anesthesia along with local intercostal nerve block is used for optimal postoperative pain management.

Morbidity and Complication Management

The reported complication rates for thoracoscopy are less than 10% and the missed injury rates are less than 1%.[24,31] The perioperative complications include intrathoracic bleed (parietal, intercostal, or parenchymal), recurrent pneumothorax, and hemothorax. Other complications include intercostal neuritis and iatrogenic lung laceration. Conversion to open thoracotomy is reported to be less than 8% and usually results from pleural adhesions or uncontrollable bleed.[31] This underscores the importance of the timing of the procedures, within 5–7 days—early enough to avoid pleural adhesions and fibrosis, and late enough to ensure adequate hemostasis. Persistent air leak in the postoperative period is attributed to underlying lung pathology such as emphysema or apical bleb disease. Late complications are rare and include the development of pneumonia, pleural edema, and empyema.[9,31] Airway complications from malpositioned dual-lumen endotracheal tubes or the development of tension pneumothorax during one lung ventilation have also been reported.[32]

DIAGNOSTIC AND THERAPEUTIC ROLE OF BRONCHOSCOPY

Attempts to directly visualize the interior of the airway date as far back as the time of Hippocrates. However, the first recorded bronchoscopy was performed by Gustav Killian of Frieburg, Germany in 1887. The only available instrument at that time was a rigid bronchoscope and the principal indications were therapeutic, the commonest being removal of inhaled foreign objects. The field was advanced by Chevalier Jackson, the father of American bronchoesophagology, who designed modern rigid bronchoscopes. In 1963, Shigeto Ikeda introduced the flexible fibroptic bronchoscope, primarily as a diagnostic instrument.[33] Flexible bronchoscopes were much easier to use, and flexible bronchoscopy became a diagnostic tool with wide application. The only therapeutic indication that persisted was removal of foreign bodies from within the tracheobronchial tree. Recent technical advances in the instrument itself and in the availability of other therapeutic tools such as stents, electrocautery, lasers, and so on, are allowing bronchoscopy to regain a role in therapy and also broadening its well established diagnostic role. While in some very limited situations rigid bronchoscopy may offer some advantages, the ease of use and greater experience in the use of flexible bronchoscopes have made rigid bronchoscopy rare in trauma settings.

Basic Technique of Flexible Fibroptic Bronchoscopy

Almost all bronchoscopies for trauma patients, whether performed in the acute setting soon after trauma or later on for pulmonary complications, are performed on patients that have endotracheal tubes in place and are mechanically ventilated.

Preparation

The patient should be placed on 100% oxygen, and the ventilator rate set at 10–12 breaths per minute. Adequate sedation is essential to avoid inducing stress. This is especially important in head injured patients as an acute rise in intracranial pressure (ICP) is well documented during bronchoscopy.[34] We use a benzodiazepine (Ativan or Versed 2–4 mg intravenously) and a narcotic analgesic (morphine 4–8 mg intravenously). While bronchoscopy can be performed without paralysis, we have found that, to be able to perform it comfortably, temporary paralysis using vecuronium (10 mg intravenously) is very helpful. Adequate time should be given to allow the patient to get preoxygenated and the medications to take effect before starting the procedure. Recently, bispectral EEG monitoring (BIS) is being used to determine optimal sedation. Extra medications should be available to be given whenever needed to avoid stress to the body.

The commonly used flexible bronchoscopes have a uniplanar direction control. To be able to manipulate the scope in the other planes, the whole scope needs to be rotated along its longitudinal axis. To achieve this, the outside end of the scope is rotated. The rotational movements will not be transmitted to the tip unless the scope is straight, and hence the height of the bed should be adjusted to keep the scope as straight as possible.

Technique

The basic technique of bronchoscopy is the same irrespective of indication. However, there are minor variations and adjunctive procedures used for various indications. After the height of the bed has been adjusted, the patient preoxygenated, and adequate sedation and paralysis achieved, a lubricated scope is inserted thought a right angled adaptor that allows some ventilation to continue while the scope is within the endotracheal tube. Once the tip of the scope is beyond the end of the tube, and the carina is visualized, the two main stem bronchi can be identified by (1) position of the tracheal rings—deficient posteriorly, (2) length of the bronchus—left being longer, and (3) angle of take-off—right being straighter. A basic knowledge of the lobar anatomy on the two sides and the bronchopleural segments in each of the lobes is essential for successful scopy. Depending on the patient body habitus, the scope can be inserted into III/IV order bronchioles. It is important to understand that while suctioning and clearing the airway of secretions is an important part of bronchoscopy, it does lead to derecruitment by collapsing alveoli; hence, like any other medical procedure, the risks and benefits should be carefully weighed before embarking on a bronchoscopy and also in deciding how much should be done at a given time.

Monitoring

The patient undergoing bronchoscopy under sedation and paralysis needs to be carefully monitored for adequate sedation, and also for any cardiorespiratory compromise that may occur during the procedure. The monitoring is best left to another person who should record vital signs continuously. The most important signs to be monitored are (1) heart rate, (2) blood pressure, (3) arterial oxygen saturation by pulse oximetry, and (4) ICP, if the patient has a monitor in place. If the patient is experiencing stress, the heart rate and blood pressure will increase. The procedure should be stopped and adequate sedation achieved before continuing. If the pulse oximeter shows a decline below 90%, the scope should be removed so that the patient can be adequately ventilated and oxygenated, except in very rare situations. Last, it is possible for the patient to maintain adequate oxygen saturation yet develop arrhythmia, usually bradyarrhythmia, and even cardiac arrest. This happens because even though oxygenation is maintained by high alveolar oxygen content achieved by preoxygenation, ventilation during the procedure is severely compromised, leading to an acute rise in $PaCO_2$ and severe respiratory acidosis. This becomes particularly important in patients with head injury as it can lead to an acute and severe rise in ICP with possible deleterious effects on the injured brain. If the patient develops any arrhythmia, the scope should immediately be removed, and adequate ventilation ensured. Resuscitative drugs should be immediately available to treat any arrhythmia that does not resolve spontaneously. A reevaluation of the risks and benefits of the scopy should occur before proceeding with the procedure.

Complications of Bronchoscopy

A large number of complications have been described after flexible fibroptic bronchoscopy (Table 2). The incidence of complications is higher the longer the procedure, the sicker the patient, and when the bronchoscopy is performed for therapeutic indications rather than diagnostic. However, in experienced hands and when the above precautions of technique and monitoring are observed, fibroptic flexible bronchoscopy is a fairly safe procedure.

Table 2: Complications of Bronchoscopy

Hypoxemia	Hypercapnia
Barotrauma	Hypotension
Hypertension	Hemorrhage
Aspiration	Intracranial hypertension
Infection	Laryngospasm
Damage to scope	Cardiac arrhythmias

Diagnostic Role of Flexible Fibroptic Bronchoscopy

Acute Trauma

Tracheobronchial injury

Tracheobronchial injury following trauma is very rare; however, the consequences of missed injuries can be significant. While some injuries can be managed nonoperatively and will heal, if an injury does require repair, delaying the repair significantly increases the chances of failure. Fibroptic bronchoscopy should be performed early in any patient who may potentially have a tracheobronchial injury.[35] In some instances, if the patient is not acutely hypoxic and tracheobronchial injury is suspected, in addition to its diagnostic role, bronchoscopy can be an invaluable aid to intubation and correct tube placement. In such situations, bronchoscopy should be performed by an experienced bronchoscopist with the endotracheal tube prepositioned over the scope.[36] There is a role for rigid bronchoscopy in patients with injury to the cervical trachea where the rigid scope can identify the distal ruptured end and align it with the proximal end allowing the patient to be intubated and the balloon of the tube passed beyond the site of injury. Once an injury has been diagnosed, the bronchoscopic findings are useful in planning appropriate therapy—nonoperative management, open surgery, or bronchoscopic placement of stent. In a report by Lin et al.,[37] bronchoscopy was useful in management decisions in one-third of the instances.

Acute or late onset bleeding in the tracheobronchial tree

Bleeding within the tracheobronchial tree following trauma is usually caused by pulmonary contusion and rarely by injury to the tree. In later stages, hemoptysis may be caused by pulmonary embolism, infections, tracheobronchial erosions, or tracheoinnominate fistula. Fibroptic bronchoscopy is useful for diagnosing the cause of the bleeding and to localize the site. It may help temporarily control the hemorrhage, isolate the site to avoid flooding the nonbleeding areas of the lung, and, in selected cases, provide definitive control of the bleeding[2] (see following section).

Inhalational injury

Fibroptic bronchoscopy plays an invaluable role in the diagnosis and management of patients suspected of inhalational injury. Any patient suspected of having suffered inhalational burns to the tracheobronchial tree should undergo early diagnostic evaluation. If signs of impeding loss of airway are present and the patient does not have an endotracheal tube, the bronchoscope may be used as a guide for safe intubation. The bronchoscopic signs of inhalational injury are observed within a few hours of the injury and may be classified as acute, subacute, and chronic.[38] In the acute stage, the most prominent finding is airway edema with soot deposition within the mucosa. As the injury progresses to the subacute phase, necrosis of the lining mucosa, and hemorrhagic tracheobronchitis are prominent. The subacute phase may last from several hours to days, and in this stage the patient may demonstrate massive bronchorrhea. Repeated broncho-

scopic toileting may be necessary to maintain airway patency. Finally, in the chronic phase formation of granulation tissue with stenosis, scarring, and obliterative bronchiolitis are observed. The initial bronchoscopic appearance is poorly correlated with the need and duration of mechanical ventilatory requirements and also the final outcome. Hence, repeated examinations may be required to accurately plan therapy.[39]

Ventilator-Associated Pneumonia

Ventilator-associated pneumonia (VAP) is one of the most common nosocomial infections in the modern intensive care unit (ICU). It is associated with high morbidity and mortality, and each incidence of VAP significantly increases the cost of care.[40] Early appropriate antimicrobial therapy has been shown to improve outcomes.[41] Despite its relative frequency, the diagnosis of VAP can be challenging, especially in the trauma patient. The reasons for this are primarily that the diagnostic criteria for pneumonia (fever with productive cough and leukocytosis, new or changing infiltrate on chest radiograph, and sputum culture demonstrating predominant growth of a single organism) are either nonspecific or falsely positive because of tracheobronchial colonization in the ICU. Quantitative examination of a lower respiratory specimen (lavage or brush) has been suggested as one method of accurately differentiating between nonpathogenic tracheobronchial colonization and VAP. Bronchoalveolar lavage (BAL) specimens from the lower respiratory tree can be easily obtained through the bronchoscope. This method has been proven to be safe and accurate in not only diagnosing VAP, but in also ruling it out so that patients are spared unnecessary antimicrobial therapy.[42] A simple scheme practiced at the authors' institution is outlined in Figure 2. Institution of this scheme, in which bronchoscopy plays a central role has significantly reduced the use of antimicrobials, and related to that, reduced microbial resistance within our ICU.

The technique of obtaining BAL specimen through a flexible bronchoscope is simple. The scope is passed into a tertiary level bronchiole and wedged in it. Suction is avoided during insertion to maintain sterility of the working channel of the scope. The site is selected by using one or more of the following criteria: (1) site of new infiltrate on chest radiograph, (2) site of maximum purulence as observed through the scope, and (3) most common site of VAP, the right lower lobe. Once the scope has been wedged in the selected bronchiole, five aliquots of 20-ml, sterile nonbacteriostatic saline are instilled through the working port and immediately aspirated. A good specimen is indicated by aspirating more than 50% of the instilled saline and observing floating froth (evidence of surfactant) in the aspirate. This specimen is then sent to the laboratory for quantitative culture and empiric antimicrobials are initiated based on the prevailing flora in the ICU. When the final quantitative culture results are available (usually in 48–72 hours), the antimicrobial therapy is tailored to the culture and sensitivity profile. In our ICU, a threshold of more than 10^5 colony-forming units per milliliter (CFU/ml) of bronchoalveolar lavage alteration (BAL) is used for the diagnosis of VAP. Other ICUs use a smaller number. An alternative to lavage is the protected specimen brush where a special brush-tipped catheter is passed through the scope and used to scrape the lining of the bronchiole. A diagnostic threshold of 10^3 CFU/ml is often adopted when the brush is used. Although nonbronchoscopic methods of obtaining the lower respiratory specimen are available, no comparative trials have been performed to compare the bronchoscopic and nonbronchoscopic methods.[40]

Stricture

Most causes of stricture within the tracheobronchial tree are related to neoplasia. In the trauma setting, strictures may be caused by prolonged intubation, scarring at the site of previous injury, or following inhalational injury. Bronchoscopy has both a diagnostic and therapeutic role in the management of strictures. Initially, bronchoscopy can confirm the presence of the stricture and localize its site. In

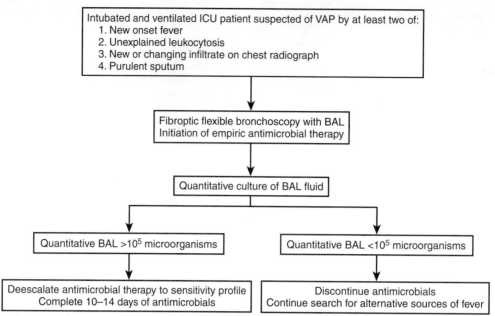

Figure 2   Simplified algorithm for evaluating a patient with new onset fever suspected of being caused by ventilator-associated pneumonia. *ICU,* Intensive care unit; *BAL,* bronchoalveolar lavage.

addition, the bronchoscopic features in terms of site, length, and character of the tissue can help with the planning of appropriate treatment. Also bronchoscopy can help with management of the atelectasis of the pulmonary segments beyond the stricture and to treat the infections in these atelectic segments.

Therapeutic Role of Flexible Fibroptic Bronchoscopy

Control of Acute or Late Onset Hemoptysis

Massive hemoptysis is defined as when the volume of blood in the tracheobronchial tree leads to a life-threatening situation by causing airway obstruction. Bronchoscopy has been used to not only diagnose the source of hemorrhage, but also to remove the blood, thereby overcoming the airway obstruction. In addition, in some selected cases, bronchoscopic techniques can provide either temporary control of hemorrhage until preparations for definitive control, by surgery or bronchial artery embolization, are made. In selected patients, bronchoscopic techniques can even provide definitive therapy. The therapeutic tools to control hemorrhage include ice-cold saline lavage, injection of 1:20,000 epinephrine, instillation of fibrin glue or other topical hemostatics, balloon tamponade, electrocautery, and laser coagulation. While most reports about the use of such techniques are from the medical literature, the same techniques are being used for acute hemorrhage following trauma or late onset hemoptysis in the surgical ICU patient.[4]

Stent Repair of Acute Airway Trauma

Major disruptions of tracheobronchial tree are rare, but life threatening. In the past the only available treatment was major surgery. Recently, covered expandable metallic stents have been developed that can be deployed under bronchoscopic control. This offers a low risk alternative of repairing these potentially devastating injuries. When injury to the tracheobronchial tree is suspected early evaluation by bronchoscopy is very helpful in diagnosing or ruling out the injury and then planning therapy. Bronchoscopy can define the site of injury, and help with safe placement of the endotracheal tube. Once the patient's airway is secured, a careful assessment should be made of

the characteristics of the injury especially the site in relation to branches, and the size of the injury. While open repair has been the traditional method of therapy, consideration should be given for stent repair if the injury is so amenable and especially if the patient's other injuries make him/her a poor surgical candidate. If none of the shelf stent is available, customized stents can be ordered to suit the anatomy of the specific injury. A recent case at the authors' institution exemplified this point. An 18-year-old man presented after a high speed motor vehicle collision with the chest CT demonstrating aortic transection. In addition, because of his massive pneumothorax and persistent high volume air leak through the chest tube, airway injury was suspected and confirmed at the distal trachea by bronchoscopy. A custom-made stent was placed via the bronchoscope, and the air leak stopped. A few days later the patient underwent successful repair of his aortic injury via a thoracotomy. Subsequent bronchoscopies revealed that the tracheal injury had healed with formation of granulation tissue around the stent. The stent was removed intact after 8 weeks, and 2 weeks following that mucosa was found to be covering the injury site.[43]

Removal of Foreign Body

Before the availability of bronchoscopy, foreign body removal from the tracheobronchial tree carried high morbidity and mortality. Availability of bronchoscopy revolutionized the care of such patients as it offered a very low-risk alternative to major surgery. Although the first removals were performed using a rigid scope, currently the large majority of such cases are performed with flexible scopes that can be inserted into more distal airways and that have a working channel through which instruments can be passed.[44,45] When inhalation of a foreign body is suspected and the patient has survived the acute obstruction, careful planning should go into any further intervention as poor planning can lead to airway obstruction and death. The procedure should be performed by an experienced endoscopist with the availability and facility with both rigid and flexible scopes.[44] While the procedure can be performed with the patient awake, often general anesthesia is required. Careful consultation between the endoscopist and the anesthesiologist as to how the airway shall be safely managed is essential. Once the airway plan is safely in place, endoscopy is carried out. Besides the availability of the two types of scopes, accessory instruments are very helpful in safely removing various bodies that may have become embedded into the mucosa.[45] These instruments include balloon catheters, special grasping forceps, and wire baskets. In addition, other adjunctive techniques have been developed to safely remove the foreign body. These include the cryo-probe that can cause the body to adhere to the end of the instrument or neodymium-ytterium-aluminum-garnet (Nd:YAG) laser to break up the foreign body, vaporize the surrounding granulation tissue to dislodge it, and blunting the sharp edges for safe removal.[44,45]

Toilet for Pulmonary Collapse, Massive Secretions, and Aspiration

Flexible bronchoscopy has become an invaluable tool for managing atelectasis and complete or partial pulmonary collapse resulting from tenacious mucoid secretions. There is an immediate benefit observed in patients with tenacious mucoid secretions obstructing central airways. In such patients, bronchoscopic suctioning for whole lung collapse or lobar atelectasis has been shown to improve oxygenation.[46] In other patients, however, the benefits of bronchoscopic clearing of airways over traditional chest percussion therapy are less clear.[47] In trauma patients, though, it may not be possible to provide good percussion therapy at times because of other injuries, and bronchoscopy may be the only effective method of clearing secretions. For patients who have suffered large-volume aspiration of gastric contents, early bronchoscopy and lavage of the airways can help clear the airways and possibly limit chemical damage. Although bronchoscopy in such settings is often used for this aim, no studies have conclusively shown its benefits. Based on anecdotal evidence, a reasonable approach may be to perform bronchoscopy and lavage on patients suspected of large volume aspiration if they are already intubated or require intubation immediately after the episode. If the patient does not require intubation, he or she should be carefully monitored and managed with aggressive percussion therapy and other measures to encourage pulmonary toilet. As with all procedures it is necessary to balance potential harm with benefit. Extensive suctioning within the airways during bronchoscopy leads to derecruitment of alveoli that can lead to problems with oxygenation and also extensive washing within the airways can cause diffusion problems further worsening oxygenation (see previous discussion of complications).

Percutaneous Dilatational Tracheostomy

Percutaneous dilatational tracheostomy has gained in popularity as an alternative to open tracheostomy that can be performed in the ICU at lower cost. While it is possible to perform the procedure without bronchoscopy, many believe that the addition of bronchoscopic control adds to the safety of the procedure.[48] The procedure consists of placing a needle within the trachea, and passing a guide wire through the needle. Once a guide wire has been placed the tract from the skin to the trachea is sequentially dilated and finally a tracheostomy tube, preloaded over the final dilator, is passed into the trachea via the established tract. When the procedure is performed under bronchoscopic control, it is possible to ensure that the needle, guide wire, and dilators are indeed passing into the trachea, as they are supposed to, and not into a false passage within the soft tissues of the neck.

Indications of percutaneous tracheostomy are the same as for open tracheostomy. Skin infection, unstable cervical spine and elevated ICP are absolute contraindications to the procedure while obesity, high ventilatory requirements, coagulopathy, and any anatomical abnormality in the area are relative contraindications.[49] Reported complications include mucosal tears, submucosal placement of tube, perforation of the posterior tracheal wall with formation of a tracheoesophageal fistula, paratracheal placement, barotrauma, and damage to the endotracheal tube and bronchoscope. Like the open procedure there is an incidence of late tracheo-innominate fistula and subglottic stenosis.[49] There have been retrospective meta-analyses and prospective studies to compare open and percutaneous tracheostomy. The results suggest that percutaneous tracheostomy has a steep learning curve; however, in experienced hands the percutaneous technique has equivalent perioperative results and possibly improved long-term results as compared with open tracheostomy.[50]

Management of Bronchopleural Fistula

Bronchopleural fistulae present as a persistent air leak from a thoracostomy tube. When conservative measures, including maintaining continuous negative pleural pressure and chemical pleurodesis, fail to close the fistula by 1–3 weeks, surgical correction may be necessary. Bronchoscopy can be useful in identifying the offending segment from which the fistula emanates. Passing the scope into different bronchopleural segments of the lung with the suspected fistula and observing for telltale granulation tissue through which bubbles are emanating is fairly accurate in diagnosing the site of the fistula. After identification a balloon-tipped catheter can be passed with the help of the bronchoscope and the balloon inflated to occlude the site. If this results in cessation of the air leak, the diagnosis and site are confirmed.[51] Once the diagnosis is confirmed and site identified, a number of substances including fibrin glue, gel foam, and lead-shot plugs have been used to temporarily seal the site prior to surgery, and, in selected cases, even offer permanent control obviating the need of major surgery. Fresh autologous blood clot delivered to the site by pasting it onto the balloon of a balloon tipped catheter has also been used. When blood clot is used, an antifibrolytic agent (e.g., epsilon aminocaproic acid), tetracycline, or doxycycline instillation can enhance the success rate.[51]

Dilatation/Laser Therapy of Tracheobronchial Strictures

Tracheobronchial strictures in trauma patients are usually related to prolonged intubation. However, they can also be caused by granulation tissue resulting from infections and occur after surgical or stent repairs of airway injuries. While surgical excision and repair of the strictured area has a high success rate,[52] bronchoscopic dilatation, with or without laser vaporization, of the stricture is a lower risk alternative that can offer temporary relief till surgical repair can be carried out or in some cases lead to permanent cure.[53] The technical details of the procedure are beyond the scope of this text, but careful consideration has to be given to plan optimal therapy in each individual situation. The important considerations include the anatomy of the stricture—site, length, and type of tissue—and, if laser therapy is opted for, the type of laser to be used—Nd:YAG, CO_2, or potassium-titanil-phosphate (KTP). In addition, local expertise and experience are important considerations. Adjunctive techniques that can be used along with laser vaporization include balloon dilatation, placement of a stent, and infusion of mitomycin C to reduce the recurrence rate following laser therapy. No comparative trials have been performed comparing surgical resection with laser therapy; a multidisciplinary approach to the management of each individual patient is the best way to obtain optimal results.[53]

Drainage of Lung Abscess

Lung abscess is a serious complication following chest trauma or pneumonia following any trauma, with high morbidity and mortality. Traditional methods of treatment include adequate early antibiotic therapy and postural drainage. Failing this, surgical drainage was the only available option, but it carried high morbidity and mortality. Interventional radiological techniques have allowed drainage of the abscess without high-risk surgery. However, radiologically placing drainage catheters deep within the lung in proximity of major airways runs the risk of developing persistent bronchopleural fistulas. Transbronchial approach via the bronchoscope is an additional technique that can be used for aspirating such abscesses, and by leaving a drainage catheter the technique allows for irrigation of the cavity and continuous drainage. Good results have been reported but care should be exercised to minimize spillage of pus into the airways.[54]

CONCLUSION

Endoscopic techniques including VATS and fibroptic bronchoscopy are increasingly being used as diagnostic and therapeutic tools in patients with chest trauma or pulmonary complications following any trauma. In carefully selected patients, these techniques can offer a lower risk alternative to open surgery both in the acute and non-acute settings. As technical advances improve instrumentation, both bronchoscopy and VATS are likely to play greater roles in the management of chest trauma and pulmonary complications following any trauma.

REFERENCES

1. LoCicero J III, Mattox KL: Epidemiology of chest trauma. Surg Clin North Am 69:15–19, 1989.
2. Shapiro MB, Anderson III HL, Bartlett RH: Surg Clin North Am 80: 871–883, 2000.
3. Karmy-Jones R, Jurkovich GJ, Shatz DV, et al: Management of traumatic lung injury: a Western Trauma Association multicenter review. J Trauma 51:1049–1053, 2001.
4. Karmy-Jones R, Cuschieri J, Vallieres E: Role of bronchoscopy in massive hemoptysis. Chest Surg Clin North Am 11:873–906, 2001.
5. Allen JN: Self-expanding metallic stents in interventional pulmonary medicine. Lung Biol Health Dis 189:239–257, 2004.
6. Karmy-Jones R, Jurkovich GJ: Blunt chest trauma. Curr Prob Surg 41: 1223–1380, 2004.
7. Jacobaues HC: The practical importance of thoracoscopy in surgery of the chest. Surg Gynecol Obstet 34:289–293, 1922.
8. Branco JMC: Thoracoscopy as a method of exploration in penetrating injuries of the chest. Dis Chest 12:330–335, 1946.
9. Meyer DM, Jessen ME, Wait MA, Estrera AS: Early evacuation of traumatic retained hemothoraces using thoracoscopy: a prospective, randomized trial. Ann Thorac Surg 64:1396–1401, 1997.
10. Manlulu AV, Lee TW, Thung KH, Wong R, Yim APC: Current indications and results of VATS in the evaluation and management of hemodynamically stable thoracic injuries. Eur J Cardiothorac Surg 25:1048–1053, 2004.
11. Rodriguez-Morales G, Rodriguez A, Shatney CH: Acute rupture of the diaphragm in blunt trauma: analysis of 60 patients. J Trauma 26:438–444, 1986.
12. Rosati C: Acute traumatic injury of the diaphragm. Chest Surg Clin North Am 8:371–379, 1998.
13. Johnson CD: Blunt injuries of the diaphragm. Br J Surg 75:226–230, 1988.
14. Martinez M, Britz JE, Carrillo EH: Delayed thoracoscopy facilitates the diagnosis and treatment of diaphragmatic injuries safely and expeditiously. Surg Endosc 15:28–32, 2001.
15. Carrillo EH, Richardson JD: Thoracoscopy for the acutely injured patient. Am J Surg 190:234–238, 2005.
16. Fabian T, Croce M, Stewart B, et al: A prospective analysis of diagnostic laparoscopy in trauma. Ann Surg 217:557–565, 1993.
17. Livingston DH, Tortella B, Blackwood J, et al: The role of laparoscopy in abdominal trauma. J Trauma 33:471–475, 1992.
18. Ivatury RR, Oschner MG, Simon R, et al: Cavitary endoscopy. In Ivatury RR, Gayten CG, editors: The Textbook of Penetrating Trauma. Media, PA, Williams & Wilkins, 1996, pp. 416–428.
19. Eddy AC, Luna GK, Copass M: Empyema thoracis in patients undergoing emergent closed tube thoracostomy for thoracic trauma. Am J Surg 157:494–497.
20. Heniford BT, Carrillo EH, Spain DA, et al: The role of thoracoscopy in the management of retained thoracic collections after trauma. Ann Thorac Surg 63:940–943, 1997.
21. Coselli JS, Mattox KL, Beal AC: Reevaluation of early evacuation of clotted hemothorax. Am J Surg 148:786–790, 1984.
22. Graham JM, Mattox KL, Beall AC Jr: Penetrating trauma of the lung. J Trauma 19:665–669, 1979.
23. Helling TS, Gyles NR III, Eisenstein CL, et al: Complications following blunt and penetrating injuries in 216 victims of chest trauma requiring tube thoracostomy. J Trauma 29:1367–1370, 1989.
24. Villavicencio RT, Aucar JA, Wall MJ: Analysis of thoracoscopy in trauma. Surg Endosc 13:3–9, 1999.
25. Landreneau RJ, Kennan RJ, Hazelrigg SR, et al: Thoracoscopy for empyema and hemothorax. Chest 109:18–24, 1995.
26. Smith RS, Fry WR, Tsoi EKM, et al: Preliminary report on videothoracoscopy in the evaluation and treatment of thoracic injury. Am J Surg 166: 690–695, 1993.
27. Kern JA, Tribble CG, Spotnitz WD, et al: Thoracoscopy in the subacute management of patient with thoracoabdominal trauma. Chest 104: 942–945, 1993.
28. Carillo EH, Schmacht DC, Gable DR, et al: Thoracoscopy in the management of posttraumatic persistent pneumothorax. J Am Coll Surg 186: 636–640, 1998.
29. Shremer CR, Matterson BD, Demarest GB III, et al: A prospective evaluation of video-assisted thoracic surgery for persistent air leak due to trauma. Am J Surg 177:480–484, 1999.
30. Pons F, Lang-Lazdunski L, Kerangal X, et al: The role of videothoracoscopy in the management of precordial thoracic penetrating injuries. Eur J Cardiothorac Surg 2:7–12, 2002.
31. Krasna MJ, Deshmukh S, Mclaughlin JS: Complications of thoracoscopy. Ann Thorac Surg 61:1066–1069, 1996.
32. Weng W, DeCrosta DJ, Zhang H: Tension pneumothorax during one-lung ventilation: a case report. J Clin Anesth 14:529–531, 2002.
33. Herth FJF, Ernst A, Beamis JF Jr: History of rigid bronchoscopy in interventional pulmonary medicine. Lung Biol Health Dis 189:1–12, 2004.
34. Kerwin AJ, Croce MA, Timmons SD, et al: Effects of fiberoptic bronchoscopy on intracranial pressure in patients with brain injury: a prospective clinical study: J Trauma 48:876–882, 2000.
35. Barmada H, Gibbons JR: Tracheobronchial injury in blunt and penetrating chest trauma. Chest 106:74–78, 1994.
36. Baumgartner F, Sheppard B, De Virgilio C, et al: Tracheal and main bronchial disruptions after blunt chest trauma: presentation and management. Ann Thorac Surg 50:569–574, 1990.
37. Lin MC, Lin HC, Lan RS, et al: Emergent flexible bronchoscopy for the evaluation of acute chest trauma. J Bronchol 1:188–193, 1995.
38. Prakash UBS: Chemical warfare and bronchoscopy. Chest 100:1486, 1991.
39. Hunt JL, Agee RN, Pruitt BA Jr: Fibroptic bronchoscopy in acute inhalation injury. J Trauma 15:641–649, 1975.
40. American Thoracic Society, Infectious Diseases Society of America: guidelines for the management of adults with hospital-acquired, ventilator-associated, and healthcare-associated pneumonia. Am J Respir Crit Care Med 171:388–416, 2005.
41. Kollef MH, Sherman G, Ward S, et al: Inadequate antimicrobial treatment of infections: a risk factor for hospital acquired mortality among critically ill patients. Chest 115:462–474, 1999.
42. Croce MA, Fabian TC, Schurr MJ, et al: Using bronchoalveolar lavage to distinguish nosocomial pneumonia from systemic inflammatory response syndrome: a prospective analysis. J Trauma 39:1134–1140, 1995.
43. Chambers AS, Shepherd RW, Moses L, et al: Novel tracheal injury management with aortic transaction. J Bronchol 13:32–34, 2006.
44. Rafanan AL, Mehta AC: Adult airway foreign body removal. Clin Chest Med 22:319–330, 2001.
45. Kelly SM, Marsh BR: Airways foreign bodies. Chest Surg Clin North Am 6:253–276, 1996.
46. Stevens RP, Lillington GA, Parsons GH: Fibroptic bronchoscopy in the intensive care unit. Heart Lung 10:1037–1045, 1981.
47. Marini J, Pierson D, Hudson L: Acute lobar atelectasis: a prospective comparison of bronchoscopy and respiratory therapy. Am Rev Respir Dis 119:971–978, 1979.
48. Lee P, Mehta AC: Therapeutic flexible bronchoscopy: overview in interventional pulmonary medicine. Lung Biol Health Dis 189:49–87, 2004.
49. Noppen N: Percutaneous dilatational tracheostomy. In Bollinger CT, Mathur PN, editors: Interventional Bronchoscopy. Basel, Karger, 2000, pp. 215–225.
50. deBoisblanc BP: Percutaneous dilatational tracheostomy in interventional pulmonary medicine. Lung Biol Health Dis 189:567–583, 2004.
51. McManigle JRE, Fletcher GL, Tenholder MF: Bronchoscopy in the management of bronchopleural fistula. Chest 97:1235–1238, 1990.
52. Rea F, Callegaro D, Loy M, et al: Benign tracheal and laryngotracheal stenosis: surgical treatment and results. J Cardiovasc Surg Eur J Cardiovasc Surg 22:352–356, 2002.
53. Shapshay SM, Valdez TA: Bronchoscopic management of benign stenosis. Chest Surg Clin North Am 11:749–768, 2001.
54. Schmitt GS, Ohar JM, Kanter KR, et al: Indwelling transbronchial catheter drainage of pulmonary abscess. Ann Thorac Surg 45:43–47, 1988.

PULMONARY CONTUSION AND FLAIL CHEST

Carl J. Hauser and **David H. Livingston**

Pulmonary contusion and flail chest are the two most common anatomic complications of major blunt chest trauma. Each will directly alter pulmonary physiology in a specific and unique fashion, and thus contribute to pulmonary dysfunction and failure after trauma. Pulmonary contusion was probably first described by Morgagni in the 18th century, but Laurent's description in the Lancet in 1883[1] appears to be the first to recognize the possibility that plasticity of the chest wall, most notably in the young, can allow injury to the underlying lungs without disruption of the bony thorax. Conversely, flail chest is predominantly a disease of the elderly, with most patients being in the sixth decade of life and beyond and older patients having the worst outcomes.[2–4] Pulmonary contusion and flail chest commonly coexist but their degree of association changes and they may exist entirely separately under specific circumstances in specific patient groups. Yet because of their close association, their effects on pulmonary pathophysiology are often confused. Such confusion can lead to misapplication of studies aimed at one entity or the other and eventually to inappropriate treatment.

INCIDENCE

Pulmonary hemorrhage and contusion were noted to be common at autopsy of patients dying from battlefield and blast injuries during World War I.[5,6] Similar findings were noted in World War II,[7,8] and the term "pulmonary concussion" appears to have been coined by Hadfield describing civilian injuries from bomb blasts sustained during the Battle of Britain.[9] Reports in the 1960s first noted that pulmonary contusions occurred frequently after civilian motor vehicular trauma and were seen in up to 10% of thoracic injuries.[10]

Currently, the incidence of "pulmonary contusion" varies markedly depending on how aggressively it is sought and diagnosed. In some large series, about 15% of major blunt injuries[11] are found to have a pulmonary contusion. Using closer computed tomography (CT) evaluation, up to 25% of patients with chest trauma may be noted to have some form of contusion.[12] Yet a 10-year registry review of approximately 20,000 blunt trauma patients seen at the New Jersey State Trauma Center in Newark performed in preparation for this review showed that only 2.6% of all patients arriving at our Level I trauma center were diagnosed as having a pulmonary contusion.

So the "denominator" patient population examined will clearly affect the disease incidence reported in administrative databases, as will the tendency to identify and report less severe injuries. Yet our experience over the last several years indeed shows that the diagnosis of pulmonary contusion is increasing alongside our increased use of CT diagnosis for chest trauma (Figure 1).

The extent to which these previously subclinical injuries will turn out to predispose patients to complications remains to be seen, but these considerations suggest that future scaling systems for thoracic trauma will need to take into account the fact that modern imaging may find contusions that are either physiologically insignificant or that may "prime" the lung for secondary injury rather than lead to immediate dysfunction.

The relative frequency of flail chest as compared with pulmonary contusion will also vary depending upon the denominator population. Pediatric reviews find that the majority of major thoracic trauma presents with pulmonary contusions whereas flail chest is very rare, even where multiple fractures exist.[13,14] In contrast, in a large contemporary descriptive series examining adult blunt chest trauma, flail chest was diagnosed in about half of all patients with significant pulmonary contusions.[11] Moreover, the diagnosis of flail chest is often missed or delayed in sicker patients that require mechanical ventilation.[4] This results from the synchronous expansion of the lungs and "splinting" of the chest wall by positive intrathoracic pressure. Thus, it is clear that the proportions change and flail chest becomes increasingly common with advancing age and brittleness of the thoracic cage. Consequently, the frail elderly frequently sustain a flail chest with relatively minor chest trauma and little or no pulmonary contusion. Similarly, flail chest has been reported in newborns with osteogenesis imperfecta.[15]

Physical Mechanisms of Injury

The overwhelming majority of significant blunt chest trauma in civilian life occurs as a result of motor vehicle crashes and motor vehicle versus pedestrian injuries. Falls are another common cause of pulmonary contusion and flail chest. Thoracic compression injuries are not as common as vehicular trauma and falls, and although they may produce similar syndromes, the slower speed of impact makes contusion less likely than flail chest. Rather, these patients may manifest traumatic asphyxia. In military practice, blast injuries from high explosives can occur both in air and underwater. These produce specific and recognizable diffuse contusion patterns resulting from the concentration of energy at interfaces between denser tissues and tissues that contain gas, like the lung and bowel. Although these injuries have been rare in civilian life for the last 60 years, the advent of international terrorism as a mode of political action within the last 10 years has led to a resurgence of such injuries in civilian life—first in the Middle East, and now in the West.[16]

All blunt injuries result from the physical transfer of energy to the patient, but because of the rigidity of the bony thorax, all pulmonary contusions and most flail chest injuries are high-energy injuries, with the primary exception being occasional chest wall injuries in the frail elderly. Thus, they are seen primarily in motor vehicular trauma, perhaps most classically where unrestrained drivers strike the steering column. Pedestrian trauma and falls from a distance are frequent causes. Interpersonal violence leading to blows with blunt objects or kicking are occasional causes of pulmonary contusion. Flail chest however, is rare in our experience, first because assaults are most common in young adults and second because biomechanically they are unlikely to result in segmental injuries of multiple contiguous ribs. The physician should also bear in mind that rib fractures in infants and small children occur most commonly as a result of child abuse, and that any rib fracture in a child is a marker for severe trauma.[17]

The transfer of energy typically leads directly to hemorrhage into the lung. Pulmonary lacerations are uncommon but can occur (Figure 2) and in our experience are seen with increasing frequency when routine CT imaging is used. On rare occasions, tangential gunshot injuries will cause contusions of the underlying pulmonary parenchyma without actually entering and lacerating the lung. These injuries are usually very limited in their extent and cause little or no physiologic effects. Another potential mechanism of pulmonary dysfunction after trauma is the activation of pulmonary vascular endothelium by percussive cellular deformation per se. This phenomenon is much better documented in cerebrovascular endothelial beds,[18,19] but it is likely to exist in the pulmonary bed as well (see Figure 2).

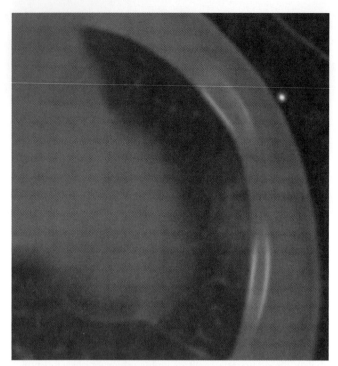

Figure 1   Subclinical "computed tomography–only" pulmonary contusion.

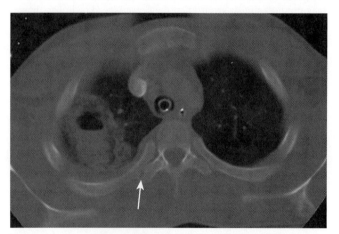

Figure 2   The admitting chest CT of 14-year-old patient in high-speed crash. Contusion with pulmonary laceration is evident. There was no significant pneumothorax or hemothorax. No rib fractures were found, but the transverse processes of T4–T7 on the right were fractured *(arrow).* In our experience, costovertebral joint separations like this are not uncommon on CT, and are the biomechanical equivalents of posterior rib fractures. *CT,* Computed tomography.

Mechanisms of Physiologic Injury

Studies done toward the end of World War I suggested that blast injury predominantly resulted in pulmonary hemorrhage,[5] and it was felt that pulmonary failure reflected the effects of blood filling the air spaces. Whereas this effect undoubtedly contributes to the increased pulmonary shunting (Qs/Qt) seen after injury, many other pathophysiologic processes are at work. There is now little doubt that the majority of pulmonary dysfunction seen after chest trauma results from secondary injury processes rather than direct injury to the lung. It is most convenient to divide the various

pathophysiologic influences on pulmonary function into those that result in increased Qs/Qt and hypoxemia, and those that alter the work of breathing and can lead to ventilatory failure. Either can result from chest wall or parenchymal pathology. It is important to note that associated intrapleural collections of air and blood may also impact mechanical chest wall function and pulmonary aeration as well as systemic hemodynamic performance, although these considerations are outside the scope of this review.

Shunting and Hypoxemia

Systemic shock and ischemia/reperfusion (I/R) are well-known activators of immune system attacks on the lung, causing shunting and hypoxia. This is perhaps most clearly evident in lung transplantation,[20] but is also seen in systemic I/R[21] as well as intestinal I/R.[22] All will activate the innate immune system and cause systemic inflammatory response syndrome (SIRS), which contributes to acute lung injury (ALI) and pulmonary dysfunction after chest trauma. Inadequately treated pain resulting from chest wall injury and splinting is a common cause of splinting and hypoventilation. The resultant atelectasis is a common cause of increased Qs/Qt and hypoxemia after trauma. The use of mechanical ventilation, although necessary, can result in ventilator-induced lung injury (VILI) through a number of mechanisms.[23] Immunologic injury can be induced by leukocytes in the presence activating cytokines, resulting in increased lung water and decreased diffusion capacity of the lung (D_L). Thus, secondary immune attack on the "primed" lung can be initiated by pneumonia, shock, injudicious ventilation strategies, or the release of cytokines into the circulation, as may happen in long-bone fixation.[24,25]

Increased Work of Breathing and Ventilatory Failure

Ventilatory failure, hypercarbia, and respiratory acidosis after injury are most commonly the result of increased work of breathing. Such increases in work of breathing seen are typically multifactorial. Chest wall injuries can lead to decreased compliance of the chest wall as well as deficits in neuromuscular chest wall function. The pain and splinting associated with chest wall injuries will also lead to decreased tidal volume. Because decreased tidal volume per se results in relatively increased anatomic dead space (Vd/Vt), patients with chest injuries need to increase minute ventilation simply to achieve normal alveolar ventilation. This can be difficult or impossible to achieve in the presence of musculoskeletal chest wall dysfunction.

In the presence of a flail chest, CO_2 retention has commonly been attributed to the pendelluft phenomenon, where to-and-fro flow of gas has been postulated to exist between the two hemithoraces in the presence of a unilateral flail segment. This concept is intuitively appealing, and the re-breathing of airway gas does create a pathologic dead space. Yet direct application of this concept to clinical chest injury is probably simplistic. In practice, elevated shunt fractions and hypoxemia are more common in flail chest and in trauma in general than is hypercarbia. Moreover, pendelluft occurs in acute lung injury even without chest wall instability. This results from the heterogeneous viscoelastic properties of the injured lung itself, which leads to gas movements between lung segments of differing compliance.[26] Clearly though, flail segments do make ventilation both painful and increasingly inefficient.

Last, in any major trauma with secondary acute lung injury the same immune attack on the pulmonary parenchyma that leads to ALI-ARDS and hypoxemia will also lead to "stiff lungs" and increased work of breathing. Such decreases in pulmonary compliance may persist even after the chest wall has resumed normal configuration and biomechanics. A final, extra-pulmonary cause of decreased pulmonary compliance that should always be sought in acute situations is abdominal compartment hypertension.

Inflammatory Lung Injury

Deteriorating pulmonary function after chest trauma is commonly related to systemic inflammation after injury. Acute lung injury (ALI) and adult respiratory distress syndrome (ARDS) are terms widely used to reflect the increasing severity of secondary lung injury after trauma. Such injury is widely believed to result from polymorphonuclear neutrophil (PMN)–endothelial cell (EC) interactions that injure pulmonary capillary endothelial membranes, causing interstitial and alveolar edema, and resulting in diminished compliance and gas diffusion. ALI/ARDS are usually defined as a diagnosis of exclusion where hypoxemia exists in the absence of other discrete causes of pulmonary failure such as pneumonia or congestive heart failure. In fact, ALI/ARDS probably exists in all major chest trauma to some extent. Although management of ALI/ARDS is to date supportive, an understanding of the pathogenesis is important because the lung should be understood to be "primed" for secondary insults after chest trauma and at risk for marked deterioration in the event of secondary insults like shock and sepsis. There is increased risk of pneumonia after chest trauma, and pneumonia, of course, can act both as a primary cause of pulmonary dysfunction and as a trigger for "second-hit" organ failure. A special problem is that chest trauma is often accompanied by long-bone fractures and patients with chest injuries are clearly at special risk for pulmonary deterioration after fracture fixation.[27] Fractures are reservoirs for inflammatory mediators in the early post-injury period which can be mobilized to the bloodstream by operation and potentially contribute to ALI/ARDS.[24,26,28,29] Prospective studies will be needed to determine whether orthopedic management of these patients should be tailored to the protection of lung function.

Extravascular Lung Water

Before the routine clinical use of pulmonary artery (PA) catheters, it was widely believed that fluid overload and subsequent increases in extravascular lung water were the primary cause of pulmonary dysfunction after trauma. In contrast, modern concepts emphasize that hypovolemia, hypoperfusion, and reperfusion can lead to inflammatory organ injury. Also, impaired right-to-left blood flow leads to preferential perfusion of the dependent (West Zone III) lung segments that are poorly ventilated, thus also increasing shunt. Chest injury may be associated with myocardial dysfunction as well, but this is typically right ventricular in nature, and resolves quickly.[30] Shock and resuscitation do in fact lead to some expansion of extravascular water, but pulmonary lymphatics protect the lung from interstitial overload remarkably well.[31] We therefore stress maintaining euvolemia and circulatory adequacy in patients with chest injuries. In patients with underlying cardiac, renal, or hepatic disease, however, extravascular lung-water accumulation may be a significant issue. These patients may require inotropes, diuretics, or oncotic support.

DIAGNOSIS

Physical Examination

The diagnosis of flail chest is best made by visual inspection or palpation of asymmetric chest wall movement in the spontaneously breathing patient. Palpation is often the more sensitive test. It is rapid and informative but is often overlooked. Mobile segments of chest wall and sternum can often be palpated even when not visible on inspection. Clinical flail chest is associated with worse outcomes and greater need for intubation than pulmonary contusion alone.[32] Spontaneously breathing patients are often best examined by placing both hands on the two hemithoraces and palpating the symmetry of chest wall motion. Crepitance is also a common finding and point tenderness over the costochondral junctions may point to dislocations or cartilaginous fractures that are not visible on radiographs.

Auscultation of the chest is usually suboptimal in trauma, and will play little role in the diagnosis of pulmonary contusion and flail chest except to diminish concern for lesions (such as pneumothoraces) that may deteriorate acutely.

Chest X-Rays

Chest x-ray (CXR) and computed tomography (CT) of the chest play key roles in the diagnosis of chest trauma. The initial anteroposterior/supine chest x-rays that are typically done in seriously injured patients may show pulmonary contusion or suggest flail chest (Figure 3).

But CXRs are of low sensitivity and will miss many very important intrathoracic lesions. Although rib fractures may also be apparent, plain x-rays show many fewer fractures than CTs. Thus, in addition to underestimating pain and disability, CXRs will rarely suggest whether rib fracture patterns are likely to be mechanically unstable. So, although the initial CXR remains crucial in the early diagnosis of immediately life-threatening lesions, it often fails to diagnose pulmonary contusions, hemothoraces, pneumothoraces, and lung lacerations that may require specific interventions. This is especially true where anterior pneumothoraces and posterior fluid collections coexist (Figure 4).

Chest Computed Tomography

Chest CT typically reveals many more rib fractures than CXR, and the distribution of the injuries may sometimes suggest the likelihood of their causing chest wall musculoskeletal dysfunction (Figure 5). Significant flail segments most commonly occur in the setting of segmental fractures of three or more contiguous ribs. CT scans will sometimes demonstrate contiguous rib fractures in a pattern that suggests geographic instability or a dysfunctional area of the chest wall where physical exam is unrevealing.

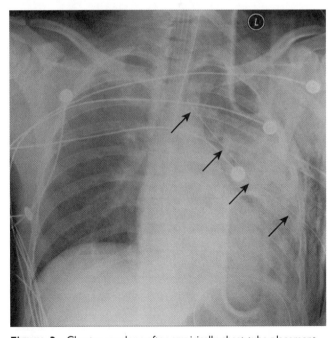

Figure 3 Chest x-ray done after empirically chest tube placement in a patient with subcutaneous emphysema and arterial desaturation. Note the left lower-lobe pulmonary contusion, the apparently ideal placement of the chest tube (*arrows*) and the absence of a visible residual pneumothorax. Fractures of the left ribs four, five, and six were visible laterally.

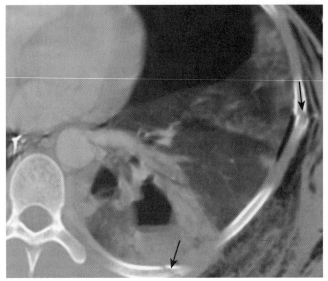

Figure 4 Initial chest computed tomography of same patient as in Figure 3. Multiple segmental rib fractures *(arrows)* were not seen on CXR. A posterior contusion-laceration and an anterior pneumothorax are present despite the chest tube laterally and the apparent expansion of the lung on CXR. This reflects the superimposition of air and fluid densities. *CXR,* Chest x-ray.

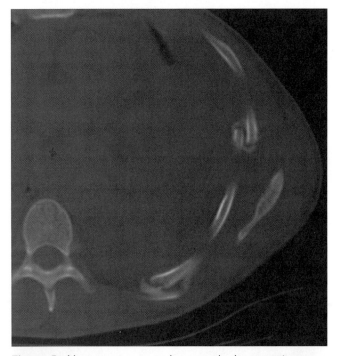

Figure 5 Noncontrast computed tomography demonstrating fractures extending over more than three contiguous rib segments. In this location (underneath the fractured scapula) such injuries are rarely found on clinical examination.

Contusions are often seen as infiltrative lesions that underlie fractures and are nonanatomic in their distribution on chest CT. But dependent infiltrates on the CT may reflect processes like aspiration, atelectasis, and later, pneumonia. These can be difficult to tell apart from contusions. In contrast, nonanatomic and antidependent distributions of infiltrative lung lesions on a chest CT may be pathognomonic for pulmonary contusion (Figure 6). A pleural-based

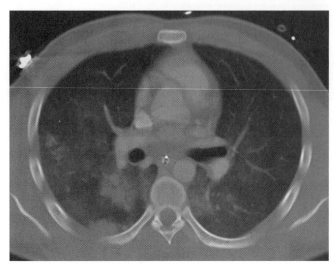

Figure 6 Admitting chest computed tomography of a 19-year-old patient after high-speed car crash with severe pulmonary contusions. The only thoracic bony injury was a fractured clavicle. The patient developed severe acute lung injury/acute respiratory distress syndrome 3 days later.

"blast-wave" pattern seen on CT is pathognomonic (see Figure 1). Early chest CT can also aid in the evaluation of pulmonary contusions by determining their extent and allowing prediction of respiratory deterioration.[12]

More heavily muscled areas of the chest are less likely to sustain flail injuries. Moreover, such areas can remain mechanically stable despite the presence of fractures. Thus, typically, visible flail segments are anterior or inferolateral in the chest. But symmetric bilateral multiple fractures in the anterior chest will also commonly cause flail injuries (Figure 7), especially in elderly persons striking a steering wheel. This mechanism can lead to a flail sternum, or if in the axillary lines, a flail of the entire anterior chest wall *en cuirasse* (i.e., like a shield).

Physiologic Studies

Radiologic imaging is often of little importance from a functional point of view because multiple nonanatomic, physiologic causes of lung injury tend to coexist. Nonetheless, the CXR and chest CT must be evaluated for evidence of pulmonary and pleural pathology amenable to direct treatment both initially and when deterioration occurs in the patient with pulmonary contusion or flail chest. In general, though, the functional physiologic diagnosis of pulmonary contusion and flail chest will rely on analysis of vital signs, arterial blood gases, and hemodynamic and bedside pulmonary function studies.

The hallmark of pulmonary contusion is hypoxemia and increased pulmonary shunting resulting from the perfusion of poorly ventilated lung. This may be defined by decreasing arterial saturation on a stable F_IO_2 or by an increasing need for inspired oxygen support to maintain saturation. This is often expressed as a decreasing PaO_2/F_IO_2 (P/F) ratio. In ventilated patients, increasing positive end-expiratory pressure (PEEP), plateau pressures, or reversed I/E ratios may all indicate a high Qs/Qt. Injury of the pulmonary parenchyma often results in decreased compliance. This may manifest as decreased tidal volume and tachypnea in spontaneously ventilating patients or in patients treated with pressure ventilation modes, or as increased peak airway pressures in ventilated patients on volume-controlled ventilator settings.

In truly isolated flail chest injuries, there is little initial hypoxemia. Rather, these patients present early with rapid shallow respiration,

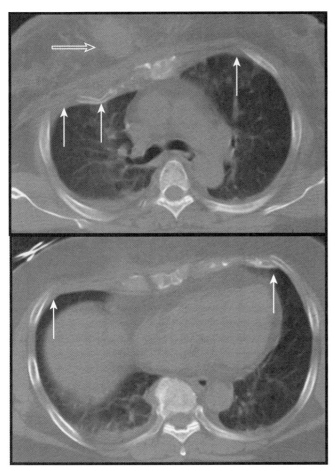

Figure 7 Computed tomography of an elderly obese woman with steering wheel injury and an anterior flail "en cuirasse." Note that multiple rib fractures *(solid arrows)* in both anterior axillary lines in this case involved every rib. There is atelectasis and a small amount of pleural fluid, but considering the degree of rib injury this patient has little pulmonary contusion. There is an arterial hematoma in the anterior chest wall *(open arrow)*. This patient was easily managed with pain medication and had no clinical pulmonary dysfunction.

and they may develop hypercarbia as ventilation fails. More often, though, they do have some element of pulmonary contusion, or they develop hypoxemia over time because of atelectasis or poor clearance of secretions. Ventilated patients may show little pulmonary dysfunction resulting from the flail chest component of their injury as long as their pressure or volume support is sufficient to splint the chest wall and cause it to move in synchrony.

ANATOMIC LOCATION OF INJURY AND INJURY GRADING

The American Association for the Surgery of Trauma-Organ Injury Scale (AAST-OIS) for chest trauma as reviewed by Moore and colleagues[33] is shown in Tables 1 and 2. It should be noted that the scores for chest wall and pulmonary injury are separated, but injuries may overlap and interact. For instance, the association of a flail chest with pulmonary contusion results in worse outcomes and greater need for intubation than pulmonary contusion only.[32] Conversely, many of the small pulmonary contusions now found on CT scan alone may be of little predictive value, or their significance may be limited to situations where patients are expected to undergo long-bone fixa-

tion.[34] Thus, these scales must clearly be in evolution at the time of CT diagnosis of intrathoracic injury (see Tables 1 and 2).

MANAGEMENT

Pulmonary contusion/flail chest can be viewed as leading to four common and important sequelae: (1) pain, (2) mechanical chest wall instability, (3) direct lung injury, and (4) secondary (immune) lung injury. To differing extents, these all contribute directly or indirectly to pulmonary gas exchange dysfunction and thus can be important contributors to the morbidity and mortality of multisystem injuries.

Immediate Management

Before the early 1980s, the major controversy in early management of pulmonary contusion/flail chest was whether early endotracheal intubation should be emphasized or whether attempts should be made to avoid intubation. This controversy reflected the early perception that patients who were intubated had a worse prognosis. Richardson and colleagues[35] were the first to show that, rather than being a causal relationship, this difference in outcomes reflected worse overall injuries in the intubated than the nonintubated group. Over time, the established approach (as reflected in ATLS and other algorithms) became early elective use of endotracheal intubation in patients presenting with any hypoxemia. Flail chest injuries in particular are associated with a tendency to early ventilatory failure requiring emergency intubation resulting from unrecognized high work of breathing.[32] This approach is controversial, however, and other workers have suggested aggressive attempts to avoid intubation.[36,37] Analysis of the available data, however, suggests that there are no true prospective series available comparing early intubation to "intubation on demand" in equivalent groups, and that in all reports the intubated patients were simply sicker. Such sicker patients simply require intubation more often. Thus, in our judgment arguments that elective intubation per se leads to worse outcomes are unsupported. Our approach has been the use of early rapid-sequence intubation and ventilation to facilitate diagnosis and management wherever there are severe injuries, with early extubation of patients who will tolerate it. Patients who have progressive deterioration of respiratory function despite intubation will require prolonged ventilation and intensive care unit (ICU) management.

Intensive Care Unit Management

Pulmonary contusion decreases parenchymal compliance and increases QS/QT. Flail chest causes chest wall dysfunction, pain, and inefficient mechanical ventilation. These two injuries contribute synergistically to hypoventilation and ventilatory failure. Pain and impaired coughing contribute to atelectasis and mucus plugging, and decreased chest wall expansion under flail segments decreases functional residual capacity (FRC).[38] Associated systemic injury, shock, and pulmonary infections contribute to secondary pulmonary parenchymal injury. All will contribute to shunting and hypoxemia. Thus, management of flail chest–pulmonary contusion is one of the most important and challenging aspects of intensive care in trauma.

General Principles of Ventilator Management

The management of flail chest/pulmonary contusion consists in great measure of the support of failing pulmonary function by the use of a ventilator. In the case of minor injuries, supplemental oxygen can be given by mask as needed. True continuous positive airway pressure (CPAP) delivered by a tight-fitting mask has been used to

Table 1: Chest Wall Injury Scale

Grade	Injury Type	Description of Injury	ICD-9	AIS-90
I	Contusion	Any size	911.0/922.1	1
	Laceration	Skin and subcutaneous	875.0	1
	Fracture	<3 ribs, closed; nondisplaced clavicle, closed	807.01 807/02 810.00/810.03	1–2 2
II	Laceration	Skin, subcutaneous, and muscle	875.1	1
	Fracture	>3 adjacent ribs, closed	807.03/807.09	2–3
		Open or displaced clavicle	810.10/810.13	2
		Nondisplaced sternum, closed	807.2	2
		Scapular body, open or closed	811.00/811.18	2
III	Laceration	Full thickness including pleural penetration	862.29	2
	Fracture	Open or displaced sternum	807.2	2
		Flail sternum	807.3	
		Unilateral flail segment (<3 ribs)	807.4	3–4
IV	Laceration	Avulsion of chest wall tissues with underlying rib fractures	807.10/807.19	4
	Fracture	Unilateral flail chest (>3 ribs)	807.4	3–4
V	Fracture	Bilateral flail chest (>3 ribs on both sides)	807.4	5

Note: This scale is confined to the chest wall alone and does not reflect associated internal or abdominal injuries. Therefore, further delineation of upper versus lower or anterior versus posterior chest wall was not considered, and a grade VI was warranted. Specifically, thoracic crush was not used as a descriptive term; instead, the geography and extent of fractures and soft tissue injury were used to define the grade.

AIS, Abbreviated Injury Scale.

Source: Adapted from Moore EE, Cogbill TH, Malangoni MA, et al: Organ injury scaling. *Surg Clin North Am* 75(2):293–303, 1995.

improve oxygenation and support the functional residual capacity, but the natural history of significant flail chest/pulmonary contusion is the gradual worsening of pulmonary function over the first few days. Thus, in our experience, CPAP is most commonly a marker for the later need for emergent intubation with its attendant problems. Moreover, because CPAP predisposes to gastric distention and thus to aspiration, we have found that using CPAP as a bridge to delay intubation in major chest trauma is usually unwise and may risk significant complications. Because endotracheal intubation will be required at some point in most patients with significant injuries, intubation should be considered early, before deterioration, and when considered is usually warranted.

Ventilatory Support

Ventilating chest trauma patients can be different from ventilating other patients. Intubated patients with lesser injuries may require some support for air exchange, but generally should be allowed to spontaneously ventilate to whatever degree is possible. We find that pressure support ventilation (PSV) mode is very satisfactory for such spontaneously breathing patients. But care should be taken using PSV in the presence of significant flails. In these cases, the negative pressures that trigger the ventilator may destabilize the chest wall[39] and should be minimized. Such motion may also be painful and delay stabilization. We often prefer to begin treatment using a volume mode like synchronized intermittent mandatory ventilation (SIMV), keeping minute ventilation high enough to raise arterial pH slightly above 7.4, thus suppressing spontaneous ventilation without undue sedation. The flail segments are allowed to stabilize over about a week, with thicker chest walls often

stabilizing more quickly. Patients are then ventilated using PSV and weaned progressively.

Chest trauma, pulmonary contusion, and ARDS can cause the chest to be noncompliant. In such cases, relatively high airway pressures are needed to sustain the traditional high tidal volumes (10–15 ml/kg) used before the ARDS-Net studies. High airway pressures ($\leq$35 cm H_2O) should be avoided where possible, and using lower tidal volumes (6–8 ml/g) will decrease peak airway pressures. Limiting airway pressures is especially important in cases of bronchopleural fistulas. Also, "normal" $PaCO_2$ values are not needed in sedated patients, and permissive hypercapnia is often useful in the treatment of hypoxemia after chest trauma.[40,41]

Oxygenation Support

Patients with significant chest trauma all manifest some degree of hypoxemia. This may be managed initially by increasing FIO_2, but prolonged high FIO_2 can be harmful in itself. The longer-term management of hypoxemia therefore entails measures to increase mean airway pressure to maintain and improve oxygenation. This may include PEEP or reversed inspiratory/expiratory (I/E) times that can be delivered by any of several ventilator strategies. These interventions can recruit alveoli and diminish alveolar and interstitial water. The reversal of I/E time is limited by the need to excrete CO_2 and stacking or auto-PEEP at high I/E ratios. Traditional high tidal volume ventilation (10–15 ml/kg) does not contribute to pulmonary expansion, nor does it improve oxygenation in the majority of cases. Rather, it has been known for many years to lead to unequal ventilation, alveolar overdistension, and VILI.[42] We began using low tidal volume ventilation in the early 1990s (then known as "the kinder,

Table 2: Lung Injury Scale

Grade[a]	Injury Type	Description of Injury	ICD-9	AIS-90
I	Contusion	Unilateral, <1 lobe	861.12 861.31	3
II	Contusion	Unilateral, single lobe	861.20 861.30	3
	Laceration	Simple pneumothorax	860.0/1	3
III	Contusion	Unilateral, >1 lobe	861.20 861.30	3
	Laceration	Persistent (>72 hours) air leak from distal airway	860.0/1 860.4/5 862.0	3–4
	Hematoma	Nonexpanding intraparenchymal	861.30	
IV	Laceration	Major (segmental or lobar) air leak	862.21 861.31	4–5
	Hematoma	Expanding intraparenchymal		
	Vascular	Primary branch intrapulmonary vessel disruption	901.40	3–5
V	Vascular	Hilar vessel disruption	901.41	4
		Total uncontained transection of pulmonary hilum	901.42	
VI	Vascular		901.41 901.42	4

[a]Advance one grade for bilateral injuries up to grade III. Hemothorax is scored under thoracic vascular injury scale.

AIS, Abbreviated Injury Scale.

Source: Adapted from Moore EE, Cogbill TH, Malangoni MA, et al: Organ injury scaling. *Surg Clin North Am* 75(2):293–303, 1995.

gentler vent breath"). Since that time, low tidal volume ventilation has been shown to improve the survival of general ICU patients in prospective studies,[43] and we extend these principles to chest trauma in most cases.

Many other therapies with little or no evidentiary support are in common use as salvage therapies in refractory hypoxemic patients. These include rotating or oscillating beds, differential lung ventilation, inhaled nitric oxide, partial liquid ventilation, hypertonic saline, red blood cell transfusions, or inotropic support to raise mixed venous oxygen saturation, and other modalities. All may have some effect in individual patients and may on occasion "buy some time" for the primary process to abate. None has been prospectively validated.

Tracheobronchial toilet in the intubated chest trauma patient should have a high priority because of the frequent coexistence of early particulate aspiration, blood casts or lobar collapse resulting from retained secretions. Both macroaspiration at the time of injury and the continued microaspiration that accompanies endotracheal intubation can increase secretions and allow airway colonization by oropharyngeal flora. Excessive secretions will also lead to lobar collapse, shunting and hypoxemia, diminished compliance, and postobstructive airway infections. Blood may accumulate in the airway after pulmonary contusion and form bronchial casts. Intubated patients cannot cough and are completely dependent upon suctioning for airway toilet. N-acetylcysteine may be used as a mucolytic if secretions are thick, but it causes bronchospasm and should be used with bronchodilators. Also, prolonged N-acetylcysteine therapy can cause bronchorrhea. Chest physiotherapy is helpful, but the percussion of injured ribs is often painful. Thus, removal of secretions or particulates frequently requires bronchoscopy. The removal of blood casts may require retrieval with snares or morcellation (Figure 8).

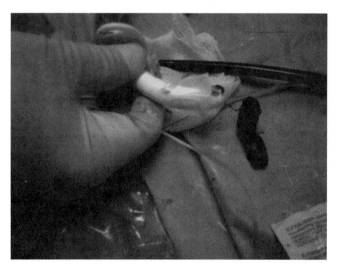

Figure 8 Airway cast due to endobronchial bleeding. The cast was too hard to be morcellated. When snared bronchoscopically it was larger than the tracheostomy and could not be removed without removing and replacing the tracheostomy.

Pain Management

The control of chest wall pain is a key consideration in management of chest injuries. Immobility of the chest wall due to splinting resulting from pain is often thought a major contributor to the development of pneumonia after rib fractures. This has never been proven and recent studies suggest that pneumonia in trauma patients, in fact, reflects the suppression of innate immunity.[44,45] Nonetheless, good pain control is an important contribution to patient care in general, and probably improves pulmonary toilet. Chest wall pain can be treated with appropriate systemic analgesic regimens or with intercostal, intrapleural, subpleural, or paravertebral blocks. Epidural blocks are probably the optimal form of analgesia where possible and not contraindicated.[46,47] There is no scientific support for the historic practice of using chest taping or strapping to relieve pain.

Steroids

As noted previously, all blunt chest injuries will have some element of ALI/ARDS, and as yet no intervention or pharmaceutical agent has been proven of significant value in treating post-traumatic ARDS. Some small series, however, have suggested that the late fibroproliferative stage of ARDS may respond in some measure to systemic corticosteroids. Nonetheless, considering the well-established dangers of steroid use, we await prospective data before using them routinely in late ARDS.

Tracheostomy

As with endotracheal intubation, it is often apparent early in patients with severe injuries that tracheostomy will be critical. Also, later deterioration often makes tracheostomy hazardous. Thus, experienced clinicians will often look for an early window of opportunity to move airway access from the endotracheal tube to a tracheostomy in sicker patients. Early tracheostomy (generally defined as at <7 days) improves access to the tracheobronchial tree for toilet and allows for better oropharyngeal hygiene. While controversy persists, this approach has been suggested to result in fewer episodes of pneumonia and more rapid weaning from mechanical ventilation.[48,49] Last, current studies have shown convincingly that low volume/low pressure ventilation is less injurious to the lung than higher ventilator volumes and pressures. Tracheostomy diminishes the anatomic dead space, and reliably lowers peak airway pressures at equivalent levels of alveolar ventilation. This is especially helpful in patients with refractory pulmonary failure who require aggressive ventilator settings to support oxygenation.

Operative Stabilization of Flail Chest

Most physiologically significant flail chest injuries are satisfactorily managed by selective intubation and mechanical ventilation. Nonetheless, several groups have advocated the operative management of flail chest injuries.[50,51] Evidence that rib fracture stabilization is useful in major chest trauma is scanty. The existing series are highly selected, and in all published series the patients with the most severe pulmonary dysfunction were not considered surgical candidates. Voggenreiter and colleagues[52] showed that patients who had flail chests and also had significant pulmonary contusions did not benefit from operation. Thus, chest wall fixation permitted early extubation only in a highly selected group of patients that had ventilatory insufficiency without pulmonary contusion, and presumably therefore without hypoxemia. Consequently, fixation can stabilize flail segments, but the significant physiologic deficits in chest trauma patients relate to underlying contusions and acute lung injury. In summary, the literature currently supports the concept that operative chest wall stabilization will not benefit the vast majority of patients with flail chest. Moreover, it has significant potential for causing mischief in sick patients. The net risk-to-benefit ratio may therefore be most favorable in the subset of patients with large unstable flail segments who already must undergo a thoracic procedure (such as a decortication) for related injuries.

MORTALITY

Most deaths after pulmonary contusion/flail chest result from associated injuries like head trauma, but major chest wall trauma can be an independent cause of death. In these instances, death is usually due to ARDS, respiratory failure, sepsis, and multiple organ failure. So these outcomes are covariant with other conditions that predispose to SIRS, respiratory failure, and MOF. These may include associated injuries, increasing ISS or APACHE scores, and increasing numbers of blood transfusions.[3,53] Where pulmonary contusions are visible on the admitting chest x-ray of a patient with a flail chest, the need for mechanical ventilation is far higher and mortality is more than doubled when compared with either condition alone.[54,55] The number of ventilator days, ICU days, and overall length of stay, as well as pneumonia and mortality, are all clearly higher in older patients with rib fractures.[56–58] Similarly, the mortality of patients with a flail chest increases with age.[59] Last, ventilator-associated pneumonia is an independent risk factor for death in chest trauma,[60] although pneumonia itself may simply be a marker for greater systemic trauma.[44,61] In summary, flail chest and pulmonary contusion are highly morbid and may contribute significantly to mortality in multisystem trauma or in patients with underlying comorbidities. Nonetheless, with good ICU treatment death from flail chest and pulmonary contusion alone should be uncommon.

CONCLUSION

- Pulmonary contusion and flail chest are common and life-threatening sequelae of blunt chest trauma.
- Pulmonary contusion and flail chest commonly coexist.
- Isolated flail chest tends to occur in older patients with brittle ribs.
- Isolated pulmonary contusions tend to occur in younger patients with flexible ribs.
- Pulmonary contusion and flail chest are each associated with pulmonary dysfunction resulting from shock, SIRS, and inflammatory ALI.
- Impairment of oxygenation in pulmonary contusion and flail chest usually reflects the effects of contusion and ALI on intrapulmonary shunting.
- Impairment of ventilation in pulmonary contusion/flail chest usually reflects the effects of chest wall injury and pain on respiratory mechanics and on the work of breathing.
- The management of significant pulmonary contusion and flail chest often entails mechanical ventilator support for 5–10 days.
- Selected minor injuries can be managed without endotracheal intubation.
- Selected major injuries should be considered for early tracheostomy.

REFERENCES

1. Laurent EA: Rupture of both lungs without external injury. *Lancet* 2:25, 1883.
2. Athanassiadi K, Gerazounis M, Theakos N: Management of 150 flail chest injuries: analysis of risk factors affecting outcome. *Eur J Cardiothorac Surg* 26(2):373–376, 2004.
3. Freedland M, Wilson RF, Bender JS, Levison MA: The management of flail chest injury: factors affecting outcome. *J Trauma* 30(12):1460–1468, 1990.
4. Landercasper J, Cogbill TH, Strutt PJ: Delayed diagnosis of flail chest. *Crit Care Med* 18(6):611–613, 1990.
5. Hooker DR: Physiological effects of air concussion. *Am J Physiol* 67:219, 1924.
6. Lockwood AL: Surgical experiences in the last war. *BMJ* 1:356, 1940.
7. Savage O: Pulmonary concussion ("blast") in non-thoracic battle wounds. *Lancet* 424, 1945.
8. Burford TH, Burbank B: Traumatic wet lung. *J Thorac Surg* 14:415, 1945.
9. Hadfield G, Christie RV: A case of pulmonary concussion ("blast") due to high explosive. *BMJ* 1:77, 1941.

10. Demuth WE Jr, Smith JM: Pulmonary contusion. *Am J Surg* 109:819–823, 1965.
11. Galan G, Penalver JC, Paris F, et al: Blunt chest injuries in 1696 patients. *Eur J Cardiothorac Surg* 6(6):284–287, 1992.
12. Miller PR, Croce MA, Bee TK, et al: ARDS after pulmonary contusion: accurate measurement of contusion volume identifies high-risk patients. *J Trauma* 51(2):223–228; discussion 229–230, 2001.
13. Balci AE, Kazez A, Eren S, et al: Blunt thoracic trauma in children: review of 137 cases. *Eur J Cardiothorac Surg* 26(2):387–392, 2004.
14. Reinberg O, Mir A, Genton N: Characteristics of thoracic injuries in children. *Chir Pediatr* 31(3):139–145, 1990.
15. Cardenas N, Manrique TA, Catlin EA: Flail chest in the newborn. A complication of osteogenesis imperfecta. *Clin Pediatr (Phila)* 27(3):161–162, 1988.
16. Argyros GJ: Management of primary blast injury. *Toxicology* 121(1):105–115, 1997.
17. Garcia VF, Gotschall CS, Eichelberger MR, et al: Rib fractures in children: a marker of severe trauma. *J Trauma* 30(6):695–700, 1990.
18. Orfeo T, Doherty JM, Adey G, et al: Sublethal percussion trauma in vitro causes a persisting derangement in the nonthrombogenic properties of brain endothelial cells. *J Trauma* 37(3):347–357, 1994.
19. Gourin CG, Shackford SR: Influence of percussion trauma on expression of intercellular adhesion molecule-1 (ICAM-1) by human cerebral microvascular endothelium. *J Trauma* 41(1):129–135, 1996.
20. de Perrot M, Liu M, Waddell TK, et al: Ischemia-reperfusion-induced lung injury. *Am J Respir Crit Care Med* 167(4):490–511, 2003.
21. Brackett DJ, McCay PB: Free radicals in the pathophysiology of pulmonary injury and disease. *Adv Exp Med Biol* 366:147–163, 1993.
22. Turnage RH, Guice KS, Oldham KT: Pulmonary microvascular injury following intestinal reperfusion. *New Horiz* 2(4):463–475, 1994.
23. Dos Santos CC, Slutsky AS: Invited review: mechanisms of ventilator-induced lung injury: a perspective. *J Appl Physiol* 89(4):1645–1655, 2000.
24. Hauser CJ, Zhou X, Joshi P, et al: The immune microenvironment of human fracture/soft-tissue hematomas and its relationship to systemic immunity. *J Trauma* 42(5):895–903, 1997.
25. Pape HC, van Griensven M, Rice J, et al: Major secondary surgery in blunt trauma patients and perioperative cytokine liberation: determination of the clinical relevance of biochemical markers. *J Trauma* 50(6):989–1000, 2001.
26. Pelosi P, Cereda M, Foti G, et al: Alterations of lung and chest wall mechanics in patients with acute lung injury: effects of positive end-expiratory pressure. *Am J Respir Crit Care Med* 152(2):531–537, 1995.
27. Shorr RM, Crittenden M, Indeck M, et al: Blunt thoracic trauma. Analysis of 515 patients. *Ann Surg* 206(2):200–205, 1987.
28. Hauser CJ, Desai N, Fekete Z, et al: Priming of neutrophil [Ca2 +]i signaling and oxidative burst by human fracture fluids. *J Trauma* 47(5):854–858, 1999.
29. Pape H-C, Aufmkolk M, Paffrath T, et al: Primary intramedullary femur fixation in multiple trauma patients with associated lung contusion—a cause of posttraumatic ARDS. *J Trauma* 33(4):540–548, 1993.
30. Harley DP, Mena I, Narahara KA, et al: Traumatic myocardial dysfunction. *J Thorac Cardiovasc Surg* 87(3):386–393, 1984.
31. Erdmann AJ 3rd, Vaughan TR, Brigham KL, et al: Effect of increased vascular pressure on lung fluid balance in unanesthetized sheep. *Circ Res* 37(3):271–284, 1975.
32. Velmahos GC, Vassiliu P, Chan LS, et al: Influence of flail chest on outcome among patients with severe thoracic cage trauma. *Int Surg* 87(4):240–244, 2002.
33. Moore EE, Cogbill TH, Malangoni MA, et al: Organ injury scaling. *Surg Clin North Am* 75(2):293–303, 1995.
34. Pape H-C, Regal G, Dwenger A, et al: Influences of different methods of intramedullary femoral nailing on lung function in patients with multiple trauma. *J Trauma* 35(5):709–716, 1993.
35. Richardson JD, Adams L, Flint LM: Selective management of flail chest and pulmonary contusion. *Ann Surg* 196(4):481–487, 1982.
36. Bolliger CT, Van Eeden SF: Treatment of multiple rib fractures. Randomized controlled trial comparing ventilatory with nonventilatory management. *Chest* 97(4):943–948, 1990.
37. Vidhani K, Kause J, Parr M: Should we follow ATLS(R) guidelines for the management of traumatic pulmonary contusion: the role of non-invasive ventilatory support. *Resuscitation* 52(3):265–268, 2002.
38. Gyhra A, Torres P, Pino J, et al: Experimental flail chest: ventilatory function with fixation of flail segment in internal and external position. *J Trauma* 40(6):977–979, 1996.
39. Cappello M, Legrand A, De Troyer A: Determinants of rib motion in flail chest. *Am J Respir Crit Care Med* 159(3):886–891, 1999.
40. Eisner MD, Thompson T, Hudson LD, et al: Efficacy of low tidal volume ventilation in patients with different clinical risk factors for acute lung injury and the acute respiratory distress syndrome. *Am J Respir Crit Care Med* 164(2):231–236, 2001.
41. Bigatello LM, Patroniti N, Sangalli F: Permissive hypercapnia. *Curr Opin Crit Care* 7(1):34–40, 2001.
42. Slutsky AS: Lung injury caused by mechanical ventilation. *Chest* 116(1 Suppl):9S–15S, 1999.
43. ARDS-Network: Ventilation with lower tidal volumes as compared with traditional tidal volumes for acute lung injury and the acute respiratory distress syndrome. The Acute Respiratory Distress Syndrome Network. *N Engl J Med* 342(18):1301–1308, 2000.
44. Tarlowe MH, Duffy A, Kannan KB, et al: Prospective study of neutrophil chemokine responses in trauma patients at risk for pneumonia. *Am J Respir Crit Care Med* 23:23, 2004.
45. Perl M, Gebhard F, Bruckner UB, et al: Pulmonary contusion causes impairment of macrophage and lymphocyte immune functions and increases mortality associated with a subsequent septic challenge. *Crit Care Med* 33(6):1351–1358, 2005.
46. Mackersie RC, Karagianes TG, Hoyt DB, et al: Prospective evaluation of epidural and intravenous administration of fentanyl for pain control and restoration of ventilatory function following multiple rib fractures. *J Trauma* 31(4):443–449; discussion 449–451, 1991.
47. Mandabach MG: Intrathecal and epidural analgesia. *Crit Care Clin* 15(1):105–118, vii, 1999.
48. Moller MG, Slaikeu JD, Bonelli P, et al: Early tracheostomy versus late tracheostomy in the surgical intensive care unit. *Am J Surg* 189(3):293–296, 2005.
49. Griffiths J, Barber VS, Morgan L, et al: Systematic review and meta-analysis of studies of the timing of tracheostomy in adult patients undergoing artificial ventilation. *BMJ* 330(7502):1243, 2005. Epub May 18, 2005.
50. Lardinois D, Kreuger T, Dusmet M, et al: Pulmonary function testing after operative stabilisation of the chest wall for flail chest. *Eur J Cardiothorac Surg* 20(3):496–501, 2001.
51. Ahmed Z, Mohyuddin Z: Management of flail chest injury: internal fixation versus endotracheal intubation and ventilation. *J Thorac Cardiovasc Surg* 110(6):1676–1680, 1995.
52. Voggenreiter G, Neudeck F, Aufmkolk M, et al: Operative chest wall stabilization in flail chest—outcomes of patients with or without pulmonary contusion. *J Am Coll Surg* 187(2):130–138, 1998.
53. Gaillard M, Herve C, Mandin L, et al: Mortality prognostic factors in chest injury. *J Trauma* 30(1):93–96, 1990.
54. Johnson JA, Cogbill TH, Winga ER: Determinants of outcome after pulmonary contusion. *J Trauma* 26(8):695–697, 1986.
55. Clark GC, Schecter WP, Trunkey DD: Variables affecting outcome in blunt chest trauma: flail chest vs. pulmonary contusion. *J Trauma* 28(3):298–304, 1988.
56. Holcomb JB, McMullin NR, Kozar RA, et al: Morbidity from rib fractures increases after age 45. *J Am Coll Surg* 196(4):549–555, 2003.
57. Taylor MD, Tracy JK, Meyer W, et al: Trauma in the elderly: intensive care unit resource use and outcome. *J Trauma* 53(3):407–414, 2002.
58. Bulger EM, Arneson MA, Mock CN, et al: Rib fractures in the elderly. *J Trauma* 48(6):1040–1046; discussion 1046–1047, 2000.
59. Albaugh G, Kann B, Puc MM, et al: Age-adjusted outcomes in traumatic flail chest injuries in the elderly. *Am Surg* 66(10):978–981, 2000.
60. Magnotti LJ, Croce MA, Fabian TC: Is ventilator-associated pneumonia in trauma patients an epiphenomenon or a cause of death? *Surg Infect (Larchmt)* 5(3):237–242, 2004.
61. Tarlowe MH, Kannan KB, Itagaki K, et al: Inflammatory chemoreceptor cross-talk suppresses leukotriene b(4) receptor 1–mediated neutrophil calcium mobilization and chemotaxis after trauma. *J Immunol* 171(4):2066–2073, 2003.

Tracheal and Tracheobronchial Tree Injuries

Preston Roy Miller   and   J. Wayne Meredith

For most of history, acute tracheobronchial injuries have been considered uniformly fatal. In 1871, Winslow observed a healed left mainstem bronchus in a canvasback duck that was taken while hunting. This showed that the animal had survived the rupture and demonstrated the potential of the airways for healing. In 1927, Krinitzki reported the first long-term human survivor. Autopsy findings of a 31-year-old woman, who had been injured at age 10 years when a keg of wine fell on her chest, suggested that humans with tracheobronchial disruption may have the same healing potential as the canvasback duck. The autopsy demonstrated a completely occluded right mainstem bronchus. In the modern era, understanding of anatomy, injury mechanisms, and surgical repair technique has led to improved outcomes in the face of such injuries. Although tracheobronchial injuries still may be lethal, most are treatable. A high index of suspicion is required to make a timely diagnosis and to provide appropriate intervention, both of which are essential if the patient is to have the best opportunity for recovery.

INCIDENCE AND MECHANISMS OF INJURY

Injury to the tracheobronchial tree is an uncommon but well-recognized complication of both penetrating and blunt chest trauma. Many victims die before emergency care from associated injuries to vital structures, hemorrhage, tension pneumothorax, or respiratory insufficiency. Thus, a substantial number of diagnoses are established only after death. At other times, the diagnosis is not readily apparent and is not made until late symptoms indicating tracheobronchial injury have developed. Thus, the true incidence of injury to the tracheobronchial tree is difficult to discern. In a review of autopsies of 1178 persons dying from blunt trauma to the chest, Bertelsen and Howitz found that tracheobronchial disruptions occurred in only 33 patients, for an incidence of 2.8%; 27 of these died immediately. In a review of survivors and non survivors, Campbell reported on 15,136 patients diagnosed with blunt chest trauma. Forty-nine (0.3%) had a tracheobronchial injury. This series showed an extremely high mortality (67%) but did not describe the severity of associated injuries. In a review of the literature, Asensio described the incidence in penetrating neck trauma with 331 of 4193 patients (8%) presenting with laryngotracheal injuries. More than 80% of blunt tracheobronchial ruptures occur within 2.5 cm of the carina. Mainstem bronchi are injured in 86% of patients and distal bronchi in only 9.3%, while complex injuries are seen in 8%.

Penetrating injury is a straightforward mechanism and consists basically of the hole created by the path of a knife or bullet. Knife wounds occur almost exclusively in the cervical trachea, whereas gunshot wounds occur at any point along the tracheobronchial tree. Intrathoracic injury to the tracheobronchial tree occurs more commonly from blunt trauma but may also result from bullet wounds. These injuries occur at a higher incidence when the projectile crosses the mediastinum. Associated injuries to other mediastinal structures, including the heart, great vessels, and esophagus, are common and contribute significantly to the morbidity and mortality.

There are several mechanisms by which blunt trauma may injure the trachea and bronchus, including direct blows, sheer stress, and burst injury. A direct blow to the neck may produce a "clothesline"-type injury, crushing the cervical trachea against the vertebral bodies and transecting the tracheal rings or cricoid cartilage. Shear forces on the trachea create damage at its relatively fixed points, the cricoid and the carina. A common factor in burst injury along the tracheobronchial tree is rapid anteroposterior compression of the thorax. This compression causes a simultaneous expansion in the lateral thoracic diameter, and the negative intrapleural pressure stretches the lungs laterally along with the chest wall, thereby placing traction on the carina. When the plasticity of the tracheobronchial tree is exceeded, the lungs are pulled apart and the bronchi avulsed. Closure of the glottis before impact may convert the trachea into a rigid tube with increased intratracheal pressure, which may cause a linear tear or blowout of the membranous portion of the trachea or cause a complex disruption of the trachea and bronchi. As predicted by the Law of LaPlace, this type of burst injury occurs where the airway diameter is greatest, usually within 2.5 cm of the carina, but may occur anywhere along the airway. A combination of these mechanisms is probably responsible for producing most injuries. Given the protected nature of these structures, a significant amount of high-energy transfer is usually required to create these injuries.

DIAGNOSIS

Presentation

A variety of clinical presentations result after injury to the tracheobronchial tree, with most depending on the severity and the location of the injury. Patients with cervical tracheal injuries may present with stridor and severe respiratory distress or with hoarseness, hemoptysis, or cervical subcutaneous emphysema. The presentation of thoracic tracheobronchial injury depends on whether the injury is confined to the mediastinum or communicates with the pleural space. Thoracic tracheobronchial injuries confined to the mediastinum usually present with massive pneumomediastinum. Pneumopericardium is occasionally described. Injuries that perforate into the pleural space usually create an ipsilateral pneumothorax that may or may not be under tension. A pneumothorax that persists despite adequate placement of a thoracostomy tube and has a continuous air leak is suggestive of tracheobronchial injury and bronchopleural fistula. Dyspnea may actually worsen after insertion of the chest tube due to the loss of total volume via the tube. In 1969, Oh and colleagues described a highly specific finding of bronchial rupture, which they termed the "fallen lung" sign. Its characteristic radiographic features show the lung falling away from the hilum, laterally and posteriorly, in contrast to the usual simple pneumothorax, which collapses toward the hilum. This sign results from the disruption of the normal central anchoring attachments of the lung and, although pathognomonic, it is rarely seen. Other radiographic clues to possible airway injury are seen with endotracheal intubation and show abnormal migration of the tube tip or overdistension of the endotracheal tube balloon outside the confines of the normal tracheal diameter.

Some retrospective reports show that up to two thirds of these intrathoracic tracheobronchial tears will go unrecognized longer than 24 hours and up to 10% of tracheobronchial tears will not produce any initial clinical or radiological signs and are recognized months later after stricture occurs. Immediate intubation of patients with multisystem trauma can mask laryngeal or high cervical tracheal injuries and contribute to a delay in the diagnosis. After tracheobronchial transection, the peribronchial connective tissues may remain intact and allow continued ventilation of the distal lung analogous to the way perfusion is maintained after traumatic aortic transection. If unrecognized, this injury heals with scarring and granulation tissue and may possibly create bronchial stenosis or obstruction such as in the duck reported by Winslow. After a latent period, granulation tissue and stricture of the bronchus will develop. Distal to the stricture, pneumonia, bronchiectasis, abscesses, and even empyema can result. Complete obstruction without infection leads to prolonged atelectasis and diminished pulmonary function.

While concomitant injury is the rule rather than the exception, patterns of associated injuries vary widely. Major vascular, cardiac, pulmonary, esophageal, bony thoracic, and neurologic injuries are common and reflect the site, magnitude, and mechanism of the trauma. The mechanisms of trauma may alert one to search for the presence of injury. For example, transcervical and transmediastinal penetrating injuries pose particular danger to the respective traversing structures. Associated injuries may be severe, and in at least one series, were responsible for all of the deaths. It has been suggested that corresponding rib fractures would be seen in all patients over 30 years old who had a rupture of the tracheobronchial tree, but this is not always true. The absence of a chest wall injury does not exclude serious chest trauma, but the presence of such an injury should alert one to investigate further for a major underlying injury. A high index of suspicion must be maintained in order to diagnose and treat an injury promptly and appropriately.

Evaluation

Diagnosis should be suspected based on the clinical history and the constellation of signs and symptoms previously listed. Evaluation of the patient with a suspected injury to the tracheobronchial tree is shown in the algorithm in Figure 1. The advent of spiral computed tomography (CT) has created interest in evaluation of injury with this technique. Three-dimensional reconstruction has been used to elegantly demonstrate the site and extent of injuries in case reports. While tracheobronchial injury may be well demonstrated on CT in some cases, there is no evidence that CT is adequate to exclude an injury and obviate the need for diagnostic bronchoscopy. CT scans suggesting injury should prompt bronchoscopy for definitive diagnosis. In addition to visualization of possible tracheal injury on CT, indications for bronchoscopy include large pneumomediastinum, refractory pneumothorax, large air leak, persistent atelectasis, or, occasionally, marked subcutaneous emphysema. Bronchoscopy, whether rigid or flexible, is the best-studied means of establishing the diagnosis and determining the site, nature, and extent of the tracheobronchial disruption. A potential disadvantage of rigid bronchoscopy is that it requires general anesthesia, as well as a stable ligamentous and bony cervical spine. A rigid scope has the advantage of direct visualization and the ability to provide ventilation. Flexible bronchoscopy may be performed without general anesthesia, and offers the potential for controlled insertion of a nasal or orotracheal tube while maintaining cervical stabilization. The most critical determinant seems to be the experience and comfort level of the endoscopist. It has been shown that, in the hands of an experienced bronchoscopist, either technique can be performed with a high degree of accuracy. Lesions may be missed initially or their severity may be underestimated. These lesions may evolve into more obvious or severe injuries, and for this reason bronchoscopy should be liberally repeated as needed.

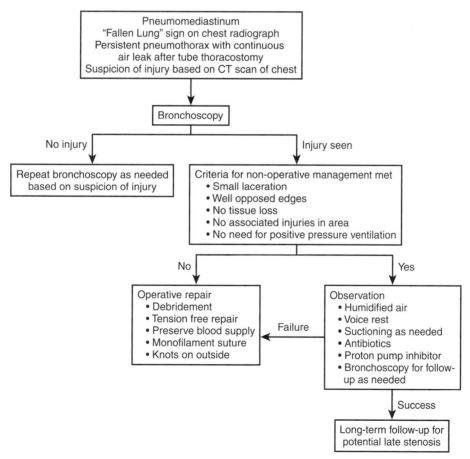

Figure 1 Algorithm for evaluation and management of suspected tracheobronchial injury.

MANAGEMENT

Initial Management

Airway management, as in all injuries, is the first priority in the management of a patient with injury to the tracheobronchial tree. If the patient is maintaining his or her own airway and is ventilating adequately, a cautious approach of nonintervention is probably the best initial choice until further diagnostic work-up can be completed or other life-threatening injuries can be stabilized. Careless handling or mishandling of the airway, such as inadvertently placing an endotracheal tube through a transected or ruptured airway into the soft tissue, may compound the injury. If the injury is suspected, the airway should be evaluated carefully with the patient awake in order to plan for appropriate intervention. A bronchoscope may be passed into the trachea to evaluate for injury. In the case of less severe injuries, an endotracheal tube may be carefully passed distal to the injury over the bronchoscope. Blind nasal intubation or use of standard rapid sequence intubation (RSI)/endotracheal intubation should not be attempted in the case of known or suspected laryngotracheal injury because of the danger of creating a complete tracheal transection by pushing the tube against or through the injury.

Tracheostomy performed in the operating room is advocated by many as the safest and securest way to obtain airway control. This may be done in the awake patient to avoid airway loss in those with adequate airway protection. If the trachea is completely transected, the distal trachea can usually be found in the superior mediastinum and grasped for insertion of a cuffed tube. The approach taken must vary with the resources and expertise available at each institution. One must also be aware that even though the airway is secured, the injury may still be exacerbated with mechanical ventilation if the injury is distal to the tube. Tube thoracostomies should be appropriately placed at this time and connected to suction. After the airway is controlled, there is time for an orderly identification of concurrent injuries, performance of interventions such as esophagoscopy, laryngoscopy, arteriography, celiotomy as necessary, and transport to definitive care areas. Guidelines for the management of tracheobronchial injuries are given in Figure 1.

Nonoperative Management

On occasion, asymptomatic tracheobronchial injuries will be found incidentally on bronchoscopy or other imaging. Nonoperative management is reserved only for these highly selected patients with unexpected small tracheobronchial tears. Lesions selected for observation must involve less than one-third the circumference of the tracheobronchial tree. For patients to be candidates for nonoperative care, tube thoracostomy must fully re-expand the lung, and air leaks should stop soon after insertion of the tube. Prophylactic antibiotics, humidified oxygen, voice rest, frequent suctioning, and close observation for sepsis and airway obstruction are required.

Small stab wounds with no evidence of loss or devitalization of tracheal tissue and with well-opposed edges may be treated effectively with temporary endotracheal intubation. The cuff of the endotracheal tube should be inflated below the level of injury and left undisturbed for 24 to 48 hours while the wound seals. Bronchoscopy should be liberally repeated to evaluate the conservatively managed patient whose clinical condition deteriorates. Even small tears may heal but produce an excess of granulation tissue, which will require late endobronchial excision.

Operative Management

As with emergency management of the airway, intraoperative management requires substantial coordination with the anesthesiologist. All of the same principles apply. After the airway is initially secured, manipulation during the repair creates additional challenges. A sterile anesthesia circuit and tube may be needed to pass off the table after regaining control of the airway at the level of transection once the peritracheal connective tissue has been disrupted or entered for repair. If orotracheal intubation is performed, a single- or double-lumen endotracheal tube may be used. A double-lumen tube offers the benefit of independent lung ventilation but, because of the large size, it may create further disruption and is less desirable. A long, single-lumen tube may be passed beyond the area of injury for proximal levels of rupture, or for distal injuries, may be advanced into the contralateral mainstem bronchus for single-lung ventilation. Intubation over a flexible bronchoscope adds safety and diagnostic capability to the procedure. If a tracheostomy is performed, it should be placed two to three rings caudally to high tracheal or laryngeal injuries and brought out through an incision separate from the surgical repair wound. Tracheostomy proximal to an injury is probably not necessary to protect the suture lines after repair of the thoracic trachea or major bronchus, and its prophylactic use is discouraged for distal tracheobronchial injuries. In the most difficult cases, in which airway management is unsatisfactory, or during complex repairs, cardiopulmonary bypass may be instituted. The potential risks and benefits of this procedure must be weighed, including the need for systemic anticoagulation, especially in the multitrauma patient.

After repair, airway management ideally should be accomplished by removal of the endotracheal tube immediately after the operation. Otherwise, it should be removed and spontaneous respirations resumed as soon as the patient can breathe effectively. Occasionally, the patient will require ongoing positive pressure ventilation, which may require creative techniques of critical care and ventilation, such as positioning of the endotracheal tube distal to the repair, dual-lung ventilation, high-frequency jet ventilation, or extracorporeal membrane oxygenation. Every effort must be made to improve lung compliance by providing good pulmonary toilet, appropriate fluid management, and aggressive treatment of pneumonia.

Most extrathoracic airway injuries can be approached through a transverse collar incision. Occasionally, for added exposure, this incision may be extended up the neck for carotid repair or teed off down the sternum, with partial or complete sternotomy being performed for more central exposure. Intrathoracic tracheal, right bronchial, and proximal left mainstem bronchus injuries are best repaired through a right posterolateral thoracotomy at the fourth or fifth intercostal space. This approach avoids the heart and aortic arch. Complex or bilateral injuries should be approached through the right chest for this same reason. Distal left bronchial injuries more than 3 cm from the carina are approached through a left posterolateral thoracotomy in the fifth intercostal space.

Optimal repair includes adequate debridement of devitalized tissue, including cartilage, and primary end-to-end anastomosis of the clean tracheal or bronchial ends. This anastomosis can be accomplished free of tension by mobilizing anteriorly and posteriorly, thereby preserving the lateral blood supply. Tension may also be released with cervical flexion. This may be maintained postoperatively by securing the chin to the chest with a suture. Many investigators have recommended completion of the anastomosis with interrupted absorbable suture. We have found, however, that the use of a running, continuous, absorbable monofilament suture offers a secure repair and better visibility during construction of the anastomosis. The membranous portion may be repaired without tension and then brought together as the cartilaginous portion is begun. Sutures may be placed around or through the cartilage but must ensure approximation of mucosa to mucosa. Tying the suture knots on the outside of the lumen helps prevent suture granulomata and subsequent stricture. To prevent subsequent leak and fistula formation, the suture line may be reinforced with a patch of pericardium, a vascularized pedicle from the pleura, intercostal muscle, strap muscles, omentum, or vascularized pleura in late repairs to protect the repair and to aid in bronchial healing. During early repairs, the pleura is flimsy and usually not suitable as reinforcement. The vascularized pedicle of intercostal muscle offers both better protection and added healing potential for the repair. For this reason, the intercostal muscle should routinely be preserved during thoracotomy with the corresponding vein, artery, and nerve. This is accomplished by entering the chest through the bed of the rib. The rib may be preserved or sacrificed. An incision is made directly over the rib and the periosteum stripped off. At the superior border of the rib, the incision is carried through the posterior layer of the periosteum to enter the pleural space. The intercostal muscle is then divided from the ribs above and below and used as a flap to be wrapped around and tacked to the trachea. In this manner, viable tissue is placed between the repair and surrounding vital structures and blood supply in the area of the repair is increased, facilitating healing (Figure 2).

Injuries to the cervical trachea may be managed by repair with or without tracheostomy. Simple anterior lacerations may undergo primary repair without tracheostomy if possible. Tracheostomy alone, without repair, occasionally may serve as the sole source of treatment in patients with isolated injuries to the anterior cervical trachea. Such circumstances are uncommon owing to the presence of exit wounds and the variable level at which the trachea may be injured. For these reasons, anterior tracheal injuries are generally repaired. Placement of a tracheostomy through these injuries should be avoided except in the case of short term need for airway control via such a maneuver. In patients with severe injury to the proximal trachea, immediate repair with protective distal tracheostomy should be performed. Consideration should be given to stenting laryngeal injuries. Occasionally, the injury may cause extensive devitalization of the trachea and contamination of the field. In these rare instances, end tracheostomy, oversewing of the proximal trachea, and drainage may be the most prudent course of action. This allows for possible definitive repair later, after resolution of scarring and inflammation. However, attempts at primary repair should be exhausted first.

OUTCOMES

The best results are obtained with early identification, debridement, and early primary repair of tracheobronchial injuries. Excellent anatomic and functional results should be expected with normal pulmonary function and voice characteristics after early repair. Early repair also results in fewer tracheal revisions to correct stenosis.

Reported mortality varies from 3.5% to 67% with most modern series reporting less than 30%. Most of the early mortality results from lack of airway control and to multiple associated injuries (e.g., vascular and esophageal injuries).

If there is delay in diagnosis, repair should proceed as soon as the diagnosis is made or when practical after treatment of other life-threatening injuries. Regardless of the length of delay, reconstruction of the tracheobronchial tree should be attempted if there is no distal suppuration. Total bronchial disruption, if unrecognized, leads to complete occlusion and sterile atelectasis that may be amenable to repair later. The occluded segment is resected and repaired in a manner similar to that of the acute injury or as one would treat a benign stenosis. While pulmonary function suffers with such delayed treatment, it can be expected to improve with repair. Incomplete bronchial obstruction ultimately leads to suppuration and irreversible pulmonary parenchymal destruction. Therapy in this case may require lobectomy or pneumonectomy depending on the patient and degree of parenchymal damage. Thus, although bronchial rupture can be treated successfully in the acute or delayed phase, early diagnosis and treatment minimize the risk of infection and other complications.

While uncommon, tracheobronchial injuries will be encountered at most busy centers. These are challenging cases in which outcome depends on successful initial airway management as well as the level of suspicion by the astute clinician in investigating patients with signs and symptoms of the injury. These may range from severe presentations such as airway disruption or pneumothorax unresponsive to adequate tube thoracostomy, to mediastinal emphysema or subtle findings on chest computed tomography. Airway management efforts must be appropriate with overly aggressive techniques such as blind nasal intubation or RSI in those suspected of tracheal injury having potentially disastrous outcomes. With well-thought-out airway management and early operative intervention, good results can be expected in most cases.

SUGGESTED READINGS

Angood PB, Attia EL, Brown RA, Mulder DS: Extrinsic civilian trauma to the larynx and cervical trachea—important predictors of long-term morbidity. *J Trauma* 26:869, 1986.

Asensio JA, Valenziano CP, Falcone RE, Grosh JD: Management of penetrating neck injuries: the controversy surrounding zone II injuries. *Surg Clin North Am* 71(2):267, 1991.

Cornwell EE, Kennedy F, Ayad IA, et al: Transmediastinal gunshot wounds: a reconsideration of the role of aortography. *Arch Surg* 131:949, 1996.

Demetriades D, Theodorou D, Cronwell E, Asensio J: Transcervical gunshot injuries: mandatory operation is not necessary. *J Trauma* 40:758, 1996.

Dowd NP, Clarkson K, Walsh MA: Delayed bronchial stenosis after blunt chest trauma. *Anesth Analg* 82:1078, 1996.

Edwards WH, Morris HA, DeLozier JB, Adkins RB: Airway injuries—the first priority in trauma. *Am Surg* 53(4):192, 1987.

Flynn AE, Thomas AN, Schecter WP: Acute tracheobronchial injury. *J Trauma* 29:1326, 1989.

Grewal H, Rao PM, Mukerji S, Ivatury RR: Management of penetrating laryngotracheal injuries. *Head Neck* 17:494, 1995.

Griffith JL: Fracture of the bronchus. *Thorax* 4:105, 1949.

Kaiser AC, O'Brien SM, Detterbeck FC. Blunt tracheobronchial injuries: treatment and outcomes. *Ann Thorac Surg* 71(6):2059–2065, 2001.

Mills SA, Hudspeth AS, Myers RT: Clinical spectrum of blunt tracheobronchial disruption illustrated by seven cases. *J Thorac Cardiovasc Surg* 84:49, 1982.

Minard G, Kudsk KA, Croce MA, et al: Laryngotracheal trauma. *Am Surg* 58: 181, 1992.

Noyes L, McSwain NE, Markowitz IP: Penendoscopy with arteriography versus mandatory exploration of penetrating wounds of neck. *Ann Surg* 204: 21, 1986.

Oh KS, Fleischner FG, Wyman SM: Characteristic pulmonary finding in traumatic complete transection of a main-stem bronchus. *Radiology* 92:371, 1969.

Sands DEL, Ledgerwood AM, Lucas CE: Pneumomediastinum on a surgical service. *Am Surg* 54:434, 1988.

Spencer JA, Rogers CE, Westaby S: Clinico-radiological correlates in rupture of the major airways. *Clin Radiol* 43:371, 1991.

Symbas PN, Justicz AG, Ricketts RR: Rupture of the airways from blunt trauma: treatment of complex injuries. *Ann Thorac Surg* 54:177, 1992.

Winslow WH: Rupture of bronchus from wild duck. *Philadelphia Medical Times*, April 15, 1871, p. 255.

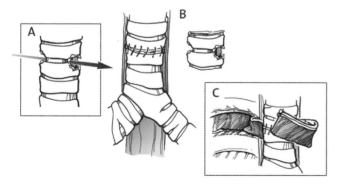

Figure 2 Injuries to thoracic trachea **(A)** are best repaired by debridement of devitalized tissue and repair with absorbable suture **(B)**. Debridement may include removal of several rings if necessary. The repair is protected with a vascularized pedicle of intercostal muscle **(C)**.

OPERATIVE MANAGEMENT OF PULMONARY INJURIES: LUNG-SPARING AND FORMAL RESECTIONS

Juan A. Asensio,   Luis Manuel García-Núñez,
Patrizio Petrone,   David King,   Ricardo Castrellon,
Dominic Duran,   Alexander D. Vara,   John S. Weston,
Donald Robinson,   and   Louis R. Pizano

Chest injuries were reported in the *Edwin Smith Surgical Papyrus*[1] as early as 3000 BC. Ancient Greek chronicles reveal examples of penetrating chest wounds and pulmonary injuries; the Greeks had anatomic knowledge and were cognizant of the thoracic structures and the position of the lungs inside the hemithoracic cavities. In Homer's *Iliad*,[2] there is a vivid description of the death of Sarpedon by Patroclus: "[H]e penetrated him with his spear and while taking it out, his diaphragm came along with it...." Homer[2] emphasized the importance of the diaphragm, anatomically related to the lungs and the "beating heart." While pneumothorax was a well-known entity, the Greeks realized the special problems related to thoracic penetration and considered open chest wounds fatal. Although the success of these early treatment modalities remains unknown, it seems that during Olympic competitions, physicians in ancient Greece were at least able to identify potential lethal chest injuries, and most likely attempt their treatment.[1–3]

Pausanias,[3] a Greek traveler during the height of Roman rule, described a penetrating injury to the chest, inflicted to Creugas of Epidamnus by Damoxenus of Syracuse, with the presence of what seems to be an obvious pulmonary injury. Eusebious described in *Evangelical Preparation*, the match of Cleomedes of Astypalaia against Ikkos of Epidauros: "Why did they deify Cleomedes? For opening his opponent's rib, inserting his hand inside and eviscerating his lung..."[1–3]

Galen (130–200 AD), one of the most prominent physicians of antiquity described packing of chest wounds in gladiators with thoracic and possibly lung injuries.[1,4] A description of a lung injury was found in a treatise of Theodoric, in 1226: "[W]hile I was living in Bolonia, a certain Domicellus, a Bolognan of normal birth was, cured by the hand of Master Hugo, part of his lung being torn away and Master Roand was there to witness it..."[5,6]

Even in the ancient world, most of the therapeutic modalities for chest wounds and traumatic pulmonary injuries were developed during wartime. In 1635, Alvar Nuñez Cabeza de Vaca,[4] a Spaniard, while traveling from the Mexican northern territory to the capital of Nueva España (Mexico City), was captured by Indians. A wounded member of the tribe was brought to Cabeza de Vaca. With his assistant Esteban, Cabeza de Vaca made an incision to remove an arrowhead embedded in the man's chest, and sutured the wound. His innovation in surgical management won freedom from his captors for him and his friend.

During the 16th century, a few contributions were made to the management of traumatic pulmonary injuries. Ambroise Paré[5] treated penetrating thoracic injuries by placing a scalding mixture of oil and treacle in the wound as the first dressing. John Hunter's[5] initial experience dealing with penetrating thoracic injuries, caused by smooth-bore muskets firing round lead balls, led him to recognize that projectile velocity is a determinant factor dictating severity of the injury. Jean-Dominique Larrey and Pierre Joseph Desault[5,6] made important contributions to the surgical procedure known as "débridement" for the management of chest wall lacerations; however, the surgical treatment of intracavitary injuries did not evolve significantly during this time. Although Larrey[5,6] described operative techniques for dealing with penetrating cardiac injuries, his contributions to the management of pulmonary injuries are not remarkable.

In 1822, William Beaumont, better known for "Beaumont's gastric fistula observations" than for his management of life-threatening chest injuries, treated a patient that sustained a gunshot wound to the chest and described the nature of the injury: "fracturing and carrying away the anterior half of the 6th rib, lacerating the lower portion of the left lobe of the lung, diaphragm and penetrating the stomach."[6] During the 18th century, controversies emerged surrounding the benefit of surgical manipulation in the treatment of traumatic thoracic and pulmonary injuries. In Germany, Auenbrugger[6] said: "opening the chest caused asphyxia because the lung collapsed." Dupuytren,[6] a famous French surgeon, in 1835 personally developed empyema. Although prepared to undergo a surgical intervention for its treatment, he decided, based on knowledge about Auenbrugger's description of "open-chest asphyxia" that "he would rather die at the hands of God than of the surgeons"; he survived for 12 days.

In the 1840s, the French Academy of Medicine[6] studied the treatment of empyema to produce guidelines for its treatment based on war experiences. In the 18th century, Hewson[6] called attention to the mechanism of pulmonary rupture after blunt trauma to the chest, while in 1886, Ashurt[6] described rupture of thoracic viscera without rib fractures. In 1889, Holmes, consulting surgeon to St. George's Hospital in London, said: "All penetrating wounds to the chest, if small, should be closed at once and dressed antiseptically. If the wound is large and the lung evidently extensively injured, it is a better plan not to close the external wound completely, but to insert a large drainage tube to carry off the blood into an antiseptic dressing and so prevent its accumulation in the pleural cavity."[6] In 1897, Duval[6–8] described median sternotomy incision, which he described as a thoracolaparotomy, while in 1906, Spangaro,[6–8] an Italian surgeon, described the left anterolateral thoracotomy incision. These incisions remain important contributions to the trauma surgical armamentarium to manage traumatic pulmonary injuries.

In 1916, Mentz[6,8] reported removal of foreign matter from the lung and pointed out the relative safety of thoracotomy. The treatment of thoracic wounds in World War I started with many of the basic principles described in the 19th century. Specifically, hemothoraces were treated expectantly. Hemothoraces were not aspirated in the belief that tamponade of the injured lung had occurred. However, when surgery was required for thoracic injury, it was aggressive and largely successful following principles of air-tight closure for wounds and removal of foreign bodies. In contrast to their surgical counterparts in the German Army, American surgeons with the Allied Expeditionary Force used positive-pressure anesthesia and a nitrous oxide/oxygen mixture, while practicing early thoracotomies following the principles for good exposure injuries, resection of affected anatomic structures, suture ligature, and irrigation of the thoracic cavity.[7,8] Thoracotomies were closed air tight, traumatic wounds excised, and no drains were placed. This technique was associated with a 9% decrease in mortality.[7,8] During this time Grey-Turner, Miles, Gask, Duval, and Bastianelli[9] defined the technique of pulmonary decortication for the treatment of retained hemothorax after traumatic lung injuries.

In World War II, because of increased awareness of the high incidence of complications associated with hemothorax after wounding, an approach of aggressive conservatism for the management of hemothorax was adopted.[7,8] Thoracentesis was used repeatedly, until the thoracic cavity was totally evacuated. No air was permitted to enter the thoracic cavity. The injured lung was allowed to re-expand and tamponade bleeding, in hopes of returning pulmonary function to normal levels. Water-sealed intercostal catheters were placed in patients with tension pneumothoraces. Thoracotomy was reserved for continued hemorrhage or significant air leaks; additional indications included thoracoabdominal wounds, mediastinal injuries, traumatic thoracotomy, "the sucking chest wound," and removal of foreign bodies. Overall mortality with this treatment of war chest wounds was reported as 8%.[7,8]

The Korean conflict created newer challenges for surgeons.[7,8] Terrain characteristics and unfavorable tactical conditions, coupled with numerous incoming casualties, overloaded mobile army surgical hospitals (MASH units). Conservative management of traumatic hemothorax was thus a therapeutic strategy extremely suited to these conditions. Eighty percent of casualties from the Korean War were managed by repeated thoracentesis alone; however, there was limited experience with the use of chest tubes for drainage of hemothorax. The introduction of more advanced resuscitative techniques helped to compensate somewhat for the problems encountered with forward treatment.[7,8]

In the Vietnam conflict, chest tube drainage for pulmonary injuries and hemothorax was widely practiced. Casualties were evacuated early at the hospital directly from combat. Well-organized "trauma centers," with cardiothoracic surgical capabilities operated under strict resuscitative protocols.[4,5,7,8] Given the success of tube thoracostomy in this setting, early thoracotomy was indicated for fewer patients with hemothorax, although the former indications for its use remained. Tube thoracostomy remains the cornerstone for the treatment of traumatic hemothorax or pneumothorax, as well as for most traumatic injuries to the lung.[10]

Recent awareness based on civilian and military experience has led to the recognition that complex procedures, such as anatomic resections and pneumonectomy in unstable patients, are poorly tolerated and potentially daunting.[7] Critically injured patients often develop hypothermia, acidosis, coagulopathy,[11] and dysrhythmias,[12–14] resulting in irreversible physiologic injury. Control of such damage is also part of the trauma surgeon's armamentarium to deal with thoracic injuries.[15–18] Progress in treating severe pulmonary injuries in critical patients has thus far relied on finding shorter, simpler, lung-sparing techniques, such as wedge and nonanatomic resections, and pneumonorrhaphy stapled and clamp tractotomy.[4,7,19–25] In 1994, Wall et al.[7] described clamp pulmonary tractotomy to maximize pulmonary parenchymal salvage. Asensio and colleagues in 1997[19] described the technique of stapled pulmonary tractotomy. The applicability of stapled pulmonary tractotomy was subsequently confirmed as a safe, valuable, lung-sparing procedure in a series of 40 patients. Subsequently, Cothren and associates[22] reported that lung-sparing techniques are associated with an improved morbidity and mortality compared with resectional techniques.

Rapid progress and advancement in technology, including endoscopic instrumentation anesthetic techniques, have revolutionized thoracic surgery and ushered in the era of video-assisted thoracoscopic surgery (VATS).[26] VATS has provided the trauma surgeon with an alternative method for accurate and direct evaluation of the lung parenchyma, mediastinum, and diaphragmatic injuries, with the advantage of simultaneously allowing definitive treatment of such injuries. VATS also has been demonstrated to be an accurate, safe, and reliable operative therapy for complications of lung trauma, including post-traumatic pleural collections.[27]

▮ INCIDENCE

The true incidence of pulmonary injuries is unknown, and difficult to estimate from the literature.[28–35] The chest, in forming such a large and exposed part of the body, is particularly vulnerable to injury. The anatomic complex formed by the lungs, pulmonary vessels, and bronchial tree so completely fills the thorax that penetration or contusion of the chest rarely occurs without injury.[36–38] The reported incidence of pulmonary injuries in the civilian arena varies according to authors and institutions. In 1979, Graham et al.[36] reported a 1-year experience, consisting of 373 patients sustaining penetrating pulmonary injuries; of these, 91 patients (24%) underwent thoracotomy, although operative interventions on the lung itself were only required in 45 (12%) patients. In this series, the mere presence of post-traumatic hemothorax or pneumothorax was considered by the authors as clear evidence of traumatic pulmonary injury, which justified the inclusion of these cases in the study.

In 1988, Robison et al.[39] described a 13-year civilian experience in the management of penetrating pulmonary injuries in 1168 patients sustaining penetrating chest injuries; however, only 68 patients required thoracotomy to manage traumatic lung injury. In 1988, Thompson et al.[40] reported a 5-year experience of 2608 patients with thoracic trauma. Of the total, 1663 patients sustained injuries from blunt trauma and only 11 (0.7%) required thoracotomy; 945 sustained penetrating injuries and 15 (1.6%) required thoracotomy. Wiencek and Wilson[35] reported a series consisting of 161 patients requiring thoracotomy for civilian penetrating pulmonary injuries during a 7-year period, which translates to 23 cases per year. Wagner et al.[37] described a 4-year experience of 104 patients with significant blunt chest trauma; 115 pulmonary lacerations were detected in 75 patients, for an incidence of 72%; 86% of these injuries were diagnosed by computed tomography (CT) scan, and 14% were detected by surgery. Based on both radiological and surgical findings, the authors reported a higher incidence of traumatic pulmonary injuries compared with other clinical series that report their results based only in surgical findings.

In 1993, Tominaga and colleagues[41] described a 7-year single institutional experience of 2934 patients sustaining both blunt and penetrating chest trauma; 347 patients (12%) required thoracotomy, and 12 (3.5%) in this subgroup required pulmonary resections. The mechanism of injury was blunt in 25%, and penetrating in 75% of cases, for an incidence of 0.04%, translating into 1.7 cases per year. Wagner and associates[42] in 1996 described an 8-year experience of 1804 patients admitted with chest trauma; 269 (15%) underwent thoracotomy, with 55 requiring operative interventions specifically for their pulmonary injuries, for an incidence of 3%, and an average of 6.9 patients per year.

In 1997, Stewart et al.[43] reported a 10-year experience consisting of 2455 patients with both penetrating and blunt chest trauma; 183 (7.4%) patients required thoracotomy, and 32 (17.4%) required pulmonary resection, which translates to 3.2 cases per year. Inci and colleagues[44] in 1998 reported a 5-year experience consisting of 755 patients sustaining penetrating chest trauma, of whom 61 (8.1%) required thoracotomy; however, specific operative interventions for penetrating pulmonary injuries were required in only three patients (4.9%), for an incidence of 0.6 cases per year.

In 1998, Wall et al.[4] described a 3-year experience of 236 patients requiring thoracotomy for penetrating chest trauma; 90 (38%) required repair or resection to manage their pulmonary lacerations, for an average of 30 patients per year. In 2001, Karmy-Jones and colleagues[21,45] reported the findings of a multicenter 4-year review of five Level I trauma centers. A total of 43,119 patients were admitted for penetrating thoracic trauma, and 290 (2.8%) required thoracotomy; surprisingly, 115 patients (40%) in this subgroup underwent some type of lung resection. In a series of 4087 patients admitted for chest trauma, Cothren and associates[22] reported that 416 patients (10%) patients required thoracotomy and 36 (9%) required surgical interventions on the lung, for an incidence of 1% and an average of 3.3 patients per year.

In the most recent report dealing with complex civilian lung injuries, in 2006, Asensio et al.[46] described 101 patients requiring thoracotomy for complex penetrating pulmonary injuries. In the military arena, Zakharia et al.[47] in 1985 reported 1992 casualties during the fighting in Lebanon; 1422 patients underwent thoracotomy for hemodynamic instability secondary to penetrating chest trauma, and pulmonary injuries were present in 210 (15%) patients, for an incidence of 11%. In 1997, Petricevic and associates[48] reported on 2547 casualties from the most recent Balkan war experience. During a period of 4 years, 424 patients (16%) sustained both blunt and penetrating chest wounds; among these patients, 81 (19%) underwent thoracotomy for pulmonary injury, for an incidence of 20 cases per year.

ETIOLOGY

Most patients requiring thoracotomy for pulmonary injuries will have suffered penetrating mechanisms of injury—gunshot wounds, stab wounds, and shotgun wounds. Much less common are blunt thoracic injuries requiring operative intervention. In 2003, Huh et al.[24] reported a gradual rise in the incidence of blunt thoracic injuries, mostly from motor vehicle collisions requiring operative intervention, from 3% before 1994, to 12% in the latter period. In the series by Tominaga and colleagues,[41] blunt mechanism of injury accounted for 25% of all pulmonary injuries requiring surgical treatment. In the civilian arena, gunshot wounds represent the major penetrating mechanism for patients requiring surgical treatment; several authors[4,21,22,35–37,39–41,43–46] have reported that gunshot wounds account for 33%–80% of cases with penetrating pulmonary injuries, while stab wounds account for 17%–67% of these injuries. Karmy-Jones et al.,[21,45] in a multicenter study on managing traumatic lung injuries, reported an increasing rate of thoracotomy among these patients. Other mechanisms such as impalement and shotgun wounds are reported with a lower frequency of 1%–5% of cases.[44,46]

In a series from 2006, Asensio et al.[46] reported on 101 patients who required thoracotomy for treatment of civilian penetrating pulmonary injuries. In this series, gunshot wounds accounted for most cases (72% of cases); stab wounds and other mechanisms (e.g., impalement, shotgun wounds) accounted for 33% and 5% of cases, respectively. In the military arena, Zakharia et al.[47] reported from the experience in Lebanon that high-velocity gunshot wounds and shelling in urban battles were the major mechanisms of pulmonary injuries. Petricevic and colleagues[48] reported the etiology of pulmonary injuries during the war in Croatia, where explosive wounds prevailed (59%), followed by gunshot wounds (both high and low velocity, 37%), whereas other types of wounds—stabbing and falling—accounted for only 4% of cases.

CLASSIFICATION

The American Association for the Surgery of Trauma Organ Injury Scaling Committee (AAST-OIS) described the lung injury scale in 1994.[49] This scale facilitates clinical research and provides a common nomenclature by which trauma surgeons may describe lung injuries and their severity. The grading scheme is fundamentally an anatomic description, scaled from 1 to 5, describing the least to the most severe injury. Thus far, studies have correlated injury grade with mortality for this study (Table 1).

DIAGNOSIS

The diagnosis of traumatic pulmonary injuries is established by physical examination and adjunctive diagnostic modalities.[37,38,50–74]

Physical Examination

The clinical presentation of patients who sustain pulmonary injuries ranges from hemodynamic stability to cardiopulmonary arrest.[50] Physical examination yields a wealth of diagnostic infor-

Table 1: Lung Injury: Organ Injury Scaling, American Association for the Surgery of Trauma

Grade[a]	Injury Type	Description[b]
I	Contusion	Unilateral, <1 lobe
II	Contusion	Unilateral, single lobe
	Laceration	Simple pneumothorax
III	Contusion	Unilateral, >1 lobe
	Laceration	Persistent (>72 hours), air leak from distal airway
	Hematoma	Nonexpanding intraparenchymal
IV	Laceration	Major (segmental or lobar) air leak
	Hematoma	Expanding intraparenchymal
	Vascular	Primary branch intrapulmonary vessel disruption
V	Vascular	Hilar vessel disruption
VI	Vascular	Total, uncontained transection of pulmonary hilum

[a]Advance one grade for multiple injuries up to grade III. Hemothorax is scored under thoracic vascular organ injury scale.
[b]Based on most accurate assessment at autopsy, operation, or radiological study.

mation, which is used to indicate emergent interventions on these patients.[51]

Patients with pulmonary injuries may present with symptoms and signs of pneumohemothorax or an open pneumothorax with partial loss of the chest wall.[50,52] They may also present with a tension hemothorax or pneumothorax, or rarely, with a pneumomediastinum upon auscultation. Hamman's crunch—a systolic crunch—may be detected upon auscultation in these patients. Similarly, they may also present with a pneumopericardium detected by auscultating Brichiteau's windmill bruit (bruit de moulin). Patients with penetrating pulmonary injuries may rarely present with true hemoptysis. Occasionally, these patients present with symptoms and signs of an associated cardiac injury.[30,31,50,65,68]

During the evaluation of these patients, the trauma surgeon must be cognizant that the thoracic cavity is composed of both right and left hemithoracic cavity as well as the anterior, posterior, and superior mediastinum; as often missiles or other wounding agents may traverse one or more of these cavities.[50,53–57] Similarly, missile trajectories are often unpredictable and frequently create secondary missiles if they impact on hard bony structures (ribs, sternum, spine), thus creating the potential for associated injuries and greater damage.

Adjunctive Diagnostic Modalities

Adjunctive diagnostic modalities are divided into noninvasive diagnostic modalities and invasive diagnostic modalities.

Noninvasive Diagnostic Modalities

These diagnostic modalities include trauma ultrasound (focused assessment with sonography for trauma [FAST]), chest x-ray (CXR), CT, and electrocardiogram (EKG).

Trauma ultrasound

Trauma ultrasound is performed as part of the secondary survey of the trauma patient, and remains a valuable diagnostic modality used to detect associated cardiac injuries as well as the presence of associated abdominal injuries in patients sustaining isolated chest trauma and multiply injured patients.[58,59] In 2004, Kirkpatrick et al.[60] reported the use of sonography for detecting traumatic pneumothoraces and described this diagnostic strategy as extended FAST (EFAST). Normal thoracic sonograms reveal comet-tail artifacts, originating from the sliding and reapposition of the visceral onto the parietal pleura during the ventilatory effort; post-traumatic pneumothoraces are diagnosed when comet-tail artifacts are absent. The authors enrolled 225 patients in this study, and concluded that EFAST has comparable specificity (99.1% vs. 98.7%) to CXR, but was more sensitive (58.9% vs. 48.8%) for the detection of post-traumatic pneumothoraces. Knudson and colleagues[61] in 2004 performed 328 thoracic evaluations in trauma patients and described thoracic sonography having a specificity of 99.7%, a negative predictive value of 99.7%, and an accuracy of 99.4% when used for diagnosing post-traumatic pneumothorax. However, thoracic sonography was noted to be more sensitive (100% vs. 88.9%) and with a higher positive-predictive value (100% vs. 88.9%) when used to diagnose post-traumatic pneumothoraces in patients sustaining penetrating versus blunt trauma, although the specificity (100% vs. 99.7%), negative-predictive value (100% vs. 99.7%), and accuracy (100% vs. 99.3%) are comparable. On the basis of these findings, Knudson et al.[61] concluded that ultrasound is a reliable modality for the diagnosis of pneumothorax in the injured patient, and thus, it may serve as an adjunct or precursor to routine chest radiography in the evaluation of injured patients.

Sonography has also been employed to detect the presence of traumatic hemothorax. The technique for this examination is similar to evaluate the upper quadrants of the abdomen. The transducer is advanced to identify the hyperechoic diaphragm and to evaluate both right and left supradiaphragmatic spaces for the presence or absence of fluid. Sisley and associates[62] in 1998 evaluated 360 patients with suspected blunt or penetrating torso trauma, with 40 post-traumatic effusions, 39 (98%) of which were detected by sonography and 37 (93%) by CXR. The authors concluded that sonography is more sensitive (97.5 vs. 92.5%) than CXR for detecting post-traumatic effusions; however, a specificity of 97.5% in both studies is comparable. On the basis of these data the authors concluded that surgeon-performed thoracic sonography is as accurate as, but significantly faster than, supine portable chest radiography for the detection of traumatic effusion.

Chest X-Ray

A standard supine posteroanterior CXR is the most frequently used diagnostic modality in patients who sustain traumatic lung injury.[6,10,15,23,30,31,36–38,44,50,52,59,63] Radiological diagnosis of traumatic pulmonary injuries by CXR is based on the presence of pneumothorax, pleural fluid collections, intrapulmonary hematomas, traumatic pneumatoceles, and pulmonary parenchymal contusions. Although CXR has been demonstrated to be 99% specific, it is a relatively insensitive test (49%) for the detection of post-traumatic pneumothorax; CXR has been demonstrated to possess a sensitivity of 93% and a specificity of 99.7% to detect post-traumatic pleural effusions.

When compared with CT, the conventional CXR underestimates or overlooks both parenchymal and pleural injuries, and has poor ability to determine the magnitude of pulmonary parenchymal compromise or pneumothorax size.[37,38,63] Wagner et al.[37] demonstrated that pulmonary parenchymal lacerations are frequently missed by CXR.

Computed tomography

Computed tomography is found to be more sensitive than CXR for diagnosing traumatic pulmonary injuries.[37,38,63] The most common types of abnormalities seen on CT scans include parenchymal lacerations, post-traumatic hemothorax, post-traumatic pneumothorax, atelectasis, subcutaneous emphysema, pneumopericardium and hemopericardium, and chest wall fractures. Additional diagnostic information related to the traumatic injury to the lung is usually supplied by CT scans, which can reliably detect the presence and extent of subtle or considerable parenchymal contusion.

As described by Karaaslan et al.[38] in 1995, CT scans are also able to detect the presence of associated thoracic and mediastinal vascular injuries, injuries to other thoracic great vessels, and extrathoracic injuries, associated cervical spine injuries, and intra-abdominal injuries in about 30% of cases.

Electrocardiogram

Nonspecific EKG abnormalities are often seen in trauma patients[64–70]; some of these changes such as sinus tachycardia, and ventricular and atrial extrasystoles are related to systemic factors such as pain, decreased intravascular volume, hypoxia, abnormal concentration of serum electrolytes, and changes in sympathetic or parasympathetic tone; however, in some cases, EKG may exhibit changes caused by associated injuries—most commonly penetrating or blunt cardiac trauma consisting of findings related to myocardial injury like new Q waves, ST-T segmental elevation or depression, conduction disorders such as right-bundle branch block, fascicular block, AV nodal conduction disorders, and other arrhythmias (atrial fibrillation, ventricular tachycardia, ventricular fibrillation, sinus bradycardia, and atrial tachycardia).[69–72]

Electrocardiogram findings may suggest the presence of pericardial tamponade in patients sustaining chest trauma and traumatic lung injuries. Low QRS voltage is closely associated with the presence of a large or moderate pericardial tamponade (sensitivity of 0%–42%, specificity of 86%–97%),[69,70] although PR segment depression and electrical alternans commonly are also present in this setting.[71,72]

Invasive Diagnostic Modalities

Chest tubes

Chest tube placement may be diagnostic as well as therapeutic.[10] After entering the pleural cavity, a finger is inserted, and depending on the position of the tract, the trauma surgeon may palpate the lung surface for the presence of contusion, the surface of the diaphragm for lacerations, and the pericardial sac to detect the presence of tamponade.

The nature and amount of the material draining from the tube is also important. The amount of blood evacuated upon initial placement of the chest tube may indicate the need for thoracotomy; persistent drainage of blood through the tube thoracostomy obligates the trauma surgeon to reassess the need for surgical intervention.[56,57] Drainage of gastrointestinal contents implies an esophageal,[54,55] gastric, or intestinal injury[53] associated with a diaphragmatic laceration.[73] An air leak implies an underlying lung laceration, and large air leaks may indicate bronchial disruption.[10,34,35,40,52,53,56,57,74]

ASSOCIATED INJURIES

Associated injuries are commonly seen in conjunction with penetrating pulmonary injuries.[46] Five to 65% of patients sustaining traumatic injuries to the lung present thoracic- or extrathoracic-associated injuries[20,22,24,25,35,36,39,41,43,45,46,48]; the average number of associated injuries reported in the literature ranges from 0.5 to 1.9 injuries per patient. The presence of an associated injury is an important determinant of outcome. Gasparri et al.[25] reported the presence of associated cardiac injury and the need for laparotomy for associated abdominal injuries as factors determining the mortality, while Asensio et al.[46] determined that the presence of an associated cardiac injury is an independent predictor of outcome.

Graham et al.[36] reported the presence of 73 associated thoracic injuries among 91 patients requiring thoracotomy for the management of penetrating pulmonary injuries, for an average of 0.8 associated thoracic injuries per patient; the most commonly injured organs included the heart, at 27%; intercostals, 16%; subclavian vessels, 9%;

and superior vena cava, 7%. The authors also reported the presence of 175 associated abdominal injuries among 89 of the patients requiring laparotomy, for an average of 1.9 associated abdominal injuries per patient; the most frequently injured organs were the liver, 21%; spleen, 19%; stomach, 14%; and colon, 10%.

Robison and colleagues[39] described the presence of 14 associated injuries in 11 of 28 patients sustaining traumatic lung injuries requiring thoracotomy and pulmonary resection or hilar repairs. In this series, the authors reported a morbidity rate of 39% and an average number of 1.3 injuries per patient. Cardiac injuries were present in 11% of cases; the remaining associated injuries follow: thoracic great vessel injuries, 7%; spinal cord injuries, 7%; hepatic injuries, 7%; pancreatic, 4%; colonic, 4%; spleen, 4%; gastric, 4%; and peripheral nerve, 4%.

Wiencek et al.[35] described the presence of 35 major associated injuries among 19 of 25 patients with central lung injuries, for an incidence of 76% and an average number of 1.4 injuries per patient, with the heart (26%) and thoracic great vessels (21%) as the most frequently injured organs. Associated abdominal injuries requiring laparotomy were found in 58% of cases. Tominaga and associates[41] reported 10 associated injuries among 12 patients that required thoracotomy and lung resection for traumatic pulmonary injuries, for an average of 0.8 injuries per patient. Associated injuries included head injuries at 17%; intra-abdominal injuries requiring laparotomy, 33%; cardiac injuries, 25%; and great vessel injury, 8%. Petricevic et al.[48] reported a 4.5% incidence of associated injuries to visceral organs in patients sustaining chest trauma during the war in Croatia. Stewart and colleagues[43] described the presence of 30 associated injuries in 21 of 32 patients (65%) requiring thoracotomy and pulmonary resection for traumatic injuries to the lung, for an average of 1.4 injuries per patient; these injuries were stratified into abdominal, 30%; musculoskeletal, 30%; neurologic, 17%; cardiac, 7%; and other injuries, 17%.

Gasparri et al.[25] reported associated injuries in 41 (58%) of 70 patients requiring thoracotomy for penetrating lung injuries, with cardiac (20%), diaphragmatic (17%), and hepatic (11%) as the most common organs involved. Karmy-Jones and colleagues[45] reported 42 associated thoracic injuries among 115 patients requiring thoracotomy and lung resection for penetrating chest trauma, for an average of 0.36 injuries per patient.

Cothren et al.[22] reported 27 associated injuries in a series of 36 patients requiring thoracotomy for severe pulmonary injuries, for an average of 0.75 injuries per patient. Associated thoracic injuries were present in 33% of patients, while associated extrathoracic injuries represented 66% of the total. Huh and colleagues[24] reported that 28% of patients requiring operative interventions on the lung required a concomitant laparotomy for intra-abdominal injuries.

Asensio and associates[46] in 2006 reported a 169-month, single-center experience consisting of 101 patients requiring thoracotomy for penetrating pulmonary injuries. In this series, there were 193 associated injuries for an average of 1.9 injuries per patient. There were 39 (22%) associated injuries to the thoracic organs, and 154 (79.7%) associated extrathoracic injuries. The most common thoracic organs involved were the heart (23.7%) and thoracic great vessels (14.8%), while the most common extrathoracic organs were the diaphragm (42.5%), liver (25.7%), and stomach (18.8%).

ANATOMIC LOCATION OF INJURY

The anatomic location of pulmonary injuries is not commonly reported in either clinical or radiological series.[24,35,36,39,46] Graham et al.[36] reported a predominance of left-sided lung injuries at 52% compared with right-side lung injuries at 36%, with bilateral injuries present in 12% of patients. Wiencek et al.,[35] in a series focusing on central/hilar traumatic lung injuries, reported an incidence of 15% of hilar traumatic disruptions among 161 patients sustaining penetrating lung trauma. Robison and colleagues[39] described the anatomic

location of traumatic lung injuries requiring resective techniques for surgical management as follows: left lower lobe, 28%; right middle lobe, 22%; left upper lobe, including lingula, 22%; right upper lobe, 17%; and right lower lobe, 17%. The left pulmonary artery (25%) was the most commonly injured pulmonary vessel, followed by the right pulmonary artery (14%), right pulmonary vein (11%), and left pulmonary vein (7%). The results of this series showed that traumatic injuries presented a slight right versus left preference, although left-sided vascular injuries were more common compared with right-sided pulmonary vascular injuries, at 56% and 44%, respectively.

Huh and associates[24] reported that the location of the traumatic pulmonary injuries requiring operative intervention showed a slight predilection for the left side (50%), followed by the right side (47%) and bilateral injuries (3%). Asensio et al.,[46] in a report consisting of 101 patients requiring thoracotomy for complex penetrating pulmonary injuries, found the left lung to be a predominant location of penetrating injuries compared with the right lung (65% vs. 35%, respectively). The authors also reported the specific location of these injuries: left lower lobe, 40%; left upper lobe, 21%; right middle lobe, 19%; right lower lobe, 11%; lingula, 5%; and right upper lobe, 5%.

MANAGEMENT

Although recent reports of thoracic injuries in military actions have advocated early thoracotomy and aggressive management of pulmonary injuries with resection as opposed to the more conservative and traditional treatment with tube thoracostomy,[35,39,40,44,47,48,77-81] the vast majority of thoracic trauma patients—75%–85%—are successfully managed with placement of chest tubes and supportive measures.[4,7,10,21,22,24,36,39,41,43,45] The combination of lung expansion, low intravascular pressures, and high concentration of tissue thromboplastin provides adequate hemostasis in most instances[20]; however, 9%–15% of patients require thoracotomy to achieve surgical hemostasis or effect necessary repairs.[35,39,40,44,47,48,77-81] Of patients undergoing thoracotomy for hemorrhage, 3%–30% have been shown to require lung resection for control of injuries.[20,21,23,24,26,32,35,36,39-45,48]

The indications for thoracotomy in patients sustaining penetrating pulmonary injuries include the following[35,36,39,40,44,47,48,74-85]:

- Cardiopulmonary arrest[39,75,76]
- Impeding cardiopulmonary arrest upon arrival at the emergency department (ED)[39,75,76]
- Evacuation of 1000–1500 ml of blood upon initial placement of chest tube[33,35,36,39,47,48]
- Evacuation of more than 1000 ml of blood upon placement of chest tube and ongoing blood loss[33,35,36,39,47,48]
- Tension hemothorax[36,39,75,76,79-81]
- Large retained hemothorax[44,82-85]
- Massive air leak from the chest tube[36,39,40,74]

Surgical Decisions

For patients who present in cardiopulmonary arrest, it is mandatory to proceed to ED thoracotomy.[75,76] The placement of a chest tube in the right hemithoracic cavity is required. This may need to be extended into bilateral anterolateral thoracotomies.[75,76] For patients who present with systolic blood pressure lower than 80 mm Hg, it is mandatory to insert bilateral chest tubes and resuscitate per the Advanced Trauma Life Support protocol. If the patient remains unstable, he or she should be immediately transported to the operating room (OR). If the patient stabilizes, a thorough work-up should be instituted.[75,76] For patients presenting with thoracoabdominal injuries, insertion of a chest tube or tubes is recommended. In patients who sustain abdominal and thoracic or thoracoabdominal injuries and require exploratory laparotomy, the trauma surgeon should reassess the need for thoracotomy in the OR.[53–55,66–68,73–76]

Operative Management

Emergency Department Thoracotomy

If the patient arrives at the ED in cardiopulmonary arrest, it is necessary to immediately proceed to ED thoracotomy.[75,76] The objectives of ED thoracotomy follow:

- Resuscitation of agonal patients with penetrating cardiothoracic injuries
- Evacuation of pericardial tamponade if there is an associated cardiac injury
- Direct repair of cardiac lacerations if there is an associated cardiac injury[65–68]
- Control of thoracic hemorrhage
- Prevention of air embolism
- Perform cardiopulmonary resuscitation, which may produce up to 60% of the normal ejection fraction
- Control of the pulmonary hemorrhage
- Cross-clamp pulmonary hilum
- Cross-clamp descending thoracic aorta[75,76]

The technique for ED thoracotomy is described as it pertains to its use for patients sustaining penetrating pulmonary injuries arriving in cardiopulmonary arrest, and should only be performed by surgeons that have had appropriate training in the performance of this procedure[75,76]:

1. Immediate endotracheal intubation and venous access are performed; and simultaneous use of rapid infusion techniques complements the resuscitative process. Chest tube insertion in the right hemithoracic cavity is also simultaneous.[75,76]
2. The left arm is elevated and the thorax is prepped rapidly with an antiseptic solution.[75,76]
3. A left anterolateral thoracotomy commencing at the lateral border of the left sternocostal junction and inferior to the nipple is carried out and extended laterally to the latissimus dorsi. In females, the breast is retracted cephalad.[75,76]
4. The incision is carried rapidly through skin, subcutaneous tissue, and the pectoralis major and serratus anterior muscles until the intercostal muscles are reached.[75,76]
5. The three layers of these interdigitated muscles are sharply transected with scissors. The pleura is then opened.[75,76]
6. Occasionally, the left fourth and fifth costochondral cartilages are transected to provide greater exposure.[75,76]
7. A Finochietto retractor is then placed to separate the ribs. At this time, the trauma surgeon should evaluate the extent of hemorrhage present within the left hemithoracic cavity. An exsanguinating hemorrhage with almost complete loss of the patient's intravascular volume is a reliable indicator of poor outcome.[13,14,65–68,75,76]
8. The left lung is then elevated medially and the descending thoracic aorta is located immediately as it enters the abdomen vita the aortic hiatus. The aorta should be palpated to assess the status of the remaining blood volume.[75,76]
9. The descending thoracic aorta can be temporarily occluded against the bodies of the thoracic vertebrae.[75,76]
10. Before cross-clamping the descending thoracic aorta, a combination of sharp and blunt dissection commencing at both the superior and inferior borders of the aorta is performed, so that the aorta may be carefully encircled between the thumb and index fingers.[75,76]
11. Inexperienced surgeons usually commit the error of clamping the esophagus, which is located superior to the aorta. A nasogastric tube previously placed can serve as a guide in distinguishing the esophagus from the often somewhat empty thoracic aorta.[75,76]
12. A Craafoord-DeBakey aortic cross-clamp should then be placed to occlude the aorta.[75,76]
13. If a cardiac injury is present, the pericardium is then opened longitudinally above the phrenic nerve; pericardial clot and blood are evacuated and the cardiac injury repaired.[65–68,75,76]
14. If a pulmonary hilar hematoma or active hemorrhage is present, cross-clamping of the pulmonary hilum with a Craafoord-DeBakey cross-clamp may be necessary.[33,35,40,42,75,76,86–90]
15. If a parenchymal laceration is detected, it should be clamped with Duval clamps.[15–17,19,23,41,44,75,77,80,86]
16. If the initial injury is located in the right hemithoracic cavity, or the previously inserted chest tube returns large quantities of blood, or pathology is encountered in the contralateral hemithoracic cavity, the sternum is transected sharply and the left anterolateral thoracotomy is then converted to a bilateral anterolateral thoracotomies.[75,76]
17. Ligation of one or both internal mammary arteries may be necessary if the left anterolateral thoracotomy has been extended to the right hemithoracic cavity.[75,76]
18. Aggressive ongoing resuscitation is needed with warm, pressure-driven fluids via rapid infusers while this procedure is ongoing.[75,76,87,88,91,92]
19. Defibrillation with internal paddles may be needed, delivering 10–50 joules.[66–68,75,76,89]
20. Epinephrine may also be administrated into the right or left ventricle or systemically.[66–68,75,76,89]
21. If air embolism is suspected, the ventricles will need to be aspirated with 16-gauge needles.[66–68,75,76]
22. Occasionally the use of a temporary pacemaker might be needed but outcomes are very poor.[66–68,75,76]
23. If the patient is successfully resuscitated, immediate and expedient transportation to the OR is mandated for definitive repair of the pulmonary injury or injuries.[75,76]

Effects of pulmonary hilar cross-clamping

Positive These effects include: (1) preservation and redistribution of remaining blood volume, (2) improvement in perfusion to contralateral uninjured lung, (3) control of hilar hemorrhage, and (4) prevention of air emboli.[75,76]

Negative These effects include: (1) renders cross-clamped lung ischemic, (2) imposes a great afterload onto the right ventricle (RV), and (3) decreases oxygenation and ventilation to cross-clamped lung.[75,76]

Unknown These effects include: length of safe cross-clamp time and incidence of pulmonary reperfusion injury to both the injured and uninjured lung.[75,76]

Effects of thoracic aortic cross-clamping

Positive These effects follow: (1) preservation and redistribution of remaining blood volume, (2) improvement of coronary/carotid arterial perfusion, (3) reduction of subdiaphragmatic blood flow, (4) increases in the left ventricular stroke work index (LVSWI), and (5) increased myocardial contractility.[75,76]

Negative These effects include: (1) decreases blood flow to the abdominal viscera to approximately 10%, (2) decreases renal blood flow to approximately 10%, (3) decreases blood flow to the spinal cord to approximately 10%, (4) induces anaerobic metabolism, (5) induces hypoxia/lactic acidosis, (6) imposes a great afterload onto the left ventricle (LV), and (7) may (rarely) cause paraplegia.[75,76]

Unknown These effects include: (1) length of safe cross-clamp time, and (2) incidence of reperfusion injury.[75,76]

Operating Room Thoracotomy

Instruments

Special instruments are needed to access the thoracic cavity as well as to retract, manipulate, and surgically intervene in the thoracic structures and lung (Figure 1). These instruments include the following:

- Doyen costal elevators (Figure 2)
- Alexander periostotome (see Figure 2)
- Cameron-Haight periosteal elevators (see Figure 2)
- Bethune rib shears (Figure 3)
- Stille-Horsley bone cutting rongeurs (see Figure 3)
- Lebsche Knife and mallet (see Figure 3)
- Rib raspatory
- Finochietto retractor
- Davidson scapular retractor (Figure 4)

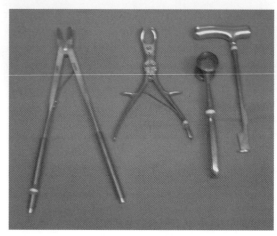

Figure 3   Bethune rib shears, Stille-Horsley bone cutting rongeurs, and Lebsche knife and mallet.

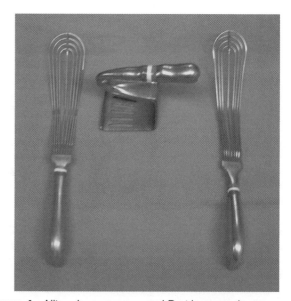

Figure 4   Allison lung retractors, and Davidson scapular retractor.

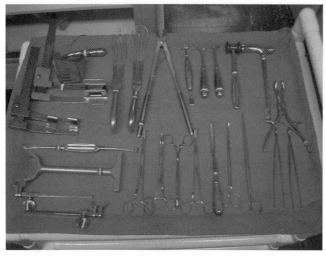

Figure 1   Thoracic instrument tray.

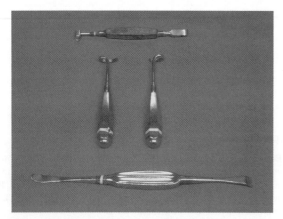

Figure 2   Alexander periostotome, right and left Doyen costal elevators, and Cameron-Haight periosteal elevator.

- Allison lung retractors (see Figure 4)
- Semb lung retractors
- Nelson lung dissecting lobectomy scissors (Figure 5)
- Metzenbaum long dissecting scissors (see Figure 5)
- Tuttle thoracic tissue forceps (see Figure 5)
- Duval lung forceps (Figure 6)
- Davidson pulmonary vessel clamps
- Sarot bronchus clamps
- Bailey's rib approximator (Figure 7)
- Berry sternal needle holder
- vascular clamps[75,76,93–95]

Adjuncts

Double-lumen tubes are invaluable adjuncts in the management of penetrating pulmonary injuries (Figure 8). Although more difficult to insert by the anesthesiologists, double-lumen tubes are designed to ventilate the right or left lung selectively.[64,75,76,78,91] There are two types of double-lumen tubes; one is designed for the left and the other for the right mainstem bronchus. By inflating the balloon that occludes either the right or left mainstem bronchus, the lung can be collapsed, thus allowing the trauma surgeon to operate on a

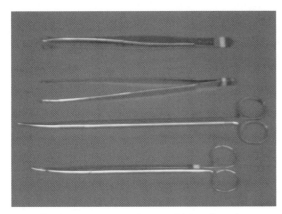

Figure 5 Tuttle thoracic tissue forceps, Nelson lung dissecting lobectomy scissors, and Metzenbaum long dissecting scissors.

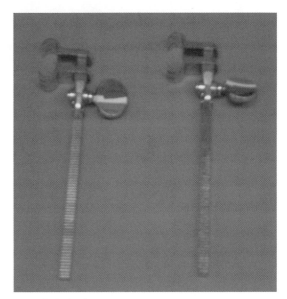

Figure 7 Bailey's rib approximator.

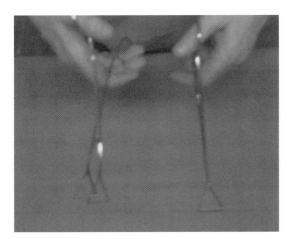

Figure 6 Duval lung forceps.

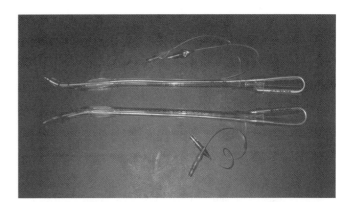

Figure 8 Double lumen endotracheal tubes.

collapsed and still lung.[64] Bronchoscopy is also an invaluable adjunct when used intraoperatively. It can serve as a diagnostic tool by locating injured bronchi at the lobar and even segmental levels. It can also be therapeutic by removing blood within the tracheobronchial tree, which tends to cause bronchospasm.[35,40,92]

Ventilation

There are two types of ventilation that can be employed in the operating room. The conventional method intermittently allows for a periodic inflation/deflation of the lung, and high-frequency jet ventilation (Figure 9), which allows the trauma surgeon to operate on a nonmoving still lung.[64]

Surgical incisions and exposures

No single incision will allow the surgeon to access all compartments of the thoracic cavity. The incisions used to access the thorax for the management of penetrating pulmonary injuries include anterolateral thoracotomy (Spangaro's incision), posterolateral thoracotomy, right posterolateral thoracotomy, left posterolateral thoracotomy, and median sternotomy (Duval-Barasty's incision).[93–95]

Anterolateral thoracotomy (Spangaro's incision) This incision is the most frequently used one to access the right or left hemithoracic cavity, as most of these patients will be transported to the operating room with some degree of hemodynamic instabil-

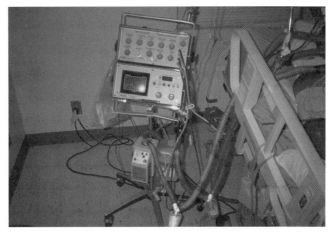

Figure 9 High-frequency jet ventilator (Percussonator™).

ity.[66–68,75,76,95] This incision allows the trauma surgeon to operate on either the right or left lung, although it provides for a very limited operating field. It does not allow access to the posterior structures of the right or left hemithoracic cavity. The left anterolateral thoracotomy will provide access to the heart and the descending thoracic aorta should cross-clamping be necessary if the patient's hemodynamic instability and/or cardiopulmonary arrest demands it.[66–68,75,76,95]

The anterolateral thoracotomy is also the incision of choice when the thoracic cavity needs to be accessed in the presence of an associated abdominal injury. Anterolateral thoracotomy may be extended into bilateral anterolateral thoracotomies if associated pathology is found in the contralateral hemithoracic cavity.[53,66–68,73,75,76,95]

Posterolateral thoracotomy This incision provides for the very best exposure for the management of penetrating pulmonary injuries. The disadvantage of this incision is that it is time consuming, as it requires a special positioning of the patient on the operating table.[93–95] Most of these patients are usually transported to the operating room with hemodynamic instability and cannot afford the luxury of being placed in this position. This incision provides suboptimal access for the management of associated cardiac injuries.[66–68,75,76,95]

Right posterolateral thoracotomy This incision provides access to the right lung, the thoracic esophagus up to its most distal portion when it crosses anterior to the thoracic aorta into the left hemithoracic cavity and superior to the descending thoracic aorta.[54,55,95] It provides access to the azygous and hemiazygous veins, and is the incision of choice for the management of most, if not all, tracheal injuries.[34,40,93–95]

Left posterolateral thoracotomy This incision provides access to the left lung, descending thoracic aorta, and the distal-most portion of the esophagus as it crosses from the right into the left hemithoracic cavity and superior to the descending thoracic aorta.[93–95]

Median sternotomy (Duval-Barasty's incision) This is the incision of choice for the management of patients with associated cardiac injuries that arrive with vital signs in the operating room.[53,66–68,73,75,76,93–95] The right or left hemithoracic cavities can be accessed if the mediastinal pleura is sharply transected. This provides access to the anterior portions of either the right or left lung although exposure of the posterior aspects of the pulmonary lobes is suboptimal. Care must be exercised when a significant portion of the lung is mobilized medially into this incision as the pulmonary hilar vessels can be rotated at a 90-degree angle, occluding both the in-flow and out-flow causing significant hemodynamic compromise to the patient. Similarly, extreme caution must be exercised when mobilizing the inferior pulmonary ligaments, as an inadvertent iatrogenic injury to the inferior pulmonary vein may ensue.[75,76,93–95]

Adjunct maneuvers

Important adjunct maneuvers used in the management of pulmonary injuries include (1) aortic cross-clamping,[75,76,95] (2) pulmonary hilar cross-clamping,[33,35,75,76,95] (3) complete in-flow occlusion (Shumacker's maneuver),[65–68,75,76,95] (4) pulmonary hilar vessel control,[33,35,75,76,95] (5) control of the main right or left pulmonary artery,[75,76,94,95] and (6) pulmonary vein control.[75,76,94,95]

Aortic cross-clamping The aorta can be cross-clamped only through a left anterolateral thoracotomy. This requires a meticulous combination of sharp and blunt dissection of this vessel before its entrance into the abdominal cavity via the aortic hiatus. The aorta should be digitally encircled; however, lateral digital dissection must be gentle and limited to prevent iatrogenic injuries to the intercostal arteries. The esophagus, which lies immediately superior to the anterior border of the aorta, must be separated before placement of a Crafoord-DeBakey aortic cross-clamp. Esophageal identification is facilitated by the prior insertion of a nasogastric tube.[75,76,95]

Pulmonary hilar cross-clamping This maneuver is used when there is a central hilar hematoma or active bleeding from the pulmonary hilum.[33,35,95] The hilum of the lung can be isolated using a meticulous combination of sharp and blunt dissection of the perihilar tissues to allow for the digital encirclement of all the structures. A Crafoord-DeBakey aortic cross-clamp is then placed as close to the pericardium as possible.[33,35,75,76,95]

Complete in-flow occlusion (Shumacker's maneuver) Shumacker's maneuver may occasionally be required if there is an associated cardiac injury either to the lateral-most aspects of the right atrium and/or atriocaval junction. This involves placement of Crafoord-DeBakey aortic cross-clamps in the intrapericardial portions of the superior vena cava as well as the inferior vena cava at the space of Gibbons. This will allow for immediate emptying of the heart. Although it is estimated that the safe period for this maneuver ranges from 1 to 3 minutes, the actual safety period is unknown.[65–68,75,76,95]

Pulmonary hilar vessel control This maneuver is necessary to control hemorrhage from the pulmonary artery or vein.[33,35,95] The dissection and ligation or stapling of pulmonary arteries and veins requires a different technique than for systemic vessels. The pulmonary vessels are thin-walled and fragile. They tear easily and cannot be clamped with standard hemostats. The dissection must be gentle and meticulous. There is almost always a perivascular plane that permits rapid and safe dissection in a vascular area. Before encirclement of either the pulmonary artery or vein, three sides of the vessels should be dissected completely before an attempt is made to pass a Mixter right-angle forceps beneath the vessel. If this is not done, perforation is likely. Pulmonary vessels should not be held with vascular forceps as they may tear; only the adventitia should be grasped. Either of these vessels may be safely held or retracted with Kittner dissectors.[33,35,75,76,95]

Control of main right or left pulmonary artery This control can be extrapleural at the hilum or intrapericardial, which requires lateral cardiac displacement and occasionally transection of the pericardium.[75,76,94,95]

Pulmonary vein control This control can be extrapleural at the hilum or intrapericardial, although the latter maneuver is quite difficult.[75,76,94,95]

Uniform approach to management of pulmonary injuries

A uniform approach to the management of traumatic pulmonary injuries has been described. This approach includes the following steps[95]:

1. Evacuate blood and clots from the thoracic cavity.
2. Expose the injured lung.
3. Pack, if necessary, to allow for restoration of depleted intravascular blood volume.
4. Evaluate for evidence of a hilar and/or central hematoma or hemorrhage.
5. Decide whether pulmonary hilar cross-clamping is necessary. If this is necessary, place a Crafoord-DeBakey aortic cross-clamp across the pulmonary hilum.
6. Proceed to identify bleeding structures within the pulmonary parenchyma and control hemorrhage proceeding to sequential declamping of the pulmonary hilum.
7. If the pulmonary parenchymal hemorrhage is away from the hilum, clamp the pulmonary injury with Duval lung forceps.
8. Evaluate pericardium and mediastinum.
9. Proceed to repair.

SURGICAL TECHNIQUES OF REPAIR AND RESECTION

The high mortality rates reported for lobectomy and pneumonectomy when performed for the management of traumatic lung injuries has served as the impetus to develop quicker and less extensive resection techniques.[4,7,19–24,33,35,36,39,41–43,95] These techniques have been denominated "lung-sparing techniques,"[4,7,19,20,22] and include suture pneumonorrhaphy,[94,95] stapled[19] and clamp[4,7] pulmonary tractotomy with selective deep vessel ligation, and nonanatomic resection.[20,94,95] In 2006, Asensio et al.[46] reported that lung-sparing techniques were used in 80% of 101 patients requiring thoracotomy for the management of traumatic pulmonary injuries. The use of adjunct intraoperative tools including the argon beam coagulator[96] and fibrin glue[97,98] are valuable adjuncts in the trauma surgeon's armamentarium.

The surgical armamentarium to manage penetrating pulmonary injuries discussed below is organized into two broad categories: tissue-sparing techniques and resectional procedures.[95]

Tissue-Sparing Procedures

These procedures include (1) suture pneumonorrhaphy,[94,95] (2) stapled pulmonary tractotomy with selective deep vessel ligation,[19,20] (3) clamp pulmonary tractotomy with selective deep vessel ligation,[4,7] and (4) nonanatomic resection.[20,94,95] It is estimated that approximately 85% of all penetrating pulmonary injuries can be managed with these techniques.[4,7,20,22,46,95]

These procedures are indicated for control of hemorrhage, control of small air leaks, and preservation of pulmonary tissue. They are also useful when the pulmonary injury is amenable to reconstruction.[4,7,19,20,22,95]

Suture Pneumonorrhaphy

The lung is stabilized with Duval lung forceps. Stay sutures of 3-0 chromic or other absorbable sutures are placed in the superior and inferior aspect of the wound as well as in the lateral aspects, and they are used to gently retract the edges. Very fine malleable ribbon retractors are placed to separate the wound and to provide for visualization of the injured vessels, which are then selectively ligated with 3-0 chromic sutures or other similarly sized absorbable sutures. The same is done for small bronchi. The edges of the wound are then approximated with a running locked suture of 3-0 chromic.[94,95]

Stapled Pulmonary Tractotomy

In 1997, Asensio et al.[19] described a technique for the management of penetrating pulmonary injuries, which included the use of a linear endo-GIA stapler (Ethicon, Somerville, NJ) to perform pulmonary tractotomy with selective vascular ligation. Clamp tractotomy was previously described by Wall et al.[7] in 1994, using aortic clamps. The lung is stabilized with Duval lung forceps and orifices of entrance and exit are defined. If need be, the overlying visceral pleura is sharply incised with Nelson scissors. A GIA 55 or 75 stapler is used to place 3.8-mm staples through the orifices of entrance and exit (Figures 10 and 11). This will open the tract traversed by the missile or other wounding agent, effectively exposing the injured vessels and bronchi, which are then selectively ligated utilizing 3-0 chromic or similarly sized absorbable sutures (Figure 12). The lung parenchyma can then be approximated with a single running locked suture of 3-0 chromic or the same size of absorbable suture. The orifices of entry and exit are left open for the egress of air and/or blood. The integrity of the suture line is tested by having the anesthesiologist inflate the lung. Air leaks are then detected and repaired.[19,95]

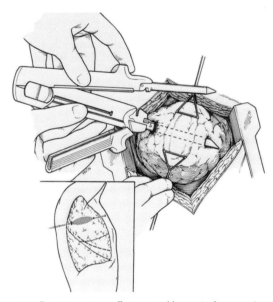

Figure 10 Depicts cavitary effect created by a missile traversing the lung. The GIA-55 is then inserted through the orifices of entry and exit. *(From Asensio JA, et al: Stapled pulmonary tractotomy: a rapid way to control hemorrhage in penetrating pulmonary injuries. J Am Coll Surg 185(5):1997.)*

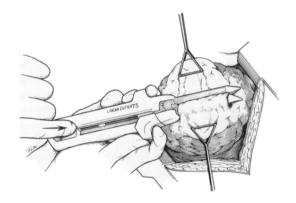

Figure 11 The GIA is then closed and fired to open up the missile tract. *(From Asensio JA, et al: Stapled pulmonary tractotomy: a rapid way to control hemorrhage in penetrating pulmonary injuries. J Am Coll Surg 185(5):1997.)*

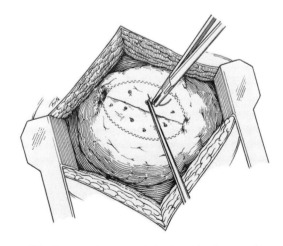

Figure 12 The tract is open and the deep bleeding vessels are ligated. *(From Asensio JA, et al: Stapled pulmonary tractotomy: a rapid way to control hemorrhage in penetrating pulmonary injuries. J Am Coll Surg 185(5):1997.)*

Clamp Pulmonary Tractotomy

The pulmonary tractotomy with selective vascular ligation described by Wall et al.[7] consists of the same technique as stapled pulmonary tractotomy; however, instead of a stapler, two Crafoord-DeBakey clamps are placed through the orifices of entrance and exit, and the pulmonary tissue between the clamps is sharply transected with either Nelson or Metzenbaum scissors.

Nonanatomic Resection

This procedure is indicated when a very small and peripheral portion of a lobe or a segment is devitalized.[20–24,36,39,41,43,94,95] The area of resection is stabilized between Duval lung forceps and a GIA 55 or 75 stapler with 3.8-mm staples is fired across, thus resecting the injured portion of the lung. The staple line may be oversewn with a running locked suture of 3-0 chromic or the same size of absorbable suture, although this is not generally necessary.[20,95,99,100] Nonanatomic resections can also be complex and require resections of major segments with complex reconstruction. This procedure will require meticulous attention in the reconstruction of an injured lobe.[94,95]

Resectional Procedures

Resectional procedures include formal lobectomy[94,95,101] and formal pneumonectomy.[28,33,35,37,42,94,95] These procedures are indicated for (1) control of hemorrhage, (2) resection of devitalized or destroyed pulmonary tissue, (3) control of major air leaks from lobar bronchi and/or mainstem bronchi not amenable to repair, and (4) control of life-threatening hemorrhage.[94,95]

Formal Lobectomy

This is indicated when there is total lobar tissue destruction, or uncontrollable hemorrhage from the lobar vessels or a large lobar bronchial injury, which is destructive and not amenable to repair.[94,95]

To perform a lobectomy the fissures must be separated. Vascular dissection should be initiated extrapleurally at the hilum through a perivascular plane to find the major pulmonary vessels. Vascular dissection in the fissures identifies the lobar vessels. Transection of the inferior pulmonary ligament distally will allow greater mobility of the lower lobes of both lungs. All pulmonary vessels, whether they be the main lobar vessels or segmental vessels, can be ligated in continuity and transfixed with nonabsorbable sutures. Alternatively, they may be stapled with a TA-30, TA-45, or TA-90, with 3.5-mm staples, or an endovascular stapler. All pulmonary vessels may also be oversewn with 4-0, 5-0, or 6-0 monofilament polypropylene sutures.[94,95]

The bronchi, whether they be the main, lobar, or segmental, should be stapled and transected with a TA-30, TA-45, or TA-90 stapler, with 4.8-mm staples.[94,95,101] This is the preferred method for handling all bronchial structures. Bronchi may also be transected utilizing Sarot lung clamps and sutured with 4-0 Tev-Dek synthetic sutures. Should a suture technique be chosen, the trauma surgeon should avoid grasping the cut end of a bronchus with any instrument. The suture technique involves clamping the bronchus distal to the intended point of transection. The bronchus is cut transversely for 4–5 mm, and the cut end is sutured with a 4-0 Tev-Dek. These sutures should be tied very carefully to avoid cutting or unnecessary devascularization. After placement of two sutures, the cut end is extended and additional sutures are placed. The sutures should be 2–3 mm apart. For a main bronchus, more than six sutures are seldom required. For a lobar bronchus, three or four sutures are usually enough. Too many sutures devascularize the transected bronchus. After closure is complete, the suture line is immersed in saline, and the lung is inflated by the anesthesiologist with up to 45 cm of inflation pressure. Additional sutures are placed if an air leak is detected.[94,95]

After a lobectomy is performed, the remaining lobes are pexed to the thoracic wall with 2-0 chromic sutures to prevent lung torsion; this is very important. The bronchial stump may be covered with a pleural flap or pericardial fat, known as Brewer's patch. These techniques are of unproven value. An intercostal pedicled muscle flap is probably superior, but it is time consuming.[94,95]

Right upper lobectomy

To perform a right upper lobectomy, both the pulmonary artery and the vein are dissected peripherally toward the right upper lobe to carefully delineate the lobe's individual blood supply. First, the anterior and apico-posterior segmental branches of the main pulmonary artery to the upper lobe are ligated in continuity with 2-0 silk sutures, divided, and transfixed proximally with 3-0 silk suture ligatures. Within the major fissure, the posterior segmental branch of the upper lobe is identified, ligated, transfixed, and divided in a similar fashion. Within the minor fissure that exists between the upper and middle lobes, the pulmonary venous drainage from the upper lobe is identified and carefully dissected. The vein is ligated in continuity with 0 silk sutures, transfixed with 2-0 silk suture, and divided. At this point, the lung is retracted forward to gain access to the posteriorly placed bronchus. The right mainstem bronchus and the carina are identified. The upper lobe bronchus is identified and transected with a TA-30 or TA-45 stapler with 4.8-mm staples.[94,95]

Right middle lobectomy

For a right middle lobectomy, the pulmonary artery branch to the middle lobe is identified, ligated with 0 silk sutures, transfixed with 2-0 silk sutures, and divided. The middle lobe division of the superior pulmonary vein is similarly ligated with 0 silk sutures, transfixed with 2-0 silk sutures, and divided. With these two vessels addressed, the trauma surgeon carefully isolates the middle lobe bronchus, which is then transected with a TA-30 or TA-45 stapler with 4.8-mm staples.[94,95]

Right lower lobectomy

To perform a right lower lobectomy, the main pulmonary artery is followed in the major fissure, and the segmental branches to the lower lobe are identified. The superior and basal segmental branches to the lower lobe are carefully identified, ligated in continuity with 0 silk sutures, transfixed with 2-0 silk sutures, and divided. Particular care is taken to avoid injury to the middle lobe arteries. Next, attention is directed to the inferior pulmonary vein, where, after the surgeon has ensured that any drainage from the middle lobe is protected, the inferior pulmonary vein is ligated in continuity with 0 silk sutures and transfixed with 2-0 silk sutures and transected. Again, within the same major fissure, the superior segmental and the basal segmental bronchi are individually identified and transected with a TA-30 or TA-45 stapler with 4.8-mm staples.[94,95]

Left upper lobectomy

To perform a left upper lobectomy, the interlobar fissure is separated by a meticulous combination of sharp and blunt dissection. If the interlobar fissure is not complete, it can be divided with a TA-30 or TA-45 with 3.8-mm staples. Arterial dissection is begun at the junction of the upper third with the middle third of the fissure. The artery is exposed. The perivascular plane is entered, and the individual segmental branches to the upper lobe are identified, carefully dissected, ligated in continuity with 0 silk sutures, and then transfixed with 2-0 silk sutures. Similarly, the superior pulmonary vein and branches to the left upper lobe are identified, ligated in continuity with 0 silk sutures, and transfixed with 2-0 silk sutures. The left upper lobar bronchus is then identified and transected with a TA-45 with 4.8-mm staples.[94,95]

Left lower lobectomy

To perform a left lower lobectomy, the same steps are taken as for a left upper lobectomy; however, the arterial and venous dissection are directed forward the appropriate left lower lobar vessels. The lingular artery or arteries, as there may be two identified, are ligated in continuity with 0 silk sutures and transfixed with 2-0 silk sutures. The left lower lobar bronchus is then identified and transected with a TA-30 or TA-45 with 4.8-mm staples.[94,95]

Pneumonectomy

Right pneumonectomy

Exploration of the right hemithoracic cavity is carried out, and the azygous vein is identified. The right pulmonary hilum is located. Using a meticulous combination of sharp and blunt dissection, the right main pulmonary artery is identified and encircled with a vessel loop; avoidance of undue traction is key. The right inferior pulmonary ligament is sharply transected. Both superior and inferior pulmonary veins are identified and encircled with vessel loops. All vessels may be either ligated in continuity or stapled individually utilizing a TA-30 or TA-45 stapler with 3.5-mm staples or an endovascular stapler. The right mainstem bronchus is then identified and encircled. The trauma surgeon must be careful not to apply undue traction to avoid tearing subcarinal structures. The bronchus is then transected with a TA-30 or TA-45 stapler with 4.8-mm staples.[28,33,35,37,42,94,95]

Left pneumonectomy

A thorough exploration of the left hemithoracic cavity is carried out. The phrenic, vagus, and left recurrent laryngeal nerves are identified and preserved. The left pulmonary hilum is located. Using a meticulous combination of sharp and blunt dissection, the left main pulmonary artery is identified and encircled with a vessel loop; avoidance of undue traction is key. The left inferior pulmonary ligament is sharply transected. Both superior and inferior pulmonary veins are identified and encircled with vessel loops. All vessels may be either ligated in continuity or stapled utilizing a TA-30 or TA-45 stapler with 3.5-mm staples or an endovascular stapler. The left mainstem bronchus is then identified and encircled. The trauma surgeon must be careful not to apply undue traction to avoid tearing subcarinal structures. The bronchus is then transected with a TA-30 or TA-45 stapler with 4.8-mm staples.[28,33,35,37,42,94,95]

Alternate technique for pneumonectomy (right or left)

If the patient is exsanguinating from a central hilar vascular injury, the pulmonary hilum may be digitally encircled and compressed to allow the anesthesiologist to replace the lost intravascular volume. A Craafoord-DeBakey aortic cross-clamp is then placed a few centimeters from the mediastinal pleura. If this maneuver controls the life-threatening hemorrhage, extrapleural dissection of hilar vessels may be carried out and individual vessels ligated. If this maneuver cannot be performed, if it does not contain the hemorrhage, or if the cross-clamp is required in a very proximal location, the pericardium may have to be opened to control the pulmonary artery and the pulmonary veins. Intrapericardial control of the pulmonary veins is quite difficult and requires lateral displacement of the heart.[28,33,35,37,42,94,95] This can be accomplished using a Satinsky clamp placed in the right auricle. It may even require total inflow occlusion with a Shumacker's maneuver.[66–68]

Alternatively, a TA-90 stapler with 4.8-mm staples may be placed across the pulmonary hilum and fired transecting the pulmonary artery, pulmonary veins, and mainstem bronchus. In most cases, this controls the hemorrhage if the injuries to the pulmonary artery or veins are found in an extrapericardial location. If this does not control the bleeding, then intrapericardial control of the pulmonary vessels will be needed.[42,94,95]

PROGNOSTIC FACTORS AND OUTCOMES

Factors associated with survival for pulmonary injuries requiring surgical intervention include the following: mechanism of injury and type of wounding agents[15,20–25,30,33,35,36,39–45,50,52,70,74,75,77,95,102–108]; prehospital transport time[42,48,65–68,95,109]; presence of shock at the scene or upon arrival[39,42,65,67,68,75,76,95]; loss of the airway[34,78,95,102,103]; presence of associated injuries[45,48,95]; complexity of the surgical procedure[40,48]; and location of the injury.[95]

Mechanism of Injury and Type of Wounding Agents

It is known that pulmonary injuries in civilian life are caused by both blunt and penetrating mechanisms.[21,45] Most commonly, penetrating pulmonary injuries are produced by knives and low-velocity missiles; although the incidence of injuries caused by high-velocity missiles is increasing.[21,45,104–108] Civilian penetrating injuries to the lung secondary to high-velocity missiles are associated with higher mortality rates than low-velocity missiles and stab wounds.[15, 20–25,30,33,35,36,39–45,50,74,75,77,95,106]

In a multicenter study dealing with traumatic pulmonary injuries in the civilian arena, Karmy-Jones and colleagues[107] reported that blunt mechanism of injury tends to provide more extensive injury to pulmonary parenchyma requiring extensive resections in case of need for surgery. Blunt trauma is associated with a 3 to 10 times greater risk of death when compared with penetrating trauma.[21,24,45,52]

In warfare, most pulmonary injuries are caused by penetrating mechanisms, such as shell fragments, shrapnel, and high-velocity missiles, although extensive damage is also observed with explosive wounds.[47,48,79–81] Zakharia et al.[47] and Petricevic and colleagues[48] reported a higher mortality rate among patients sustaining pulmonary lesions secondary to explosive devices and destructive injuries inflicted by high-velocity missiles, than in those patients sustaining stab wounds or falls.

Prehospital Transport Time

The "scoop-and-run" doctrine of Gervin and Fischer[65–68,109] might improve the survival prospects of some patients with time-related deterioration resulting from torso injuries. Wagner et al.[42] reported that rapidity of prehospital transport of patients with severe penetrating pulmonary injuries results in better outcomes, concluding that a well-organized trauma service caring for patients within the framework of well-defined protocols, increases the survival rate. This fact was also reported by Petricevic and colleagues,[48] who pointed out that the key for success in the treatment of patients sustaining traumatic pulmonary injuries during wartime, is rapid transportation of the wounded to surgical centers.

Presence of Shock at Scene or upon Arrival

Well-known physiologic factors predictive of high mortality in patients with traumatic pulmonary injuries include prehospital and ED absence of both vital signs and cardiac rhythm. Similarly, the absence of a palpable pulse in the presence of cardiopulmonary arrest is also predictive of high mortality.[75,76] Robison et al.[39] reported a mortality rate of 85% among patients presenting with cardiopulmonary arrest upon arrival to the ED, while Wagner and colleagues[42] reported that hypotensive patients sustaining penetrating pulmonary injuries with systolic blood pressures less than 90 mm Hg had a mortality rate of 90%.

Buckman et al.,[65] using the cardiovascular and respiratory components of the trauma score (CVRS) on admission of patients sustaining penetrating cardiac injuries, concluded that prospective physiologic scoring is helpful in predicting outcomes. Physiologic factors and CVRS have been further validated by Asensio et al.,[67,68] as important predictive factors of outcome, in two prospective studies dealing with this type of lethal injuries. It would be appropriate to extrapolate that these physiologic variables can play the same significant role among patients sustaining traumatic pulmonary injuries.

Loss of Airway

It is known that the highest priority in the resuscitation of the critical injured patient lies in achieving a rapid and secure airway regardless of setting wherever performed, and this dictum includes, of course, patients sustaining traumatic pulmonary injuries. Unsolved loss of the airway is uniformly fatal.[34,78,102,103] As reported by Asensio et al.,[103] the vast majority of trauma patients treated at the ED in certified trauma centers in which endotracheal intubation is indicated will have a secured airway by means of this procedure. Occasionally endotracheal intubation is unsuccessful or contraindicated, and a surgical airway is required; in this case, emergency surgical cricothyroidotomy should be performed.[34,78,102,103] Inoue and colleagues[78] reported a strategy to secure the airway in patients with traumatic pulmonary injuries, consisting of selective exclusion of the injured lung by using endotracheal tubes with a moveable bronchial occlusion cuff (Univent®, Fuji Systems Corporation, Tokyo). By means of this strategy, occlusion by blood of the airways of the noninjured lung is prevented.

Presence of Associated Injuries

The presence of associated injuries, particularly cardiac or thoracic vascular injuries, uniformly increases mortality. Similarly, the presence of complex associated abdominal injuries is also known to increase mortality in these patients.

Complexity of Surgical Procedure

Several authors have pointed out that the complexity of the surgical procedure is closely related to the mortality rate. Wall et al.,[4,7] Velmahos and colleagues,[20] and Cothren et al.[22] have established that the use of lung-sparing procedures correlates with lower rates of mortality than more extensive resective procedures. The mortality rate reported in the literature for pneumonorrhaphy, stapled tractotomy, clamp tractotomy, and wedge/nonanatomic resections varies. In contrast, the mortality rate reported for anatomic lobectomy is 40%–50%, and for pneumonectomy, 60%–100%.

Wagner and colleagues[42] reported a 50% mortality rate among patients requiring pneumonectomy for trauma, while Thompson and associates[40] reported 54.5% mortality rate for lobectomy and 100% for pneumonectomy; the overall mortality for this series was 28%, and the mortality for pneumonorrhaphy was 3%, and for tractotomy, 17%. In 1993, Tominaga et al.[41] reported an overall mortality rate of 33%; the authors correlated the complexity of the surgical procedure on the lung with mortality, reporting a rate of 20% for nonanatomic resections, 33% for lobectomy, and 50% for pneumonectomy. In 1991, Velmahos et al.[20] reported an overall mortality rate of 5% among patients requiring thoracotomy for penetrating lung injuries. In this study, the authors focused on techniques employed to deal with these injuries. The mortality rate among patients requiring lung-sparing surgery was 3%, compared with 20% for those requiring resective techniques. Stewart et al.[43] reported an overall mortality rate of 12.5% among patients requiring pulmonary resection for pulmonary injuries and concluded that the use of stapled resections could be a factor related to the low mortality in the series. Karmy-Jones et al.[45] reported that mortality increased with each step of increasing complexity of the surgical technique, with pneumonorrhaphy at 9%; stapled tractotomy, 13%; wedge resection, 30%; lobectomy, 43%; and

pneumonectomy, 50%. In 2002, Cothren et al.[22] reported an overall mortality rate of 30% among 36 patients requiring thoracotomy for severe lung injuries, and compared mortality rates for patients requiring anatomic resection at 77%, versus a 4% mortality rate for those patients that underwent nonanatomic resections. The authors reported that stapled tractotomy correlated with a significant reduction in mortality. Huh and colleagues,[24] also focusing on the level of complexity of the lung intervention, described a mortality rate of 24% for pneumonorrhaphy, 9.1% for tractotomy, 20% for wedge resection, 35% for lobectomy, and 69.7% for pneumonectomy.

Location of Injury

Wagner and associates[42] pointed out that injury to the hilar pulmonary vasculature is associated with greater than 70% of mortality. Wiencek and Wilson[35] reported a mortality rate of 63% among patients sustaining central/hilar lung injuries secondary to gunshot wounds, while the mortality rate among patients with hilar injuries resulting from stab wounds was 44%. The major causes of death in this series were exsanguination, and possibly air embolism. These authors also reported an overall mortality rate of 56% among patients with penetrating central pulmonary injuries. Petricevic and colleagues[48] pointed out that the mortality rate is much higher if lung injury is combined with one or more extrathoracic lesions (from 6% to 14% to as much as 55%).

MORBIDITY

According to Asensio et al.,[95] complications related to the presence of a traumatic pulmonary injury or surgical management are classified into three main categories: intraoperative, short-term postoperative, and long-term postoperative complications.

Intraoperative Complications

These complications comprise univentricular failure (usually right ventricular failure) and biventricular failure.

Short-Term Postoperative Complications

Technical short-term complications follow:

- Lung hernia
- Lung torsion
- Bronchopleural fistulas
- Arteriovenous fistulas
- Bronchial stump leaks
- Bronchial stump blowouts

    Physiological short-term complications follow:

- Right ventricular failure
- Pulmonary artery hypertension
- "Run-away" pulmonary artery hypertension
- Biventricular failure

Long-Term Postoperative Complications

These complications are classified as follows:

- Persistent bronchopleural fistula
- Bronchial stenosis
- Empyema
- Lung abscess
- Bronchiectasis
- Arteriovenous fistula

In 1979, Graham et al.[36] described the presence of 155 postoperative complications among 108 of 373 patients sustaining penetrating injuries to the lung, for a morbidity rate of 29% and an average number of 1.43 complications per patient. The most common causes of morbidity included postoperative hemorrhage, at 32%; atelectasis, 13%; recurrent pneumothorax, 10%; persistent air leak, 9%; wound infection, 8%; and pneumonia, 6%. Postoperative hemorrhage and persistent air leak were major indications for surgical reintervention. Robison[39] reported a morbidity rate of 70% among patients requiring thoracotomy for resective surgery of lung injuries. The most frequent postoperative complications included hemoptysis, bronchopleural fistula, air embolism, sepsis, and respiratory insufficiency.

MORTALITY

The overall mortality rate reported in the literature for patients with traumatic pulmonary injuries ranges from 1.7% to 37%. There are many factors significantly associated with mortality. The factors repeatedly mentioned in various series as outcome determinants are the physiologic status of the patient after injury, complexity of the pulmonary surgical intervention, number of associated injuries (especially cardiac injury), and need for additional surgical interventions.

In 1979, Graham et al.[36] reported an overall mortality rate of 8% among patients sustaining penetrating pulmonary injuries. The mortality rate among patients requiring only tube thoracostomy was 3%, versus 6% for those requiring thoracotomy. Major causes of death were respiratory insufficiency, at 36%; shock/hemorrhage, 32%; sepsis, 11%; central nervous system injury, 11%; air embolism, 7%; and tracheoesophageal fistula, 4%. Robison[39] in 1988 reported an overall mortality rate of 2.4%, with sepsis, the presence of associated injuries, air embolism, and exsanguination (notoriously common in central lung injuries) determined to be major causes of mortality.

In 1988, Wiencek and Wilson[35] reported a mortality rate of 56% among patients sustaining central/hilar vascular injuries to the lung and concluded that exsanguination and air embolism play a cardinal role as cause of death in these patients. In 1993, Tominaga et al.[41] reported an overall mortality rate of 33% and noticed the role that complexity of the pulmonary surgical procedure played on mortality, describing a mortality rate of 20% for nonanatomic resections, 33% for lobectomy, and 50% for pneumonectomy. Velmahos, Asensio, and colleagues[20] reported in 1999 an overall mortality rate of 5% among patients who underwent thoracotomy for penetrating lung injuries; the authors focused on the techniques employed to deal with these injuries and reported that mortality rates among patients requiring lung-sparing surgery was 3% versus 20% for those requiring resective techniques.

In 1997, Petricevic and colleagues[48] reported an overall mortality rate of 1.7% among patients sustaining traumatic pulmonary injuries during the war in Croatia; causes of death were identified as hemorrhage and irreversible shock, 30%, and septic complications, 70%. Stewart et al.[43] reported an overall mortality rate of 12.5% among patients requiring pulmonary resection for lung trauma, concluding that the use of stapled resections could be a factor related to the low mortality in the series.

In 2001, Karmy-Jones et al.,[21,45] in a retrospective multicenter 4-year study, reported an overall mortality rate of 9% among 451 patients requiring thoracotomy for traumatic pulmonary injuries. Stratified by mechanism of injury, blunt trauma accounted for 68% and penetrating trauma 19%. Mortality increased with complexity of the surgical technique required to manage these injuries: for pneumonorrhaphy, the mortality rate was 9%; stapled tractotomy, 13%; wedge resection, 30%; lobectomy, 43%; and pneumonectomy, 50%. Blunt injuries were associated with a 10 times greater risk of death compared with penetrating trauma. Factors identified by univariate analysis as being significantly associated with mortality included mechanism—blunt versus penetrating trauma, high head/neck Abbreviated Injury Score,

need for laparotomy, and presenting systolic blood pressure on arrival in operating room. When these factors were entered along with type of lung repair/resection—suture, stapled tractotomy, wedge resection, lobectomy, and pneumonectomy—into a stepwise model regression analysis, factors that retained significance were mechanism of injury, presenting systolic blood pressure on arrival in operating room, and increasing degree of pulmonary resection.

In 2001, Gasparri et al.[25] described an overall mortality rate of 16% among patients requiring pulmonary parenchymal interventions for lung trauma. Mortality was significantly higher in the presence of low systolic blood pressure, low temperature, high Injury Severity Score, large estimated blood losses, associated cardiac injuries, and the need for laparotomy. However, the authors did not find a correlation between the complexity of the operative intervention on the lung and the outcome. Cothren and colleagues[22] reported an overall mortality rate of 30% among 36 patients requiring thoracotomy for severe lung injuries. The mortality rate for patients with anatomic resection was 77%, compared with 4% among patients who underwent nonanatomic resection. The authors reported that stapled tractotomy was related with a significant reduction in mortality. Huh et al.[24] reported an overall mortality rate of 28% among patients requiring thoracotomy for traumatic pulmonary injuries, and reported that if a concomitant laparotomy was required, mortality increased to 33%. The authors focused on the level of complexity of the lung intervention, and described a mortality rate of 23.9% for pneumonorrhaphy, 9.1% for stapled tractotomy, 20% for wedge resection, 35% for lobectomy, and 69.7% for pneumonectomy. In 2006, Asensio and colleagues[46] reported an overall mortality rate of 37% among 101 patients requiring thoracotomy for penetrating pulmonary injuries; seven of these patients (19%) required an EDT and did not reach the OR.

CONCLUSIONS

Pulmonary injuries requiring thoracotomy are uncommon even in busy urban trauma centers. Their operative management requires excellent surgical technique to prevent postoperative complications. Simpler surgical techniques such as pneumonorrhaphy and wedge resections are frequently used for their management. Stapled pulmonary tractotomy has become the most frequently used lung sparing procedure and can be used effectively to manage 85% of all pulmonary injuries requiring surgical intervention. Despite recent advances in trauma surgery and surgical critical care, pulmonary injuries, particularly those requiring resective procedures, are marked by high morbidity and mortality.

REFERENCES

1. Breasted JH, editor: *The Edwin Smith Surgical Papyrus*, vol. 1. Chicago, University of Chicago Press, 1930, 369–373.
2. Homer: *The Iliad*, vol. XVI. Translated by Alexander Pope. London, George Bell & Sons, 1904, lines 588–625, p. 299.
3. Menenakos E, Alexakis N, Leandros E, Laskaratos G, Nikiteas N, Bramis J, et al: Fatal chest injury with lung evisceration during athletic games in ancient Greece. *World J Surg* 29:1348–1351, 2005.
4. Wall MJ, Villavicencio RT, Miller CC, Aucar JA, Granchi TA, Liscum KR, et al: Pulmonary tractotomy as an abbreviated thoracotomy technique. *J Trauma* 45:1015–1023, 1998.
5. Bellamy RF, Zajtchuk R: The evolution of wound ballistics: a brief history. In Bellamy RF, Zajtchuk R, editors: *Textbook of Military Medicine*. Washington, DC, Office of the Surgeon General at TMM Publications, Center of Excellence in Military Medical Research and Education, Department of the Army, 1989, pp. 83–106.
6. Molnar TF, Hasse J, Jeyasingham K, Rendeki MS: Changing dogmas: history of development in modalities of traumatic pneumothorax, hemothorax and post-traumatic empyema thoracis. *Ann Thorac Surg* 77:372–378, 2004.
7. Wall MJ, Hirshberg A, Mattox KL: Pulmonary tractotomy with selective vascular ligation for penetrating injuries to the lung. *Am J Surg* 168:665–669, 1994.

8. Fallon WF: Surgical lessons learned on the battlefield. *J Trauma* 43:209–213, 1997.
9. White H: An outstanding ISS/SIC surgeon: Gregory Grey Turner. *World J Surg* 27:511–513, 2003.
10. Mattox KL, Allen MK: Systematic approach to pneumothorax, hemothorax, pneumomediastinum and subcutaneous emphysema. *Injury* 17:309–312, 1986.
11. Stone HH, Strom PR, Mullins RJ: Management of the major coagulopathy with onset during laparotomy. *Ann Surg* 197:532–535, 1983.
12. Asensio JA, Petrone P, Roldan G, Kuncir E, Ramicone E, Chan L: Has evolution in awareness of guidelines for institution of damage control improved outcome in the management of the post-traumatic open abdomen? *Arch Surg* 139:209–214, 2004.
13. Asensio JA, Petrone P, O'Shanahan G, Kuncir E: Managing exsanguination: what we know about damage control/bailout is not enough. *Baylor U Med Ctr Proc* 16:294–296, 2003.
14. Asensio JA, McDuffie L, Petrone P, Roldan G, Forno W, Gambaro E, et al: Reliable variables in the exsanguinated patient which indicate damage control and predict outcome. *Am J Surg* 182:743–751, 2001.
15. Wall MJ, Soltero E: Damage control for thoracic injuries. *Surg Clin North Am* 77:863–878, 1997.
16. Boubolis N, Rivas LF, Kuo J: Packing the chest: a useful technique for intractable bleeding after open heart operation. *J Cardiovasc Surg* 57:856–861, 1994.
17. Urschel JD, Bertsch DJ, Takita H: Thoracic packing for postoperative hemorrhage. *J Cardiovasc Surg* 38:373–375, 1997.
18. Caceres M, Buechter K, Tillou A, Shih JA, Lui D, Steeb G: Thoracic packing for uncontrolled bleeding in penetrating thoracic injuries. *South Med J* 97:637–641, 2004.
19. Asensio JA, Demetriades D, Berne JD, Velmahos GC, Cornwell EE 3rd, Murray JA, et al: Stapled pulmonary tractotomy: a rapid way to control hemorrhage in penetrating pulmonary injuries. *J Am Coll Surg* 185:504–505, 1997.
20. Velmahos GC, Baker C, Demetriades D, Goodman J, Murray JA, Asensio JA: Lung-sparing surgery after penetrating trauma using tractotomy, partial lobectomy and pneumonorrhaphy. *Arch Surg* 134:186–189, 1999.
21. Karmy-Jones R, Jurkovich G, Shatz D, Brundage S, Wall MJ, Engelhardt S, et al: Management of traumatic lung injury: a Western Trauma Association Multicenter review. *J Trauma* 51:1049–1053, 2001.
22. Cothren C, Moore EE, Biffl WL, Franciose RJ, Offner PJ, Burch JM: Lung-sparing techniques are associated with improved outcome compared with anatomic resection for severe lung injuries. *J Trauma* 53:483–487, 2002.
23. Livingston DH, Hauser CJ: Trauma to the chest wall and lung. In Moore EE, Feliciano DV, Mattox KL, editors: *Trauma*, 5th ed. New York, McGraw-Hill, 2004, pp. 507–538.
24. Huh J, Wall MJ, Estrera AL, Soltero ER, Mattox KL: Surgical management of traumatic pulmonary injury. *Am J Surg* 186:620–624, 2003.
25. Gasparri M, Karmy-Jones R, Kralovich KA, Patton JH, Arbabi S: Pulmonary tractotomy vs. lung resection: viable options in penetrating lung injury. *J Trauma* 51:1092–1097, 2001.
26. Manlulu AV, Lee TW, Thung KH, Wong R, Yim APC: Current indications and results of VATS in the evaluation and management of hemodynamically stable thoracic injuries. *Eur J Cardiothorac Surg* 25:1048–1053, 2004.
27. Navsaria PH, Vogel RJ, Nicol AJ: Thoracoscopic evacuation of retained post-traumatic hemothorax. *Ann Thorac Surg* 78:282–286, 2004.
28. Jougon J, Dubois G, Velly JF: Techniques de pneumoniectomie (surgical techniques of pneumonectomies). *EMC Chirurgie* 2:537–564, 2005.
29. Association for Surgical Education: Surgical education: lungs, vol. 1, no. 1, 2006. . Available at http://surgicaleducation.com/reference/gray/subjects/subject?id=240.
30. Pezzella AT, Silva WE, Lancey RA: Cardiothoracic trauma. *Curr Prob Surg* 35:647–790, 1998.
31. Pezzella AT, Adebonojo SA, Hooker SG, Mabogunje OA, Conlan AA: Complications in general thoracic surgery. *Curr Prob Surg* 37:733–860, 2000.
32. Weigelt JA: Pulmonary resection for trauma. In Dudley H, Carter D, Russell RCG, editors: *Operative Surgery. Trauma Surgery Part I*, 4th ed. London, Butterworth and Co, 1983, pp. 311–317.
33. Powell RJ, Redan JA, Swan KG: The hilar snare, an improved technique for securing rapid vascular control of the pulmonary hilum. *J Trauma* 30:208–210, 1990.
34. Millhalm FH, Rajii-Khorasani A, Birkett DF, Hirsch EF: Carinal injury: diagnosis and treatment—case report. *J Trauma* 31:1420–1422, 1991.
35. Wiencek RG, Wilson RF: Central lung injuries: a need for early vascular control. *J Trauma* 28:1418–1424, 1988.
36. Graham JM, Mattox KL, Beall AC: Penetrating trauma of the lung. *J Trauma* 19:665–669, 1979.
37. Wagner RB, Crawford WO, Schimpf PP: Classification of parenchymal injuries to the lung. *Radiology* 167:77–82, 1988.
38. Karaaslan T, Meuli R, Androux R, Duvoisin B, Hessler C, Schnyder P: Traumatic chest lesions in patients with severe head trauma: a comparative study with computed tomography and conventional chest roentgenograms. *J Trauma* 39:1081–1086, 1995.
39. Robison PD, Harman PK, Trinkle JK, Grover FL: Management of penetrating lung injuries in civilian practice. *Thorac Cardiovasc Surg J Thorac Cardiovasc Surg* 95:184–190, 1988.
40. Thompson DA, Rowlands BJ, Walker WE, Kuykendall RC, Miller PW, Fischer RP: Urgent thoracotomy for pulmonary and tracheobronchial injury. *J Trauma* 23:276–280, 1988.
41. Tominaga GT, Waxman K, Scanell G, Annas C, Ott R, Gazzaniga AB: Emergency thoracotomy with lung resection following trauma. *Am Surg* 59:834–837, 1993.
42. Wagner JW, Obeid FN, Karmy-Jones RC, Casey G, Sorensen VJ, Horst HM: Trauma pneumonectomy revisited: the role of simultaneous stapled pneumonectomy. *J Trauma* 40:590–594, 1996.
43. Stewart KC, Urschel JD, Nakai SS, Gelfand ET, Hamilton SM: Pulmonary resection for lung trauma. *Ann Thorac Surg* 63:1587–1588, 1997.
44. Inci I, Ozcelik C, Tacyildiz I, Nizam O, Eren N, Ozgen G: Penetrating chest injuries: unusually high incidence of high-velocity gunshot wounds in civilian practice. *World J Surg* 22:438–442, 1998.
45. Karmy-Jones R, Jurkovich GJ, Nathens AB, Shatz DV, Brundage S, Wall MJ, et al: Timing of urgent thoracotomy for hemorrhage after trauma. A multicenter study. *Arch Surg* 136:513–518, 2001.
46. Asensio JA, García-Núñez LM, Constantinou C, Jamiana M, Petrone P, Lavery RF: Predictors of outcome in 101 patients requiring thoracotomy for penetrating pulmonary injuries. Tissue sparing rules! Abstract submitted to the American Association for the Surgery of Trauma Annual Meeting, 2006.
47. Zakharia AT: Thoracic battle injuries in the Lebanon War: a review of the early operative approach in 1,992 patients. *Ann Thorac Surg* 40:209–213, 1985.
48. Petricevic A, Ilic N, Bacic A, Petricevic M, Vidjak V, Tanfara S: War injuries of the lungs. *Eur J Cardiothorac Surg* 11:843–847, 1997.
49. Moore EE, Malangoni MA, Cogbill TH, Shackford SR, Champion H, Jurkovich GJ, et al: Organ Injury Scaling IV: thoracic vascular, lung, cardiac, and diaphragm. *J Trauma* 36:299–300, 1994.
50. Symbas PN: Cardiothoracic trauma. *Curr Prob Surg* 28:741–796, 1991.
51. Bokhari F, Brakenridge S, Nagy K, Roberts R, Smith R, Joseph K, et al: Prospective study of the sensitivity of physical examination in chest trauma. *J Trauma* 53:1135–1138, 2002.
52. Ayed AK, Shawaf EA: Diagnosis and treatment of traumatic intrathoracic bronchial disruption. *Injury* 35:484–499, 2004.
53. Asensio JA, Arroyo Jr H, Veloz W, Forno W, Gambaro E, Roldan GA, et al: Penetrating thoracoabdominal injuries: ongoing dilemma—which cavity and when? *World J Surg* 26:539–543, 2002.
54. Asensio JA, Berne J, Demetriades D, Murray J, Gomez H, Falabella A, et al: Penetrating esophageal injuries: time interval of safety for preoperative evaluation—how long is safe? *J Trauma* 43:319–324, 1997.
55. Asensio JA, Chahwan S, Forno W, MacKersie R, Wall MJ, Lake J, et al: Penetrating esophageal injuries: multicenter study of the American Association for the Surgery of Trauma. *J Trauma* 50:289–296, 2001.
56. Cornwell EE 3rd, Kennedy F, Ayad IA, Berne TV, Velmahos G, Asensio JA, et al: Transmediastinal gunshot wounds. A reconsideration of the role of aortography. *Arch Surg* 131:949–952, 1996.
57. Hanpeter DE, Demetriades D, Asensio JA, Berne TV, Velmahos GC, Murray J: Helical computed tomography scan in the evaluation of mediastinal gunshot wounds. *J Trauma* 49:689–695, 2000.
58. Rozycki GS, Dente CJ: Surgeon-performed ultrasound in trauma and surgical critical care. In Moore EE, Feliciano DV, Mattox KL, editors: *Trauma*, 5th ed. New York, McGraw-Hill, 2004, pp. 311–328.
59. Rainer TH, Griffith JF, Lam E, Lam PKW, Metreweli C: Comparison of thoracic ultrasound, clinical acumen and radiography in patients with minor chest injury. *J Trauma* 56:1211–1213, 2004.
60. Kirkpatrick AW, Sirois M, Laupland KB, Lui D, Rowan K, Ball CG, et al: Hand-held thoracic sonography for detecting traumatic pneumothoraces: the Extended Focused Assessment with Sonography for Trauma (EFAST). *J Trauma* 57:288–295, 2004.

61. Knudson JL, Dort JM, Helmer SD, Smith S: Surgeon-performed ultrasound for pneumothorax in the trauma suite. *J Trauma* 56:527–530, 2004.
62. Sisley AC, Rozycki GS, Ballard RB, Namias N, Salomone JP, Feliciano DV: Rapid detection of traumatic effusion using surgeon-performed ultrasonography. *J Trauma* 44:291–297, 1998.
63. Mann FA, Linnau KF: Diagnostic and interventional radiology. In Moore E, Feliciano DV, Mattox KL, editors: *Trauma*, 5th ed. New York, McGraw-Hill, 2004, pp. 255–310.
64. Duke JC. Anesthesia: In Moore EE, Feliciano DV, Mattox KL, editors: *Trauma*, 5th ed. New York, McGraw-Hill, 2004, pp. 329–354.
65. Buckman RF, Badellino MM, Mauro LH, Asensio JA, Caputo C, Grass JD, et al: Penetrating cardiac wounds: prospective study of factors influencing initial resuscitation. *J Trauma* 34:717–726, 1993.
66. Asensio JA, Stewart BM, Murray J, Fox AH, Falabella A, Gomez H, et al: Penetrating cardiac injuries. *Surg Clin North Am* 76:685–724, 1996.
67. Asensio JA, Murray J, Demetriades D, Berne J, Cornwell EE 3rd, Velmahos GC, et al: Penetrating cardiac injuries: a prospective study of variables predicting outcomes. *J Am Coll Surg* 186:24–34, 1998.
68. Asensio JA, Berne JD, Demetriades D, Chan L, Murray J, Falabella A, et al: One hundred five penetrating cardiac injuries. A two year prospective evaluation. *J Trauma* 44:1073–1082, 1998.
69. Eisenberg MJ, Muñoz de Romeral L, Heidenreich PA, Schiller NB, Evans GT: The diagnosis of pericardial effusion and cardiac tamponade by 12-lead ECG. *Chest* 110:318–324, 1996.
70. Bruch C, Schmermund A, Dagres N, Bartel T, Caspari G, Sack S, et al: Changes in QRS voltage in cardiac tamponade and pericardial effusion: reversibility after pericardiocentesis and after anti-inflammatory drug treatment. *J Am Coll Cardiol* 38:219–226, 2001.
71. Sybrandy KC, Cramer JM, Burgersdijk C: Diagnosing cardiac contusion: old wisdom and new insights. *Heart* 89:485–489, 2003.
72. Nagy KK, Krosner SM, Roberts RR, Joseph KT, Smith RF, Barret J: Determining which patients require evaluation for blunt cardiac injury following blunt chest trauma. *World J Surg* 25:108–111, 2001.
73. Asensio JA, Petrone P, Demetriades D: Injury to the diaphragm. In Moore EE, Feliciano DV, Mattox KL, editors: *Trauma*, 5th ed. New York, McGraw-Hill, 2004, pp. 613–636.
74. Riley RD, Miller PR, Meredith JW: Injury to the esophagus, trachea and bronchus. In Moore EE, Feliciano DV, Mattox KL, editors: *Trauma*, 5th ed. New York, McGraw-Hill, 2004, pp. 539–554.
75. Working Group, Ad Hoc Subcommittee on Outcomes, American College of Surgeons-Committee on Trauma: Practice management guidelines for emergency department thoracotomy. *J Am Coll Surg* 193:303–309, 2001.
76. Asensio JA, Petrone P, Costa D, Robin A, Pardo M, Kimbrell B: An evidence-based critical appraisal of emergency department thoracotomy. *Evidence-Based Surg* 1:11–21, 2003.
77. Gaillard M, Herve C, Mandin L, Raynaud P: Mortality prognostic factors in chest injury. *J Trauma* 30:93–96, 1990.
78. Inoue H, Suzuki I, Iwasaki M, Ogawa JI, Koide S, Shotsu A: Selective exclusion of the injured lung. *J Trauma* 34:496–498, 1993.
79. McNamara JJ, Messersmith JK, Dunn RA, et al: Thoracic injuries in combat casualties in Vietnam. *Ann Thorac Surg* 10:389–401, 1970.
80. Suleman ND, Rasoul HA: War injuries to the chest. *Injury* 16:382–384, 1985.
81. Wanebo H, van Dyke J: The high velocity pulmonary injury: relation to traumatic wet lung syndrome. *J Thorac Cardiovasc Surg* 64:537–550, 1972.
82. Heniford BT, Carrillo EH, Spain DA, Sosa JL, Fulton RL et al: The role of thoracoscopy in the management of retained thoracic collections after trauma. *Ann Thorac Surg* 63:940–943, 1997.
83. Landreneau RJ, Keenan RJ, Hazelrigg SR, Mack MJ et al: Thoracoscopy for empyema and hemothorax. *Chest* 109:18–24, 1995.
84. Vassiliu P, Velmahos GC, Toutouzas KG: Timing, safety and efficacy of thoracoscopic evacuation of undrained post-traumatic hemothorax. *Am Surg* 67:1165–1169, 2001.
85. Aboholda A, Livingston DH, Donahoo JS, Allen K: Diagnostic and therapeutic video-assisted thoracic surgery (VATS) following chest trauma. *Eur J Cardiothorac Surg* 12:356–360, 1997.
86. Biffl WL, Moore EE, Johnson JL: Emergency department thoracotomy. In Moore EE, Feliciano DV, Mattox KL, editors: *Trauma*, 5th ed. New York, McGraw-Hill, 2004, pp. 239–254.
87. Stammers AH, Murdock JD, Klayman MH, Trowbridge C, Yen BR, Franklin D, et al: Utilization of rapid-infuser devices for massive blood loss. *Perfusion* 20:65–69, 2005.
88. Rieger A, Phillippi W, Spies C, Eyrich K: Safe normothermic massive transfusions by modification of an infusion warming and pressure device. *J Trauma* 39:686–688, 1995.
89. Bartlett RL, Stewart NJ Jr, Raymond J, Anstadt GL, Martin SD: Comparative study of three methods of resuscitation: closed-chest, open-chest manual, and direct mechanical ventricular assistance. *Ann Emerg Med* 13:773–777, 1984.
90. Cryer HG, Mavroudis C, Yu J, Roberts AW, Cue JI, Richardson JD, et al: Shock, transfusion and pneumonectomy. Death is due to right heart failure and increased pulmonary vascular resistance. *Ann Surg* 212:197–201, 1990.
91. Campos JH: Lung isolation techniques. *Anesthesiol Clin North Am* 19:455–474, 2001.
92. Self ML, Mangram A, Berne JD, Villarreal D, Norwood S: Non operative management of severe tracheobronchial injuries with positive end-expiratory pressure and low tidal volume ventilation. *J Trauma* 59:1072–1075, 2005.
93. Wall MJ Jr, Huh J, Mattox KL: Thoracotomy. In Moore EE, Feliciano DV, Mattox KL, editors: *Trauma*, 5th ed. New York, McGraw-Hill, 2004, pp. 493–506.
94. Blaisdell FW: Pulmonary injury: laceration, contusion, hematoma, pneumatocele and traumatic asphyxia blast injury. In Blaisdell FW, Trunkey DD, editors: *Trauma Management III: Cervicothoracic Trauma*. New York, Thieme Medical Publishers; New York and Stuttgart, Verlag, 1994, pp. 234–261.
95. Asensio JA, García-Núñez LM, Petrone P: Injuries to the lung. In Flint L, Meredith JW, Schwab CW, Takeri P, Trunkey DD, editors: *Trauma: Contemporary Principles and Therapy*. Philadelphia, Lippincott-Williams & Wilkins, 2006.
96. Lewis RJ, Caccavale RJ, Sisler GE: VATS-argon beam coagulator treatment of diffuse end-stage bilateral bullous disease of the lung. *Ann Thorac Surg* 55:1394–1398, 1993.
97. Gagarine A, Urschel JD, Miller JD, Bennett WF, Young JE: Effect of fibrin glue on air leak and length of hospital stay after pulmonary lobectomy. *J Cardiovasc Surg* 44:771–773, 2003.
98. Fabian T, Federico JA, Ponn RB: Fibrin glue in pulmonary resection. A prospective, randomized, blinded study. *Ann Thorac Surg* 75:1587–1592, 2003.
99. Murray KD, Ho CH, Hsia JY, Little AG: The influence of pulmonary staple line reinforcement on air leaks. *Chest* 122:2146–2149, 2002.
100. Downey DM, Michel M, Harre JG, Pratt JW: Functional assessment of a new staple line reinforcement in lung resection. *J Surg Res* 131:49–52, 2006.
101. Temes RT, Willms CD, Endara SA, Wernly JA: Fissureless lobectomy. *Ann Thorac Surg* 65:282–284, 1998.
102. Salvino CK, Dries D, Gamelli R, Murphy Macabobby M, Marshall W: Emergency cricothyroidotomy in trauma victims. *J Trauma* 34:503–505, 1993.
103. Asensio JA, Ceballos JJ, Rodriguez A, Forno W, Gambaro E, Hanpeter D, et al: Emergency department cricothyroidotomy. A marker of severe injury and mortality in trauma patients. *Eur J Trauma Emerg Surg* 22:101–106, 1999.
104. Reul GJ, Mattox KL, Beall AC Jr, Jordan GL Jr: Recent advances in the operative management of massive chest trauma. *Ann Thorac Surg* 16:52–66, 1973.
105. Khan FA, Phillips W, Khan A, Seriff NS: Unusual unilateral blunt chest trauma without rib fractures leading to pulmonary laceration requiring pneumonectomy. *Chest* 66:211–214, 1974.
106. Fisher RP, Geiger JP, Guernsey JM: Pulmonary resections for severe pulmonary contusions secondary to high velocity missile wounds. *J Trauma* 14:293–302, 1974.
107. Hankins JR, McAslan TC, Shin B, Ayella R, Cowley RA, McLaughlin JG: Excessive pulmonary laceration caused by blunt trauma. *J Cardiovasc Surg* 74:519–527, 1977.
108. Bowling R, Mavroudis C, Richardson JD, Flint LM, Howe WR, Gray LA Jr: Emergency pneumonectomy for penetrating and blunt trauma. *Am Surg* 51:136–141, 1985.
109. Gervin AS, Fischer RP: The importance of prompt transport in salvage of patients with penetrating heart wounds. *J Trauma* 22:443–448, 1982.

COMPLICATIONS
OF PULMONARY
AND PLEURAL INJURY

Riyad C. Karmy-Jones and Gregory J. Jurkovich

It has been stated that chest trauma is the primary cause of death in up to 25% of fatalities following traumatic injury, and a major contributing factor in another 25%, although as few as 5%–15% require acute operative intervention. Based on these generalizations, it is accepted that overall chest injury is common, acute operative intervention uncommon, and a significant, although ill-defined, number of thoracic operations are performed for delayed complications. The actual incidence of each of these varies from center to center based on ratio of blunt to penetrating admissions as well as overall volume. The two most common complications, persistent air leak and empyema, occur roughly in 5% of patients admitted who have required tube thoracostomy.

PULMONARY

Persistent Air Leak

There are three simple scenarios that describe persistent air leak: persistent air leak after parenchyma injury, after anatomic lung resection, and in ventilated patients. Persistent air leak after parenchyma injury can occur because of penetrating injury, blunt trauma with maceration or rib penetration, or in patients with underlying predisposing parenchyma lesions, primarily bullous disease. In this setting, management has followed the algorithm for spontaneous pneumothorax. Simple tube thoracostomy suffices in more than 80% of cases as long as there is full expansion. Occasionally, placing the chest drain to water seal will actually hasten resolution as the transpleural gradient is diminished. Air leak during more than 3 days or associated with recurrent pneumothorax appear to be most efficiently managed by thoracoscopic approaches than persistent chest drainage. Schermer and colleagues reviewed the course of 39 trauma patients who, except for air leak, were ready for discharge. This was determined by air leakage over more than 3 days. Twenty-five agreed to video-assisted thoracoscopic surgery (VATS) with reduced chest tube duration (total 8 vs. 12 days) and length of stay (10 vs. 17 days). Of course, technical factors should be ruled out (tube dislodgement or disconnection). Computed tomography (CT) scans can help define local lesions that may be amenable to thoracoscopic wedge resection or glue application, which may also prompt earlier VATS. In many instances, simply breaking down soft loculations and placing a chest drain under direct vision is the primary therapeutic benefit of thoracoscopy. We prefer to not use chemical pleurodesis, but rather pleural abrasion as we feel that this reduces the risk of parenchyma trapping and the uncertain long-term impact of chemical agents in younger patients. Patients with underlying lung lesions should be managed as they would in non-trauma circumstances. A final option in patients with prohibitive operative risks or small leaks is to convert the patients to Heimlich valve and manage them outpatient. As many as 80% will seal within 3 weeks using this approach.

As lobectomy and pneumonectomy are rarely performed for traumatic injury, it follows that the incidence of air leak (broncho-pleural fistula [BPF]) is also small. However, the nature of acute lung resections is such that the risk is higher than after elective resection. Risk factors include long stumps, devascularization, and contaminated hemothorax. Ideally, after lobectomy/pneumonectomy, the stump should be reinforced either at the time of original resection or second-look exploration with pleural, intercostals, or other flap. Once it occurs, management is determined by timing (less than or more than 7 days postoperatively), degree (ventilatory compromise and whether the defect can be visualized endoscopically), physiologic status, and whether the patient is ventilated. BPF may present in stable patients as a new productive cough, with a drop in pleural fluid levels (after pneumonectomy) of two or more rib spaces, or new air–fluid level. In ventilated patients, empyema and loss of tidal volume may predominate. The primary goal is to prevent aspiration. In nonintubated patients, this is best accompanied by upright positioning or affected side down. Then, drainage should be instituted if a chest drain is not in place. If a drain is not in place, the new drain should be placed above the thoracotomy scar, as the diaphragm tends to rise to the level of the scar and adhere. If the leak is small, and endoscopically the hole cannot be clearly visualized, it is reasonable to attempt bronchoscopic glue application. Reoperation and stump closure are possible within 7 days, but the associated empyema increases the risk of failure. The longer the interval between the initial and second operation, the greater the difficulty. After pneumonectomy, the mediastinum becomes inflamed, the stump can only with difficulty be visualized, and mobilization is essentially impossible. Thus, after pneumonectomy, the best option is probably to occlude the stump with omentum, pack the chest with packs, and plan serial washouts until the leak scarifies closed. An alternative approach, particularly after right-sided pneumonectomy, is to perform trans-carinal right mainstem resection. The residual stump cannot be removed as it tends to be fixed, but the mucosa should be cauterized and omentum or other viable tissue should be used to reinforce the new stump. The empyema cavity can then be treated by the drainage procedure of the surgeon's choice. After lobectomy, similar options are possible, but further resection may be required (e.g., right middle lobectomy after right lower lobe stump leak).

Persistent air leak in a ventilated patient without a discrete lesion is better thought of as an alveolar-pleural fistula rather than a BPF. Clearly, the underlying lung injury affects outcome, with alveolar-pleural leak in adult respiratory distress syndrome patients being associated with up to 80% mortality. Whatever the underlying anatomy, air leak in ventilated patients can be a significant marker of increased mortality. Pierson and colleagues reviewed the course of 39 patients (out of a population of 1700 mechanically ventilated patients) who presented with air leak lasting more than 24 hours, of whom 27 were trauma patients. The risk factors for mortality correlated with the following: air leak not present on admission or shortly thereafter (45% early vs. 94% if developed later); leak greater than 500 ml per breath (57% if less vs. 100% if greater); and post–chest trauma (56% for trauma admissions vs. 92% for nontrauma admissions). These findings illustrate that while the course in trauma admissions is more benign, it still represents a major concern. On the other hand, the air leak itself is rarely the cause of death. These air leaks can lead to persistent or even tension pneumothorax that compromises ventilation. Pleural tubes (at times multiple) may be required. Less commonly, air leak is significant enough to affect oxygenation. The primary treatment is to minimize alveolar pressure, using end-inspiratory plateau pressure as an (admittedly crude) reflection of this. Ideally, the end-inspiratory plateau pressure should be less than 30 cm H_2O. The most common method of attaining this is to combine low tidal volume and permissive hypercapnia. Alternative methods if this approach fails are high-frequency jet ventilation or independent lung ventilation. It should be stressed that high-frequency jet ventilation, although used successfully in patients with central airway disruption and in the operating room, does not reduce mean airway pressure consistently, nor does it uniformly reduce air leak or improve oxygenation. Thus, it should not be used routinely in patients with alveolar-pleural fistula. A temporizing technique is to isolate the lobe that is the primary source of leak bronchoscopically. This is done by sequentially occluding bronchi with a Swan-Ganz or other balloon catheter. If this results in elimination or significant reduction in air leak, occlusive material (Gelfoam, fibrin glue, blood mixed with tetracycline, etc.) can be injected. In most cases, the air leak will diminish as airway pressure decreases. Surgery can be performed, but in the setting of diffuse parenchyma injury, lung inflammation, severe emphysema, and/or steroids, the risk is that staple lines will fail and the leak will be exacerbated. If surgery is felt to be needed, reinforced staple lines (i.e., with bovine strips, etc.), apical tents (mobilizing the apical pleura so that it falls onto the area of resection), and/or anatomic lobectomy (if predominantly one lobe) should be considered.

Pneumatocoele/Hematoma

Pneumatocoeles occur when disruption of lung parenchyma leads to internal rather than external leak of air and/or blood. They occur more commonly after blunt injury, but can be seen occasionally with deep stab or low-caliber missile injuries. These lesions are thus best described as a pulmonary laceration. They are usually solitary, at times multilobulated, and occasionally multiple. They are typically not apparent on initial radiographs, because small size and/or a superimposed contusion or hemorrhage obscures them. Over time, they evolve into thin-walled cavities with air and/or fluid. The location and size are affected by the mechanism. Compression leading to rupture, the most common mechanism, tends to be associated with central lesions. Compression, leading to shear forces, tends to present as an elongated paramediastinal cavity extending from hilum to diaphragm, and may be confused with loculated pneumothorax. Rib penetration forms tend to be small and peripheral. Adhesion tears are the least common. In the vast majority of cases, pneumatocoeles are benign. In rare cases, they may result in persistent air leak or become infected, in which case they are treated as abscesses.

Hematomas are formed by the same mechanisms that result in pneumatocoeles. They may remain solid, or with partial evacuation they can develop an air-fluid level or even a fibrin wall resulting in a crescent of air on the superior surface that mimics a fungus ball.

Usually these lesions resolve over 3–6 months, and recognizing the shrinking process is one method to avoid confusing these with malignant processes.

Pneumonia

Pneumonia may be the most common complication of chest trauma. Risk factors include aspiration, need for ventilation, direct injury, pulmonary contusion, and persistent atelectasis secondary to pain. The incidence is as low as 6% in nonintubated patients to as high as 44% in ventilated patients. Despite the high incidence, there are no data supporting prophylactic antibiotics. Of all patients admitted with a diagnosis of pulmonary contusion, nearly 50% will develop pneumonia, barotrauma, and/or major atelectasis. One-fourth will progress to adult respiratory distress syndrome. Ventilator-associated pneumonia (VAP), defined as pneumonia arising more than 48 hours after initiation of mechanical ventilation, is difficult to define and diagnose. At our institution, we have found that the incidence in patients ventilated for more than 7 days ranges from 20% to 30%. Clinical suspicion is often raised by new infiltrates, recurring fever, rising leukocytes, and/or a change in endotracheal secretions. However, distinguishing between colonization and infection may require specialized techniques. Quantitative cultures obtained from a variety of approaches increase the specificity (although perhaps with reduced sensitivity) of endobronchial cultures, and each institution must define cut-off values based on whether the patient is already receiving antibiotics (Table 1).

Necrotizing Lung Infection

Necrotizing lung infections comprise a triad of clinical scenarios that overlap or can be present concomitantly. These are lung abscess, necrotizing pneumonia, and lung gangrene. All three are similar in that lack of perfusion is combined with tissue devitalization. In simplistic terms, lung abscess can be described as a region of necrosis less than a lobe with viable surrounding or bordering parenchyma. Lung gangrene represents complete lobar or entire lung destruction, often with only a rim of tissue remaining. Lung necrosis is best represented by patchy, often nonanatomic, loss of perfusion with variable parenchyma destruction, often seen on radiograph as multiple small abscess-like cavities. Although the three can be discussed separately, in most cases two or three coexist and so the management can also overlap.

Table 1: Yields of Diagnostic Tests for Ventilator-Associated Pneumonia

	Threshold	Sensitivity (%)	Specificity (%)
Endotracheal aspirate	Any pathogen	70–95	<50
Endotracheal aspirate	$>10^6$ CFU/ml	25–70	70–85
Bronchoscopy			
PSB culture	$>10^3$ CFU/ml	30–100	80–100
BAL culture	$>10^4$ CFU/ml	55–95	70–100
BAL cytology	2%–7% CAB	30–85	65–100
Nonbronchoscopic			
PSB	10^3 CFU/ml	60–100	75–100
BAL	10^4 CFU/ml	70–100	65–95

BAL, Bronchoalveolar lavage; *CAB,* cell-associated bacteria; *CFU/ml,* colony-forming units per milliliter; *PSB,* protected specimen brush.
Source: Skerrett SJ: The diagnosis of ventilator-associated pneumonia. In Karmy-Jones R, Nathens A, Stern E, eds. *Thoracic Trauma and Critical Care.* Boston, Kluwer Medical Publishers, 2002, 397–402, with permission.

The cause(s) of lung abscess in the surgical intensive care unit (ICU) population include aspiration, complications of pneumonia, retained foreign body, septic emboli, and/or infected traumatic injury. More specific etiologies in the trauma population include aspiration (with or without bronchial obstruction), infected pneumatocoele, infected site of resection (in particular emergent tractotomy), and late complications of ventilator-associated pneumonia. As a whole, these are less common in trauma patients than nontrauma patients. Of 45 thoracotomies performed at our institution over 7 years for abscess, necrotizing pneumonia, and lung gangrene, only 4 were in patients initially admitted after traumatic injury.

The diagnosis of lung abscess may be relatively simple. Fever, purulent sputum production, or hemoptysis may prompt chest radiograph, which will identify an air-fluid cavity. On the other extreme, a persistently febrile patient in the ICU with dense consolidation may require CT scan before the underlying cavity can be recognized.

Over the three decades of approximately the 1950s through the 1970s, a number of advances reduced the mortality rates from approximately 50% to 10%. These advances included recognizing the importance of antibiotics, the role of aspiration, the need for pulmonary toilet (including liberal use of bronchoscopy), and finally the benefit in selected patients of operative intervention. Subsequently, the major addition to the armamentarium has been image-guided catheter drainage as an intermediate category between medical and surgical management. Percutaneous catheter drainage can be performed even in ventilated patients and has reduced the number of thoracotomies required. While there is always concern about the risk of empyema and/or bronchopleural fistula, the former can be usually easily managed by chest drainage, and the latter is rarely so significant as to impair oxygenation. Some patients will require thoracotomy, which, in the trauma population, usually results from persistent sepsis and inability or incomplete drainage, hemoptysis, or persistent or major bronchopleural fistula (see Table 1). The two primary operations are lobectomy for large central cavities, or debridement (plus muscle flap to help close the space) for smaller peripheral cavities. At operation, there are several technical points that can help reduce complications: prevent aspiration by isolating the affected lung before posterolateral positioning; expose the main pulmonary artery early in the case so that control can be achieved should hemorrhage result; place a nasogastric tube or esophagoscope in the esophagus because the anatomy may be obliterated; and refrain from resecting small abscesses (<2 cm) that are in otherwise viable parenchyma. Air leak is not uncommon, and, as will be discussed under the empyema section, a residual space can be managed with continuous postoperative irrigation.

The distinguishing characteristics of lung gangrene are central vascular thrombosis and bronchial obstruction, leading to significant cavitation and/or lobar or whole-lung liquefaction. As opposed to lung abscess, there is no firm, well-defined capsule. Both these features are defined by CT with intravenous contrast, and either one predicts the failure of medical therapy. This is because medical therapy relies on both blood supply for antibiotic therapy to be effective and on bronchial patency to allow expectoration of purulent material. Schamaun and colleagues followed 14 patients with unilateral complete lung gangrene. Four were treated medically and all died, while 10 underwent surgical resection with 100% survival. Some patients have diffuse bilateral disease. In the face of persistent signs of infection, if there is a primary target site, surgery is still possible and can be performed even if the patient cannot tolerate independent lung ventilation. Interestingly, dissection in the fissures and of the vessels is relatively easy, as the necrotic tissue tends to be easily swept aside. However, surgery resection should not be performed if the patient is pressor dependent. In this setting, it is better to temporize with pleuroscopy to treat associated empyema and percutaneous drainage of the large cavitary lesions.

Necrotizing pneumonia is characterized by areas of dense consolidation, patchy perfusion, and often multiple small cavitary changes. Percutaneous drainage does not help in this setting. Generally, parenchyma resection is not indicated. However, serial CT scans can identify areas that are developing demarcation lines, and in the setting of persistent pulmonary sepsis resection can be a reasonable option.

Bronchial Stricture

Of patients with blunt traumatic injury to the distal trachea or bronchi, 10%–20% are not diagnosed acutely, but in a delayed fashion as stricturing occurs. In approximately two-thirds of these cases, suppuration, persistent atelectasis, and/or hemoptysis develop within 1–2 weeks of injury. In the remainder, presentation may be delayed years until "asthma," dyspnea on exertion, and/or delayed parenchyma necrosis develops. Any young patient with new-onset asthma should be considered for airway evaluation if this develops 1–2 years after blunt traumatic chest injury, even if initial radiographic and bronchoscopic work-up was done and was normal. Bronchoscopy, CT scan, CT (or "virtual") bronchography, and/or flow-volume loops can help make the diagnosis depending on clinical circumstances. If postobstructive parenchyma destruction has occurred, then distal lung resection is required. If not, airway resection and reconstruction can salvage the distal lung. In chronic settings, there may be a suggestion of lack of perfusion to the affected lung. In the absence of clinical signs of sepsis and evidence of lung necrosis, attempts should be made to reconstruct the airway, as in most cases this lack of perfusion is a hypoxic vasoconstrictive response that reverses when ventilation is restored. In patients who are too unstable, airway stenting can be tried to maintain airway patency as a temporizing measure. In patients who present years later with a chronic fibrotic stricture, balloon dilation and repeat stenting may be an alternative to operative repair as well.

Pulmonary Torsion

Lobar torsion is exceedingly rare after trauma and is reported more commonly after upper lobectomy when the middle lobe can swing freely in the residual space. Recognizing this potential, stapling the middle lobe to the lower lobe can prevent this from occurring. Alternatively, the lung may torsed during thoracotomy, during retraction to expose posterior mediastinal structures, particularly if the inferior pulmonary ligament has been divided. The key to prevent this complication is to observe that the lung expands properly before closing the chest. Primary pulmonary torsion is exceedingly rare, but not unheard of. Schamaun reviewed 26 cases of torsion in the literature and found that 5 were post-traumatic. Possible mechanisms include focal injury to one lobe, in the setting of a complete fissure, resulting in a focal immediate twisting or delayed torsion as hemorrhage and edema create a lead point. The diagnosis may be suggested by lobar consolidation and the development of fever and hemoptysis, eventually developing into frank pulmonary sepsis. The diagnosis can be confirmed by bronchoscopy, which documents a "fish-mouth" appearance of the affected bronchus, occasionally with blood and/or purulent material intermittently draining. When diagnosed, immediate operation is required. If not frankly gangrenous, the lobe should be "de-torsed" to assess viability. If not viable, lobectomy is required. If viable, it should be stapled to an adjacent lobe to prevent retorsion.

Retained Parenchyma Missiles

The need for removal of parenchyma foreign objects is based on the risk of developing complications, which appear to be more common with irregularly shaped missiles compared with smooth objects. The

University of Heidelberg reviewed the course of 55 patients who had retained bullets. Thirty-four experienced recurrent hemoptysis (single episode in eight). A Finnish review of 502 patients over several years noted that 20% developed complications requiring surgery. These included chronic bronchitis (39), lung abscess (31), bronchiectasis (5), empyema (24), and/or bronchopleural fistula (10). Many contemporary recommendations are based on data from World War II and in the two decades following, including the aforementioned studies. In World War II, early removal of retained missiles was associated with 0.9% mortality, while late removal of symptomatic objects was associated with 7.3% mortality. However, it was noted then and subsequently that waiting 2–6 weeks to allow parenchyma inflammation to resolve was also associated with easier removal, with reduced complications, notably less bleeding, air leak, and empyema. The technique of removal obviously depends on the location and nature of the missile. Peripheral objects can be removed by wedge resection. Deeper objects can be retrieved via tractotomy or occasionally lobectomy if there is significant associated destruction, necrosis, or infection. Uncommonly, over time central foreign objects can erode into the bronchi, leading to obstructive pneumonitis and abscess formation. These may be retrieved endoscopically, while severe tissue destruction, if present, mandates lobectomy. Alternatively, these objects may migrate peripherally, resulting in empyema. These can be retrieved and the empyema managed by VATS or thoracotomy.

PLEURAL

Retained Hemothorax

Tube thoracostomy fails to completely evacuate hemothorax in approximately 5% of cases. Complications that may arise include empyema and/or fibrothorax. Conditions that predispose patients to both include prolonged ventilation, development of pneumonia, break in the pleura with residual blood (as is the case after tube thoracostomy), and/or other sites of infection. On the other hand, stable, nonventilated patients with small effusions (less than one-quarter hemothorax) following blunt trauma with no obvious pleural disruption usually will resolve without sequelae. In these patients the cornerstone of therapy should be observation.

The use of antibiotics, in particular with Gram-positive coverage, in many, but not all, reviews show a reduction in the risk of empyema. However, even those papers that support prophylactic antibiotics do not show an advantage to giving one dose, 24 hours worth, or keeping the antibiotic coverage until the drains are removed; all are equivalent. Thus, our practice is to give one dose only, unless there are other risk factors.

Early evacuation of hemothorax has been shown to reduce the incidence of complications preferably within 7 days when loculations begin to complicate pleural debridement. In particular, the risk of empyema is reduced. However, recognizing the extent of hemothorax can be difficult. Chest radiography can underestimate both the extent of parenchyma consolidation and the volume of retained blood, particularly in ventilated patients. Chest CT is much more accurate in this setting, but interpretation requires some individualization. Moderate effusions in ventilated patients or those with other risk factors should be aggressively drained when detected by CT.

When recognized acutely after injury, the simplest and most expeditious treatment is to place a second chest tube. When recognized after 1–2 days, this may not be helpful in that it may simply increase pain, splinting, and the risk of pneumonia with subsequent seeding of the pleural space. Intrapleural streptokinase (250,000 units) or urokinase (40,000 units) has efficacy of 65%–90%. Complications include fever and pain, but the risk of re-starting bleeding is negligible. The downside of this approach is that it takes several days longer than more direct operative drainage and will not break down

loculations. Thus, it may be more useful after debridement when it is suspected that the clot is relatively "soft."

Thoracoscopy offers the advantage of complete removal of all clots without the excess morbidity of a formal thoracotomy. Meyer et al. compared placement of a second chest tube versus thoracoscopy for treatment of retained traumatic hemothorax. Patients undergoing thoracoscopy had a shortened length of time requiring chest tube drainage, a shortened hospital stay (2.7 days less), and decreased total hospital costs ($6000 less) compared with patients treated with a second chest tube. There were no failures, no complications, and no patients who required conversion to a formal thoracotomy in the group randomized to early thoracoscopy. In contrast, a second chest tube failed to completely evacuate the retained hemothorax requiring operative treatment in over 40% of the patients.

Thoracotomies through "mini" approaches are often sufficient to allow removal of soft gelatinous visceral and pleural rind, permitting full lung expansion. Irrigation with warm saline facilitates clot removal. The denser the adhesions, the greater the exposure must be, and if a formal decortication of a formed visceral peel is anticipated, a standard approach is required. This can be facilitated by excising a rib subperiosteally to allow safe identification of the pleura.

In summary, patients with retained hemothorax, at risk of empyema, should be managed aggressively, preferably by early thoracoscopic drainage.[27] Occasionally, there are patients who present with delayed effusions, days after blunt injury, presumably partially because of missed small hemothorax and partially secondary to reactive fluid accumulation. If these patients have adequate pain control, have small effusions (less than one-fourth of the hemithorax), and have no signs of infection, tube thoracostomy does not need to be performed, as the risk of fibrothorax is negligible. Patients who present late (usually more than 3 months after injury) with an element of fibrothorax (but with no infection) should be managed nonoperatively, as at 6–9 months there is some remodeling and adaptation in most cases, and if surgery is required there is no increased difficulty if it is undertaken at a later date.

Empyema

Empyema occurs in 2%–7% of patients who undergo tube thoracostomy after trauma. Patients at risk include those with residual hemothorax noted on chest radiograph, concurrent pneumonia, pain with diminished cough, extrathoracic sites of infection, and/or possibly those who are ventilated and who have a chest tube in place. Trauma patients are at risk of developing Gram-positive empyema, characterized by early loculations and formation of dense adhesions because of hemothorax, which offers both a rich supply of bacterial nutrients as well as fibrin. These factors also tend to make empyema in trauma patients less amenable to simple drainage than the more common parapneumonic empyema seen in medical patients.

The diagnosis of empyema is based on the documentation of an exudative effusion, characterized in particular by an elevated pleural/serum lactate dehydrogenase ration (>0.6). In approximately 25%–30% of cases, cultures will be negative because of suppression but not eradication by antibiotics. It is not uncommon for patients to present with indolent courses, often characterized by a failure to wean from ventilation, with persistent fluid noted by CT or chest x-ray, despite tube drainage. Contrast CT scans often reveal a "rim sign" of enhancing pleura, indicative of ongoing inflammation. In many cases, once these "contaminated hemothoraces" are drained, the clinical picture rapidly improves.

Empyema has been described as having three stages. The first, usually within 1–7 days, is referred to as the "acute" or "serous" phase. This distinction is important because at this stage there is the best chance for draining the thin, exudative fluid by simple thoracostomy. There have been attempts to treat this early stage by simple aspiration. Evidence of vigorous inflammation (pH<7.0) almost universally predicts failure of this technique. Tapping may be appropriate in patients who have complex effusions, with or without loculations, but who have other potential sites of infection. However managed, it is imperative that complete drainage be achieved, or failing that, early operative drainage is performed before progressive pleural obliteration occurs, characteristic of progression to the second or "subacute" phase, and thence the final or "chronic" phase. Palpation at the time of thoracostomy and/or loculations noted on CT can alert the surgeon to the presence of loculations that would indicate simple tube drainage will fail.

Probably the major reason for earlier intervention is that minimally invasive approaches are more successful early, whereas with the passage of time the combined impact of pleural space obliteration and visceral peel leading to parenchyma trapping increases both the likelihood of requiring thoracotomy as well as the incidence of primary failure. As noted earlier, compared with nontrauma patients, empyema after trauma is much more likely to require operative intervention.

The primary treatment of empyema is to both completely drain the thorax and to permit full lung expansion. There are several "local" considerations that may impact operative approach and outcomes (Table 2). Predominant among these are whether loculations and/or a restrictive visceral peel have formed. In the acute setting, particularly when clinical signs suggest active infection, the primary goal is simply to drain the pleura. Evidence of loculations suggests that simple tube drainage will fail. Alternative approaches could include image-directed catheter placement, thoracoscopic drainage, and "mini" or full thoracotomy. Thrombolytic therapy has been advocated as an alternative to operative intervention, but current data suggest that when compared with thoracoscopic approaches as primary intervention, thrombolytic therapy is associated with a higher failure rate, increased length of stay, and greater cost. Thrombolytic therapy is a reasonable alternative in patients who are deemed at high risk for operative intervention, and whose loculations may be diaphanous. In essence, these criteria would be in the uncommon scenario of a patient who is clinically infected and frail but not yet intubated, as once a patient is on the ventilator, the primary complication of operative approaches (respiratory failure) has already occurred. Thrombolytic therapy does have a role in the early postoperative period after operative decortication residual loculated fluid collections are present. In this setting, the fibrinous adhesions are "soft" and may be lysed.

Thoracoscopy, both VATS and pleuroscopy (using a mediastinoscope) have been compared with thoracotomy in a variety of series, which tend to be nonrandomized. VATS appears to be associated with decreased morbidity and shorter length of stay; however, it is usually performed much earlier in the hospital course when loculations are less formed and the patients clinically more stable. VATS may not be technically possible because of high ventilator requirements precluding lung isolation and/or dense pleural symphysis. An alternative approach is "rigid" thoracoscopy or pleuroscopy. Pleuroscopy can be performed on these patients, using CT imaging to direct the initial approach. The wider port allows easier debridement and suctioning, and visceral decortication is possible except in the most fibrotic cases.

Irrigation postoperatively is a useful adjunct in certain cases. The goal of irrigation may be to wash out blood from the operation, thus preventing new, vigorous adhesions. In addition, antibiotics can be added to improve local treatment of resistant organisms (such as *Candida* or methicillin-resistant organisms). Irrigation systems can be modified according to circumstances (e.g., a Jackson-Pratt drain connected to intravenous tubing via a three-way stop cock). The actual volume of irrigation is flexible, although we usually use 100 cc/hr. To avoid excessive drainage through the incision or drain sites, these need to be closed tightly. When the pleural effluent is clear and culture negative, the irrigation can be discontinued. One potential disadvantage of postoperative irrigation is that pleural symphysis may be prevented, resulting in residual spaces. On the other hand, if a residual space is anticipated, irrigation is particularly effective. In fact, in some cases, as the chest tubes are removed, it is possible, for example, to convert the Jackson-Pratt back into a simple bulb drain, which is better tolerated by the patient.

The residual pleural space remains a problem, requiring a flexible approach, depending primarily on whether the lung is capable of expanding (Table 3). In the trauma population, the primary reason for failure of lung expansion is visceral peel, while in nontraumatic empyema, the etiology is relatively equally divided among visceral peel, parenchyma consolidation, and/or space after lung resection.

When performing thoracotomy for empyema, it may be advisable to avoid "counting ribs" beneath the scapula. This reduces contamination and the potential for a subscapular abscess. If a dense parietal pleural and/or significant pleural symphysis is anticipated, subperiosteal rib resection provides a safer avenue of entering the thorax. Visceral decortication may actually be simpler and safer with the affected lung being ventilated, as the "peel–parenchyma" interface is easier to define. Significant peripheral lung leaks are acceptable if it looks like the lung will expand and significantly fill the thorax. If the parenchyma is too consolidated to expand, or if visceral pleurectomy is proceeding poorly (technically difficult, large air leaks, bloody), it may be necessary to abandon pleurectomy in favor of a strategy aimed at treating a residual space, such as drainage, irrigation, tissue flaps, and/or open drainage.

However the empyema is drained, it is important to recognize that the underlying lung may have to be reevaluated. Once expansion has occurred, it may be apparent that there was a lung abscess or other necrotizing process that may require further intervention. In addition, in most cases the pleural space will appear radiographically much as it did before operation. This may make clinical assessment of whether there is ongoing pleural sepsis difficult. One manner in which this can be sorted out is to follow serial LDH levels form the chest tubes. A falling LDH implies a reduction in pleural inflammation and success, while a rising LDH implies the opposite.

In summary, the principles of treating empyema are as follows: drain the pleura; debride the pleura; maximize lung expansion; if lung expansion is not possible, consider either tissue flaps (if small) or chronic open drainage; and close significant bronchopleural fistulae. Earlier intervention allows less invasive procedures to be performed with higher likelihood of success. Thoracoscopy using "rigid" techniques is still possible in patients who are not VATS candidates, but thoracotomy should not be delayed.

Table 2: Considerations When Treating Empyema

Residual space
Quality of lung parenchyma
Trapped lung
Density of loculations
Patient ventilated
Air leak current or anticipated
Lung abscess

Table 3: Managing Residual Space

Irrigation plus antibiotics
Positive-pressure ventilation to expand consolidated lung
Bronchoscopy to rule out and/or treat endobronchial obstruction
Visceral decortication
Open drainage for chronic treatment, particularly if patient debilitated
Tissue flaps
Combination: Claggett procedure

Chylothorax

Primary traumatic chylothorax is exceedingly uncommon. It can occur after penetrating injuries to the thoracic inlet, transmediastinal injuries, or blunt trauma. Of interest, chylothorax is associated with spine fractures in only 20% of cases. Chylothorax can manifest in a delayed fashion with recurrent effusions, as persistent milky pleural output, or rarely as a tension chylothorax. Chylothorax is more commonly seen as a complication after repair of aortic injury or esophageal resection. The diagnosis can be established by documenting triglyceride levels greater than 110 mg/dl and/or predominant lymphocytes in the effusion. If noted acutely, it is important to consider the possibility of associated injury to adjacent structures, especially esophagus or aorta. The primary complication is nutritional and immunological compromise. Initial management includes drainage, ensuring complete lung expansion (with increased positive end-expiratory pressure in ventilated patients), and parenteral nutritional support. Although low-fat diets do reduce the flow of chyle, even oral water has been noted to increase chyle flow. How long medical therapy should be attempted is not clear, but generally 4 weeks is the maximum duration, depending on the physiological reserves of the patient. Chylothorax noted immediately after operation may be best treated by reoperation and maneuvers as described below.

Lymphangiography (via CT, nuclear studies, or formal lymphangiogram) may be helpful in determining the site of the leak, presence of collaterals, and volume of the leak, all of which may predict success or failure of medical therapy. If no specific leak is documented, and collaterals are noted to drain into the venous system, medical management has a much higher success rate. With parenteral nutrition and strict NPO, an almost immediate cessation of chyle flow is a good prognostic sign that supports medical management. Octreotide has also been used as an adjunct. If the duct can be identified, then transabdominal coil embolization has been successful. A persistent space (especially after pneumonectomy), widespread disruption (e.g., after esophagectomy), or persistent high output with medical therapy is associated with an extremely high failure rate, and earlier intervention is warranted. Ultimately, surgery should be considered if the leak persists after 2 weeks, and certainly by 4 weeks, if the patient is deteriorating immunologically or nutritionally, and clearly if there is another indication for surgery. Patients who present in a delayed fashion are managed similarly. Our bias is that if after 1 week of maximal medical therapy, the patient continues to drain more than 1500 cc in 24 hours and/or is clearly losing ground nutritionally; then in the vast majority of cases, we would try coil embolization, and if this is not possible or is unsuccessful, perform open ligation.

Surgery can be performed by thoracoscopy or thoracotomy. The site may be directly visualized, in which case direct ligation (usually with pledgeted sutures) and/or glue application should be used. Localization can be assisted by feeding the patient cream just before operation. Mass ligation at the level of the diaphragm on the right side can resolve both right and left leaks. It is critical to recognize that the duct and surrounding tissue can be very friable, and thus ligation can lead to another leak site. In addition, collaterals may exist that bypass the site of ligation. We have thus found that a critical component is to ensure complete decortication (to allow lung expansion), pleural abrasion, or decortication, and if in doubt, continue ventilation for 24 hours to assist full lung expansion. We maintain a strict NPO status for 7 days after surgery.

Fibrothorax

As mentioned in the discussion of retained hemothorax, symptomatic fibrothorax is more feared than real. Patients who have had an infected hemothorax are at the greatest risk and usually present much sooner in their hospital course. The problems with deciding whether to operate for fibrothorax associated with chronic respiratory complaints include the following: in many cases, the decision is based on CT findings of pleural thickening, and invariably the postoperative films look identical to the preoperative films; and patients who have sustained multiple chest wall injuries are actually symptomatic from that rather than fibrothorax, including chronic pain, which will be aggravated rather than relieved by thoracotomy.

Suggested Readings

Aguilar MM, Battistella FD, Owings JT, Su T: Posttraumatic empyema: risk factor analysis. *Arch Surg* 132:647–650, 1997.

Bayfield MS, Spotnitz WD: Fibrin sealant in thoracic surgery: pulmonary applications, including management of bronchopleural fistula. *Chest Surg Clin North Am* 6:567–584, 1996.

Boyd AD, Glassman LR: Trauma to the lung. *Chest Surg Clin North Am* 7:263–284, 1997.

Eddy AC, Luna GK, Copass M: Empyema thoracis in patients undergoing emergent closed tube thoracostomy for thoracic trauma. *Am J Surg* 157: 494–497, 1989.

Hagan JL, Hardy JD: Lung abscess revisited: a survey of 184 cases. *Ann Surg* 197:755–762, 1983.

Karmy-Jones R, Jurkovich GJ: Blunt chest trauma. *Curr Prob Surg* 41: 211–380, 2004.

Karmy-Jones R, Vallieres E, Harrington R: Surgical management of necrotizing pneumonia. *Clin Pulm Med* 10:17–25, 2003.

Dulchavesky SA, Ledgerwood AM, Lucas CE: Management of chylothorax after blunt chest trauma. *J Trauma* 28:1400–1401, 1988.

Meyer DM, Jessen ME, Wait MA, Estera AS: Early evacuation of traumatic retained hemothoraces using thoracoscopy: a prospective, randomized trial. *Ann Thorac Surg* 64:1396–1400, 1997.

Moon WK, Im JG, Yeon KM, et al: Complications of *Klebsiella pneumonia*: CT evaluation. *J Comput Assist Tomogr* 19:176–181, 1995.

Pierson DJ, Horton CA, Bates PW: Persistent bronchopleural air leak during mechanical ventilation: a review of 39 cases. *Chest* 90:321–323, 1986.

Richardson JD, Carrillo E: Thoracic infection after trauma. *Chest Surg Clin North Am* 7:401–428, 1997.

Schamaun M: Postoperative pulmonary torsion: report of a case and survey of the literature including spontaneous and posttraumatic torsion. *Thorac Cardiovasc Surg* 42:116–121, 1994.

Schamaun M, von Buren U, Pirozynski W: Massive lung necrosis in *Klebsiella pneumonia*. *Schweiz Med Wochenser* 110:223–225, 1980.

Schermer CR, Matteson BD, Demarest GB 3rd, et al: A prospective evaluation of video-assisted thoracic surgery for persistent air leak due to trauma. *Am J Surg* 177:480–484, 1999.

Skerrett SJ: The diagnosis of ventilator-associated pneumonia. In Karmy-Jones R, Nathens A, Stern E, editors: *Thoracic Trauma and Critical Care*. Boston, Kluwer Medical Publishers, 2002, pp. 397–402.

Stathopoulos G, Chrysikopoulou E, Kalogeromitros A, et al: Bilateral traumatic pulmonary pseudocysts: case report and literature review. *J Trauma* 53:993–996, 2002.

Taskinen SO, Salo JA, Halttunen PE, Sovijarvi AR: Tracheobronchial rupture due to blunt chest trauma: a follow-up study. *Ann Thorac Surg* 48: 846–849, 1989.

Velmahos GC, Demetriades D, Chan L, et al: Predicting the need for thoracoscopic evacuation of residual traumatic hemothorax: chest radiograph is insufficient. *J Trauma* 46:65–70, 1999.

Vogt-Moykopf MD, Krumhaar D: Treatment of intrapulmonary shell fragments. *Surg Gynecol Obstet* 123:1233–1236, 1966.

Wait MA, Sharma S, Hohn J, Dal Nogare A: A randomized trial of empyema therapy. *Chest* 111:1548–1551, 1997.

CARDIAC INJURIES

Juan A. Asensio,   Luis Manuel García-Núñez,   Patrizio Petrone,   Dominic Duran,   Alexander D. Vara,   John S. Weston,   Scott B. Gmora,   Ara Feinstein, Donald Robinson,   Nicholas Namias, and   Louis R. Pizano

PENETRATING CARDIAC INJURY

Historical Perspective

The earliest descriptions of a cardiac injury are found in the *Iliad*[1] and in the *Edwin Smith Papyrus*,[2,3] written in approximately 3000 BC. Hippocrates[4] stated that all wounds of the heart were deadly. Ambrose Pare,[5,6] the famous French trauma surgeon, described two cases of penetrating cardiac injuries, both detailed from autopsy studies. Wolf,[7] in 1642, was the first to describe a healed wound of the heart, while Senac,[8] in 1749, concluded that although all wounds of the heart were serious, some wounds might heal and not be fatal. Larrey[9,10] was the first to describe the surgical approach to the pericardium to relieve a pericardial effusion, and is credited with pioneering the technique for pericardial window. Billroth, in 1875 and in 1883, proclaimed his strong resistance to any attempt at cardiac injury repair.[11–13] Block,[14] in 1882, created cardiac wounds in a rabbit model and was successful in achieving repair, thus demonstrating successful recovery and suggesting that the same techniques could be applicable to humans. Also, Del Vecchio[15] demonstrated cardiac injury healing after suturing the heart in a canine model.

However, it took the courage of Cappelen[16] from Norway to attempt cardiac injury repair in a human; in 1895 he repaired a 2-cm left ventricular laceration including ligation of a large branch of the distal left anterior descending coronary artery. This was followed by Farina[17] in Italy in 1896, who also attempted to repair a left ventricular wound; however, both patients succumbed. Rehn[18] in Germany in 1896 was successful in repairing a wound of the right ventricle, while in the United States, Hill,[19] in 1902, was the first surgeon to successfully repair a left ventricular injury.

Duval[20] described the median sternotomy incision, and Spangaro,[21] in 1906, described the left anterolateral thoracotomy incision. Peck[22] in 1909 was the first to describe successful repair of a stab wound of the right atrium, and he reported a total of 11 patients. Smith[23] was the first to develop a comprehensive plan for cardiac injury management, and for the first time pointed out the dangers of dysrhythmias occurring during cardiac manipulation. He also described the use of an Allis clamp near the apex to stabilize and hold the heart during suture placement.

Beck[24] in 1942 described the technique of placing mattress sutures under the bed of the coronary arteries. During the same year, Griswold[25] refined the techniques in the management of cardiac injuries and recommended that every large general hospital should have available a sterile set of instruments plus an available operating room 24 hours a day. Elkin[26–28] in 1944 recommended the administration of intravenous infusions before operation and pointed to the beneficial effects of increasing blood volume and thus cardiac output. Beall and colleagues[29–32] were the first to describe the technique of emergency department (ED) thoracotomy. Meanwhile, Mattox et al.[33–35] refined and protocolized ED thoracotomy and cardiorrhaphy, inclusive of the use of emergency cardiopulmonary bypass in the management of

these injuries. These hallmark contributions have made it possible for patients sustaining penetrating cardiac injuries to survive today.

Incidence

Feliciano et al.[36] in 1983 described a 1-year experience consisting of 48 cardiac injuries at Ben Taub Hospital in Houston. Mattox and associates[37] in 1989 described a 30-year experience from the same institution reporting 539 cardiac injuries (18 cardiac injuries per year). Asensio and colleagues[38,39] reported two prospective consecutive series reporting a total of 165 cardiac injuries in a 3-year period (55 cardiac injuries per year) at Los Angeles County/USC Medical Center in Los Angeles. A recent review by Asensio et al.,[40] which focused on the National Trauma Databank (NTDB) of the American College of Surgeons (ACS), identified a total of 2016 patients sustaining penetrating cardiac injuries, and calculated the national incidence of 0.16% for these injuries. Thus, penetrating cardiac injuries are uncommon and are usually seen only in busy urban trauma centers.

Etiology

In the civilian arena, penetrating cardiac injuries are usually caused by gunshot wounds (GSWs), stab wounds (SWs), and rarely by shotgun wounds and ice picks.[41] According to a recent review,[40] 63% of all reported cardiac injuries in America are caused by gunshot wounds and 36% are caused by stab wounds, while shotgun and impalement injuries accounted for approximately 1% of these injuries. In the military arena, Rich and Spencer[42] reported 96 cardiac injuries from the Vietnam conflict. Most of these patients sustained injuries from grenade fragments or shrapnel, while a few of these patients were impaled by flechettes.

Clinical Presentation

Beck's triad—muffled heart tones, jugular venous distention, and hypotension—describes the classical presentation of a patient with pericardial tamponade.[3,41] Kussmaul's sign, described as jugular venous distention upon inspiration, is another classic sign attributed to pericardial tamponade. In reality, the presence of Beck's triad and Kussmaul's signs represent the exception rather than the rule.[3,41,43] It is estimated that Beck's triad is only present in approximately 10% of patients.[41]

The clinical presentation of penetrating cardiac injuries may range from complete hemodynamic instability to cardiopulmonary arrest; in fact, some penetrating cardiac injuries can be very deceptive in their presentation.[41,44] The clinical presentation of penetrating cardiac injuries may also be related to factors including the wounding mechanism; the length of time elapsed before arrival at a trauma center; and the extent of the injury, which if sufficiently large in terms of myocardial destruction will invariably lead to exsanguinating hemorrhage into the left hemithoracic cavity. The presentation of these injuries is also related to blood loss, as patients who lose between 40% and 50% of intravascular blood volume develop cardiopulmonary arrest. The muscular nature of the left ventricle, and to a lesser extent that of the right ventricle, may seal penetrating injuries and prevent exsanguinating hemorrhage, allowing these patients to arrive with some signs of life at a trauma center.[41,44]

The most unique presentation of a penetrating cardiac injury is pericardial tamponade. The tough fibrous nature, lack of elasticity, and noncompliance of this structure translate to acute rises in intrapericardial pressure leading to compression of the thin wall of the right ventricle, impairing its ability to accept the returning blood volume, resulting in a concomitant decrease in left ventricular filling and ejection fraction. This results in a drastic decrease in cardiac output (CO) and stroke volume (SV). The impaired ability to generate both right and left ventricular ejection fractions increases cardiac work and myocardial wall tension. This results in an increase in myocardial volume of oxygen consumption (MVO_2) which cannot be met, leading to myocardial hypoxemia and lactic acidosis.[41,44]

It is well known that the pericardium is able to accommodate gradual quantities of blood, provided that the rate of hemorrhage is slow and does not cause acute rises in intrapericardial pressures exceeding the right ventricle and subsequently the left ventricle's ability to fill. Pericardial tamponade can have both deleterious and protective effects. Its deleterious effects can lead to a rapid rise in pericardial pressure and cardiopulmonary arrest, whereas its protective effect will limit extrapericardial hemorrhage into the left hemithoracic cavity, preventing exsanguinating hemorrhage. Moreno et al.,[45] in a retrospective study consisting of 100 patients presenting with penetrating cardiac injuries, reported 77 patients who presented with pericardial tamponade. The authors reported that for patients presenting with pericardial tamponade, the survival rate was much higher—73% versus 11%—thereby ascribing tamponade a protective effect. These findings were statistically significant, leading the authors to conclude that pericardial tamponade is a critical independent factor in patient survival.

Asensio et al.,[39] in a prospective 2-year study reporting 105 patients failed to find any statistical significance to the presence of pericardial tamponade in terms of survival, and were not able to identify it as a critical independent factor for survival. What remains undefined is the actual period of time after which the protective effect of pericardial tamponade is lost, and when exactly this transition occurs causing its adverse effect on cardiac function.

Diagnosis

Physical Examination

The clinical presentation of patients with penetrating cardiac injury may range from presenting hemodynamically stable to cardiopulmonary arrest. Frequently, these patients present with associated pneumohemothoraces and decreased breath sounds in the ipsilateral hemithoracic cavity. Occasionally, patients presenting with precordial injuries are restless and refuse to lie down; this may be a subtle indicator denoting the presence of hemopericardium and/or incipient pericardial tamponade. The most dramatic presentation for a patient sustaining a penetrating cardiac injury is, of course, cardiopulmonary arrest, which will require ED thoracotomy as a life-saving intervention.[41,42] Pericardiocentesis is only mentioned to note that it currently has no role in establishing the diagnosis of cardiac injuries.

Subxiphoid Pericardial Window

The original technique of pericardial window was described by Larrey[9,10,41] in the 1800s, and only small variations in the original technique have been added to this procedure. This technique has seen a marked diminution in its role during recent times because of the advent of two-dimensional echocardiography a part of the focused assessment and sonographic examination of the trauma patient (FAST).[41] Nevertheless, the technique is still widely employed in many countries where medical personnel do not have access to ultrasound equipment.

Pericardial window must be performed in an operating room under general anesthesia. A 10-cm incision is made in the midline over the xiphoid process. Blunt and sharp dissection after digitally palpating the transmitted cardiac impulses is used to locate the pericardium, which is then isolated and grasped between two Allis clamps and placed under gentle downward traction. A longitudinal incision measuring approximately 1–2 cm is made in the pericardium sharply, with meticulous care taken to avoid an iatrogenic injury to the underlying myocardium. After this longitudinal aperture is made, fluid in the pericardium will escape,

the field is either flooded with clear straw-colored pericardial fluid, which signifies a negative window or with blood, indicative of a positive window, and thus, an underlying cardiac injury. A positive pericardial window mandates proceeding with median sternotomy. Finally, the field may remain dry, if blood has clotted within the pericardium.

The advantages of this technique are safety and reliability for the detection of penetrating cardiac injuries. This relatively simple surgical technique belongs in the surgical armamentarium of every trauma surgeon. Disadvantages consist of having to subject the patient to a general anesthetic and a surgical procedure.

Two-Dimensional Echocardiography

Echocardiography as part of FAST has become the gold standard in the evaluation of patients with penetrating thoracic injury. Major benefits of echocardiography include being noninvasive, rapid, and accurate; its ability to be repeated at any time; and most importantly, its painlessness. Data from two multicenter studies[46,47] conclusively support the role of FAST as the initial investigative tool for the evaluation of patients with penetrating cardiac injuries, given its accuracy and ease of performance. Other techniques such as transesophageal echocardiography (TEE) have no role in the immediate evaluation sustaining penetrating precordial injuries.[41]

Minimally Invasive Methods

Thoracoscopy

Morales et al.[48] reported a 31% incidence of positive windows describing a technique that was both accurate and well tolerated without any complications, and the authors recommend this technique to be used in patients also requiring evacuation of a retained hemothorax. In our opinion, thoracoscopic pericardial window has no role in the acute evaluation of penetrating cardiac injuries.

Laparoscopy

Similarly, laparoscopy has been used to detect peritoneal violation in patients sustaining penetrating abdominal trauma. It has been used to evaluate patients with thoracoabdominal injuries to evaluate presence of diaphragmatic or solid organ injuries. During laparoscopy, the pericardium can also be evaluated. Although this technique can be used, it is the opinion of the authors that it has no role in the acute evaluation of penetrating cardiac injuries.

Management

Prehospital

Emergency medical systems in large urban areas providing rapid transport to trauma centers have allowed patients with penetrating cardiac injuries an opportunity to undergo life-saving surgical procedures. Field stabilization of patients with penetrating cardiac injuries should consist of intubation and closed cardiopulmonary resuscitation for patients found in cardiopulmonary arrest. Several studies[49–52] strongly support and advocate for the need of immediate transport of patients with penetrating thoracic injuries to a trauma center, with the only predictors of outcome being the achievement of an airway via endotracheal intubation. Endotracheal intubation has been proven to increase both duration and tolerance of cardiopulmonary resuscitation administered for a period of less than 5 minutes. The return of organized cardiac electrical activity will provide the best opportunity at survival for these patients.

Emergency Department

All patients with penetrating cardiac injuries should undergo rapid initial assessment and resuscitation following Advanced Trauma Life Support (ATLS) protocols.[53] Patients will usually self-stratify into those who are hemodynamically stable and may undergo diagnostic studies, those who are hemodynamically unstable but will respond to fluid resuscitation and allow for rapid transport to the operating room (OR), and those who present in cardiopulmonary arrest and will necessitate life-saving surgical interventions such as ED thoracotomy. Patients can be initially and rapidly evaluated with FAST, chest x-ray, and optionally an electrocardiogram (EKG). Volume resuscitation with lactated Ringer and O- or type-specific blood should be initiated. An arterial blood gas to determine initial pH and base deficit and lactic acid level should also be obtained. However, a significant majority of these patients will arrive "in extremis" requiring life-saving interventions.[38,39,41,44]

Emergency department thoracotomy

Emergency department thoracotomy is a surgical procedure of great value if undertaken after strict indications for its performance. This procedure is routinely performed in urban trauma centers that receive patients "in extremis." When performed in an expedient fashion, ED thoracotomy, aortic cross-clamping, and cardiorrhaphy are successful in salvaging approximately 10% of all penetrating cardiac injuries. Open cardiopulmonary massage after definitive repair of penetrating cardiac injuries is more effective in producing a greater ejection fraction. Similarly, lacerations of major thoracic blood vessels can also be controlled by means of vascular clamps.[41,44]

Prehospital factors predictive of poor outcome include absence of vital signs, fixed and dilated pupils, absence of cardiac rhythm, absence of motion in the extremities, absence of a palpable pulse, and the presence of cardiopulmonary arrest are predictors of poor outcome.[41,44]

Generally accepted indications for this procedure include cardiopulmonary arrest secondary to penetrating thoracic injuries and profound shock with systolic blood pressures of less than 60 mm Hg because of exsanguinating hemorrhage or pericardial tamponade. Cardiopulmonary arrest secondary to blunt injury is generally a contraindication to the performance of this procedure.[41,42,44]

Objectives to be achieved with this procedure include resuscitation of agonal patients arriving with penetrating cardiothoracic injuries, evacuation of pericardial tamponade, control of massive intrathoracic hemorrhage secondary to cardiovascular injuries, prevention of air emboli, and restoration of cardiac function using open cardiopulmonary massage. Other objectives accomplished include definitive repairs of penetrating cardiac injuries and control of exsanguinating thoracic vascular injuries. Similarly, cross-clamping of the descending thoracic aorta, redistributing the remaining blood volume to perfuse the carotid and coronary arteries, is achieved with this technique.[41,42,44]

Emergency department thoracotomy should be performed simultaneously with the initial assessment evaluation and resuscitation, using the ATLS[53] protocols by trained trauma surgeons. Similarly, immediate venous access with simultaneous use of rapid infusion techniques complements the resuscitative process. A left anterolateral thoracotomy commencing at the lateral border of the left sternocostal junction and inferior to the nipple is carried out and extended laterally to the latissimus dorsi. In females, the breast is retracted cephalad. This incision is rapidly carried through skin until the intercostal muscles have been reached and sharply transected. A Finochietto retractor is then placed to separate the ribs. The lung is then elevated medially, and the thoracic aorta is located immediately as it enters the abdomen via the aortic hiatus. The aorta should then be palpated to assess the status of the remaining blood volume. It can also be temporarily occluded digitally against the bodies of the lower thoracic vertebrae. To fully cross-clamp the aorta, a combination of sharp and blunt dissection commencing at both the superior and inferior borders of the aorta is performed, so that the aorta may be encircled between the thumb and index fingers; this facilitates the aortic cross-clamp to be placed safely. Trauma surgeons should then observe the pericardium and search for the presence of an injury. The pericardium is usually tense and discolored in the presence of tamponade. A longitudinal opening in the pericardial sac is then made anterior to the phrenic nerve and extended both inferiorly and superiorly. Usually it is necessary to grasp the pericardium and then make a small incision sharply, followed by opening the pericardium with Metzenbaum scissors.

After opening the pericardium, clotted blood is evacuated. The trauma surgeon should immediately note the presence and/or absence and type of underlying cardiac rhythm as well as location of the penetrating injury or injuries. The finding of a flaccid heart, devoid of any effective forward pumping motion is a strong predictor of poor outcome. Other predictors of poor outcome are empty coronary arteries and presence of air, indicating air emboli in the coronary veins.

Digital control of penetrating ventricular injuries as they are simultaneously sutured prevents further hemorrhage. We generally recommend the use of monofilament suture, such as 2-0 polypropylene. If the injury or injuries are quite large, balloon tamponade using a Foley catheter can temporarily arrest the hemorrhage either to allow the performance of cardiorrhaphy or to gain time so that the patient may be transferred expeditiously to an OR for a more definitive surgical procedure. We do not recommend the use of bioprosthetic materials such as Teflon patches in the ED. This is a time-consuming technique that, if needed, should be performed in the OR.[41,44]

In our experience, staples do not effectively control hemorrhage, tend to enlarge the cardiac injury, and prove to be rather difficult to remove, although they have worked in the hands of others.[54]

Strict pharmacologic manipulation coupled with directly delivered countershocks of 20–50 joules is frequently needed to restore a normal sinus rhythm. At times a rhythm can be restored, but no effective pumping mechanism is observed. Progressive myocardial death can be witnessed, first by dilatation of the right ventricle with accompanying cessation of contractility and motion, followed by the same process in the left ventricle.

Outcomes of emergency department thoracotomy for penetrating cardiac injuries

Wide disparity in the reporting of outcomes exists in the literature, ranging from 0% to 72%. Most of these series are retrospective, and the patients reported have been injured because of stab wounds. Asensio, Wall, and others in the Working Group of the Committee on Trauma of the American College of Surgeons,[55] after an extensive analysis of the literature, generated practice management guidelines for ED thoracotomy (Table 1).

Techniques for Cardiac Injury Repair

Incisions

Two main incisions are used in the management of penetrating cardiac injuries. Median sternotomy described by Duval[20] is the incision of choice for patients admitted with penetrating precordial injuries that arrive with some degree of hemodynamic instability and may either undergo preoperative investigation with FAST and/or chest x-ray. The left anterolateral thoracotomy described by Spangaro[21] is the incision of choice in the management of patients who arrive "in extremis." This incision is used in the ED for resuscitative purposes, and it can also be extended across the sternum as bilateral anterolateral thoracotomies. Extension into bilateral anterolateral thoracotomies is also the incision of choice for patients who are hemodynamically unstable after incurring mediastinal-traversing injuries (Figure 1). It is important to note that upon transection of the sternum, both internal mammary arteries are also transected and must be ligated after restoration of perfusion pressure. For patients who sustain thoracoabdominal injuries, the left anterolateral thoracotomy is also the incision of choice if patients deteriorate in the OR while undergoing a laparotomy.[44,92]

Table I: EDT for Cardiac Injuries

Author and Year	Type of Study	Survivors/Penetrating Trauma	Survivors/Total Number of EDTs
Boyd 1965[56]	R	0/0	17/25
Beall 1966[29]	R	3/16	42/197
Sauer 1967[57]	R	12/0	12/13
Sugg 1968[58]	R	0/0	63/459
Yao 1968[59]	R	0/0	61/80
Steichen 1971[60]	R	7/21	35/58
Beall 1971[30]	R	29/52	42/66
Borja 1971[61]	R	0/0	24/145
Carrasquilla 1972[62]	R	8/30	20/245
Beall 1972[63]	R	0/0	67/269
Bolanowski 1973[64]	R	0/0	33/44
Trinkle 1974[65]	R	0/0	38/45
Mattox 1974[34]	R	25/37	31/62
Harvey 1975[66]	R	0/0	22/28
Symbas 1976[67]	R	0/0	50/98
Beach 1976[68]	R	0/4	26/34
Asfaw 1977[69]	R	0/0	277/323
Sherman 1978[70]	R	32/41	31/92
Trinkle 1979[71]	R	0/0	89/100
Evans 1979[72]	R	0/4	29/46
Breaux 1979[73]	R	39/44	78/197
Mandal 1979[74]	R	0/38	26/55
Gervin 1982[49]	R	4/21	4/21
Demetriades 1983[75]	R	2/16	40/125
Demetriades 1984[76]	R	1/11	0/45
Tavares 1984[77]	R	21/37	64
Feliciano 1984[36]	R	5/15	2/3
Mattox 1985[35]	R	50/119	204
Demetriades 1986[78]	R	1/18	70
Moreno 1985[45]	R	4/69	100
Ivatury 1987[51]	R	28/91	—
Jebara 1989[79]	R	4/17	—
Attar 1991[80]	R	21/55	—
Knott-Craig 1992[81]	R	5/13	—
Buchman 1992[82]	R	1/2	23
Benyan 1992[83]	R	1/13	—
Macho 1993[54]	R	12/24	—
Mitchell 1993[84]	R	7/47	—
Kaplan 1993[85]	R	2/23	
Henderson 1994[86]	R	6/122	215
Coimbra 1995[87]	R	0/20	
Arreola-Risa 1995[88]	R	11/40	
Karmy-Jones 1997[89]	R	3/6	16
Rhee 1998[90]	R	15/58	41/96
Asensio 1998[38]	P	6/37	6/37
Asensio 1998[39]	P	10/71	10/71
Tyburski 2000[91]	R	12/152	12/152
Asensio 2006[40]	R	47/830	47/830

Note: There were no survivors of blunt trauma.
EDT, Emergency department thoracotomy; *P*, prospective; *R*, retrospective.

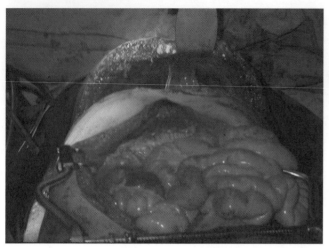

Figure 1 Bilateral thoracotomy and laparotomy in management of patients with thoracoabdominal injuries arriving "in extremis."

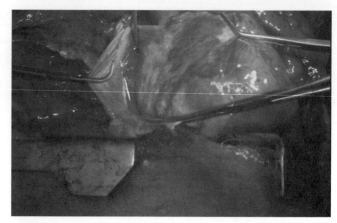

Figure 2 Both superior and inferior vena cava (SVC and IVC) clamped. The IVC is clamped at the Gibbon's space. Note the clamp on the right auricle providing better exposure.

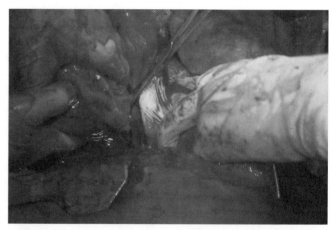

Figure 3 Vascular clamps in the pulmonary hilum. This maneuver is helpful to control penetrating pulmonary injuries with profuse bleeding or with a big hematoma in the pulmonary hilum.

Adjunct Maneuvers

Trauma surgeons must possess several maneuvers in their armamentarium to deal with penetrating cardiothoracic injuries. Total inflow occlusion to the heart is a complex maneuver which entails cross-clamping both the superior (SVC) and inferior vena cava (IVC) in their intrapericardial location to arrest total blood flow to the heart (Figure 2). It is indicated for the management of injuries in the lateral-most aspect of the right atrium and/or the superior or inferior atriocaval junction. The safe period for this maneuver is unknown, although a 1–3-minute range is often quoted in the literature as the period of time after which clamps must be released.

Cross-clamping of the pulmonary hilum is another valuable maneuver indicated for the management of associated pulmonary injuries, particularly those that present with hilar central hematomas and/or active bleeding (Figure 3). This maneuver arrests bleeding from the lung and prevents air emboli from reaching the systemic circulation. However, in the presence of acidosis, hypothermia, and ischemia, the right ventricle may not be able to tolerate this maneuver, leading to fibrillation and arrest.

At times, a trauma surgeon will need to elevate the heart out of the pericardium in order to repair certain injuries. If hemorrhage can be digitally controlled, gradual elevation of the heart by placing multiple laparotomy packs will allow better tolerance of this maneuver while decreasing the chances for development of dysrhythmias.

Repair of Atrial Injuries

Atrial injuries can usually be controlled by placement of a Satinsky partial occlusion vascular clamp. Control of the wound will allow the trauma surgeon to perform cardiorrhaphy. We recommend utilizing monofilament sutures of 2-0 polypropylene on an (MH) needle either in a running or in an interrupted fashion. It is important to visualize both sides of the atrial injury, particularly those caused by missiles, as they can cause a significant amount of tissue destruction which might require meticulous debridement before closure. The use of bioprosthetic materials in the form of Teflon pledgets is not recommended for the management of these injuries.

Repair of Ventricular Injuries

Ventricular injuries usually cause significant hemorrhage. They should be occluded digitally while simultaneously repaired by either simple interrupted or horizontal mattress sutures of Halsted. Performing cardiorrhaphy for ventricular stab wounds is usually less challenging than for gunshot wounds. Missile injuries often produce some degree of blast effect that causes myocardial fibers to retract, and frequently require multiple sutures to control significant hemorrhage. In the presence of this scenario, bioprosthetic materials such as Teflon strips and/or pledgets are often needed to buttress the suture line (Figure 4). We recommend 2-0 monofilament sutures of polypropylene on an MH needle.

Coronary Artery Injuries

The repair of ventricular injuries adjacent to coronary arteries can be very challenging. In order to avoid potential narrowing and/or occlusion of a coronary artery or one of its branches, it is recommended that sutures be placed underneath the bed of the coronary artery. Coronary arteries are usually divided into three segments: proximal, middle, and distal. Injuries to the proximal and middle segments will usually require cardiopulmonary bypass for repair, and the institution of intra-aortic balloon counterpulsation followed by aortocoronary bypass, respectively. Lacerations of the distal segment of the coronary artery, particularly in the distal-most third of the vessel, are managed by ligation.

Complex and Combined Injuries

A significant number of patients arrive harboring multiple associated injuries in addition to their penetrating cardiac injuries. Complex and combined cardiac injuries can be defined as a penetrating cardiac injury plus associated neck, thoracic, thoracic-vascular, abdominal, abdominal

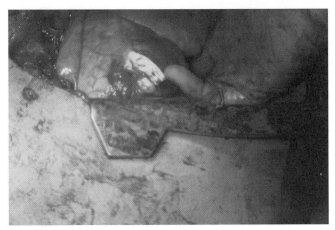

Figure 4 Gunshot wound to the left ventricle repaired with Teflon strips.

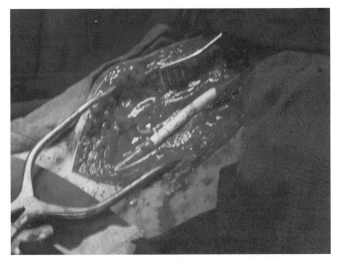

Figure 5 Patient with a femoro-femoral bypass with polytetrafluoroethylene, and after ligation of femoral vein. This patient sustained a gunshot wound to the left ventricle, and concomitantly left lung, left femur, and right hand injuries.

vascular, or peripheral vascular injuries (Figures 5 and 6). These injuries are quite challenging to manage. Priority should be given early to the injury causing the greatest blood loss or threatening the patient's life.

Anatomic Location of Injury

A great deal of variability exists in the literature when it comes to reporting the breakdown of cardiac injuries by chambers (Table 2). Ventricular injuries occur with an incidence ranging from 37% to 67% of all cardiac injuries, whereas left ventricular injuries occur with an incidence ranging from 19% to 40%. Right atrial injuries appear to occur with greater frequency ranging from 5% to 20%, whereas the left atrium, the most recessed chamber of the heart, is injured between 2% and 12% of the times.[38,39,86,88,91,93–95]

Associated Injuries

Penetrating cardiac injuries resulting from stab wounds are generally isolated and usually only involve one chamber because of their precordial penetration. However, missile injuries may injure the heart

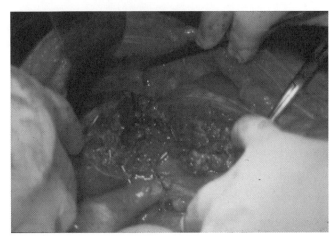

Figure 6 Liver injury American Association for the Surgery of Trauma, Organ Injury Scale grade IV concomitantly with a cardiac injury. Complex hepatotomy and hepatorrhaphy were performed. Note the clips used to control bleeding.

either from precordial as well as extraprecordial locations, and thus have a greater propensity for causing multiple-chamber and associated injuries.

Prognostic Factors

The American Association for the Surgery of Trauma and its Organ Injury Scaling (AAST-OIS)[96] committee have developed a scale to uniformly describe cardiac injuries (Table 3). This scale comprehensively describes these injuries and, although the scale has been available since 1994, few studies have correlated cardiac injury grade with mortality.

Asensio and colleagues,[39] in a 2-year prospective study of 105 patients, correlated AAST-OIS for cardiac injuries with mortality, in which 99 (94%) of the 105 patients incurred grade IV–VI injuries. Mortality progressively increased with injury grade. Grade IV injuries incurred mortality of 56%, grade V 76%, and grade VI 91%. Although findings of both these studies would appear to validate the correlation between mortality and organ injury grade, the authors feel that further work is necessary to confirm their findings. Furthermore, the authors strongly believe that all cardiac injuries should be graded according to this scale.

Prognostic factors such as mechanism of injury, physiologic parameters at the scene of the traumatic incident, during transport and upon arrival such as pupillary response, spontaneous ventilation, presence of a carotid pulse, presence of a measurable blood pressure, sinus rhythm, any extremity movement, need for intubation and cardiopulmonary resuscitation, as well as scene times greater than 10 minutes have been prospectively validated in many studies.[38,39,49,94] The presence of cardiopulmonary arrest upon arrival as a poor predictor of outcome has been confirmed.[36,37,51,86,91] Similarly, physiologic parameters upon arrival such as these measured by the cardiovascular respiratory score (CVRS) component of the trauma score (TS) have been validated by Buckman et al.[94]

BLUNT CARDIAC INJURY

Historical Perspective

The first unquestionable case of myocardial contusion was reported in 1764 by Akenside,[97] and the first recorded case of blunt cardiac chamber rupture was reported in 1679 by Borch.[98,99] According to

Table 2: Anatomic Location of Injuries

Author	Year	Span (Years)	# of Patients	Cardiac Chambers (#/%)				Multiple Chambers	Associated Coronary Arteries
				RV	LV	RA	LA		
Ivatury[93]	1987	20	228	90 (39.4%)	44 (19.2%)	15 (6.5%)	6 (2.6%)	38 (16.6%), Location NR 20 (8.8%)	11 (4.8%)
Buckman and Asensio[94]	1993	2.25	66	Single chamber 42 (63.6%)				24 (36.3%)	NR
Henderson[86]	1994	6	251	96 (38.2%)	98 (39.8%)	57 (22.7%)	31 (12.3%)	101 (40.2%)	NR
Arreola-Risa[88]	1995	7	55	29 (52%)	17 (30%)	7 (12%)	2 (3%)	11 (20%)	1 (1.5%)
Wall[95]	1997	20	711	284 (40%)	284 (40%)	171 (24%)	21 (3%)	14 (1.9%)	39 (5.4%)
Asensio[38]	1998	1	60	40 (66.6%)	15 (25%)	11 (18.3%)	3 (5%)	NR	5 (8.3%)
Asensio[39]	1998	2	105	39 (37.1%)	26 (24.7%)	8 (7.6%)	5 (4.7%)	23 (21.9%)	9 (8.5%)
Tyburski[91]	2000	17	302	121 (40%)	75 (24.8%)	17 (5.6%)	6 (1.9%)	83 (27.4%)	NR
Totals			1778	699	559	328	74	314	65

LA, Left atrium, *LV,* left ventricle; *RA,* right atrium; *RV,* right ventricle; *NR,* not reported.

Table 3: American Association for the Surgery of Trauma, Organ Injury Scale: Cardiac Injury

Grade[a]	Injury Description
I	Blunt cardiac injury with minor electrocardiographic abnormality (nonspecific T or T-wave changes, premature atrial or ventricular contraction, or persistent sinus tachycardia). Blunt or penetrating pericardial wound without cardiac injury, cardiac tamponade, or cardiac herniation.
II	Blunt cardiac injury with heart block (right or left bundle branch, left anterior fascicular, or atrioventricular) or ischemic changes (ST depression or T-wave inversion) without cardiac failure. Penetrating tangential myocardial wound up to, but not extending through, endocardium, without tamponade.
III	Blunt cardiac injury with sustained (>5 beats per minute) or multifocal ventricular contractions. Blunt or penetrating cardiac injury with septal rupture, pulmonary or tricuspid valvular incompetence, papillary muscle dysfunction, or distal coronary arterial occlusion without cardiac failure. Blunt pericardial laceration with cardiac herniation. Blunt cardiac injury with cardiac failure. Penetrating tangential myocardial wound up to, but not extending through, endocardium, with tamponade.
IV	Blunt or penetrating cardiac injury with septal rupture, pulmonary or tricuspid valvular incompetence, papillary muscle dysfunction, or distal coronary arterial occlusion producing cardiac failure. Blunt or penetrating cardiac injury with aortic or mitral valve incompetence. Blunt or penetrating cardiac injury of the right ventricle, right atrium, or left atrium.
V	Blunt or penetrating cardiac injury with proximal coronary arterial occlusion. Blunt or penetrating left ventricular perforation. Stellate wound with <50% tissue loss of the right ventricle, right atrium, or left atrium.
VI	Blunt avulsion of the heart; penetrating wound producing >50% tissue loss of a chamber.

[a]Advance one grade for multiple penetrating wounds to a single chamber or multiple chamber involvement.
Modified from Moore EE, Malangoni MA, Cogbill TH, et al: Organ injury scaling IV: thoracic, vascular, lung, cardiac, and diaphragm. *J Trauma* 36:229–300, 1994, with permission.

Warburg,[100] for almost 200 years, from 1676 to 1868, only 27 cases of blunt traumatic cardiac injuries were reported in the literature.[101]

In 1958, Parmley et al.[102] reviewed 207,548 autopsy cases from the Armed Forces Institute of Pathology (AFIP), and described 546 patients with nonpenetrating traumatic injury to the heart reporting an incidence of 0.1%. In this hallmark study, the authors reported 353 cases of cardiac chamber rupture, of which 273 were isolated and 80 associated with combined aortic ruptures. The breakdown per chamber included 66 ruptured right ventricles, 59 ruptured left ventricles, 41 ruptured right atria, and 26 ruptured left atria. A total of 106 patients sustained multiple-chamber injuries.

Mechanism, Pathophysiology, and Incidence

Establishing a firm definition for what blunt cardiac injury (BCI) is has remained somewhat elusive. In fact, this entity was for quite some time known as myocardial contusion and has even been described as myocardial concussion. The exact definition of blunt cardiac injury has remained difficult to pinpoint because it is not really a single entity but rather a spectrum of entities.

Blunt cardiac injury can range from a mild myocardial contusion to frank cardiac chamber rupture including the rare entity of "comotio cordis" described as sudden cardiac arrest from a sternal blow, leading to cardiogenic shock. Blunt cardiac injuries may occur secondary to compression, deceleration, blast, and direct forces applied to the chest, or transmitted increases in intravascular abdominal pressures associated with compression of the abdominal contents. High-speed motor vehicular collisions, causing crushing injuries to the thoracic cage or objects of great weight falling directly onto the sternum or thoracic cage will directly compress the heart against the vertebral column causing BCI. Similarly, accidental falls from great heights as well as blast injuries can also cause BCIs. The true incidence of BCIs remains difficult to estimate from the literature.[103]

Clinical Presentation

Blunt cardiac injury encompasses an entire spectrum of different processes; therefore, clinical presentation for patients sustaining BCI may range from complete hemodynamic instability to cardiopulmonary arrest. These patients may also present with the classical syndrome of pericardial tamponade. Chest pain experienced by some of these patients and its distribution may be indistinguishable from the classical pain of myocardial infarction. Physical findings may include pain and tenderness over the anterior chest wall, contusion, ecchymosis, anterior rib fractures, and even a central flail chest.[103]

Diagnosis

A number of different modalities have been employed to establish a diagnosis of BCI including chest x-ray, EKG, Holter monitoring, measurement of cardiac enzymes, transthoracic (TTE) and TEE echocardiography, and nuclear medicine scans including radionuclide angiography (RNA), thallium 201, single-photon emission computed tomography (SPECT), and multiple-gated image acquisition scans (MUGAs).[103] Chest x-rays are routinely obtained in all trauma patients; they may detect the presence of fractured ribs and flail chest and rarely may reveal a globular-shaped cardiac silhouette. EKG is used to screen patients and detect conduction disturbances. However, there is no pathonogmonic finding that can reliably establish the diagnosis of BCI.

The measurement of creatine phosphokinase (CPK) or creatine kinase (CK) with measurement of the myocardial band (MB) was for a time used to establish the diagnosis of BCI. However, more specific measurements of contractile proteins of different muscle types including troponin (cTn) have emerged as tools to diagnose BCI as both troponin T and I belong to a group of proteins of the contractile apparatus that are unique to cardiac muscle. Fulda et al.[104] prospectively evaluated 71 patients with thoracic wall injuries utilizing signal-averaged EKG, serum troponin T levels, standard EKG, and CPK-MB measurements. Patients were monitored electrocardiographically and by serial measurements of troponin-T and CPK-MB fractions. The authors reported that the sensitivity and specificity of troponin-T in predicting clinically significant abnormalities were 27% and 91%, respectively. From the findings of this study, the authors concluded that the best predictors for the development of significant electrocardiographic changes are an abnormality detected in the initial EKG as well as an elevated serum troponin T level, recommending that both of these tests be obtained to diagnose BCI.

Salim and colleagues[105] investigated the role of serum cardiac troponin I and EKG to identify patients at risk for the development of cardiac complications after blunt cardiac trauma. In this prospective 115-patient study, the authors identified patients at risk for significant BCI defined as cardiogenic shock, arrhythmias requiring treatment, or structural cardiac abnormalities directly related to blunt cardiac trauma. All patients were evaluated with EKG upon admission, which was repeated at an 8-hour interval. Cardiac troponin I was obtained at admission and also at 4 and 8 hours. Two-dimensional EKGs were obtained when clinically indicated. Nineteen patients (16.5%) had significant BCIs. In 18 of the 19, symptoms were present within 24 hours. Of the 115 patients, 58 (50%) had abnormal EKGs and 27 (23.5%) had increased cTnI. From these data, the authors concluded that the combination of EKG and troponin I reliably identified the presence or absence of significant BCIs.

The use of two-dimensional echocardiography (TTE) has been extensively used as diagnostic modality for the evaluation of patients with suspected BCI. Patients are selected for evaluation by this modality after abnormal EKG and abnormal cardiac enzymes and troponin level measurements are detected. TTE evaluates segmental wall abnormalities or valvular dysfunction.[103] However, although useful, it has not been shown to correlate with complications or eventual outcome in BCI, and whereas it may detect and identify structural defects and abnormalities with wall motion, it is limited by chest wall edema, and traumatic structural abnormalities such as fractured ribs and flail chest, but most importantly it cannot detect the electrical instability that is a hallmark for BCI.

Transesophageal echocardiography has been shown to be a useful adjunct to evaluate patients with BCI, as it is more versatile in its ability to detect BCI. However, it is an invasive procedure that is operator dependent and not always available around the clock.[106–108]

A number of different radionuclide scans have been used in the past for the diagnosis of BCI, but none were sufficiently sensitive or specific to reliably establish the diagnosis of BCI and have been abandoned.[103]

Spectrum of Blunt Cardiac Injury

Clinically, BCI can be divided into two types: acute and subacute. The acute type is usually the catastrophic injury that causes death immediately or rapidly if surgical intervention is not instituted, including cardiac chamber rupture with acute pericardial tamponade, combined chamber and pericardial rupture with hemorrhage into the pleural cavity, and acute myocardial injury with cardiogenic shock. Subacute cardiac injury may not lead to immediate death, but does impact cardiac hemodynamics, while placing the patient at risk for the development of significant arrhythmias and hemodynamic complications, and includes myocardial contusion, subacute pericardial tamponade, myocardial infarction, valvular injury, intracardiac shunts, mural thrombi, and of course, arrhythmias.

Pericardial Injury

Blunt rupture of the pericardium occurs from direct high-energy impact or from transmitted sudden and acute increases of intraabdominal pressure. The pericardium may rupture on the diaphragmatic or pleural surfaces usually parallel to the left phrenic nerve. In addition, the heart may eviscerate into the abdominal cavity; in rare cases it can cause torsion of the great vessels acutely. The clinical presentation of patients sustaining blunt pericardial rupture can range from hemodynamic instability to cardiopulmonary arrest secondary torsion of the great vessels or associated blunt cardiac chamber rupture. Patients should be investigated with a chest x-ray that may reveal displacement of the cardiac silhouette, pneumopericardium, or an abnormal gas pattern secondary to herniated hollow viscera. If hemodynamically stable, the patients may be investigated with FAST and EKG. Diagnosis can also be confirmed via a subxyphoid pericardial window, which will reveal a hemopericardium. This should then be followed by median sternotomy.

Valvular, Papillary Muscle/Chordae Tendineae, and Septal Injury

Blunt cardiac injury may rarely cause valvular injuries. The most frequently injured valves include the aortic, followed by the mitral. The classic signs associated with valvular dysfunction may not be immediately recognized because of the presence of more obvious life-threatening injuries. Important clinical findings include the presence of new cardiac murmurs, thrills, or loud musical murmurs. Similarly acute left ventricular dysfunction with cardiogenic shock and associated pulmonary edema are important clinical findings.

Rapid displacement of blood secondary to crushing or compressive forces applied to the thoracic cage during ventricular diastole may lacerate cardiac valve leaflets, papillary muscles, or chordae tendinea, leading to valvular insufficiency. From this mechanism, the aortic valve is most frequently injured. Similarly, any sudden increases in intra-aortic pressure may lead to laceration or leaflet rupture, and can also result in stretching and hematoma formation within the papillary muscle. Sudden alterations in papillary muscle anatomy will render it dysfunctional, and may cause valvular insufficiency.

Septal ruptures are also uncommon. Hewett[109] in 1847 first described the rupture of the intraventricular septum caused by blunt trauma. Bright and Beck[110] in 1935 described 11 patients with septal rupture in a series of 152 patients who sustained fatal cardiac injury.

Blunt Coronary Artery Injury

Blunt coronary artery injuries are extremely rare. Direct impacts may cause acute coronary thrombosis, and may result in intimal disruption caused by significant application of blunt energy to the chest. Blunt coronary artery injuries are usually associated with severe myocardial contusions, generally along the distribution of the left anterior descending coronary artery (LAD). The clinical presentation of these patients cannot be distinguished from acute myocardial infarction. Long-term sequelae of these injuries may lead to the development of a ventricular aneurysm with its potential complications such as rupture, ventricular failure, and production of emboli or malignant arrhythmias.[102]

Cardiac Chamber Rupture

Blunt cardiac rupture is relatively uncommon. Only a small number of patients sustaining these injuries survive to reach the hospital. Blunt chamber rupture is often the immediate cause of death at the scene of motor vehicular collisions, and is frequently encountered during autopsy. Several mechanisms for blunt cardiac rupture have been postulated, including direct precordial impacts, hydraulic effect from retrograde transmission of force through the abdomen into the venous system causing rapid rises of venous pressure transmitted to the heart particularly the atria, compression, acceleration or deceleration injuries leading to tears of the heart at its attachment to the great thoracic vessels, blast effects, and concussive blows thought to be fatal secondary to the production of malignant arrhythmias.

Blunt cardiac chamber rupture usually presents with persistent hypotension and/or pericardial tamponade. Similarly, patients may present in cardiopulmonary arrest secondary to exsanguinating hemorrhage. These patients should be rapidly evaluated by FAST to detect pericardial fluid. For those who are hemodynamically stable, subxyphoid pericardial window remains an option to confirm the results of FAST, however, for those who present cardiopulmonary arrest, ED thoracotomy may be their only chance at survival, albeit these patients have a dismal prognosis.

Türk and Tsokos[111] reported that blunt atrial injuries are more common than ventricular injuries. The most frequently injured cardiac chambers are the right atrium followed by the right ventricle. Left-sided chamber injuries occur with a smaller frequency. Several patients have been reported with multiple chamber injuries; however, none survived.

Myocardial Contusion

Out of all the BCIs, the least important and more difficult to define is myocardial contusion/concussion. The definition of myocardial contusion has evolved over several decades of discussion among trauma surgeons. This diagnosis is more often established out of proportion to its incidence, severity, and clinical relevance. Mattox et al.[112] suggested that the terms of myocardial contusion and concussion be eliminated in favor of a more reasonable definition for this entity, and proposed that they be defined as BCI either with cardiac failure, with the presence of complex arrhythmia, and those with minor EKG or enzyme abnormality. On this basis, it is recommended that asymptomatic patients with anterior chest wall injuries should not be admitted to a surgical intensive care unit for continuous EKG monitoring, serial determination of CPK-MB enzyme levels, or further cardiac imaging.

Civetta and colleagues[113] concluded that significant cardiac events are uncommon in young patients with chest trauma, and pointed out that initial EKG abnormalities are better indicators of cardiac complications in critically injured patients.

After a thorough review of the literature, Pasquale et al.[114] identified well-conducted primary studies or reviews involving the identification of BCI. On the basis of this literature review, the Eastern Association for the Surgery of Trauma (EAST) generated the following three recommendations:

Level I

An admission EKG should be performed for all patients in whom there is suspected BCI.

Level II

1. If the admission EKG results are abnormal, the patient should be admitted for continuous EKG monitoring for 24–48 hours. If the admission EKG results are normal, the pursuit of diagnosis should be terminated.
2. If the patient is hemodynamically unstable, an imaging study should be obtained. If an optimal TTE cannot be performed, then the patient should have a TEE.
3. Nuclear medicine studies add little compared with echocardiography, and are not useful if an echocardiogram has been performed.

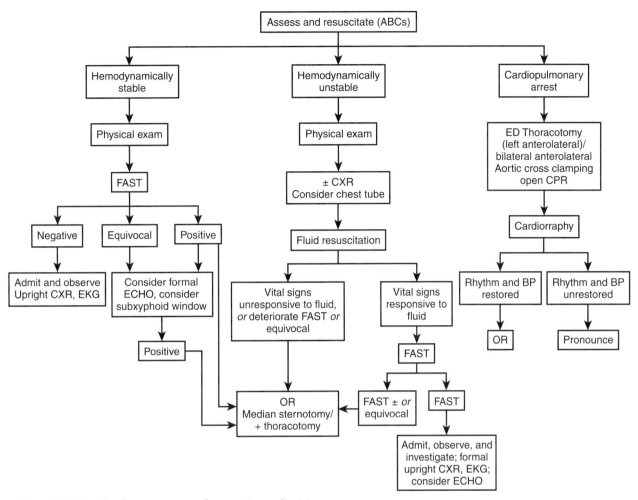

Figure 7 Algorithm for management of penetrating cardiac injury.

Level III

1. Elderly patients with known cardiac disease, unstable patients, and those with an abnormal admission EKG can be safely operated on provided that they are closely monitored. Consideration should be given to placement of a pulmonary artery catheter in such cases.
2. The presence of a sternal fracture does not predict the presence of BCI, and does not necessarily indicate that monitoring should be performed.
3. Neither CPK analysis nor measurements of circulating cardiac troponin T are useful in predicting which patients have or will have complications related to BCI.

CONCLUSIONS

Cardiac injuries continue to be both challenging and fascinating entities. Only with serious scientific inquiry based on prospective collection and analysis of data can we extend the frontiers in the management of these critical injuries (Figure 7).

REFERENCES

1. Homer: *The Iliad*, Vol. XIII. Translated by Lang, Leaf, and Myers. New York, McMillan & Co, 1922, line 442, p. 259.
2. Breasted JH: *The Edwin Smith Papyrus*, Vol. 1. Chicago, University of Chicago Press, 1930.
3. Beck CS: Wounds of the heart. The technique of suture. *Arch Surg* 13: 205–227, 1926.
4. Hippocrates: *The Genuine Works of Hippocrates*, Vol. 2. Translated by Francis Adams. New York, William Wood and Co, 1886, Sec. 6, aphorism 18, p. 252.
5. Pare A: *The works of that Famous Chirurgion Ambroise Pare*. Translated by T. Johnson. London, Cates & Co, 1634. (As cited by Beck CS: Wounds of the heart: the technique of suture. *Arch Surg* 13:205–227, 1926.)
6. Pare A: *The Apologia and Treatise of Ambroise Pare (Concerning the Voyages Made into Divers Places with Many of His Writings on Surgery)*. Edited by Keynes G. Chicago, University of Chicago Press, 1952.
7. Wolf I: Cited by Fischer G. Die Wunden des Herzens und des Herzbentels. *Arch Klin Chir* 9:571, 1868.
8. Senac JB: *Traite de la structure du Coeur, de son action, et de ses maladies*, Vol. 2. Paris, Breasson, 1749. (As cited by Beck CS. Wounds of the heart: the technique of suture. *Arch Surg* 13:205–227, 1926.)
9. Larrey DJ: *Bull Sci Med* 6:284, 1810.
10. Larrey DJ: *Chirurgie* 2:303, 1829.
11. Billroth T: Quoted by Jeger E: *Die Chirurgie der Blutgefasse und des Herzens*, Berlin, A Hirschwald, 1913, p. 295. (As cited by Beck CS: Wounds of the heart. The technique of suture. *Arch Surg* 13:205–227, 1926.)
12. Billroth T: Cited by Richardson RG, editor: *The Scalpel and the Heart*. New York, Scribner, 1970, p. 27.
13. Billroth T: Offenes Schreibner and Herr der Wittelshofer uver die erste mil gustingen susgange ausgefuhrte pylorectomie. *Wiener Med Wochensch* 31:161, 1881.
14. Block MH: Verhandlunge der Deutchsen Gesselhoff fur Chirurgie. Elfren Congress, Berlin, 1882, part I, p. 108. (As cited by Beck CS: Wounds of the heart. The technique of suture. *Arch Surg* 13:205–227, 1926.)

15. Del Vecchio S: *Sutura del cuore.* Napoli, Reforma Med, 1985, pp. xi-ii, 38. (As cited by Beck CS: Wounds of the heart. The technique of suture. *Arch Surg* 13:205–227, 1926.)

16. Cappelen A: *Vinia cordis, suture of hjertet.* Norsk, Mag. F. Laegy; Kristiania, 4, R; xi, 285, 1896. (As cited by Beck CS: Wounds of the heart. The technique of suture. *Arch Surg* 13:205–227, 1926.)

17. Farina G: Discussion. *Centralbl Chir* 23:1224, 1896. (As cited by Beck CS: Wounds of the heart. The technique of suture. *Arch Surg* 13:205–227, 1926.)

18. Rehn L: Ueber penetrerende herzwunden und herznaht. *Arch Klin Chir* 55:315, 1897.

19. Hill LL: A report of case of successful suturing of the heart, and table of 37 other cases of suturing by different operators with various terminations and conclusions drawn. *Med Record* 62:846, 1902. (As cited by Beck CS: Wounds of the heart. The technique of suture. *Arch Surg* 13:205–227, 1926.)

20. Duval P: Le incision median thoraco-laparotomie. *Bull Mem Soc Chir Paris* 33:15, 1907. (As cited by Ballana C: Bradshaw Lecture. The surgery of the heart. *Lancet* CXCVIII:73–79, 1920.)

21. Spangaro S: Sulla tecnica da seguire negli interventi chirurgici per ferrite del cuore e su di un nuovo processo di toracotomia. *Clin Chir* 14:227, 1906. (As cited by Beck CS: Wounds of the heart. The technique of suture. *Arch Surg* 13:205–227, 1926.)

22. Peck CH: The operative treatment of heart wounds. *Ann Surg* 50:100–134, 1909.

23. Smith WR: Cardiorraphy in acute injuries. *Ann Surg* 78:696–710, 1923.

24. Beck C: Further observations on stab wounds of the heart. *Ann Surg* 115:698–704, 1942.

25. Griswold A, Maguire CH: Penetrating wounds of the heart and pericardium. *Surg Gynecol Obstet* 74:406–418, 1942.

26. Elkin DC: The diagnosis and treatment of cardiac trauma. *Ann Surg* 114:169, 1941.

27. Elkin DC: Wounds of the heart. *Ann Surg* 120:817–821, 1941.

28. Elkin DC, Campbell RE: Cardiac tamponade: treatment by aspiration. *Ann Surg* 623–630, 1941.

29. Beall AC, Dietrich EB, Crawford HW: Surgical management of penetrating cardiac injuries. *Am J Surg* 112:686–692, 1966.

30. Beall AC, Gasior RM, Bricker DL: Gunshot wounds of the heart. Changing patterns of surgical management. *Ann Thorac Surg* 11:523–531, 1971.

31. Beall AC, Morris GC, Cooley DA: Temporary cardiopulmonary bypass in the management of penetrating wounds of the heart. *Surgery* 52:330–337, 1962.

32. Beall AC, Oschner JL, Morris GC, et al: Penetrating wounds of the heart. *J Trauma* 1:195–207, 1961.

33. Mattox KL, Espada R, Beall AC, et al: Performing thoracotomy in the emergency center. *J Am Coll Emerg Phys* 3:13–17, 1974.

34. Mattox KL, Beall AC, Jordan GL, et al: Cardiorraphy in the emergency center. *J Am Coll Emerg Phys* 68:886–895, 1974.

35. Mattox KL, Limacher MC, Feliciano DR, et al: Cardiac evaluation following heart injury. *J Trauma* 25:758–765, 1985.

36. Feliciano DV, Bitondo CG, Mattox KL, et al: Civilian trauma in the 1980's. A 1-year experience with 456 vascular and cardiac injuries. *Ann Surg* 199:717–724, 1984.

37. Mattox KL, Feliciano DV, Burch J, Beall AC Jr, et al: Five thousand seven hundred sixty cardiovascular injuries in 4459 patients. Epidemiologic evolution 1958 to 1987. *Ann Surg* 210:698–707, 1989.

38. Asensio JA, Murray J, Demetriades D, et al: Penetrating cardiac injuries: Prospective one year preliminary report; an analysis of variables predicting outcome. *J Am Coll Surg* 186:24–33, 1998.

39. Asensio JA, Berne JD, Demetriades D, et al: One hundred and five penetrating cardiac injuries. A two year prospective evaluation. *J Trauma* 44:1073–1083, 1998.

40. Asensio JA, García-Núñez LM, Healy M, Petrone P, Lavery R: Penetrating cardiac injuries in America—Predictors of outcome in 2016 patients from the National Trauma Data Bank. Abstract submitted to the American Association for the Surgery of Trauma Annual Meeting, 2006.

41. Asensio JA, Stewart BM, Murray JA, Fox AH, et al: Penetrating cardiac injuries. *Surg Clin North Am* 76:685–724, 1996.

42. Rich NM, Spencer FC: Wounds of the heart. In Rich NM, Spencer FC, editors: *Vascular Trauma.* Philadelphia, WB Saunders, 1978: pp. 384–424.

43. Borchdart E: *Sammlung Klin.* Leipzig, Vortrage, 1906. (As cited by Peck CH: The operative treatment of heart wounds. *Ann Surg* 50:100–134, 1909.

44. Asensio JA, Petrone P, Costa D, et al: An evidence-based critical appraisal of emergency department thoracotomy. *Evidence-Based Surg* 1:11–21, 2003.

45. Moreno C, Moore EE, Majure JA, et al: Pericardial tamponade. A critical determinant for survival following penetrating cardiac wounds. *J Trauma* 26:821–825, 1986.

46. Rozycki GS, Feliciano DV, Schmidt JA, et al: The role of surgeon-performed ultrasound in patients with possible penetrating cardiac wounds. *Ann Surg* 223:737–746, 1996.

47. Rozycki GS, Feliciano DV, Oschner MG, et al: The role of ultrasound in patients with possible penetrating cardiac wounds: a prospective multi-center study. *J Trauma* 46:543–552, 1999.

48. Morales CH, Salinas CM, Henao CA, et al: Thoracoscopic pericardial window and penetrating cardiac trauma. *J Trauma* 42:273–275, 1997.

49. Gervin AS, Fischer RP: The importance of prompt transport in salvage of patients with penetrating heart wounds. *J Trauma* 22:443–448, 1982.

50. Durham LA 3rd, Richardson RJ, Wall MJ Jr, et al: Emergency center thoracotomy: impact of prehospital resuscitation. *J Trauma* 32:775–779, 1992.

51. Ivatury RR, Nallathambi MN, Roberge RJ, et al: Penetrating thoracic injuries: in-field stabilization vs. prompt transport. *J Trauma* 27:1066–1073, 1987.

52. Millham F, Grindlinger G: Survival determinants in patients undergoing emergency room thoracotomy for penetrating chest injury. *J Trauma* 34:332–336, 1993.

53. American College of Surgeons, Committee on Trauma (ACS-COT): *Advanced Trauma Life Support Manual,* 7th ed. Chicago, American College of Surgeons, 2005.

54. Macho JR, Markinson RE, Schecter WP: Cardiac stapling in the management of penetrating injuries of the heart: rapid control of hemorrhage and decreased risk of personal contamination. *J Trauma* 34:711–716, 1993.

55. Working Group, Ad Hoc Subcommittee on Outcomes, American College of Surgeons, Committee on Trauma: practice management guidelines for emergency department thoracotomy. *J Am Coll Surg* 193:303–309, 2001.

56. Boyd TF, Strieder JW: Immediate surgery for traumatic heart disease. *J Thorac Cardiovasc Surg* 50:305–315, 1965.

57. Sauer PE, Murdock CE: Immediate surgery for cardiac and great vessel wounds. *Arch Surg* 95:7–11, 1967.

58. Sugg WL, Rea WJ, Ecker RR, et al: Penetrating wounds of the heart. *J Thorac Cardiovasc Surg* 56:530–545, 1968.

59. Yao ST, Vanecko RM, Printen K, Shoemaker WC: Penetrating wounds of the heart: a review of 80 cases. *Ann Surg* 168:67–78, 1968.

60. Steichen FM, Dargan EL, Efron G, et al: A graded approach to the management of penetrating wounds of the heart. *Arch Surg* 103:574–580, 1971.

61. Borja AR, Randsell HT: Treatment of penetrating gunshot wounds of the chest. *Am J Surg* 122:81–84, 1971.

62. Carrasquilla C, Wilson RF, Walt AJ, et al: Gunshot wounds of the heart. *Ann Thorac Surg* 13:208–213, 1972.

63. Beall AC, Patrick TD, Ikles JE, et al: Penetrating wounds of the heart: changing patterns of surgical management. *J Trauma* 12:468–473, 1972.

64. Bolanowski PS, Swaminathan AP, Neville WE: Aggressive surgical management of penetrating cardiac injuries. *J Thorac Cardiovasc Surg* 66:52–57, 1973.

65. Trinkle JK, Marcos J, Grover FL, et al: Management of the wounded heart. *Ann Thorac Surg* 17:231–236, 1974.

66. Harvey JC, Pacifico AD: Primary operative management method of choice for stab wound to the heart. *South Med J* 68:149–152, 1975.

67. Symbas PN, Harlaftis N, Waldo WJ: Penetrating cardiac wounds: a comparison of different therapeutic methods. *Ann Surg* 183:377–381, 1976.

68. Beach PM, Bognolo D, Hutchinson JE: Penetrating cardiac trauma. Experience with thirty four patients in a hospital without cardiopulmonary bypass capability. *Am J Surg* 131:411–415, 1976.

69. Asfaw I, Arbulu A: Penetrating wounds of the pericardium and heart. *Surg Clin North Am* 57:37–49, 1977.

70. Sherman MM, Saini UK, Yardoz MD, et al: Management of penetrating cardiac wounds. *Am J Surg* 135:553–558, 1978.

71. Trinkle JK, Toon R, Franz JL, et al: Affairs of the wounded heart: penetrating cardiac wounds. *J Trauma* 19:467–472, 1978.

72. Evans J, Gray LA, Payner A, et al: Principles for the management of penetrating cardiac wounds. *Ann Surg* 189:777–784, 1979.

73. Breaux EP, Dupont JB, Albert HM, et al: Cardiac tamponade following penetrating mediastinal injuries: improved survival with early pericardiocentesis. *J Trauma* 19:461–466, 1979.

74. Mandal AK, Awariefe SO, Oparah SS: Experience in the management of 50 consecutive penetrating wounds of the heart. *Br J Surg* 66:565–568, 1979.

75. Demetriades D, Vander Veen BW: Penetrating injuries of the heart: experience over two years in South Africa. *J Trauma* 23:1034–1041, 1983.

76. Demetriades D: Cardiac penetrating injuries: personal experience of 45 cases. *Br J Surg* 71:95–97, 1984.
77. Tavares S, Hankins JR, Moulton AL, et al: Management of penetrating cardiac injuries: the role of emergency thoracotomy. *Ann Thorac Surg* 38:183–187, 1984.
78. Demetriades D: Cardiac wounds. Experience with 70 patients. *Ann Surg* 203:315–317, 1986.
79. Jebara VA, Saade B: Penetrating wounds to the heart: a wartime experience. *Ann Thorac Surg* 47:250–253, 1989.
80. Attar S, Suter CM, Hankins JR, et al: Penetrating cardiac injuries. *Ann Thorac Surg* 51:711–716, 1991.
81. Knott-Craig CJ, Dalton RP, Rossouw GJ, et al: Penetrating cardiac trauma: management strategy based on 129 surgical emergencies over 2 years. *Ann Thorac Surg* 53:1006–1009, 1992.
82. Buchman TG, Phillips J, Menker JB: Recognition, resuscitation and management of patients with penetrating cardiac injuries. *Surg Gynecol Obstet* 174:205–210, 1992.
83. Benyan AKZ, Al-A'Ragy HH: The pattern of penetrating cardiac trauma on Basrah province: personal experience with seventy-two cases in a hospital without cardiopulmonary bypass facility. *Int Surg* 77:111–113, 1992.
84. Mitchell ME, Muakkassa FF, Poole GV, et al: Surgical approach of choice for penetrating cardiac wounds. *J Trauma* 34:17–20, 1993.
85. Kaplan AJ, Norcross ED, Crawford FA: Predictors of mortality in penetrating cardiac injury. *Am Surg* 59:338–342, 1993.
86. Henderson VJ, Smith SR, Fry WR, et al: Cardiac injuries: analysis of an unselected series of 251 cases. *J Trauma* 36:341–348, 1994.
87. Coimbra R, Pinto MCC, Razuk A, et al: Penetrating cardiac wounds: predictive value of trauma indices and the necessity of terminology standardization. *Am Surg* 61:448–452, 1995.
88. Arreola-Risa C, Rhee P, Boyle EM, et al: Factors influencing outcome in stab wounds of the heart. *Am J Surg* 169:553–556, 1995.
89. Karmy-Jones R, Van Wijngaarden MH, Talwar MK, et al: Penetrating cardiac injuries. *Injury* 28:57–61, 1997.
90. Rhee PM, Foy H, Kaufman C, et al: Penetrating cardiac injuries: a population based study. *J Trauma* 45:366–370, 1998.
91. Tyburski JG, Astra L, Wilson RF, et al: Factors affecting prognosis with penetrating wounds of the heart. *J Trauma* 48:587–591, 2000.
92. Asensio JA, Hanpeter D, Demetriades D, et al: The futility of the liberal utilization of emergency department thoracotomy. A prospective study. In Proceedings of the American Association for the Surgery of Trauma 58th Annual Meeting, Baltimore, MD, September 1998, p. 210.
93. Ivatury RR, Rohman M, Steichen FM, et al: Penetrating cardiac injuries: twenty-year experience. *Am Surg* 53:310–317, 1987.
94. Buckman RF, Badellino MM, Mauro LH, et al: Penetrating cardiac wounds: prospective study of factors influencing initial resuscitation. *J Trauma* 34:717–727, 1993.
95. Wall MJ Jr, Mattox KL, Chen C, Baldwin JC: Acute management of complex cardiac injuries. *J Trauma* 42:905–912, 1997.
96. Moore EE, Malangoni MA, Cogbill TH, et al: Organ injury scaling IV: thoracic, vascular, lung, cardiac and diaphragm. *J Trauma* 36:299–300, 1994.
97. Akenside M: An account of a blow upon the heart and its effects. *Philosophical Transactions*, 1764. p. 353.
98. Osborn LR: Findings in 262 fatal accidents. *Lancet* 2:277, 1943.
99. Urbach J: Die Verletzungen des Herzens durch stumple Gewalt. *Beitr Ger Med* 4:653, 1940.
100. Warburg E: *Traumatic Heart Lesions.* London, Humphrey Milford, Oxford University Press, 1938.
101. Kissane RW: Traumatic heart disease: non-penetrating injuries. *Circulation* 6:421–425, 1952.
102. Parmley LF, Manion WC, Mattingly TW: Non penetrating traumatic injury of the heart. *Circulation* 18:371–396, 1958.
103. Newman PG, Feliciano DV: Blunt cardiac injury. *New Horiz* 7:26–34, 1999.
104. Fulda GJ, Giberson F, Hailstone D, et al: An evaluation of serum troponin T and signal averaged electrocardiography in predicting electrocardiographic abnormalities after blunt chest trauma. *J Trauma* 43:304–312, 1997.
105. Salim A, Velmahos GC, Jindal A, et al: Clinically significant blunt cardiac trauma. Role of serum troponin levels combined with electrocardiographic findings. *J Trauma* 50:237–243, 2001.
106. Biffl WL, Moore FA, Moore EE, et al: Cardiac enzymes are irrelevant in the patient with suspected myocardial contusion. *Am J Surg* 169:523–528, 1994.
107. Hiatt JR, Yeatman LA Jr, Child JS: The value of echocardiography in blunt chest trauma. *J Trauma* 28:914–922, 1988.
108. King MR, Mucha P Jr, Seward JB, et al: Cardiac contusion: a new diagnostic approach utilizing two-dimensional echocardiography. *J Trauma* 23:610–614, 1983.
109. Hewett P: Rupture of the heart and large vessels: the result of injuries. *Lond Med Gaz* 1:870, 1847.
110. Bright EF, Beck CS: Non-penetrating wounds of the heart: a clinical and experimental study. *Am Heart J* 10:293, 1935.
111. Türk EE, Tsokos M: Blunt cardiac trauma caused by fatal falls from height: an autopsy-based assessment of the injury pattern. *J Trauma* 57:301–304, 2004.
112. Mattox KL, Flint LM, Carrico CJ, et al: Blunt cardiac injury (editorial). *J Trauma* 33:649–650, 1992.
113. Civetta J: The clinical significance of myocardial contusion (discussion of Cachecho R, Grindlinger GA, Lee VW). *J Trauma* 38:68–73, 1992.
114. Pasquale M, Fabian TC: Practice management guidelines for trauma from the Eastern Association for the Surgery of Trauma. *J Trauma* 44:941–957, 1998.

THORACIC VASCULAR INJURY

Danny Chu, Matthew J. Wall,
and Kenneth Mattox

One of the earliest reports of thoracic vascular injury was described by Vesalius in 1557 of a fatal, blunt traumatic rupture of the aorta in a man who was thrown from a horse.[1] In 1946, DeBakey and Simeone collectively described the morbidity and the complexity of the few battlefield thoracic vascular injuries that occurred during World War II.[2] It was not until 1959 that Passaro and Pace[3] reported the first successful primary repair of traumatic aortic rupture performed by Klassen in 1958.

Before the development of modern trauma centers, most individuals with thoracic vascular trauma died before reaching the hospital. With the advent of rapid-response trauma systems, the incidence of thoracic vascular injury that survives to the hospital is increasing and the complexity of the injuries is becoming more challenging. Mattox et al.[4] reported 1467 cardiovascular injuries in 1117 patients over a 5-year period from 1979 to 1983 in Houston, Texas.

Thoracic vascular injury presents a particular challenge to trauma surgeons because it often spans two unique anatomic areas of the body, that is, chest to neck versus chest to abdomen. Exposure for proximal and distal control of these vascular injuries is not straightforward. Poorly planned incisions can potentially lead to devastating consequences. Because of the increasing complexity of thoracic vascular injuries reaching trauma centers, it is important for the surgeons caring for them to have a systematic approach and a plan of action formulated in order to avoid the associated morbidity and mortality of such injuries.

INCIDENCE

Thoracic trauma is responsible for 50% of all trauma deaths nationally.[5] The incidence of chest trauma is reported to be 12 per million per day in the United States by Beeson and Saegesser.[6] In a large series of thoracic trauma patients, the aorta and great vessels were injured in 4% of cases.[7] Furthermore, thoracic vascular injuries are often associated with other nonvascular injuries because of their anatomic location and mechanism of injury.

Vascular injuries of the chest often include named vessels such as aorta, innominate artery, and proximal common carotid and subclavian arteries. Right-sided vascular injuries such as pulmonary artery, inferior/superior vena cava, innominate vein, and azygos veins are also important to recognize and treat. The anatomic location of the ascending aorta makes it the most commonly injured large thoracic vessel from stab wounds, whereas gunshot wounds usually cause descending aortic injury. The vessels commonly injured in blunt trauma are the descending thoracic aorta and proximal aortic-arch vessels. With penetrating trauma, all thoracic vessels are potentially susceptible to injury.

MECHANISM OF INJURY

A large number of thoracic great-vessel injuries are caused by penetrating or iatrogenic trauma.[4] The mechanism of injury for penetrating thoracic vascular trauma is usually direct laceration or penetration of blood vessels. This type of injury can often present with external or internal hemorrhage, vascular thrombosis from intimal flap, or pseudoaneurysms. Because of the various types of missiles involved in penetrating vascular trauma, all thoracic vascular structures are at risk. External bleeding from skin tracts usually occurs with injuries to vessels at the thoracic inlet, whereas internal hemorrhage commonly occurs with aortic and caval injuries. Intrathoracic great-vessel injuries can present with internal bleeding into the mediastinum, pleural space, or pericardial sac. It is important to note that the presence of a normal palpable distal pulse does not rule out a proximal vascular injury. Penetrating vascular injuries can be completely contained by perivascular adventitia with blood flow preserved distally.

The absence of a significant amount of bleeding does not rule out vascular injury from penetrating trauma. Vascular injuries from stab wounds can often cause an intimal flap or dissection which may eventually lead to partial or complete thrombosis of injured vessels. Small vascular disruptions may not present initially with bleeding, but can present with delayed formation of a pseudoaneurysm. Gunshot blast vascular injuries are often underestimated because intimal disruption sometimes extends beyond external signs of injury. For this reason, meticulous intimal inspection from inside of the blood vessel is helpful during thoracic vascular reconstruction.

Because of the large diameter of thoracic vessels, bullets can directly enter vessels and migrate distally (Figure 1). The diagnosis of bullet embolism is often delayed because the course of the bullet may not be obvious. Bullet embolism for thoracic missiles usually lodges in the iliac and femoral vessels. The site of entry should be controlled for hemorrhage first, followed with attempts at removing the bullet emboli with endovascular intervention or separate arteriotomy.

The great vessel that is the most commonly injured in blunt thoracic trauma is the descending aorta. These injuries usually involve the proximal descending aorta near the isthmus. There are two proposed mechanisms for such injuries. During anteroposterior impact in the thorax, the aorta and its branched vessels may be "pinched" between the sternum and the vertebral column, resulting in vascular disruption. In rapid-deceleration thoracic injuries from either frontal or side-impact motor vehicle accidents, the point of attachment of pulmonary veins, vena cava, and the relative immobility of the descending aorta at the level of the ligamentum arteriosum and diaphragm increase their susceptibility to rupture.

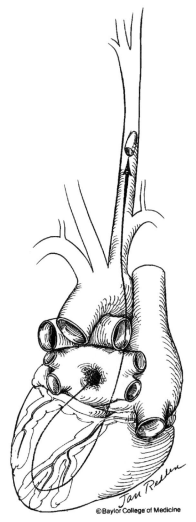

Figure 1 Bullet embolism from the left atrium to the left carotid artery. *(Courtesy Jan Redden, Baylor College of Medicine, 1980.)*

DIAGNOSIS

Patients with penetrating thoracic vascular trauma often present with hemodynamic instability from uncontrolled hemorrhage into the mediastinum, pleural space, or pericardial sac, and are taken emergently to the operating room for surgical management. These injuries are typically diagnosed intraoperatively during resuscitative thoracotomy. In contrast, patients with blunt thoracic trauma are often initially hemodynamically stable with multiple other injuries that may mask a significant concomitant vascular injury.

Focused history and physical examination in the trauma room are helpful in arriving at a specific vascular injury diagnosis. In penetrating trauma, it can be helpful to note the type of instrument used, length of the knife, caliber of the gun, and patient's distance from the firearm. While often unreliable, this information may help the surgeon to develop a mental picture of the trajectory of penetrating missile injury and to formulate a surgical treatment plan. In blunt thoracic trauma, the mechanism of injury is of particular importance to allow the surgeon to estimate the amount of kinetic energy transferred as it relates the geometry of the patient's body upon impact. Emergency medical personnel can also provide information regarding amount of blood loss in the field and hemodynamic stability during transport.

Indicators of possible thoracic vascular injury are outlined in Table 1. The single most important screening tool for thoracic vascular trauma is the anteroposterior chest radiograph. There are numerous

Table 1: Indicators of Possible Thoracic Vascular Injury

Mechanism of Injury

Severe deceleration caused by falls, motor vehicle accidents, and pedestrian versus motor vehicle

Crush injuries

Penetrating injuries to chest with suggestive trajectories, including mediastinal traverse gunshot wounds

Suggestive Physical Signs

Thoracic outlet hematoma

Unequal peripheral pulses or blood pressures

Steering wheel contusion on anterior chest

Palpable sternal fracture

Focal neurologic deficits

Findings on Chest Radiographs

Abnormal or widened mediastinum

Obliteration of aortic knob contour

Lateral deviation of trachea or nasogastric tube

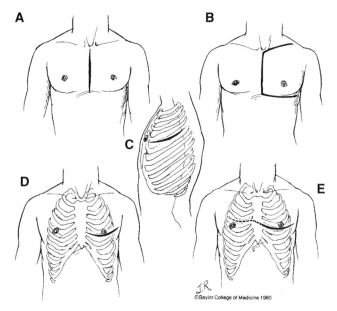

Figure 2 Various thoracic incisions that may be employed to manage thoracic vascular injuries. **(A)** Median sternotomy. **(B)** Combined anterolateral thoracotomy and supraclavicular incision (less commonly with sternotomy to form "trapdoor" thoracotomy). **(C)** Posterolateral thoracotomy. **(D)** Anterolateral thoracotomy (the universal incision for patients in extremis). **(E)** Extension of left anterolateral thoracotomy to right from clamshell incision. *(Courtesy Jan Redden, Baylor College of Medicine, 1980.)*

radiographic findings suggesting thoracic vascular injury as outlined in Table 2. One of the most reliable radiographic findings suggestive of blunt thoracic vascular injury is alteration of the aortic knob contour on chest radiograph.

Arteriography remains the "gold standard" imaging study for evaluation of suspected thoracic vascular injury. It is important to note that preoperative angiography is never indicated in hemodynamically unstable patients with suspected thoracic vascular injury. In hemodynamically stable patients with suspected penetrating injury to the innominate, carotid, or subclavian arteries, preoperative arteriography is indicated to provide information on the type of incisions to make for proximal control of these branched aortic vessels (Figure 2). Furthermore, the proximity of missile trajectory to brachiocephalic vessels is an indication for arteriography in order to definitively rule out an injury. In blunt thoracic trauma, the need for arteriography is determined by mechanism of injury, physical examination, and screening chest radiograph. Fifty percent of patients with blunt thoracic vascular injury present without any external signs of injury.[8] Seven percent of patients with blunt injury to the

Table 2: Radiological Findings Suggesting Great Vessel Injury

Widening of the superior mediastinum >8 cm

Depression of the left mainstem bronchus >140 degrees

Loss of the aortic knob

Deviation of nasogastric or endotracheal tubes, or trachea to the right

Fracture of the first or second rib, scapula, or sternum

Left apical pleural cap

Obliteration of the aortopulmonary window on lateral chest radiograph

Anterior displacement of trachea on lateral chest radiograph

Fracture dislocation of thoracic spine

Calcium layering in aortic knob area

Obvious double contour of aorta

Multiple left rib fractures

Massive hemothorax

aorta and its branched vessels have a normal-appearing mediastinum on screening chest radiograph.[9] Therefore, additional imaging studies are indicated in patients with either physical examination or chest radiograph suggesting thoracic vascular injury.

In patients with a significant mechanism of injury, but a benign physical examination and normal admission chest radiograph, it is reasonable to repeat a delayed chest radiograph to screen for radiographic evidence of thoracic vascular injury with a follow-up arteriography for a definitive diagnosis. Contrast-enhanced spiral computed tomography (CT) of the chest is being used more frequently for evaluating thoracic trauma. The sensitivity of chest CT scan for thoracic vascular injury ranges from 54% to 80%.[10–16] The negative predictive value of a chest CT scan is close to 100% in evaluating thoracic vascular injury.[10–16] Therefore, it is also reasonable to use chest CT scan as a screening tool in stable patients with significant mechanism of injury, normal-appearing admission chest radiograph, and benign physical examination to rule out an underlying thoracic vascular injury. However, any positive findings on CT scan should be followed by the "gold standard" arteriography for definitive diagnosis of thoracic vascular injury before operative intervention.

Magnetic resonance angiography (MRA) has been used in sporadic case reports for thoracic vascular injury. Its application in acutely injured trauma patients is neither ideal nor practical because of the difficulty in monitoring and managing patients in the magnetic resonance coil suites. To date, the use of MRA in evaluating thoracic vascular trauma has not been studied.

Transesophageal echocardiography (TEE) offers several potential advantages to arteriography in evaluating thoracic vascular injury. Avoidance of intravenous contrast, the concomitant information gained on cardiac function, and its portability are potential advantages compared with arteriography. However, published literature reports sensitivity and specificity of 85.7% and 92.0% for TEE compared with 89.0% and 100% for arteriography, respectively, in diagnosing aortic injury.[17] TEE is also heavily technician and operator dependent. Furthermore, the ascending aorta, proximal aortic arch, and branch aortic vessel are extremely difficult to visualize with TEE. Therefore, its use in evaluating thoracic vascular injury is not routinely recommended.

AMERICAN ASSOCIATION FOR THE SURGERY OF TRAUMA, ORGAN INJURY SCALE

The American Association for the Surgery of Trauma (AAST) designates an organ injury scale for thoracic vascular injury from grade I to VI as outlined in Table 3, based on the size and severity of the injury.

Grade I injuries generally involve small thoracic vessels. Grade II injuries involve named venous tributaries of the superior vena cava such as the innominate vein, internal jugular veins, subclavian veins, and azygos vein. Branched aortic vessels such as innominate artery, carotid arteries, and subclavian arteries make up grade III injuries. Grade IV injuries include large-size named extrapericardial vascular structures, whereas grade V injuries include major named intrapericardial vascular structures. Grade VI injuries are uncontained, complete transection of the thoracic aorta or pulmonary hilum.

SURGICAL MANAGEMENT

Indications for urgent surgical intervention for thoracic vascular injuries are outlined in Table 4. The choice of incisions varies depending on the location of injury (see Figure 2). For unstable patients

Table 3: American Association for the Surgery of Trauma, Thoracic Vascular Injury Scale

Grade[a]	Description of Injury
I	Intercostal vessels Internal mammary vessels Bronchial vessels Esophageal vessels Hemiazygos vein Unnamed vessels
II	Azygos vein Internal jugular vein Subclavian vein Innominate vein
III	Carotid artery Innominate artery Subclavian artery
IV	Descending thoracic aorta Intrathoracic inferior vena cava Pulmonary artery/vein, primary intraparenchymal branch
V	Ascending aorta Aortic arch Superior vena cava Main pulmonary artery trunk Pulmonary vein, main trunk
VI	Uncontained complete transaction of thoracic aorta or pulmonary hilar vessels

[a]Increase one grade for multiple grade III injuries or >50% circumference involvement in grade IV injuries. Decrease one grade for grade IV injuries if <25% circumference involvement.
Modified from American Association for the Surgery of Trauma (AAST).

Table 4: Indications for Operative Repair of Thoracic Great Vessel Injury

Initial loss of 1500 ml of blood from chest tube

Continuing hemorrhage >200 ml/hr from tube thoracostomy

Posttraumatic hemopericardium

Pericardial tamponade

Expanding hematoma at thoracic outlet

Exsanguinating hemorrhage presenting from supraclavicular penetrating wound

Imaging evidence of acute thoracic great vessel injury

Radiographic or other imaging evidence of chronic thoracic great vessel injury complications

with presumed but undiagnosed thoracic vascular injury, the most appropriate incision is a left anterolateral thoracotomy in the supine position. This incision allows excellent exposure to the heart and aorta for resuscitative efforts. Furthermore, it can easily be converted to a clamshell incision by extending transternally to the contralateral side to provide exposure to the right lung hilum, ascending aorta, and right subclavian vessels. Median sternotomy is the incision of choice for innominate, right subclavian, right carotid, and proximal left carotid arterial injuries. Oblique cervical or transverse supraclavicular extensions can be added to provide further exposure. Left posterolateral thoracotomy in the lateral decubitus position provides the best exposure for known injuries to the descending thoracic aorta and left lung hilum.

Patients with ascending/transverse aortic injury rarely survive long enough to be transported to the trauma center. Most of these blunt injuries require the use of interposition grafts and cardiopulmonary bypass for repair. In selected patients with penetrating trauma small anterior or lateral lacerations of the ascending aorta can be primarily repaired without the use of cardiopulmonary bypass. Complex injuries involving posterior aspects of the ascending aorta and pulmonary artery are also repaired with cardiopulmonary bypass. Exposure of the transverse arch can be improved by extending the median sternotomy incision to the neck and dividing the innominate vein.

Innominate artery and proximal left common carotid artery injuries are best approached via median sternotomy incision with cervical extension if necessary. Division of the innominate vein provides excellent exposure to the transverse aortic arch for proximal control. In patients with small, partial tears of the distal innominate artery, primary repair with 4-0 polypropylene suture is often possible. In most cases, innominate artery injuries are best managed using the bypass exclusion technique[18] (Figure 3). This approach allows management without the use of systemic heparinization, cardiopulmonary bypass, or hypothermic circulatory arrest. A 10-mm knitted tube graft is used to create a proximal ascending aorta to distal innominate artery bypass. After the bypass is completed, the injury at the origin of the aortic duct is oversewn. Injuries to the proximal left common carotid artery can also be managed in a similar fashion.

Known isolated injuries to the descending thoracic aorta are best approached through a left posterolateral thoracotomy incision in the fourth intercostal space. Most patients with descending thoracic aortic injuries have concomitant injuries in other body compartments. Prioritizing surgical treatment for each of these compartmental injuries can be a challenge. In general, for patients with a stable mediastinal hematoma and unstable intra-abdominal injury, exploratory laparotomy should be performed first.

The principles of managing descending thoracic aortic injuries are proximal/distal control, addressing the injured segment, and reestablishing continuity of blood flow. Most blunt traumatic injuries in the descending thoracic aorta originate medially at the level

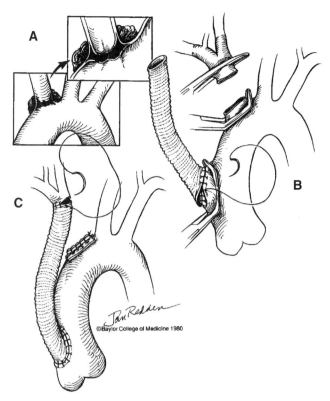

Figure 3 Bypass-exclusion technique for management of innominate artery injuries. **(A)** Severe intimal disruption may be associated with minimal external hematoma. **(B)** A site is selected for aortotomy along the ascending aorta, and a prosthetic graft is sewn end to side. A partial occluding vascular clamp is placed at the origin of the innominate artery and a vascular clamp is placed across the distal innominate artery. The artery is divided between the clamps. **(C)** The repair is completed by an end-to-end anastomosis of the graft to the distal innominate artery and by oversewing the native origin of the innominate artery on the aorta.   *(Courtesy Jan Redden, Baylor College of Medicine, 1980.)*

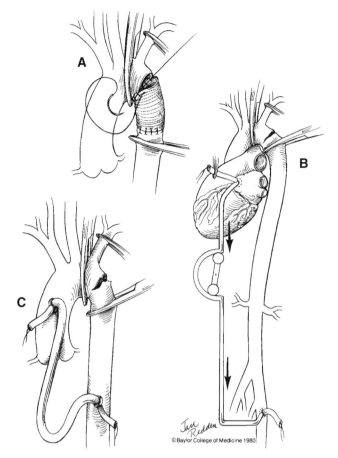

Figure 4 Adjuncts in the management of descending thoracic aortic injuries. **(A)** Simple clamp and sew technique with proximal and distal control using vascular clamps. **(B)** Active left atriofemoral bypass with partial left-heart bypass. **(C)** Passive ascending to descending thoracic aorta with shunt.   *(Courtesy Jan Redden, Baylor College of Medicine, 1980.)*

of the ligamentum arteriosum. The most expeditious way of obtaining proximal control is to follow the left subclavian artery proximally to the aortic arch and place an umbilical tape around the aortic arch between the takeoff of the left common carotid artery and the left subclavian artery. An umbilical tape is also passed around the left subclavian artery. Care should be taken to try to avoid injury to the left recurrent laryngeal nerve as it courses posteriorly around the aortic arch near the ligamentum arteriosum. The next maneuver is to achieve vascular control distal to the anticipated injury. It is important to examine the entire length of the descending thoracic aorta in order to identify any additional tears, especially at the level of the diaphragm. There are several approaches to the basic vascular repair of the descending thoracic aorta. First is the simple clamp-and-sew technique without the use of shunts or left heart bypass. Second is the use of a passive shunt, which is less commonly used. Some surgeons advocate the use of active partial left heart bypass for repairing descending thoracic aortic injuries (Figure 4). All of these adjunct techniques should be familiar to surgeons managing this type of injury. The hematoma is entered after proximal and distal control is established. Intercostal vessels are not routinely oversewn. The extent of the injury is inspected from both external and internal aspects of the aorta. Simple partial lacerations of the aorta can be primarily closed with running sutures using 4-0 polypropylene. Complex injuries often require an interposition graft.

Heated debate continues in the literature on whether active distal perfusion decreases the dreaded morbidity of paraplegia in the management of descending thoracic aortic injuries. There are reports supporting both sides of the argument. The length of aortic cross clamp time has been argued as an independent factor contributing to increased incidence of postoperative paraplegia. Numerous studies, however, have shown that the incidence of postoperative paraplegia is multifactorial and cannot be attributed to any single cause.[19–26] All distal perfusion techniques have potential complications including those from cannulation sites or from systemic heparinization. Regardless of the technique used, the overall incidence of postoperative paraplegia averages 8% according to various studies.[23,27–30] To date, no prospective randomized trial has documented the superiority of any single technique.

Median sternotomy with right-sided cervical extension is the incision of choice for right subclavian artery injury. Proximal left subclavian artery injury is best repaired through a left posterolateral thoracotomy in the fourth intercostal space. Exposure of the distal left subclavian artery can be obtained through a left supraclavicular incision with proximal control via a third interspace anterolateral incision. While seldom needed, injury to multiple segments of the left subclavian artery can be managed by combining the two incisions to create a "trapdoor" incision. Injury to the phrenic nerve, lying anterior to the scalenus anticus muscle, should be avoided during exposure of the subclavian artery. The left clavicle can be divided or resected to provide better exposure if necessary. After obtaining proximal and distal control, either primary repair or interposition knitted or polytetrafluoroethylene grafts may be used depending on the extent of injury. Because of the soft nature of the subclavian artery, mobilization for end-to-end anastomosis is generally difficult. Subclavian artery injuries are often associated with concomitant brachial plexus injuries; therefore, it is helpful to note the preoperative neurological examination. Subclavian venous injuries are exposed similarly as subclavian artery injuries. Venous injuries are repaired by either primary venorrhaphy or ligation.

Intrapericardial pulmonary artery injuries are best approached with a median sternotomy incision. Main pulmonary artery and proximal right pulmonary artery are readily accessible upon opening the pericardium. The proximal left pulmonary artery is exposed by dissecting between the superior vena cava and the ascending aorta. Small anterior injuries are primarily repaired with running 4-0 polypropylene sutures with the use of a partial occluding vascular clamp. More complex and posterior injuries may require the use of cardiopulmonary bypass. Distal extrapericardial pulmonary artery injuries are approached with thoracotomy incisions. In selected patients, pneumonectomy may be the life-saving procedure of choice for major hilar injuries.

Injuries to the thoracic vena cava are extremely difficult to manage surgically because of its anatomic location. A median sternotomy incision provides optimal exposure. Simple anterior lacerations can be primarily repaired with a partial occluding vascular clamp. Posterior injuries may require the use of total cardiopulmonary bypass. Subsequent repair is accomplished from inside the right atrium. Occasionally, an intracaval shunt may be a useful adjunct.

Intrapericardial pulmonary venous injuries are rare and diagnosed intraoperatively during an empiric emergent thoracotomy. The optimal incision is a left anterolateral thoracotomy that allows access to the posterior aspect of the heart. Extrapericardial pulmonary venous injuries in stable patients are approached from posterolateral thoracotomy incisions. Simple lacerations can be closed primarily. Massive hemorrhage can be controlled with temporary hilar occlusion. If a pulmonary vein must be ligated for life-saving measures, appropriate pulmonary lobectomy should follow.

Because the azygous vein drains directly into the superior vena cava, injuries to the azygous veins can be potentially fatal. This type of injury is rarely diagnosed or suspected preoperatively. When seen in the operating room, azygous venous injuries are best managed by primary repair or division and suture ligation of both ends. Similarly, internal mammary arterial and venous injuries can cause massive hemorrhage and are often diagnosed intraoperatively. The best treatment option is simple ligation and proper documentation in the operative notes in order to eliminate the possibility of using internal mammary arteries as conduits for potential future coronary artery bypass operations.

In a dying patient with thoracic vascular injury, damage control thoracotomy is a treatment option. A left anterolateral thoracotomy incision provides the best initial exposure. The principle of damage control thoracotomy consists of the use of simpler techniques to achieve expeditious control of hemorrhage in a single setting, or temporary measures for hemorrhage control with planned second operation for definitive repair as the patient's physiologic status is restored to a more survivable level.[31] Hilar vascular injuries can be controlled quickly by performing pneumonectomy or lobectomy with a stapling device. For vessels greater than 5 mm, synthetic grafts may be used to avoid delays in harvesting vein grafts. Temporary ligation and placement of intravascular shunts can control hemorrhage until the patient's physiologic status is restored to a more appropriate level for definitive repair. Ligation of the subclavian artery is often well tolerated and can be used in a damage control setting. Thoracotomy incisions can be closed quickly with towel clips; however, en-mass closure using large needles encompassing all muscle layers are more hemostatic. A "Bogotá bag" or patch closure can also be used as temporary closures in patients with cardiac dysfunction in order to prevent compression of the heart.

Young patients usually have very soft medium and large size named arteries in the chest without atherosclerotic disease. During surgical repair of thoracic vessels, any slight lateral deviation from the natural curve of the suture needle translates to increasing hemorrhage from needle holes, which on some occasions may lead to further tears in the artery and result in a fatal outcome. Gentle, precise technique provides the best repairs.

MORBIDITY AND MANAGEMENT COMPLICATIONS

Neurologic deficits often accompany injuries to thoracic vascular structures either as additional associated injuries or as postoperative morbidities. Therefore, proper preoperative documentation of the patient's neurologic status is important. As mentioned previously, the overall average incidence of postoperative paraplegia is 8% for descending thoracic aortic repair. The anatomic proximity of the brachial plexus to the subclavian vessels is the reason for the high incidence of brachial plexopathy associated with subclavian vessel injuries. Detailed discussion with the patient and family members of these associated neurologic morbidities is warranted. Some patients experience persistent post-thoracotomy pain, which can be socially and emotionally devastating. Thus, early mobility and rehabilitation are important adjuncts to the care of these patients. In selected patients, intercostal nerve blocks may be beneficial.

A majority of patients with thoracic vascular trauma have associated multiorgan injury. As a result, a significant portion of these patients remain critically ill in the intensive care unit setting. Various pulmonary complications such as atelectasis, pneumonia, and acute respiratory distress syndrome are becoming some of the most common complications in the early postoperative period. Patients with concomitant pulmonary contusions are at an increased risk of developing acute respiratory distress syndrome. Aggressive pulmonary toilet, adequate pain control, and detailed critical care are all essential elements in preventing these complications.

MORTALITY

Thoracic vascular injuries have one of the highest mortality rates of any organ system because of the high incidence of other concomitant injuries in other body compartments. Patients with ascending aortic injuries rarely reach the hospital alive. The mortality rate remains as high as 50% for patients with ascending aortic injuries with stable vital signs on arrival to trauma centers.[8] Injuries to the central pulmonary artery and vein are highly lethal with mortality rates in excess of 70%.[8] Similarly, thoracic vena cava injuries are infrequent but extremely difficult to control and carries a mortality rate greater than 60%.[8] Regardless of the surgical technique used, the mortality rate of descending thoracic aortic injuries ranges from 5% to 25%.[30] The overall mortality for innominate artery injuries is reported to be 25% from 1960 to 1992.[18] Subclavian artery injuries have the best prognosis with an overall mortality rate of less than 5% as reported by Graham et al.[32]

CONCLUSIONS

Managing patients with thoracic vascular injuries requires technical expertise and excellent surgical judgment. For this reason, taking care of patients with this type of injury can be both extremely challenging and rewarding.

Unlike abdominal injuries where midline vertical incision is the standard exploratory incision, patients with stable thoracic vascular injuries require careful preoperative planning. Because of the rigid chest wall, ill-placed incisions and incorrect intercostal space entry significantly compromise exposure for proximal/distal control of hemorrhage from thoracic vascular injuries. Although thoracic vascular injuries have one of the highest mortality rates of any trauma, superb surgical judgment along with operative precision will translate to improved patient care and outcome.

REFERENCES

1. Vesalius A: In *Beonetus T. Sepulchretaum sive Anataomia Practica ex Cad ak Veribus Morbo Denatis.* Geneva, 1700, sec. 2:290.
2. DeBakey ME, Simeone FA: Battle injuries of the arteries in WWII. *Ann Surg* 123:534, 1946.
3. Passaro E, Pace WG: Traumatic rupture of the aorta. *Surgery* 41:787, 1959.
4. Mattox KL, Feliciano DV, Burch J, Beall AC Jr, Jordan GL Jr, DeBakey ME: Five thousand seven hundred sixty cardiovascular injuries in 4459 patients—epidemiological evolution 1958 to 1987. *Ann Surg* 209:698, 1989.
5. Trunkey DD: Thoracic trauma. In Trunkey DD, Lewis FR, editors: *Current Therapy of Trauma.* St. Louis, CV Mosby, 1984, p. 85.
6. Beeson A, Saegesser F: *Color Atlas of Chest Trauma and Associated Injuries.* Oradell, NJ, Medical Economics Books, 1983.
7. Bickell WH, Wall MJ Jr, Pepe PE, Martin RR, Ginger VF, Allen MK, Mattox KL: Immediate versus delayed fluid resuscitation for hypotensive patients with penetrating torso injuries. *N Engl J Med* 331:1105–1109, 1994.
8. Mattox KL: Approaches to trauma involving the major vessels of the thorax. *Surg Clin North Am* 69:77, 1989.
9. Woodring JH: The normal mediastinum in blunt traumatic rupture of the thoracic aorta and brachiocephalic arteries. *J Emerg Med* 8:467, 1990.
10. Wintermark M, Wicky S, Schnyder P: Imaging of acute traumatic injuries of the thoracic aorta. *Eur Radiol* 12(2):431–442, 2002.
11. Parker MS, Matheson TL, Rao AV, et al: Making the transition: the role of helical CT in the evaluation of potentially acute thoracic aortic injuries. *Am J Roentgenol* 176(5):1267–1272, 2001.
12. Dyer DS, Moore EE, Ilke DN, et al: Thoracic aortic injury: how predictive is mechanism and is chest computed tomography a reliable screening tool? A prospective study of 1,561 patients. *J Trauma* 48(4):673–682, 2000.
13. Dyer DS, Moore EE, Mestek MF, et al: Can chest CT be used to exclude aortic injury? *Radiology* 213(1):195–202, 1999.
14. Tello R, Munden RF, Hooton S, Kandarpa K, Pugatch R: Value of spiral CT in hemodynamically stable patients following blunt chest trauma. *Comput Med Imaging Graph* 22(6):447–452, 1998.
15. Mirvis SE, Shanmuganathan K, Buell J, Rodriguez A: Use of spiral computed tomography for the assessment of blunt trauma patients with potential aortic injury. *J Trauma* 45(5):922–930, 1998.
16. Durham RM, Zuckerman D, Wolverson M, et al: Computed tomography as a screening exam in patients with suspected blunt aortic injury. *Ann Surg* 220(5):699–704, 1994.
17. Ben-Menachem Y: Assessment of blunt aortic-brachiocephalic trauma: should angiography be supplanted by transesophageal echocardiography? *J Trauma* 42:969, 1997.
18. Johnston RH Jr, Wall MJ Jr, Mattox KL: Innominate artery trauma: a thirty-year experience. *J Vasc Surg* 17:134, 1993.
19. Crawford ES, Rubio PA: Reappraisal of adjuncts to avoid ischemia in the treatment of aneurysm of descending thoracic aorta. *J Thorac Cardiovasc Surg* 85:98, 1983.
20. Culliford AT, Ayvaliotic B, Shemin R, et al: Aneurysms of the descending aorta. *J Thorac Cardiovasc Surg* 85:98, 1983.
21. Laschinger JC, Cunningham JN Jr, Nathan IM, et al: Experimental and clinical assessment of the adequacy of partial bypass in maintenance of spinal cord flow during operations on the thoracic aorta. *Ann Thorac Surg* 36:417, 1983.
22. Mattox KL: Fact and fiction about management of aortic transection. *Ann Thorac Surg* 48:1, 1989.
23. Mattox KL, Holtzman M, Pickard LR, et al: Cmap/repair: a safe technique for treatment of blunt injury to the descending thoracic aorta. *Ann Thorac Surg* 40:456, 1985.
24. Williams TE, Vasco JS, Kakos GS, et al: Treatment of acute and chronic traumatic rupture of the descending thoracic aorta. *World J Surg* 4:545, 1980.
25. Moore EE, Burch JM, Moore JB: Repair of the torn descending thoracic aorta using the centrifugal pump for partial left heart bypass. *Ann Surg* 240(1):38–43, 2004.
26. Coselli JS, LeMaire SA, Conklin LD, Adams GJ: Left heart bypass during descending thoracic aortic aneurysm repair does not reduce the incidence of paraplegia. *Ann Thorac Surg* 77(4):1298–1303, 2004.
27. Cowley RA, Turney SZ, Hankins JR, et al: Rupture of thoracic aorta due to blunt trauma: a 15 year experience. *J Thorac Cardiovasc Surg* 100:652, 1990.
28. Hilgenberg AD, Logan KL, Akins CW, et al: Blunt injuries of the thoracic aorta. *Ann Thorac Surg* 53:233, 1992.
29. Pate JW, Fabian TC, Walker WA: Acute traumatic rupture of the aortic isthmus: repair with cardiopulmonary bypass. *Ann Thorac Surg* 59:90, 1995.
30. Von Oppell UO, Dunne TT, De Groot MK, et al: Traumatic aortic rupture: twenty-year meta-analysis of mortality and risk of paraplegia. *Ann Thorac Surg* 58:585, 1994.
31. Wall MJ Jr, Soltero E: Damage control for thoracic injuries. *Surg Clin North Am* 77:863, 1997.
32. Graham JM, Feliciano DV, Mattox KL, et al: Management of subclavian vascular injuries. *J Trauma* 20:537, 1980.

TREATMENT OF ESOPHAGEAL INJURY

A. Britton Christmas and J. David Richardson

The treatment of esophageal perforations remains controversial, with uncertainty surrounding several aspects of surgical management: the preferred method of surgical repair, the management of injuries recognized late, and the role of cervical esophagostomy for diversion, among others. Much of this controversy stems from the uncommon nature of these injuries. The relative infrequency of esophageal injury may be attributed to the deep location of this collapsed structure that is surrounded by vital organs. Many penetrating wounds injure the heart or aorta and result in death at the scene.

Blunt injuries to the esophagus are very unusual. Anatomic features, with the lack of serosa, contribute to the difficulty in treatment. Given the frequency of delay in diagnosis and the complexity of operative treatment, injuries of the esophagus remain among the most difficult injuries to manage without major morbidity or mortality. Even the busiest trauma centers often encounter fewer than five esophageal injuries per year.

INCIDENCE

The incidence of esophageal injuries is low with most resulting from penetrating trauma. Esophageal trauma received little notice until the completion of World War II, with only 18 esophageal injuries recorded in the military records reviewed from that war and the Korean and Vietnam Wars combined. Numerous reports in the literature document the incidence of esophageal trauma to be less than 1% with the most common cause being penetrating injuries sustained from stab and gunshot wounds. The cervical esophagus represents the most common site of injury followed by thoracic and abdominal esophageal injuries. While these wounds occur relatively infrequently, they continue to be associated with high mortality ranging from 20% to 30%. Virtually all patients who sustain an esophageal injury also incur associated injuries to other respiratory, gastrointestinal, and vascular injuries. As a result, surgeons must maintain a high index of suspicion so that untoward diagnostic delays may be avoided.

Penetrating injuries of the esophagus far outnumber blunt esophageal injuries. The predominant mechanism of esophageal trauma or injury is gunshot wounds (70%–80%) followed by stab wounds (15%–20%) and shotgun wounds (3%–5%). Esophageal injuries resulting from blunt trauma account for less than 1% of all esophageal injuries. These injuries are most often located in the cervical esophagus as the result of an anterior blow with the neck in a hyperextended position. An acute blow to a distended stomach may produce tears of the distal esophagus.

DIAGNOSIS

Diagnostic delays are often cited as significant factors in the high morbidity and mortality associated with injuries to the esophagus. Several factors contribute to this diagnostic delay including the uncommon occurrence of these injuries. Because associated injuries are common, delays may occur before the initiation of specific diagnostic tests to evaluate the esophagus. All the while, even a "simple" perforation elicits a massive inflammatory response with mediastinal tissue destruction that may further complicate the repair.

Esophageal injuries must be suspected in penetrating neck injuries that violate the platysma, in transmediastinal gunshot wounds, and with significant chest trauma with associated tracheobronchial injuries. The clinical findings most commonly associated with cervical esophageal injuries include neck pain and dysphagia. Tenderness to palpation and with passive motion, dyspnea, and/or hoarseness may be present. Hematemesis, hemoptysis, or bloody nasogastric tube aspirate in the absence of obvious oral or pharyngeal trauma should suggest the possibility of esophageal injury. Expanding cervical hematoma is certainly a cause for concern as are the subsequent development of fever, cough, and stridor. Palpable crepitus or air within the soft tissues or a wide prevertebral shadow on neck or cervical spine radiographs may be the initial suggestion of an esophageal injury. Computed tomography examination may demonstrate subcutaneous emphysema within the soft tissues or in the upper mediastinum.

The clinical findings associated with thoracic esophageal injuries may be nonspecific and initially absent. They may include abdominal tenderness and/or rigidity, cervical crepitation from tracking of mediastinal emphysema, and Hamman's sign (mediastinal crunch on auscultation). The presence of mediastinal emphysema and pleural effusion in the face of penetrating thoracic trauma should elevate awareness for the possibility of a thoracic esophageal injury.

Subdiaphragmatic esophageal injuries often present with abdominal tenderness and/or rigidity. Patients frequently complain of abdominal pain and may progress to signs of frank peritonitis. Upright chest radiographs or computed tomography scans may demonstrate pneumoperitoneum.

While penetrating neck or thoracic wound with hemodynamic instability will often necessitate immediate exploration for associated injuries, the hemodynamically stable patient often presents a diagnostic challenge. In the past, all penetrating neck wounds that violated the platysma were routinely explored. However, many trauma centers now practice selective management of neck wounds. Selective management necessitates some type of study to exclude esophageal injury. We recommend a water-soluble contrast esophagogram in stable patients. If no injury is seen with this technique, addition of dilute barium adds a measure of safety in excluding an injury. Because contrast studies yield a false-negative rate of up to 25%, esophagoscopy may be added in patients regarded as high risk for injury. The specificity of a negative esophagogram accompanied by

negative esophagoscopy approaches 100%. Even in hemodynamically stable patients with cervical hematomas who will undergo exploration, we advocate esophagoscopy, as the injury may be localized by the appreciation of blood or hematoma within the esophagus. It is often difficult to identify an esophageal injury during exploration due to extensive blood staining of the tissues. All studies should be obtained in an expeditious manner as prolonged time to diagnosis has been widely correlated to increased morbidity and mortality. Once an esophageal injury has been diagnosed, all oral intake is held, nasogastric tube decompression is performed, and intravenous fluid resuscitation and broad-spectrum antibiotics are initiated before prompt surgical intervention.

SURGICAL TREATMENT

While some penetrating cervical wounds may be managed nonoperatively, all confirmed esophageal injuries should be managed operatively in expedient fashion. The preferred surgical management of esophageal injuries is dictated by the location of the injury, stability of the patient, time to diagnosis, and associated injuries.

In our opinion, all esophageal injuries should be treated by general unifying principles regardless of location. These principles include (1) attempted closure of all defects by some method; (2) the use of onlay flaps, preferably muscular, as a buttress or for primary closure; and (3) tube drainage near the repair. Given the lack of a serosa, primary healing is not uniform. Therefore, the use of a buttress often enhances healing without fistula development. Local muscle flaps, in particular, are useful for either buttress or as a primary onlay repair.

Injuries to the cervical esophagus may be approached either by a collar incision or by an incision anterior to the sternocleidomastoid. An anterior unilateral incision should be made for unilateral cervical and single injuries, whereas a collar incision is indicated for midline, multiple, or bilateral cervical injuries. The esophagus is located deep to the trachea and placement of a nasogastric tube often facilitates localization by palpation. Throughout the dissection, great care must be taken to identify and avoid injury to the recurrent laryngeal nerves which are located in the tracheoesophageal groove. If further exposure is needed, the omohyoid muscle may be divided. After blunt dissection, the esophagus should be encircled by a Penrose drain in order to further facilitate the dissection.

Thoracic esophageal injuries are best approached through thoracotomy incisions based on the suspected level of the injury. Following initial studies, the decision for the incision should be determined by the presence of pleural effusion or defined leak identified on esophagogram. Injuries to the upper two-thirds of the thoracic esophagus are best approached through a right posterolateral thoracotomy though the fifth intercostal space. Injuries to the lower third of the thoracic esophagus are best approached through an incision in the left sixth intercostal space.

Injuries to the most distal portion of the esophagus should be approached through a laparotomy incision, with the left chest prepped into the operative field should a thoracic approach be necessitated. Additional exposure can be achieved by placing the patient in the Trendelenburg position and by mobilizing the left lobe of the liver. The midline incision can be extended superiorly and to the left of the xiphoid process for an additional 1–2 cm of exposure. The esophagus should be exposed with blunt manual dissection at the gastroesophageal junction and encircled with a Penrose drain. The hiatus can be widened, if necessary, to expose wounds near the gastroesophageal junction.

Most injuries of the esophagus can be primarily repaired if promptly diagnosed. Small injuries may be closed transversely, whereas injuries larger than 2–3 cm can be closed longitudinally in order to avoid undue tension. Unfortunately, diagnostic delay often creates a situation associated with significant mediastinal inflammation and sepsis. Furthermore, the lack of a serosal layer complicates primary reapproximation as the esophageal tissues are extremely friable especially under these circumstances. Numerous strategies have been proposed including non-operative management with drainage, esophageal resection, and diversion with exclusion. The use of pleural and pericardial flaps has been widely described for buttressing primary repairs. More recently, various muscle flaps have been advocated for primary repair of esophageal defects. However, adequate esophageal tissue debridement, tension-free repairs, and effective drainage remain the mainstays of successful operative management.

CERVICAL ESOPHAGUS

The presence of a cervical esophageal injury usually mandates exploration of the neck. Careful examination of the esophagus should be performed to locate the site of esophageal injury as well as possible concomitant injuries to the trachea or vascular structures. Once identified, any nonviable or necrotic tissue should be debrided until viable edges are obtained. The defect should be closed in two layers if possible. An absorbable mucosal repair is preferable with a non-absorbable suture closure of the muscular layer. If significant inflammation has occurred, a single layer closure may be the only feasible option. All wounds of the cervical esophagus may be buttressed or closed primarily by a sternocleidomastoid muscle flap. The muscle flap is created by mobilizing the sternal attachment of the sternocleidomastoid and positioning it over the suture line. Absorbable sutures are used to secure the muscle flap over the defect or repair. All repairs should be drained with either Penrose or silastic tube drains. In the presence of associated carotid artery injuries, drainage should be performed from the opposite side of the neck so as to divert leakage and avoid late vascular complications.

Occasionally, diagnostic delays of an injured esophagus cause intense inflammation in the neck. If the site of injury is not obvious, the esophagus may be insufflated with air under a layer of sterile water. Methylene blue may also be instilled into the esophagus in an attempt to localize the injury. If the injury cannot be localized, then drainage and broad-spectrum antibiotics will often provide satisfactory results.

The delayed diagnosis of cervical esophageal injuries necessitates adequate debridement, irrigation, and drainage. In these instances, primary repair will often not suffice. Therefore, the defect may be primarily closed with a sternocleidomastoid muscle flap. The paraesophageal and precervical planes must also be inspected, irrigated, and drained to decrease contamination. We have treated several patients with large defects that could not be closed primarily with muscle flaps. Likewise, we have treated several patients with delayed recognition of an injury with onlay sternocleidomastoid flaps.

THORACIC ESOPHAGUS

Once the diagnosis of a thoracic esophageal injury has been identified, surgical exploration should ensue through an appropriate thoracotomy as previously described. These injuries are frequently associated with acute coagulation necrosis, diffuse tissue hemorrhage, and significant inflammation. The mediastinum should be opened and thoroughly irrigated. Occasionally, the inflammation is so severe that the defect is difficult to identify. In such cases, the esophagus can be encircled in an area remote from the injury. The esophagus can then be mobilized toward the area of injury. Diligent exploration should be performed until the injury is identified. Both mucosal and muscular layers should be identified, and one should recognize that the mucosal tear is usually larger than the muscular defect. Subsequently, it is often necessary to open the muscular layer more proximally and distally to fully appreciate the mucosal defect. Failure to completely expose the mucosal defect may result in incomplete closure of the defect and subsequent leakage from the site of repair. If possible, a double-layered closure

should be performed with reapproximation of both mucosa and muscularis. The repair should always be buttressed with adjacent tissue for additional reinforcement.

Primary repairs of the thoracic esophagus tend to fail in a significant percentage of cases. The lower esophageal blood supply and the lack of a serosal layer make primary closure much more tenuous. As a result, several adjacent tissues have been used to buttress or primarily repair these injuries with variable success. Pleural flaps have been widely used but are often too friable and sometimes provide inadequate tissue coverage. Pleural flaps are more reliable if there have been inflammatory changes to thicken the pleura. The use of pericardial flaps seems unwise, as this would expose the pericardial sac to contamination. In our experience, we have found muscle flaps to be more reliable both in terms of buttressing and primary repair of esophageal defects.

Adequate tissue coverage is especially important in close proximity to the trachea in order to reduce the incidence of later fistula development. If both trachea and esophagus are injured, we attempt to interpose a muscle flap between the suture lines of the two injuries. Muscle flaps tend to be less friable and provide greater bulk of tissue coverage of the defect. Intercostal bundles are frequently mentioned as muscle flaps but we often find they provide inadequate tissue for buttress and especially for primary repair.

We have demonstrated that injuries to the esophagus involving up to two-thirds of the circumference can be adequately closed with muscle flaps without increased incidence of stricture. The rhomboid muscle may be mobilized for repair of upper- and mid-esophageal injuries (Figure 1). The muscle is dissected from its attachment of the scapula through a parascapular incision and transferred as a pedicle flap into the thoracotomy. For distal esophageal lesions that are too proximal to be buttressed with the gastric fundus, we advocate the use of a diaphragm muscle flap (Figure 2). The central portion of the diaphragm is excised as a pedicle flap and sutured over the defect or buttressed to the repair. The flap should be posteriorly based and great care should be taken to avoid the phrenic nerve. Diaphragm pedicle flaps may reach to the level of the azygous vein. The edges of the diaphragm are then reapproximated with heavy nonabsorbable sutures. A two layer closure is performed if feasible. This has the additional benefit of plicating the diaphragm.

Delayed diagnosis of thoracic esophageal injuries presents a significant surgical challenge. Prolonged perforations are often difficult to visualize secondary to mediastinitis and subsequent empyema. Successful management of uncontained esophageal leaks requires debridement of necrotic tissue, copious irrigation, and complete mediastinal and pleural drainage. Often, a decortication must also be performed at the time of operation if the diagnosis has been delayed for several days. While primary repair remains the preferred method of management, we have found that this is essentially futile after delayed diagnosis and treatment.

All thoracic esophageal injuries should be widely drained. The mediastinal pleura should be widely incised, and a large bore chest tube should be placed in the mediastinum adjacent to the repair. In those with large esophageal injuries, delayed diagnosis of the injury, or those believed at high risk for failure, we support the routine placement of a gastrostomy tube for gastric decompression. The placement of a jejunostomy tube for distal feeding should also be considered in order to maintain adequate nutrition.

ABDOMINAL ESOPHAGUS

Injuries to the abdominal esophagus are often accompanied by extensive intra-abdominal or intrathoracic injuries. These injuries are best approached through a laparotomy incision with the left chest prepped into the operative field should a thoracotomy be necessitated. Perforations or injuries to the distal esophagus should be closed primarily

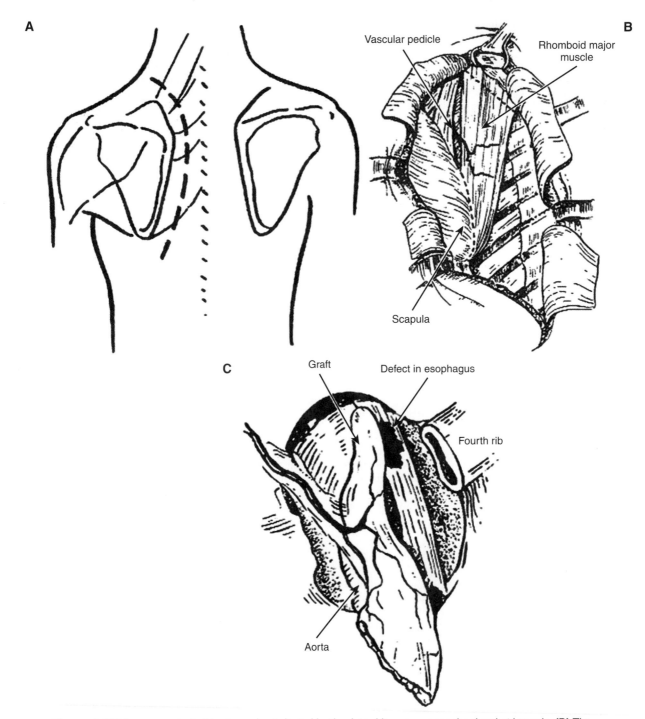

Figure 1 **(A)** A parascapular incision is used as indicated by the dotted lines to expose the rhomboid muscle. **(B)** The rhomboid muscle is isolated and carefully dissected to preserve its vascular pedicle. **(C)** A rib resection allows the muscle to be transposed into the thoracic cavity where it is sutured over the esophageal defect as an onlay flap. *(From Richardson JD, Tobin GR: Closure of esophageal defects with muscle flaps. Arch Surg 129:541–548, 1994.)*

in two layers with nonabsorbable sutures. The layered closure should then be buttressed with either a Nissen fundoplication over a 50–60 French bougie, a "Thal" patch, or with a diaphragm flap. Injuries that are not amenable to primary closure should be primarily closed with the diaphragm flap. The area of repair should be adequately drained with a silastic tube drain. A gastrostomy tube should be placed for gastric decompression, and a jejunostomy tube should be placed for distal enteric feeding.

DEVASTATING INJURIES

Occasionally, devastating injuries of the esophagus occur. If repair is not feasible, there are several less than desirable options, including resection, T-tube placement, and cervical esophagostomy with or without esophageal exclusion.

Esophageal resection may be indicated in some unusual circumstances, but the senior author has never been forced to resect the

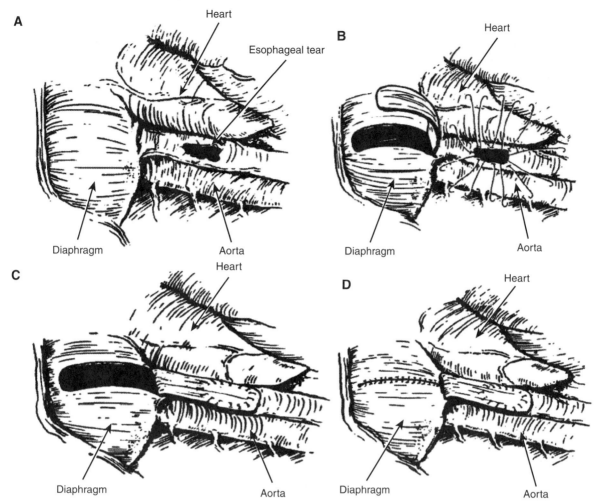

Figure 2 **(A)** Defects in the distal one-third of the esophagus are generally in close proximity to the diaphragm. The diaphragm can be used to close midthoracic defects. **(B)** The edges of the esophageal defect are debrided and a diaphragm flap is elevated. Double-armed sutures can be passed through the defect and then sutured to muscle to ensure a complete onlay graft. **(C)** The flap is then sutured in position. **(D)** The diaphragmatic defect is closed in two layers with heavy sutures. *(From Richardson JD, Tobin GR: Closure of esophageal defects with muscle flaps. Arch Surg 129:541–548, 1994.)*

esophagus for trauma in 30 years of experience. Clearly, injuries to a damaged esophagus or caustic injuries may require emergency esophagectomy. If this unusual circumstance arises, delayed reconstruction using stomach or colonic bypass would likely be the treatment of choice.

Occasionally, large defects in the esophagus are encountered that cannot be closed. Although we attempt to cover such injuries with an onlay muscle flap, creation of a controlled fistula with a T-tube has been reported. In this technique, the short limb of the T-tube is placed in the defect and the long limb is brought out through the chest. In our experience, if a perforation is amenable to closure around a tube, it can be closed with a tissue flap even if the treatment is delayed.

Cervical esophagostomy should not be used routinely because it represents extremely difficult problems to reconstruct. In our experience, a diversion should be performed for an uncontrolled leak that results in sepsis or a life-threatening problem. If possible, a loop esophagostomy should be performed. This permits the possibility of a one-stage closure of the esophagostomy if and when the esophageal injury has healed. End esophagostomy invariably requires complex reconstruction.

If diversion is performed, we rarely use esophageal exclusion in which the distal esophagus is ligated. This creates a distal obstruction and permits bacterial overgrowth in an organ whose only egress is through the original injury. For this reason, we do no attempt to exclude the esophagus even if a proximal diversion is performed. An esophagus damaged badly enough to require exclusion is best treated by resection. Using muscle flaps, we have been able to preserve esophageal function in many patients with complex injuries.

MANAGEMENT OF COMPLICATIONS

The morbidity associated with cervical esophageal injuries has been estimated as high as 16%, with most complications related to the duration of diagnostic delay and subsequent contamination from esophageal contents. Gunshot wounds exhibit a greater preponderance for complications, whereas stab wounds often fare better secondary to less tissue destruction.

Increased morbidity from diagnostic delays and subsequent delays in operative treatment has been well established. However, little literature exists addressing long-term complications and esophageal function after traumatic esophageal injuries. Certainly, the most concerning complications associated with esophageal injuries are major vascular or airway injuries producing massive hemorrhage or acute respiratory decompensation. The development of anastomotic leaks with subsequent mediastinitis, sepsis, and pulmonary failure presents significant management challenges. Shock, extensive mobilization, inadequate debridement, and tension are well-known risk factors for suture line breakdown and subsequent esophageal leakage. Approximately 50% of esophageal leaks are asymptomatic being noticed only on post-operative esophagograms. Once a leak is identified, the initiation of adequate drainage, wide-spectrum antibiotics, parenteral or distal enteral nutrition, and limited oral intake are the mainstays of therapy. The development of interventional radiological techniques with the advent of percutaneous drainage has certainly assisted in the management of these complicated injuries. Most leaks will subsequently resolve without the need for further operative intervention. Increasingly, endoluminal stents have been used to manage esophageal leaks. We have no experience using stents as primary treatment, but we have used them on two occasions for the treatment of delayed leaks resulting from trauma.

CONCLUSIONS

Esophageal injuries, while uncommon, mandate a high degree of suspicion especially for penetrating injuries to the neck or thorax. Many of these patients have concomitant vascular, airway, or intra-abdominal injuries that often require emergent operative intervention. For those who remain hemodynamically stable, prompt diagnostic evaluation should ensue to avoid delays in treatment. A water-soluble esophagogram should be performed followed by dilute barium if no leak is visualized. A false-negative rate as high as 25% has been reported with esophagogram alone. Therefore, radiographic studies should be complemented with esophagoscopy for verification. The combination of esophagography in combination with esophagoscopy approaches a specificity of nearly 100%. In the presence of cervical hematoma, we advocate the use of intraoperative esophagoscopy to localize the injury before operative exploration. This should be performed in the operative suite in the event of hemorrhage, loss of airway, or hemodynamic collapse. After diagnosis, wide-spectrum antibiotics, meticulous surgical technique with ade-

quate debridement, and wide drainage comprise the mainstays of successful management.

SUGGESTED READINGS

Andrade-Alegre R: T-tube intubation in the management of late esophageal perforations: case report. *J Trauma* 37:131–132, 1994.
Asensio JA, Berne J, Demetriades D, et al: Penetrating esophageal injuries: time interval of safety for preoperative evaluation—how long is safe? *J Trauma* 43:319–324, 1997.
Asensio JA, Chawan S, Forno W, et al: Penetrating esophageal injuries: multi-center study of the American Association for the Surgery of Trauma. *J Trauma* 50:289–296, 2001.
Back MR, Baumgartner FJ, Klein SR: Detection and evaluation of aerodigestive tract injuries caused by cervical and transmediastinal gunshot wounds. *J Trauma* 42:680–686, 1997.
Bufkin BL, Miller JI, Mansour KA: Esophageal perforation: emphasis on management. *Ann Thorac Surg* 61:1447–1452, 1996.
Cheadle W, Richardson JD: Options in the management of trauma to the esophagus. *Surg Gynecol Obstet* 155:380–384, 1982.
Cohn HE, Hubbard A, Patton G: Management of esophageal injuries. *Ann Thorac Surg* 48:309–314, 1989.
Glatterer MS Jr, Toon RS, Ellestad C, et al: Management of blunt and penetrating external esophageal trauma. *J Trauma* 25:784–792, 1985.
Grillo HC, Wilkins EW Jr: Esophageal repair following late diagnosis of intrathoracic perforation. *Ann Thorac Surg* 20:387–399, 1975.
Karmy-Jones RC, Wagner JW, Lewis JW Jr: Esophageal injury. In Trunkey DD, Lewis FR, editors: *Current Therapy of Trauma*, 4th ed. St. Louis, MO, Mosby, 1999, pp. 209–216.
Pass LJ, LeNarz LA, Schreiber JT, Estrera AS: Management of esophageal gunshot wounds. *Ann Thorac Surg* 44:253–256, 1987.
Popovsky J, Lee YC, Berk JL: Gunshot wounds of the esophagus. *J Thorac Cardiovasc Surg* 72:609–612, 1976.
Port JL, Kent MS, Korst RJ, et al: Thoracic esophageal perforations: a decade of experience. *Ann Thorac Surg* 75:1071–1074, 2003.
Richardson JD: Management of esophageal perforations: the value of aggressive surgical treatment. *Am J Surg* 190:161–165, 2005.
Richardson JD, Flint LM, Snow NJ, et al: Management of transmediastinal gunshot wounds. *Surgery* 90:671–676, 1981.
Richardson JD, Tobin GR: Closure of esophageal defects with muscle flaps. *Arch Surg* 129:541–548, 1994.
Riley RD, Miller PR, Meredith JW: Injury to the esophagus, trachea, and bronchus. In Moore EE, Feliciano DV, Mattox KL, editors: *Trauma*, 5th ed. New York, McGraw-Hill, 2004, pp. 539–552.
Triggiani E, Belsey R: Oesophageal trauma: incidence, diagnosis and management. *Thorax* 32:241–249, 1977.

DIAPHRAGMATIC INJURY

Charles E. Lucas and Anna M. Ledgerwood

ANATOMY AND PHYSIOLOGY

The diaphragm is a musculotendinous organ that separates the thoracic cavity from the abdominal cavity.[1,2] This important organ arises from the confluence of the abdominal peritoneum and the parietal pleural during the first trimester of pregnancy. The muscular ingrowth represents an extension from the circumference of the thoracic inlet, specifically the posterior sternal border, the inner surfaces of the lower six costal cartilages, and the posterior

lumbocostal arches. These three muscular groups join together as a central tendon, which has three leaflets, namely, left, right, and central leaflets (Figures 1 and 2). The most medial posterior margins are formed by the crura. The central leaflet is located posterior to the sternum and inferior to the heart; it contributes to the pericardial fibers. The right and left leaflets are located posterolaterally in each hemithorax. Incomplete closure of this posterior lateral leaflet results in herniation in the posterior lateral foramen of Bochdalek. Partial closure may result in pleural and peritoneal apposition without union as a central tendon.[3] This results in an eventration that may be an important consideration in the differential diagnosis of blunt diaphragmatic injury (Figures 3 and 4).[3]

The diaphragm, as a muscular organ, varies widely in contour during the ventilatory cycle.[1] During full expiration, the diaphragmatic dome extends high into the thoracic cavity. When the dia-

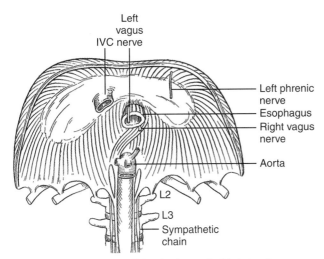

Figure 1 Inferior view of the diaphragm highlighting the posteriorly located foramina and central tendon. *IVC,* Inferior vena cava. *(From Asensio AA, et al:* Diaphragmatic Injuries: Operative Techniques in General Surgery. *Philadelphia, WB Saunders, 2000, with permission.)*

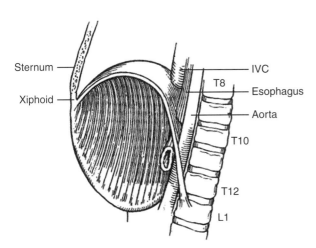

Figure 2 Lateral view of the diaphragm. Note xiphoid and sternal attachments anteriorly and the extension of the crus posteriorly. *IVC,* Inferior vena cava. *(From Asensio AA, et al:* Diaphragmatic Injuries: Operative Techniques in General Surgery. *Philadelphia, WB Saunders, 2000, with permission.)*

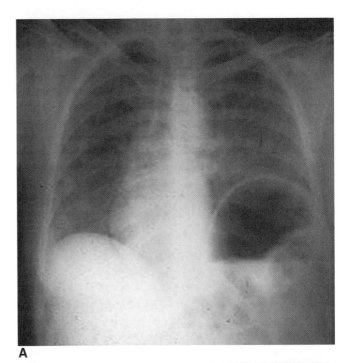

A

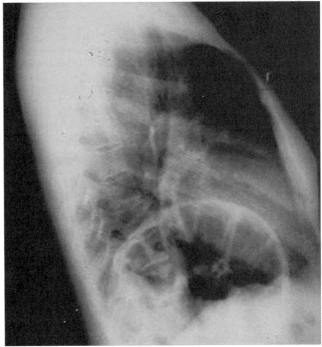

B

Figure 3 Preoperative, anteroposterior **(A)** and lateral **(B)** views of eventration misdiagnosed as ruptured diaphragm after motor vehicle collision.

phragm contracts during forced inspiration, the central tendon is pulled inferiorly and becomes more plate-like.[1] This reduces the intrathoracic pressure and raises the intra-abdominal pressure. The excursion of the diaphragm during forced expiration is great; the dome of the diaphragm elevates to the level of the fourth intercostal space at the sternal junction on the right side and to about the level of the fifth intercostal space on the left side.[1,2] The diaphragm may extend inferiorly at least three intercostal spaces during full inspiration. The most inferior extension posteriorly occurs at the crura. The right crus arises from the bodies and fibrocartilages of the lumbar vertebrae one through three, whereas the smaller left crus arises from the first and second lumbar vertebrae. They join superiorly to encompass the esophagus at the esophageal foramen. The posterior lateral sulcus or recess of the diaphragm is directly posterior to many of the intra-abdominal

organs. Consequently, the posterior sulcus extends inferiorly to the midportion of the kidneys. This inferior extension is often not appreciated when patients with upper abdominal gunshot wounds or stab wounds are treated for intra-abdominal injuries; thus, perforation of the diaphragm in this area is easily overlooked. The resultant hemothorax is diagnosed postoperatively. Careful inspection followed by repair and tube thoracostomy precludes the development of this complication.

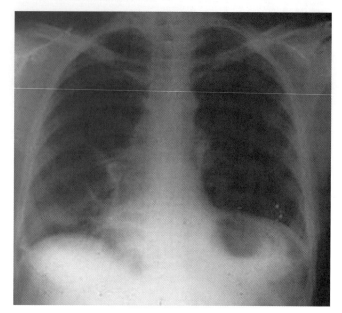

Figure 4 Postoperative view after placation of eventration misdiagnosed as ruptured diaphragm.

The diaphragm has three major foramina (see Figure 1). The aortic hiatus is the most posterior, located between the diaphragmatic muscle and the 12th vertebra. The esophageal hiatus is bordered by the strong muscular crura; the left crus encircles the esophagus and forms an important part of the lower esophageal sphincter. Immediately posterior to the esophagus, sinuous fibers from each hemidiaphragm join as the median arcuate ligament, which is anterior to the aorta and superior to the celiac axis. Immediately posterior to the esophageal foramen on the right side is the foramen for the inferior vena cava (see Figure 1). There are also lesser diaphragmatic apertures. The anterior foramen of Morgagni is in the retroxiphoid space; the internal mammary arteries pass through this foramen while coursing from the mediastinum before dividing into the superior epigastric arteries and the subcostal arteries.[4] The accompanying veins follow the same course.

The median plane of the diaphragm extending from the foramen of Morgagni to the esophageal foramen, the so-called median raphe, is less vascular than the more lateral muscular portions of the diaphragm (see Figure 2). This plane can be divided to provide better exposure to the inferior mediastinum. Care must be taken, however, to prevent injury to the phrenic vein, which may cross this median plane about 1 cm above the esophageal hiatus. This vein, if not controlled while dividing the median raphe between the foramen of Morgagni and esophageal hiatus, can lead to major hemorrhage.

The diaphragm is innervated by the phrenic nerve with arises from the cervical portion of the spinal cord, namely, C3, C4, and C5 (see Figure 1).[1] After these nerves pass inferior through the mediastinum to the medial portion of the diaphragm, they curve laterally, like a fan, from the central medial portion of the diaphragm to the anterior, lateral, and posterior attachments (see Figure 1). In theory, one should protect these nerves while performing surgery on the diaphragm; this is accomplished by detachment of the diaphragm from the peripheral thorax. This is seldom necessary for most patients with diaphragmatic injury. When the origins of the diaphragm are to be relocated for treatment of unusual injuries, however, care should be taken to protect the neural innovation as much as is practical.

INCIDENCE OF DIAPHRAGMATIC INJURIES

The reported incidence of diaphragmatic injury varies widely. Asensio et al.,[2] in a multicenter review, identified a 3% incidence of diaphragmatic injuries for all patients sustaining torso trauma with a range of 0.8%–5.8%; this wide range reflects the different types of injuries treated at each institution and the diligence one places on confirming a diaphragmatic perforation. Rural trauma centers are more likely to treat patients with blunt diaphragmatic injury, whereas penetrating diaphragmatic injury predominates in patients presenting to inner city trauma centers.[5]

The reported incidence of diaphragmatic rupture may also reflect the different therapeutic approaches to patients with both blunt and penetrating abdominal wounds.[6] Most patients with penetrating stab wounds to the abdomen are now being treated nonoperatively when the patient exhibits no signs of peritonitis or hemoperitoneum.[7,8] This is also true for patients with lower thoracic stab wounds causing hemopneumothorax which, based on prior experiences with a more liberal approach to exploratory laparotomy, would be associated with a high incidence of confirmed diaphragmatic penetration.[8] This includes some patients who have hemothorax treated by tube thoracostomy; many of these patients have unrecognized diaphragmatic perforation (Figure 5). Moreover, patients with through-and-through anterior to posterior right upper quadrant gunshot wounds near the liver and associated right-sided hemopneumothorax are being treated by tube thoracostomy alone, even though there are at least two diaphragmatic perforations. The missile in this setting would pass through the lower rib cage anteriorly, enter the anterior hemithorax, pass through the anterior portion of the diaphragm, transit the liver, re-enter the chest through the posterior portion of the diaphragm, and exit through the posterior chest wall.[9] When treated only with right tube thoracostomy for hemothorax, the diaphragmatic perforations are not diagnosed, and therefore, not coded in the trauma registry.[8] When diagnostic peritoneal lavage (DPL) was performed routinely for patients with penetrating wounds of the lower rib cage, the effluent would be pink with a red cell count less 100,000/cm³ in patients with isolated diaphragmatic perforation.[8] Laparotomy in these patients would confirm a diaphragmatic perforation that was sutured.[10] The current trend for routine ultrasonography (US) in patients with abdominal injury has replaced DPL; US is less sensitive for identifying small amounts of blood. Consequently, clinically insignificant diaphragmatic perforations are not being recognized and are not coded in the trauma registry. Penetrating diaphragmatic perforation after upper abdominal wounds may also go unrecognized despite laparotomy for repair of other intra-abdominal visceral injuries. The perforation may be missed because the missile is thought to have penetrated only the transversalis abdominus muscle. When a subsequent hemothorax appears postoperatively, the treating physician, hopefully, will recognize that there was a missed diaphragmatic injury. Patients with blunt injury are less likely to have a diaphragmatic injury that is not recognized during the same hospitalization (Figure 6). There are, however, a number of patients who present with a diaphragmatic hernia years after major blunt torso trauma when diaphragmatic injury was not recognized initially.

During the 1970s, when routine laparotomy was performed for all penetrating abdominal wounds and careful examination of the inferior diaphragmatic extensions was routine, the incidence of diaphragmatic perforation was approximately 19% for upper abdominal gunshot wounds and 11% for upper abdominal stab wounds.[8] Now that laparotomy for penetrating abdominal wounds is performed more selectively, the incidence of confirmed diaphragmatic perforation is about 8% for gunshot wounds and 2% for stab wounds. In contrast, the recent incidence of diaphrag-

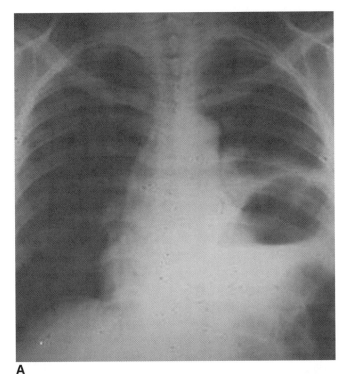

A

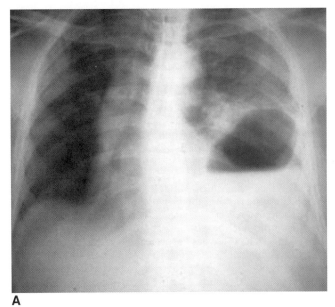

A

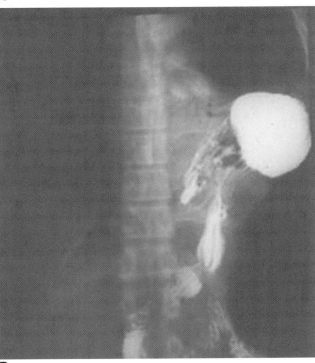

B

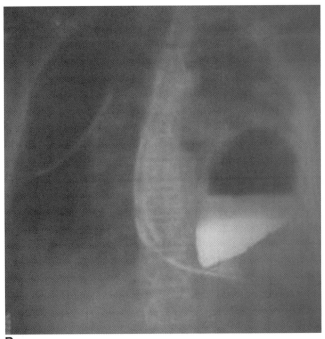

B

Figure 6   **(A)** Anteroposterior chest x-ray demonstrates an apparent gastric bubble in the left hemothorax after blunt trauma. **(B)** Injection of contrast agent through the nasogastric tube confirms the gastric filling.

Figure 5   **(A)** Anteroposterior view of chest showing diaphragmatic hernia in patient treated 18 months earlier by tube thoracostomy for stab wound of left chest. **(B)** Gastrografin confirms the presence of stomach in the left hemithorax.

matic injury in patients admitted after blunt torso injury is less than 1%; most patients with blunt rupture of the liver or spleen are treated nonoperatively. Patients requiring laparotomy for blunt abdominal injury have about a 3% incidence of diaphragmatic rupture.[5,8]

MECHANISM AND LOCATION OF INJURY

The location of diaphragmatic perforation varies with mechanism of injury.[2,8] The classic scenario for blunt diaphragmatic injury is a head-on motor vehicle collision or a T-bone impact causing a marked increase in the intra-abdominal pressure, thereby stretching the diaphragm to the point of rupture. The rupture typically occurs in the posterior lateral segment in the central tendon of the left diaphragm, often with extension into the muscular portion of the diaphragm. Blunt rupture can also occur after assaults, stompings, falls from a height, and explosions.[11] Although the posterior lateral location is the most common site for injury, rupture may occur adjacent to the esophageal hiatus, near the bare area of the liver on the right side, and in a subxyphoid location on either side.

After blunt injury, most ruptures occur in the left hemidiaphragm.[12] A review of 32 published series with 1589 patients by Asensio et al.[2] showed a distribution of left-sided rupture in 1187 patients (75%), right-sided rupture in 363 patients (23%), and bilateral rupture in 39 patients (2%). This observation parallels the authors' experience. The relative protection of the right hemidiaphragm, historically, has been attributed to the protective effects of the liver, which blunts the rapid rise in the intra-abdominal against the right hemidiaphragm.[13] A less common explanation may reflect a weaker left hemidiaphragm that undergoes a later intrauterine closure[14]; an inherent tendinous or muscular weakness, however, has not been demonstrated with carefully constructed bursting tests.[15] The site of injury with penetrating wounds may be anywhere. Bilateral perforations are more likely with missiles. Stab wounds are more commonly located along the periphery of the diaphragm.[8]

SEVERITY OF INJURY

The severity of diaphragmatic rupture or injury is best judged by the organ injury scale for diaphragmatic injury developed by the American Association for the Surgery of Trauma.[16] This scale identifies five grades of injury. Grade I injury is a contusion or hematoma without rupture. Grade II injury is a laceration less than 2 cm in diameter. Grade III rupture is a laceration greater than 2 cm but less that 10 cm in magnitude. Grade IV rupture is greater than 10 cm or has loss of diaphragmatic tissue, which is less than 25 cm^2. Grade V injury is an extensive tear with tissue loss greater than 25 cm^2.

Patients with penetrating stab wounds and gunshot wounds likely have minor ruptures (grades I and II); some patients with low-velocity missile perforations will have grade III perforations. Patients with blunt injury are more likely to have grade III or grade IV lacerations. The massive injuries with extensive tissue loss (grade V) are more likely to be caused by a close-range shotgun blast, high-velocity rifle perforation, or explosions.[17,18]

DIAGNOSIS OF DIAPHRAGMATIC INJURY

The diagnosis of diaphragmatic rupture after blunt injury is usually made on the basis of a chest x-ray that demonstrates the gastric bubble in the left hemithorax (see Figure 6). This can easily be confirmed to be the gastric bubble by showing that the nasogastric tube will pass up into the thorax and contrast agent injected through this tube will fill the gastric bubble. Because a routine chest x-ray is obtained in all patients with significant blunt injury, this provides the simplest and quickest method of diagnosis.[2,7,19] Patients with multisystem injuries involving the chest and pelvis in the presence of hypotension, are more likely to have an associated diaphragmatic injury.[20] When the diaphragmatic perforation is not appreciated on the initial chest x-rays, a subsequent computed tomography (CT) scan of the trunk may show the injury; the diagnosis of diaphragmatic rupture by CT, however, is not very sensitive.[21] The features which lead to the diagnosis being made or suspected by chest x-ray include obfuscation of the costal phrenic angle, apparent elevation of the hemidiaphragm, and the presence of the gastric bubble in a location that is too superior to be intra-abdominal (see Figure 6). Although not readily apparent, the spleen and splenic flexure of the colon, with or without omentum,

are also commonly relocated into the left thorax after blunt diaphragmatic rupture.[2,8]

When the blunt injury occurs on the right side, the liver may prevent abdominal viscera from entering the right hemithorax with the result that the injury may be overlooked.[7] Patients presenting with blunt trauma and significant bleeding from a right-sided pneumothorax, however, should be suspected of having a right-sided hemidiaphragmatic tear in the bare area of the liver, which is also injured and is the source of bleeding (Figure 7).

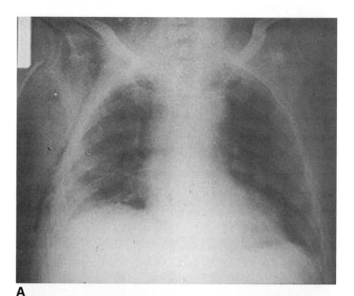

A

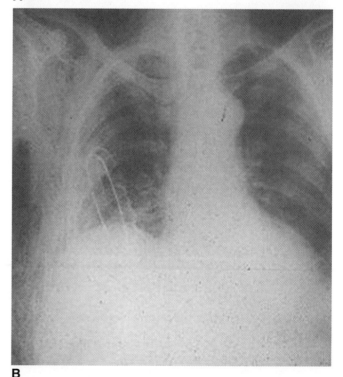

B

Figure 7 **(A)** This 86-year-old man was hit by a bus, sustaining right rib fractures, subcutaneous emphysema, and hemothorax. Note lack of clarity of the right costal phrenic angle. **(B)** Right chest tube yielded 500 ml of blood with continued bleeding of 300 ml during the next hour. Laparotomy revealed a large rent in the dome of the diaphragm and a type IV liver injury that was repaired.

Bilateral diaphragmatic rupture is much less frequent but, when present, may lead to a delay in diagnosis resulting from the apparent lack of diaphragmatic elevation on either side. Both costophrenic angles, however, show lack of clarity (Figure 8). Repeat chest x-rays in such patients will typically show further elevation of one or both hemidiaphragms (see Figure 8). The elevation on the left side would be more likely to show an intrathoracic gastric bubble even in patients after a delay in diagnosis. When the chest x-ray shows what appears to be a large rupture of the left hemidiaphragm in a patient who has minimal symptoms, one should obtain a good history to rule out previous anatomic changes of the left hemidiaphragm and, if possible, obtain old chest x-rays that might identify the presence of an eventration (see Figure 8).

When the chest x-ray does not confirm a diaphragmatic rupture, a number of other studies may be obtained. As indicated, CT is not highly accurate in patients with diaphragmatic injury.[21] Laparoscopy has become more popular for identifying diaphragmatic injury but this has been used primarily in patients with penetrating wounds.[22,23] Likewise, technetium scanning has been employed but has not been that helpful.[24] DPL may lead to suspicion of diaphragmatic injury in patients with associated penetrating wounds to the lower thorax, but has not been too reliable in patients with blunt torso injuries.[8,25] Thorascopy has also been used in patients with late manifestations of a previously missed diaphragmatic injury.[26] Finally, magnetic resonance imaging has been attempted but is of limited value.[27]

The diagnosis of a diaphragmatic injury after a penetrating wound is usually made at the time of laparotomy performed for the treatment of other organ injuries.[2,8] As indicated previously, many diaphragmatic perforations are not currently being diagnosed because of the nonoperative treatment of highly selected patients with torso stab wounds and torso gunshot wounds. When a patient has a stab wound to the lower chest associated with hemothorax, however, a DPL yielding a small amount of hemoperitoneum strongly suggests diaphragmatic perforation.[8,25] This can be confirmed by means of laparoscopy, which will also allow for the small grade II perforation to be repaired.[22,23] A missed diaphragmatic injury is more likely to occur now that patients with these asymptomatic penetrating wounds associated with hemothorax no longer undergo laparotomy (see Figure 5). These missed injuries are more complicated to repair because of associated adhesions; this repair, however, can usually be accomplished through a transabdominal approach.[8,28] When the perforation occurs along the medial portion of the diaphragm, near the esophageal foramen, the herniated viscus may also extend into the pericardium, which makes the diagnosis somewhat more difficult.[29]

The location of diaphragmatic rupture along the more medial portion of the diaphragm increases the likelihood that the rupture will be missed when laparotomy is performed for repair of other injuries (Figure 9). After completing therapy for associated intra-abdominal injuries, the surgeon should carefully examine all of the diaphragm, including the posterior portions of the diaphragm behind the triangular ligaments, especially on the left side.

MANAGEMENT OF DIAPHRAGMATIC INJURY

The severity of diaphragmatic injury plus the magnitude of the associated injuries determines the optimal approach to surgical treatment.[2,8] The decisions regarding resuscitation and prioritization of specific organ injury treatment are discussed elsewhere in this text. Antibiotics should be administered.[30] Most patients with grade II injury, contusion or hematoma, are diagnosed at the time of laparotomy or thoracotomy performed for some other reason.[2,8] These injuries require no special surgical treatment. The surgeon should make sure that the hematoma or contusion is not hiding a full-thickness perforation. When a full-thickness perforation is seen, it is small and can be treated by simple closure. When diagnosed by laparoscopy, isolated grade I perforation may be repaired through the scope.[22,23] The type of suture used for closure of diaphragmatic perforations varies according to surgical preference; the authors prefer 2-0 or 1-0 absorbable polyglycolic sutures,[8] while others prefer 2-0 polypropylene sutures, either in an interrupted fashion using Halsted horizontal mattress sutures or in a running fashion.

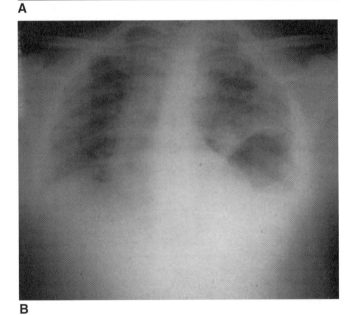

Figure 8 **(A)** Chest x-ray after steering wheel impact in an elderly man shows obfuscation of the left costal phrenic angle without diaphragmatic elevation when compared with the right side. **(B)** Two hours later, both hemidiaphragms are elevated and both costal phrenic angles are obfuscated. Laparotomy revealed bilateral hemidiaphragmatic rupture.

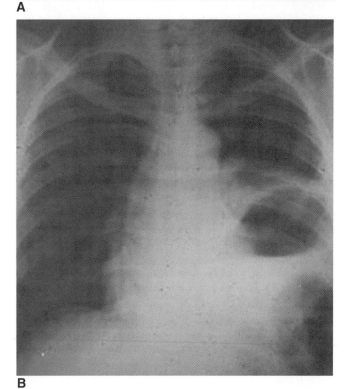

A

B

Figure 9 **(A)** Postoperative chest x-ray, 1 day after laparotomy and repair of a grade III blunt liver injury, shows an air bubble in the left chest thought to be an eventration. **(B)** This air bubble increased 1 day later resulting in re-operation, which demonstrated a missed 4-cm vertical tear of the diaphragm posterior to the left triangular ligament and adjacent to the esophageal foramen.

Grade II injuries with full perforation less than 2 cm in size result from stab wounds or small-caliber gunshot wounds. These are treated with primary closure (Figure 10). When the perforation is located posteriorly, suture placement may be difficult. This can be facilitated by hooking the diaphragm through the perforation with a long right-angle clamp. This permits the first suture to be placed and tied. The first suture then becomes the handle to expose the diaphragm for placement of subsequent sutures (Figure 11).

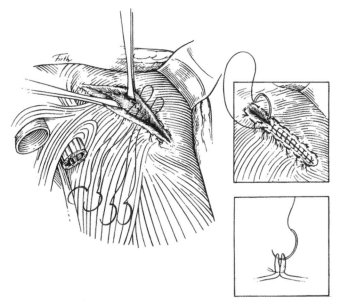

Figure 10 Most minor diaphragmatic ruptures can be repaired with a running or an interrupted suture technique. The authors prefer a running O absorbable polyglycolic suture for most minor injuries. This is reinforced with strategically placed interrupted sutures for major injuries. *(From Asensio AA, et al: Diaphragmatic Injuries: Operative Techniques in General Surgery. Philadelphia, WB Saunders, 2000, with permission.)*

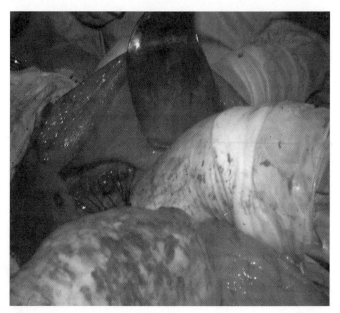

Figure 11 Running O nonabsorbable suture repair shown for grade III perforation after blunt injury.

Larger grade III rents of 2–10 cm can be closed primarily using the same techniques described previously when the tear is linear, as might be caused by a large knife or, in some patients, after blunt injury (see Figure 11). The grade III tears that are seen after large high velocity missile impact or with blunt injury, however, are often irregular. Once the perforation is exposed, meticulous debridement of devitalized tissue is in order, followed by initial placement of strategic sutures designed to reapproximate the irregular borders, which helps with the subsequent closure. Minimal debridement of irregular fragments may help with the approximation. The authors prefer to use interrupted 1-0 absorbable suture for approximation of irregular borders, followed by the placement of running 1-0 absorbable sutures for the definitive closure.

The reconstruction of grade IV lacerations greater than 10 cm in size and associated with modest tissue loss is more challenging.[2,8] These larger injuries often are associated with herniation of abdominal viscera into the left hemithorax. Classically, the stomach, spleen, and colon are inherniated; omentum and small bowel may also be in the thorax.[2,8] Once exposed, these organs need to be relocated within the abdomen. Gentle traction should be tried initially. If the viscera resist gentle traction, the surgeon should place a hand within the thorax, cup the spleen, and gently relocate the viscera into the peritoneal cavity. When the diaphragmatic rent is too tight around the herniated viscera, opening the rent further in a radial direction will allow the surgeon's hand to get superior to the viscera to successfully restore them into the abdomen. This precaution protects the herniated spleen which, surprisingly, is often not injured in these patients. Most grade IV injuries, however, can be closed primarily without using mesh or fascia lata and without altering diaphragmatic attachments. The diaphragm has significant redundancy in the relaxed state so that this approximation can be achieved without tension. Although there will be decreased excursion of the repaired hemidiaphragm after primary closure in this setting, there is seldom long-term impairment. When approximation of ragged borders is difficult, a modified Z-plasty is helpful. In theory, the incisions made in creating the Z-plasty should be radial, extending from the medial plane to the periphery to maximally preserve the branches of the phrenic nerve; however, the long-term result of successful approximation of a viable diaphragm is almost always excellent, even when branches of the phrenic nerve are severed.[2,8] When repairing large defects, one should reapproximate the midportions of the defect so that the lateral portions can be accurately reapposed without creating a dog-ear type of irregular closure.

The grade V diaphragmatic injury with tissue loss exceeding 25 cm^2 presents a major surgical challenge. Many of these large defects with major tissue loss, however, can be closed, primarily if the adjacent chest cage and abdominal wall are intact. When the central defect precludes a tension-free approximation, even in the relaxed state, the peripheral diaphragmatic attachments can be severed anteriorly, laterally, and posteriorly from their costal origins so that the defect can be closed and the diaphragmatic edges reattached two or three interspaces more cephalad.[17] This permits generous advancement of healthy tissue and allows a tension-free primary closure. The long-term results are good.[17]

not unusual. In contrast, patients presenting with penetrating wounds to the diaphragm often have associated injuries to the lung and a number of intra-abdominal viscera. When these injuries involve major vessels, the mortality rate is extraordinarily high.

Asensio and colleagues[2] collectively reviewed 33 published reports on diaphragmatic injury with an overall mortality rate that ranged from 4.3% to 41%, with the average morality rate being 13.7%. The total number of patients included in this review was 1799. The lower mortality rate was reported by Aronoff et al.,[19] who treated patients with mostly penetrating diaphragmatic wounds; the higher mortality rate was reported by Boulanger and colleagues,[12] who treated patients, primarily, with blunt rupture. The reason that the patients with blunt diaphragmatic rupture have a higher mortality rate than the patients with penetrating wounds is related to the magnitude of associated injury involving the rib cage, lungs, and brain.[8,12]

The observed mortality rate will also reflect different therapeutic approaches to treating patients with torso injuries after both penetrating wounds and blunt injury. When all stable patients with penetrating wounds to the abdomen undergo exploratory laparotomy despite the lack of evidence of hypotension or peritoneal irritation, many diaphragmatic perforations will be identified and closed.[2,8,19] The vast majority of these patients would have done well without operation. During the period of time when this approach to penetrating abdominal wounds was followed, the authors observed a mortality rate of well under 4% in patients treated with penetrating diaphragmatic wounds.[8] This same phenomenon was seen in patients with gunshot wounds who had stable vital signs, no evidence of blood loss, and no clinical evidence of hollow viscus perforation. Over the past generation, there have been major changes in the approach to penetrating wounds to the torso. Despite known penetration, patients who are stable and have no evidence of peritonitis are watched overnight and discharged home the next day. Many of these patients likely have perforated diaphragms that are not diagnosed, not treated, and not included in the statistical review of diaphragmatic injuries. In contrast, those patients who do undergo operation for penetrating wounds of the torso have evidence of hypotension and/or peritonitis; these patients have life-threatening injuries to other organs so the repair of a diaphragmatic perforation represents the minor part of their total treatment. Consequently, the mortality rate now exceeds 30% for penetrating diaphragmatic injuries; the deaths are related to hemorrhage from associated injuries, particularly for those patients sustaining thoracoabdominal injuries.

The mechanism of injury also affects the manner of treatment and the likelihood for life-threatening associated injuries after blunt trauma. Patients presenting after high-speed motor vehicle collisions are the most likely candidates for life-threatening injuries to the lung, brain, and pelvis. In contrast, patients presenting after a fall or a stomping brought about by not repaying drug-related loans are more likely to have isolated injuries. This is reflected in the reduced mortality rate for patients treated for blunt rupture of the diaphragm. The authors found no deaths in 11 patients treated for blunt diaphragmatic rupture in 2004.

MORTALITY

The reported morbidity and mortality after diaphragmatic injury vary depending on the etiology, severity of injury, and the extent of injury to other organs.[2,8] Most complications and deaths are caused by the associated injuries. Patients sustaining blunt diaphragmatic rupture often have associated injury to the liver, spleen, or more importantly, the underlying lung. The association of multiple rib fractures and pulmonary contusion with diaphragmatic rupture often causes severe pulmonary contusion resulting in respiratory compromise and prolonged ventilatory support; a fatal outcome is

MORBIDITY

Like mortality, the observed morbidity after diaphragmatic injury results, primarily, from injuries to other organs. Pulmonary insufficiency resulting from atelectasis, pneumonia, and contusion is more likely in patients with multiple rib fractures. An intrapulmonary hematoma that becomes infected and develops into a lung abscess is more commonly seen after a gunshot wound. Occasionally, there will be a surgical disruption of a diaphragmatic repair after one has performed extensive mobilization to achieve primary closure for a grade IV or grade V injury. Breakdown of the diaphragmatic repair, however, is an unusual occurrence. Other complications that occur with diaphragmatic injury include phrenic nerve paralysis, supradiaphragmatic empyema, and subdiaphragmatic abscess. Rodriguez-Morales et al.[5] reported a 65% incidence of atelectasis and a 5% incidence of empyema. Wiencek and colleagues[32] reported a 31% complication rate primarily caused by atelectasis; most complications were not life threatening.

COMPLICATED DIAPHRAGMATIC REPAIR WITH THORACIC INJURY

The greatest technical challenge with the treatment of grade V diaphragmatic injuries occurs when there are associated injuries to the chest wall and/or abdominal wall.[17,18] These massive injuries are usually caused by close-range shotgun blast or high-velocity rifle wounds. There are few descriptions of the technical challenges associated with these rare injuries, probably because the mortality rate is extraordinarily high. Successful care of these huge defects requires the combined reconstruction of the diaphragm and the torso wall; this may take place in multiple phases.

These patients typically present in shock because of associated injuries to major vessels, lung or intraperitoneal viscera, and especially the liver.[17,18] During rapid resuscitation, the surgeon must remember that a complicated repair of the torso wall in conjunction with a large diaphragmatic rupture is facilitated by having separate airway control of both mainstem bronchi. Intubation with a double-lumen tube allows for the injured lung to be deflated while the abdominal or thoracic wall reconstruction is performed in conjunction with the diaphragmatic repair.[17,18] Likewise, the double-lumen airway tube prevents blood from flowing, by gravity, from the injured side, across the carina into the dependent uninjured side; this results in respiratory insufficiency and is likely to be lethal. The primary intraoperative objective is to get rapid control of hemorrhage, which may require pulmonary lobectomy for a massively injured lung (Figure 12). This is followed by debridement of devitalized tissues of the chest wall and diaphragm (Figure 13). Often the resultant defect after massive injury

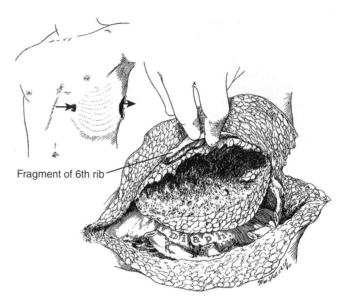

Figure 13 After left lobectomy for hemostasis and debridement of extensive chest wall tissue, he was left with a full-thickness chest wall defect.

precludes successful closure. When the wound occurs solely in the abdomen, the abdominal wall pack technique can be used.[32] However, when the wound involves the thorax, it is impossible to pack the thorax open, so some type of imaginative reconstruction must take place. Sometimes, it is possible to relocate the diaphragm to a more superior position in the thorax (Figure 14). This is accomplished by detaching the anterior, lateral, and posterior attachments from their peripheral origins and reattaching them, superiorly, to an inner space that is above the destroyed chest wall (Figure 15). This allows for the thoracic cavity to be closed and the defect, which is now in the rib cage that covers

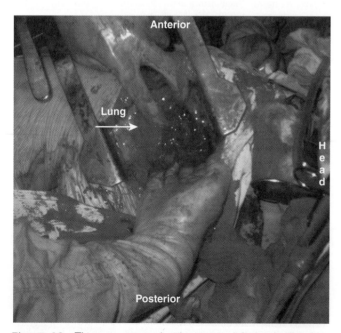

Figure 12 This man presented with a massive left chest wall and left lower lung injury from a close-range shotgun blast.

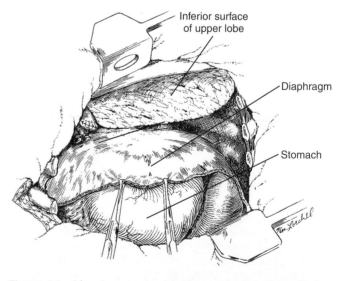

Figure 14 After the extensive debridement shown in Figure 13, the diaphragm was detached anteriorly, laterally, and posteriorly so that it could be reattached three inner spaces higher, thereby converting a chest wall defect into an abdominal defect.

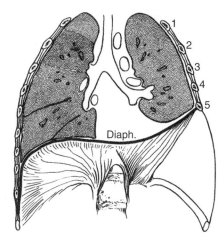

Figure 15 Relocation of the diaphragm to an inner space superior to the full-thickness chest wall defect converts the chest wall defect into an abdominal wall defect, which is then packed.

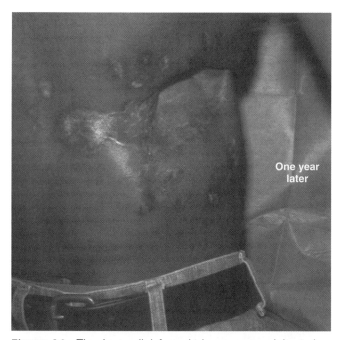

Figure 16 The chest wall defect, which now covers abdominal viscera, has been successfully skin grafted; later reconstruction is performed after the patient has recovered from his underlying insult, which is best judged by restoration of normal activity and weight gain.

only the abdominal cavity, can be treated by the abdominal wall packed technique.[31] Continued dressing changes will allow for granulation tissues to develop, after which a split-thickness skin graft can be placed over the granulation tissues (Figure 16). Later construction of the defect can be accomplished by rotating fascial grafts after the patient has recovered from the underlying insult.

The diaphragm is a large muscular organ with an excellent medially based blood supply, thereby facilitating easy detachment and resuturing. Being native tissue, there is less risk of infection. Even if

the diaphragm has been partially destroyed by the blast, the redundancy should allow for relocation. This technique is ideally suited for lower thoracic full-thickness chest wall defects.[17] The technique reported herein is not suited for superiorly located chest wall defects. More superiorly located full-thickness defects from shotgun blasts can be managed by upper lobectomy combined with wound coverage by a thoracoplasty or rotation of a latissimus dorsi muscle flap. An anteriorly located wound that dismembers the ipsilateral breast and underlying chest wall can be managed by relocation of the uninjured contralateral breast.

COMBINED CHEST WALL AND ABDOMINAL DEFECT WITH DIAPHRAGMATIC RUPTURE

The challenge is greater when both the chest wall and abdominal wall are associated with diaphragmatic rupture. The technical challenges of successful treatment of such an injury are best illustrated by the care provided to a young man who presented minutes after sustaining a close-range shotgun blast of the right inferior and lateral chest wall plus the superior and lateral abdominal wall (Figure 17). During rapid resuscitation, a double-lumen endotracheal tube was inserted to prevent blood aspiration into the left lung. The presence of a large combined injury of the abdominal wall, chest wall, and hemidiaphragm should not influence the surgeon to minimize debridement of devitalized tissue in order to achieve primary closure. The likely result will be ischemia, infection, and an exposed lung; this result is fatal. When mature and proper debridement results in a huge defect of the chest and abdomen walls, unusual techniques must be used to achieve a tension-free closure. Different types of mesh may be tried, but are doomed to failure if there is associated colon spill. Successful closure of this combined defect may be achieved with native tissues by a number of rotation flaps of chest wall with rib fragments and abdominal wall musculature (Figures 18, 19, and 20). The primary concern is coverage; resultant hernias can be repaired later when the patient has recovered. The exposed tissues without skin coverage are treated with frequent dressing changes until later skin graft coverage (Figure 21). After removal of the skin graft and primary closure, the patient shown herein elected not to have his full-thickness abdominal wall defect repaired (Figure 22).

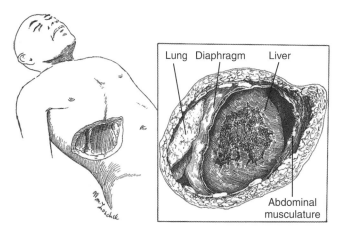

Figure 17 This young man sustained a close-range shotgun blast to the right upper quadrant and right lower chest wall. After debridement of nonviable liver, diaphragm, right lower lobe, and chest wall, the combined defect measured 25 × 18 cm.

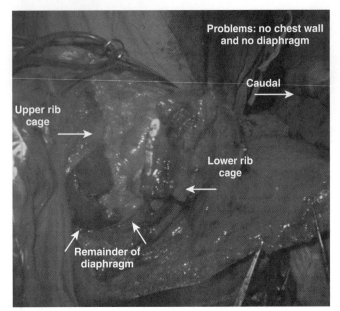

Figure 18 Part of the chest defect was closed by detaching the anterior confluence of ribs 7 through 10 from the sternum and rotating it to superiorly and laterally to approximate a portion of the diaphragm. The posterior segment of diaphragm that remained was relocated to a higher inner space, thereby allowing for diaphragmatic closure. The remaining chest wall and abdominal defect was closed by rotating a full-thickness abdominal wall musculature flap off of the linea alba medially to a superior and lateral location. The right-sided abdominal defect was covered with the skin and subcutaneous tissue.

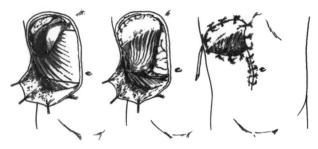

Figure 19 The full-thickness, right-sided abdominal wall muscular flap with preserved blood supply laterally is rotated superiorly to cover the abdominal visceral and create a new costal arch.

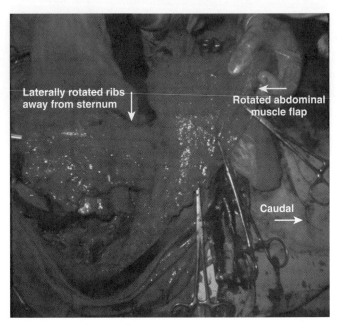

Figure 20 This rotated abdominal wall muscular flap allows for a tension-free closure of the exposed lower thorax and upper abdomen.

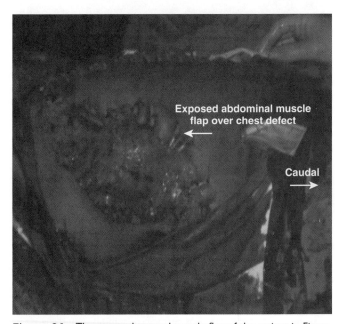

Figure 21 The exposed rotated muscle flap of the patient in Figure 16 was treated with frequent dressing changes and later skin grafted.

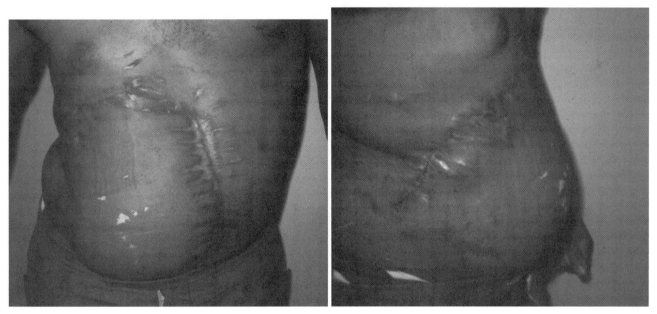

Figure 22 One year later, split graft was removed and skin was closed primarily. The patient declined to have repair of his full-thickness abdominal wall defect, preferring a corset.

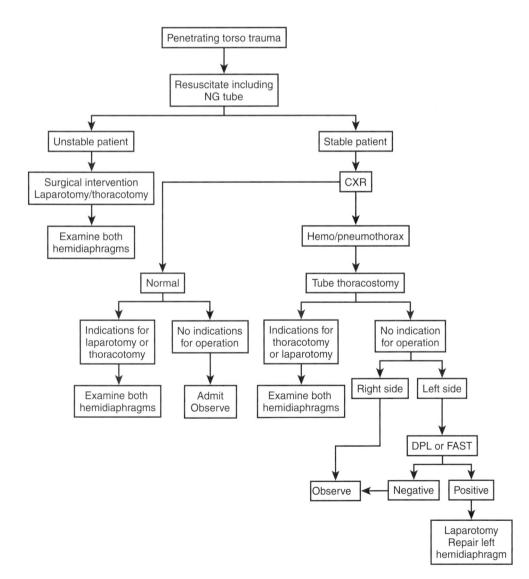

Figure 23 Algorithm for acute penetrating thoracoabdominal trauma.

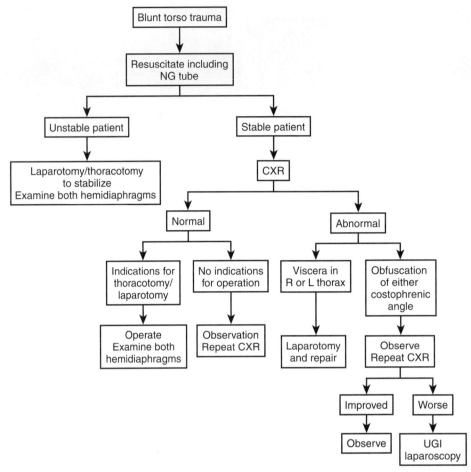

Figure 24 Algorithm for blunt torso trauma.

REFERENCES

1. Williams PL, Bannister LH, editors: *Gray's Anatomy*, 38th ed. Edinburgh, New York, Churchill Livingstone, 1995.
2. Asensio JA, Petrone P, Demetriades D: Injury to the diaphragm. In Zietlow SP, Feliciano DV, editors: *Trauma Surgery*. Philadelphia, WB Saunders, 2000, pp. 613–634.
3. Michelson E: Eventration of the diaphragm. *Surgery* 49:410, 1961.
4. Morgagni GB: *Seats and Causes of Diseases. Monograph on Hernia of the Diaphragm*. London, Zellts 54, 1769.
5. Rodriguez-Morales G, Rodriguez A, Shatney CH: Acute rupture of the diaphragm in blunt trauma: analysis of 60 patients. *J Trauma* 26:438, 1986.
6. Murray JA, Demetriades D, Asensio JA, et al: Occult injuries to the diaphragm: prospective evaluation of laparoscopy in penetrating injuries to the lower left chest. *J Am Coll Surg* 187(6):626–630, 1998.
7. Payne JH, Yellin AE: Traumatic diaphragmatic hernia. *Arch Surg* 117:18, 1982.
8. Lucas CE, Ledgerwood AM: Diaphragmatic injury. In Cameron JL, editor: *Current Surgical Therapy*, 6th ed. St. Louis, MO, Mosby, 1998, pp. 944–952.
9. Murray JA, Demetriades D, Cornwell EE, et al: Penetrating left thoracoabdominal trauma: the incidence and clinical presentation of diaphragm injuries. *J Trauma* 43(8):824, 1997.
10. Pagliarello G, Carter J: Traumatic injury to the diaphragm: timely diagnosis and treatment. *J Trauma* 33:194, 1992.
11. Voeller GR, Reisser JR, Fabian TC, et al: Blunt diaphragm injuries. *Am Surg* 56:28,1990.
12. Boulanger BR, Milzman DP, Rosato C, et al: A comparison of right and left blunt traumatic diaphragmatic rupture. *J Trauma* 35:255, 1993.
13. Somers JM, Gleeson FV, Flower CDR: Rupture of the right hemidiaphragm following blunt trauma: the use of ultrasound in diagnosis. *Clin Radiol* 42:97,1990.
14. Andrus CH, Morton JH: Rupture of the diaphragm after blunt trauma. *Am J Surg* 119:686, 1970.
15. Brown LG, Richardson DJ: Traumatic diaphragmatic hernia: a continuing challenge. *Ann Thorac Surg* 39:170, 1984.
16. Moore EE, Malangoni MA, Cogbill T, et al: Organ injury scaling. IV: thoracic, vascular, lung, cardiac and diaphragm. *J Trauma* 36:299, 1994.
17. Bender JS, Lucas CE: Management of close-range shotgun injuries to the chest by diaphragmatic transposition: case reports. *J Trauma* 30(12):1581–1584, 1990.
18. Carrasquilla C, Watts J, Ledgerwood AM, Lucas CE: Management of massive thoracocoabdominal wall defect from close-range shotgun blast. *J Trauma* 11(8):715–717, 1971.
19. Aronoff RJ, Reynolds J, Thal ER: Evaluation of diaphragmatic injuries. *Am J Surg* 144:671, 1982.
20. Beal SL, McKennan M: Blunt diaphragmatic rupture: a morbid injury. *Arch Surg* 123:828, 1988.
21. Chen JC, Wilson SE: Diaphragmatic injuries: recognition and management in sixty-two patients. *Am Surg* 57:810, 1991.
22. Ivatury RR, Simon RJ, Stahl WM: A critical evaluation of laparoscopy in penetrating abdominal trauma. *J Trauma* 34:822, 1993.
23. Salvino CK, Esposito TJ, Marshall WJ, et al: The role of diagnostic laparoscopy in the management of trauma patients: a preliminary assessment. *J Trauma* 34:506, 1993.
24. Ramirez JS, Moreno AJ, Otero C, et al: Detection of diaphragmatic disruptions by peritoneoscintigraphy using technetium-99M diethylenetriamine pentaacetic acid. *J Trauma* 28(6):818–822, 1988.

25. Merlotti G, Marcel G, Sheaff EM, et al: Use of peritoneal lavage to evaluate abdominal penetration. *J Trauma* 25:228, 1985.
26. Ochsner MG, Rozycki GS, Lucente F, et al: Prospective evaluation of thoracoscopy for diagnosing diaphragmatic injury in thoracoabdominal trauma: a preliminary report. *J Trauma* 34:704, 1993.
27. Boulanger BR, Mirvis SE, Rodriguez A: Magnetic resonance imaging in traumatic diaphragmatic rupture: case reports. *J Trauma* 32:89, 1992.
28. Feliciano DV, Cruse PA, Matox KL, et al: Delayed diagnosis of injuries to the diaphragm after penetrating wounds. *J Trauma* 28:1135, 1988.
29. de Rooiwj PD, Haarman HTM: Herniation of the stomach into the pericardial sac combined with cardiac luxation caused by blunt trauma: a case report. *J Trauma* 34:453,1993.
30. Jones RJ, Thal ER, Johnson NA, et al: Evaluation of antibiotic therapy following penetrating abdominal trauma. *Surgery* 201:576, 1985.
31. Lucas CE, Ledgerwood AM: Autologous closure of giant abdominal wall defects. *Am Surg* 64(7):607–610, 1998.
32. Wiencek RG, Wilson RF, Steiger Z: Acute injuries of the diaphragm: analysis of 165 cases. *J Thorac Cardiovasc Surg* 92:989, 1986.

Abdominal Injuries

Surgical Anatomy of the Abdomen and Retroperitoneum

Grant Bochicchio and **Thomas M. Scalea**

The abdominal cavity and the retroperitoneum lie immediately adjacent to one another. Some organs such as the small bowel and the colon have portions within the abdominal cavity while other parts are within the retroperitoneum. Vascular structures such as the superior mesenteric artery and vein course through both body compartments as well. A thorough knowledge of the anatomy of both the abdomen and retroperitoneum is critical for a rational operative approach to torso injuries.

Injuries to both the abdomen and retroperitoneum are generally approached via the same incision. Some structures such as the supraceliac aorta or the pelvic vasculature may require a counter incision such as a thoracotomy, a groin exploration, or a direct retroperitoneal incision to identify and repair specific injuries. In this chapter, we review the pertinent anatomic considerations of both the abdomen and retroperitoneum. In particular, we will stress functional anatomic considerations that are important during operative trauma surgery.

MAKING THE INCISION

The abdomen and retroperitoneum are generally explored via a generous midline incision. The incision should be made from the xiphoid to pubis, unless a specific already-diagnosed injury is to be treated. This gives the greatest access to all of the structures in the abdomen and retroperitoneum. Several additional options exist in order to reach specific areas. A thoracoabdominal approach gives access to certain structures high in the abdomen. This generally involves a seventh or eighth interspace anterolateral thoracotomy that is brought down to the sternum. The ribs are divided flush with the sternum. The diaphragm is then taken down off the chest wall radially. Approximately one to two inches should be left on the chest wall for diaphragmatic reconstruction later. On the left side, the diaphragm should be taken down all the way to the aorta. A left-sided thoracoabdominal approach is probably the best exposure for the supraceliac aorta. A right-sided thoracoabdominal incision increases the exposure of the posterior portion of the right lobe of the liver. Exposure of the retrohepatic cava is also enhanced with the use of a right-sided thoracoabdominal approach.

Occasionally, the midline incision is extended up into a medium sternotomy. This gives access to the anterior mediastinal structures. If an atriocaval shunt is to be used to treat a retrohepatic caval injury, a sternotomy is probably the best approach. In addition, if one wishes to control the inferior vena cava within the pericardium to achieve complete vascular isolation of the liver, a sternotomy or a right-sided thoracoabdominal incision will give the surgeon adequate access to perform that maneuver.

Exposure of the deep pelvic vasculature can also be difficult through a standard laparotomy. Several options exist to increase that exposure. A groin incision allows for vascular control of the common femoral artery and vein at the level of the inguinal ligaments. A combination of a full laparotomy and groin incision can aid in repair of a vascular injury immediately adjacent to the inguinal ligaments. Another option is to perform a retroperitoneal incision similar to those used for renal transplant. This hockey stick incision comes down through the retroperitoneum and exposes the distal iliac artery and vein. Distal pelvic vascular repair can then be accomplished via the combined incisions. While rare, if a transplant incision is combined with a midline incision, the bridge of skin, subcutaneous tissue, and fascia between the two incisions can become ischemic and infarct.

EXPLORING THE ABDOMEN

As the fascia is divided at the time of laparotomy, it is helpful to look at the peritoneum. If it is bulging, and has a bluish discoloration, that generally means there is a tense hemoperitoneum that will be released as the peritoneum is opened. Blood should be aspirated into a cell saver circuit. The most commonly injured organs after blunt trauma are the liver and spleen. They can be quickly assessed for injury by palpating the right upper quadrant and left upper quadrant. The surgeon can then sweep the small bowel and colon medially, which identifies any large retroperitoneal hemorrhage. If the base of the small bowel mesentery is examined, any mesenteric injury can be identified.

It is imperative to fully mobilize the spleen in order to be able to fully inspect all surfaces. This allows for intelligent decision making as to whether splenectomy or splenorrhaphy will be wise (Figure 1). All of the ligamentous attachments must be divided in order to get the spleen up to the anterior abdominal wall.

A similar strategy is important when inspecting the injured liver. The falciform ligament should be taken down all the way to the level of the vena cava. Both triangular ligaments must be completely incised. This leaves the liver suspended only on the hepatic veins and the portal structures. This allows the surgeon to rotate the liver up out of the deep recesses of the right upper quadrant, which is especially important when evaluating injuries to the posterior right lobe. In addition, one should evaluate whether sternotomy and/or right

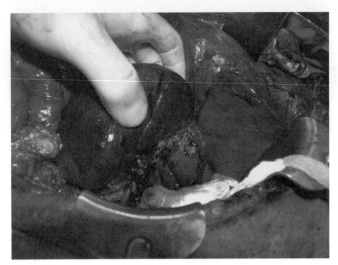

Figure 1   Full mobilization of the spleen, allowing for inspection of all surfaces.

thoracotomy with takedown of the diaphragm will be needed for added exposure.

Most blunt liver injuries are now treated nonoperatively. Bleeding from higher-grade liver injury is often persistent and of significant volume. In these cases, manual compression by direct pressure or packing will often temporize the bleeding. The Pringle maneuver is often diagnostic, and it achieves temporary hemostasis. The Pringle maneuver involves placing a non-crushing vascular clamp across the hepaticoduodenal ligament, thereby occluding both portal venous and hepatic arterial inflow. Once the clamp is applied, the liver can be reinspected and repair undertaken under better circumstances. If bleeding persists despite portal compression, the surgeon must suspect a retrohepatic inferior vena cava injury, hepatic vein injury, or anomalous hepatic arterial anatomy (10%–25%). The main or right hepatic artery comes off the superior mesenteric artery (SMA) in 10%–20% of cases, as the accessory right hepatic artery comes off the SMA in about 5% of cases. In addition, an anomalous left hepatic artery comes off the left gastric artery in nearly 5% of cases.

While often quite effective, the Pringle maneuver has some drawbacks. The Pringle maneuver produces global ischemia of the liver, potentially worsening hepatic function in the postoperative period. While there is some evidence that the liver can withstand several hours of warm ischemia during elective hepatic resection, the same may not be true for the patient in shock. The Pringle maneuver can also be cumbersome, limiting exposure. In addition, in severe liver injuries there almost always is a component of hepatic venous injury limiting the utility of the Pringle maneuver.

In more severe cases of liver injury, one may also consider the Heaney maneuver, which involves complete vascular isolation of the liver. In this technique, vascular clamps are placed on the cava, above and below the liver. When combined with the Pringle maneuver and/or supraceliac aorta clamping, this should provide for a relatively dry field in order to attempt to definitively repair the liver, and the hepatic venous injury. While this can be effective, it may be difficult to dissect out the suprahepatic vena cava in order to place a clamp, unless the diaphragm has been divided or the pericardium opened via a thoracotomy or sternotomy. The infrahepatic cava must be occluded distal to the junction of the renal vein. If the clamp is placed too low, flow from the renal vein into the cava will perpetuate bleeding and continue to make exposure extremely difficult. Occasionally, complete vascular isolation can be combined with a venous bypass circuit to allow for venous return to the heart (Figure 2).

Perhaps the greatest downside to the use of complete vascular isolation is the rapid and profound decrease in venous return to the

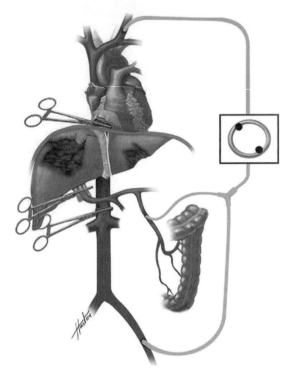

Figure 2   Hepatic venous exclusion and venovenous bypass.   *(Courtesy of ATOM, L. Jacobs, MD, Cine-Med, 2004.)*

heart. In these critically ill patients, this can occasionally produce cardiovascular collapse and/or cardiac arrest. If the technique is to be used, all resuscitation lines must be placed in the upper extremity or the mediastinal veins.

An intermediate solution to injuries with a hepatic vein component is manual compression medial to the injury. This should control all inflow to the injured segment. The injured liver can then be debrided. The hepatic vein can then be identified and ligated when pressure is relaxed. The more central hepatic arterial and portal venous branches can be ligated as well using the same temporary relaxation of hand held pressure (Figure 3).

The anterior portions of the duodenum and the head of the pancreas are in the abdomen. The posterior portion of the duodenum

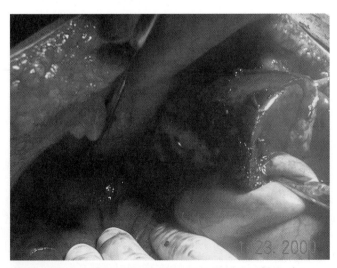

Figure 3   Liver after right debridement hepatectomy. Note the hemoclips on the cut surface.

and the head of the pancreas are in the retroperitoneum. A full Kocher maneuver (incising the lateral peritoneal reflection and completely mobilizing the duodenum and pancreas) is necessary to evaluate both structures for injuries. The body of the pancreas lies within the lesser sac. It is necessary to widely open the lesser sac to examine the posterior stomach, as well as the anterior aspect of the body of the pancreas. This is best accomplished by dividing the gastrocolic omentum.

The gastrocolic omentum can be divided all the way up the greater curvature of the stomach to the level of the gastroesophageal (GE) junction. This requires taking the short gastric vessels adjacent to the spleen. When the gastrocolic omentum has been completely divided, the surgeon has good access to the lesser sac, allowing inspection of the posterior wall of the stomach. It is necessary to carefully inspect the stomach, particularly around the area of the GE junction in order to avoid missing small injuries. If necessary, the intra-abdominal portion of the esophagus can be mobilized on a Penrose drain to aid in exposure. We attempt to triangulate the stomach using sponge sticks to flatten out both the anterior and posterior aspect of the stomach adjacent to the GE junction. This allows for complete inspection and avoids missing a subtle injury high up on the stomach.

The area of the porta contains the hepatic artery, portal vein, and common bile duct. The portal structures are covered with peritoneum. When the peritoneum is opened, the common bile duct is generally the first structure encountered. The hepatic artery can be identified by its palpable pulse and the thrill usually present within it. The portal vein lies posterior to the common bile duct. Each of these can be individually isolated and examined for injury.

It is necessary to completely evaluate the small intestine to avoid missing an injury. Complete evaluation of the bowel involves running the small bowel using a hand over hand technique. The bowel should be flipped with each inspection to be sure both sides have been completely evaluated. Spreading the bowel out allows for inspection of the corresponding mesentery. Once major vascular injuries and solid visceral injuries are controlled, the small bowel should be examined next. We generally re-examine the small bowel before closing to avoid missing an injury.

EXPLORING THE RETROPERITONEUM

The retroperitoneum is generally divided into three zones (Figure 4). Zone one is the central portion of the retroperitoneum containing the aorta, vena cava, and the major branch vessels, as well as the superior mesenteric vein and splenic vein. Any retroperitoneal hematoma in zone one is generally explored.

Zone two is the lateral perinephric area above the pelvis. Zone two houses the kidney, ureters, and renal artery and vein. In general, zone two hematomas are explored after all penetrating injuries. Zone two hematomas in blunt trauma can be managed expectantly unless there is a known injury requiring operation such as a ruptured ureter or if the hematomas are expanding or pulsatile.

Zone three houses all pelvic organs. This includes the common and external iliac artery as well as the hypogastric artery. The lower portion of the sigmoid colon is in zone three as well as the distal ureters. Zone three hematomas are explored in penetrating injury only. In general, surgical exploration of a pelvic retroperitoneal hematoma after blunt trauma is discouraged. The hypogastric artery is short and branches into a large number of small vessels. Unroofing the pelvic hematoma risks loss of tamponade. Other techniques such as external compression or angiographic embolization generally are a wiser course to treat bleeding in zone three following blunt trauma.

There are several surgical maneuvers to allow access to the retroperitoneum. These involve medial visceral rotation on either the left or right side. The viscera can be rotated medially by incising the white line of Toldt. A small incision can be made in the white line and

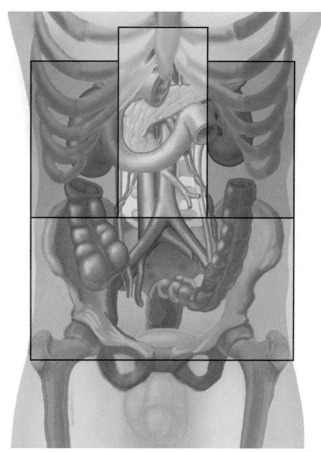

Figure 4 Retroperitoneal hematoma. Zone one: mandatory exploration. Zone two: explore in all penetrating injury and blunt injury with expanding or pulsatile hematoma. Zone three: explore in penetrating injury only. *(Courtesy of ATOM, L. Jacobs, MD, Cine-Med, 2004.)*

then the white line may be divided using the cautery or a pair of scissors over a finger inserted into the retroperitoneum to protect the deeper structures. The incision should be brought around the hepatic or splenic flexure of the colon. We generally hold the colon up with a hand and then sweep the retroperitoneal contents downward either with a laparotomy sponge, sponge stick, or hand. This protects the mesentery of the colon and allows for raid access to the retroperitoneum.

The original left medial visceral rotation maneuver was described by Creech and DeBakey in 1956. It involves taking down the white line of Toldt of the left colon all the way to the splenic flexure and sweeping the spleen, tail of the pancreas, and stomach medially to the hip or the aorta, celiac axis, and superior mesenteric artery.

The so-called "Mattox maneuver" involves medial visceral rotation on the left side (Figure 5). The left colon is mobilized as described previously. This brings the surgeon down into the retroperitoneum. At the base of the mesentery, the surgeon will then encounter the aorta. The aorta can be followed up on its lateral margin at 3:00 quickly as there are no branches until one encounters the left renal artery and vein.

The Mattox maneuver involves mobilizing the kidney with the remainder of the viscera (see Figure 5). We generally prefer to leave the kidney in situ and mobilize it later if necessary. The splenic flexure must be completely mobilized into the lesser sac. The spleen and tail of pancreas can be mobilized which exposes the aorta up to the level of the hiatus. This is our preferred method of achieving aortic control at the level of the diaphragm. Often, the

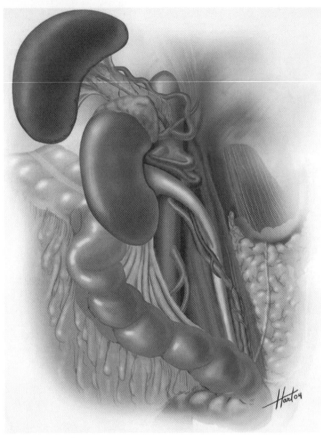

Figure 5   Aortic exposure: Mattox maneuver.   *(Courtesy of ATOM, L. Jacobs, MD, Cine-Med, 2004.)*

diaphragmatic crura come down lower than the surgeon expects. It may be necessary to divide the diaphragmatic fibers to control the supraceliac aorta.

We strongly believe that supraceliac aorta control must be accomplished by completely encircling the aorta. Blindly placing a clamp either from the anterior or lateral aspect of the aorta almost certainly results in the clamp slipping off. We mobilize the esophagus off the aorta anteriorly and insert a finger from the left side around to the right. It is then possible to bluntly dissect the fibers holding the aorta down to the spine. With a finger completely encircling the aorta, it is then possible to gently place the cross-clamp around the aorta and clamp the aorta. The left-sided medial rotation also provides good access to the left renal artery and vein. If exploring a patient for a penetrating injury to the pelvis, left-sided medial visceral rotation allows aortic control above the bifurcation. This is also a reasonable exposure to control the superior mesenteric artery at its origin. If one must expose a longer length of the supermesenteric artery, we generally combine a lesser sac exposure with the left-sided medial rotation.

Supraceliac aortic control can also be obtained via a lesser sac approach (Figure 6). The lesser sac is opened widely by dividing the gastrohepatic ligament or lesser omentum, and then dissects down onto the superior aspect of the pancreas. The pancreas is mobilized and the esophagus and stomach bluntly dissected. This will bring the surgeon down onto the aorta. Again the diaphragmatic crura may have to be divided in order to gain good access to the aorta. With the aorta exposed, a cross-clamp can be applied.

We prefer the left-sided visceral rotation for several reasons. There are a number of esophageal branches coming off of the anterior aorta. The lesser sac approach risks injuring these as the dissection is somewhat blind. In addition, we have found it more difficult to completely encircle the aorta through the lesser sac. Using this approach, the clamp is generally applied somewhat blindly down onto the aorta and risks slipping off.

A right-sided medial visceral rotation, the so called Cattel-Braasch maneuver, exposes the right-sided retroperitoneal structures

PROXIMAL AORTIC CONTROL

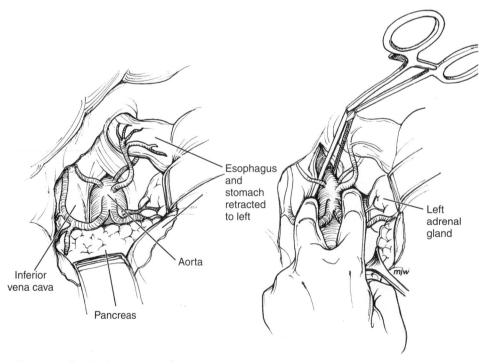

Esophagus and stomach retracted to left

Left adrenal gland

Inferior vena cava

Pancreas

Aorta

Figure 6   Proximal aortic control.

(Figure 7). The right colon is mobilized in a technique exactly similar to what was described on the left side. Similarly, the dissection should be brought around the hepatic flexure and into the lesser sac. The duodenum and head of pancreas should be completely mobilized via a Kocher maneuver. This brings the surgeon down onto the inferior vena cava (IVC). The IVC can be controlled and traced up to the confluence of the left and right renal vein. There is a short suprarenal segment of the cava and then the vena cava becomes retrohepatic in location.

The Cattel-Braasch maneuver is ideal exposure for the vena cava and the right kidney with its vasculature. When combined with the Kocher maneuver, the duodenum and head of the pancreas can be completely explored. In addition, the right-sided pelvic vasculature can be exposed via this maneuver. The Cattel-Braasch maneuver gives better access to the pelvic vasculature than does a left-sided approach. The mesentery of the left colon can limit exposure with the Mattox maneuver. As there is no mesentery to obscure the view, the Cattel-Braasch maneuver gives wider exposure.

The mesentery of the small bowel can also be incised and lifted up off the aorta and vena cava in a maneuver similar to that used by vascular surgeons during aortic surgery. When combined with the Cattel-Braasch maneuver, it gives the widest exposure of the retroperitoneal vasculature from the aorta and cava down into the pelvis.

Retroperitoneal arterial injuries are handled using the standard technique. Proximal and distal control must be obtained, and a decision made about direct repair, bypass grafting, or shunting. Injuries to the external iliac artery at the junction with the common iliac and hypogastric arteries can sometimes be managed by using the proximal hypogastric artery as a conduit. The hypogastric artery is mobilized out of the pelvis and ligated. An end-to-end anastomosis then can be performed between the hypogastric and the external iliac artery.

Retroperitoneal venous injuries can be among the most difficult to treat, particularly if located at the confluence of the vena cava and external iliac vein or in the juxtarenal IVC. Many techniques have been described for temporary vascular control including the use of sponge sticks, vascular clamps, and direct finger pressure to control bleeding. We have preferred the use of intestinal Allis clamps (Figures 8, 9, and 10). The vascular injury is first controlled with digital pressure and an Allis clamp is applied at the apex of the injury vessel. The clamps are then sequentially stacked for the length of the injury. The clamps can then be lifted. This allows for restoration of venous return to the heart. A decision can be made about ligation or repair. Vascular ligation can be accomplished by running a suture onto the clamp.

Exposure of the superior mesenteric vein (SMV) within the lesser sac can be extraordinarily problematic. The SMV courses behind the pancreas and joins the splenic vein to become the short portal vein. SMV injuries often present with torrential blood loss.

Occasionally, the pancreas can be mobilized up off the SMV and the injury isolated. There are many small branches off the SMV that must be individually ligated. If these are torn, the bleeding only becomes more difficult to control. Occasionally, identification of the location of an SMV injury is impossible, particularly if it is directly behind the pancreas or adjacent to the confluence of the splenic vein. In those cases, we generally divide the pancreas at the level of the SMV. This is done by gently inserting a finger

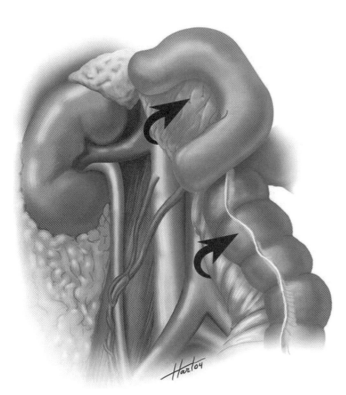

Figure 7 Cattel-Braasch maneuver or right-sided medial visceral rotation. Kocher maneuver. Mobilize the right colon along the equivalent of the white line of Toldt. *(Courtesy of ATOM, L. Jacobs, MD, Cine-Med, 2004.)*

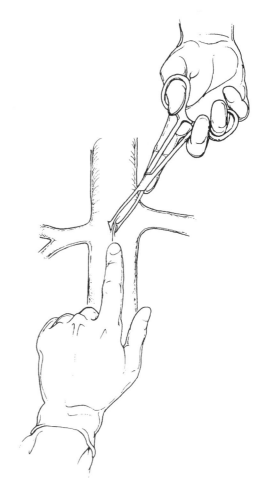

Figure 8 Temporary venous control is obtained with digital pressure. Intestinal Allis clamps are stacked and the vein repaired by running a suture under them. *(From Henry SM, Duncan AO, Scalea TM: Intestinal allis clamps as temporary vascular control for major retroperitoneal venous injury. J Trauma 51:170–172, 2001.)*

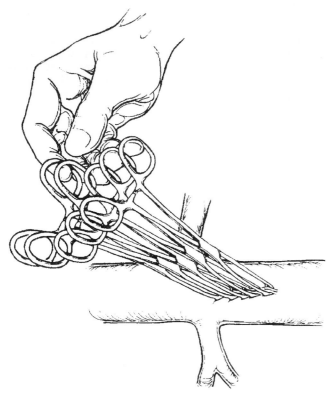

Figure 9 Temporary venous control is obtained with digital pressure. Intestinal Allis clamps are stacked and the vein repaired by running a suture under them. *(From Henry SM, Duncan AO, Scalea TM: Intestinal allis clamps as temporary vascular control for major retroperitoneal venous injury. J Trauma 51:170–172, 2001.)*

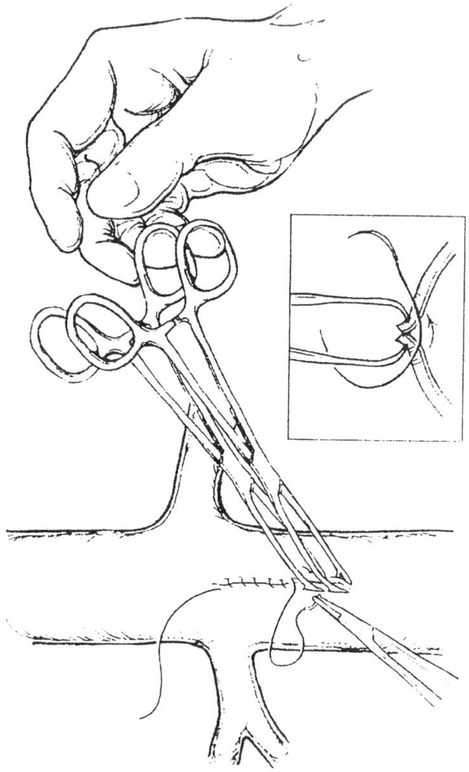

Figure 10 Temporary venous control is obtained with digital pressure. Intestinal Allis clamps are stacked and the vein repaired by running a suture under them. *(From Henry SM, Duncan AO, Scalea TM: Intestinal allis clamps as temporary vascular control for major retroperitoneal venous injury. J Trauma 51:170–172, 2001.)*

behind the pancreas and mobilizing the pancreas off the SMV. A GIA stapler can be guided using a Penrose drain and the pancreas divided. This gives excellent exposure to the SMV proper and its junction with the splenic and portal veins. Virtually any injury can be identified and repaired. The distal pancreatic remnant can be resected later or inserted into a loop of jejunum depending on the surgeon's preference.

Exposing the pelvic vasculature is a particular challenge (Figure 11). It is essential to identify the aorta proximally and be sure of its identification. Young patients in profound hemorrhagic shock can become intensely vasospastic. The common iliac artery may be mistaken for the external iliac artery or even the aorta. With the aorta and cava clearly identified and controlled, the surgeon must sequentially expose the common, external and hypogastric arteries. All of these should be individually controlled. The ureter runs through the retroperitoneum and into the pelvis at the confluence of the iliac arteries. This is a constant anatomic relationship. The ureter should be identified and protected during any pelvic exposure.

The pelvic veins are very large and fragile. They generally course behind the arteries. Iatrogenic injury to these can be devastating. Even if patients are in deep shock, the surgeon must be deliberate enough to avoid adding to the problem. Temporary venous control can be obtained by packing and the veins individually identified and looped.

FUTURE CHALLENGES

Operative trauma cases are declining. Nonoperative management has become the norm for the vast majority of blunt solid visceral injuries. Even operative cases following penetrating injury are fewer

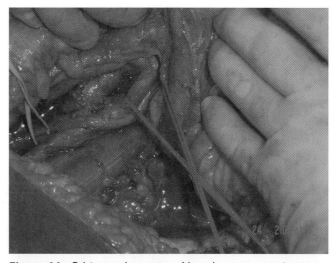

Figure 11 Pelvic vascular anatomy. Note the ureter coursing over the iliac bifurcation.

in number and are concentrated in a few centers. How then will we train the surgeons of the future to understand these complex anatomic relationships and operative techniques?

The average general surgeon spends little time in the retroperitoneum, the lesser sac, or near the GE junction. Conditions that were once treated operatively are now treated nonoperatively because of better pharmacological agents and minimally invasive endoscopic techniques. General surgical procedures are increasingly being performed via a laparoscope. Finally, the average general surgery resident finishes his or her residency with fewer than 700 operative cases, a number far fewer than residents performed in the past. While community surgeons may opt to transfer moderately injured patients to a higher level of care, it simply is not feasible if the patient is hemodynamically unstable.

Clearly we must devise a different training scheme so that surgeons of the future are prepared to deal with operative trauma. A number of solutions have been proposed. Simulators offer some advantages, although the technology is not yet robust enough to replace hands-on operating. Cadaver courses can be helpful, allowing the surgeon to understand anatomic relationships. Unfortunately, cadaveric tissues handle much differently than in a hemorrhaging trauma patient. The cadaver course is a static experience; it has none of the urgency of operating on a real-life trauma surgery.

We have embraced the Advanced Trauma Operative Management course (ATOM). This was developed in Hartford, Connecticut, by Dr. Lentworth Jacob. The students must repair injuries in a 50-kg swine. These injuries encompass all organ systems in the abdomen and some in the chest. For instance, the student must successfully repair the bladder, ureter, and the pancreas as well as more common liver, spleen, and bowel injuries. The final two scenarios involve a large injury to the inferior vena cava and a right ventricular stab wound.

The course is conducted in a full operating room atmosphere with real instruments, drapes, and scrub tech. It does not take long to forget that this is an animal exercise and fall into the rhythm of repairing injury. While other options will almost certainly occur in the future, we believe that at present the ATOM course is the best option available.

SUMMARY

A complete knowledge of anatomic relationship in the abdomen and retroperitoneum is absolutely essential to being able to rapidly and effectively control hemorrhage and repair injuries. It is critical that the general surgeon understand these and be comfortable with them before being called to see a patient with a serious torso injury. Operative trauma case volume is shrinking. Thus, surgical residents are exposed to fewer and fewer trauma operations. Other training paradigms exist, and we strongly urge that these be incorporated into residency training and special courses at postresidency to be sure that surgeons of tomorrow are adequately prepared to meet the challenge of operative trauma surgery.

SUGGESTED READINGS

Asensio JA, Forno W, Roldan G, Petrone P, Rojo E, Ceballos J, Wang C, Costaglioli B, Romero J, Tillou A, Carmody I, Shoemaker WC, Berne TV: Visceral vascular injuries. *Surg Clin North Am* 82(1):1–20, xix, 2002.

Feliciano DV: Management of traumatic retroperitoneal hematoma. *Ann Surg* 211:109–123, 1990.

Fry WR, Fry RE, Fry WJ: Operative exposure of the abdominal arteries for trauma. *Arch Surg* 126(3):289–291, 1991.

Golocovsky M: Retroperitoneal vascular trauma. In Champion H, Robbs JV, Trunkey D, editors: *Rob and Smith's Operative Surgery: Trauma Surgery,* 4th ed. London, Butterworths, 1998, pp. 555–557.

Hoyt D, Mileski W: Gallbladder and biliary tract. In Carrico C, Thal E, Weigelt J, editors: *Operative Trauma Management: An Atlas.* New York, Appleton and Lange, 1998, pp. 144–155.

Scalea TM, Rodriguez A: Initial surgical care of the trauma patient. In Corson JD, Williamson R, editors: *Surgery.* St. Louis, Mosby, 2001, Chapter 4.

Wilson R, Walt A: Injuries to the liver and biliary tract. In Wilson R, Walt A, editors: *Management of Trauma: Pitfalls and Practice,* 2nd ed. Baltimore, Williams and Wilkins, 1996, pp. 457–458.

DIAGNOSTIC PERITONEAL LAVAGE AND LAPAROSCOPY IN EVALUATION OF ABDOMINAL TRAUMA

R. Stephen Smith, John A. Aucar, and William R. Fry

Before 1965, lavage of the peritoneal cavity had a recognized role for the diagnosis and treatment of acute peritonitis, treatment of chronic renal failure, and treatment of drug overdosage. In 1965, Root published a landmark article describing the use of peritoneal lavage to diagnose occult intra-abdominal hemorrhage in 28 patients. Lavage of the abdominal cavity with 1 liter of an isotonic solution dramatically improved the sensitivity for detecting intra-abdominal hemorrhage compared with four quadrant paracentesis, which carried false negative rates of 17%–36%. In the period before 1965, blunt abdominal trauma mortality was over 45%, with two-thirds of deaths attributed to undiagnosed intra-abdominal hemorrhage or visceral injury. Root established the basic principles pertaining to diagnostic peritoneal lavage (DPL) that would be followed for over 20 years.

These include controlling skin bleeding before catheter insertion to reduce contamination of the fluid, attempting aspiration of free blood before infusing fluid, mild rocking of the patient to improve the chance of a mixed sample, retrieving a large proportion of the infusate, and examining the lavage fluid for hemoglobin concentration, amylase, and bacteria. Root did not specify criteria for hemoglobin concentration or cell counts, but noted the subjective criterion of "more than a faint salmon pink tinge of blood in the retrieved perfusate is an indication of intra-peritoneal hemorrhage requiring laparotomy...." He noted the excellent sensitivity and found no false positives, but one case was reported as a possible complication because an isolated bowel perforation was encountered.

From 1966 to September 2005, there were 2445 Medline-indexed articles, which referred to "peritoneal lavage" as a medical subject heading (MESH) or in the title or abstract. Of these, 931 articles also map to the MESH term "wounds and injuries," or mention "trauma" in the title or abstract. After eliminating review articles and those that do not pertain to humans, 791 remained that relate to diagnostic peritoneal lavage in the context of trauma. There are no randomized prospective clinical trials comparing DPL to other diagnostic maneuvers. However, there are nine randomized clinical trials comparing at least two distinct DPL techniques. While the transitions are indistinct, some generalizations can be made about observable patterns in the literature. Publications in the first decade following Root's article consisted mainly of case reports and case series showing the adoption of DPL as a diagnostic maneuver for blunt abdominal trauma. The second decade (1976–1985) brought larger case series, describing variations in technique, defined specific criteria for a positive lavage, and compared DPL to computed tomography (CT) and ultrasound (US) for diagnosing abdominal injury. During this period, DPL was regarded as the gold standard to which developing technologies were compared. Comparisons were not randomized, but based on selection by hemodynamic stability. Many studies used a cross-over design, where patients underwent two studies and the results were compared. By the third decade (1986–1995), CT scanning emerged as the preferred modality for diagnosing traumatic abdominal injuries. US was being evaluated as a viable and less invasive substitute for DPL, and DPL was mentioned passively, predominantly as one of several modalities by which abdominal injuries were being diagnosed in larger retrospective series. Of the 205 articles mentioning DPL since 1996, only 42 were coded as having a focus on the subject. Seven of these pertain to an article and six comments entitled "Diagnostic Peritoneal Lavage—An Obituary." Despite the implications of the article, there remains support for a limited role for DPL in trauma.

DPL can be performed by either an "open" or "closed" technique. It can also be considered in the context of three distinct portions of the examination: initial aspiration, visual examination of the lavage fluid, and microscopic examination of lavage fluid. In addition, consideration has been given to the potential role of (1) delayed DPL, when an extended time interval has passed since the occurrence of injury; and (2) repeat DPL for clarification of initially ambiguous findings. Unfortunately, these additional roles are not well defined and are unlikely to be studied in the future. The technique of DPL is the only aspect compared in a randomized clinical trial (RCT) model. Of the nine RCTs performed between 1980 and 1991, two compared catheter types or the position for access. The remaining seven compared open and closed techniques. One article provides evidence for a lower complication rate with the open technique. Six articles indicate an equal or lower complication rate with the percutaneous or closed technique. General conditions for keeping the closed technique safe include decompression of the stomach and bladder, exclusion of patients with major pelvic fracture or pregnancy, absence of prior abdominal surgery, and experience of the surgeon. The closed technique is recognized to be faster. It is performed by sterile preparation, infiltration of local anesthetic, creation of a small skin incision, and the insertion of a multiholed catheter over a trocar or the use of a Seldinger needle–guide-wire technique. Initial aspiration of 10 cc–20 cc of gross blood is considered an indication of intra-abdominal injury. If aspiration is negative, 1 liter of saline or lactated Ringers is infused and recovered by the siphon effect. It is expected that 60%–90% of the instilled volume must be recovered to provide a reliable sample, although some claim that recovery of 200 ml is adequate. The open technique is preferred in cases in which gastric and bladder decompression is not practical, the patient is pregnant, or a pelvic fracture is present. Similar preliminary preparations are made; however, the open procedure is facilitated by two operators or an assistant. Performing a 2-cm incision

in the supraumbilical position avoids potential injury to the gravid uterus or decompression of a suprapubic hematoma. The fascia is sharply incised under direct visualization, and the peritoneum is drawn upward and incised between clamps. A catheter can then be directly inserted into the peritoneal cavity and directed toward the pelvis. Aspiration and lavage are then performed as in the closed technique. Technical complications are reported to occur in less than 1%–5%, with the most common occurrence being failure to recover the desired volume of fluid. Iatrogenic perforation of the bladder, stomach, small bowel, or colon occurs rarely. Traditionally, such perforations, indicated by retrieval of luminal contents rather than blood, were considered an indication for abdominal exploration. It is recognized that these needle and catheter size injuries can be selectively managed nonoperatively in the stable patient.

Options for diagnostic evaluation of the ambiguous abdomen include serial clinical exam, DPL, US, and CT. Clinical exam is notoriously unreliable, particularly when confounded by distracting injuries and altered sensorium resulting from intoxication, head injury, or both. Serial exam and repeat hemoglobin measurement continues to be a viable approach for stable, alert patients, with a low suspicion for abdominal injury. Some advocate a more definitive objective evaluation for the sake of shortening hospital stay and reducing resource utilization. DPL emerged as the standard for resolving the ambiguous abdominal exam. Its primary advantages and disadvantages are noted in Table 1. When considered as a diagnostic tool for hemoperitoneum, DPL is highly sensitive, specific, and accurate. However, according to current concepts in the management of abdominal trauma, hemoperitoneum alone does not constitute an indication for operative exploration. Thus, DPL is too sensitive and leads to a high incidence of nontherapeutic laparotomy. When used to indicate the need for laparotomy, the specificity is low and accuracy is limited. Given that low-grade splenic and hepatic injuries are the most common cause of hemoperitoneum after blunt trauma, and that most of these can be successfully managed nonoperatively, DPL has been largely replaced by focused assessment with sonography for trauma (FAST) and CT as the preferred diagnostic modalities by which therapeutic decisions are made.

In an effort to refine the diagnostic value of DPL, attention was directed toward microscopic examination of lavage fluid. Rather than merely characterizing the color of the fluid as "salmon pink," the inability to "read newsprint" through the fluid was used as a predictive criteria. This evolved into the use of automated cell counts with varying thresholds. Greater than 100,000 red blood cells per cubic millimeter of lavage fluid or greater than 500 white blood cells per cubic millimeter became commonly accepted as an indication for abdominal exploration following blunt injury. By these criteria, Nagy achieved a sensitivity of 100% and specificity of 96% for 2500 patients. However, like much of the literature pertaining to DPL, the

Table 1: Primary Advantages and Disadvantages of DPL

Advantages of DPL	Disadvantages of DPL
Rapid to perform	Potential for inadequate exam
Relatively easy to teach	Potential to produce visceral injury
Does not require high technology	Requires element of training and skill
Highly sensitive for hemoperitoneum Highly specific for hemoperitoneum	Oversensitive for hemoperitoneum leading to high rate of nontherapeutic laparotomy
Can detect hollow viscus injury	May miss retroperitoneal injuries
Can be used for blunt or penetrating injuries	May lead to rupture and decompression of retroperitoneal hematoma
Can be performed in emergency room or operating room during other emergency procedures	

DPL, Diagnostic peritoneal lavage.

incidence of nontherapeutic laparotomy is not reported. Although the criteria are variable, nontherapeutic laparotomy rates associated with DPL are reported as high as 36%. In cases of penetrating trauma, a lower red cell count, 10,000/mm^3–50,000/mm^3, are used as criteria to establish penetration of the abdominal wall. A similar dilemma exists regarding the incidence of nontherapeutic laparotomy, because penetration is not always accompanied by visceral perforation. For both blunt and penetrating trauma, if one accepts that the amount of blood in the peritoneal cavity is proportional to the severity of the injury, then an inverse relationship can be predicted between the quantified cell counts and the likelihood of nontherapeutic laparotomy. If one lowers the threshold to designate DPL as positive, then the sensitivity for hemoperitoneum will be high, but the incidence of nontherapeutic operations will rise.

Other maneuvers used to improve the accuracy of DPL include the measurement of amylase and bilirubin and microscopic examination for particulate matter. These maneuvers are aimed at adding sensitivity for hollow viscus injury, which may occur in the presence or absence of significant hemoperitoneum. In addition, the use of the "cell count ratio," defined as the ratio between white blood cell count and red blood cell count in the lavage fluid divided by the ratio of the same parameters in the peripheral blood, was reported to yield a sensitivity of 100% and specificity of 97% for hollow viscus perforation when the cell count ratio was greater than 1. A special consideration arises when DPL is employed in the presence of diaphragmatic rupture or intraperitoneal bladder rupture. Failure to recover the lavage fluid may indicate that the fluid has found another route to egress the abdomen. A sudden increase in clear or bloody drainage through a chest tube or urinary catheter is practically diagnostic of injury to those structures.

The general acceptance of CT and FAST exams as the mainstay for abdominal evaluation in preference to DPL has led to the perhaps premature publication of its obituary. Despite the advantage of providing sufficient anatomic detail to grade the severity of liver and spleen injuries, and the ability to evaluate retroperitoneal structures, early implementation of the CT scan required an extended visit to the radiology suite and was practical only for stable patients. In addition, early generation scanners provided limited anatomic detail. Improvements in resuscitation techniques and advancing technology have dramatically increased the applicability of CT scans to the multiply injured patient. Fast, high-resolution scanners, strategically located in proximity to the resuscitation bay, have made it practical to evaluate the abdomen in conjunction with the head, neck, chest, and pelvis, with virtually no exclusions.

Because the CT is relatively expensive and carries the disadvantage of radiation exposure, an alternative method for screening the abdomen is desirable. FAST by surgeons and emergency physicians has flourished in common practice as a means to detect intra-abdominal free fluid, which is presumed to be blood until proven otherwise. Despite its popularity, there are few instances where the FAST exam leads directly to the decision to operate without obtaining an additional study. A recent systematic review of randomized prospective studies by the Cochrane Collaboration was unable to establish a clear advantage for US-based evaluation algorithms to affect the frequency of CT scans, DPL, or mortality. Yet, the FAST exam has been reported to carry a lower rate of nontherapeutic laparotomy (13%) than DPL (36%); however, statistical significance was not reached in this sample. The question remains whether there is a residual role for DPL in contemporary trauma care. Given the propensity for injuries to occur across a broad spectrum of combinations, severity, and demographic and geographic circumstances, and given the complex nature of resuscitation and treatment decisions applicable to trauma, it is unlikely that a single diagnostic maneuver will address all situations. The acceptability of nonoperative management in the face of mechanisms and patterns of injury that previously called for compulsory surgical exploration has placed a burden of diagnostic accuracy on trauma surgeons that DPL will never again satisfy. However, not all cases hinge on the

decision of whether to operate on the hemodynamically stable patient. When an unstable patient presents with more than one potential source of hypotension, a negative DPL may sway the decision to explore the abdomen first, and thus preserve a transient opportunity for timely angiography, thoracotomy, decompressive craniotomy, or pelvic fixation. A case can be made for the application of the FAST exam under those circumstances. However, the FAST exam requires availability of the technology and an operator with experience and skill. It can also be confounded easily by body habitus, bowel gas, nonhemorrhagic abdominal fluid, and other factors. Less dramatic circumstances where DPL may still have a role include the early identification of hollow viscus injury resulting from either blunt or penetrating trauma. Both US and CT are notoriously weak in identifying small bowel and colon injuries, although it remains a difficult decision to consider when a DPL might be appropriate in favor of serial examination and specialized radiographic techniques, such as triple-contrast CT scan.

Ultrasound-guided paracentesis is a technique which combines principles of DPL and FAST. In performing US examinations for the diagnosis of intra-abdominal, intra-thoracic, or cardiac injury, it is assumed that the hypoechoic areas seen on the video screen represent blood. In most instances, this assumption is correct. Trauma victims, to some degree, reflect the population as a whole with respect to underlying disease processes. Thus, incidental nonhemoglobin-containing fluid collections will be identified. Fluid collections from infection, chronic organ dysfunction (such as cirrhosis), end-stage renal disease, cardiomyopathy, and malignancy will be encountered.

Ultrasound-guided paracentesis is within the ability of the trained surgeon. The procedure is already well within the skill set of those that perform US-guided biopsy or US-guided central line insertion. Like other US-guided needle placement procedures, the procedure is done in two parts. First, the fluid collection is identified and localized using routine scanning windows. Care should be taken to select a sonographic window and needle path that will cause the least amount of collateral damage to other structures such as bowel, solid organs, and intercostal vessels. Care should also be taken to select a pathway to minimize traversing the pleura, if not necessary, to decrease the chances of creating an iatrogenic pneumothorax. Once the sonographic window and needle pathway have been chosen, the area is prepped and draped in the standard fashion. Local anesthesia should be used to anesthetize the intended needle pathway. For US-guided diagnostic fluid sampling, we have found that prepping the US probe along with the use of sterile US gel is adequate aseptic technique and that a sterile probe cover is not necessary. The access window can be located where there is a clear access to the fluid without traversing solid or hollow viscera. Locating or creating dependent fluid collections can be accomplished by changing the patient's position. This is accomplished by allowing the fluid to pool by placing the patient in a lateral decubitus or semi-Fowler position.

Many recently trained surgeons have little or no experience in performing DPL or in exercising the complex decision making that might lead to its appropriate application in special circumstances. For many, exposure to DPL is limited to animal or mannequin practice during the Advanced Trauma Life Support (ATLS) course. Fortunately, both the open and closed techniques are paralleled by the common practice of laparoscopic port placement. In addition, the burgeoning interest in virtual simulation technology has created an opportunity to demonstrate its potential usefulness to teach uncommon procedures through the development of a DPL training simulator. While advanced imaging techniques have been extremely beneficial for trauma care and are likely to dominate the diagnostic approach in the future, it would benefit surgical science to preserve and teach DPL techniques and strategies. Although the opportunity to use it may be rare, understanding its historical development and limitations parallels our understanding of the anatomic and pathologic implications of abdominal trauma. Even if the technique of DPL is considered to be retired, it should not be buried.

LAPAROSCOPY IN TRAUMA

Evaluation of the abdomen in potentially injured patients remains one of the greatest challenges faced by surgeons. None of the current diagnostic modalities available to the trauma surgeon are completely accurate. All of the available techniques, including DPL, sonography, CT, and laparoscopy, have advantages and disadvantages. At present, laparoscopy is not considered a frontline method for evaluation of the abdomen, but it is an important adjunct.

Laparoscopy has been used sporadically over the past four decades in the evaluation of patients at risk for abdominal injury. Utilization of laparoscopy in the trauma setting has increased dramatically over the past 15 years. This increase in utilization corresponds to the greater availability of high-quality laparoscopic equipment and the greater penetration of laparoscopy into general surgery training programs. At present, laparoscopy holds the greatest promise in evaluating a select group of patients with penetrating injury. A number of recent series have documented the utility of laparoscopy in the evaluation of the diaphragm in hemodynamically stable patients with a history of thoracoabdominal wounds. The use of laparoscopy in the blunt trauma setting is much less frequent and its indications remain controversial in this group of patients.

Sporadic reports of novel uses of laparoscopy, for example, laparoscopically guided blood salvage and laparoscopic decompression of abdominal compartment syndrome, have appeared more recently. In some centers, laparoscopy is used for the assessment of the hollow viscera in patients who are suspected of having a seat-belt injury that cannot be ruled out with other diagnostic modalities. Therapeutic laparoscopy for a select group of isolated patients, that is, those with small diaphragmatic lacerations, is used more frequently and may be applicable for a small subset of patients. In addition, some centers have reported repair of small enterotomies with laparoscopic techniques, if these injuries are isolated.

Sound surgical judgment must be used in choosing patients for laparoscopic evaluation after injury. Any injured patient with hemodynamic instability or obvious complex intra-abdominal injury, is not a candidate for laparoscopy, but instead requires immediate laparotomy. Several large series performed by experienced groups have demonstrated that only about 15% of patients with suspected intra-abdominal injury are reasonable candidates for adjunctive

laparoscopic evaluation or treatment. For patients with gunshot wounds to the abdomen, laparoscopy has proved most useful for evaluation of the diaphragm in patients with thoracoabdominal wounds (Figure 1). In addition, laparoscopy has proven useful to determine if peritoneal penetration has occurred from tangential gunshot wounds or stab wounds.

The use of laparoscopy is not without risk in these patients. In patients with a diaphragmatic injury, production of tension pneumothorax upon insufflation of CO_2 for creation of pneumoperitoneum has been reported. Although this does not occur in every patient with diaphragmatic laceration, it is estimated that this will occur in 10% of patients with diaphragmatic injury. The surgeon who uses laparoscopy for evaluation of potential diaphragmatic wounds must be prepared to immediately decompress the pneumoperitoneum and place a tube thoracostomy if signs and symptoms of tension pneumothorax develop. Patients with gunshot wounds of the abdomen are not candidates for laparoscopy, as this group of patients has a very high incidence of significant intra-abdominal injury that must be treated at laparotomy.

Victims of stab wounds are somewhat more likely to benefit from laparoscopic examination (Figure 2). In this group of patients, as many as 50% will not have significant intra-abdominal injury. Laparoscopy can be used to reduce the number of negative and nontherapeutic laparotomies in patients with minimal injuries. Laparoscopic repair of small diaphragmatic injures and limited hollow viscus injuries secondary to stab wounds has been reported in the literature and appears to be a viable technique in the hands of a skilled laparoscopic surgeon. The use of laparoscopy in most trauma centers has been associated with a small decrease in the incidence of negative and nontherapeutic laparotomy.

A very small percentage of patients with blunt abdominal trauma may benefit from laparoscopic evaluation. Previous reports using laparoscopy for the examination of hepatic and splenic lacerations are not pertinent at this time. The increasing trend toward nonoperative treatment of these injuries and the emergence of arteriography and embolization has made this approach to solid organ injury less viable. An area of potential benefit in the blunt trauma setting is examination of the entire small bowel and colon in a patient at risk for the so-called "seat-belt" syndrome. With moderately developed laparoscopic skills, the vast majority of the

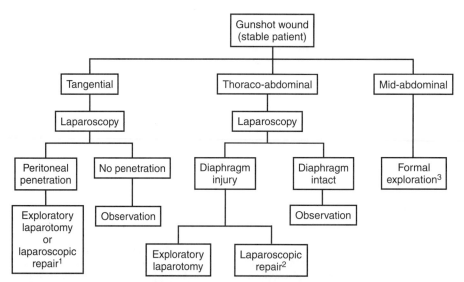

Figure 1   Algorithm for management of a gunshot wound in a stable patient. (1) Laparoscopic repair may be performed for limited injuries, depending on the capabilities of the surgeon. (2) Posterior wounds may be more easily identified and repaired with a thoracoscopic approach. Identification of injuries of associated abdominal organs may necessitate laparotomy. (3) Gunshot wounds in this location have a greater than 90% probability of producing wounds that require definitive surgical repair.

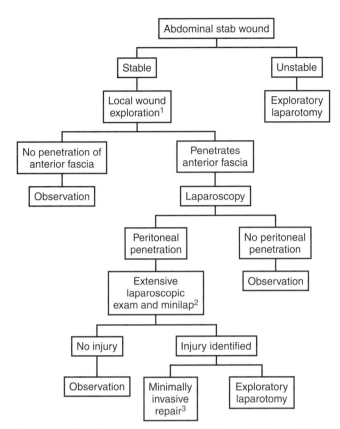

Figure 2 Algorithm for management of abdominal stab wounds. (1) Local wound exploration performed in the emergency room. (2) Majority of examination is performed by laparoscopy; examination of the small bowel is performed via a 4-cm minilaparotomy incision. (3) Limited injuries may be repaired laparoscopically depending on the capability of the surgeon.

small bowel and colon can be examined with laparoscopic techniques. Large injuries to hollow viscera are easily detected; however, small enterotomies may still be missed. Therefore, a very low threshold for conversion to laparotomy must be maintained in the patient at risk for hollow viscus injury. Unfortunately, the literature does not clearly delineate or document the efficacy of laparoscopy in the blunt trauma setting.

Standard laparoscopic equipment is used for examination of the trauma patient. Laparoscopic exploration of the abdomen in the trauma setting is similar to patients who present with an acute abdomen. In most cases, the laparoscope is inserted through a periumbilical incision to provide optimal visualization of all quadrants of the abdomen. Additional small operating ports are located to permit the use of other laparoscopic instruments. Location of these ports should allow the greatest manipulation of abdominal contents in the area of interest. A nasogastric tube and urinary catheter should be inserted before the laparoscopic examination for trauma. Most trauma surgeons who use laparoscopy prefer a 30-degree angled lens, as this provides enhanced visualization of areas that are difficult to examine, such as posterior aspects of the diaphragm.

Carbon dioxide pneumoperitoneum is used in the trauma setting just as for elective laparoscopy. Initial insufflation may be conducted with either a Veress needle or a Hasson cannula. In the trauma setting, initial insufflation pressures should be limited to 8–0 mm Hg. This threshold is maintained to minimize the risk of the development of tension pneumothorax in patients with diaphragmatic defects, and to minimize the onset of hypotension in a patient with less than optimal intravascular volume. If insufflation to this level is

tolerated, then the limit may be increased to 15 mm Hg to enhance exposure. Gas embolism is also a theoretical risk in patients with intra-abdominal venous injury, but is rarely encountered.

If significant enteric spillage or hemorrhage is found on the initial laparoscopic assessment, then laparoscopy should be halted and conversion to a laparotomy should be performed without delay. In most trauma centers that use laparoscopy, significant penetration of the peritoneum secondary to a gunshot wound is an indication for conversion to exploratory laparotomy. Peritoneal penetration secondary to a stab wound allows a more selective approach to further exploration. Certainly, not all injuries identified at the time of laparoscopy require conversion to laparotomy. For example, if an isolated injury to the liver without significant bleeding is encountered, conversion to laparotomy is contraindicated.

If the trauma surgeon possesses laparoscopic suturing skills, isolated small diaphragmatic lacerations may be repaired readily with laparoscopic techniques. Posterior areas of the diaphragm are somewhat more difficult to visualize and injuries in this area are difficult to repair with laparoscopic techniques. The liver and spleen are relatively easy to visualize during laparoscopic techniques, but this may require rotating the operating table to the right or left and placing the patient in reverse Trendelenburg position for full visualization of the spleen. Visualization of the pancreas is accomplished by dividing the gastrocolic ligament with laparoscopic vascular clips, staplers, or other devices, such as the harmonic scalpel, which are used for vessel ligation.

Approximately 5% of all patients who undergo laparoscopic examination are candidates for therapeutic intervention. These patients most commonly have small diaphragmatic lacerations or a very limited, isolated enterotomy. Sporadic reports of laparoscopic repair of the colon, as well as hepatorrhaphy and splenorrhaphy, have appeared in the literature, but cannot be advocated based on the present evidence.

In summary, laparoscopy is a useful adjunct for the evaluation of a select group of injured patients. Laparoscopic techniques are limited to hemodynamically stable patients without clear indication for laparotomy. At present, the best indication for laparoscopy is in patients with a penetrating mechanism of injury who have either tangential injuries of the abdominal wall or injuries to the thoracoabdominal region in which the diaphragm is at risk.

SUGGESTED READINGS

Adkinson C, Roller B, Clinton J, Ruiz E, Bretzke M: A comparison of open peritoneal lavage with modified closed peritoneal lavage in blunt abdominal trauma. *Am J Emerg Med* 7(4):352–356, 1989.

Bain IM, Kirby RM, Tiwari P, McCaig J, Cook AL, Oakley PA, Templeton J, Braithwaite M: Survey of abdominal ultrasound and diagnostic peritoneal lavage for suspected intra-abdominal injury following blunt trauma. *Injury* 29(1):65–71, 1998.

Bowyer CM, Liu AV, Bonar JP: Validation of SimPL—a simulator for diagnostic peritoneal lavage training. *Stud Health Technol Inform* 111:64–67, 2005.

Brams DM, Cardoza MD, Smith RS: Laparoscopic repair of a traumatic gastric perforation using a gasless technique. *J Laparoendosc Surg* 3: 587–591, 1993.

Brown GR Jr, Burnett WE: Evaluation of peritoneal lavage in the treatment of severe, diffuse peritonitis. *Surg Forum* 7:166–168, 1957.

Cochran W, Sobat WS: Open versus closed diagnostic peritoneal lavage. A multiphasic prospective randomized comparison. *Ann Surg* 200(1):24–28, 1984.

Cue JI, Miller FB, Cryer HM 3rd, Malangoni MA, Richardson JD: A prospective, randomized comparison between open and closed peritoneal lavage techniques. *J Trauma Inj Infect Crit Care* 30(7):880–883, 1990.

DeMaria EJ: Management of patients with indeterminate diagnostic peritoneal lavage results following blunt trauma. *J Trauma Inj Infect Crit Care* 31(12):1627–1631, 1991.

Esposito TJ: Laparoscopy in blunt trauma. *Trauma Q* 10:260–272, 1993.

Fabian TC, Croce MA, Stewart RM, Pritchard FE, Minard G, Kudsk KA: A prospective analysis of diagnostic laparoscopy in trauma. *Ann Surg* 217: 557–565, 1993.

Fang JF, Chen RJ, Lin BC: Cell count ratio: new criterion of diagnostic peritoneal lavage for detection of hollow organ perforation. *J Trauma Inj Infect Crit Care* 45(3):540–544, 1998.

Felice PR, Morgan AS, Becker DR: A prospective randomized study evaluating periumbilical versus infraumbilical peritoneal lavage: a preliminary report. A combined hospital study. *Am Surg* 53(9):518–520, 1987.

Fryer JP, Graham TL, Fong HM, Burns CM: Diagnostic peritoneal lavage as an indicator for therapeutic surgery. *Can J Surg* 34(5):471–476, 1991.

Gou DY, Jin Y, Chen LY, Wei Q: ICU management of patients with suspected positive findings of diagnostic peritoneal lavage following blunt abdominal trauma. *Chin J Traumatol* 8(1):46–48, 2005.

Ivatury RR, Simon RJ, Stahl WM: A critical evaluation of laparoscopy in penetrating abdominal trauma. *J Trauma* 34:822–828, 1993.

Ivatury RR, Simon RJ, Stahl WM: Selective celiotomy for missile wounds of the abdomen based on laparoscopy. *Surg Endosc* 8:366–370, 1994.

Ivatury RR, Simon RJ, Weksler B, Bayard V, Stahl WM: Laparoscopy in the evaluation of the intrathoracic abdomen after penetrating injury. *J Trauma* 33:101–109, 1992.

James JA, Kimbell L, Read WT: Experimental salicylate intoxication. I. Comparison of exchange transfusion, intermittent peritoneal lavage, and hemodialysis as means for removing salicylate. *Pediatrics* 29:442–447, 1962.

Jansen JO, Logie JR: Diagnostic peritoneal lavage—an obituary. *Br J Surg* 92(5):517–518, 2008.

Lopez-Viego MA, Mickel TJ, Weigelt JA: Open versus closed diagnostic peritoneal lavage in the evaluation of abdominal trauma. *Am J Surg* 160(6):594–596, discussion 596–597, 1990.

Moore JB, Moore EE, Markovchick V, Rosen P: Peritoneal lavage in abdominal trauma: a prospective study comparing the peritoneal dialysis catheter with the intracatheter. *Ann Emerg Med* 9(4):190–192, 1980.

Nagy KK, Roberts RR, Joseph KT, Smith RF, An GC, Bokhari F, Barrett J: Experience with over 2500 diagnostic peritoneal lavages. *Injury* 31(7):479–482, 2000.

Perry JF Jr: A five-year survey of 152 acute abdominal injuries. *J Trauma Inj Infect Crit Care* 147:53–61, 1965.

Root HD, Hauser CW, McKinley CR, Lafave JW, Mendiola RP Jr: Diagnostic peritoneal lavage. *Surgery* 57:633–637, 1965.

Sicilia LS, Barber ND, Mulinari AS, Kolff WJ: Automatic device for peritoneal lavage in chronic renal failure. *Ohio State Med J* 60:839–843, 1964.

Smith RS, Fry WR: Alternative techniques in laparoscopy for trauma. *Trauma Q* 10:291–300, 1994.

Smith RS, Fry WR, Morabito DJ, Koehler RH, Organ CH Jr: Therapeutic laparoscopy in trauma. *Am J Surg* 170:632–637, 1995.

Smith RS, Fry WR, Tsoi EK, et al: Gasless laparoscopy and conventional instruments: the next phase of minimally invasive surgery. *Arch Surg* 128:1102–1107, 1993.

Smith RS, Meister RK, Tsoi EKM, Bohman HR: Laparoscopically-guided blood salvage and autotransfusion in splenic trauma: a case report. *J Trauma* 34:313–314, 1993.

Stengel D, Bauwens K, Sehouli J, Rademacher G, Mutze S, Ekkernkamp A, Porzsolt F: Emergency ultrasound-based algorithms for diagnosing blunt abdominal trauma. *Cochrane Database Syst Rev* (2):CD004446, 2005.

Troop B, Fabian T, Alsup B, Kudsk K: Randomized, prospective comparison of open and closed peritoneal lavage for abdominal trauma. *Ann Emerg Med* 20(12):1290–1292, 1991.

Wilson WR, Schwarcz TH, Pilcher DB: A prospective randomized trial of the Lazarus-Nelson vs. the standard peritoneal dialysis catheter for peritoneal lavage in blunt abdominal trauma. *J Trauma Inj Infect Crit Care* 27(10):1177–1180, 1987.

Zantut LF, Ivatury RR, Smith RS, et al: Diagnostic and therapeutic laparoscopy for penetrating abdominal trauma: a multicenter experience. *J Trauma* 42:825–831, 1997.

Zantut LF, Rodrigues AJ, Birolini D: Laparoscopy as a diagnostic tool in the evaluation of trauma. *Pan Am J Trauma* 2:6, 1990.

NONOPERATIVE MANAGEMENT OF BLUNT AND PENETRATING ABDOMINAL INJURIES

Matthew J. Martin and **Peter M. Rhee**

BLUNT ABDOMINAL INJURY

The evaluation and management of the abdominal cavity in the blunt trauma patient has undergone radical change over the past several decades, resulting from both significant technological advances as well as a critical reappraisal of management techniques and their outcomes. Early and rapid diagnosis of injuries coupled with the application of modern trauma-care principles has made successful nonoperative management of most blunt abdominal injuries the rule rather than the exception. Although select patients may require immediate or delayed surgical intervention, nonoperative management can now safely be extended to most patients with blunt abdominal injury regardless of age or associated injuries.

Incidence

The incidence of intra-abdominal injury after blunt trauma will vary widely by the patient population, mechanism of injury, and the diagnostic studies employed by the particular center. Approximately 12% of all blunt trauma patients who are screened with computed tomography (CT) have one or more intra-abdominal injuries, with 46% of these being major injuries and 30% requiring surgical or angiographic intervention.[1,2] The vast majority of these will be solid organ injuries to the spleen and/or liver, followed by injury to the kidney, mesentery, small bowel, colon, and pancreas. These injuries may be categorized as solid organ (liver, spleen, kidney), hollow viscus (stomach, duodenum, small bowel, colon, ureter, bladder), endocrine (pancreas, adrenal), or vascular. Overall, greater than 95% of these injuries may be managed without surgical intervention and with similar or lower complication rates compared with operative management.[3]

Mechanism of Injury

Blunt trauma may produce abdominal injuries through a variety of mechanisms, including direct transmission of energy to abdominal structures causing tissue disruption or hollow viscus blowout, shearing from rapid deceleration, direct compression of abdominal organs against the vertebral column, and puncture or laceration from associated rib fracture, spine fracture, or foreign bodies. Although there is not a linear relationship between the degree of force and the amount of abdominal injury, mechanisms involving higher velocity and/or forces will result in more significant and extensive injuries to the abdominal organs. Direct transmission of force to the abdomen will predominantly be absorbed by the large solid organs, such as liver, spleen, and kidney, resulting in parenchymal disruption. Rapid deceleration forces tend to affect fixed or tethered structures such as the kidneys, duodenum, and bowel mesentery, resulting in lacerations or pedicle avulsion. Although seat-belt use has resulted in a decrease in traumatic brain injury and death, there is a twofold increase in the incidence of hollow viscus injuries resulting from the use of seat-belts.[3] Organs that are fixed to or in close proximity to the vertebral column may also be injured by direct compression, such as the distal duodenum, pancreas, and great vessels. Fractures of the lower rib cage may directly lacerate upper abdominal structures including the diaphragm, liver, spleen, and kidneys.

Diagnosis

The diagnosis of intra-abdominal injury in the blunt trauma patient begins with the primary survey and focused examination of the abdomen. Hypotension should be assumed to result from hemorrhage from an abdominal injury until proven otherwise. Physical examination of the abdomen may be limited by distracting injuries or depressed mental status, but should focus on the elicitation of peritoneal signs, localized tenderness, external bruising or evidence of a "seat-belt sign," and distension.[4] Peritonitis should never be attributed to a solid organ injury, as isolated hemoperitoneum should not cause diffuse peritoneal irritation. Focused abdominal sonography for trauma (FAST) is now commonly performed as part of the initial evaluation. While a "positive" FAST exam reliably identifies the presence of free fluid in the abdominal cavity suggestive of injury, a negative study does not exclude significant abdominal injury and should not be considered a definitive evaluation. Although ultrasound has been used to identify and grade specific organ injuries (i.e., liver and spleen), its reliability and reproducibility in this capacity has not been well demonstrated. Diagnostic peritoneal lavage (DPL) has largely been replaced by the FAST exam and CT scan and is rarely indicated, although it may be useful in select cases where there is suspicion for hollow viscus perforation with a compromised physical examination and equivocal CT scan findings. However, a diagnostic peritoneal aspirate (DPA) looking for the presence of gross blood only, can be very useful in the patient who is hypotensive with a negative FAST exam. A urinalysis should be obtained on all patients, and evaluation of the complete urinary tract (kidneys, ureters, bladder) should be performed in the presence of significant hematuria.

Computed tomography has become the standard of care for the definitive diagnosis of most blunt abdominal injuries, and should be used liberally. Missed intra-abdominal injuries, typically resulting from an incomplete diagnostic evaluation, represent the most common cause of preventable deaths from trauma.[5] Modern generation helical CT scanners provide excellent detailed imaging of the abdominal organs, including retroperitoneal structures and major vasculature. It has a sensitivity and specificity approaching 100% for solid organ injuries, and provides anatomic detail that is invaluable for injury grading.[1,3] The abdominal CT scan should always be performed using intravenous contrast if possible, as a "contrast blush" can provide evidence of active bleeding or arteriovenous fistula. Although some older series have characterized CT as unreliable for hollow viscus perforation or duodenal/pancreatic injury, more recent experience demonstrates that a high-quality CT scan will correctly identify most of these injuries. However, repeat CT imaging (if no other indication for laparotomy is present) or DPL should be considered in those infrequent situations with a high index of suspicion for missed injury or equivocal findings on the initial CT scan. We perform the abdominal CT scan with intravenous contrast only,

as oral contrast has been shown to add little value in the trauma setting and may create undue delay as well as risk aspiration. Oral contrast may be useful when obtaining a delayed CT scan to evaluate for hollow viscus perforation, or to better delineate known or suspected pancreatic or duodenal injuries.

Anatomic Location of Injury and AAST-OIS Grading

The abdominal cavity can be divided into two main compartments, the peritoneal cavity and the retroperitoneum. Most injuries after blunt trauma are to the intraperitoneal structures, such as the liver, spleen, small bowel, and mesentery, and frequently result in clinical signs/symptoms such as pain, tenderness, and distension. The main retroperitoneal structures of concern to the trauma surgeon are the kidneys, duodenum, pancreas, great vessels, and portions of the colon. Clinical signs and symptoms with retroperitoneal injuries may frequently be absent or significantly delayed, even in the presence of a severe injury. Fortunately, retroperitoneal hollow viscous injuries are relatively rare.

Abdominal injuries identified by CT should be graded according to the American Association for the Surgery of Trauma–Organ Injury Scale (AAST-OIS system) (Table 1). This provides a commonly understood language for discussion and study of these injuries, and may be used to guide the level and duration of monitoring for nonoperative management. Although higher-grade injuries are associated with higher rates of morbidity and failure of nonoperative management, the grade of injury should not be the primary factor in this decision. All grades of injury may be successfully managed nonoperatively in the appropriate clinical setting. Additional factors such as the amount of hemoperitoneum, presence of associated injuries, and presence of a contrast "blush" should be noted and factored into subsequent management decisions.

Management

Initial management decisions in patients with a known or suspected intra-abdominal injury should be based on the clinical examination and hemodynamic status. Patients with peritonitis or hemodynamic instability that persists despite adequate fluid resuscitation should undergo prompt exploratory celiotomy. Fluid resuscitation in the early evaluation period should be administered judiciously and only if necessary. Overzealous volume resuscitation with elevation of the mean arterial pressure may exacerbate hemorrhage from the injured organ or may cause an iatrogenic drop in the hemoglobin by hemodilution, which may be difficult to differentiate from active bleeding. We prefer small-volume boluses with immediate assessment of the patient's response by an experienced trauma surgeon. There is a mounting body of evidence that supports the positive resuscitation and immunomodulatory benefits of hypertonic crystalloid solutions over standard crystalloid or colloid formulas.[6] Administration of small boluses of hypertonic fluid (100 cc–250 cc of 3%–7.5% saline) will result in decreased tissue edema with improved gas exchange, a decreased systemic and organ-specific inflammatory response, with an excellent safety profile. In patients with associated traumatic head injury, hypertonic saline has the added benefit of lowering intracranial pressure while volume resuscitating the patient.

The primary components of safely managing these injuries are appropriate monitoring and frequent reassessments of the patient's clinical exam and laboratory values. The level of inpatient care (intensive care unit [ICU] versus ward) and the frequency of monitoring should be dictated by the patient's clinical status, associated injuries, and the severity of the organ injury. All personnel caring for the patient should be made aware of the presence and type of abdominal injury, and a clear plan for monitoring and alerting the trauma team to any changes should be in place. Most injuries that fail nonoperative

Table 1: American Association for the Surgery of Trauma–Organ Injury Scale (AAST-OIS) Grading Scales for Selected Abdominal Organs

	Spleen*			Pancreas*
I	Laceration <1 cm		I	Superficial laceration, no duct injury
	Subcapsular hematoma <10% surface area			Minor contusion, no duct injury
II	Laceration 1–3 cm		II	Major laceration, no duct injury
	Subcapsular hematoma 10%–50% surface area			Major contusion, no duct injury
	Intraparenchymal hematoma <5 cm diameter			
III	Laceration >3 cm or involving trabecular vessels		III	Distal transaction or parenchymal injury with duct injury
	Subcapsular hematoma >50% surface area or expanding/ruptured			
	Intraparenchymal hematoma >5 cm or expanding/ruptured			
IV	Laceration of segmental or hilar vessels with major devascularization (>25% of spleen)		IV	Proximal transaction or parenchymal injury involving ampulla
V	Shattered spleen Hilar vascular injury with complete devascularization		V	Massive disruption of pancreatic head

	Liver*			Abdominal Vascular
I	Laceration <1 cm deep		I	Non-named branches; phrenic, lumbar, gonadal, or ovarian artery/vein
	Subcapsular hematoma <10% surface area			
II	Laceration 1–3 cm deep, <10 cm in length		II	Hepatic, splenic, gastric, gastroduodenal, inferior mesenteric or primary named mesenteric arteries/veins requiring ligation or repair
	Subcapsular hematoma 10%–50% surface area			
	Intraparenchymal hematoma <10 cm diameter			
III	Laceration >3 cm deep		III	Superior mesenteric vein, infrarenal vena cava
	Subcapsular hematoma >50% surface area or expanding/ruptured			Renal, iliac, or hypogastric artery/vein
	Intraparenchymal hematoma >10 cm diameter or expanding/ruptured			
IV	Parenchymal disruption involving 25%–75% of hepatic lobe or 1–3 Couinaud's segments within a single lobe		IV	Superior mesenteric artery, celiac axis, suprarenal vena cava, infrarenal aorta
V	Parenchymal disruption >75% of lobe or >3 Couinaud's segments		V	Portal vein, extraparenchymal hepatic vein
	Juxtahepatic venous injuries to vena cava or major hepatic veins			Retrohepatic or suprahepatic vena cava
VI	Hepatic avulsion			Suprarenal subdiaphragmatic aorta

	Kidney*			Duodenum*
I	Hematuria with normal urologic studies		I	Hematoma involving single portion
	Subcapsular hematoma			Laceration, partial thickness
II	Laceration <1 cm deep without urinary extravasation		II	Hematoma involving more than one portion
	Nonexpanding perirenal hematoma			Laceration <50% of circumference
III	Laceration >1 cm deep without collecting system rupture or urinary extravasation		III	Laceration 50%–75% circumference of D2 or 50%–100% of D1, D3, or D4
IV	Laceration through renal cortex, medulla, and collecting system		IV	Laceration >75% circumference of D2
	Main renal artery or vein injury with contained hemorrhage			Involvement of ampulla or distal common bile duct
V	Completely shattered kidney		V	Massive disruption of duodenopancreatic complex
	Renal hilar avulsion with devascularized kidney			Devascularization of duodenum

*Advance one grade for multiple injuries, up to grade III.

Modified from Moore EE, Cogbill TH, Jurkovich GJ, et al: Organ injury scaling: spleen and liver (1994 revision). *J Trauma* 38:323–324, 1994; Moore EE, Cogbill TH, Jurkovich GJ, et al: Organ injury scaling III: Chest wall, abdominal vascular, ureters, bladder, and urethra. *J Trauma* 33:337–339, 1992; Moore EE, Cogbill TH, Malangoni MA, et al: Organ injury scaling, II: pancreas, duodenum, small bowel, colon, and rectum. *J Trauma* 30:1427–1429, 1990; and Moore EE, Shackford SR, Pachter HL, et al: Organ injury scaling: spleen, liver, and kidney. *J Trauma* 29:1664–1666, 1989, with permissions.

management will declare themselves within 48 hours of injury, and this should be the period of most intensive monitoring.

Additional important factors to be considered in guiding management are the age of the patient and the presence of comorbidities and associated injuries. Traditionally, nonoperative management of abdominal solid organ injuries was contraindicated in elderly patients and those with multiple associated injuries, particularly severe traumatic brain injuries. However, with improvements in imaging technology and monitoring capabilities, many centers are reporting favorable results of nonoperative management in these more difficult patient populations.[7,8] Success rates for nonoperative management of over 90% have been reported among patients with multiple associated injuries, with similar complication rates to those with isolated injuries.[9,10] This should only be attempted at centers with experience and expertise in managing complex, multisystem trauma and requires coordination and cooperation between the involved surgical services, such as neurosurgery and orthopedics.

Spleen and Liver

Patients with any identified injury of the spleen and/or liver should be admitted to the hospital for a minimum of 24–48 hours of observation. We recommend ICU or intermediate-level (step-down) admission for all high-grade injuries (grades III through V) (Figures 1 and 2). The primary purpose of observation is to identify the presence of any associated abdominal injuries and to monitor for ongoing or recurrent bleeding from the liver or spleen. The overall incidence of missed injuries in these patients appears to be low (around 2%), and should not influence the decision for nonoperative management.[5,11] Serial physical examinations should focus on the patient's hemodynamic status and any evidence of worsening abdominal tenderness, distension, or the development of peritonitis. Serial laboratory evaluations should include a complete blood count at the minimum. Some measure of global tissue perfusion and acidosis, such as the lactate or base deficit, may be useful in making management and treatment decisions in these patients. The timing and appropriateness of blood transfusion in these patients remains an area of controversy. Although the need for transfusion was previously used as a guideline for operative intervention, this is no longer the case. For spleen injuries, we favor a low threshold for operative or angiographic intervention if the patient requires more than one to two units of transfused blood. We accept a higher threshold for surgical intervention on liver injuries that require transfusion, typically after four to six units of transfused blood. Ideally it would be preferred if one could avoid transfusion and surgery, but the exact timing of

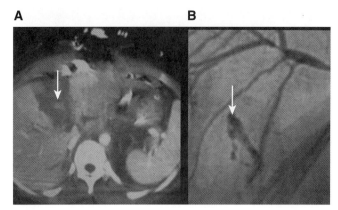

Figure 2   **(A)** Abdominal computed tomography scan demonstrating intraparenchymal liver laceration (grade III) with an area of contrast extravasation or "blush" *(white arrow)*. **(B)** Hepatic angiogram of the same injury demonstrating contrast extravasation from the right hepatic arterial system *(white arrow)*.

transfusion, surgery, or both for patients with solid organ injuries remains more an art than science. It requires the expert judgment of an experienced trauma surgeon to avoid the error of delaying a needed laparotomy until the patient is on the verge of hemodynamic collapse.

Bed rest and activity restriction have traditionally been recommended for these injuries, but there is no clinical data or science to support this practice. Prolonged immobility should be avoided, and patients should be allowed to mobilize as early as possible. Although routine repeat imaging of all injuries with ultrasound or CT does not appear to be beneficial or cost-effective, we recommend re-imaging in select patients such as those with high-grade injuries or those with above-average activity levels, such as athletes, fire fighters, and police officers, among others. Age-appropriate immunizations against encapsulated organisms should be considered for all patients with grade IV or V splenic injuries as they may be functionally asplenic. Immunizations should be administered before patient discharge to ensure compliance.

Kidney

The kidneys are highly amenable to nonoperative management of most blunt injuries, with successful nonoperative management reported in over 90% of injuries and even in up to 50% of grade V injuries.[12,13] This is particularly important for preserving renal function, as a significant number of surgical explorations for blunt renal injury will result in nephrectomy. Tamponade of hemorrhage from the renal parenchyma is enhanced by the tough, fibrous capsule of the kidneys (Gerota's fascia) and their retroperitoneal location. The principles of hospital admission, monitoring, and serial evaluations are the same as for liver and spleen injuries. In addition to serial hemoglobin assessments for bleeding, measures of renal function (blood urea nitrogen, creatinine, creatinine clearance) should be obtained at admission and intermittently throughout the hospital stay. A urinary catheter should be placed to quantify urine output and the degree of hematuria (if present) in the initial observation period. We recommend liberal use of repeat imaging, including renal function studies, in patients with grades III through V injuries to assess the extent of injury and amount of functional renal parenchyma remaining (Figure 3).

Duodenum and Pancreas

Injury to the duodenum or pancreas is rare after blunt trauma, and appears to occur more frequently in children compared with adults. Diagnosis of these injuries is difficult because of their retroperitoneal location, often subtle clinical signs, and frequent poor visualization

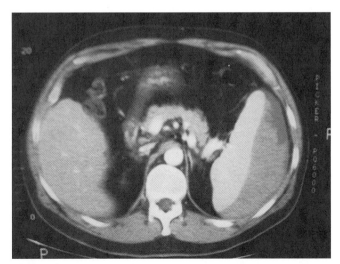

Figure 1   Abdominal computed tomography scan demonstrating large subcapsular splenic hematoma (grade III) with no evidence of active contrast extravasation.

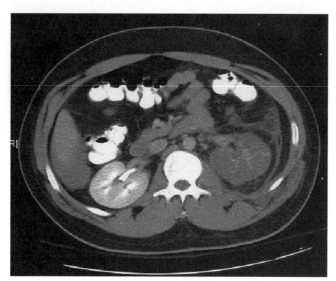

Figure 3   Abdominal computed tomography scan demonstrating a blunt left renal artery injury with an ischemic left kidney and normal, contrast-enhancing right kidney.

by CT scan. Unlike other abdominal organ injuries, most identified duodenal and pancreatic injuries will require operative exploration for repair and drainage. However, select lower-grade injuries may be amenable to successful nonoperative management. Most grade I injuries of the duodenum (hematoma or partial-thickness laceration) do not require laparotomy and will resolve spontaneously. Patients with a large intramural hematoma, particularly children, may experience obstructive symptoms and require hospitalization for nutritional management until the hematoma shrinks and obstruction resolves. Repeat imaging with oral contrast may be helpful in these patients to assess the degree of luminal obstruction and resolution or progression of the lesion.

The primary determinant of the need for operative intervention in pancreatic injuries will be the extent of parenchymal disruption and the presence or absence of ductal injury. Grades I and II injuries (contusions and lacerations without ductal injury) identified by CT scan may be managed by observation alone in the hemodynamically stable patient with minimal clinical symptoms. Serial physical examinations and measurement of pancreatic enzymes (amylase and lipase) should be performed to monitor the progression or resolution of pancreatic injury and inflammation. Repeat imaging with a contrast-enhanced, dedicated pancreatic CT should be performed in the face of clinical deterioration or laboratory evidence of worsening pancreatic injury. If a localized fluid collection or pancreatic abscess is identified, percutaneous drainage may be attempted in lieu of operative drainage. If ductal injury is suspected, endoscopic retrograde cholangiopancreatography (ERCP) may be performed to both diagnose the injury and perform a therapeutic intervention (stenting, sphincterotomy). However, laparotomy should be strongly considered if there is evidence of a significant ductal disruption.

Role of Angiographic Interventions

The increased abilities and availability of interventional radiology are now being widely applied to the management of traumatic abdominal injuries, and may offer significant benefit in the nonoperative management of select injury types.[14] The most common application of these techniques in the abdomen is to control active hemorrhage from the spleen or liver by angioembolization of either the bleeding vessel (selective) or the proximal main vessel supplying the bleeding area (nonselective). Patients with a contrast blush seen on the initial CT scan or evidence of ongoing hemorrhage should be considered

for angiographic embolization if they remain hemodynamically stable enough to undergo the procedure. Although there are no well-defined criteria for prophylactic embolization, we recommend it in the nonoperative management of complex hepatic injuries (grades IV and V) that have a high rate of recurrent bleeding and failure of nonoperative management. Angiographic embolization is currently performed with either coil placement, which causes permanent clotting of the vessel, or with absorbable Gelfoam. Gelfoam usually only provides temporary occlusion of the vessel, and as recanalization can occur in 8–96 hours, the patient should be monitored for recurrent hemorrhage.

Angiographic interventions such as catheter-directed clot lysis and vessel stenting may also have a role in the management of selected blunt vascular injuries, particularly injury to the renal vasculature, if performed within several hours of injury. Although angiography is increasingly being integrated as a component of nonoperative management, it is an invasive procedure with a well-defined complication profile that should be factored in to any management decisions or algorithms. Further study and experience with these techniques are needed to clarify the indications and treatment-associated outcomes as this is an evolving field.

Morbidity and Complications Management

The amount and degree of morbidity associated with nonoperative management of blunt abdominal injuries will be a function of the specific organ injured, the presence and degree of associated injuries, and patient factors such as age and comorbid disease. Avoiding a laparotomy does not equate to avoiding any morbidities, and in some cases may be associated with equal or greater morbidity than operative management. Although hemorrhage from a missed solid organ injury has classically been described as the most common cause of preventable morbidity and mortality in trauma patients, this should be an extremely rare occurrence in a modern, dedicated trauma center. Approximately 25% of patients with abdominal organ injuries managed nonoperatively will develop a complication requiring some form of intervention, and over 80% of these can be successfully managed without surgical intervention.[2,9,11]

The most common sources of morbidity in this patient population will be those seen in any injured and hospitalized patient population. These include local and systemic infections, single and multiple organ failures, venous thromboembolism, prolonged hospital stay, and functional disability. Other complications specific to the injured organ may also be seen, such as delayed hemorrhage, organ necrosis or abscess formation, pseudoaneurysm or arteriovenous fistula, bile or pancreatic leak, hemobilia, urinary extravasation, and end-organ ischemia from arterial or venous thrombosis.

The key to optimizing patient outcomes after blunt abdominal injury is anticipation of the commonly associated complications, and institution of a multidisciplinary approach to diagnosis and management. Any change in the patient's clinical status or complaints suggestive of an abdominal complication (pain, fever, emesis, ileus, bleeding, jaundice) should prompt immediate investigation. CT is the study of choice for diagnosing most of these organ-specific complications, and can readily visualize organ necrosis or ischemia, fluid collections (abscess, biloma, urinoma, pseudocyst), biliary ductal dilation, and progression or resolution of the primary organ injury.[15] The addition of intravenous contrast can delineate most vascular complications, such as pseudoaneurysm, arteriovenous (or portovenous) fistula, intimal dissection, and thrombosis. Arteriography should be performed if the diagnosis is unclear by CT or to perform interventional therapy. Fluoroscopic contrast studies such as intravenous pyelography and retrograde urethrography may be indicated to evaluate the urinary tract for injury or urine leak. Suspected biliary or pancreatic pathology (leaks, fistulae) should be further studied using ERCP or percutaneous transhepatic cholangiography (PTC).

The management of these complications will depend on the nature of the complication, the patient's clinical status, and the availability of resources and expertise. However, most of these complications may also be managed nonoperatively or with minimally invasive techniques. Although there is no role for prophylactic antibiotics in the nonoperative management of abdominal injuries, appropriate antibiotics should be started immediately when infection is diagnosed or strongly suspected. Percutaneous drainage of abdominal fluid collections can be performed using CT or ultrasound guidance and the fluid should be sent for gram staining and appropriate microbiologic cultures. Additional studies such as bilirubin, creatinine, and amylase levels may assist the diagnosis in cases of suspected biloma, urinoma, or pancreatic leak, and can be followed serially to assess for resolution. Major hepatic injuries with persistent biliary leak should undergo ERCP or PTC with biliary stent placement. Stenting across the ampulla may also decrease or resolve pancreatic ductal leaks. Similarly, persistent urinary extravasation can usually be treated successfully with percutaneous drainage and ureteral stent placement. Repeat imaging studies should be obtained to assess the efficacy of these interventions and the timing of drain or stent removal.

Parenchymal injury to any abdominal organ will result in some degree of tissue necrosis, which is usually followed by tissue regeneration, remodeling, or scar formation. A large volume of necrotic tissue or necrotic tissue that becomes secondarily infected may result in local and systemic complications. This may be particularly pronounced in patients who have decreased organ perfusion after angioembolization. Most patients can be managed successfully with intravenous fluids and antibiotics, and percutaneous drainage should be considered if there is a significant component of liquefied necrosis. However, select patients will require laparotomy with surgical debridement of all necrotic and infected tissue (Figure 4). Finally, vascular complications after blunt abdominal trauma may manifest at any time after the injury, with many being identified years later. Small, asymptomatic pseudoaneurysms and arteriovenous fistulae may be managed by observation and repeat imaging. Any significant or symptomatic lesion is best managed by angiographic embolization (Figure 5). Hemobilia should be suspected in any patient with evidence of upper GI bleeding after a blunt hepatic injury, and is also best managed by angiographic embolization.

Mortality

The mortality rates for nonoperative management of abdominal injuries will vary widely by the patient population being studied, the specific organ or organs involved, and the grade of organ injury. Death in these patients will most commonly be a result of associated injuries and comorbid conditions, and not directly attributable to

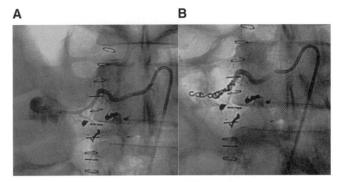

Figure 5 **(A)** Arteriogram obtained 10 days after liver injury demonstrating a hepatic artery pseudoaneurysm. **(B)** Repeat arteriogram after embolization demonstrating coils in position and obliteration of the pseudoaneurysm.

the abdominal organ injury. Over half of all deaths in this patient population are attributable to other associated injuries, most commonly closed head and thoracic injuries, with only about 10% of deaths related to hemorrhage from the injured organ.[2,9] The overall mortality rate for nonoperative splenic injuries in modern series is approximately 6%, with the mortality doubling for patients older than 55 years.[8,11] Failure of nonoperative management is also associated with increased mortality rates of 12%–30%. Nonoperatively managed liver injuries are associated with higher rates of nonoperative failure, continued hemorrhage, and associated injuries, and thus a higher overall mortality compared with splenic injuries. There is an approximate 12% mortality rate for all liver injuries managed nonoperatively, with increased death rates of up to 80% reported for high-grade liver injuries (IV and V).[5,12] Failure of nonoperative management, continued organ-related hemorrhage, and overall mortality among these patients doubles when additional abdominal organ injury (spleen, kidney) is present. Similar mortality rates have been reported for renal and other blunt abdominal injuries managed nonoperatively, but again are mainly a function of patient factors and associated injury patterns.[13]

Conclusions

The overwhelming majority of trauma in most modern civilian settings is from blunt, high-velocity mechanisms that commonly result in abdominal organ injury. All emergency and trauma physicians must be well versed in the epidemiology, diagnostic modalities, and modern management strategies to achieve optimal outcomes in the care of these often complex patients. The multiplicity of factors and decision points that must be taken into account when performing nonoperative management of these injuries precludes a simple algorithmic approach and requires the skill and constant vigilance of an experienced physician. Once hemodynamic stability has been determined, nonoperative management may be extended to most patients with blunt abdominal organ injuries with a low rate of failure and adverse outcomes. The most important factor for maximizing the success and outcome among this patient population is management by an expert and dedicated trauma team.

PENETRATING ABDOMINAL INJURY

There are few situations in the field of surgery that generate as much excitement and adrenaline as a "crash celiotomy" in the trauma patient with a penetrating abdominal injury. Despite the omnipresence of these scenarios in movies and television programs, the overall incidence of penetrating trauma in both the civilian and military

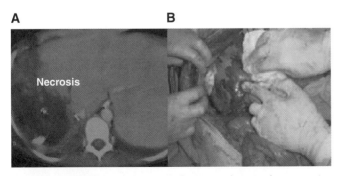

Figure 4 **(A)** Abdominal computed tomography scan demonstrating necrosis of the lateral portion of the right hepatic lobe which required operative debridement. **(B)** Intraoperative findings demonstrate segmental area of necrosis in right hepatic lobe.

setting has sharply declined over recent decades. This has resulted in a paucity of experience with penetrating abdominal injuries among surgeons and residents in all but a few select, high-volume urban centers. In contrast to the revolutions seen in blunt trauma management, there has been relatively little change in the general approach to most penetrating injuries over the past 50 years. While penetrating abdominal trauma with suspicion or evidence of peritoneal violation has traditionally mandated an exploratory celiotomy, there is a small but growing body of experience with selective nonoperative management of civilian penetrating abdominal injuries. While this approach has been well described and is becoming more widely accepted for stab wounds, the selective nonoperative approach to abdominal gunshot wounds remains an area of active study and controversy.

Incidence

The overall incidence of penetrating trauma has declined sharply in modern times because of multiple factors. Penetrating mechanisms now account for less than 10% of all trauma presentations, even at most dedicated and high-volume trauma centers in the United States. Only a select few urban trauma centers continue to see penetrating trauma as a high (40%–50%) proportion. The overall incidence of penetrating mechanisms among over 850,000 civilian trauma patients in the 2005 report from the National Trauma Data Bank[TM] was 5.85% for gunshot wounds and 4.6% for stab wounds, with the highest percentages documented in the 15–35-year-old age groups. Recent military experience has shown that the widespread use of body armor has resulted in a shift away from chest and abdominal injuries and toward a predominance of extremity injuries. However, U.S. military surgeons can still expect to treat penetrating abdominal injuries as they often care for the civilian population and enemy forces that do not have access to body armor.

The most important issue when discussing the validity of selective nonoperative management of penetrating abdominal wounds is the incidence and type of intra-abdominal organ injury. Approximately half of all patients with anterior abdominal stab wounds and up to 30% of patients with proven peritoneal violation will not have any significant intra-abdominal injury.[16,17] The incidence of intra-abdominal and retroperitoneal injury is significantly lower for flank or back stab wounds.[18] Although there is an alleged greater than 90% incidence of organ injury requiring laparotomy after abdominal gunshot wounds, this mainly applies to high-velocity injuries often seen in military combat, which will not be specifically addressed in this chapter. Approximately 30%–40% of patients with anterior abdominal gunshot wounds and up to 70% with posterior wounds do not have clinically significant intra-abdominal injuries that require surgical therapy.[19] Successful selective nonoperative management offers the benefit of avoiding the morbidity of an unnecessary celiotomy, but must always be weighed against the risk of missed or delayed treatment of a significant intra-abdominal injury. Approximately 20%–40% of abdominal gunshot wounds and more than 50% of stab wounds can be successfully and safely managed without celiotomy.

Mechanism of Injury

Tissue and organ injury from penetrating wounds may occur by a variety of mechanisms, and will vary significantly by the type of weapon involved. Stab wounds are very low velocity and produce injury through primary tissue disruption or devascularization at the point of contact. The degree of tissue injury and clinical significance will largely depend on the exact location and depth of the wound. They produce relatively uniform injuries (punctures, lacerations) with little or no damage to surrounding tissue. Although the vast majority of stabbing injuries are direct and linear with forceful insertion and extraction of the blade, one must be aware that on occasion, there can be a pivoting and twisting motion during the injury. The

point of pivot is at the skin and this "jug" maneuver can cause seemingly minor injury at the skin but can have a larger lacerating injury within the abdomen (Figure 6).

In contrast, missile wounds may vary widely in the mechanisms of injury and the amount of tissue involved. Projectiles typically create a tract or cavity as they travel through tissue, producing primary injury by mechanical disruption and laceration. Fragmentation of the missile after impact (or secondary to striking bone) may produce multiple smaller projectiles that increase the cavity size and area of tissue injured, and explains the larger wounds produced by unjacketed bullets. Bullet deformation or spin upon impact will also significantly increase the extent of the primary wound cavity produced. In addition to the primary tissue injury, the energy imparted by the bullet to surrounding tissues creates a "shock wave" or temporary cavitation that may result in tissue injury and devitalization over a much greater area.

Despite the long published experience with civilian and military gunshot injuries, there are many misconceptions regarding wound ballistics that have become widely propagated. Although high-velocity types of weapons do impart greater force to the involved tissue, the amount of tissue injury and cavitation will depend more on the properties of the missile (jacketing, deformities, amount of spin and yaw) than the velocity. As an example, a high-velocity jacketed round may pass cleanly through a tissue bed producing little injury, while a low-velocity unjacketed round, which easily deforms and fragments, may produce a significantly larger wound and greater tissue destruction. In addition, the size and clinical significance of the "temporary cavity" has been largely overstated, and appears to be much less than the oft-quoted 20 or 30 times the bullet diameter (Figure 7).[20] The dictum that all high-velocity wounds require extensive debridement of the temporary cavity area is not supported by animal or clinical data, and the corollary that all low-velocity wounds require little debridement is equally unsupported.

Diagnosis

The diagnostic approach to the hemodynamically normal patient with a penetrating abdominal wound is controversial, and will vary by the injury mechanism, wound location, and the patient's clinical status. The diagnostic paradigm has rightly shifted away from determining whether the peritoneum has been violated, to determining whether there has been an injury that needs surgical therapy. The

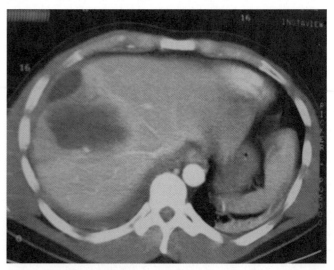

Figure 6   Abdominal computed tomography scan following an anterior abdominal stab wound demonstrates a grade III parenchymal injury to right lobe of liver.

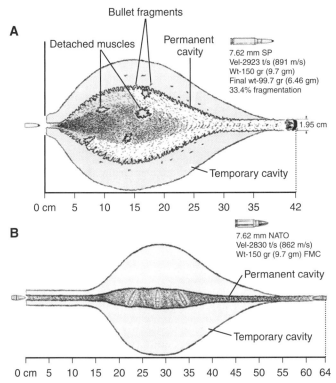

A

Bullet fragments

Detached muscles

Permanent cavity

7.62 mm SP
Vel-2923 t/s (891 m/s)
Wt-150 gr (9.7 gm)
Final wt-99.7 gr (6.46 gm)
33.4% fragmentation

1.95 cm

Temporary cavity

0 cm   5   10   15   20   25   30   35   42

B

7.62 mm NATO
Vel-2830 t/s (862 m/s)
Wt-150 gr (9.7 gm) FMC

Permanent cavity

Temporary cavity

0 cm 5   10   15   20   25   30   35   40   45   50   55   60 64

Figure 7 Wound profiles created by the **(A)** 7.62-mm NATO cartridge loaded with a soft-point hunting bullet that expands and fragments upon impact. **(B)** 7.62-mm NATO standard rifle bullet. Note that despite having similar masses and velocities, the soft-point bullet in panel **A** produces a significantly larger primary wound cavity than the standard military round in panel **B**. *(Modified from Fackler ML: Civilian gunshot wounds and ballistics: dispelling the myths. Emerg Med Clin North Am 16:17–28, 1998, with permission.)*

Flank or back stab wounds should undergo contrast-enhanced CT scan of the abdomen and pelvis unless they are clearly superficial in nature. Although some of the literature does recommend triple-contrast CT (IV, oral, rectal), there are other studies that refute the necessity of oral and rectal contrast.[18] We have not found that triple-contrast CT is required and prefer to use only intravenous enhanced CT of the abdomen and pelvis. The role of CT scan for anterior abdominal stab wounds is not well-defined, but should be considered if there is a high suspicion for solid organ injury based on wound location, a positive FAST exam, or hematuria. However, most patients who are hemodynamically stable, have an intact mental status and clear sensorium, and have no evidence of peritonitis do not require any further imaging studies. Although local wound exploration is used by some groups, we do not recommend this strategy as the decision point for celiotomy should be based on the patient's clinical status and not on evidence of fascial penetration alone.

Anatomic Location of Injury and AAST-OIS Grading

The anatomic location of injury will depend primarily on the wounding mechanism and the tract of injury. Stab wounds will most often be anatomically limited to one area or zone of the abdomen and usually involve only one organ or structure. Gunshot wounds may involve multiple areas of the abdomen, and frequently cross into separate body cavities (thoracic, pelvis) and may also be transaxial (across the midline). Injuries or tracts that involve the upper abdomen or lower chest, defined as the area from the inferior border of the costal margin to the nipple line circumferentially, should be assumed to have penetrated the diaphragm until proven otherwise.[21] Organ injuries should be assessed and scored according to the AAST-OIS scheme in the same manner as previously described for blunt abdominal trauma (see Table 1). Although anatomic delineation of the missile tract by CT scan should not be the primary determinant of therapy, it may increase or lower the threshold for performing an exploratory celiotomy.

Management

The most important factors in safe and successful selective nonoperative management for penetrating abdominal injuries are proper patient selection and supervision by an experienced surgeon.[19,22] Once the diagnostic evaluation has been completed as outlined above, the patient should be admitted to an area where close observation and monitoring can be easily accomplished for at least 24 hours. Serial laboratory evaluations and examinations should be performed as outlined in the section on blunt abdominal injuries. It is preferable that the serial physical examinations are performed by the same physician (attending or supervised resident) so that subtle changes can be more easily appreciated. Immediate celiotomy is performed at the first indicator of clinical deterioration or development of peritoneal signs. Other factors that should prompt consideration for celiotomy are persistent tachycardia, fever, and rising white blood cell count or worsening metabolic acidosis (base deficit or lactate). Although surgeons are classically taught that the physical examination is unreliable and can miss injuries, we have found that the physical exam is accurate and reliable in determining who requires surgical therapy.

Pain medication may be administered but should be given judiciously and the patient immediately re-evaluated in the presence of increasing abdominal pain. Clear liquids may be administered shortly after admission and prolonged periods of fasting in anticipation of a possible celiotomy should be avoided. There appears to be no benefit (and significant detriment) to prolonged immobility, so early ambulation is encouraged. The duration of intensive monitoring will vary by the type of abdominal injury and associated conditions, but any significant problems such as bleeding or the development of

evaluation should focus on rapidly identifying those patients with injuries requiring immediate or urgent laparotomy, such as hollow viscus perforation or ongoing hemorrhage, and evaluation for significant extra-abdominal injuries.

The diagnostic evaluation of abdominal gunshot wounds has traditionally been minimal, with the diagnosis of most injuries occurring in the operating room during exploratory celiotomy. In the emergency department, a thorough external survey should be performed to identify and mark the location of all wounds, and a radiologic survey (chest, abdomen, and pelvis x-ray) can rapidly identify the number and location of retained missiles or fragments. Despite the oft-repeated entreaty to never probe a penetrating wound, we will liberally (and gently) probe penetrating abdominal wounds to clarify the direction of the tract. This is often useful in determining whether the course of the missile is superficial or if it tracks into the abdominal cavity. Patients who are hemodynamically stable, awake and alert, have a reliable physical exam (no intoxication or significant distracting injuries), and have no other indication for operation or general anesthesia are candidates for nonoperative management. These patients should then undergo an urgent CT scan of the abdomen, which we perform with fine cuts through the area of injury or wound tract. In addition to delineating solid organ and other injuries, the CT scan can be used to reconstruct the missile tract and determine the likelihood of injury to surrounding structures. Close monitoring by an experienced surgeon during the entire radiological evaluation is important to identify any change in clinical status that will mandate urgent operative intervention.[19]

Upper abdominal stab wounds should have a chest x-ray performed, and any evidence of thoracic involvement (pneumothorax, hemothorax) should be considered diagnostic of a diaphragm injury.

peritonitis will almost always occur within 24–48 hours of injury. Criteria for hospital discharge and instructions should be the same as previously described for blunt organ injuries. Outpatient follow-up and arrangements for emergency care if needed must be ensured before hospital discharge.

The role of angiography and other minimally invasive techniques in penetrating abdominal injuries has not been well studied. The indications and utility of interventional techniques such as angioembolization in the management of hemorrhage from solid organ injuries should be essentially the same as previously described for blunt injuries (Figures 8 and 9). In addition, angiography and embolization should be considered for all high-grade liver injuries (grades IV and V) or if angiography is already being performed for other reasons.[22] Even after the successful nonoperative management of a penetrating injury, laparoscopic or thoracoscopic evaluation of the diaphragm may be required for select high-risk injury locations (as outlined in the previous section).[21]

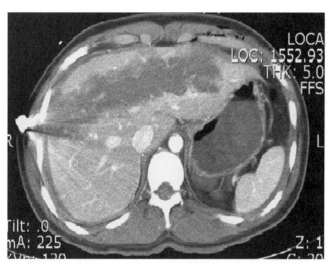

Figure 8   Abdominal computed tomography scan showing a transhepatic gunshot wound (grade IV) that was successfully managed nonoperatively.

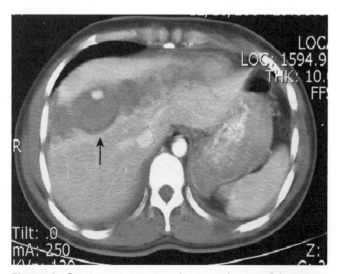

Figure 9   Routine repeat computed tomography scan of the injury depicted in Figure 8 at 1 week postinjury demonstrates a large pseudoaneurysm with central contrast enhancement (*black arrow*) that was managed by angiographic embolization.

However, this should be considered an elective procedure and should not be done until the patient has been observed for long enough to ensure clinical stability and no other indication for celiotomy develops.

Morbidity and Complications Management

The most significant concern among this patient cohort is the incidence and outcome of failures of nonoperative management. Although there is an overall high incidence of injuries requiring celiotomy with penetrating abdominal wounds, there is an extremely low incidence of these injuries among the cohort of patients who qualify for selective nonoperative management as previously described. For both abdominal stab and gunshot wounds, approximately 4% of patients initially managed nonoperatively go on to require celiotomy, most commonly for the development of peritoneal signs. The morbidity and mortality rates associated with delayed celiotomy are low, and are comparable to those undergoing immediate celiotomy. However, there is a significant benefit of selective nonoperative management in reducing the incidence of nontherapeutic laparotomies from 30%–50% down to 5%–10%.[19] This will translate into a significant reduction in resource utilization, patient morbidity, and costs to the hospital and health-care system.

The development of infectious and organ-specific complications and their management among patients managed nonoperatively are essentially the same as previously described for blunt injuries, and will not be repeated here. The role of routine repeat imaging to identify important but clinically silent complications after penetrating solid-organ injuries has not been well defined, and is at the discretion of the managing physician. Delayed imaging (7–10 days postinjury) after severe solid organ injury will identify organ-related complications in up to 50% of patients, with half of these being among asymptomatic patients. Until further data is available on the natural history of these injuries, we recommend liberal use of routine repeat imaging with abdominal CT, which we perform before hospital discharge and at several months postinjury. The majority of identified complications such as fluid collections or vascular pathologies (pseudoaneurysms, arteriovenous fistulae) can be managed nonoperatively, using interventional or minimally invasive adjuncts (see Figure 9). Although the movement toward nonoperative management may be disappointing to surgeons, in most cases it will be beneficial in improving patient outcomes.

Mortality

In the 2005 National Trauma Data Bank™ report, the overall case-fatality rate for gunshot wounds was 16%, and for stab wounds was significantly lower at 1.88%. Mortality will mainly be a reflection of the severity of injuries, patient factors (age, comorbid conditions), and the appropriate postinjury management. Several large series of abdominal stab wounds have reported no deaths among patients initially selected for nonoperative management, even including those who failed and required celiotomy.[16,17] Similarly, the reported mortality rates for nonoperative management of abdominal gunshot wounds is less than 1%, and is significantly lower than the 10%–20% mortality among patients managed surgically.[19,22] The most important factors for avoiding any preventable mortality from selective nonoperative management are proper patient selection and adherence to strict criteria for monitoring and conversion to operative management.

Although death resulting from a missed intra-abdominal injury has been a primary concern among skeptics of nonoperative management, the collective experience to date confirms that properly performed selective nonoperative management is safe and effective.

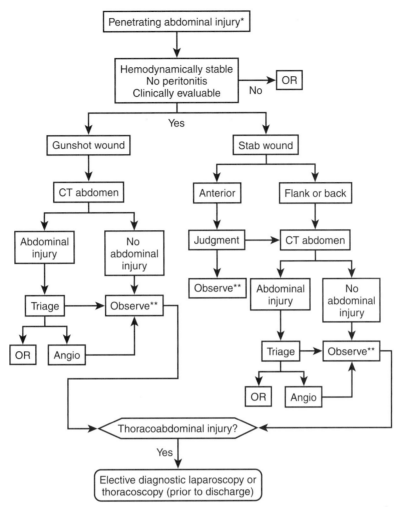

Figure 10 Algorithm for the initial evaluation and selective nonoperative management of patients with penetrating abdominal trauma. *Evaluation and decision for nonoperative management made by attending trauma surgeon. **Observation in monitored setting with serial laboratory and clinical evaluations for at least 24 hours.

In fact, it appears that the overall morbidity and resultant mortality rates will be significantly lowered by avoiding the high rates of nontherapeutic celiotomy associated with a policy of liberal celiotomy for penetrating injury.

Conclusions and Algorithm

While the nonoperative management of most blunt abdominal organ injuries has become routine at all modern trauma centers, there is a very limited experience and willingness to extend this option to penetrating abdominal injuries. Selective nonoperative management can be performed safely in appropriate candidates, but should only be considered if adequate resources and experienced supervision are present. Strict adherence to the principles outlined above is particularly critical to the safe nonoperative management of patients with abdominal gunshot wounds. We believe that as further experience is gained and published, there will be increased acceptance and utilization of selective nonoperative management. The avoidance of the costs and morbidities associated with nontherapeutic laparotomies will benefit the individual patient as well as the entire health-care system.

Figure 10 outlines our current algorithm used for the triage of patients with penetrating abdominal trauma without peritonitis.

REFERENCES

1. Hoff WS, Holevar M, Nagy KK, et al: Practice management guidelines for the evaluation of blunt abdominal trauma. *J Trauma* 53(3):602–615, 2002.
2. Knudson MM, Maull KI: Nonoperative management of solid organ injuries: past, present, and future. *Surg Clin North Am* 79(6):1357–1371, 1999.
3. Alonso M, Brathwaite C, Garcia V, et al: Practice management guidelines for the nonoperative management of blunt injury to the liver and spleen. Eastern Association for the Surgery of Trauma, 2003. http://www.east.org/tpg/livspleen.pdf.
4. Poletti PA, Mirvis SE, Shanmuganathan K, et al: Blunt abdominal trauma patients: can organ injury be excluded without performing computed tomography? *J Trauma* 57(5):1072–1081, 2004.
5. Miller PR, Croce MA, Bee TK, et al: Associated injuries in blunt solid organ trauma: implications for missed injury in nonoperative management. *J Trauma* 53(2):238–244, 2002.
6. Kramer GC: Hypertonic resuscitation: physiologic mechanisms and recommendations for trauma care. *J Trauma* 54(5 Suppl):S89–S99, 2003.

7. Cocanour CS, Moore FA, Ware DN, et al: Age should not be a consideration for nonoperative management of blunt splenic injury. *J Trauma* 48(4):606–612, 2000.
8. Harbrecht BG, Peitzman AB, Rivera L, et al: Contribution of age and gender to outcome of blunt splenic injury in adults: multicenter study of the Eastern Association for the Surgery of Trauma. *J Trauma* 51(5): 887–895, 2001.
9. Malhotra AK, Latifi R, Fabian TC, et al: Multiplicity of solid organ injury: influence on management and outcomes after blunt abdominal trauma. *J Trauma* 54(5):925–929, 2003.
10. Nix JA, Costanza M, Daley BJ, et al: Outcome of the current management of splenic injuries. *Trauma* 50(5):835–842, 2001.
11. Haan JM, Bochicchio GV, Kramer N, et al: Nonoperative management of blunt splenic injury: a 5-year experience. *J Trauma* 58(3):492–498, 2005.
12. Sartorelli KH, Frumiento C, Rogers FB, et al: Nonoperative management of hepatic, splenic, and renal injuries in adults with multiple injuries. *J Trauma* 49(1):56–62, 2000.
13. Toutouzas KG, Karaiskakis M, Kaminski A, et al: Nonoperative management of blunt renal trauma: a prospective study. *Am Surg* 68(12): 1097–1103, 2002.
14. Carrillo EH, Spain DA, Wohltmann CD, et al: Interventional techniques are useful adjuncts in the nonoperative management of hepatic injuries. *J Trauma* 46(4):619–624, 1999.
15. Demetriades D, Karaiskakis M, Alo K, et al: Role of postoperative computed tomography in patients with severe liver injury. *Br J Surg* 90(11):1398–1400, 2003.
16. Robin AP, Andrews JR, Lange DA, et al: Selective management of anterior abdominal stab wounds. *J Trauma* 29(12):1684–1689, 1989.
17. Demetriades D, Rabinowitz B: Indications for operation in abdominal stab wounds. A prospective study of 651 patients. *Ann Surg* 205(2): 129–132, 1987.
18. Hauser CJ, Huprich JE, Bosco P, et al: Triple-contrast computed tomography in the evaluation of penetrating posterior abdominal injuries. *Arch Surg* 122(10):1112–1115, 1987.
19. Velmahos GC, Demetriades D, Toutouzas KG, et al: Selective nonoperative management in 1,856 patients with abdominal gunshot wounds: should routine laparotomy still be the standard of care? *Ann Surg* 234(3):395–403, 2001.
20. Fackler ML: Civilian gunshot wounds and ballistics: dispelling the myths. *Emerg Med Clin North Am* 16(1):17–28, 1998.
21. Murray JA, Demetriades D, Asensio JA, et al: Occult injuries to the diaphragm: prospective evaluation of laparoscopy in penetrating injuries to the left lower chest. *J Am Coll Surg* 187(6):626–630, 1998.
22. Demetriades D, Gomez H, Chahwan S, et al: Gunshot injuries to the liver: the role of selective nonoperative management. *J Am Coll Surg* 188(4): 343–348, 1999.

GASTRIC INJURIES

Lawrence N. Diebel

The stomach is a relatively thick-walled, well-vascularized organ that is variably positioned in the peritoneal cavity. Although partially protected by the lower rib cage, its size and location put the stomach at risk for injury, particularly with injury from penetrating trauma to the abdomen or lower chest.

The generous blood supply to the stomach includes (1) the left gastric artery, a branch of the celiac axis; (2) the right gastric artery, a branch of the common hepatic artery; (3) the right gastroepiploic artery, a branch of the gastroduodenal artery; (4) the left gastroepiploic artery, a branch of the splenic artery; and (5) the short gastric arteries, which also arise from the splenic artery. Because of the plentiful blood supply, gastric injuries can cause significant bleeding and require precise hemostasis in their repair. However, the excellent blood supply to the stomach contributes to the good results of the surgical repair of most gastric injuries in even the worst clinical circumstances.

The stomach has a number of important anatomic relationships, including the diaphragm, liver, spleen, pancreas, and transverse colon and mesocolon. Concomitant injuries to these adjacent structures often dictate the priority of management of the ultimate outcome for both blunt and penetrating gastric trauma.

INCIDENCE

Gastric injuries usually result from penetrating trauma and occur in approximately 20% of gunshot wounds and 10% of stab wounds.[1-3] Blunt gastric trauma is much less common. The American Association for the Surgery of Trauma (East) multi-institutional study on hollow viscus injury reported that the prevalence of blunt gastric rupture was 0.06% in patients undergoing evaluation for blunt abdominal trauma and 2.1% of all patients found to have hollow viscus injury.[4]

MECHANISM OF INJURY

The stomach is at risk for injury after stab wounds to the left thoracoabdominal region of the body. A single perforation occurs in over 50% of these cases.[2] However, injury to adjacent organs is common. Gunshot wounds result in two or more gastric wounds in 90% of cases.[2] Although often associated with some surrounding tissue damage to the stomach, this is usually only significant with high-velocity missiles. Shotgun wounds at close range (<15 feet) are often associated with massive destruction of the abdominal wall, stomach, and other intra-abdominal organs.

Blunt injury to the stomach is most often the result of motor vehicle crashes, or motor vehicle–pedestrian trauma.[5-7] Less common causes include falls, assaults, and improperly performed cardiopulmonary resuscitation. Blunt gastric injuries include linear lacerations and complete gastric rupture. The postulated mechanisms for blunt gastric injury include sudden increases in intraluminal pressure resulting in a balloon-bursting type of phenomenon of a full stomach, compression against the spine (seat-belt injury), or a deceleration injury with shearing forces resulting in a laceration of the anterior stomach wall.

DIAGNOSIS

Gastric perforations caused by blunt forces are often large, and intraperitoneal contamination is usually significant. Peritoneal signs are usually obvious, leading to early surgical intervention. Patients with blunt gastric rupture are frequently in shock related to other significant injuries including spleen and/or liver wounds.

Patients with stab wounds and hypotension, peritonitis, or both should undergo laparotomy immediately. Asymptomatic patients without central nervous system injury (brain or spinal cord injury) or drug or alcohol involvement may be observed with repeated physical exams. In other patients, local wound exploration, diagnostic peritoneal lavage (DPL), or laparoscopy are alternatives. Laparoscopy is most helpful with thoracoabdominal stab wounds in identifying associated injuries to the diaphragm.[8] Focused assessment with sonography for trauma (FAST) may not identify the small amount of fluid initially associated with hollow viscus injury, and thus may be misleading with isolated gastric injuries.

Early operation is indicated for symptomatic gunshot wounds to the abdomen. Occasionally, a tangential gunshot wound in a stable patient may be observed, or such a wound may be found after the patient undergoes either DPL or laparoscopy. Abdominal CT is also helpful in this situation. In patients suspected to have either blunt or penetrating gastric injury, the placement of a nasogastric tube is helpful. Not only does proper placement of a nasogastric tube minimize the risk of aspiration, but a bloody aspirate when present is highly suspicious for a gastric injury. In patients with blunt gastric injury and no obvious peritoneal signs, a supine film of the abdomen discloses free air in less than 50% of cases. In this situation, abdominal CT is more sensitive in identifying free air.

SURGICAL MANAGEMENT

The abdomen is explored through a midline incision. Visualization of the stomach is facilitated by nasogastric tube decompression. Control of hemorrhage is the first priority, followed by control of enteric spill. Gastric wounds may be rapidly initially controlled by a running locking full-thickness closure with absorbable sutures. A seromuscular layer of nonabsorbable sutures is placed later in the operation. This not only affords hemostasis, but also controls further peritoneal contamination by gastric contents. Alternatively a TA-stapler or Allis or Babcock clamp may be used for temporary control.

After attention to the more life-threatening injuries, the stomach wound may be addressed. The stomach should first be carefully inspected for ecchymosis or hematomas along either the lesser or greater curvature. Certain areas of the stomach are particularly difficult to assess: the gastroesophageal junction, high in the gastric fundus, the lesser curvature, and the posterior wall. Perixiphoid extension of the midline incision, the use of a self-retaining retractor, and positioning of the hemodynamically stable patient in the reverse Trendelenburg position may aid in exposure of these problematic areas. The gastroesophageal junction area may also be better exposed by division of the left triangular ligament and mobilization of the lateral segment of the left lobe. The posterior wall of the stomach is exposed by opening the gastrocolic ligament just outside the gastroepiploic arcade along the greater curvature of the stomach. Division of the short gastric vessels may be necessary to adequately expose the proximal gastric fundus. Occasionally, air insufflated into the stomach via the nasogastric tube with the stomach submerged in saline may help identify an occult injury to the stomach. Tangential wounds and/or single perforations of the stomach do occur, but this is a diagnosis of exclusion.

Gastric injuries thus identified are treated according to their severity (Table 1, Figure 1). Most intramural hematomas (grades I and II) are treated by careful evacuation, hemostasis, and closure with seromuscular sutures made of nonabsorbable material. Small grade I and II perforations can be closed in one or two layers. Because of the vascularity of the stomach, I prefer a two-layer closure after hemostasis is achieved.

Table 1: AAST Organ Injury Scale for Stomach

AAST Grade	Characteristics of Injury
I	Intramural hematoma <3 cm, partial thickness laceration
II	Intramural hematoma >3 cm; small (<3 cm) laceration
III	Large (>3 cm) laceration
IV	Large laceration involving vessels of greater or lesser curvature
V	Extensive (>50%) rupture; stomach devascularization

AAST, American Association for the Surgery of Trauma.
Modified from American Association for the Surgery of Trauma (AAST).

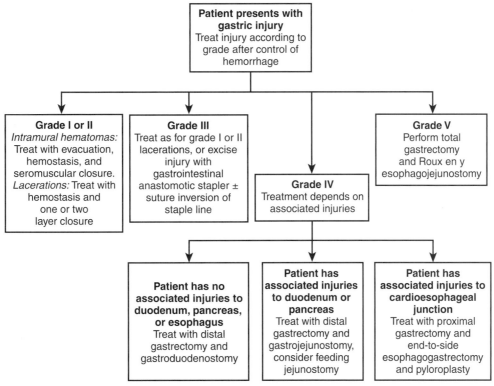

Figure 1   Algorithm for treatment of gastric injury.

Large (grade III) injuries near the greater curvature can be closed by the same technique or by the use of a GIA stapler. Certain defects may also be closed using a TA stapler. The staple line may be protected with a seromuscular closure using nonabsorbable sutures. Care must be taken to avoid stenosis in the gastroesophageal and pyloric area. A pyloric wound may be converted to a pyloroplasty to avoid possible stenosis in this area. Extensive wounds (grade IV) may be so destructive that a proximal or distal gastrectomy is required. Reconstruction with either a Billroth I or II anastomosis is dictated by the presence or absence of an associated duodenal injury. In rare cases, a total gastrectomy and a Roux-en-Y esophojejunostomy are necessary for severe injuries (grade V).

If a diaphragm injury occurs in association with a gastric perforation, contamination of pleural cavity with gastric contents can be problematic.[9] Under most circumstances, it is sufficient to clear the pleural space through the diaphragmatic rent after closure of the gastric perforation. It may be necessary to enlarge the diaphragmatic injury to achieve complete evacuation of the pleural contamination. After surgical repair of the stomach, the diaphragm injury is closed, and a chest tube is placed. Occasionally, the contamination may be so severe, particularly if operation is delayed, that a separate thoracotomy to provide adequate drainage of the pleural space is necessary. Thoracoscopic evacuation of the gastric contamination of the pleural space followed by chest tube placement is another option.

MORTALITY

Mortality after gastric injury is related to the mechanism of injury and the presence of shock and transfusion requirements, as well as the number of associated injuries. The mortality associated with blunt gastric rupture has been reported to range from 0% to 66% and averages around 30%.[4–8] Associated intra- and extra-abdominal injuries are usually present. The intra-abdominal organs most frequently injured include the spleen, liver, small bowel, and pancreas. The most frequent extra-abdominal injuries include chest, extremity, and head. Hemorrhagic shock and complications related to the associated injuries account for the vast majority of deaths.

The overall mortality rate for penetrating gastric injuries is 14%–20%.[1–3] Early deaths are related to irreversible hemorrhagic shock from associated injuries. Mortality increases dramatically with the number of organs injured. The most common associated injuries include the liver, diaphragm, colon, lung, and small bowel. Injuries to the spleen, pancreas, and major blood vessels in the abdomen are also common. Mortality after either penetrating or blunt gastric injury rarely is the result of injury to the stomach. When it occurs, it is related to anastomotic dehiscence, abscess or fistula formation, and subsequent organ failure.

MORBIDITY

Major morbidity after gastric injury includes intra-abdominal abscess formation, bleeding, anastomotic breakdown, and empyema formation.[3,6] The severity of gastric injury and degree of contamination contribute to the development of intra-abdominal abscess formation. Intra-abdominal contamination is often significantly greater after blunt gastric injury.

After penetrating trauma, the incidence of intra-abdominal abscess formation and surgical site infection is similarly low for both isolated gastric and colonic injury. The low incidence of intra-abdominal abscess formation with either isolated stomach or colon injury increases dramatically when concomitant injuries to the liver, kidney, pancreas, or duodenum are present.[10,11] There is even a greater synergistic effect on intra-abdominal abscess formation with combined stomach and colon injuries. The risk of empyema increases significantly when there is a diaphragm injury in association with penetrating injuries to the stomach. Bleeding can occur from the surgical site or gastric suture line, and may require reoperation. Occasionally suture line bleeding may be controlled using endoscopic techniques. In the rare instances of gastric injuries that require resection and anastomosis, anastomotic stenosis may require revision.

CONCLUSION

Most gastric injuries require debridement and closure. On rare occurrences more complex procedures, including gastric resection and anastomosis, are required. Shock and associated injuries dictate overall outcome.

REFERENCES

1. Nicholas JM, Parker Rix E, Esley KA, et al: Changing patterns in the management of penetrating abdominal trauma: the more things change, the more they stay the same. *J Trauma* 55:1095–1110, 2003.
2. Durham RM, Olson S, Weigelt JA: Penetrating injuries to the stomach. *Surg Gynecol Obstet* 172:298–302, 1991.
3. Coimbra R, Pinto MCC, Aguir JR, Rasslan S: Factors related to the occurrence of postoperative complications following penetrating gastric injuries. *Injury* 26:463–466, 1995.
4. Watts DD, Fakry SM: EAST Multi-Institutional Hollow Viscus Injury Research Group. Incidence of hollow viscus injury in blunt trauma: an analysis from 275,557 trauma admissions from the EAST multi-institutional trial. *J Trauma* 54:289–294, 2003.
5. Shinkawa H, Yasuhara H, Nika S, et al: Characteristic features of bdominal organ injuries associated with gastric rupture in blunt abdominal trauma. *Am J Surg* 187:394–397, 2004.
6. Bruscagin V, Coimbra R, Rasslan S, et al: Blunt gastric injury: a multicentre experience. *Injury* 32:761–764, 2001.
7. Nanji SA, Mock C: Gastric rupture resulting from blunt abdominal trauma and requiring gastric resection. *J Trauma* 47:410–412, 1999.
8. Ivatury RR, Simon RJ, Stahl WM: A critical evaluation of laparoscopy in penetrating abdominal trauma. *J Trauma* 34:827–828, 1993.
9. Zellweger R, Navsaria PH, Hess F, Omoshoro-Jones J, Kahn D, Nicol A: Transdiaphragmatic pleural lavage in penetrating thoracoabdominal trauma. *Br J Surg* 91:1619–1623, 2004.
10. Croce MA, Fabian TC, Patton JH, et al: Impact of stomach and colon injuries on intraabdominal abscess and the synergistic effect of hemorrhage and associated injury. *J Trauma* 45:649–655, 1998.
11. O'Neill PA, Kirton OC, Dresner LS, Tortella B, Kestner MM: Analysis of 162 colon injuries in patients with penetrating abdominal trauma: concomitant stomach injury results in a higher rate of infection. *J Trauma* 56:304–313, 2004.

SMALL BOWEL INJURY

Kimball Maull

Injuries to the intestines have been described since antiquity. The statement "a slight blow will cause rupture of the intestines without injury to the skin" is attributed to Aristotle, and Hippocrates was the first to describe intestinal injury from penetrating trauma. In 1275, De Salicet was the first to report lateral suture repair of an intestinal wound. In 1686, Bonet described blunt intestinal injury in a hunter who was thrown violently against a tree by a stag. Autopsy showed rupture of the terminal ileum and cecum. In 1761, Morgagni reported several instances of blunt trauma to the small intestine caused by direct blows to the abdomen. He emphasized the slow and insidious nature of abdominal signs, an observation clinically pertinent to this day. The first long term survivor after repair of a traumatic totally divided small intestine was reported in 1889 by Croft. In the early 20th century, the experience of Bedroitz during the Russo-Japanese War confirmed the advantage of early operative intervention for abdominal injuries. She positioned her operating theatre close to the frontlines and, by being able to treat casualties within 4 hours, showed improved outcomes. In the late 20th century, awareness of the benefits of early repair, coupled with the technologic advances in diagnosis, led to significant improvements in outcome. However, they also led to controversy and loss of consensus regarding both diagnostic and therapeutic approaches to patients at risk. As a result, there continue to be missteps in both diagnosis and management that require surgical vigilance.

INCIDENCE

Injuries to the small intestine must be differentiated by their means of wounding. Because the small intestine occupies the largest portion of the peritoneal cavity, injuries to the small intestine are over-represented after penetrating trauma. Most series cite an incidence of involvement of the small bowel or its mesentery in 80% or greater after gunshot wounds and 25%–30% after stab wounds. In blunt trauma, although the small bowel is acknowledged as the third most common organ injured, after the liver and spleen, the incidence has recently been shown to be much less than previously thought (Table 1). The 1% incidence after blunt trauma increases to 3% in patients with blunt abdominal trauma, with the incidence of free perforation after blunt abdominal trauma still less than 1%. These figures may be misleading. Nance et al., using data from the Pennsylvania Trauma System database, showed a strong statistical correlation between the number of solid organs injured and the likelihood of associated hollow viscus injury.[1] The overall incidence was 9.6%, but climbed appreciably as the number of solid organs increased, reaching 34% with three or more solid organ injuries. Isolated injury to the pancreas was associated with a 33% incidence of hollow viscus injury. Only hollow viscus injuries with an Abbreviated Injury Score (AIS) of 3 or greater were included, but the database also included injuries to the gall bladder and urinary bladder.

MECHANISM OF INJURY

There are few anatomic areas, other than the hollow viscera, where the mechanism of injury plays as important a role in determining the ease or difficulty of diagnosis or where the treatment is so well defined or confused. The small bowel may be injured by penetrating forces, including gunshot or shotgun wounds, stabbings, or impalements. Although there are recent reports attesting to the validity of nonoperative management of gunshot wounds, most surgeons hold to the belief that operation is mandated for gunshot wounds of the abdomen or where the abdomen is in jeopardy, that is, lower thoracic entry or buttock wounds. Because the likelihood of surgically significant injury exceeds 80% for gunshot wounds of the abdomen, celiotomy is indicated. Further, even when penetration of the peritoneal cavity can be excluded, blast effect leading to perforation has been described from proximity wounds, especially if the offending firearm is of high velocity (>2000 ft/sec).[2] The injurious nature of shotgun wounds is directly related to the shot size and distance between the victim and the muzzle of the shotgun, with large shot size and close-range wounds being the most damaging. Stab wounds are considerably less lethal, but because most are managed selectively, the risk of missed injury is increased compared with those where protocol demands operation.

The small bowel may be injured by nonpenetrating forces. High-speed modes of transport and the omnipresent use of safety restraints have enhanced the risk of blunt small bowel injury. Whereas traffic casualties died at the scene or sustained rapidly fatal central nervous system injuries in the past, road safety efforts have reduced traffic fatalities and created different patterns of injury, one of which is the seat-belt syndrome, which includes small bowel injuries. In fact, in the multi-institutional report of Fakhry et al., a seat-belt mark was associated with an increased risk of perforated small bowel injury.[3] In many cases, the mark represented incorrect usage of the safety belt, that is, too loose, too high, or poor geometry related to body size, as in children restrained by adult belts.

The pathogenesis of small bowel rupture from blunt forces is still speculative, but has variously been ascribed to crushing, shearing, or bursting forces. A violent force directly applied to the abdomen can crush the intestines between the external force and the spine. This mechanism is commonly accompanied by injuries to other organs. Shearing injuries occur from sudden deceleration with typical injuries occurring at points of relative fixation such as the ligament of Treitz and terminal ileum or at sites of adhesive bands. Some investigators have minimized this as an injury mechanism, citing the relatively even distribution of small bowel injuries in some series. The small bowel may burst if force is applied to a distended segment where ends may be temporarily closed. This explains how the small bowel may rupture after relatively minimal force, and has actually been demonstrated in the canine model. In summary, gaping small bowel disruptions with mesenteric mutilation and extensive small bowel contusion suggests a crush injury mechanism (Figure 1). Small bowel injuries with isolated clearly defined points of rupture probably represent burst injuries and shredding injuries, especially if near the ligament of Treitz, cecum, or other points of fixation, and are probably caused by shearing forces (Figures 2 and 3).

DIAGNOSIS

The diagnostic approach to penetrating wounds of the abdomen is slowly evolving based on newer technologies and minimally invasive surgical techniques. In 1960, Shaftan created controversy by suggesting that surgical judgment rather than mandatory celiotomy was the preferred approach to patients with penetrating trauma.[4] His initial efforts slowly gained support in the management of stab wounds. Stab wounds follow the rule of thirds: one-third do not penetrate the peritoneal cavity, one-third penetrate the peritoneal cavity but do not create injury, and one-third cause injury requiring operative repair. Recognizing that a mandatory policy of celiotomy resulted in

Table 1: Prevalence of Blunt Small Bowel Injury

	Blunt Trauma Admissions (n=227,972)		Blunt Abdominal Trauma (n=85,643)	
	Any Injury	Perforating Injury	Any Injury	Perforating Injury
All small bowel	1.1	0.3	2.9	0.8
Jejunum/ilium	0.9	0.3	2.5	0.7

Adapted from Fakhry SM, Brownstein M, Watts DD, et al: Relatively short diagnostic delays (<8 hours) produce morbidity and mortality in blunt small bowel injury: an analysis of time of operative intervention in 198 patients from a multicenter experience. *J Trauma* 48:408–415, 2000.

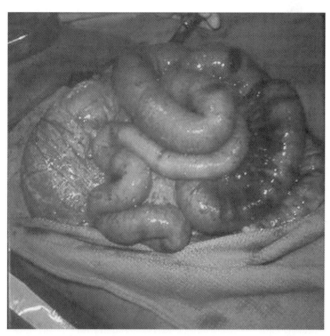

Figure 1 Small bowel injury from crushing force. Note extensive areas of nonviability.

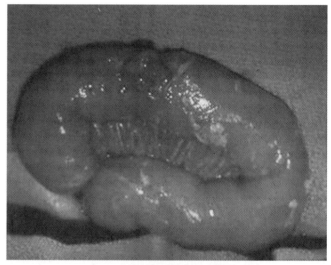

Figure 2 Small bowel segment showing burst injury.

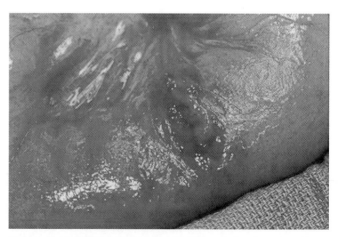

Figure 3 Small bowel demonstrating linear perforation, suggesting shear injury mechanism.

negative or nontherapeutic celiotomy in two-thirds of patients, selective management is now a common practice. In 2001, Scalea et al.[5] reported a prospective series of hemodynamically stable patients with penetrating trauma studied by triple-contrast computed tomography (CT). There were 75 consecutive patients and 60% sustained gunshot or shotgun wounds. Nonoperative management was successful in 96% of patients with a negative CT scan. Despite this impressive series, most surgeons employ celiotomy for the treatment of gunshot wounds and accept a 15% negative or nontherapeutic celiotomy rate. In some institutions, both operative and selective management coexist, with surgical judgment prevailing in instances where the suspicion of intraperitoneal penetration or injury is low, that is, flank wounds and wounds confined to the liver.

Indications for operation follow generally accepted algorithms (Figures 4 and 5). When criteria are met, most surgeons proceed with operative treatment. The emergence of experienced minimally invasive surgeons is beginning to modify indications for celiotomy after penetrating trauma, especially in wounds that potentially injure the hemidiaphragm or where abdominal penetration is in doubt. These enhanced skills have supported the evolution of laparoscopy from a primary diagnostic modality to both a diagnostic and therapeutic tool.[6] Wounds to the diaphragm can be seen and repaired; wounds to other organ systems can be detected, characterized as to injury severity and, in many instances, repaired or controlled with hemostatics.

Small bowel wounds remain problematic. Injuries obvious to the laparoscopic surgeon are probably detectable by other simple or less invasive techniques, that is, physical examination, CT, and diagnostic peritoneal lavage (DPL). Occult injuries may be initially missed regardless of the diagnostic approach, but exclusion of peritoneal penetration is useful whether by local wound exploration or direct visualization via a laparoscope.

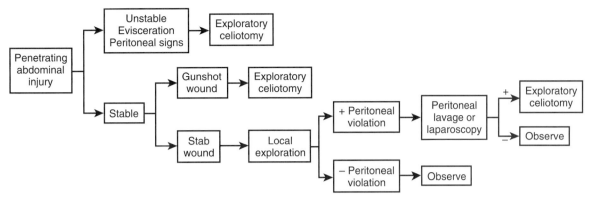

Figure 4   Algorithm for penetrating injuries to small bowel.

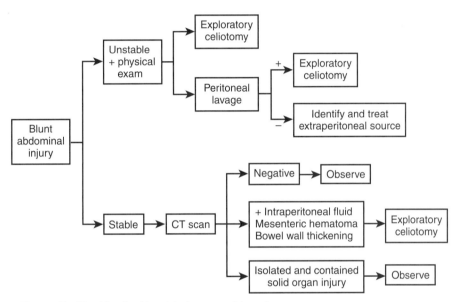

Figure 5   Algorithm for blunt injuries to small bowel.

Diagnosis of blunt small bowel injury is less obvious. Blunt small bowel injury ranges from contusion with or without serosal tear to intramural hematoma to loss of integrity of the bowel wall. The latter usually occurs immediately as a direct result of the injury, but there are many examples of delayed perforation, presumably as a result of post-traumatic ischemia leading to bowel wall necrosis. Trauma to the mesentery can have similar consequences or resolve only to cause post-traumatic stricture and delayed symptoms of intestinal obstruction. Injured patients with free perforation almost always present with abdominal pain and usually have signs of peritoneal irritation including percussion tenderness, tenderness to deep palpation, and direct and referred rebound tenderness. Operation is indicated in such situations without additional diagnostic studies. In many injured patients, the physical examination may be obscured by concurrent head injury, use of alcohol or other drugs, or associated injuries that distract the patient.[7] In these instances, diagnostic studies, including CT, ultrasonography, DPL, or laparoscopy may play a role. The algorithm for the diagnosis of small bowel injury rests on certain caveats:

1. The alert patient is subject to reliable interpretation of physical findings.
2. There is no single diagnostic test, other than celiotomy, that can diagnose a small bowel injury with certainty.
3. There are injuries to the small bowel and mesentery that do not cause free perforation but still require operative management.

The reliability of CT scanning in the diagnosis of small bowel injury is subject to great debate. The technique of performing the CT, that is, whether or not oral contrast adds to the accuracy of the scan, is debated. What to do in the patient with free intraperitoneal fluid without solid organ injury is debated. The role of DPL as a complementary study to CT is debated.[8] What is not debated, however, is the fact that patients can have a normal CT scan and still have significant small bowel injury, including perforation. CT findings suggesting small bowel injury occur in less than 50% of cases in some series (Figure 6). Because abdominal CT has become the most widely used test to detect intra-abdominal injury, there is great potential, in the patient with a negative CT, to miss the diagnosis and delay appropriate operative therapy. In 2000, Malhotra et al. cited the difference in the generations of CT scanners as impacting the ability to identify blunt small bowel injuries.[9] Compared with early-generation scans, the newer helical scanners appeared to be more sensitive. Yet, there were 7 of 47 patients (15%) in his series who had negative scans and had small bowel or mesenteric injuries requiring operation. Malhotra's experience parallels that from the EAST multi-institutional trial, which demonstrated a 13% false negative rate for CT in the diagnosis of small bowel injury. In 2004, Allen et al. reported sensitivity and specificity of 95 and 99%, respectively, for abdominal CT scans performed with intravenous contrast alone in the diagnosis of blunt small bowel and mesentery injuries.[10] However, their sample of patients with actual injury was small. In 2001,

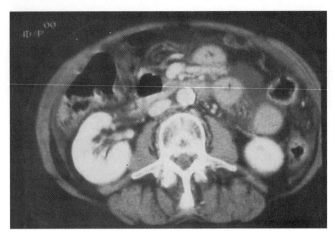

Figure 6 Positive computed tomography findings of wall thickening and adjacent free intraperitoneal fluid in patient with ruptured small bowel.

Gonzalez et al. reported the use of pre-CT DPL in a series of patients and compared the study group with a like group randomized to CT only.[11] If red blood cells per millimeter cubed were higher than 20,000, a CT was performed. Those undergoing CT only and found to have free fluid without solid organ injuries were explored. Using this protocol of screening DPL, they found a low nontherapeutic celiotomy rate and improved cost-effectiveness. CT scanning has also been combined with laparoscopy in an attempt to improve diagnostic accuracy. In 2005, Mitsuhide et al. reported the use of selective laparoscopy in patients suspected of small bowel injury, either by physical examination or CT scanning.[12] The laparoscopic finding of bowel perforation or ischemia mandated conversion to open operation. They concluded that CT combined with laparoscopy could prevent nontherapeutic celiotomy and reduced delay in diagnosis. In 2000, a report of the American Association for the Surgery of Trauma (AAST) membership regarding diagnosis and management of small bowel injuries showed a lack of confidence in any of the available diagnostic approaches.[13] There was considerable variation in how to manage the neurologically impaired patient with free fluid on CT in the absence of solid organ injury (Table 2). Options ranged from observation to operation with a plurality using DPL when in doubt. In children, the presence of abdominal tenderness and isolated free intraperitoneal fluid was highly predictive of small bowel perforation.

INJURY GRADING

The grading of small bowel injuries is uncomplicated, but the consequences of the injury are not. The reason for this is simple—bowel injuries occur and some are not initially diagnosed. Many proceed to heal without incident, some necrose and present as an intra-abdominal catastrophe, and others cause delayed symptoms, often requiring late operative treatment.[14] The AAST–Organ Injury Scale is depicted in Table 3. Note that grades 2–4 correspond to free perforation and are likely to be encountered immediately or soon after presentation. Grade 5 injuries, transection with segmental tissue loss and/or devascularization, may be apparent or occult, but both cause loss of bowel integrity and require small bowel resection. Somewhere in the scheme of things, but still unclassified, rests the partial devascularization injury without full thickness necrosis that heals by stricture and causes delayed obstructive symptoms. Operation is almost always required to deal with this problem.

SURGICAL MANAGEMENT

In most instances, surgical management means operative management. Nonetheless, there is a definite role for surgical judgment to decide the need for resection, the extent of resection, and the method of repair and/or resection. Small bowel injuries occur as isolated injuries but they more commonly coexist with other intra-abdominal injuries from both penetrating or blunt injury mechanisms. Surgical decision making is critical in the management of associated injuries and whether to employ damage control. In 2000, Hackam et al. compared small bowel–injured patients both with and without other intra-abdominal injuries.[15] Although the presence of other injuries led to earlier diagnosis and celiotomy, associated injuries adversely affected mortality, length of hospital stay (LOS), and intra-abdominal complications.

Injuries to the small bowel that require operative management include perforation, intramural hematoma, crush injury with loss of viability, laceration, and mesenteric trauma causing tears or avulsions of the mesentery, hemorrhage, expanding hematoma, and small bowel ischemia. The decision to repair, resect, or employ damage control techniques is based on the patient's clinical condition, the anatomy of the injury, whether the injuries are localized to a single wound site or intestinal segment, or if multiple wounds are dispersed over several segments of intestine. The surgeon should beware the finding of a single perforation or an odd number of intestinal wounds. While this may be explained by a tangential wound or the finding of an intraluminal missile, perforation of the intramesenteric small bowel wall is more likely and easy to miss. All juxtaintestinal mesenteric hematomas should be opened to ensure integrity of the intestinal wall.

Repair is best performed by direct suture. If resection is indicated, stapler and hand-sewn techniques of anastomosis appear to be

Table 2: Patient Management: No Solid Organ Injury, Free Fluid, Unreliable Exam

	Head Injury %	Intoxication %
Observe	28	51
Repeat computed tomography	12	11
Diagnostic peritoneal lavage	42	26
Operate	16	10

Adapted from Brownstein MR, Bunting T, Meyer AA, Fakhry SM: Diagnosis and management of blunt small bowel injury: a survey of the membership of the American Association for the Surgery of Trauma. *J Trauma* 48: 402–407, 2000.

Table 3: Small Bowel Injury

Grade[a]	Type of Injury	Description of Injury	AIS
I	Hematoma	Contusion or hematoma without devascularization	2
	Laceration	Partial thickness, no perforation	2
II	Laceration	Laceration <50% of circumference	3
III	Laceration	Laceration 50% of circumference without transaction	3
IV	Laceration	Transection of small bowel	4
V	Laceration	Transection of small bowel with segmental tissue loss	4
	Vascular	Devascularized segment	4

[a]Advance one grade for multiple injuries up to grade III.
AIS, Abbreviated Injury Score.

equally effective. However, both forms of resection have higher complication rates than repair. Therefore, injuries amenable to suture repair should be repaired rather than resected unless there are multiple proximity wounds that are technically easier to include in a limited resection than repair individually. In the damage control mode, wounds and lacerations are closed rapidly with a stapler to prevent continued soiling. No definitive anastomoses are performed.

Celiotomy for trauma must include an initial exploration to control active hemorrhage followed by a systematic inspection to identify all injuries. Injuries missed at celiotomy are the most lethal missed injuries. Therefore, every effort should be made to identify all intra-abdominal injuries, especially in a damage control situation where continued contamination predicts poor outcome. Soiling from hollow viscus injuries should be isolated with noncrushing intestinal clamps or controlled with the assistant's thumb and forefinger. Alternately, Babcock clamps can be applied. After the intestinal tract is examined from gastroesophageal junction to rectum, injuries should be counted and mentally noted or identified with tag sutures. Areas of hematoma should be carefully inspected. Most are limited to serosal injuries and are best treated by imbricating the bordering serosal margins. True intramural hematomas require surgical judgment. If limited in extent and nonexpanding, the hematoma will likely resolve on its own and does not require specific therapy. Large or expanding intramural hematomas, or those in which the viability of the involved intestinal segment cannot be determined, require intervention. Both hematoma evacuation and resection of the involved segment have been recommended. This author favors the latter. Perforations should be carefully debrided back to viable tissue, splayed with corner stay sutures and closed transversely in two layers (Figures 7, 8, and 9). Perforations that are closely opposed should be converted to a single defect and closed in like manner (Figure 10). Multiple perforations within a short segment are best treated by resection and anastomosis (Figure 11). The mesenteric defect should be closed in continuity (Figure 12).

Injuries to the mesentery vary from small hematomas to extensive life-threatening avulsion injuries. Large or expanding mesenteric hematomas and those adjoining the intestinal wall should be

explored and direct vascular control established by suture ligature (Figure 13). The integrity of the intestinal wall should be confirmed or repaired, as needed. Mesenteric tears may cause ischemia of the involved intestinal segment and resection may be necessary (Figure 14). All tears must be closed with sutures (Figure 15).

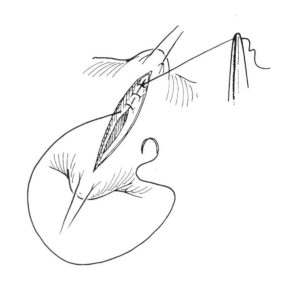

Figure 8 Perforations splayed with corner stay sutures. *(From Maull KI: Stomach, small bowel and mesentery injury. In Champion HR, Robbs JV, Trunkey DD, editors: Rob and Smith's Operative Surgery: Trauma Surgery, 4th ed. London, Butterworth-Heinemann, London, pp. 401–413.)*

Figure 7 Perforations carefully debrided back to viable tissue. *(From Maull KI: Stomach, small bowel and mesentery injury. In Champion HR, Robbs JV, Trunkey DD, editors: Rob and Smith's Operative Surgery: Trauma Surgery, 4th ed. London, Butterworth-Heinemann, London, pp. 401–413.)*

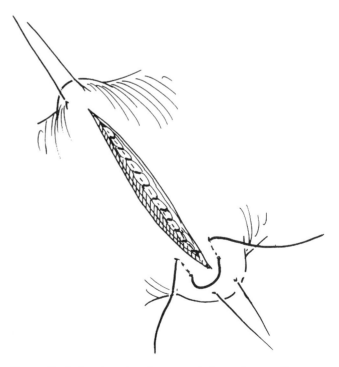

Figure 9 Perforations closed transversely in two layers. *(From Maull KI: Stomach, small bowel and mesentery injury. In Champion HR, Robbs JV, Trunkey DD, editors: Rob and Smith's Operative Surgery: Trauma Surgery, 4th ed. London, Butterworth-Heinemann, London, pp. 401–413.)*

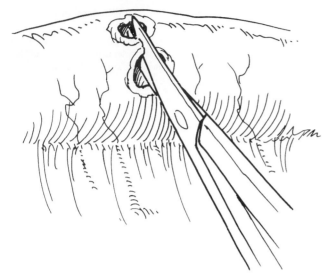

Figure 10 Perforations that are closely opposed should be converted to a single defect and closed in like manner. *(From Maull KI: Stomach, small bowel and mesentery injury. In Champion HR, Robbs JV, Trunkey DD, editors: Rob and Smith's Operative Surgery: Trauma Surgery, 4th ed. London, Butterworth-Heinemann, London, pp. 401–413.)*

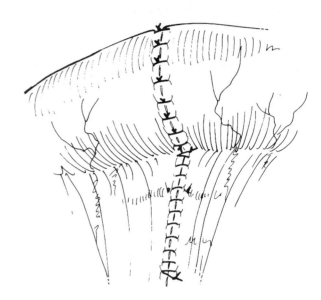

Figure 12 The mesenteric defect should be closed in continuity. *(From Maull KI: Stomach, small bowel and mesentery injury. In Champion HR, Robbs JV, Trunkey DD, editors: Rob and Smith's Operative Surgery: Trauma Surgery, 4th ed. London, Butterworth-Heinemann, London, pp. 401–413.)*

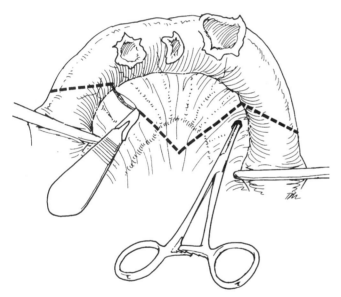

Figure 11 Multiple perforations within a short segment are best treated by resection and anastomosis. *(From Maull KI: Stomach, small bowel and mesentery injury. In Champion HR, Robbs JV, Trunkey DD, editors: Rob and Smith's Operative Surgery: Trauma Surgery, 4th ed. London, Butterworth-Heinemann, London, pp. 401–413.)*

▇ COMPLICATIONS

Complications after small bowel injury differ by injury mechanism. In blunt trauma, the principal concern is delay in diagnosis. In 2000, Fakhry et al., in a multicenter study of eight trauma centers, reported a statistically significant increased risk of wound infection, wound dehiscence, intra-abdominal abscess, adult respiratory distress syndrome (ARDS), and sepsis in patients with isolated small bowel perforations operated on more than 24 hours after injury compared with those undergoing operation less than 8 hours after injury.[16] Fang et al. reported a dramatic increase in complications if surgery was delayed more than 24 hours.[17] In children sustaining blunt small

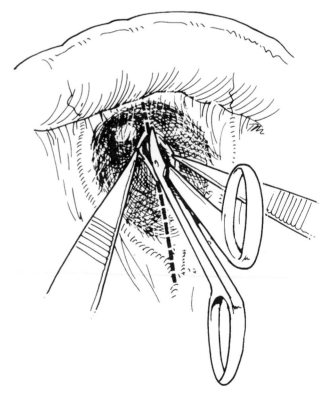

Figure 13 Large or expanding mesenteric hematomas and those adjoining the intestinal wall should be explored and direct vascular control established by suture ligature. *(From Maull KI: Stomach, small bowel and mesentery injury. In Champion HR, Robbs JV, Trunkey DD, editors: Rob and Smith's Operative Surgery: Trauma Surgery, 4th ed. London, Butterworth-Heinemann, London, pp. 401–413.)*

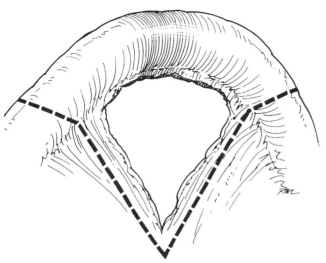

Figure 14 Mesenteric tears may cause ischemia of the involved intestinal segment, and resection may be necessary. *(From Maull KI: Stomach, small bowel and mesentery injury. In Champion HR, Robbs JV, Trunkey DD, editors: Rob and Smith's Operative Surgery: Trauma Surgery, 4th ed. London, Butterworth-Heinemann, London, pp. 401–413.)*

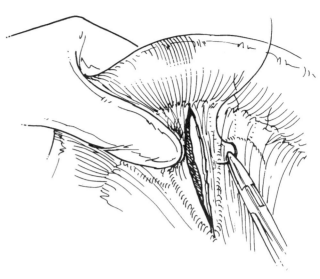

Figure 15 All mesenteric tears must be closed with sutures. *(From Maull KI: Stomach, small bowel and mesentery injury. In Champion HR, Robbs JV, Trunkey DD, editors: Rob and Smith's Operative Surgery: Trauma Surgery, 4th ed. London, Butterworth-Heinemann, London, pp. 401–413.)*

bowel rupture, delay in diagnosis more than 24 hours did not result in increased morbidity or mortality as reported by Bensard et al.[18]

Complications are also related to associated injuries and to whether management of the small bowel injury requires repair or resection. Associated multisystem injuries occur in as many as 70% of cases after blunt trauma, and often dictate not only the occurrence of complications, but also the eventual outcome[19](Figure 16). Anastomosis-related complications include leaks, enterocutaneous fistula, and intra-abdominal abscess.[20] These complications are uncommon but exceed the incidence after simple repair. Damage control predicts an increased likelihood of anastomosis-related complications.

Late complications of bowel obstruction relate to adhesions and ischemic stenosis from unrecognized small bowel or mesenteric

injury. In the latter circumstance, symptoms usually appear within 6 weeks postinjury and vary from vague abdominal pain to frank obstruction.[21] Resection is necessary to relieve the obstruction.

MORTALITY

Although reported mortalities have reached 25% or higher in some series, the consensus mortality after blunt small bowel injury is approximately 10%. In the multicenter study reported by Fakhry et al., there was no difference in mortality between patients with isolated small bowel injury and those who incurred small bowel injury in the setting of multiple other injuries.[16] Delays in diagnosis were directly

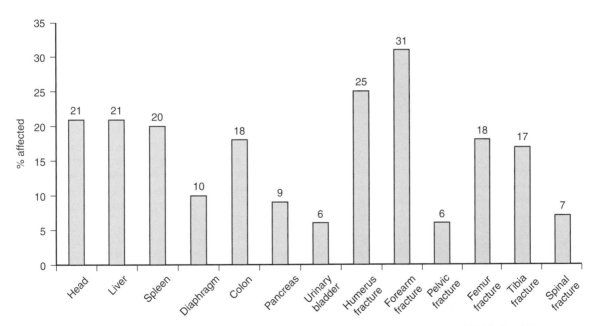

Figure 16 Typical injuries accompanying blunt small bowel trauma. *(Adapted from Neugebauer H, Wallenboeck E, Hungerford M: Seventy cases of injury of the small intestine caused by blunt abdominal trauma: a retrospective study from 1970 to 1994. J Trauma 46:116–121, 1999.)*

related to almost half the deaths in this series. In fact, delays exceeding as little as 8 hours resulted in increased morbidity and mortality.

Mortality after penetrating injury is most commonly related to injury to other intraperitoneal and/or retroperitoneal injuries.[22]

CONCLUSIONS

Small bowel injuries may follow blunt or penetrating trauma. The major concern in the patient who sustains blunt small bowel injury is recognizing the presence of the injury. In patients with associated injuries requiring operation or in those sustaining gunshot wounds, small bowel injuries are promptly discoverable. The trend toward CT-based nonoperative management and the inaccuracy of early postinjury CT places patients with isolated blunt small bowel injury at risk of delayed diagnosis and increased morbidity and mortality. The importance of injury mechanism and physical findings is often overlooked. Patients who are neurologically intact will demonstrate abdominal tenderness; many will have peritoneal findings at presentation. The presence of a seat-belt contusion should elevate concern. Injuries that can be repaired by lateral enterorrhaphy rarely cause postoperative complications, which are more commonly related to associated injuries after both blunt and penetrating trauma. Surgical judgment is required to ensure early diagnosis and appropriate operative management.

REFERENCES

1. Nance ML, Peden GW, Shapiro MB, et al: Solid viscus injury predicts major hollow viscus injury in blunt abdominal trauma. *J Trauma* 43: 618–623, 1997.
2. Velitchkov NG, Losanoff JE, Kjossev KT, et al: Delayed small bowel injury as a result of penetrating extraperitoneal high-velocity ballistic trauma to the abdomen. *J Trauma* 48:169–170, 2000.
3. Fakhry SM, Watts DD, Luchette FA: Current diagnostic approaches lack sensitivity in the diagnosis of perforated small bowel injury: analysis from 275,557 trauma admissions form the EAST multi-institutional HVI trial. *J Trauma* 54:295–306, 2003.
4. Shaftan GW: Indications for operation in abdominal trauma. *Am J Surg* 99:657–664, 1960.
5. Chiu WC, Shanmuganathan K, Mirvis SE, Scalea TM: Determining the need for laparotomy in penetrating torso trauma: a prospective study using triple-contrast enhanced abdominopelvic computed tomography. *J Trauma* 51:860–869, 2001.
6. Sinha R, Sharma N, Joshi M: Laparoscopic repair of small bowel perforation. *J Soc Laparoendosc Surg* 9:399–402, 2005.
7. Maull KI, Reath DB: Impact of early recognition on outcome in nonpenetrating wounds of the small bowel. *South Med J* 77:1075–1077, 1984.
8. Brasel KJ, Olsen CJ, Stafford RE, Johnson TJ: Incidence and significance of free fluid on abdominal computed tomographic scan in blunt trauma. *J Trauma* 44:889–892, 1998.
9. Malhotra AK, Fabian TC, Katsis SB, et al: Blunt bowel and mesenteric injuries: the role of screening computed tomography. *J Trauma* 48: 991–1000, 2000.
10. Allen TL, Mueller MT, Bonk T, et al: Computed tomographic scanning without oral contrast solution for blunt bowel and mesenteric injuries in abdominal trauma. *J Trauma* 56:314–322, 2004.
11. Gonzalez RP, Ickler J, Gachassin P: Complementary roles of diagnostic peritoneal lavage and computed tomography in the evaluation of blunt abdominal trauma. *J Trauma* 51:1128–1136, 2001.
12. Mitsuhide K, Junichi S, Atsushi N et al: Computed tomography scanning and selective laparoscopy in the diagnosis of blunt small bowel injury: a prospective study. *J Trauma* 58:696–703, 2005.
13. Brownstein MR, Bunting T, Meyer AA, Fakhry SM: Diagnosis and management of blunt small bowel injury: a survey of the membership of the American Association for the Surgery of Trauma. *J Trauma* 48:402–407, 2000.
14. Kaban G, Somani RA, Carter J: Delayed presentation of small bowel injury after blunt abdominal trauma. *J Trauma* 56:1144–1145, 2004.
15. Hackam DJ, Ali J, Jastaniah SS: Effects of other intra-abdominal injuries on the diagnosis, management and outcome of small bowel injuries. *J Trauma* 49:606–610, 2000.
16. Fakhry SM, Brownstein M, Watts DD, et al: Relatively short diagnostic delays (<8 hours) produce morbidity and mortality in blunt small bowel injury: an analysis of time of operative intervention in 198 patients from a multicenter experience. *J Trauma* 48:408–415, 2000.
17. Fang JF, Chen RJ, Lin BC, et al: Small bowel perforation: is urgent surgery necessary? *J Trauma* 47:515–520, 1999.
18. Bensard DD, Beaver B, Besner GE, Cooney DR: Small bowel injury in children after blunt abdominal trauma: is diagnostic delay important? *J Trauma* 41:476–483, 1996.
19. Neugebauer H, Wallenboeck E, Hungerford M: Seventy cases of injury of the small intestine caused by blunt abdominal trauma: a retrospective study from 1970 to 1994. *J Trauma* 46:116–121, 1999.
20. Maull KI: Stomach, small bowel and mesentery injury. In Dudley H, Carter D, Russell RC, editors: *Operative Surgery.* London, Butterworths, 1989, pp. 401–413.
21. Kirkpatrick AW, Baxter KA, Simons RK, et al: Intra-abdominal complications after surgical repair of small bowel injuries: an international review. *J Trauma* 55:399–406, 2003.
22. Stevens SL, Maull KI: Small bowel injuries. *Surg Clin North Am* 70: 541–560, 1990.

DUODENAL INJURIES

Gregory J. Jurkovich

Duodenal injuries are uncommon, but not so rare as to preclude a comprehensive understanding of treatment strategies by general surgeons. A 6-year statewide review in Pennsylvania documented a 0.2% incidence of blunt duodenal injury (206 of 103,864 trauma registry entries), and only 30 of these patients had full-thickness duodenal injuries.[1] Blunt duodenal injuries are the result of a direct blow to the epigastria, which in adults is usually from a steering wheel injury in an unrestrained driver, and in children is the result of a direct blow from a bicycle handlebar, fist, or similar mechanism. Penetrating wounds are more common causes of duodenal injury, with about 75% of patients in published reports sustaining penetrating trauma.[2] This figure may primarily be a reflection of the experience of urban trauma centers where penetrating mechanism are more prevalent, and of academic centers that publish their results. Penetrating duodenal wounds are usually rapidly diagnosed as part of a laparotomy and evaluation of the tract of the offending agent. But blunt duodenal injuries are often more insidious in their presentation, making the initial diagnosis difficult. Despite this well-known observation, delays in the diagnosis of duodenal trauma continue to plague trauma surgeons and seriously compromise patient care.[3]

DETERMINANTS OF OUTCOME

Directly attributable duodenal mortality ranges from 2%–5%, and is the result of the common complications of wound dehiscence, sepsis, and multiple organ failure.[4-11] Associated causes of mortality in patients with a duodenal injury can be garnered from large series of duodenal injuries reported during the late 20th century. These reports demonstrated an average mortality in patients with a duodenal injury of 18%, but with great individual report variability, ranging from 6%–29%.[6,12–14] Morbidity rates after duodenal injury range from 30%–63%, although only about a third of these are directly related to the duodenal injury itself.[6,9,12] Reasons for this variability in morbidity and mortality statistics include the mechanism of injury, associated injuries, and time to initial diagnosis. For example, Ivatury and colleagues' review of 100 consecutive penetrating duodenal injuries documented a 25% mortality rate,[6] compared with mortality rates of 12%–14% in patients with blunt injury mechanisms.[3,9]

Early death from a duodenal injury, particularly with penetrating wounds, is caused by exsanguination from associated vascular, liver, or spleen injuries.[15,16] The proximity of the duodenum to other vital structures makes isolated injuries uncommon, but not unheard of. While exsanguinating hemorrhage and associated injuries are responsible for early deaths, infection and multiple-system organ failure are responsible for most late deaths. Up to one-third of patients who survive the first 48 hours develop a complication related to the duodenal injury. Anastomotic breakdown, fistula, intra-abdominal abscess, pneumonia, septicemia, and organ failure are the common complications. Late deaths in patients with a duodenal injury typically occur 1–2 weeks or more after the injury, with about one-third of the late deaths attributable to the injury itself.[9,12]

The time from injury to definitive treatment is also an important factor in the development of late complications and subsequent mortality. Roman and colleagues[17] identified 10 patients in whom the diagnosis of duodenal injury was delayed over 24 hours; 4 of the 10 died, and 3 of the 10 had duodenal fistulas. In a true trauma classic report, Lucas and Ledgerwood[18] demonstrated the remarkable importance (and frequency) of a delay in diagnosis of duodenal injury. In their report, a delay in diagnosis of more than 12 hours occurred in 53% of their patients, and a delay of more than 24 hours in 28%; mortality was 40% among the patients in whom the diagnosis was delayed greater than 24 hours, as opposed to 11% in those undergoing surgery within 24 hours. Snyder and coworkers[9] confirmed these observations, noting that of the four patients with blunt duodenal trauma in their series in whom the diagnosis was delayed, two died and the other two developed duodenal fistula. Cuddington and associates[3] also noted that 100% of the deaths directly attributable to duodenal injury occurred in patients in whom there was a delay in diagnosing such injury.

The implication of these observations is that the first priority in managing duodenal trauma should be control of hemorrhage. The next priority is limiting bacterial contamination from colon or other bowel injury to prevent late infections. A clear identification of the extent of the duodenal injury should follow as the next priority, with an emphasis on determining the status of the pancreas as well, as this affects definitive treatment plans.[13,19]

ANATOMY AND PHYSIOLOGY

The duodenum is the first portion of the small intestine, beginning just to the right of the spine at the level of the first lumbar vertebra and extending from the pyloric ring to the duodenojejunal flexure, commonly known as the ligament of Treitz. The duodenum is named from the Latin word *duodeni*, which means "twelve each," because it is in total 25 to 30 cm, or about 12 fingerbreadths, in length. For convenience of description, the duodenum is arbitrarily divided into four divisions, differentiated by the alteration in direction of the organ.[20] The *superior* or first portion of the duodenum passes backward and upward toward the neck of the gallbladder, and most of this portion is intraperitoneal. The *descending* (vertical) or second portion forms an acute angle with the first portion and descends 7–8 cm. It contains the bile and pancreatic duct openings. This

portion (and the remainder of the duodenum) is entirely retroperitoneal; this is the segment mobilized by a Kocher maneuver. The *transverse* or third portion of the duodenum runs 12 cm horizontally to the left in front of the ureter, inferior vena cava, lumbar column, and aorta, and ends at just at the left edge of the third lumbar vertebra. The superior mesenteric artery runs downward over the anterior surface of the third portion of the duodenum. The *ascending* or fourth portion of the duodenum runs upward and slightly to the left for only a short distance (2–3 cm) alongside the spine to the duodenal suspensory ligament of Treitz.

The arterial blood supply of the duodenum is derived from the pancreaticoduodenal artery. The superior branch comes off the hepatic artery, and the inferior branch from the superior mesenteric artery. These two arteries run in a groove between the descending (second) and transverse (third) portions of the duodenum and the head of the pancreas, with well-developed collateralization via a continuous marginal artery. The venous drainage parallels the arterial supply, with the posterosuperior arcade draining into the portal vein and the anteroinferior arcade draining into the gastrocolic trunk.[21]

The duodenal mucosa resembles that of the remainder of the small bowel, with the characteristic histologic feature of the submucosal Brunner's glands in the most proximal (first) portion. The viscous, mucoid, alkaline secretion of these glands probably affords some protection to the duodenum from gastric acid and serves to begin neutralization of this acid. The mixing of pancreatic and bile juices with the gastric efflux also normally occurs in the duodenum. The duodenum sees an average of 2500 ml gastric juice, 1000 ml of bile, 800–1000 ml of pancreatic juices, and 800 ml of saliva, for a total of about 5 liters of combined flow through the duodenum per day. Such massive flow volumes make it clear that duodenal integrity is crucial, and help to explain why duodenal fistulae can be such a difficult complication of injury to this organ.

DIAGNOSTIC ADJUVANTS

The radiologic signs of duodenal injury on the initial plain abdominal or upright chest radiograph are often quite subtle, with mild spine scoliosis or obliteration of the right psoas muscle being occasionally all that suggests a retroperitoneal duodenal injury. The presence of air in the retroperitoneum is a clear sign of duodenal injury, but this is often difficult to distinguish from the overlying transverse colon. Computed tomography (CT) at the current time is the best method of early diagnosis of a duodenal injury, but it is not infallible. In a 1997 report describing a 6-year statewide experience with duodenal injuries, Ballard et al.[1] reported that of 30 documented blunt duodenal injuries, the initial CT scan missed 27%. The (CT) scan must be performed with both oral and intravenous contrast (Figure 1). The exam must be interpreted with great suspicion for injury, and uncertainty in interpretation is adequate justification for operative exploration. False-negative exams are known to occur.[22] In one careful study of the accuracy of CT in diagnosing duodenal and other small bowel injuries, only 59% (10 of 17) scans were prospectively (preoperatively) interpreted as suggestive for bowel injury, which increased to 88% (15 of 17 injuries) when evaluated retrospectively.[23] These investigators emphasized that using CT for the diagnosis of blunt bowel rupture requires careful inspection and technique to detect the often-subtle findings.

A more cumbersome alternative to CT is upper gastrointestinal series with water-soluble contrast medium followed by barium if the initial exam is negative. Some have advocated this study if the initial CT is difficult to interpret, but I would argue that subtle findings on CT are adequate justification for operative exploration. In a series of 96 patients with CT findings suspicious for duodenal injury, the sensitivity of a subsequent duodenography was 54% with a specificity of 98%.[24] For those injuries requiring operative repair, the sensitivity was only 25%, with a 25% false-negative rate. Allen et al.[25] demonstrated that 83% of the patients with a delay in the diagnosis

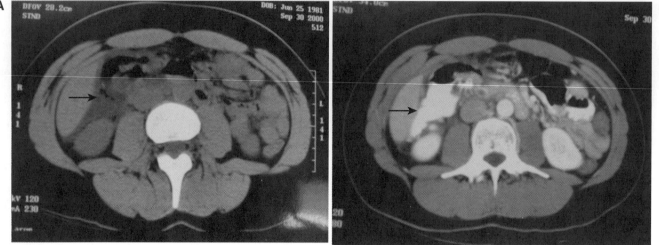

Figure 1 Duodenal perforation. Nineteen-year-old female dropped a 185-lb barbell on abdomen, presented to emergency department 4 hours later with mild abdominal pain and nausea. Afebrile, hemodynamics stable, persistent epigastric tenderness without peritoneal signs, WCC 16 K, amylase 114. Arrow points to nonluminal air in the retroperitoneum and free extravasation of contrast.

of blunt duodenal injury had subtle CT findings, including pneumoperitoneum, unexplained fluid, and unusual bowel morphology that were dismissed. These authors emphasized the point that subtle findings of duodenal injury on abdominal CT should mandate laparotomy.

Diagnostic peritoneal lavage (DPL) is unreliable in detecting *isolated* duodenal and other retroperitoneal injuries. Nevertheless, DPL is often helpful because approximately 40% of patients with a duodenal injury have associated intra-abdominal injuries that will result in a positive peritoneal lavage. The findings of amylase or bile in the lavage effluent are more specific indicators of possible duodenal injury. Serum amylase levels are nondiagnostic as well, but if elevated additional investigation (CT or celiotomy) for the possibility of pancreatic or duodenal injury is warranted. At celiotomy, the presence of *any* central upper abdominal retroperitoneal hematoma, bile staining, or air mandates visualization and a thorough examination of the duodenum. Asensio and colleagues[26] have published the technical details of exposing the entire duodenum and pancreas.

TREATMENT

Treatment principles are governed by the severity of duodenal injury and the likelihood of postrepair complications. Approximately 70% of duodenal wounds can be safely repaired primarily, and the remaining 30% are "severe" injuries that require more complex procedures. Snyder and colleagues[9] are credited with cataloging the factors that determine whether a duodenal wound can be primarily repaired. In their review of 247 patients treated for duodenal trauma, they reported an overall duodenal fistula rate of 7% and a mortality rate of 10.5% in the 228 patients surviving for greater than 72 hours. These investigators felt that five of the factors listed in Table 1 most significantly correlate with the severity of duodenal injury and subsequent morbidity and mortality. A more recent addition, as noted in the table, is the presence of a pancreatic injury, a significant predictor of late morbidity and mortality. Each of these factors, either individually or in combination, has been used to develop a variety of duodenal injury classification systems. Snyder and colleagues[9] demonstrated that patients with "mild" duodenal trauma had 0% mortality and 2% duodenal fistula rate, as compared with 6% mortality and 10% fistula rate among those with severe duodenal injuries. In general, patients with a "mild" duodenal injury and no pancreatic injury can be primarily repaired. Patients with more severe duodenal injuries may require more complex treatment strategies. A useful algo-

Table 1: Determinants of Duodenal Injury Severity

	Mild	Severe
Determinants of Injury Severity		
Agent	Stab	Blunt or missile
Size	<75% wall	≥75% wall
Duodenal site	3, 4	1, 2
Injury-repair interval (hr)	<24	≥24
Adjacent injury	No CBD	CBD
	No pancreatic injury	Pancreatic injury
Outcome		
Mortality (%)	6%	16%
Duodenal morbidity (%)	6%	14%

CBD, Common bile duct.

rithm approach to the management of duodenal injuries is provided in Figure 2.[27] A classification system for all organ injuries has been developed by the American Association for the Surgery of Trauma (AAST) and is known as the Organ Injury Scale (OIS).[28] This classification for duodenal wounds is listed in Table 2, with duodenal injuries graded from I to V, minor to major injury. In a review of 164 duodenal trauma patients managed at eight trauma centers and to whom the AAST/OIS classification scheme was applied, there were 38 class I, 70 class II, 48 class III, four class IV, and four class V injuries. Primary repair alone was performed in 71% (117) of all cases.[4] Primary duodenal repair was performed in 90 of 108 patients with class I or II injuries. More complex duodenal treatment strategies, including pyloric exclusion, duodenoduodenostomy, duodenojejunostomy, or pancreatoduodenectomy, were employed in 26 of 56 (46%) patients with class III to V injuries, or 29% of the total population.

Primary repair is usually the simplest, fastest, and most appropriate way to manage duodenal injuries.[29] Primary repair is appropriate for complete transection of the duodenum if there is little tissue loss, if the ampulla is not involved, and if the mucosal edges can be debrided and closed without tension. The repair is done as with any

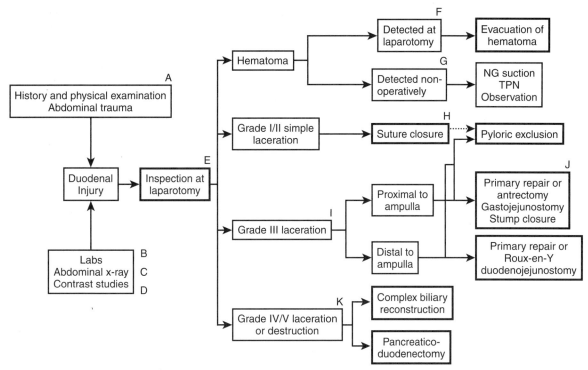

Figure 2 Algorithm for the management of duodenal injuries. *(From Jurkovich G: Duodenal injury. In McIntyre R, Van Stiegmann G, Eiseman B, editors:* Surgical Decision Making, *5th ed. Philadelphia, Elsevier, 2004, pp. 512–513.)*

Table 2: AAST-OIS Grading of Duodenal Injury Severity

Grade	Type	Description
I	Hematoma	Single portion of duodenum
	Laceration	Partial thickness
II	Hematoma	More than one portion
	Laceration	<50% circumference
III	Laceration	50%–75% D2
		50%–100% D1, D3, D4
IV	Laceration	≥75% D2
		Involves ampulla or distal CBD
V	Laceration	Massive disruption of duodeno-pancreatic complex
		Devascularization

AAST-OIS, American Association for the Surgery of Trauma Organ Injury Severity scoring system.
Modified from American Association for the Surgery of Trauma (AAST).

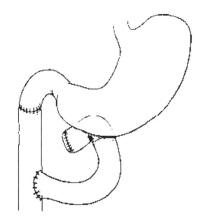

Figure 3 Extensive disruptions of the duodenum may be treated by resection with end-to-end Roux-en-Y duodenojejunostomy. *(From Asensio J, Feliciano D, Britt L, Kerstein M: Management of duodenal injuries.* Curr Probl Surg *11, 1993, p. 1064, figure 9.)*

small bowel repair. I prefer a two-layer closure, but a watertight, serosa-approximating single layer repair is equally acceptable. However, if adequate mobilization for a tension-free repair is impossible, or if the injury is very near the ampulla and mobilization risks common bile duct injury, a Roux-en-Y jejunal limb anastomosis to the proximal duodenal injury with oversewing of the distal duodenal injury is the most reasonable option (Figure 3). Mucosal jejunal patch repair as depicted in Figure 4 is rarely, if ever, used, and was not used in any patient in the most recent multicenter trial in which only five patients (3%) had duodenoduodenostomy or duodenojejunostomy repairs.[4] While historically utilized, a 1985 report by Ivatury et al.[30] demonstrates why this is generally a poor solution to manag-

ing a duodenal wound. In this report of 60 patients with penetrating duodenal injuries, there was a 64% incidence of abdominal sepsis and a 27% death rate in 11 patients with duodenal gunshot wounds, compared with a 7% abdominal sepsis and 0% mortality in 30 patients who had either primary repair of Roux-en-Y anastomotic repair of similar injuries. In 17 patients from that same series with duodenal stab wounds, the complication rate was also higher if the "sucker patch" repair of a duodenal wound was used. It is usually preferable to fully debride the wound and transect the duodenum, mobilize the edges, and perform a direct end-to-end duodeno–duodeno anastomosis. Because the duodenal mesentery is short, this is usually readily accomplished. Pancreatoduodenectomy is only

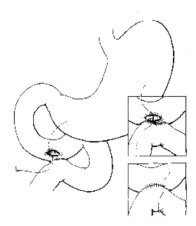

Figure 4 Injuries in which loss of duodenal wall has occurred that cannot be repaired, primarily without severe narrowing of the lumen, may be repaired by use of a serosal patch technique. The serosa of a loop of jejunum is sutured to the edges of the duodenal defect. Experimental studies have demonstrated that the serosa exposed to the duodenal lumen rapidly undergoes complete mucosal resurfacing. *(From Asensio J, Feliciano D, Britt L, Kerstein M: Management of duodenal injuries. Curr Probl Surg 11, 1993, p. 1060, figure 6.)*

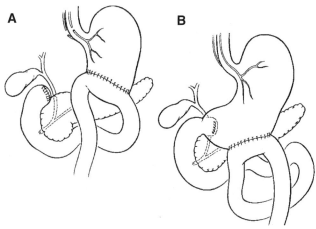

Figure 5 **(A)** Berne diverticulization and **(B)** pyloric exclusion. *(From Jurkovich GJ: Duodenum and pancreas. In Moore EE, Feliciano DV, Mattox K, editors: Trauma, 5th ed. New York, McGraw-Hill, 2004, p. 717.)*

required for duodenal injuries if there is uncontrollable pancreatic hemorrhage or combined duodenal and distal common bile duct or pancreatic duct injury. Most often this represents the completion of a debridement initiated by the injury forces.

Several techniques may help protect a tenuous duodenal repair. Buttressing the repair with omentum (my preference) or a "serosal patch" from a loop of jejunum seems logical, although the benefit of such techniques is unproven.[6,31] Diversion of gastric contents is another option, most commonly accomplished by the Vaughan/Jordan pyloric exclusion technique.[32] Probably first described by Summers in 1904 as an adjunct to treatment of duodenal wounds,[33] pyloric exclusion is a less disruptive procedure than true duodenal "diverticulization" advocated by Berne and Donovan and colleagues[34,35] (Figure 5).

Duodenal "diverticulization" employs primary closure of the duodenal wound, antrectomy, vagotomy, end-to-side gastrojejunostomy, T-tube common bile duct drainage, and lateral tube duodenostomy. The concept is to completely divert both gastric and biliary contents away from the duodenal injury, provide enteral nutrition via the gastrojejunostomy, and convert a potential uncontrolled lateral duodenal fistula to a controlled fistula. A less formidable and less destructive alternative is the "pyloric exclusion," which does not employ antrectomy, biliary diversion, or vagotomy[32,34,36,37] (Figure 6). This procedure is performed through a gastrotomy and consists of grasping the pylorus with a Babcock clamp and suturing closed the pylorus with absorbable size 0 polyglycolic acid or polyglactin, or Maxon® (polyglyconate) or PDS® (polydioxanone) suture and construction of loop gastrojejunostomy. This diverts gastric flow away from the duodenum for several weeks while the duodenal and pancreatic injuries heal. The pylorus eventually opens (2 weeks to 2 months) and the gastrojejunostomy functionally closes. Fang and colleagues[38] at Chang-Gung Memorial Hospital in Taiwan have described a technical method of a controlled release of the pyloric exclusion knot and thereby timing the opening of the pyloric occlusion. Marginal ulceration at the site of gastrojejunostomy has been reported in 5%–33% of patients, prompting some to add truncal vagotomy to the procedure.[14,32,36,38] Most surgeons do not add a truncal vagotomy to pyloric exclusion, however, because nearly all of the pyloric closures open within a few weeks, regardless of the type of suture material used, and the occasional marginal ulcer can be medically managed in the interim. The data supports the use of pyloric exclusion and gastrojejunostomy in "severe" duodenal injuries[7,14] or in cases of delayed diagnosis,[36] although no prospective, randomized trial has proven the true benefit of gastric diversion. In addition, the added operating time and the extra anastomosis suggest a good deal of selectivity should be applied to its use.

Mortality directly related to the duodenal injury is the result of duodenal dehiscence, uncontrolled sepsis, and subsequent

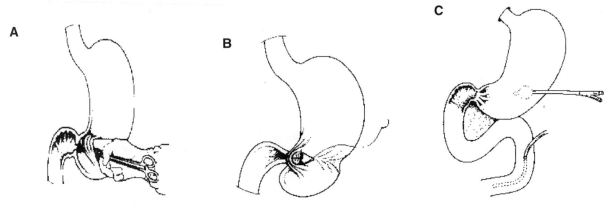

Figure 6 Pyloric exclusion technique.

multiple-system organ failure. Knowledge of the lethal nature of duodenal dehiscence and duodenal fistula certainly tempts the operating surgeon to add pyloric exclusion, anastomosis buttressing, and duodenostomy to the repair of class III or IV duodenal injuries. As noted previously, concomitant pancreatic injury should also be included as a high-risk confounder that might warrant pyloric exclusion added to the duodenal repair. In one report of 40 patients with penetrating duodenal injuries, there were 14 patients with combined duodenal and pancreatic wounds. Five patients with this combination of injuries had primary duodenal repair alone, and two incurred duodenal leaks. Three of the patients with combined injuries had pyloric exclusion as a treatment adjunct, and none had duodenal leaks.[39]

An alternative or addition to gastric diversion is duodenal decompression via retrograde jejunostomy. Stone and Fabian[10] reported a fistula rate of less than 0.5% (1 in 237 patients) in a variety of duodenal injuries all treated by retrograde jejunostomy tube drainage, in contrast to a 19.3% incidence of duodenal complications when decompression was not used. Retrograde duodenodenal drainage is preferred to lateral duodenostomy. Direct drainage with a tube through the suture line results in a high dehiscence or fistula rate of 23%. Hasson and colleagues[40] reviewed the literature up to 1984 on penetrating duodenal trauma and tube duodenostomy, evaluating eight retrospective series and over 550 patients. They reported overall mortality of 19.4% and a fistula rate of 11.8% without decompression, compared with 9% mortality and 2.3% fistula rate with decompression. They too concluded that tube drainage should be performed either via stomach or retrograde jejunostomy, as these methods had a lower fistula rate and less overall mortality than lateral tube duodenostomy. Nonetheless, as is the case of pyloric exclusion for gastric diversion, there has been no prospective, randomized analysis of the efficacy of tube duodenal drainage techniques, and not all surgeons support use of decompression techniques.

In very massive injuries of the proximal duodenum and head of the pancreas, destruction of the ampulla and proximal pancreatic duct or distal common bile duct may preclude reconstruction. In addition, because the duodenum and the head of the pancreas have a common arterial supply, it is essentially impossible to entirely resect one without making the other ischemic. In this situation, a pancreatoduodenectomy is required. Between 1961 and 1994, 184 Whipple procedures were reported for trauma, with 26 operative deaths (14%) and 39 delayed deaths, for a 64% overall survival rate.[41] With appropriate selection criteria, pancreatoduodenectomy for injury can be performed with similar morbidity and mortality as described in resections done for cancer.[42–44]

DUODENAL HEMATOMA

Duodenal hematoma is generally considered an injury of childhood play or child abuse, but can occur in adults as well. In one report, 50% of the cases of duodenal hematoma in children resulted from child abuse.[45] Remarkably, the duodenum is the fourth most commonly injured intra-abdominal organ after blunt abdominal trauma, occurring in 2%–10% of children.[46] Nearly one-third of the patients present with obstruction of insidious onset at least 48 hours after injury, presumably the result of fluid shift into the hyperosmotic duodenal hematoma. Duodenal hematoma in general represents a nonsurgical injury, in that the best results are obtained with conservative or nonsurgical management.[47] It can be diagnosed either by contrast-enhanced CT scan or upper gastrointestinal (UGI) study (Figure 7). The initial water-soluble contrast (meglumine diatrizoate) exam should be followed by barium to provide the greater detail needed to detect the so-called "coiled spring" or "stacked coin" sign. Although characteristic of intramural duodenal hematoma, this finding is present in only approximately one-quarter of patients with hematoma.

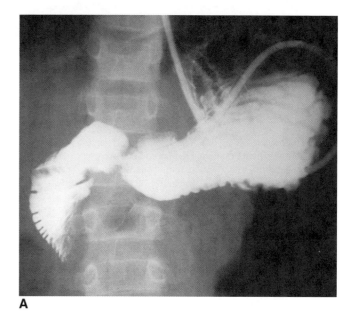

A

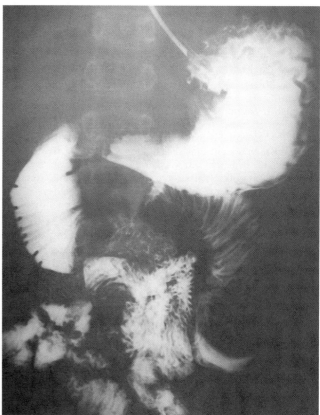

B

Figure 7 Duodenal hematoma. The two images are sequential. **(A)** Initial showing near total duodenal obstruction. **(B)** Portrays contrast passage into the jejunum. The hematoma has infiltrated the wall, producing fold thickening, loop narrowing, and displacement. The mesentery is also involved, and there is a pronounced hematoma component nearly occluding the first jejunal loop. This case shows the characteristic involvement of the duodenum as it traverses the spine, sparing, but obstructing, the proximal duodenal (1 and 2) segments.

Although the initial treatment is nonoperative, associated injuries should be excluded, particularly pancreatic injury. Desai et al.[46] reported that 42% of pediatric patients with a duodenal injury (perforation or hematoma) had a concomitant pancreatic injury, and Jewett et al.[47] found a 20% incidence of pancreatic injury in patients with a duodenal hematoma. Continuous nasogastric suction should be employed and total parenteral nutrition begun. The patient should be re-evaluated with UGI contrast studies at 5–7-day intervals if signs of obstruction do not spontaneously abate. Ultrasound has also been used to follow a resolving duodenal hematoma.[48] Percutaneous drainage of an unresolving duodenal hematoma has been reported,[49,50] but operative exploration and evacuation of the hematoma is usually recommended after 2 weeks of conservative therapy to rule out stricture, duodenal perforation, or injury to the head of the pancreas as factors that might be contributing to the obstruction.[51] One review of six cases of duodenal and jejunal hematomas resulting from blunt trauma demonstrated resolution with nonoperative management in five of the six patients, with an average hospital stay of 16 days (range, 10–23 days), and total parenteral nutrition of 9 days (range, 4–16 days). The sixth case had evidence of complete bowel obstruction on UGI series, which failed to resolve after 18 days of conservative management. Laparotomy revealed jejunal and colonic strictures with fibrosis, which were successfully resected.[52] Another report included 19 cases of duodenal hematoma in children, 17 (89%) managed nonoperatively and 2 patients in operative incision and drainage occurred within the first 24 hours and never attempted nonoperative management.[46] Nasogastric decompression and total parenteral nutrition were employed for an average of 9.3 (±7.7) days (range, 2–29 days), with an average hospital stay of 16.4 (±17.8) days (range, 2–37 days).

If a duodenal hematoma is incidentally found at celiotomy, a thorough inspection must ensue to exclude perforation. This will require an extended Kocher maneuver, which usually successfully drains the subserosal hematoma. It is unclear whether the serosa of the duodenum should intentionally be incised along its extent to "evacuate" the hematoma, or whether this in fact increases the likelihood of converting a partial duodenal wall tear into a complete perforation. Unless my index of suspicion is very high for a full-thickness duodenal wall injury, I generally do not open a duodenal hematoma found incidentally, although I do inspect it carefully. A feeding jejunostomy should be placed, because an extended period of gastric decompression will likely be required.

REFERENCES

1. Ballard RB, Badellino MM, Eynon CA, Spott MA, Staz CF, Buckman RF Jr: Blunt duodenal rupture: a 6-year statewide experience. *J Trauma* 43(2): 229–232discussion 33, 1997.
2. Asensio J, Feliciano D, Britt L, Kerstein M: Management of duodenal injuries. *Curr Probl Surg* 11:1021, 1993.
3. Cuddington G, Rusnak C, Cameron R, Carter J: Management of duodenal injuries. *Can J Surg* 33(1):41–44, 1990.
4. Cogbill T, Moore E, Feliciano D, et al: Conservative management of duodenal trauma: a multicenter perspective. *J Trauma* 30(22):1469–1475, 1990.
5. Flint L, McCoy M, Richardson J, Polk H: Duodenal injury: analysis of common misconceptions in diagnosis and treatment. *Ann Surg* 191(6):697–702, 1980.
6. Ivatury R, Nallathambi M, Gaudino J, Rohman M, Stahl W: Penetrating duodenal injuries: an analysis of 100 consecutive cases. *Ann Surg* 202(2):154–158, 1985.
7. Kashuk J, Moore E, Cogbill T: Management of the intermediate severity duodenal injury. *Surgery* 92:758–764, 1982.
8. Levison M, Petersen S, Sheldon G: Duodenal trauma: experience of a trauma center. *J Trauma* 24(6):475–480, 1984.
9. Snyder W, Weigelt J, Watkins W, Bietz D: The surgical management of duodenal trauma. *Arch Surg* 115:422–429, 1980.
10. Stone H, Fabian T: Management of duodenal wounds. *J Trauma* 19(5): 334–339, 1979.
11. Vasquez JC, Coimbra R, Hoyt DB, Fortlage D: Management of penetrating pancreatic trauma: an 11-year experience of a level-1 trauma center. *Injury* 32(10):753–759, 2001.
12. Shorr R, Greaney G, Donovan A: Injuries of the duodenum. *Am J Surg* 154(7):93–98, 1987.
13. Jurkovich GJ, Bulger E: Duodenum and pancreas. In Moore EE, Feliciano DV, Mattox K, editors: *Trauma*, 5th ed. New York, McGraw-Hill, 2004, pp. 709–733.
14. Martin T, Feliciano D, Mattox K, Jordon G: Severe duodenal injuries: treatment with pyloric exclusion and gastrojejunostomy. *Arch Surg* 118: 631–635, 1983.
15. Heitsch R, Knutson C, Fulton R, et al: Delineation of critical factors in the treatment of pancreatic injury. *Surgery* 80(4):523–529, 1976.
16. Sukul K, Lont H, Johannes E: Management of pancreatic injuries. *Hepatogastroenterology* 39:447–450, 1992.
17. Roman E, Silva Y, Lucas C: Management of blunt duodenal injury. *Surg Gynecol Obstet* 132:7–14, 1971.
18. Lucas C, Ledgerwood A: Factors influencing outcome after blunt duodenal injury. *J Trauma* 15(10):839–846, 1975.
19. Smego DR, Richardson JD, Flint LM: Determinants of outcome in pancreatic trauma. *J Trauma* 25(8):771–776, 1985.
20. Anatomy and physiology of the duodenum. In Shackelford R, Zuidema G, editors: *Surgery of the Alimentary Tract*. Philadelphia, WB Saunders, 1981, pp. 38–45.
21. Edwards E, Malone P, MacArthur J: *Operative Anatomy of Abdomen and Pelvis*. Philadelphia, Lea & Febiger, 1975.
22. Sherck J, Oakes D: Intestinal injuries missed by computed tomography. *J Trauma* 30(1):1–5, 1990.
23. Mirvis S, Gens D, Shanmuganathan K: Rupture of the bowel after blunt abdominal trauma: diagnosis with CT. *Am J Roentgenol* 159(6): 1217–1221, 1992.
24. Timaran CH, Daley BJ, Enderson BL: Role of duodenography in the diagnosis of blunt duodenal injuries. *J Trauma* 51(4):648–651, 2001.
25. Allen G, Moore F, Cox CJ, Mehall J, Duke J: Delayed diagnosis of blunt duodenal injury: an avoidable complication. *J Am Coll Surg* 187:393–399, 1998.
26. Asensio JA, Demetriades D, Berne JD, et al: A unified approach to the surgical exposure of pancreatic and duodenal injuries. *Am J Surg* 174(1):54–60, 1997.
27. Jurkovich G: Duodenal injury. In McIntyre R, Van Stiegmann G, Eiseman B, editors: *Surgical Decision Making*, 5th ed. Philadelphia, Elsevier, 2004, pp. 512–513.
28. Moore E, Cogbill T, Malangoni M, et al: Organ injury scaling II: pancreas, duodenum, small bowel, colon, and rectum. *J Trauma* 30(11):1427–1429, 1990.
29. Asensio J, Feliciano D, Britt L, Kerstein M: Management of duodenal injuries. *Curr Probl Surg* 11:1021–1100, 1993.
30. Ivatury R, Gaudino J, Ascer E, Nallathambi M, Ramirez-Schon G, Stahl W: Treatment of penetrating duodenal injuries: primary repair vs. repair with decompressive enterostomy/serosal patch. *J Trauma* 25(4):337–341, 1985.
31. McInnis W, Aust J, Cruz A, et al: Traumatic injuries of the duodenum: a comparison of primary closure and the jejunal patch. *J Trauma* 15: 847–858, 1975.
32. Vaughan G, Grazier O, Graham D, et al: The use of pyloric exclusion in the management of severe duodenal injuries. *Am J Surg* 134:785–790, 1977.
33. Summers JJ: The treatment of posterior perforations of the fixed portions of the duodenum. *Ann Surg* 39:727, 1904.
34. Berne C, Donovan A, White E, et al: Duodenal "diverticulization" for duodenal and pancreatic injury. *Am J Surg* 127:503–505, 1974.
35. Donovan A, Hagen W, Berne D: Traumatic perforations of the duodenum. *Am J Surg* 111:341–350, 1966.
36. Buck JR, Sorensen VJ, Fath JJ, Horst HM, Obeid FN: Severe pancreaticoduodenal injuries: the effectiveness of pyloric exclusion with vagotomy. *Am Surg* 58(9):557–560discussion 561, 1992.
37. Cogbill T, Moore E, Kashuk J: Changing trends in the management of pancreatic trauma. *Arch Surg* 117:722–728, 1982.
38. Fang JF, Chen RJ, Lin BC: Controlled reopen suture technique for pyloric exclusion. *J Trauma* 45(3):593–596, 1998.
39. McKenney MG, Nir I, Levi DM, Martin L: Evaluation of minor penetrating duodenal injuries. *Am Surg* 62(11):952–955, 1996.
40. Hasson J, Stern D, Moss G: Penetrating duodenal trauma. *J Trauma* 24(6):471–474, 1984.
41. Delcore R, Stauffer J, Thomas J, Pierce G: The role of pancreatogastrostomy following pancreatoduodenectomy for trauma. *J Trauma* 37(3): 395–400, 1994.

42. Heimansohn DA, Canal DF, McCarthy MC, Yaw PB, Madura JA, Broadie TA: The role of pancreaticoduodenectomy in the management of traumatic injuries to the pancreas and duodenum. *Am Surg* 56(8):511–514, 1990.

43. McKone T, Bursch L, Scholten D: Pancreaticoduodenectomy for trauma: a life saving procedure. *Am Surg* 54(6):361–364, 1988.

44. Oreskovich M, Carrico C: Pancreaticoduodenectomy for trauma: a viable option? *Am J Surg* 147(5):618–623, 1984.

45. Wooley M, Mahour G, Sloan T: Duodenal hematoma in infancy and childhood. *Am J Surg* 136:8–14, 1978.

46. Desai KM, Dorward IG, Minkes RK, Dillon PA: Blunt duodenal injuries in children. *J Trauma* 54(4):640–645, discussion 645–646, 2003.

47. Jewett TJ, Caldarola V, Karp M, Allen J, Cooney D: Intramural hematoma of the duodenum. *Arch Surg* 123(1):54–58, 1988.

48. Megremis S, Segkos N, Andrianaki A, et al: Sonographic diagnosis and monitoring of an obstructing duodenal hematoma after blunt trauma: correlation with computed tomographic and surgical findings. *J Ultrasound Med* 23(12):1679–1683, 2004.

49. Gullotto C, Paulson EK: CT-guided percutaneous drainage of a duodenal hematoma. *Am J Roentgenol* 184(1):231–233, 2005.

50. Kortbeek JB, Brown M, Steed B: Percutaneous drainage of a duodenal haematoma. *Injury* 28(5–6):419–420, 1997.

51. Touloukian R: Protocol for the nonoperative treatment of obstructing intramural duodenal hematoma. *Am J Surg* 145:330–335, 1983.

52. Czyrko C, Weltz C, Markowitz R, O'Neill J: Blunt abdominal trauma resulting in intestinal obstruction: when to operate? *J Trauma* 30(12):1567–1571, 1990.

PANCREATIC INJURIES

Louis J. Magnotti   and   Martin A. Croce

The pancreas is relatively protected deep within the confines of the retroperitoneum. As such, injuries to the pancreas are uncommon, but not rare, and can present a diagnostic dilemma. In fact, despite advances in modern trauma care, there remains significant morbidity and mortality, with mortality rates ranging from 9%–34%.[1] Frequent complications are also common following pancreatic injuries, occurring in 30%–60% of patients. The high complication rate associated with these injuries is primarily secondary to diagnostic delays and missed injuries. When identified early, the treatment of most pancreatic injuries is straightforward. It is the delayed recognition and/or treatment of these injuries that can result in devastating outcomes.

There are few well-documented historical accounts about the management of pancreatic injuries. The first documented case of pancreatic trauma was an autopsy report from St. Thomas Hospital in London in 1827 in which a patient struck by the wheel of a stagecoach suffered a complete pancreatic body transection.[2] Over the next several decades, reports of pancreatic injuries were scattered. In 1903, after extensive review of the literature, only 45 cases of pancreatic trauma, 21 resulting from penetrating injuries and 24 from blunt trauma could be identified.[3] The occurrence of complications following pancreatic injury was also noted early. In 1905, Korte[4] reported a case of an isolated pancreatic transection with resultant pancreatic fistula. The fistula closed spontaneously and the patient survived.

The following chapter attempts to clarify the anatomic and physiologic basis for the concerns over injuries to the pancreas as well as elucidate specific diagnostic and therapeutic interventions after traumatic injuries to the pancreas.

ANATOMY

A complete understanding of pancreatic relational anatomy is essential for providing appropriate treatment and understanding the potential for associated injuries. The pancreas is about 15–20 cm in length, 3.1 cm wide, and 1–1.5 cm thick. The average mass is 90 g (ranging from 40 to 180 g).[5] The inferior vena cava, aorta, left kidney, both renal veins, and right renal artery lie posterior to the pancreas. The head of the pancreas is nestled in the duodenal sweep, with the body crossing the spine and the tail resting within the hilum of the spleen. The splenic artery and vein can be found along the superior border of the pancreas. The superior mesenteric artery and vein reside just behind the neck of the pancreas and are enclosed posteriorly by the uncinate process. This process can be absent or can almost completely encircle the superior mesenteric artery and vein.

The head of the pancreas is suspended from the liver by the hepatoduodenal ligament and is firmly fixed to the medial aspect of the second and third portions of the duodenum. A line extending from the portal vein superiorly to the superior mesenteric vein inferiorly marks the division between the head and the neck of the gland. The neck of the pancreas measures approximately 1.5–2 cm in length and lies at the level of the first lumbar vertebra. It overlies the superior mesenteric vessels and is fixed between them and the celiac trunk superiorly. The body of the pancreas is technically defined as that portion of the pancreas that lies to the left of the superior mesenteric vessels. There is no true anatomic division between the body and the tail, nor is there any imaginary dividing line as in the case of the head and neck.

The main pancreatic duct of Wirsung originates in the tail of the pancreas and typically traverses the entire length of the gland and joins the common bile duct before emptying into the duodenum. Throughout its course in the tail and body, the duct lies midway between the superior and inferior margins and slightly more posterior. The accessory duct of Santorini usually branches out from the pancreatic duct in the neck of the pancreas and empties separately into the duodenum. A significant number of anatomic variants exist and must be recognized: (1) in 60% of individuals, the ducts open separately into the duodenum; (2) in 30%, the duct of Wirsung carries the entire glandular secretion and the duct of Santorini ends blindly; and (3) in 10%, the duct of Santorini carries the entire secretion of the gland and the duct of Wirsung is either small or absent. In all cases, the ducts lie anterior to the major pancreatic vessels.

The arterial and venous blood supply of the pancreas is relatively constant. The arterial blood supply of the pancreas originates from both the celiac trunk and the superior mesenteric artery. The blood supply to the head of the pancreas appears to be the greatest, with less flow to the body and tail and the least to the neck. The veins, like the arteries, are found posterior to the ducts, lie superficial to the arteries, and parallel the arteries for the most part throughout their course. The venous drainage of the pancreas is to the portal, splenic, and superior mesenteric vein.

PHYSIOLOGY

The pancreas is a compound tubuloalveolar gland with both endocrine (insulin, glucagon, somatostatin) and exocrine (digestive enzyme precursors, bicarbonate) function. The endocrine cells are separated histologically into nests of cells known as the islets of

Langerhans. There are three predominant subtypes of islet cells: alpha cells (which produce glucagon), beta cells (which produce insulin), and delta cells (which produce somatostatin). Although these cells are distributed throughout the substance of the pancreas, most reside primarily within the tail. Consequently, it would seem that a distal pancreatectomy would be poorly tolerated in terms of endocrine function. However, it is well known that resection of more than 90% of the pancreas must occur before endocrine insufficiency develops, provided the remainder of the gland is normal. In fact, partial resection induces hypertrophy and increased activity of the residual islet cells. In animal studies, Dragstedt[6] was the first to show that removal of 80% of the pancreas did not significantly alter carbohydrate or fat metabolism or the digestion and/or absorption of food, provided that the remaining gland is normal and that pancreatic secretions still have access to the upper digestive tract via the ductal system.

DIAGNOSIS

It is important to remember that whenever there is trauma to the pancreas, particular attention must be given to the possibility of a major ductal injury for this is the single most important determinant of outcome after pancreatic injury. In fact, this concept was first recognized as early as 1962.[7] Subsequent investigators have confirmed and reemphasized the necessity of determining the status of the pancreatic duct. In fact, Heitsch et al.[8] found that distal resection of ductal injuries significantly lowered postoperative morbidity and mortality when compared with drainage alone. This finding was confirmed over a decade later when investigators documented a drop in mortality rate from 19%–3% after pancreatic resection proximal to the site of ductal injury.[9]

Successful diagnosis of a pancreatic injury requires a high index of suspicion. The mechanism of injury, need for laparotomy, and time interval following initial abdominal insult will direct the trauma surgeon to the most appropriate procedures and tests. Those patients with need for immediate laparotomy require little or no preoperative evaluation, as the diagnosis of pancreatic injury can be made at the time of exploration. Conversely, patients without clear need for operative exploration may require extensive efforts to establish the presence of a pancreatic injury.

Pancreatic injuries typically result from high-energy transfer to the upper abdomen. In adults, motor vehicle accidents are the primary cause of pancreatic injuries, usually secondary to impact of the steering wheel. In children, the typical scenario involves a handlebar injury to the epigastrium. In any case, the energy of impact is directed at the upper abdomen (epigastrium or hypochondrium), resulting in crushing of the retroperitoneal structures. Typical findings suggestive of retroperitoneal injury include contusion/bruising to the upper abdomen with epigastric pain out of proportion to physical examination.

Elevated serum amylase is not a reliable indicator of pancreatic trauma. In fact, the use of amylase as a screening tool in blunt trauma carries a negative predictive value of 95%.[10] Measurement of the pancreatic isoamylase fraction has failed to substantially improve both the sensitivity and specificity of this value as a marker of pancreatic injury.

Asymptomatic patients with elevated serum pancreatic isoamylase require observation and repeat amylase determination. Persistently elevated serum amylase or the development of abdominal symptomatology warrants further investigation and may include computed tomography (CT) scan, endoscopic retrograde cholangiopancreatography (ERCP), or operative exploration. Abdominal CT scans have a reported sensitivity and specificity as high as 80% in diagnosing pancreatic injury.[11] Patton and colleagues[12] reported that in 26 patients that sustained blunt pancreatic trauma, early CT scan was suspicious for injury in 15. CT failed to demonstrate injury in four patients (21%), resulting in a delay in operative intervention (mean, 3.8 days). The remaining patients had other indications for exploration.

Computed tomography findings diagnostic of pancreatic injury include parenchymal disruption, intrapancreatic hematoma, fluid in the lesser sac or separating the splenic vein and body of the pancreas, peripancreatic edema, thickened left anterior renal fascia, and retroperitoneal hematoma and/or fluid. Clearly, certain findings are more reliable than others and rarely are all present in a single patient. In fact, some of the CT signs of pancreatic injury may not be immediately apparent following injury, but rather require time to develop postinjury. It is important to remember this when evaluating the patient with worsening abdominal symptoms and an unimpressive initial CT scan.

Endoscopic retrograde cholangiopancreatography can be useful in the diagnosis of pancreatic duct rupture. In addition, it can aid in the diagnosis of and occasionally the management of the complications of missed pancreatic injuries. A report from the University of Louisville documents ERCP as a useful diagnostic tool in the evaluation of the pancreatic duct in the early postinjury period in hemodynamically stable patients with elevated amylase levels, persistent abdominal pain, and abnormal or questionable abdominal CT findings.[13] ERCP is also extremely helpful in the evaluation of patients in whom the diagnosis of pancreatic injury was missed during the initial evaluation. It is in these patients that ERCP can aid in diagnosing the injury, planning the surgical approach if necessary, determining internal transpancreatic stent placement, and transductal drainage of a pancreatic abscess. However, ERCP may not always be available and should not delay operation in patients with progressive clinical deterioration.

Magnetic resonance (MR) imaging, specifically MRCP (magnetic resonance cholangiopancreatography), has emerged as an alternative technique for evaluating the pancreatic duct. Although primarily used in elective circumstances, MRCP has been reported as a viable option for evaluating the status of the duct in those patients with pancreatic injuries.[14] However, it frequently is not practical for use in trauma patients.

In order to successfully diagnose the presence and extent of a potential pancreatic injury, the surgeon must recognize those findings associated with pancreatic injury and adequately visualize the entire gland. In addition, it is also imperative to determine the integrity of the pancreatic parenchyma and status of the major pancreatic duct. Pancreatic injuries are classified based on the status of the duct and the anatomic location of the injury within the gland. Associated injuries often complicate pancreatic evaluation. The presence of a central retroperitoneal hematoma or a hematoma overlying the pancreas, retroperitoneal saponification or bile staining mandates complete pancreatic exploration.

Once again, it must be stressed that, if possible, it is important to determine the status of the duct at the time of exploration. Most of these injuries can be diagnosed by local exploration. Injuries to the duct occur in approximately 15% of pancreatic trauma and are generally the result of penetrating injury.[15] Blunt injury can also result in transection of the major duct with or without complete transection of the gland. Minor contusions and/or lacerations of the pancreatic parenchyma usually do not require further evaluation of the duct. However, an intact pancreatic capsule does not eliminate the possibility of complete transection of the pancreatic duct.[9]

The use of intraoperative observations such as direct visualization of ductal disruption, complete transection of the substance of the gland, free leakage of pancreatic fluid, lacerations involving more than one-half of the diameter of the gland, central perforations, and severe lacerations with or without massive tissue disruption can predict the presence of a major ductal injury with a high degree of accuracy. However, in those instances in which the status of the duct is uncertain, intraoperative pancreatography has been used as a technique for visualization of the main pancreatic duct. While intraoperative pancreatography may sound appealing, it is frequently impractical.

Nevertheless, pancreatography can be performed either by directly cannulating the ampulla of Vater through a duodenotomy or the main pancreatic duct through the amputated tail of the pancreas.

A 5F pediatric feeding tube is used along with 2–5 ml of contrast. Cannulating the ampulla of Vater entails creating a duodenotomy unless there is an associated duodenal injury. It should be stressed that identifying the ampulla can be difficult and that resection of the tail does not always ensure visualization of the pancreatic duct.

The simplest technique is a needle cholecystocholangiogram. In this technique, a purse-string suture is placed in the gallbladder just proximal to the cystic duct. An 18-gauge angiocatheter is then introduced into the gallbladder. The remainder of the gallbladder can be excluded with a bowel clamp. Water-soluble contrast is injected into the gallbladder under direct fluoroscopy. A cholecystectomy is not necessary following this procedure.

CLASSIFICATION OF PANCREATIC INJURIES

Although a number of classification systems have been devised to categorize pancreatic injuries, the American Association for the Surgery of Trauma (AAST) Committee on Organ Injury Scaling addresses the key issues of treatment of parenchymal disruption and major pancreatic ductal injury by focusing on the anatomic location of the injury (Table 1). Proximal duct injuries require different management than do distal duct and parenchymal injuries. The difficulty arises in those patients with parenchymal disruption and major duct injury. This classification scheme provides a useful management guide by focusing on the anatomic location of the duct and parenchymal injury (proximal vs. distal).

SURGICAL MANAGEMENT OF PANCREATIC INJURIES

As with any case of abdominal trauma, the primary operative focus is control of ongoing hemorrhage and gastrointestinal contamination. Once these have been addressed, systemic abdominal exploration should include recognition and evaluation of the possibility of pancreatic injury.

Proper evaluation of the pancreas requires complete exposure of the gland. Access to the pancreas is best accomplished by opening the lesser sac. That is, by dividing the gastrocolic omentum inferior to the gastroepiploic vessels, the anterior surface and the superior and inferior borders of the body and tail of the pancreas can be visualized. The transverse colon is retracted inferiorly and the stomach superiorly (Figure 1). The nasogastric tube may be advanced along the greater curvature of the stomach and can be used as a handle for retraction of the stomach. An adequate Kocher maneuver will allow complete visualization of the pancreatic head and uncinate process.

Table 1: Pancreatic Organ Injury Scale: American Association for the Surgery of Trauma

Grade		Injury Description
I	Hematoma	Minor contusion without duct injury
	Laceration	Superficial laceration without duct injury
II	Hematoma	Major contusion without duct injury or tissue loss
	Laceration	Major laceration without duct injury or tissue loss
III	Laceration	Distal transection or parenchymal injury with duct injury
IV	Laceration	Proximal (right of superior mesenteric vein) transection or parenchymal injury
V	Laceration	Massive disruption of pancreatic head

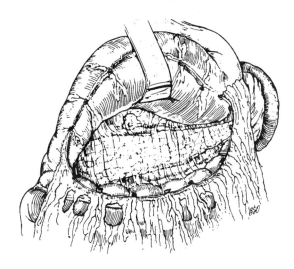

Figure 1   Transection of the gastrocolic ligament with superior retraction of the stomach and inferior retraction of the transverse colon allows complete visualization of the body and tail of the pancreas.   *(From Asensio JA, Demetriades D, Berne JD, et al: A unified approach to the surgical exposure of pancreatic and duodenal injuries. Am J Surg 174:54–60, 1997.)*

This is accomplished by incising the lateral peritoneal attachments of the duodenum and sweeping the second and third portions medially with a combination of both blunt and sharp dissection (Figure 2). If a large retroperitoneal hematoma is encountered, the nasogastric tube should be advanced through the pylorus and used as a palpable guide to avoid iatrogenic injury to the duodenal wall. The Kocher

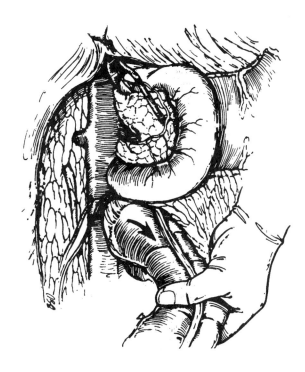

Figure 2   The Kocher maneuver is performed by incising the lateral attachments of the duodenum and sweeping the second and third portions medially.   *(From Asensio JA, Demetriades D, Berne JD, et al: A unified approach to the surgical exposure of pancreatic and duodenal injuries. Am J Surg 174:54–60, 1997.)*

maneuver should be extensive enough that the left renal vein is easily identified. Occasionally, mobilization of the hepatic flexure is necessary to adequately evaluate the pancreatic head. If the tail of the pancreas is involved, exposure of the splenic hilum is necessary. Division of the peritoneal attachments lateral to the spleen and colon facilitate mobilization. A plane is then created between the spleen, colon and pancreas anteriorly and the kidney posteriorly. This maneuver allows for inspection of the posterior surface of the pancreas (Figure 3).

Approximately 60% of all pancreatic injuries consist of minor contusions, hematomas, and capsular lacerations (Figure 4). Lacera-

tions of the pancreatic parenchyma without major ductal disruption or tissue loss account for an additional 20% of pancreatic injuries (Figure 5). These injuries require only hemostasis and adequate external drainage.[12] The temptation to repair capsular lacerations should be resisted, as this tends to lead to pseudocyst formation, whereas a controlled pancreatic fistula is usually self-limited. Closed-suction drains should be used for drainage of any pancreatic injury. These drains are better tolerated by the patient in terms of decreased intra-abdominal abscess formation, more reliable collection of the effluent and less skin excoriation.[16] Typically, these drains are left in place for a minimum of 10 days, because if a fistula is going to develop, it should be evident by that time.

Nutritional support can be provided via either the oral or gastric route almost immediately. However, with more severe injuries, prolonged gastric ileus and potential pancreatic complications may preclude standard feeding. In addition, the majority of tube feed formulations increase pancreatic stimulation and, in turn, pancreatic effluent and amylase concentration. Elemental diets (low fat, higher pH) are less stimulating to the pancreas, and may be useful in these situations.[17] Intraoperative placement of a feeding jejunostomy at the time of initial exploration should be considered for all patients with grade III–V injuries. These allow for early postoperative enteral feeding and avert the need for total parenteral nutrition in those patients unable to tolerate either oral or gastric feedings.

Distal parenchymal transection, especially with disruption of the main pancreatic duct (Figure 6), is best treated with distal pancreatectomy. In general, the anatomic distinction between proximal and distal pancreas is defined by the superior mesenteric vessels passing behind the pancreas at the junction of the head and body. Provided that the proximal duct is normal, the transected duct should be closed with either a "U" stitch or a "figure of eight" with direct suture ligation.[18] Although normal endocrine and exocrine function has been reported after 90% pancreatectomy, efforts should be made to leave at least 20% residual pancreatic tissue to minimize postoperative complications.

The technique of pancreatic transection depends on individual preference. Interlocking "U" stitches with nonabsorbable sutures placed through the full thickness of the gland from anterior to posterior capsule help minimize potential leak from the transected parenchyma. Others prefer to use stapling devices for closure of the pancreatic parenchyma[19] (Figure 7). Whatever technique is used for resection and closure of the pancreatic parenchyma, the duct itself (if

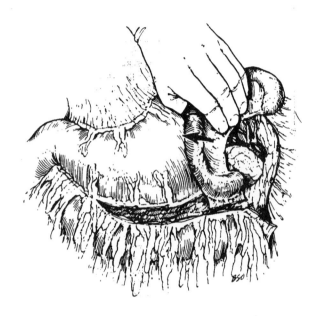

Figure 3   Mobilization of the spleen from a lateral to a medial position to visualize the spleen and posterior aspects of the tail of the pancreas.   *(From Asensio JA, Demetriades D, Berne JD, et al: A unified approach to the surgical exposure of pancreatic and duodenal injuries. Am J Surg 174:54–60, 1997.)*

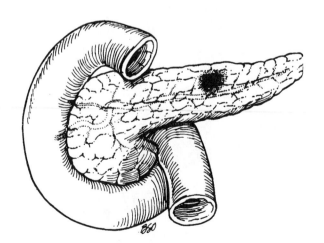

Figure 4   Pancreatic contusion or minor hematoma does not violate the capsule.   *(From Asensio JA, Demetriades D, Berne TV: Atlas and Textbook of Techniques in Complex Trauma Surgery. Philadelphia, Saunders, 2005.)*

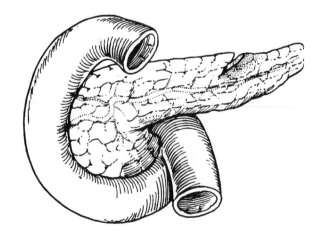

Figure 5   Pancreatic parenchymal injury without ductal injury.   *(From Asensio JA, Demetriades D, Berne TV: Atlas and Textbook of Techniques in Complex Trauma Surgery. Philadelphia, Saunders, 2005.)*

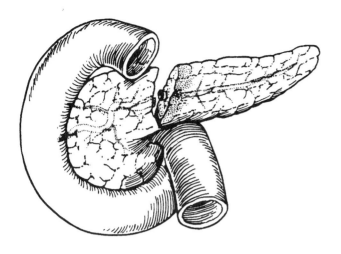

Figure 6 Pancreatic parenchymal disruption with ductal injury. *(From Asensio JA, Demetriades D, Berne TV: Atlas and Textbook of Techniques in Complex Trauma Surgery. Philadelphia, Saunders, 2005.)*

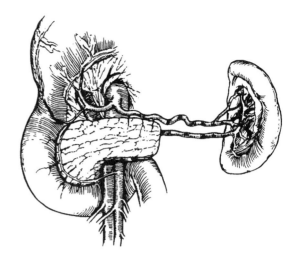

Figure 8 Distal pancreas resection with preservation of the spleen. *(From Asensio JA, Demetriades D, Berne TV: Atlas and Textbook of Techniques in Complex Trauma Surgery. Philadelphia, Saunders, 2005.)*

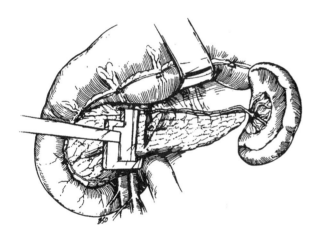

Figure 7 Distal pancreatectomy with the TA stapler. The splenic vessels should be ligated before transection of the pancreas. *(From Asensio JA, Demetriades D, Berne TV: Atlas and Textbook of Techniques in Complex Trauma Surgery. Philadelphia, Saunders, 2005.)*

visible) should be identified and individually ligated. If available, a small omental patch can be placed over the area of resection to buttress stump closure. A closed-suction drain should be left near the transection line, similar to injuries undergoing external drainage.

Distal pancreatectomy can be performed with or without splenectomy. The technical challenge in pancreatectomy without splenectomy involves isolating splenic branch vessels and avoiding injury to the splenic hilum (Figure 8). These, in turn, lead to increased operative time and potential blood loss. Nevertheless, the decision to proceed with splenic salvage requires a completely hemodynamically stable normothermic patient. The risk for postsplenectomy sepsis must also be considered. Generous mobilization of the entire pancreatic gland and spleen must be accomplished before even attempting splenic salvage. Transection of the gland just proximal to the point of injury is followed by elevation of the distal body with meticulous

attention to individual ligation of the numerous arterial and venous tributaries found along the superior border of the gland.

The most challenging management problems arise with injuries to the pancreatic head. Although important with all pancreatic injuries, it is essential to define ductal anatomy for all proximal pancreatic injuries. Intraoperative pancreatography is an important technique for these situations. If local inspection and exploration of the defect fails to exclude ductal injury and intraoperative pancreatography is not an option, wide external drainage with postoperative ERCP is a viable alternative. In fact, because of the high morbidity associated with proximal pancreatic duct injury, closed-suction drainage should be used in virtually all cases of proximal pancreatic injury.[12]

The importance of adequate external drainage cannot be stressed enough. In fact, the pancreas, when injured, can be an unforgiving organ. Uncontrolled leakage of pancreatic juice (especially pancreatic enzymes) normally used for digestion either into the retroperitoneum or intraperitoneally can cause significant injury to the patient by digesting the retroperitoneum and suture lines used to repair bowel and/or blood vessels.

Adequate external drainage is effective for injuries to the pancreatic head and neck in the absence of major ductal injury. Similarly, if the patient is hemodynamically unstable and the status of the proximal duct is uncertain, wide external drainage with postoperative ERCP is recommended. Patton and colleagues report the effectiveness of drainage alone for proximal pancreatic injuries.[12] Of the 37 patients with proximal pancreatic injuries managed with closed-suction drainage, only 13.5% developed either a fistula or abscess.

In the case of incomplete pancreatic parenchymal transection, some surgeons have described an end jejunum to side pancreas anastomosis. This technique is mentioned for historical interest only and is not recommended because of the difficulty in ensuring the integrity of the anastomosis and potential for a high output pancreatic fistula from the posterior aspect of the injury. Stone and coworkers[20] have illustrated the high complication rate associated with this dated technique. Of the 7 patients out of 238 in whom this technique was used, 5 (71%) developed a fistula and 3 (43%) died.

Fortunately, severe combined pancreatic head and duodenal injuries are rare. These injuries are most commonly caused by penetrating wounds and occur in association with multiple intra-abdominal injuries. Because of the large number of possible injury patterns, no single therapeutic intervention is right for all patients. The best treatment option is determined by the integrity of the distal common bile duct and ampulla, coupled with the severity of the duodenal injury. For that reason, any patient with a combined injury to the pancreas and duodenum must, at a minimum, have an intraoperative cholangiogram performed before an adequate treatment decision can be made.

The primary cause of mortality in those patients with combined pancreatic and duodenal injuries is secondary to major vascular injury. Once vascular control is obtained, Whipple resection remains the preferred option in that select group of patients with combined massive destruction of the duodenum and pancreatic head for whom pancreaticoduodenectomy is the completion of surgical debridement of devitalized tissue.

During a 6-year period, 10 of 117 patients at Harborview Medical Center in Seattle underwent Whipple resection for nonreconstructible injury to the ampulla or severe combined pancreaticoduodenal injuries. Postoperative complications included four intra-abdominal abscesses, two cases of pancreatitis, and one pancreatic fistula. More importantly, all patients survived.[21]

Morbidity and Complications Management

Although most complications related to pancreatic injury are self-limiting and/or treatable, the possibility of sepsis and multiple organ failure leading to death is real and results in nearly 30% of the deaths after pancreatic trauma.[22]

A fistula is the most common complication after pancreatic injury, with an incidence of 7%–20%.[11] For the most part, these are minor (<200 ml/day) and resolve spontaneously with adequate external drainage.[23] However, those with output greater than 700 ml/day (high output) generally require longer periods of external drainage and may require operative intervention. During this period, nutritional support is paramount. Low-fat, higher pH elemental formulas result in less pancreatic stimulation and should be tried before total parental nutrition.[17] Placement of a feeding jejunostomy at the time of initial or subsequent exploration is extremely helpful in those patients with prolonged fistula output in order to provide enteral nutrition.

The use of the long-acting somatostatin analog, octreotide acetate, has been reported in the management of postoperative complications after elective pancreatic resections.[24] The use of this synthetic analog has been extended to the treatment of posttraumatic pancreatic fistulas, but there are few data in the literature documenting its efficacy. In fact, the reports that do exist are contradictory.[25,26]

Abscess formation after pancreatic trauma depends on the number and type of associated injuries and ranges from 10%–25%. The intra-abdominal abscess is often subfascial or peripancreatic. Although a true pancreatic abscess is rare, it is usually the result of inadequate debridement of dead tissue and/or initial drainage and often requires open debridement and drainage. In any case, the mortality rate in this group of patients remains about 25%[27] underscoring the need for prompt drainage (either percutaneous or open).

Another common complication after operative management of pancreatic trauma is pancreatitis, occurring in 8%–18% of patients.[20] This type of pancreatitis, characterized by transient abdominal pain and a rise in serum amylase, is amenable to bowel rest, with or without nasogastric decompression and nutritional support. In these cases, the course is usually self-limited and resolves spontaneously. A less common complication is hemorrhagic pancreatitis, occurring in less than 2% of postoperative patients.[28]

Secondary hemorrhage after operative management of pancreatic trauma may occur in 5%–10% of patients.[29] This is particularly common with inadequate external drainage after pancreatic debridement or in the face of a postoperative intra-abdominal abscess. These patients often require re-exploration for hemorrhage but angioembolization remains a viable option.

Pseudocyst formation after nonoperative management of unrecognized pancreatic trauma is not uncommon. It is important to remember that, as stated earlier, the major determinant of outcome and primary indicator of optimal treatment after pancreatic trauma is the status of the duct. In fact, if the duct is intact, percutaneous drainage is often all that is needed for resolution of a pseudocyst. In contrast, if the duct is injured, percutaneous drainage will not provide definitive therapy but will instead create a fistula. Clearly, if there is any question as to the status of the duct, an endoscopic retrograde pancreatogram should be performed before percutaneous drainage.

Neither exocrine nor endocrine insufficiency after pancreatic injury is commonly observed. In fact, in both animal and human studies, it has been shown that only 10%–20% of normal pancreatic tissue is needed for normal pancreatic function.[6] Thus, distal resection should be well tolerated with little if any physiologic sequelae. This conclusion was confirmed by a multicenter study in which there was only one case of endocrine insufficiency and no exocrine abnormalities were identified.[23]

CONCLUSIONS

Injuries to the pancreas after trauma are relatively uncommon. As a result, they are easily missed, even by the experienced clinician. Consequently, they represent a significant source of morbidity and mortality relative to their overall incidence. This is primarily related to the accuracy and timing of diagnosis, the completeness of the operative procedure and the meticulous attention to detail that is required in the postoperative period to identify and treat potential complications associated with pancreatic injury. Prompt diagnosis requires a high index of suspicion (both preoperatively as well as intraoperatively) and appropriate tests performed in a timely fashion. Subsequent operative treatment is dictated by the pattern and severity of injury.

REFERENCES

1. Wilson R, Moorehead R: Current management of trauma to the pancreas. *Br J Surg* 78:1196–1202, 1991.
2. Travers B: Rupture of the pancreas. *Lancet* 12:384, 1827.
3. Mickulicz-Radecki JV: Surgery of the pancreas. *Ann Surg* 38:1–27, 1903.
4. Korte W: Quoted by Robson AVM, Cambridge PJ: *The Pancreas: Its Surgery and Pathology.* Philadelphia, Saunders, 1907.
5. Innes J, Carey L: Normal pancreatic dimensions in the adult human. *Am J Surg* 167:261–264, 1994.
6. Dragstedt LR: Some physiologic problems in surgery of the pancreas. *Ann Surg* 118:576–593, 1943.
7. Baker R, Dippel W, Freeark R: The surgical significance of trauma to the pancreas. *Trans West Drug Assoc* 70:361–367, 1962.
8. Heitsch RC, Knutson CO, Fulton RL, Jones CE: Delineation of critical factors in the treatment of pancreatic trauma. *Surgery* 80:523–529, 1976.
9. Smego DR, Richardson JD, Flint LM: Determinants of outcome in pancreatic trauma. *J Trauma* 25:771–776, 1985.
10. Olsen W: The serum amylase in blunt abdominal trauma. *J Trauma* 13:200, 1973.
11. Peitzman A, et al: Prospective study of computed tomography in initial management of blunt abdominal trauma. *J Trauma* 26:585–592, 1986.
12. Patton JH Jr, et al: Pancreatic trauma: a simplified management guideline. *J Trauma* 43:234–239, 1997.
13. Harrell D, Vitale G, Larson G: Selective role for endoscopic retrograde cholangiopancreatography in abdominal trauma. *Surg Endosc* 12:400–404, 1998.
14. Soto JA, et al: Traumatic disruption of the pancreatic duct: diagnosis with MR pancreatography. *Am J Roentgenol* 176:175–178, 2001.
15. Graham J, Mattox K, Jordan G: Traumatic injuries of the pancreas. *Am J Surg* 136:744–748, 1978.
16. Fabian TC, et al: Superiority of closed suction drainage for pancreatic trauma. A randomized, prospective study. *Ann Surg* 211:724–728, 1990.
17. Kellum J, Holland G, McNeill P: Traumatic pancreatic cutaneous fistula: comparison of enteral and parenteral feedings. *J Trauma* 28:700–704, 1988.

18. Fitzgibbons T, et al: Management of the transected pancreas following distal pancreatectomy. *Surg Gynecol Obstet* 154:225–231, 1982.
19. Anderson D, et al: Management of penetrating pancreatic injuries: subtotal pancreatectomy using the auto suture stapler. *J Trauma* 20:347–349, 1980.
20. Stone H: Experiences in the management of pancreatic trauma. *J Trauma* 21:771–776, 1981.
21. Oreskovich M, Carrico C: Pancreaticoduodenectomy for trauma: a viable option? *Am J Surg* 147:618–623, 1984.
22. Leppaniemi A, et al: Pancreatic trauma: acute and late manifestations. *Br J Surg* 75:165–167, 1988.
23. Cogbill TH, et al: Distal pancreatectomy for trauma: a multicenter experience. *J Trauma* 31:1600–1606, 1991.
24. Buchler M, Friess H, Klempa I, et al: Role of octreotide in the prevention of postoperative complications following pancreatic resection. *Am J Surg* 163:126–131, 1992.
25. Amirata E, Livingston DH, Elcavage J: Octreotide acetate decreases pancreatic complications after pancreatic trauma. *Am J Surg* 168:345–347, 1994.
26. Nwariaku FE, et al: Is octreotide beneficial following pancreatic injury? *Am J Surg* 170:582–585, 1995.
27. Feliciano D, et al: Management of combined pancreatoduodenal injuries. *Ann Surg* 205:673–679, 1987.
28. Jones R: Management of pancreatic trauma. *Am J Surg* 150:698–704, 1985.
29. Campbell R, Kennedy T: The management of pancreatic and pancreaticoduodenal injuries. *Br J Surg* 67:845–850, 1980.

LIVER INJURY

Manish S. Parikh and H. Leon Pachter

The liver is the most commonly injured intra-abdominal organ with an incidence of 30%–40%. The overwhelming majority of liver injuries, however, are minor, with spontaneous cessation of hemorrhage almost always the rule, and operative intervention is rarely required. On the other hand, complex hepatic injuries continue to challenge even the most experienced trauma surgeons.

Perhaps the single greatest advance in the management of hepatic trauma over the past two decades has been the nonoperative management of blunt hepatic injuries. Other advances include the combination of portal triad occlusion, finger-fracture technique (hepatotomy) and omental packing for complex hepatic injuries, and perihepatic packing with planned re-exploration in trauma patients demonstrating signs of the "triad of death" (acidosis, coagulopathy, and hypothermia).

In the new millennium, a "multidisciplinary approach" concept has evolved as the standard of care in the treatment of complex hepatic trauma. In addition to prompt surgical intervention, when indicated, adjunctive interventional techniques such as hepatic angiography, endoscopic retrograde cholangiopancreatography (ERCP), biliary stenting, and percutaneous computed tomography (CT) scan–guided drainage have become a part of the trauma surgeon's armamentarium.

INCIDENCE

Hepatic injury occurs in approximately 5% of all trauma admissions. Nationwide, there has been a steady decline in the incidence of penetrating liver injuries. However, blunt injuries seem to be on the rise predominantly because their presence has been more readily detected by the almost routine use of CT scanning in patients sustaining blunt trauma. The incidence of complex hepatic injuries, however, has remained relatively stable over the past 25 years, ranging from 12% to 15%.[1]

Motor vehicle crashes (MVCs) continue to account for most (approximately 80%) blunt hepatic injuries, followed by pedestrian and car collisions, falls, assaults, and motorcycle crashes. Most patients with blunt hepatic trauma have associated injuries, both intra-abdominal and extra-abdominal. Concomitant chest trauma is the most common associated injury encountered with blunt hepatic trauma, occurring in over 50% of patients. Patients with right-sided lower rib fractures, particularly ribs 9–11, have at least a 20% chance of sustaining an underlying hepatic injury. In spite of the high aforementioned incidence of associated chest trauma, injury to the brain remains the single most significant determinant in overall survival outcome.[2] In the era of nonoperative management of blunt trauma, the risk of a missed injury, especially to the diaphragm or small bowel, is of major concern. Adherence to meticulous interpretation on imaging studies by experienced personnel should limit this pitfall to 1%–2%.

Penetrating thoracoabdominal trauma has been noted to be associated with injuries to the liver in 30%–40% of such injuries. The extent of the injury is directly related to the type of weapon used. Associated intra-abdominal injuries (e.g., stomach, duodenum, colon, and pancreas) are common but rarely detected preoperatively.

MECHANISM OF INJURY

Blunt Hepatic Injury

In MVCs, those most susceptible to hepatic injury are unrestrained front-seat passengers. These passengers are particularly vulnerable to a compression injury from the steering wheel especially during periods of rapid deceleration.[3] Although the anterior abdominal wall stops, the posterior abdominal wall continues to move forward, and the intra-abdominal organs are "trapped" and compressed resulting in stretching/tearing of the liver at its vascular and structural attachments. As the liver is only partially protected by the rib cage, liver injury from steering wheel contact is one of the most important contributing factors to driver injury.

In lateral impact ("T-bone") collisions, the target vehicle is hit on its side and accelerated rapidly at 90 degrees to its previous direction of travel. The unrestrained passenger is subject to both compression and shear injuries that cause stretching/tearing and, at times, result in avulsion of the liver. Furthermore, in lateral impact injuries, because the spine/posterior abdominal wall is not in the line of impact in contradistinction to frontal impact injuries, more relative motion of the intra-abdominal organs ensues resulting in a greater likelihood of injury.

Penetrating Hepatic Injury

Damage caused by a penetrating injury is based on the kinetic energy of the projectile and the density and elasticity of the tissue. Low-energy weapons such as knives only cut and do not create a temporary cavity. Medium-energy and high-energy firearms damage not only the tissue directly in the path of the missile but also the tissue on each side of the missile's path. As a missile passes through the relatively inelastic liver parenchyma, a temporary cavity (three to six times the size of the missile's front surface area, lasting for a fraction of a second) and a permanent cavity (visible to the examiner) are created. The higher-energy firearms create larger temporary and permanent cavities, resulting in far more extensive tissue damage; the vacuum created by this larger cavity pulls clothing, bacteria, and other debris from the surrounding area into the wound as well.

DIAGNOSIS

Hemodynamically Unstable Patients

Patients who arrive with hemodynamic instability (systolic blood pressure <90 mm Hg) and who do not immediately respond to appropriate fluid resuscitation are expeditiously taken to the operating room without delay, irrespective of mechanism of injury. Further diagnostic evaluation at this point is contraindicated, as unnecessary delays inevitably follow and are often responsible for the ensuing fatalities.

In the hemodynamically unstable patient with pelvic fractures from blunt trauma, diagnostic peritoneal lavage (DPL) and focused abdominal sonography for trauma (FAST) are currently the diagnostic modalities used to detect the presence of intraperitoneal blood. DPL is 96% accurate in detecting intraperitoneal blood and a grossly positive aspiration (>10 ml) mandates immediate operative intervention. In most trauma centers, FAST has replaced DPL as the preferred diagnostic modality for the determination of hemoperitoneum in the unstable bluntly injured patient. Although FAST has a 97% sensitivity for hemoperitoneum greater than 1 liter, the location of the parenchymal injury

often cannot be reliably identified. One's ability to assess the source of the hemorrhage will continue to increase as experience with FAST increases. The sensitivity of FAST drops precipitously when the quantity of intraperitoneal fluid is less than 400 ml.

Hemodynamically Stable Patients

The hemodynamically stable blunt-trauma patient, on the other hand, may undergo further diagnostic studies. Hemodynamic stability, however, should not lull the trauma surgeon into a false sense of security, as significant intra-abdominal injuries may be present despite normal vital signs and a normal abdominal exam. The ability to accurately assess the presence or absence of significant intra-abdominal injuries by physical examination alone in the blunt trauma patient is notoriously poor, as up to 20%–30% of patients with a "benign" abdomen on physical examination have been shown to subsequently have significant intra-abdominal injuries on imaging or at laparotomy.

CT scanning is the preferred initial diagnostic modality in the hemodynamically stable patient with blunt abdominal or lower thoracic cage injuries. High-speed resolution scanning with a spiral scanner is employed after the administration of intravenous and oral (when feasible) contrast. Five-millimeter cuts are obtained after 120 ml of noniodinated contrast (Omnipaque) is injected at a rate of 2 ml/sec. Scanning commences 50 seconds after injection, a delay that corresponds to the portal venous phase of liver imaging.

Scans should immediately be interpreted and classified according to the American Association for the Surgery of Trauma liver injury scale[4] (Table 1) by the CT fellow or attending radiologist, always in

Table 1: American Association for the Surgery of Trauma Liver Injury Scale

	Grade[a]	Injury Description	ICD-9	AIS-90
I	Hematoma	Subcapsular, <10% surface area	864.01 864.11	2
	Laceration	Capsular tear, <1 cm parenchymal depth	864.02 864.12	2
II	Hematoma	Subcapsular, 10%–50% surface area; intraparenchymal, <10 cm in diameter	864.01 864.11	2
	Laceration	1–3 cm parenchymal depth, <10 cm in length	864.03 864.13	2
III	Hematoma	Subcapsular, >50% surface area or expanding; ruptured subcapsular or parenchymal hematoma. Intraparenchymal hematoma >10 cm or expanding		3
	Laceration	>3 cm parenchymal depth	864.04 864.14	3
IV	Laceration	Parenchymal disruption involving 25%–75% of hepatic lobe or 1–3 Couinaud's segments within a single lobe	864.04 864.14	4
V	Laceration	Parenchymal disruption involving >75% of hepatic lobe or >3 Couinaud's segments within a single lobe		5
	Vascular	Juxtahepatic venous injuries, i.e., retrohepatic vena cava/central major hepatic veins		5
VI	Vascular	Hepatic avulsion		6

[a]Advance one grade for multiple injuries, up to grade III.
From Moore E, Cogbill T, Jurkovich G, et al: Organ injury scaling: spleen and liver (1994 revision). *J Trauma* 38:323–324, 1995.

the presence of the chief trauma resident and trauma attending. The senior trauma attending in presence makes the final decision as to the appropriateness of nonoperative therapy. It should be noted that the grade of injury or degree of hemoperitoneum on CT does *not* determine the need for operative intervention, as this decision is based primarily on the patient's hemodynamic stability and the absence of peritoneal signs. Instead, the CT scan merely provides the surgeon with a general anatomic overview of the injury, identifies associated abdominal injuries requiring operative intervention, and can be used as a base for comparing future healing of the hepatic injury and resorption of intraperitoneal blood. CT can also identify injuries involving the bare area of the liver, which commonly present with minimal intra-abdominal bleeding, a paucity of abdominal signs, and often a negative DPL.

The role of FAST as a screening exam in hemodynamically stable patients is evolving and in the near future may eliminate the need for CT scan. Currently, many trauma centers forgo CT scanning in stable patients with negative initial FAST exams and merely repeat the FAST in 6 hours. However, scanning for only free fluid has its diagnostic limitations because not all blunt hepatic injuries result in hemoperitoneum. In a recent study looking specifically at sonographic detection of blunt hepatic trauma, Richards et al.[5] determined the overall sensitivity of FAST for blunt hepatic injuries (all grades) to be 67%, based on the detection of free fluid alone. On the other hand, it is clear that most solid organ injuries without intraperitoneal fluid on FAST are, in general, of minimal clinical significance.[6] At present, most trauma surgeons agree that those patients who are hemodynamically stable and who have either intraperitoneal blood on their initial FAST exam or positive findings on physical exam over the lower chest and upper abdomen should have a CT to specifically identify a hepatic or splenic injury that can be managed nonoperatively. Once identified, the hepatic injury may be followed with ultrasound if necessary.

Diagnostic laparoscopy (DL) is a safe procedure that has had a major impact in avoiding unnecessary abdominal explorations in patients with stab wounds or gunshot wounds that may not have penetrated the peritoneal cavity. The role of diagnostic laparoscopy in patients with blunt hepatic injury is less clear. DL should allow for an accurate assessment of most hepatic injuries and, as advances in laparoscopic instrumentation progress, perhaps allow for repair of some liver injuries. However, reports of missed enteric and other intra-abdominal injuries with DL are sufficiently significant to warrant further evaluation of DL in blunt trauma patients.

ANATOMIC LOCATION OF INJURY AND INJURY GRADING—AAST-OIS

Comprehensive knowledge of hepatic anatomy is essential to the proper management of traumatic liver injuries. Couinaud has described the functional anatomy of the liver, based on the hepatic venous drainage (Figure 1). The ligamentous attachments of the liver are depicted in Figure 2.

The American Association for the Surgery of Trauma (AAST) created the Organ Injury Scaling (OIS) Committee to standardize injury severity scores for individual organs to facilitate clinical investigation and outcomes research. The liver injury scale devised by the AAST is shown in Table 1.

MANAGEMENT

Nonoperative Management/Blunt Hepatic Trauma

Currently, nonoperative management of adult blunt hepatic injuries is the standard of care. Initial hemodynamic stability or hemodynamic stability achieved and maintained with moderate fluid resus-

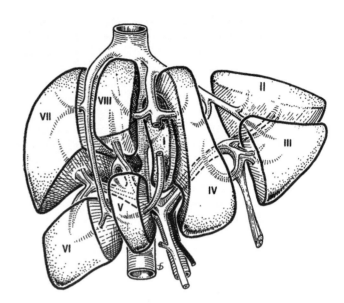

Figure 1 Functional division of the liver, according to Couinaud's nomenclature. *(From Mattox KL, Feliciano DV, Moore EE, editors: Trauma, 4th ed. New York, McGraw-Hill, 1999, figure 30-1. Originally appeared in Blumgart LH, editor: Surgery of the Liver and Biliary Tract. New York, Churchill Livingstone, 1988.)*

citation is the single most crucial prerequisite qualifying patients for nonoperative management. Once hemodynamic stability has been ascertained, the following criteria must be met:

- Absence of peritoneal signs
- Precise CT scan delineation and AAST grading (see Table 1)
- Absence of associated intra-abdominal or retroperitoneal injuries on CT scan that require operative intervention
- Avoidance of excessive hepatic-related blood transfusions

Previously cited inclusion criteria such as neurological integrity are no longer valid, as neurologically impaired patients can be safely managed nonoperatively in a monitored setting.[7] Furthermore, mandatory repeat CT scans to document improvement or stabilization of injury are unnecessary and contribute little to patient outcome. Rather, the patient's clinical course should dictate the need for additional evaluation.

Most (80%–90%) blunt hepatic trauma patients can be successfully managed nonoperatively. Although nonoperative management was initially limited to AAST grades I–III injuries, it is now clear that the hemodynamic status of the patient, rather than AAST grade of injury, is the most significant factor in determining the need for operative intervention. Up to 20% of select patients with grades IV and V injuries can be managed nonoperatively. However, many grade IV and most grade V injuries will usually present with hemodynamic instability or concomitant injuries mandating surgery, thus precluding nonoperative intervention. In a multi-institutional study, grades IV and V injuries were responsible for 67% of all patients who failed nonoperative management and subsequently required operative intervention.[8] Therefore, although hemodynamic stability determines which patients can be managed nonoperatively, the subgroup of patients with complex hepatic injuries (grades IV and V) are at substantially higher risk for treatment failure and should therefore be closely monitored in a critical care unit.

Conversely, the same basic standards apply to patients with lower AAST-grade injuries (i.e., I–III). In these instances, the initial injury may be deemed as "not significant," and thus it becomes tempting to avoid surgical intervention despite hemodynamic instability or a decreasing hematocrit, relying instead on further fluid and blood transfusions. This course of action is fraught with

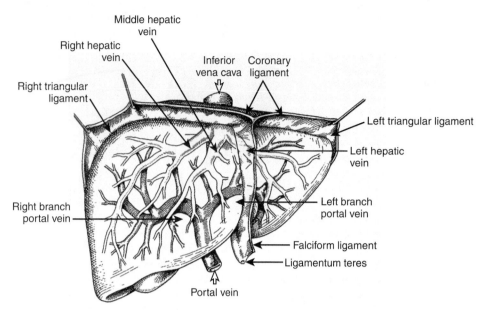

Figure 2   Surgical anatomy of the liver. *(From Mattox KL, Feliciano DV, Moore EE, editors: Trauma, 5th ed. New York, McGraw-Hill, 2004, figure 30-2.)*

pitfalls and should be avoided to minimize the morbidity and mortality of nonoperative management. To summarize, of all the variables monitored, hemodynamic stability appears to be the most crucial and is considered the watershed for nonoperative or operative intervention.

Contrast "Blush" on CT

Specific cause for concern is the presence on the initial CT scan, after the administration of intravenous contrast, of a contrast "blush" or "pooling" of contrast material within the hepatic parenchyma. This finding indicates active bleeding. Even in the context of hemodynamic stability and irrespective of AAST grade of injury, preparation for possible surgical intervention should promptly be made, as patients can suddenly and unpredictably decompensate clinically. If the patient remains hemodynamically stable, angiography with the intent of embolizing the lacerated vessel should be attempted (with an operating room on standby secured). An experienced interventional radiologist will usually have little difficulty in selectively catheterizing and embolizing the injured vessel, most often with stainless steel coils and/or Gelfoam. Successful embolization will then permit further nonoperative management. As the natural history of these lesions is unknown, they are best dealt with immediately so that sudden bleeding, false aneurysm formation, and late hemobilia may be avoided.

Persistent and prolonged attempts at controlling the bleeding vessel through angiographic means should be discouraged. In the rare event in which angioembolization fails to control ongoing bleeding, surgical intervention using the angiogram as an anatomic marker to more rapidly achieve intrahepatic hemostasis should promptly be undertaken.

Nonoperative Management/Penetrating Hepatic Trauma

Most penetrating civilian injuries to the liver result in a lesser degree of parenchymal damage than do those incurred by blunt trauma, at least by AAST criteria. Therefore, it seems logical that nonoperative management of a penetrating isolated hepatic injury would be successful in hemodynamically stable patients without evidence of peritonitis.

Renz et al.[9] nonoperatively managed 13 patients with penetrating right thoracoabdominal gunshot wounds. The authors stressed the importance of serial abdominal exams and contrast-enhanced CT scanning in their successful nonoperative management. Demetriades et al.[10] substantiated this concept with their successful management of select patients with isolated gunshot injuries to the liver. These authors concluded that hemodynamically stable patients with grades I and II liver injuries and no evidence of peritonitis can be safely managed nonoperatively. However, it should be noted that this approach failed in nearly one-third ($5/16$) of the patients in the "observed group" who eventually required delayed laparotomy. More recently, Omoshoro-Jones et al.[11] described successful nonoperative management in 31 of 33 patients with gunshot wounds to the liver, including grades III–V injuries. Although the higher-grade injuries were associated with more complications (most of which were managed nonoperatively), the overall success of nonoperative management did not depend on the AAST grade of liver injury.

Clearly, the most difficult aspect in the nonoperative management of penetrating hepatic trauma is patient selection, as only up to 30% of those with gunshot wounds to the liver are eligible for nonoperative management to begin with. At the very least, hemodynamic stability, an intact level of consciousness to allow serial abdominal exams, absence of peritoneal signs, and no evidence of active bleeding on CT are required for successful nonoperative management.

Operative Management/General Principles

The four basic principles in the management of liver trauma requiring surgery are hemostasis, adequate exposure, debridement, and drainage. With hepatic injuries, these objectives can be reached by the use of the finger-fracture technique (hepatotomy) to incise hepatic parenchyma, often combined with temporary occlusion of the portal triad for hemostasis (discussion follows). Extensive debridement of injured hepatic tissue can then be done, followed by application of a viable pedicled omental pack and closed-suction drainage.

Before the incision is made, the patient should receive a dose of antibiotics to cover aerobic and anaerobic microbes and is placed on a warming blanket. The surgeon must keep in mind that hypothermia is a frequent complication of resuscitation and operation in patients with major hepatic injuries. Appropriate maneuvers to decrease hypothermia are shown in Table 2.[12] Adherence to these ma-

Table 2: Maneuvers to Prevent/Decrease Hypothermia in Patients with Major Hepatic Injuries

Resuscitation with warm (37° C–40° C) crystalloid solutions

Resuscitation with high-flow blood warmers

Covering the patient's head with plastic bags

Placing the patient on a heating blanket

Use of a Bair Hugger on the lower extremities and on chest if thoracotomy is not needed

Irrigation of open body cavities with warm saline

Use of heating cascade on anesthesia machine

Adapted from Pachter H, Liang H, Hofstetter S: Liver and biliary tract trauma. In Feliciano DV, Moore EE, Mattox KL, editors: *Trauma*, 4th ed. Stamford, CT, Appleton and Lange, 2000, p. 637.

neuvers will usually prevent the development of intraoperative co-agulopathies and fatal arrhythmias.

The skin is prepped from the chin to the knees and a standard midline incision is made. The midline incision not only affords excellent exposure of the entire liver but also provides wide access to all peritoneal and retroperitoneal structures. The combination of a long midline incision and the use of large "upper-hand" retractors have, for the most part, eliminated the need for thoracic extension of the abdominal exposure. It should be kept in mind that extending the midline incision to the sternal notch (i.e., completing a median sternotomy) exposes the patient to two open cavities with the attendant increased risks of hypothermia and coagulopathy.

Exsanguinating hemorrhage continues to remain the most immediate cause of death in patients sustaining hepatic trauma. The initial incision into the peritoneal cavity can be accompanied by profuse hemorrhage once the tamponading effect has been lost. At this time, all efforts should be directed toward intraoperative resuscitation. Attempts at definitive surgical hemostasis without proper intraoperative resuscitation usually results in systemic hypothermia and profound coagulation defects with their dire consequences. This fundamental pitfall should be avoided at all costs. Irrespective of the severity of hepatic injury, almost all liver injuries can be initially managed by manually compressing the injury overlap pads (Figure 3), while hemodynamic and metabolic stability are restored by the anesthesia team. Failure to correct hypovolemia and acidosis before attempts at surgical control will likely lead to cardiac arrest and subsequent death. Once intraoperative resuscitation has been achieved, manual compression of the liver is slowly released so that a more accurate assessment of the injury can be made.

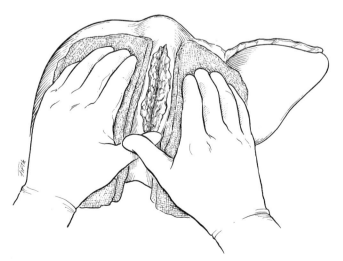

Figure 3 Manual compression of a severe liver injury overlap pads.

In order to better visualize injuries on the superior or lateral aspects of an injured hepatic lobe, it is often necessary to mobilize the liver into the midline wound. Division of the falciform ligament allows for placement of an "upper-hand" self-retaining retractor in the incision. Once this is done, careful traction on its hepatic end can aid in exposing the dome of the liver and the suprahepatic inferior vena cava. Additional exposure is obtained by placing laparotomy pads behind the posterior surface of the liver. Mobilization of the right and left lobes proceeds with division of the triangular ligaments (Figure 4). If there is a hematoma within the leaves of the triangular ligament, a hepatic vein or venal caval injury is most likely. Extreme caution must be taken because traction may disrupt a stable hematoma and can create massive bleeding.

Operative Management/Minor Injuries (Grades I and II)

Simple techniques of controlling hemorrhage include: a 5–10-minute period of compression, application of topical agents including fibrin glue, electrocautery/Argon beam electrocoagulation, and suture hepatorrhaphy (Figure 5). In many patients with superficial lacerations of the capsule, a 5–10-minute period of compression will frequently control any hemorrhage. If there is no visible leakage of bile, no further therapy is indicated. Topical agents such as Surgicel, Avitene, and fibrin glue are useful when avulsion of Glisson's capsule is present. Five minutes of compression with lap pads is performed after the application of a topical agent to the raw surface. After releasing compression, the electrocautery can be used for any remaining bleeders. Drainage is not necessary in the absence of further hemorrhage or obvious bile leakage.

Suture hepatorrhaphy has historically been the mainstay of hepatic hemostasis in grade II and some grade III injuries. It is important to first enter the hepatic wound and selectively ligate any open/avulsed bile ducts or blood vessels. Figure-of-eight 2-0 or 3-0 Prolene sutures are usually employed. Small defects in the hepatic parenchyma can be closed with simple interrupted 0-chromic or 2-0 chromic liver sutures with blunt-nosed needles (Figure 6). For deeper lacerations, attempts at primary closure of the hepatic defect should not be undertaken. Instead, a tongue of omentum on a pedicle is placed within the hepatic parenchymal defect and is then held in place with interrupted liver sutures (Figure 7). It is important to loosely approximate the edges because portions of the liver beneath can become necrotic in the postoperative period if the sutures are tied too tightly.

Operative Management/Complex Injuries (Grades III to V)

If significant hemorrhage continues after the release of manual compression of the liver, the portal triad should be occluded with an atraumatic vascular clamp (the "Pringle" maneuver; Figure 8). In over 85% of patients with complex hepatic injuries, occlusion of the portal triad will temporarily stop the bleeding. This maneuver, coupled with the finger fracture technique to expose lacerated blood vessels for direct repair, is responsible for the dramatic decrease in mortality from exsanguination.

Complex hepatic injuries (grades III to V) can best be managed by adhering to five sequential crucial steps:

1. Portal triad occlusion (Pringle maneuver)
2. Finger fracture of the hepatic parenchyma (hepatotomy), exposing lacerated vessels and bile ducts for direct ligation/repair
3. Debridement of nonviable hepatic tissue
4. Placement of an omental pedicle, with its blood supply intact, into the injury site
5. Closed-suction drainage

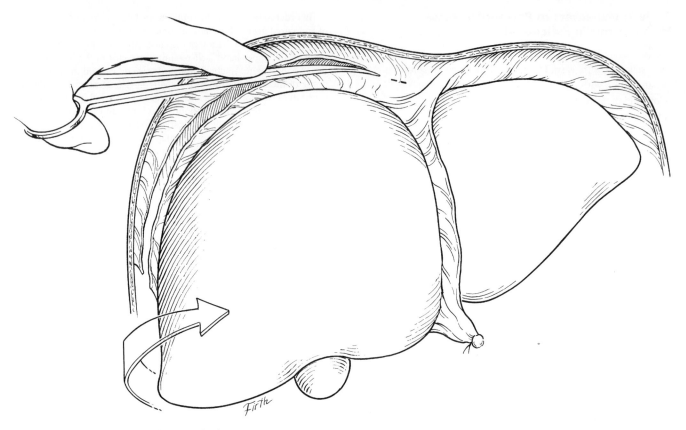

Figure 4   Mobilization of right triangular ligament.

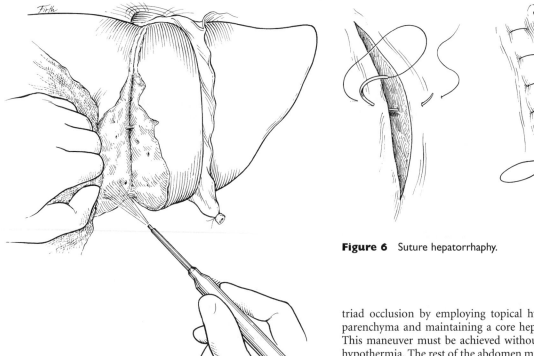

Figure 5   Use of argon beam to control hemorrhage.

Figure 6   Suture hepatorrhaphy.

Much controversy has surrounded the normothermic ischemic time produced by the Pringle maneuver. The data are clear that complex hepatic injuries can be managed with continuous cross clamping of the porta hepatis for up to 75 minutes without adverse sequelae.[13] We prefer to achieve hepatocyte protection before portal

triad occlusion by employing topical hypothermia to the hepatic parenchyma and maintaining a core hepatic temperature of 32° C. This maneuver must be achieved without contributing to systemic hypothermia. The rest of the abdomen must be packed off with multiple lap pads, and topical hypothermia with iced Ringer's lactate is achieved by intermittently pouring the solution directly onto the liver. Essential to this approach is the use of an intrahepatic digital temperature probe so that core hepatic parenchymal temperature can be seen at all times.

With portal triad occlusion achieved by an atraumatic vascular clamp, the surgeon then opens the liver parenchyma (hepatotomy) in the direction of the injury (Figure 9). Although it initially seems

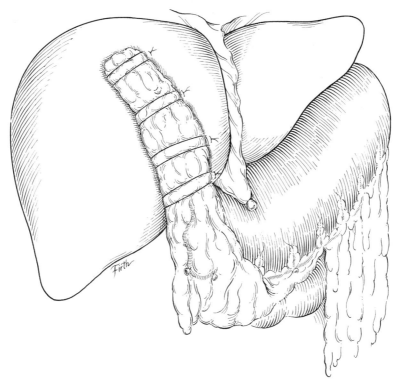

Figure 7 Omental packing.

crude, the finger-fracture technique constitutes the benchmark of obtaining rapid, adequate exposure. Specifically, using the electrocautery, Glisson's capsule is incised in the direction of the injury. Normal hepatic parenchyma is then crushed between the surgeon's thumb and index finger (or a neuro-tipped suction device), thereby rapidly exposing injured blood vessels and bile ducts, which are repaired or ligated under direct vision. Narrow Deaver retractors can be inserted into the hepatotomy tract for better intrahepatic exposure (Figure 10). Large lacerated intralobar branches of the portal vein or hepatic veins can be repaired in a lateral fashion using 5-0 Prolene sutures (Figure 11).

After intrahepatic hemostasis has been achieved, thorough debridement of devascularized hepatic tissue is essential to avoid postoperative septic complications. The use of omentum is extremely beneficial in the management of complex hepatic injuries, as it provides viable tissue to fill dead space, tamponades minor venous oozing, and provides a rich source of macrophages that may help combat infection.

The preferred method of drainage is with closed-suction Jackson-Pratt drains anterior and posterior to the injury. The data rendering drains unnecessary in elective hepatic resection cannot be applied to complex hepatic trauma, where blood loss, hypotension, and the frequent need to terminate surgery are the usual order of the day. In addition, the "zone" of injury may extend centimeters beyond what appears to be normal hepatic parenchyma, leading to eventual necrosis and abscess formation. While routine drainage after elective hepatic resection may be superfluous, enough variables exist in the trauma setting to merit the routine use of closed suction drains for complex hepatic injuries.

Juxtahepatic Venous Injuries (Grade V)

Juxtahepatic venous injuries, especially from blunt trauma, are often fatal, with mortality rates up to 50%. Failure to control hemorrhage from a deep laceration, missile tract, or stab wound with

a Pringle maneuver still in place strongly suggests the presence of a juxtahepatic venous injury. Regardless of the technique used to manage these devastating injuries, early recognition is essential because prompt modification of the surgical approach is necessary.

In the past, in order to try to salvage these patients, trauma surgeons inserted an atriocaval shunt with a resultant prohibitively high mortality (60%–100%). Currently, the use of atriocaval shunting has been virtually abandoned, and these difficult injuries have been, at times, successfully managed using a variety of approaches.

At present, there is a general consensus among trauma surgeons that if a retrohepatic caval injury or a hepatic venous injury (grade V) can be adequately controlled with perihepatic packing, no attempts at further repair should be initiated. When adequate resuscitation has been accomplished, there may be a role for endovascular stenting of the injury before pack removal.[14] Even without endovascular stenting, when planned re-exploration is undertaken, no further bleeding is often noted. If bleeding occurs after pack removal, definitive treatment can then be undertaken with the knowledge that the patient's hemodynamic status has been optimized and that adequate personnel are available if a vascular shunt is necessary.

Another approach is direct hepatotomy through normal hepatic parenchyma to reach the injured retrohepatic cava or hepatic veins.[15] After manual compression, vigorous resuscitation and prolonged portal triad occlusion, mobilization of the liver is performed with medial rotation, thus providing access to the retrohepatic cava and hepatic veins. Rapid and extensive finger fracture should be directed toward the site of injury until the lacerated retrohepatic cava or hepatic vein is found and repaired under direct vision. The surgeon must be prepared to finger fracture the hepatic parenchyma through normal and frequently nonanatomic planes. Because these patients usually have injured hepatic parenchyma as well, portal triad occlusion serves two purposes: it contributes to controlling hemorrhage from intrahepatic branches of

A

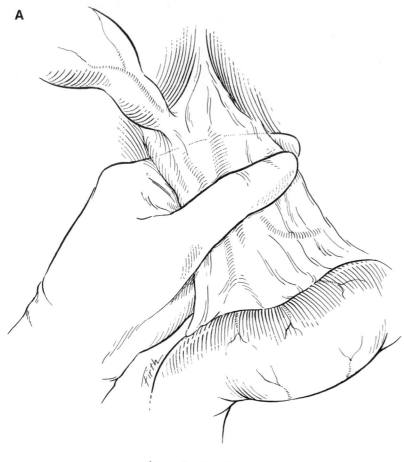

B

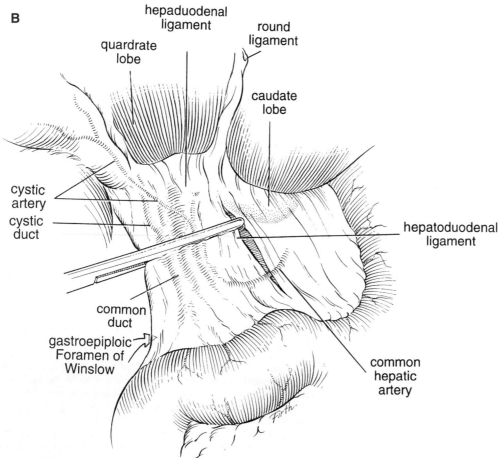

hepaduodenal
ligament

round
ligament

quardrate
lobe

caudate
lobe

cystic
artery

cystic
duct

hepatoduodenal
ligament

common
duct

gastroepiploic
Foramen of
Winslow

common
hepatic
artery

Figure 8 "Pringle" maneuver.

A

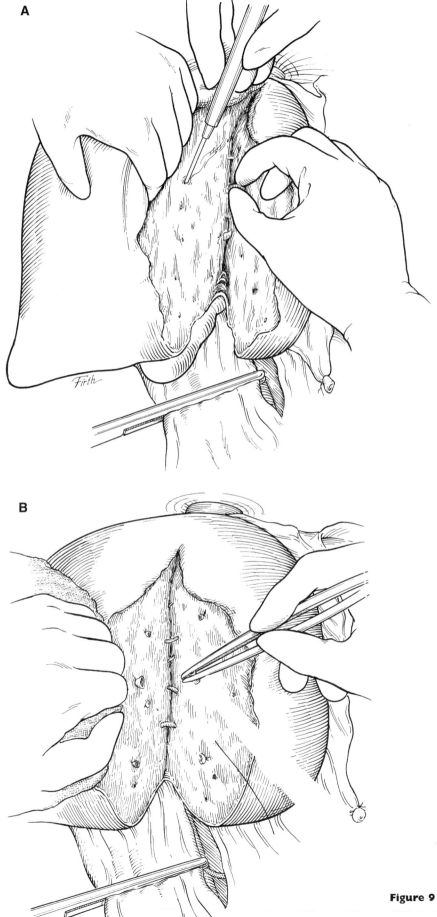

B

Figure 9   Finger-fracture technique.

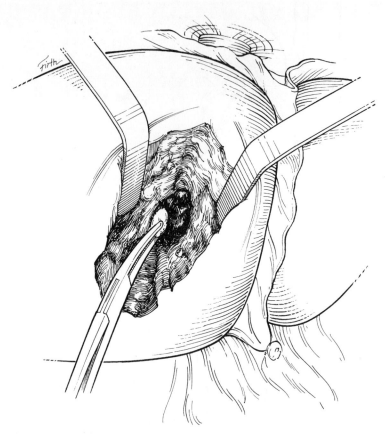

Figure 10 Placing Deaver retractors for better exposure.

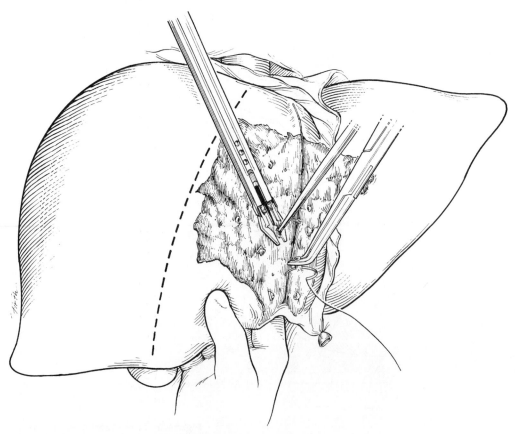

Figure 11 Ligating large branches with Prolene sutures or clips.

the hepatic artery and portal vein, and it decreases the inflow to the liver, thereby aiding finger fracture while minimizing blood loss.

Venovenous bypass, vascular exclusion, and primary repair[16] comprise a third approach. Total vascular isolation of the liver via venovenous bypass (combined with the Pringle maneuver and clamping of the suprarenal and suprahepatic cava) permits direct suture repair of the venous injury. The advantage here is that vascular isolation with venovenous bypass obviates the need for an intracaval shunt. Cannulation for bypass can be done peripherally via saphenous vein and axillary vein cutdowns. Venovenous bypass has been used in a small number of severe retrohepatic liver injuries with an overall survival rate of 88%.

Next is total hepatic resection and delayed liver transplantation.[17] Total hepatectomy and second-stage hepatic transplantation can be a drastic yet life-saving maneuver for devastating liver injuries that have failed all conventional treatments. Perihepatic packing and total hepatectomy with portacaval shunting can be performed in the primary hospital; the anhepatic patient can then be transferred to a transplant center for eventual liver transplant. Although this radical maneuver can be associated with high morbidity and mortality, the prognosis is better if the decision to proceed with total hepatectomy and portacaval shunting is made before the development of intractable multiorgan failure.

Portal Triad Injuries

As exsanguination is the most common (85%) cause of death in these highly lethal and complex injuries, the first priority in portal triad trauma is hemorrhage control, specifically manual compression followed by the Pringle maneuver. A wide Kocher maneuver and mobilization of the hepatic flexure will allow medial rotation of the ascending colon to better expose the portal structures. Exposure of a retropancreatic portal vein injury may require pancreatic transection with distal pancreatectomy after the vascular repair is complete. Although portal vein ligation can be used to expeditiously manage portal vein injuries, the preferred treatment is lateral venorrhaphy, as most series report a 51%–60% survival with this approach.[18]

Hepatic artery injuries should generally be managed with ligation. However, the hepatic parenchyma must be evaluated for ischemia after ligation, especially in the presence of portal vein injury or shock. In addition, the gallbladder should be removed if the hepatic artery is ligated. Partial extrahepatic bile duct injuries (less than 50% circumference) may be primarily repaired, with or without stenting. However, complete or complex bile duct injuries are best managed by Roux-en-Y biliary-enteric anastomosis. For the unstable patient, ligation with external drainage and delayed reconstruction is a reasonable approach.

Damage Control/Perihepatic Packing and Planned Re-Exploration

Perihepatic packing has emerged as an essential life-saving maneuver in patients with complex injuries refractory to conventional methods of treatment and usually complicated by brisk bleeding, hypothermia (less than 34° C), acidosis (pH < 7.2), and coagulation defects from massive transfusion (over 10 units). The effectiveness of perihepatic packing is directly related to the tamponading effect of the packs on the hepatic injury. Specifically, the packs raise intra-abdominal pressure, causing tamponade of low-pressure venous and nonmechanical capillary bleeding. The key to the success of perihepatic packing is to insert the packs early in the course of the operation before the onset of repeated episodes of hypotension.

Primary indications for perihepatic packing follow:

Onset of intraoperative coagulopathy
Extensive bilobar injuries in which bleeding cannot be controlled
Large, expanding subcapsular hematomas or ruptured hematomas
The necessity to terminate surgery as a result of profound hypothermia, which usually results in hemodynamic instability
Failure of other maneuvers to control hemorrhage
Patients who require transfer to Level I trauma centers
Juxtahepatic venous injuries

As a general rule, the liver should be mobilized before packing to help establish a tamponading effect. If, however, a significant hematoma is encountered in the triangular ligament (indicative of a vena caval or hepatic vein injury), further mobilization is contraindicated as massive and uncontrollable bleeding may follow. Most often, dry multiple-lap pads are placed on top of the injured liver until the ipsilateral hemidiaphragm is reached (Figure 12). In order to lessen the degree of bleeding when lap pads are peeled off the raw liver surface, we routinely place a Steri-Drape (3M, St. Paul, MN) directly upon the liver surface to serve as an interface between the injured liver and the lap pads.

Resorting to packing is usually synonymous with a dire situation. Under these circumstances, we prefer rapid closure of the abdomen with towel clips. Several large Steri-Drapes impregnated with Betadine cover the entire incision, encompassing all towel clips. Towel-clip closure takes minutes to perform and facilitates rapid patient transfer to a critical care setting where the patient's metabolic status can be optimized. Alternatively, prosthetic abdominal wall closure with an IV bag can also be employed.

Because perihepatic packing raises intra-abdominal pressure (IAP), monitoring IAP in the perioperative period is critical to avoid the development of an abdominal compartment syndrome. Pack removal should be dictated by the reversal of the patient's hypothermia, acidosis, and coagulopathy. These goals can usually be achieved within 36–48 hours. Packing has been historically associated with a 20%–30% incidence of perihepatic sepsis. However, early pack removal, the evacuation of intraperitoneal clots and the thorough debridement of necrotic hepatic tissue have lessened the incidence of this complication.

Adjuncts to Operative Management

Asensio et al.[19] advocate early hepatic angiography and angioembolization (AE) in all patients with grades IV and V hepatic injuries. These authors reported an improved survival with immediate surgery to control life-threatening hemorrhage, the institution of early hepatic packing when necessary, and subsequent patient transport directly from the operating room to the angiography suite for immediate hepatic angioembolization. Clearly, AE is essential in the management of complex hepatic injuries, whether they arise from blunt or penetrating mechanisms.

Early AE may also be useful in the multiply injured patient whose hepatic injury is being managed nonoperatively but whose serial hematocrits are noted to be dropping. Under these circumstances, the patient should immediately undergo repeat CT scanning, rather than arbitrarily receive incremental blood transfusions. If the repeat CT scan confirms that the liver injury has deteriorated and the patient remains hemodynamically stable, then AE should be attempted. Failure of AE to arrest ongoing hemorrhage or hemodynamic instability at any given time should prompt immediate laparotomy.

Late angiography is therapeutic in the presence of hemobilia, bleeding emanating from abdominal drains in the postoperative period, or vascular abnormalities noted when follow-up CT scan is indicated.

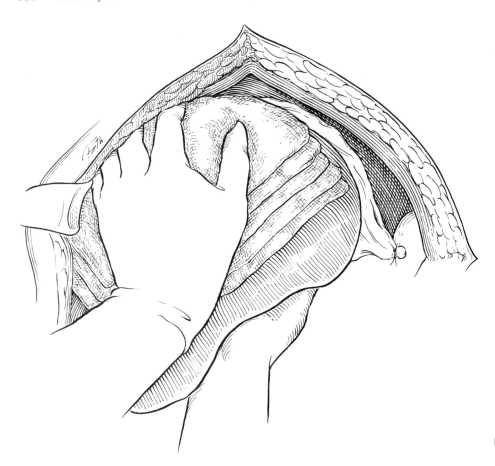

Figure 12 Perihepatic packing.

MORBIDITY AND COMPLICATIONS MANAGEMENT

Failure of Nonoperative Management

Nonoperative management of adult blunt hepatic injuries has resulted in an overall success rate of 95%. Fears concerning excessive blood transfusions in patients managed nonoperatively have not materialized, as the mean transfusion rate in most large series is approximately two units. Failure of nonoperative management of blunt hepatic injuries is usually associated with the presence of a "contrast blush" on the initial CT scan, indicating active hemorrhage and mandating intervention irrespective of the patient's hemodynamic status. If stable, AE has emerged as the adjunctive treatment modality of choice. When hemodynamic instability unresponsive to fluid resuscitation manifests itself initially or after the documentation of a contrast blush, operative intervention should be undertaken without delay. For this clinical picture to emerge, a significant injury has likely occurred and often necessitates damage control laparotomy.

Most failures of nonoperative management (with lack of contrast blush on initial CT) result from associated abdominal injuries rather than the liver per se. In a recent series reported by Velmahos et al.,[20] the grade of injury did not correlate with failure of nonoperative management. Most impressive was their reported liver-related failure rate of 0%. Although their series was too small to determine independent predictors of failure, they found that patients who failed had a higher Injury Severity Score, required greater volumes of initial fluid resuscitation and blood transfusion, and had other associated abdominal injuries.

Hemorrhage

Hemorrhage complicating the nonoperative management of hemodynamically stable patients with blunt injuries occurs at a frequency of less than 5%, particularly when a helical contrast-enhanced CT scan fails to show an active blush. For the most part, these cases follow a predictable pattern of gradual hemorrhage and hematoma formation, rather than sudden decompensation. The reported incidence of delayed hemorrhage requiring laparotomy is well under 2%–3%.

Bleeding after operative management of hepatic injuries is usually not subtle as evidenced by brisk bleeding from intraperitoneal drains. However, a more subtle presentation is the hemodynamically stable patient with a partially distended abdomen accompanied by a decreasing hematocrit. In the past, reoperation to control bleeding from within the injured liver was promptly undertaken after correction of acidosis, hypothermia, and coagulation defects. Currently, in the absence of hemodynamic instability, AE is the preferred treatment.

In the hemodynamically unstable postoperative patient, re-exploration is warranted. The same techniques apply, namely manual compression of the liver with concomitant intraoperative resuscitation, the Pringle maneuver, and finger fracture, if necessary, through the repaired area. If there is a concern that extensive hepatotomy may sever major vascular structures or hepatic bile ducts, persistent bleeding may be controlled by extralobar hepatic arterial ligation or balloon tamponade with Penrose and red rubber catheters. If a diligent search has failed to reveal a mechanical source of bleeding, a transfusion-related coagulopathy is the most likely culprit. Under these circumstances, packing of the injured liver should rapidly be undertaken, following the guidelines for packing removal as described earlier.

Perihepatic Sepsis/Abscess

The predominant cause of the late morbidity and mortality associated with complex hepatic injuries is perihepatic sepsis (3%–5%). Perihepatic sepsis, especially in the multiply injured patient, can lead to septic shock formation, systemic inflammatory response syndrome, and multiple organ failure. Noninfectious factors can also initiate severe inflammatory responses that may culminate in multiple organ failure and death.

A variety of risk factors for postoperative abscesses after hepatic trauma have been identified, including associated enteric injuries, extent of parenchymal damage, transfusion requirements, and inadequate debridement/drainage at the initial operation. For the most part, the rate of hepatic abscess formation can be significantly reduced with meticulous hemostasis, adequate debridement of nonviable hepatic parenchyma, and avoiding open-suction drainage.

Most abscesses can be drained percutaneously. Failure of the septic patient to improve within 24–36 hours after percutaneous drainage is a compelling reason to repeat the CT scan to determine if the catheter needs to be readjusted or whether operative intervention is needed. If surgery is required, the abscess cavity should be unroofed, devitalized tissue debrided, and closed-suction drainage established. Rarely, resectional debridement or frank lobectomy may be required to eradicate either an infected biloma or abscess cavity.

Bile Collections/Fistula

The second most common late complication encountered with the nonoperative management of blunt hepatic injuries is either the development of a collection of bile (biloma) or the formation of a biliary fistula. Although leakage of bile from lacerated biliary radicals after hepatic injuries occurs commonly, the reported incidence of clinically significant bile leaks is low (2%–3%). Extravasation of bile demonstrated on nuclear imaging (HIDA scan) rarely requires operative intervention, as percutaneous drainage is usually successful. The key to the management of bile leaks is adequate closed suction drainage. Even a biliary fistula (>50 ml/day over 14 days) that is adequately drained usually closes spontaneously. When biliary fistulas fail to resolve, ERCP with stent and/or sphincterotomy should be performed.

Thoracobiliary fistula is a rare complication of penetrating thoracoabdominal trauma. The responsible mechanism is usually a missed or deliberate non-repair of small diaphragmatic lesion. Percutaneous drainage of the chest collection combined with endoscopic sphincterotomy is almost always curative. It should be stressed, however, that early diagnosis is critical to avoid the corrosive effect of bile on the lungs and pleural space.

Hemobilia

Hemobilia is an uncommon complication of hepatic trauma, occurring at most in 1%. Hemobilia may result from blunt or penetrating trauma or iatrogenically induced by deep suture hepatorrhaphy. Signs and symptoms of gastrointestinal hemorrhage, right upper quadrant pain, and jaundice (Sandbloom's triad) may occur 4 days to 1 month postinjury. Repeat endoscopy is usually unrevealing. In this setting, a history of trauma mandates celiac angiography. If hemobilia is the cause of the bleeding, angiography will demonstrate a hepatic artery pseudoaneurysm that can be embolized with steel coils, Gelfoam, or acrylate glue. Surgical intervention is rarely necessary unless hemobilia is either associated with a large intrahepatic cavity or angiography is not available. If surgery is required, the optimal treatment is hepatic resection encompassing the large cavity and the pseudoaneurysm. Vascular control (by intraoperative Pringle maneuver or direct ligation of the hepatic artery) is essential before attempting to debride or resect large intrahepatic cavities associated with hepatic artery pseudoaneurysms.

Injury to the Intrahepatic Bile Ducts and Late Stricture

Injuries to the intrahepatic bile ducts are rare. The long-term sequelae of spontaneous healing of the injured hepatic parenchyma surrounding both normal and disrupted intrahepatic bile ducts are presently unknown. While disruption of secondary and tertiary biliary radicals within the liver occurs often, late intrahepatic bile duct stricture formation is an exceedingly rare occurrence.

Postobservational CT Scanning

The physiology of hepatic repair after blunt injury progresses in a predictable fashion that results in virtually complete restoration of hepatic integrity at the end of 3 months. There is general agreement that postobservational scanning in patients with grades I and II injuries contributes little to the clinical management of asymptomatic patients. In patients with grades III to V injuries, repeat CT scan or ultrasound, showing resolution of the injury, can serve as an invaluable guide in identifying patients for whom critical care monitoring may no longer be necessary. The optimal time frame for follow-up CT scan in these patients, if necessary, is 7–10 days after the original injury.

Resumption of Normal Activities

Dulchavsky et al.[21] demonstrated in experimental models that hepatic wound bursting strength at 3 weeks after injury was comparable and often exceeded wound bursting strength of normal hepatic parenchyma. Moreover, healing by secondary intention resulted in wound bursting strength equal or greater than hepatorrhaphy or hepatorrhaphy and omental packing at 3 and 6 weeks. The healing mechanism responsible for the increased wound bursting strengths appears to be the proliferative fibrosis throughout the injured hepatic parenchyma and the overlying Glisson's capsule. Hepatic parenchymal healing appears to be virtually complete at 6 to 8 weeks postinjury. A reasonable and safe approach to pursue would be to allow patients with grade III or greater injury to resume normal activities after CT scan documentation, at 3 months, of major injury resolution.

MORTALITY

The overall liver-related mortality in most large series of nonoperatively managed blunt hepatic injuries is 0.5%. When blunt hepatic injuries are stratified by severity, it is clear that with the exception of grades IV and V injuries, it is the associated organ injuries, specifically brain and cardiopulmonary injury, which ultimately affect mortality rates. In most large series of blunt hepatic injuries, associated brain injuries account for most (60%–70%) of the deaths.

Most liver-related mortalities result from complex hepatic trauma (grades IV and V), especially juxtahepatic venous injuries and portal triad injuries, which often result in prohibitively high mortality rates. Over the past two decades, the mortality of complex hepatic injuries has decreased, predominantly because of a reduction in deaths from liver hemorrhage. Responsible contributing factors include: prolonged inflow occlusion times, hepatotomy with selective vascular ligation, early packing and re-exploration, and adjunctive interventional procedures, especially hepatic artery angioembolization.

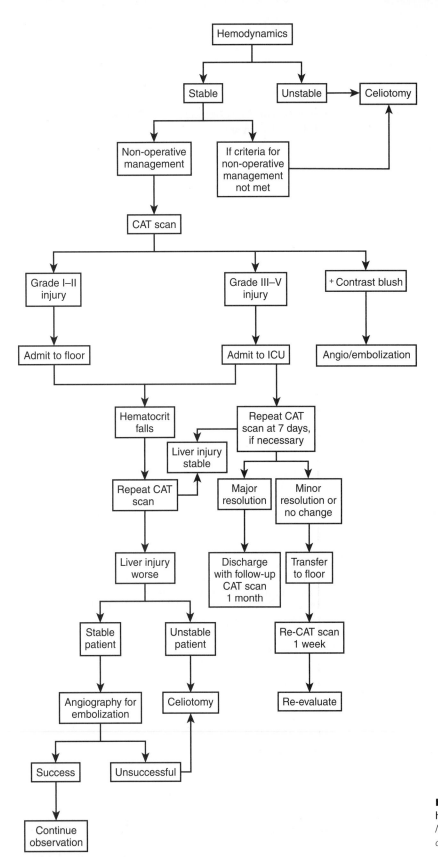

Figure 13 Algorithm for management of blunt hepatic injury. *(Adapted from Feliciano DV, Moore EE, Mattox KL, editors: Trauma, 3rd ed. Stamford, CT, Appleton and Lange, 1996, p. 643.)*

CONCLUSIONS/ALGORITHM

Nonoperative management can be used to successfully manage most blunt hepatic trauma patients and a select group of penetrating hepatic trauma patients. The cornerstone of nonoperative management is hemodynamic stability. An active "blush" on con-

trast-enhanced CT mandates immediate angiography, irrespective of CT grade of injury. Successful embolization of the lesion usually permits continued nonoperative management. Should the patient under observation become hemodynamically unstable or develop peritoneal signs, operative intervention should be undertaken without the slightest hesitation.

When the liver injury requires operative intervention, four essential maneuvers should be kept in mind, which can be life-saving, even in the hands of those with limited experience in this area: (1) manual compression of the injury, (2) resuscitation, (3) assessment of the injury, and (4) the Pringle maneuver (inflow occlusion).

Complex hepatic injuries (grades IV and V) continue to challenge trauma surgeons and tax the resources of trauma centers. Most of these patients are hemodynamically unstable, have multiple associated injuries, require massive blood transfusions, and have a significant mortality rate. Nevertheless, surgeons should be familiar with five critical approaches if patients are to be salvaged:

- Hepatotomy and hepatorrhaphy
- Packing and planned re-exploration
- Nonanatomic and anatomic resection
- Angioembolization
- Endoscopic retrograde cholangiography, papillotomy, and endostenting

Algorithms for the management of hepatic injuries are shown in Figures 13 and 14.

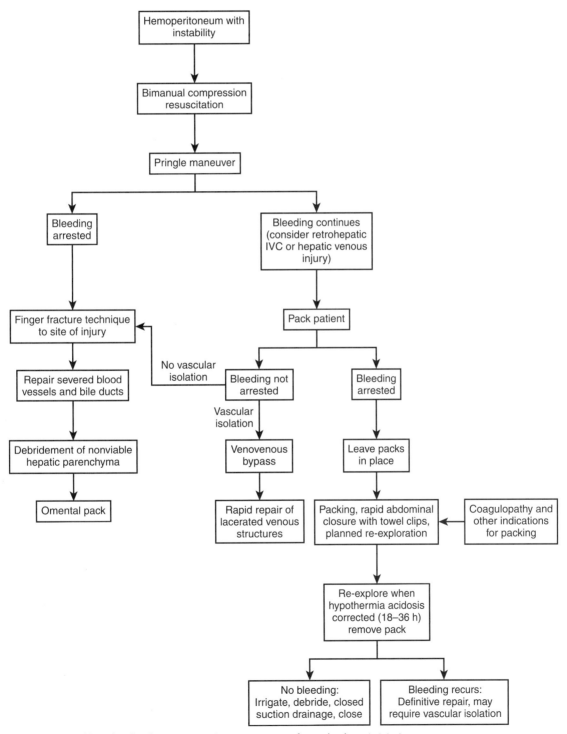

Figure 14 Algorithm for the intraoperative management of complex hepatic injuries.

REFERENCES

1. Richardson J, Franklin G, Lukan J, et al: Evolution in the management of hepatic trauma: a 25-year perspective. *Ann Surg* 232:324–330, 2000.
2. Rivkind A, Siegel J, Dunham M: Patterns of organ injury in blunt hepatic trauma and their significance for management and outcome. *J Trauma* 29:1398–1415, 1989.
3. Lau I, Horsch J, Viano D, et al: Biomechanics of liver injury by steering wheel loading. *J Trauma* 27:225–235, 1987.
4. Moore E, Cogbill T, Jurkovich G, et al: Organ injury scaling: spleen and liver (1994 revision). *J Trauma* 38:323–324, 1995.
5. Richards J, McGahan P, Pali M, et al: Sonographic detection of blunt hepatic trauma hemoperitoneum and parenchymal patterns of injury. *J Trauma* 47:1092–1097, 1999.
6. Ochsner M, Knudson M, Pachter H, et al: Significance of minimal or no intraperitoneal fluid visible on CT scan associated with blunt liver and splenic injuries: a multicenter analysis. *J Trauma* 49:505–510, 2000.
7. Archer L, Rogers F, Shackford S: Selective nonoperative management of liver and spleen injuries in neurologically impaired adult patients. *Arch Surg* 131:309–415, 1996.
8. Pachter H, Knudson M, Esrig B, et al: Status of nonoperative management of blunt hepatic injuries in 1995: a multicenter experience with 404 patients. *J Trauma* 40:31–38, 1996.
9. Renz B, Feliciano D: Gunshot wounds to the right thoracoabdomen: a prospective study of nonoperative management. *J Trauma* 37:737–744, 1994.
10. Demetriades D, Gomez H, Chahwan S, et al: Gunshot injuries to the liver: the role of selective nonoperative management. *J Am Coll Surg* 188:343–348, 1999.
11. Omoshoro-Jones J, Nicol A, Navsaria P, et al: Selective non-operative management of liver gunshot injuries. *Br J Surg* 92: 890–895, 2005.
12. Pachter H, Liang H, Hofstetter S: Liver and biliary tract trauma. In Mattox KL, Feliciano DV, Moore EE, editors: *Trauma*, 4th ed. New York: McGraw-Hill Companies, 2000, pp. 633–682.
13. Pachter H, Spencer F, Hofstetter S, et al: Significant trends in the treatment of hepatic trauma: experience with 411 injuries. *Ann Surg* 215:492–502, 1992.
14. Denton J, Moore G, Coldwell D: Multimodality treatment for grade V hepatic injuries: perihepatic packing, arterial embolization, and venous stenting. *J Trauma* 42:964–968, 1997.
15. Pachter H, Spencer F, Hofstetter S, et al: The management of juxtahepatic venous injuries without an atriocaval shunt: preliminary clinical observations. *Surgery* 99:569–575, 1986.
16. Rogers F, Reese J, Shackford S, et al: The use of venovenous bypass and total vascular isolation of the liver in the surgical management of juxtahepatic venous injuries in blunt hepatic trauma. *J Trauma* 43:530–533, 1997.
17. Ringe B, Pichlmayr R: Total hepatectomy and liver transplantation: a lifesaving procedure in patients with severe hepatic trauma. *Br J Surg* 82:837–839, 1995.
18. Jurkovich G, Hoyt D, Moore F, et al: Portal triad injuries. *J Trauma* 39:426–433, 1995.
19. Asensio J, Roldan G, Petrone P, et al: Operative management and outcomes in 103 AAST-OIS grades IV and V complex hepatic injuries: trauma surgeons still need to operate but angioembolization helps. *J Trauma* 54:647–653, 2003.
20. Velmahos G, Toutouzas K, Radin R, et al: High success with nonoperative management of blunt hepatic trauma. *Arch Surg* 138:475–481, 2003.
21. Dulchavsky S, Lucas C, Ledgerwood A, et al: Efficacy of liver wound healing by secondary intent. *J Trauma* 30:44–48, 1990.

SPLENIC INJURIES

David H. Wisner and Glenn S. Tse

The spleen has had a prominent role in medical theory and practice throughout history. The Greeks and Romans believed that the spleen played a role in filtering the humors of the body, mirroring some of our modern concepts. During the middle of the last millennium, the Thuggee was a cult that worshipped Kali, a Hindu goddess of destruction. The members were professional assassins, and the act of murder for pay was an act of worship for their goddess. They were most famous for their use of the noose, but also targeted the left upper quadrant where, often fragile and swollen from malaria, the spleen lay. A well-placed blow leading to splenic rupture and bleeding in the absence of available transfusion and modern surgery might well prove fatal.

During the past 50 years, there has been increasing interest in the notion that not all splenic injuries require splenectomy. Our understanding of splenic injury has increased and our management of ruptured spleens has evolved. Although that evolution has steadily moved us away from routine aggressive operative management, it is important to always keep in mind that splenic injuries can be deadly and that patients with damage to the spleen can bleed to death.

INCIDENCE AND MECHANISM OF INJURY

The spleen is listed, along with the liver, as either the first or second most commonly injured solid viscus in the abdomen after blunt trauma. Because splenic injuries have a tendency to demonstrate themselves clinically more often than do hepatic injuries, splenic injury was listed as the most commonly injured intra-abdominal solid viscus before the advent of computed tomography (CT) scanning. After the advent of CT scanning and our ability to better diagnose clinically silent intra-abdominal injuries, it became apparent that the liver is also commonly injured and some series now list hepatic injuries as more common than splenic injuries. One large, multi-institutional study showed a 2.6% incidence of splenic injuries (6308 of 227,656 patients) for all patients evaluated for trauma, with splenic injury confirmed by either laparotomy or computed tomography.[1]

For penetrating trauma, retrospective reviews of two large centers, Grady Memorial Hospital and Ben Taub General Hospital, showed the incidence of splenic injury from abdominal gunshot wounds to be 7%–9%, far less than for the hollow organs and the liver.[2,3] Injuries to the spleen from stab wounds are even more infrequent.

Splenic bleeding can also occur on a delayed basis, a phenomenon of obvious importance in patients treated nonoperatively. The incidence of delayed bleeding, leading to failure of nonoperative therapy, varies depending on the grade of the injury. The failure rate of nonoperative management in aggregate for a large multi-institutional study was 10.6%, but varied from 4.8% for grade I injuries to 75% for grade V injuries.[1] One hypothesis for the pathophysiology leading to delayed rupture and bleeding is that as subcapsular clot breaks down several days after injury into its component parts, the number of osmotically active particles in the area increases and draws more fluid into the area of injury. The resultant increase in size of the area may then rupture the capsule, leading to renewed bleeding. Even without being trapped under the capsule of the spleen, the inflammation and fibrinolysis in and around the healing injury and clot may weaken the clot enough to result in renewed hemorrhage.

DIAGNOSIS

As with any other trauma patient, the initial management of the patient with splenic injury should follow the ABCs of trauma resuscitation. A particularly important general comment relative to initial resuscitation is that it is important to recognize refractory shock early and treat it with an appropriate operative response.

In the initial history taking, it is important to note any previous operations the patient has undergone, especially a history of splenectomy. History of direct blows to the lower left chest or left upper abdomen, with concomitant pain, may engender suspicion for splenic injury. Any pre-existing conditions that might predispose the spleen to enlargement or other abnormalities also should be ascertained if possible. The patient or significant others should be asked about the presence of liver or portal venous disease, ongoing anticoagulation, propensity for bleeding, or a recent history of aspirin or nonsteroidal anti-inflammatory drug use.

On physical examination, it is important to determine if the patient has left rib pain or tenderness. The left lower ribs are particularly important in that they overlie the spleen, especially posteriorly. In children, the plasticity of the chest wall allows for severe underlying injury to the spleen without the presence of overlying rib fractures. Older patients may not report lower rib pain and may not have particularly noteworthy findings on physical examination in spite of severe chest wall trauma and an underlying splenic injury. Examination of the abdomen can demonstrate localized tenderness in the left upper quadrant or generalized abdominal tenderness, but not all patients with splenic injury will reliably manifest peritoneal or other findings on physical examination. Bleeding without clot formation may not generate peritonitis that can be easily elicited. The unreliability of the physical examination is obvious in patients with altered mental status. As a consequence, imaging of the abdomen in hemodynamically stable patients has become an important element of diagnosis and management.

Diagnostic peritoneal lavage (DPL), once a mainstay diagnostic technique after abdominal trauma, is much less frequently used now. Its role as an initial diagnostic maneuver to dictate subsequent testing or operative intervention has been supplanted in many institutions by ultrasonography and CT scanning of the abdomen. Peritoneal lavage remains useful when ultrasonography is not available or reliable, in that it is a quick way of determining whether a hemodynamically unstable patient is bleeding intraperitoneally.

Ultrasound of the abdomen for free fluid, the so-called FAST (focused assessment with sonography for trauma) examination, is being used increasingly as a means of diagnosing hemoperitoneum in blunt trauma patients. Like DPL, it is most useful in unstable patients. Also, as with peritoneal lavage, the ability of ultrasound to determine exactly what is bleeding in the peritoneal cavity is limited. Attempts to image specific organ injuries using ultrasound have met with limited success. The most common method of using FAST examinations is for detection of intraperitoneal fluid and as a determinant of the need for either further imaging of the abdomen or for emergency surgery (Figure 1).

CT of the abdomen is the dominant means of nonoperative diagnosis of splenic injury (Figures 2, 3, and 4). Patients are sent either directly for abdominal CT scanning after initial resuscitation or are screened by abdominal ultrasonography as reasonable candidates for subsequent CT. When abdominal CT scanning is done, intravenous contrast is quite helpful in diagnosis; oral contrast is less helpful and does not measurably increase the sensitivity of CT for splenic injury detection.

A CT finding in the spleen that has received a great deal of attention is the presence in the disrupted splenic parenchyma of a "blush," or hyperdense area with a collection of contrast in it. When present, a blush is thought to represent ongoing bleeding with active extravasation of contrast. There is reasonably convincing evidence that the presence of a blush correlates with an increased likelihood of continued or

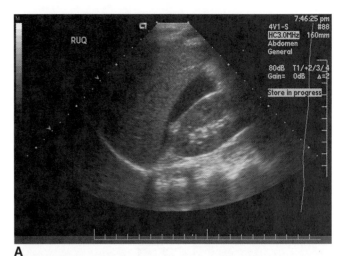

A

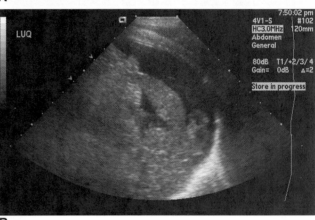

B

Figure 1 Focused assessment with sonography for trauma (FAST). Fluid in Morrison's pouch. The fluid is the dark area between the posteriorly located kidney and the anteriorly located liver **(A)**. Fluid around the spleen in the left upper quadrant. The fluid is the dark area located laterally **(B)**.

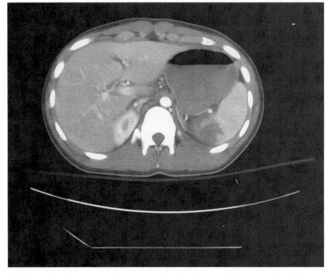

Figure 2 Computed tomography findings in blunt splenic injury, grade III. The posterior and inferior aspect of the splenic parenchyma is disrupted with the formation of a subcapsular hematoma.

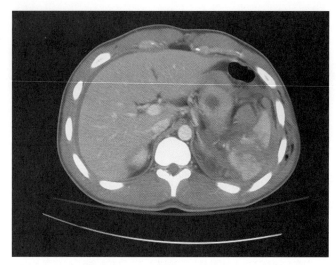

Figure 3 Computed tomography findings in blunt splenic injury, grade IV. A laceration through the parenchyma of the spleen with disruption of the capsule.

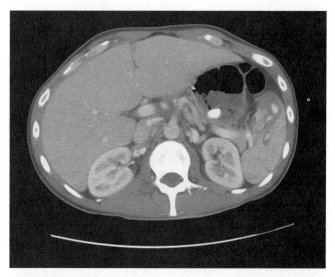

Figure 4 Computed tomography findings in blunt splenic injury, grade III. A laceration through the anterior portion of the spleen with a "blush" in the parenchyma.

delayed bleeding from the splenic parenchyma. Such a finding therefore has important implications with respect to either operative intervention or the use of angiographic splenic embolization to stop ongoing bleeding (Figure 5).

Anatomic Location of Injury and Injury Grading: American Association for the Surgery of Trauma Organ Injury Scale

Histologically, the spleen is divided into what has been termed *red pulp* and *white pulp*. The red pulp is a series of large passageways that filter old red blood cells and also catch bacteria. The filtering of bacteria in the interstices of the red pulp allows the antigens of the bacterial walls to be presented to lymphocytes in the adjacent white pulp. The white pulp is filled largely with lymphocytes located such that they can be exposed to antigens either on microorganisms or moving freely in the circulation. Lymphocyte exposure to antigens

results in the production of immunoglobulins, the most common of which is IgM.

The spleen develops initially as a bulge on the left side of the dorsal mesogastrium and begins a gradual leftward migration to the left upper quadrant. It changes in relative size during maturation. As the child's bone marrow matures, the spleen becomes relatively less important and diminishes in size relative to the rest of the body. There are also some important differences between pediatric and adult spleens with respect to the splenic capsule and the consistency of the splenic parenchyma. The capsule in children is relatively thicker than it is in adults, and there is also some evidence that the parenchyma is firmer in consistency in children than it is in adults. These two differences have implications for the success of nonoperative management; pediatric patients are more likely to succeed with nonoperative therapy.

It is perhaps not intuitive from the anteroposterior views depicted in anatomy textbooks, but the spleen is normally located quite posteriorly in the upper abdomen. It is covered by the peritoneum except at the hilum. Posteriorly and laterally, the spleen is related to the left hemidiaphragm and the left posterior and posterolateral lower ribs. The lateral aspect of the spleen is attached to the posterior and lateral abdominal wall and the left hemidiaphragm (splenophrenic ligament) with a variable number of attachments; these require division during mobilization of the spleen. Posteriorly, the spleen is related to the left iliopsoas muscle and the left adrenal gland. Posteriorly and medially, the spleen is related to the body and tail of the pancreas, and it is quite helpful to mobilize the tail and body of the pancreas along with the spleen when elevating the spleen out of the left upper quadrant. Medially and to some extent anteriorly, the spleen is related to the greater curvature of the stomach. Posteriorly and inferiorly, the spleen is related to the left kidney. There are attachments between the spleen and left kidney (splenorenal ligament) that require division during mobilization. Finally, the spleen is related inferiorly to the distal transverse colon and splenic flexure. The lower pole of the spleen is attached to the colon (splenocolic ligament), and these attachments require division during splenic mobilization. The main arterial blood supply emanates from the celiac axis through the splenic artery, whose course can be somewhat variable along the upper border of the body and tail of the pancreas. The branch points of the splenic artery in the hilum as well as the number of splenic artery branches are also variable. The other sources of arterial blood supply for the spleen are the short gastric vessels that connect the left gastroepiploic artery and the splenic circulation along the greater curvature of the stomach. The venous drainage of the spleen is through the splenic vein and the short gastric veins.

A number of different grading systems have been devised to quantify the degree of injury to the spleen. These systems have been created based both on the computed tomographic appearance of ruptured spleens as well as the intraoperative appearance of the spleen. The best known splenic grading system is the one created by the American Association for the Surgery of Trauma (AAST) (Table 1).[4] Implicit in the AAST grading system are the perhaps fairly obvious concepts that grade increases with an increase in either the length or depth of parenchymal injury, injury to the hilum, or injuries to multiple areas of the spleen.

The CT and intraoperative appearances of a splenic injury are often different from one another. Some of these differences might be because of evolution of the injury between the time of CT scanning and operation, but it is also likely that CT scanning is imperfect in describing the pathologic anatomy of a splenic rupture. Splenic injury scores based on CT scans can both overestimate and underestimate the degree of splenic injury seen at surgery. It is possible to have a CT appearance of fairly trivial injury but at surgery find significant splenic disruption. Conversely, it is possible to see what looks like a major disruption of the spleen on CT scanning and not see the same kind of severity of injury at surgery. In general, the CT scan and associated scores tend, if anything, to underestimate the degree of splenic injury compared with what is seen at surgery.[5]

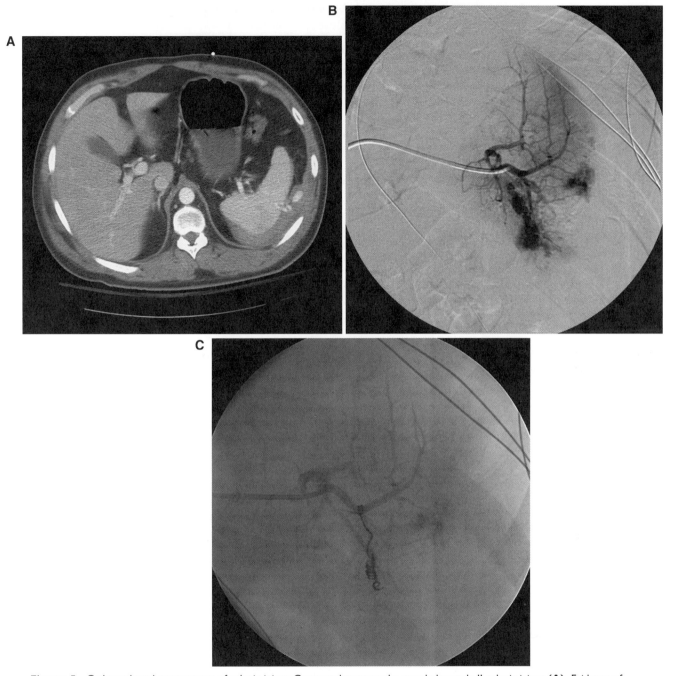

Figure 5   Catheter-based management of splenic injury. Computed tomography revealed a grade II splenic injury **(A).** Evidence of continued bleeding led to angiography. The angiogram demonstrated active extravasation **(B),** and the injured area was treated with embolization **(C).**

An important point about CT-based grading systems is that clinical outcome does not tightly correlate with the degree of injury seen on CT. Although there is a rough correlation between the grade of splenic injury seen on CT scanning and the frequency of operative intervention, exceptions are common. It is possible to have what looks like a fairly trivial injury on CT scan turn out to require delayed operative intervention. In contrast, severe looking splenic injuries on CT scan quite often follow a benign post injury course and are successfully managed nonoperatively.

Probably the major usefulness of splenic organ injury grading, particularly when the AAST Organ Injury Scale is used, is to allow for objective standardization of terminology and to ensure that individual injuries are described in precise terms understandable to oth-

ers. Standardized organ injury scaling is also useful for describing populations of splenic injury patients and for construction of treatment algorithms.

MANAGEMENT

Nonoperative Management

Appropriate patient selection is the most important element of nonoperative management. Although it is certainly true that nonoperative management is possible in a large number of patients

Table 1: American Association for the Surgery of Trauma Organ Injury Scaling: Splenic Injury Grading

Grade[a]	Injury Type	Description of Injury
I	Hematoma	Subcapsular, <10% surface area
	Laceration	Capsular tear, <1 cm parenchymal depth
II	Hematoma	Subcapsular, 10%–50% surface area
	Laceration	Capsular tear, 1–3 cm parenchymal depth that does not involve a trabecular vessel
III	Hematoma	Subcapsular, >50% surface area or expanding; ruptured subcapsular or parenchymal hematoma; intraparenchymal hematoma 5 cm or expanding
	Laceration	>3-cm parenchymal depth or involving trabecular vessels
IV	Laceration	Laceration involving segmental or hilar vessels producing major devascularization (>25% of spleen)
V	Laceration	Completely shattered spleen
	Vascular	Hilar vascular injury which devascularizes spleen

[a]Advance one grade for multiple injuries, up to grade III.
Adapted from Moore EE, Cogbill TH, Jurkovich GJ, et al: Organ injury scaling: spleen and liver. *J Trauma*, 38:323, 1995.

with splenic injury, emergency surgery is still sometimes necessary to stop life-threatening hemorrhage. Of paramount importance in the determination of the suitability of nonoperative management is the hemodynamic stability of the patient. *Hemodynamic stability* can be a somewhat illusory concept and one for which there is no consensus definition, but hypotension (systolic blood pressure <90 mmHg in an adult) is generally considered worthy of concern. Prehospital or emergency department hypotension is worrisome, and a high index of suspicion for ongoing hemorrhage should be maintained when either is present. In most instances, those patients that remain hemodynamically unstable are inappropriate candidates for abdominal CT scanning. They require either a direct trip to the operating room or, more commonly, abdominal ultrasonography or DPL to determine the presence or absence of intraperitoneal fluid and help guide the initial decision-making process.

Assuming hemodynamic stability, the other important prerequisite for consideration of nonoperative management is the patient's abdominal examination. In patients who are alert and can provide feedback on physical examination, it is important that they not have diffuse, persistent peritonitis. Although patients with splenic injury often will have abdominal findings secondary to intraperitoneal blood, and localized pain and tenderness in the left upper quadrant are common, obvious diffuse peritoneal signs can be a sign of intestinal injury and warrant abdominal exploration. If a patient with splenic injury is selected for CT scanning and subsequent nonoperative management, it is important to continue to follow the physical examination. If the examination worsens, the possibility of a blunt intestinal injury should be increasingly considered. The most common CT finding in patients with blunt intestinal injury is free fluid in the peritoneal cavity. In patients with damage to the spleen, the free fluid can be mistakenly attributed solely to the splenic injury, and the presence of an associated bowel injury can be missed; the physical examination becomes of even greater importance in such circumstances.

Reported success rates for nonoperative management are 95% or higher for pediatric patients and approximately 80% or higher in adults.[6,7] These high success rates can be misleading, however, in that they apply only to the group of patients in whom nonoperative management was chosen rather than all patients with splenic injury. When immediate splenectomy patients are included, the

overall nonoperative management rates tend to be around 50%–60% in adult patients.[1,8] It is also important to remember that these series generally do not include patients in whom the initial impetus was for nonoperative management but in whom emergency surgery was necessary when the patient got into trouble either in the emergency department or during the acquisition of CT scans. The published series of nonoperatively managed spleens generally include only patients who were stable enough to undergo CT scanning and in whom the scan showed a ruptured spleen.

Beyond hemodynamic stability and abdominal findings in the determination of the appropriateness of nonoperative management, other important considerations are the medical environment and some specific characteristics of the patient. Nonoperative management should only be undertaken if it will be possible to closely follow the patient. If close inpatient follow-up is simply not possible, abdominal exploration may be appropriate. Similarly, if rapid mobilization of the operating room and quick operative intervention in the case of ongoing or delayed bleeding is impossible, initial operative intervention may be appropriate.

For patients who are stable enough to undergo CT scanning and in whom a ruptured spleen is seen, nonoperative management is reasonable if they continue to remain stable. In addition to vital signs, one of the other commonly followed parameters in such patients is the hematocrit. A common practice is to determine a cut-off value below which the hematocrit will not be allowed to fall. If the hematocrit drops to that level or below, operative intervention is undertaken. Such an approach works best if there are no associated injuries; when other injuries are present, it can be difficult to know if the spleen is continuing to bleed or if the fall in hematocrit is secondary to bleeding from sites other than the spleen. When contemplating transfusion in patients with splenic injury who are being managed nonoperatively, it should be kept in mind that there is increasingly convincing evidence that transfusion has harmful immunologic effects and is an independent predictor of poor outcome after trauma.[9]

There is some evidence that older patients (>55 years old) might have a worse prognosis with respect to nonoperative management than do younger patients, but there are other reports concluding that outcomes are the same in older versus younger patients.[10,11] Although the evidence in this area is mixed, a relatively recent large multicenter study showed that older patients are more likely to fail nonoperative management, and older patients undergoing nonoperative therapy would likely benefit from earlier conversion to invasive therapy if their condition worsens.[12]

The presence of severe associated injuries, particularly head injury, has been suggested as another relative contraindication to nonoperative management of splenic injury. As previously noted, following the hematocrit in a patient with multiple severe injuries can be problematic. Furthermore, there are concerns about the effects of ongoing or delayed splenic bleeding on the prognosis of a severe head injury. While these factors do not mandate operative intervention in all patients who fall into these groups, they should lower the threshold for operative intervention on an individual basis.

There is little scientific evidence to dictate the specifics of how nonoperative management of splenic injury should be done, and most recommendations are simply matters of common sense and opinion. Most patients should be admitted to an intensive care unit setting for their initial course, including those with grade II or above splenic injuries and patients with multiple associated injuries that make following serial hematocrit levels and physical examinations difficult.

Patients should initially be kept with nothing by mouth in case nonoperative management fails because of significant ongoing bleeding and they require rapid operative intervention, most likely to occur in the early post injury period. Nasogastric suction is not necessary unless needed for other reasons. Bed rest for the patient is somewhat controversial; there is little empirical evidence that it makes a difference. Early mobilization is generally beneficial for trauma patients and should be the practice in patients with splenic injury. Patients should be followed closely hemodynamically, and the urine output should be monitored. Serial hematocrits should be obtained and compared with each other as well as with the admission hematocrit.

Vaccines for meningococcal and streptococcal infection prevention should be given while the patient is observed nonoperatively. There are some theoretical reasons to believe that the vaccinations are more effective if given before splenectomy. It is therefore preferable to vaccinate patients who are managed nonoperatively early in their course rather than waiting to vaccinate them after they have required splenectomy.

The appropriate length of stay in the intensive care unit is not clearly defined. Most centers keep patients with splenic injury in the intensive care unit for 24–72 hours and then transfer them to a ward bed if they have been stable and other injuries permit. At this point, patients are allowed to eat unless other injuries preclude oral intake.

The optimal hospital length of stay is also poorly defined, and there is a variety of practice in this regard. A large multi-institutional study showed that most failures of nonoperative management occur within the first 6–8 days after injury.[1] Our institutional approach is to keep patients in the hospital for an arbitrary 7 days, picking up the vast majority of delayed bleeding episodes during the inpatient stay.

The issue of follow-up CT scans in patients with nonoperatively managed splenic injuries is also controversial. Most series indicate either they are not necessary or that the frequency with which they alter management is extremely low. Our policy is to study only patients who have persistent abdominal signs and symptoms after a week of observation. On occasion such patients have developed pseudoaneurysms of the spleen, even if the initial CT did not demonstrate a blush. It is difficult to know exactly what the natural history of these pseudoaneurysms would be if left untreated, but they can be impressive in appearance and are amenable to angiographic embolization.

When patients are discharged to home, they should be counseled not to engage in contact sports or other activities where they might suffer a blow to the torso. The best length of time to maintain this admonition is unknown, but typical recommendations range from 2 to 6 months. There is experimental evidence that most injured spleens have not recovered their normal integrity and strength until at least 6–8 weeks post injury, so the recommendation to avoid contact sports for 2–6 months seems reasonable.

Transcatheter Embolization

Embolization of bleeding areas in a ruptured spleen can be an important adjunct to successful nonoperative management. As with nonoperative management in general, patient selection is of paramount importance. Hemodynamic stability is a prerequisite, in that the patient has to be able to tolerate a possibly lengthy diagnostic and therapeutic procedure. There are no consensus guidelines at present for when angiography and embolization are indicated,[13–16] but current trends generally reserve catheter-based interventions for higher grade injuries as well as those with CT evidence of a contrast blush, pseudoaneurysm, arteriovenous fistula, or active extravasation, regardless of the grade of injury.

Operative Management

The best incision for splenic injury, as well as for most trauma operations on the abdomen, is through the midline. Such an approach is versatile, can be extended easily both superiorly and inferiorly, and is also the quickest incision if speed of intervention is important. For operations on an injured spleen, it is often helpful to extend the incision superiorly and to the left of the xiphoid process. This maneuver improves exposure of the left upper quadrant, particularly in large patients and those with a narrow costal angle.

As with all trauma celiotomies, it is important to rapidly examine and pack all four quadrants of the abdomen in patients who are grossly unstable. The initial investigation of the abdomen should not be definitive and should be used only for a quick look at all four quadrants and for packing. While the quadrants are being packed, it is helpful to look for clotting. Clotting tends to localize to the site of injury, whereas defibrinated blood will spread diffusely in the abdomen.

Once attention has been directed to the left upper quadrant, all of the structures in that quadrant should be inspected. There should be an initial look at the greater curvature of the stomach and the left hemidiaphragm. The left hemidiaphragm should be inspected again once the spleen is mobilized if mobilization is necessary. The left lobe of the liver and left kidney should be looked at as well, as should the tail of the pancreas. If the spleen is to be mobilized, inspection of the tail of the pancreas is easier after mobilization has been accomplished.

Splenic mobilization should be done in a stepwise fashion, and the stepwise approach helps in providing adequate mobilization while minimizing the chance of iatrogenic splenic or pancreatic injury. The sequence of splenic mobilization is also important in that it allows for splenic salvage and splenorrhaphy up until the final step of hilar ligation.

The first step in mobilization of the spleen is to cut the lateral attachments of the spleen, the splenophrenic and splenorenal ligaments. This step should be started with sharp dissection and can then be continued with a combination of blunt and sharp dissection. The lateral and superior attachments should be cut to near the level of the esophageal hiatus. Cutting the lateral attachments is sometimes facilitated by putting a finger or clamp underneath them and then bluntly developing the underlying plane before dividing the peritoneum. In large patients and in those with a spleen that is very posterior, it may be necessary to do some of the sharp dissection by feel.

After the lateral attachments have been divided, the next step is to mobilize the spleen and tail of the pancreas as a unit from lateral to medial. One of the easier ways to do this is to place the back of the fingernails of the right hand underneath the spleen and tail of the pancreas so that they are adjacent to the underlying left kidney. The kidney can be palpated easily because it is firm and provides an excellent landmark for the proper plane of dissection. A common error is to try to mobilize the spleen alone without the adjacent pancreas, thus limiting the degree of splenic mobility and making it more difficult to avoid iatrogenic injury to the spleen and pancreatic tail. The splenic hilum can be injured during mobilization from lateral to medial; the pancreatic tail can be inadvertently included in the hilar clamping of the spleen. Both problems are minimized with optimal mobilization and visualization.

After the spleen and pancreas have been mobilized as a unit, it is generally apparent that the next constraining attachments of the spleen are the short gastric vessels. Because of the dual blood supply of the spleen though its hilum and also through the short gastric vessels, it is possible to divide the short gastric vessels without compromising splenic viability. The best way to divide the short gastric vessels is to have an assistant elevate the spleen

and tail of the pancreas into the operative field and then to securely clamp the vessels starting proximally on the greater curvature of the stomach. The short gastric vessels, as the name implies, are short. It is therefore not uncommon to be concerned about a clamp on the gastric portion of a short gastric vessel having included a small portion of stomach. In such cases, the tie on the short gastric vessels and nubbin of stomach can necrose the stomach, leading to a delayed gastric leak. This concern can be addressed by oversewing any gastric areas in question.

The final step necessary for full mobilization of the spleen is division of the splenocolic ligamentous attachment between the lower pole of the spleen and the distal transverse colon and splenic flexure (Figure 6). During division of both the short gastric vessels and the splenocolic ligament, bleeding from the spleen can be controlled using digital compression of the hilum. If the patient is exsanguinating and the bleeding is massive, a clamp can be placed on the hilum during the later steps of mobilization. Mass clamping should only be done in extreme circumstances, however, because it increases the chances of injury to the tail of the pancreas (Figure 7).

After the spleen has been fully mobilized, it is possible to inspect it in its entirety. It is also possible to examine the posterior aspect of the body and tail of the pancreas. It is helpful after

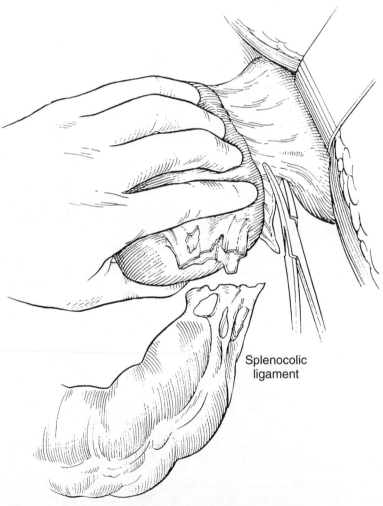

Splenocolic
ligament

Figure 6   The spleen is grasped and the lateral peritoneal ligaments are divided. The splenocolic ligaments have been divided to release the splenic flexure.   *(From Khatri V, Asensio JA: Operative Surgery Manual. Philadelphia, WB Saunders, 2002, p. 189.)*

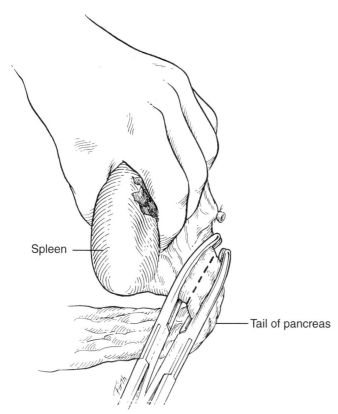

Figure 7 After complete mobilization of the spleen, the vessels at the hilum are clamped and divided, avoiding injury to the tail of the pancreas. *(From Khatri V, Asensio JA: Operative Surgery Manual. Philadelphia, WB Saunders, 2002, p. 189.)*

mobilization to pack the splenic fossa to tamponade any minor bleeding and also to help keep the spleen and distal pancreas elevated into the field. During this packing maneuver, the left adrenal gland can be inspected and the left hemidiaphragm re-examined.

If the injury is small and bleeding minimally, topical hemostatic agents can be used and the spleen returned to its normal position. Electrocautery is rarely helpful. Argon beam coagulators have shown promise in animal models of splenic injury. If the injury is more severe and the patient's overall condition is not too serious, splenorrhaphy can be done, although with the advent of nonoperative management the number of splenic injuries found at surgical intervention that are amenable to repair has decreased. The spleen can be sutured, especially when there is an intact capsule, but it does not hold sutures particularly well and it is advisable therefore to use pledgets. Wrapping of either all or part of an injured spleen with absorbable mesh can also be done, but these techniques are moderately time consuming. Partial splenectomy has been described and is possible because of the segmental nature of the splenic blood supply. The blood supply to the damaged portion can be ligated and the spleen observed for its demarcation. The nonviable portion is removed with the exposed parenchyma made hemostatic either with suture or mesh wrapping.

Splenectomy should be done in patients who are unstable or who have serious associated injuries. It should also generally be done for the highest grades of splenic injury (IV to V) if operative management has been chosen. The hilar structures should be addressed with serial dissection and division. Suture ligation should be used for large vessels.

Drains should not be routinely placed after either splenectomy or splenorrhaphy and may actually increase the rate of postoperative

complications. Drainage is reasonable if there is associated pancreatic injury or an associated renal injury when there is concern about postoperative urine leak.

MORBIDITY AND COMPLICATIONS OF MANAGEMENT

The most common complication of nonoperative management of the spleen is continued bleeding. Another potential complication is delayed diagnosis of an associated intra-abdominal injury that requires operative intervention, most commonly an injury to the bowel or pancreas. The frequency with which serious associated injuries are present in patients who are good candidates for nonoperative management is fairly low, at most in the 5%–10% range, but the possibility of an injury to either the bowel or the pancreas should always be kept in mind when the decision is made to treat a splenic injury nonoperatively. The physical examination of the abdomen is helpful in the diagnosis of an initially missed injury, as are pancreatic enzymes, serial complete blood cell counts, and peritoneal lavage.

There are also potential complications of transcatheter therapy. A failed embolization with persistent bleeding is the most common problem. Arterial injuries may occur during vascular access. Necrotic spleen, either from injury or from embolization, can evolve into a splenic abscess. Finally, missed injury remains a concern for this set of patients.[15]

As with any surgical procedure, there is a risk of bleeding after splenectomy or splenorrhaphy. The source may be from the splenic parenchyma after repair, the splenic bed, the short gastric vessels, or the hilar vessels. Coagulopathy should be addressed, but the possibility of surgical bleeding in the postoperative period should always be entertained when the patient is not doing well. As described previously, short gastric ligatures can result in necrosis of a portion of the greater curvature of the stomach, leading to leakage. Gastric distention may occur after splenectomy and is easily treated with nasogastric decompression if the diagnosis is entertained. Pancreatic injury may be the result of operative dissection or initial injury.

Venous thromboembolic complications are always a concern after trauma, and may be worsened with a splenic injury. Timely anticoagulation or mobilization can be hampered by nonoperative management or splenorrhaphy. Splenectomy can cause thrombocytosis, but there is no definitive evidence that postsplenectomy thrombocytosis leads to an increased incidence of deep venous thrombosis.

Although commonly mentioned, overwhelming postsplenectomy sepsis is a rare entity. The actual rate at which overwhelming sepsis in asplenic patients occurs is unknown, but one estimate is a 0.026 lifetime risk for adults and a 0.052 lifetime risk for children.[17] Pneumococcus and meningococcus are the most common pathogens, and protection against *H. influenzae* may also be helpful. Given the extremely low incidence of overwhelming postsplenectomy sepsis, it is difficult to prove the efficacy of vaccination. Nevertheless, vaccination has become the standard of care in patients who have had splenectomy.

MORTALITY

Mortality from splenic injury alone should be fairly low given careful selection and monitoring of nonoperative management and the definitively curative nature of splenectomy. In a study of a national database involving nearly fifteen thousand patients with splenic injury, the mortality was approximately 1%–3%.[18] Much of the mortality in patients with splenic injury results from associated injuries, especially head injury.

CONCLUSIONS AND ALGORITHM:

Patients with abdominal trauma and possible splenic injury should be managed initially with the ABC's of initial trauma resuscitation (Figure 8). If hemodynamically unstable, ultrasound or diagnostic peritoneal lavage should be done to determine if there is intraperitoneal hemorrhage. If the patient remains hemodynamically unstable and there is intraperitoneal hemorrhage, the patient should be explored. If splenic injury is found, splenectomy should be done if the splenic injury is of high grade or the patient has severe associated injuries and/or hemodynamic instability (Figure 9).

If the patient on initial presentation is hemodynamically stable, abdominal CT scanning should be done. If there is a splenic blush on CT, angiography with embolization should be done. If there is no blush and the patient remains hemodynamically stable, a course of nonoperative management should be undertaken. If the patient develops diffuse or worsening peritonitis or shows signs of ongoing bleeding (falling hematocrit, hemodynamic instability), abdominal exploration should be done and the splenic injury managed operatively (Figure 10).

Throughout the management of patients with splenic injury, from the initial resuscitation in the emergency department through the subsequent course of operative or nonoperative management, it should always be borne in mind that splenic injuries can bleed significantly and can lead to major morbidity and even mortality if they are not handled appropriately.

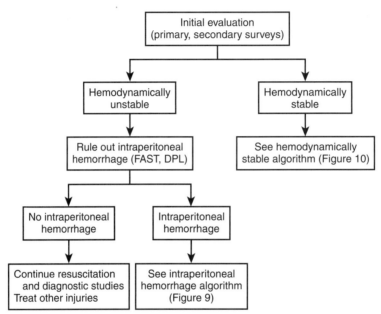

Figure 8 Algorithm for initial evaluation of patients with abdominal trauma and possible splenic injury.

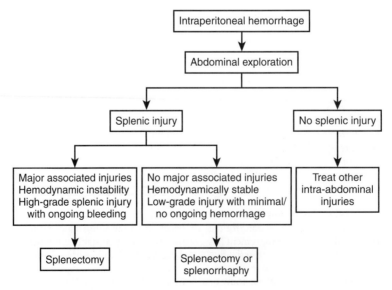

Figure 9 Algorithm for management of hemodynamically unstable patients with intraperitoneal hemorrhage.

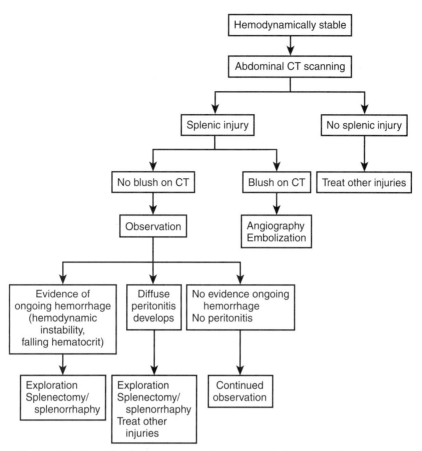

Figure 10 Algorithm for management of hemodynamically stable patients.

REFERENCES

1. Peitzman AB, Heil B, Rivera L, et al: Blunt splenic injury in adults: multi-institutional study of the Eastern Association for the Surgery of Trauma. *J Trauma* 49:177, 2000.
2. Feliciano DV, Burch JM, Spjut-Patrinely V, et al: Abdominal gunshot wounds: an urban trauma center's experience with 300 consecutive patients. *Ann Surg* 208:903, 1988.
3. Nicholas JM, Rix EP, Easley KA, et al: Changing patterns in the management of penetrating abdominal trauma: the more things change, the more they stay the same. *J Trauma* 55:1095, 2003.
4. Moore EE, Cogbill TH, Jurkovich GJ, et al: Organ injury scaling: spleen and liver (1994 revision). *J Trauma* 38:323, 1995.
5. Shapiro MJ, Krausz C, Durham RM, et al: Overuse of splenic scoring and computed tomographic scans. *J Trauma* 47:651, 1999.
6. Nix JA, Costanza M, Daley BJ, et al: Outcome of the current management of splenic injuries. *J Trauma* 50:835, 2001.
7. Buyukunal C, Danismend N, Yeker D: Spleen-saving procedures in paediatric splenic trauma. *Br J Surg* 74:350, 1987.
8. Pachter HL, Hofstetter SR, Spencer FC: Evolving concepts in splenic surgery. *Ann Surg*194:262, 1981.
9. Robinson WP, Ahn J, Stiffler A, et al: Blood transfusion is an independent predictor of increased mortality in nonoperatively managed blunt hepatic and splenic injuries. *J Trauma* 58:437, 2005.

10. Godley CD, Warren RL, Sheridan RL, et al: Nonoperative management of blunt splenic injury in adults: age over 55 years as a powerful indicator for failure. *J Am Coll Surg* 183:133, 1996.
11. Cocanour CS, Moore FA, Ware DN, et al: Age should not be a consideration for nonoperative management of blunt splenic injury. *J Trauma* 48:606, 2000.
12. Harbrecht BG, Peitzman AB, Rivera L, et al: Contribution of age and gender to outcome of blunt splenic injury in adults: multicenter study of the Eastern Association for the Surgery of Trauma. *J Trauma* 51:887, 2001.
13. Omert LA, Salyer D, Dunham CM, et al: Implications of the "contrast blush" finding on computed tomographic scan of the spleen in trauma. *J Trauma* 51:272, 2001.
14. Cloutier DR, Baird TB, Gormley P, et al: Pediatric splenic injuries with a contrast blush: successful nonoperative management without angiography and embolization. *J Pediatr Surg* 39:969, 2004.
15. Haan JM, Biffl W, Knudson MM, et al: Splenic embolization revisited: a multicenter review. *J Trauma* 56:542, 2004.
16. Haan JM, Bochicchio GV, Kramer N, Scalea TM: Nonoperative management of blunt splenic injury: a 5 year experience. *J Trauma* 58:492, 2005.
17. Luna GK, Delinger EP: Nonoperative observation therapy for splenic injuries: a safe therapeutic option? *Am J Surg* 153:462, 1987.
18. Todd SR, Arthur M, Newgard C, et al: Hospital factors associated with splenectomy for splenic injury: a national perspective. *J Trauma* 57:1065, 2004.

ABDOMINAL VASCULAR INJURIES

Thomas J. Goaley   and   David V. Feliciano

Abdominal vascular injuries remain among the most lethal of injuries that the trauma surgeon will encounter. The successful management of these injuries requires a well-organized trauma system capable of swiftly transporting the patient to the appropriate facility, a trauma center capable of rapidly mobilizing an appropriate surgical team, and a trauma surgeon capable of expeditiously resuscitating the patient, localizing the injury, and controlling the source of hemorrhage.

EPIDEMIOLOGY

All patients sustaining either blunt or penetrating abdominal trauma are at risk for hemorrhage from multiple sites, including the viscera (especially from blunt trauma), the mesentery (from blunt or penetrating trauma), or blood vessels (especially from penetrating trauma). The term abdominal vascular injury, however, is generally reserved for injury to one of the major (named) vessels in the abdominal cavity.

Penetrating abdominal injuries are the most common cause of abdominal vascular injuries, accounting for 67%–91%.[1] Abdominal vascular injuries are treated much more commonly in today's urban trauma centers than in recent military conflicts.[2] Indeed, in DeBakey and Simeone's[3] classic review of 2471 arterial injuries from World War II, only 49 (2%) were abdominal arterial injuries. Similarly, Hughes[4] reported on 304 arterial injuries from the Korean conflict and found 7 (2.3%) occurred in the iliac arteries. Finally, Rich and colleagues[5] reviewed 1000 arterial injuries from the Vietnam conflict and found that only 29 (2.9%) involved abdominal vessels. In contrast, a 30-year review of 5760 cardiovascular injuries from Ben Taub General Hospital in Houston found 1947 (33.8%) abdominal vascular injuries.[6] The Emory University trauma service at Grady Memorial Hospital consistently treats over 30 patients per year with abdominal vascular injuries. The marked difference between the two settings is believed to reflect the increased wounding power of military firearms, delayed transport to appropriate surgical facilities and, more recently, the protection of torso body armor.

Patients undergoing laparotomy after sustaining abdominal gunshot wounds will be found to have an injury to a major vessel 20%–25% of the time,[7] while penetrating stab wounds will produce a major abdominal vascular injury in only 10% of patients.[8] In contrast, only 5% of patients with blunt abdominal trauma are found to have an injury to a major abdominal vessel at laparotomy.[9] Blunt trauma to the abdominal vasculature typically arises from either rapid deceleration or anterior crush injuries. Deceleration injuries result either in the avulsion of small branches from major vessels (such as avulsion of intestinal branches from the superior mesenteric artery) or in a proximal intimal tear with secondary thrombosis (i.e., renal artery thrombosis).[10] Anterior crush injury also results in two different types of vascular trauma including an intimal flap resulting in secondary thrombosis (superior mesenteric artery, infrarenal abdominal aorta and iliac artery) or a direct blow that completely disrupts an exposed vessel (left renal vein over the aorta).[11]

Abdominal vascular injuries rarely occur in isolation because of a predominantly posterior-central location of a majority of the vasculature. Approximately two to four associated intra-abdominal injuries occur with abdominal vascular injuries, and patients with an injured abdominal vessel have an approximately 50% chance of having injured multiple vessels.[6,12]

INITIAL RESUSCITATION

Physical findings in patients with abdominal vascular trauma depend on the degree of containment of the injury. Patients with contained hematomas in the retroperitoneum, base of the mesentery, or hepatoduodenal ligament frequently present with transient hypotension that responds to an initial bolus of a crystalloid solution. These patients may remain hemodynamically stable with minimal physical findings until the hematoma is opened in the operating room. Conversely, patients presenting with free intraperitoneal hemorrhage have marked hypotension that does not respond to crystalloid boluses and may have a rigid abdomen on physical examination. Comparing patients with abdominal vascular injuries who had hypotension (a lowest emergency department systolic blood pressure of <100 mm Hg) with those without hypotension, it was noted in one study that patients with active bleeding had worse physiologic parameters (mean base deficit of −14.7 compared with −7.2), required more transfusions (15.1 units compared with 8.6 units of blood in the operating room), and had a worse survival rate (43% vs. 96%).[13]

Initial resuscitation for patients with suspected blunt or penetrating injuries to abdominal vessels includes basic airway maneuvers and optimizing pulmonary function. Peripheral intravenous lines should be inserted to start resuscitation with crystalloid solutions. There is no consistent evidence to definitively support either the prehospital administration of crystalloid solutions[14] or the "delayed resuscitation" practice of withholding fluid.[15]

In patients arriving with blunt abdominal trauma, hypotension, and a positive surgeon-performed FAST (focused assessment with sonography for trauma) or in patients arriving with penetrating abdominal trauma, hypotension, and peritonitis, a less than 5-minute time limit in the emergency department resuscitation area is mandatory. Measures to limit heat loss need to be an integral part of each resuscitation, including warmed intravenous fluids, warm blankets, and a dry environment.

Agonal patients presenting to the trauma bay with a rigid abdomen secondary to penetrating trauma may require an emergency department thoracotomy with cross-clamping of the descending thoracic aorta in order to maintain cerebral and coronary arterial blood flow.[16] This maneuver will clearly complicate the patient's intraoperative course, and the need for performing this maneuver is predictive of a less than 5% survival rate.[17]

When transferred to the operating room, standard maneuvers need to be used to prevent hypothermia, including warming the room to more than 85° F (24.9° C), covering the head and exposed upper and lower extremities with a heating unit, using a heating cascade on the anesthetic circuit, and irrigating the body cavities with warm saline.[18] If the patient's systolic pressure is less than 70 mm Hg, some centers use a preliminary operating room thoracotomy with cross-clamping of the descending thoracic aorta before beginning a celiotomy. Even though this maneuver can assist in maintaining cerebral and cardiac blood flow, it has little effect on intra-abdominal vascular injuries because of the significant back flow. Persistent shock (systolic blood pressure <90 mm Hg) after placing a cross-clamp on the descending thoracic aorta portends a universally fatal prognosis.[19]

GENERAL OPERATIVE MANEUVERS

Exposure is obtained through a standard midline abdominal incision, and all clots and free blood are manually evacuated. An initial inspection is conducted in order to identify areas of ongoing hemorrhage, contained hematomas or evidence of ischemia (such as the "black bowel," which is a sign of occlusion of the proximal superior mesenteric artery). Active hemorrhage from solid organs is contained with abdominal packing. Hemorrhage from intra-abdominal vessels is controlled with standard vascular techniques of digital pressure, pressure with laparotomy pads, or hand-held sponge sticks, grabbing the injured vessel with a hand (common or external iliac artery), or formal proximal and distal control. When the active bleeding has been controlled or if the hematoma is initially contained, the surgeon can quickly control enteric or colonic sources of contamination by placing intestinal clamps or bowel staplers across perforations, followed by irrigation of the abdomen and changing gloves before completion of the necessary vascular repair.

CLASSIFICATION OF INJURIES

Major abdominal vascular injuries are best classified as occurring in one of four zones as follows:

Zone 1: Midline retroperitoneum
Supramesocolic region: Suprarenal aorta, celiac axis, proximal superior mesenteric artery, proximal renal artery, and superior mesenteric vein
Inframesocolic region: Infrarenal aorta and infrahepatic inferior vena cava
Zone 2: Upper lateral retroperitoneum
Renal artery and renal vein
Zone 3: Pelvic retroperitoneum
Common, external, and internal iliac arteries and veins
Porta hepatis/retrohepatic inferior vena cava
Portal vein, hepatic artery, and retrohepatic inferior vena cava

INJURIES IN SUPRAMESOCOLIC REGION OF ZONE 1

An abdominal hematoma or hemorrhage in the supramesocolic region of zone 1 typically results from an injury to the suprarenal aorta, celiac axis, proximal superior mesenteric artery, or proximal renal artery. Suprarenal aortic injuries carry reported survival rates ranging from 10%–50%.[20] Proximal vascular control of the aorta should be obtained at the aortic hiatus of the diaphragm. This can be achieved either by manual compression with an aortic compressor (which is correctly positioned by dividing the lesser omentum and retracting the stomach and esophagus to the left; formal cross-clamping at this level will mandate separating the crura from the supraceliac aorta with the electrocautery) or by performing a formal left-sided medial visceral rotation (reflecting all left-sided intra-abdominal viscera, including the colon, kidney, spleen, tail of the pancreas, and fundus of the stomach) (Figure 1). The advantage of the latter is that it provides exposure of the entire abdominal aorta from the hiatus to the aortic bifurcation. This is achieved at a cost of 5 minutes of exposure time and a significant risk of injury to the spleen, left kidney, or left renal artery.[21,22] Supraceliac exposure can be improved by dividing the left crus of the diaphragm at the 2 o'clock position and exposing the distal descending thoracic aorta.[23] An aortic cross-clamp can be applied quickly at this level with minimal dissection. Prolonged cross-clamping of the supraceliac aorta can lead to hepatic hypoperfusion, which may induce a primary fibrinolytic state[24] and severe ischemia of the lower extremities. The lower extremities should be examined at the end of the

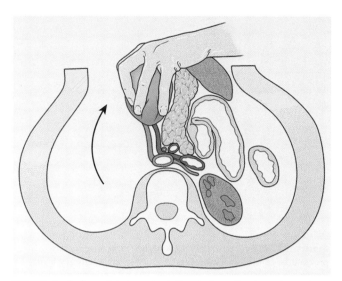

Figure 1 Left medial visceral rotation. Left medial visceral rotation performed with sharp and blunt dissection to elevate the left colon, left kidney, spleen, tail of the pancreas, and gastric fundus. *(From Feliciano DV: Injuries to the great vessels of the abdomen. ACS Surgery: Principles and Practice, 7(10), figure 3, p. 3. WebMD, 2004.)*

procedure and compartment pressures measured below the knee; bilateral below-knee, two-skin incision, four-compartment fasciotomies should be considered for pressures over 30–35 mm Hg.

Aortic injuries at this level can be repaired with 3-0 polypropylene suture in a transverse fashion. When a significant defect is present, a patch aortoplasty can be performed using a patch of polytetrafluoroethylene (PTFE). Resection of a short segment and end-to-end anastomosis at this level are nearly impossible because of the limited mobility of the aorta, so an interposition PTFE graft is necessary for segmental defects.

Asensio and colleagues[25] recently reviewed 13 celiac axis injuries with an overall survival rate of 38% (5 of 13). Four of the five survivors were managed with ligation of the celiac axis. This is well-tolerated because of extensive collateral circulation, especially in the splenic and left gastric arterial beds. Injuries to the common hepatic artery proximal to the gastroduodenal artery are also amenable to ligation. Ligation of the celiac axis may result in necrosis of the gallbladder, however, and a cholecystectomy should be strongly considered.[26] Graham et al.[27] reported a series of patients with injuries to the celiac axis and noted a 100% survival in those with isolated injuries, 33% survival in those with one associated vascular injury, and 100% mortality in those with three associated vascular injuries.

Mesenteric arterial injuries occur in only 12% of penetrating vascular injuries and are associated with 33%–57% mortality.[28] Fullen and colleagues[29] described four anatomic zones of the superior mesenteric artery which dictate options for repair. Fullen zone I injuries lie beneath the pancreas. Exposure requires either transection of the neck of the pancreas between Glassman clamps or a left medial visceral rotation in order to control bleeding. Fullen zone II injuries lie between the pancreaticoduodenal and the middle colic branches of the artery and lie between the pancreas and the base of the transverse mesocolon. Repairs at this level will lie adjacent to the pancreas and are susceptible to pancreatic leaks. Therefore, these lesions and those in zone I in hemodynamically unstable patients are best temporized with the insertion of a temporary intraluminal shunt until the patient is stabilized. Definitive repair can then be accomplished in a more stable patient by performing a saphenous vein or PTFE bypass from the distal infrarenal aorta through the posterior aspect of the small bowel mesentery to the distal superior mesenteric artery in an end-to-side fashion[30] (Figure 2). The aortic suture line must then be protected with retroperitoneal fat or omentum in order

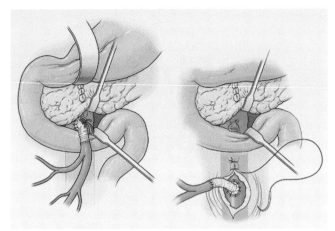

Figure 2 SMA reconstruction. **(A)** When complete grafting procedures to the superior mesenteric artery are necessary, it may be dangerous to place the proximal suture line near an associated pancreatic injury. **(B)** The proximal suture line should be in the lower aorta, away from the upper abdominal injuries, and should be covered with retroperitoneal tissue. *(From Feliciano DV: Injuries to the great vessels of the abdomen. ACS Surgery: Principles and Practice, 7(10), figure 8, p. 5. WebMD, 2004.)*

to avoid the formation of an aorto-enteric fistula. Fullen zone III injuries lay beyond the middle colic branch, and Fullen zone IV injuries lay at the level of the enteric branches. These injures must be primarily repaired to preserve adequate blood flow to the affected regions of small bowel.

The superior mesenteric vein lies to the right of the superior mesenteric artery, and proximal injuries are difficult to manage. Injuries behind the pancreas will also require pancreatic transection to expose and repair. The perforation may also lie inferior to the lower border of the pancreas. These injuries can be digitally controlled by the surgeon and repaired by an assistant with a continuous row of 5-0 polypropylene sutures. In a damage control setting, the superior mesenteric vein can be ligated with reported survival rates ranging up to 85%.[31] If ligation is required, Stone et al.[32] recognized the ongoing need for vigorous postoperative fluid resuscitation lasting up to 3 days. Because these patients often develop massive edema of the small bowel, the abdomen should be left open under a temporary silo.

INJURIES IN INFRAMESOCOLIC REGION OF ZONE I

Injuries to the infrarenal abdominal aorta and the inferior vena cava are the most common vascular injuries in the inframesocolic area of the central abdomen. Exposure at this level is similar to that required for repair of an abdominal aortic aneurysm. With the transverse mesocolon elevated and the small bowel eviscerated to the right, the retroperitoneum is opened at the ligament of Treitz and the opening is extended superiorly to expose the left renal vein. When the aortic injury is underneath a large central retroperitoneal hematoma inferior to the transverse mesocolon, one option is to manually split the hematoma at its highest point and advance the fingers down to identify and compress the point of injury. The injury is always found under the highest point of the hematoma ("Mt. Everest phenomenon"). After obtaining proximal and distal control, the aorta can be repaired primarily with 3-0 polypropylene sutures, with a PTFE patch angioplasty or with an interposition tube graft. The aorta in young trauma patients will usually accommodate a 12–16 mm graft. The gastrocolic omentum should be mobilized and used to cover the graft to prevent a postoperative aortoduodenal fistula.[33]

Injuries to the inferior vena cava present with an inframesocolic hematoma that is more extensive on the right and may have active hemorrhage coming through the base of the mesentery of the ascending colon or at the hepatic flexure. Exposure of the entire abdominal vena cava (from the confluence of the iliac veins to the inferior hepatic margin) is best provided by performing a right medial visceral rotation. This involves mobilization of the right colon and C-loop of the duodenum, leaving the right kidney in situ (Figure 3). The site of hemorrhage can be identified only after stripping the loose retroperitoneal tissue around the inferior vena cava. The injury in this vessel may be harder to identify than one in the adjacent aorta, and sponge sticks may be used to occlude the vessel proximal and distal to the site of hemorrhage until all the fatty tissue is dissected free and the injury is identified. An anterior injury can be controlled using Allis clamps to pull the wound margins into a Satinsky clamp. An extensive injury may require the placement of proximal and distal DeBakey aortic clamps. Another useful adjunct can be the placement of a 5-ml or 30-ml balloon catheter into the caval lumen at the site of laceration and inflating the balloon until better exposure can be obtained or the repair completed.[34] Repair can then be accomplished with a continuous 4-0 or 5-0 polypropylene suture with meticulous bites used to avoid an "hourglass" effect on the vessel at the site of repair.

The two most difficult locations to obtain vascular control of the infrahepatic vena cava are (1) at the junction of the renal veins, and (2) at the confluence of the common iliac veins. Perforations at the junction of the renal veins require proximal and distal compression of the vena cava while vessel loops are passed around the right and left renal veins. If this dissection is not possible, the right kidney can be mobilized from lateral to medial allowing for visualization and placement of a side-biting clamp at the junction of the right renal vein and inferior vena cava. Exposure of perforations at the confluence of the iliac veins is limited by the overlying aortic bifurcation. If necessary, the right common iliac artery can be temporarily divided between vascular clamps, allowing the

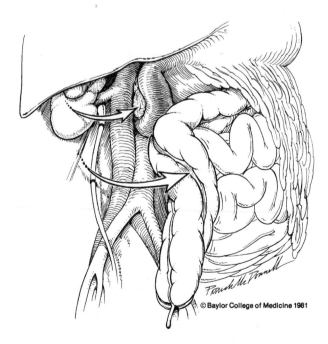

Figure 3 Right medial visceral rotation. Medial rotation of the right sided abdominal viscera (except the kidney) allows for visualization of the entire infrahepatic inferior vena cava. *(From Feliciano DV: Abdominal vascular injury. In Moore EE, Feliciano DV, Mattox KL, editors: Trauma, 5th ed. New York, McGraw-Hill, 2004, figure 36-5, p. 765. Copyright Baylor College of Medicine, 1981.)*

surgeon to mobilize the aortic bifurcation to the left, primarily repair the venous injury, and then reanastomose the right common iliac artery.[35] Alternatively, the ipsilateral internal iliac artery may be ligated, which allows greater mobilization of the right iliac artery away from the vein.

In a young patient who is exsanguinating, the infrarenal inferior vena cava can be ligated. This maneuver is well tolerated with the appropriate perioperative management which includes the following: (1) immediate bilateral below-knee, four-compartment fasciotomies; (2) possible bilateral thigh fasciotomies within the first 48 hours; (3) aggressive, appropriate postoperative fluid resuscitation; (4) application of elastic compression wraps to both lower extremities; and (5) elevation of both lower extremities for 5–7 days postoperatively. When ambulating, the patient should continue to wear the compression wraps and be fitted for full-length, custom-made support hose. Most patients, if treated properly, will have minimal long-term edema of the lower extremities. Current studies indicate survival rates of 22%–56% for injuries to the inferior vena cava, depending on the location.

INJURIES IN ZONE 2

Blunt injuries to the kidney identified on CT rarely require exploration. Stable patients who have a penetrating injury to the flank are evaluated by CT and, if found to have a minor renal injury, can also be observed.[36] In addition, patients undergoing abdominal exploration for other blunt injuries do not need to have a stable hematoma in zone 2 opened, especially if a preoperative CT scan has visualized a reasonably intact kidney. Conversely, in patients who have not undergone a preoperative CT and who are undergoing celiotomy for penetrating abdominal injury, any hemorrhage or hematoma in the lateral upper retroperitoneal area suggests injury to the renal artery, renal vein, or the kidney itself and should be explored. Preliminary vascular control of the renal hilum has not been shown to have an impact on the rate of nephrectomy, transfusion requirements, or blood loss; its use is, therefore, quite variable among trauma centers.[37] Exposure of the traumatized kidney is best obtained by dividing the retroperitoneum lateral to the affected kidney, manually elevating the kidney into the wound, and placing a large vascular clamp proximal to the hilum.

Injuries to the renal artery are difficult to manage because of the small size of the vessel and its location deep in the retroperitoneum. In an unstable patient with two kidneys, multiple intra-abdominal injuries, or a long preoperative period of ischemia, a nephrectomy is clearly warranted. In stable patients, renal arterial injuries can be managed with a lateral arteriorrhaphy or with resection and end-to-end anastomosis. Interposition grafts and borrowed arterial repairs (splenic or right hepatic) have been reported, but are rarely indicated.[38] Survival for patients with isolated injuries to the renal arteries ranges from 56%–74%.

INJURIES IN ZONE 3

The iliac artery and iliac veins lie in the lateral pelvis and can be injured by blunt or penetrating forces. Blunt injuries to branches of the iliac artery, with or without associated pelvic fractures, are typically evaluated and embolized with arteriography. Penetrating injury to the pelvic vessels requires urgent laparotomy. Initial control of hemorrhage can be accomplished with digital or sponge-stick compression until formal proximal and distal control can be achieved by opening the retroperitoneum over the aortic bifurcation and passing vascular tapes around the common, external, and internal iliac vessels. Injuries to the common or external iliac artery should be repaired. In patients with multiple injuries or severe shock, a temporary Argyle shunt may be placed to allow for

damage control. Once the patient is stabilized, options for primary repair include lateral arteriorrhaphy, end-to-end anastomosis, insertion of a saphenous vein or PTFE interposition graft, mobilization and rotation of the internal iliac artery as a replacement, and transposition of one iliac artery to the side of the contralateral iliac for wounds close to the bifurcation.[39] Primary arterial repair in the pelvis (especially with synthetic grafts) is contraindicated in the presence of significant enteric or fecal contamination. In this situation, the proximal and distal artery around the site of injury should be ligated with a double running row of 4-0 polypropylene suture and buried in the retroperitoneum or in an omental pedicle. If the patient is unstable, a four-compartment fasciotomy should be performed on the affected side, and resuscitation continued. When the patient is stable, an extra-anatomic femoro-femoral crossover graft should be performed with an externally ringed, 8-mm PTFE graft. The overall survival for injuries to the common or external iliac artery depends on whether associated vascular injuries or free bleeding into the peritoneal cavity is present. In recent series, survival rates after injury to the external iliac artery has been approximately 65%.

Injuries to the common and external iliac veins can be repaired with 4-0 or 5-0 polypropylene suture or ligated. If repaired and narrowed, postoperative anticoagulation should be administered to avoid thrombotic complications. If ligated, the extremity should be managed as described after ligation of the inferior vena cava.[40] In recent series, survival rates after injuries to the common or external iliac veins were 60% and 72%, respectively.

INJURIES IN PORTA HEPATIS OR TO RETROHEPATIC INFERIOR VENA CAVA

Hematoma and hemorrhage in the area of the portal triad result from injury to the portal vein and/or the hepatic artery with or without an injury to the common bile duct. Before entering the hematoma, a Pringle maneuver is applied by placing a vascular tape or clamp around the hepatoduodenal ligament. Injuries to the hepatic artery are difficult to repair at this level because of the small size and proximity to the portal vein and common bile duct. The vascular injury should be well-delineated before attempted repair. If portal flow is maintained and the patient is in extremis, the hepatic artery can be ligated at this level with a chance of hepatic ischemia. Again, this will necessitate a cholecystectomy.

Injuries to any portion of the portal vein are more difficult to manage than those to the hepatic artery. The portal vein is located more posterior in the hepatoduodenal ligament; it is more friable and has a greater blood flow. The anterior vein is exposed as described previously; however, the posterior portions of the vein require an extensive Kocher maneuver. If the injury appears to be located behind the pancreas, it will be necessary to obtain vascular control by manually occluding the proximal superior mesenteric vein and clamping the portal vein in the hepatoduodenal ligament. The retropancreatic tunnel overlying the anterior wall of the portal vein then needs to be defined and opened. Preferably, the vein can be repaired with running 4-0 polypropylene suture. Major injuries are ligated, a silo is applied, vigorous fluid resuscitation is instituted, and the midgut is inspected at a reoperation in 12–18 hours. The overall survival rate for injuries to the portal vein is 50%.

INJURY GRADING

The American Association for the Surgery of Trauma (AAST) has advanced the Abdominal Vascular Organ Injury Score (AAST-OIS) in order to better describe and define abdominal vascular injuries located more than 2 cm from an organ parenchyma (Table 1).[41] Overall mortality has been shown by Asensio and colleagues[1] to

Table 1: Abdominal Vascular Injury Scale

Grade[a]	Description of Injury	ICD-9	AIS-90
I	Non-named superior mesenteric artery or superior mesenteric vein branches	902.20/.39	NS
	Non-named inferior mesenteric artery or inferior mesenteric vein branches	902.27/.32	NS
	Phrenic artery or vein	902.89	NS
	Lumbar artery or vein	902.89	NS
	Gonadal artery or vein	902.89	NS
	Ovarian artery or vein	902.81/.82	NS
	Other non-named small arterial or venous structures requiring ligation	902.90	NS
II	Right, left, or common hepatic artery	902.22	3
	Splenic artery or vein	902.23/.34	3
	Right or left gastric arteries	902.21	3
	Gastroduodenal artery	902.24	3
	Inferior mesenteric artery, or inferior mesenteric vein, trunk	902.27/.32	3
	Primary named branches of mesenteric artery (e.g., ileocolic artery) or mesenteric vein	902.26/.31	3
	Other named abdominal vessels requiring ligation or repair	902.89	3
III	Superior mesenteric vein, trunk	902.31	3
	Renal artery or vein	902.41/.42	3
	Iliac artery or vein	902.53/.54	3
	Hypogastric artery or vein	902.51/.52	3
	Vena cava, infrarenal	902.10	3
IV	Superior mesenteric artery, trunk	902.25	3
	Celiac axis proper	902.24	3
	Vena cava, suprarenal and infrahepatic	902.10	3
	Aorta, infrarenal	902.00	4
V	Portal vein	902.33	3
	Extraparenchymal hepatic vein	902.11	3 (hepatic vein), 5 (liver + veins)
	Vena cava, retrohepatic or suprahepatic	902.19	5
	Aorta suprarenal, subdiaphragmatic	902.00	4

[a]This classification system is applicable to extraparenchymal vascular injuries. If the vessel injury is within 2 cm of the organ parenchyma, refer to specific organ injury scale. Increase one grade for multiple grade III or IV injuries involving >50% vessel circumference. Downgrade one grade if <25% vessel circumference laceration for grades IV or V.

NS, Not scored.

From Moore EE, et al: Organ injury scaling. III: chest wall, abdominal vascular, ureter, bladder, and urethra. *J Trauma* 33(3):337–339, 1992.

correlate well with the grade of injury: grade II 25%, grade III 32%, grade IV 65%, and grade V 88%.

■ CONCLUSIONS

Injuries to the great vessels of the abdomen are relatively common in busy urban trauma centers. Improving the high morbidity and mortality of patients sustaining abdominal vascular injuries requires a commitment to (1) development of a trauma system in order to minimize transport times, (2) specialized trauma centers, and (3) continued educational efforts to maintain the skill level of practicing trauma surgeons. Still, with the techniques reviewed in this chapter, many of these critically injured patients can be saved.

KEY BIBLIOGRAPHY

Asensio JA, Chahwan S, Hanpeter D, Demetriades D, et al: Operative management and outcomes of 302 abdominal vascular injuries. *Am J Surg* 180: 528–534, 2000.

Asensio JA, Forno W, Roldan G, et al: Abdominal vascular injuries. *Surg Clin North Am* 81(6):1395–1416, 2001.

Davis TP, Feliciano DV, Rozycki GS, et al: Results with abdominal vascular trauma in the modern era. *Am Surg* 67:565–571, 2001.

Feliciano DV, Burch JM, Spjut-Patrinely V, et al: Abdominal gunshot wounds: an urban trauma center's experience with 300 consecutive patients. *Ann Surg* 208:362–370, 1988.

Feliciano DV, Rozycki GS: The management of penetrating abdominal trauma. *Adv Surg* 28:1–39, 1995.

Feliciano DV: Vascular exposure: aorta and vena cava, renal artery and vein, iliac artery and vein, hepatic artery, and portal vein. In Zietlow SP,

Feliciano DV, editors: *Operative Techniques in General Surgery.* Philadelphia, WB Saunders, 2000, pp. 253–264.

Feliciano DV: Abdominal vascular injury. In Moore EE, Feliciano DV, Mattox KL, editors: *Trauma*, 5th ed. New York, McGraw-Hill, 2004, pp. 755–777.

Feliciano DV: Injuries to the great vessels of the abdomen. In Souba WW, Fink MP, Jurkovich GJ, et al, editors: *ACS Surgery: Principles and Practice.* WebMD, 2006, pp. 1250–1261.

Mattox KL, Feliciano DV, Burch J, Beall AC Jr, Jordan GL Jr, Debakey ME: Five thousand seven hundred sixty cardiovascular injuries in 4459 patients. Epidemiologic evolution 1958 to 1987. *Ann Surg* 209:698–707, 1989.

Stone HH, Fabian TC, Turkleson ML: Wounds of the portal venous system. *World J Surg* 6:335–341, 1982.

REFERENCES

1. Asensio JA, Chahwan S, Hanpeter D, et al: Operative management and outcome of 302 abdominal vascular injuries. *Am J Surg* 180:528–534, 2000.
2. Asensio JA, Forno W, Roldan G, et al: Abdominal vascular injuries. *Surg Clin North Am* 81(6):1395–1416, 2001.
3. DeBakey ME, Simeone FA: Battle injuries of the arteries in World War II: an analysis of 2471 cases. *Ann Surg* 123:534–579, 1946.
4. Hughes CW: Arterial repair during the Korean War. *Ann Surg* 147:555–561, 1958.
5. Rich NM, Baugh JH, Hughes CW: Acute arterial injuries in Vietnam: 1,000 cases. *J Trauma* 10:359–369, 1970.
6. Mattox KL, Feliciano DV, Burch J, et al: Five thousand seven hundred sixty cardiovascular injuries in 4459 patients. Epidemiologic evolution 1958 to 1987. *Ann Surg* 209:698–707, 1989.
7. Feliciano DV, Burch JM, Spjut-Patrinely V, et al: Abdominal gunshot wounds: an urban trauma center's experience with 300 consecutive patients. *Ann Surg* 208:362, 1988.
8. Spjut-Patrinely V, Feliciano DV: Trauma Data from Ben Taub General Hospital, Houston, Texas, July 1985 to June 1988.
9. Cox CE: Blunt abdominal trauma. A 5-year analysis of 870 patients requiring celiotomy. *Ann Surg* 199:467–474, 1984.
10. Haas CA, Dinchman KH, Nasrallah PF, et al: Traumatic renal artery occlusion: a 15-year review. *J Trauma* 45:557–561, 1998.
11. Feliciano DV: Abdominal vascular injuries. *Surg Clin North Am* 68:741–755, 1988.
12. Feliciano DV: Abdominal vessels. In Ivatury R, Cayten CG, editors: *The Textbook of Penetrating Trauma.* Baltimore, Williams and Wilkins, 1996, pp. 702–716.
13. Ingram WI, Feliciano DV, Renz BM, et al: Blood pressure in the emergency department in patients with abdominal vascular injuries: effect on management and prognostic value. Presented at the 55th Meeting of American Association for the Surgery of Trauma, Halifax, Nova Scotia, Canada, September 27–30, 1995.
14. Kaweski SM, Sise MJ, Virgilio RW: The effect of prehospital fluids on survival in trauma. *J Trauma* 30:1215–1218, 1990.
15. Bickell WH, Wall MJ Jr, Pepe PE, et al: Immediate versus delayed fluid resuscitation in patients with penetrating torso injuries. *N Engl J Med* 331:1105–1109, 1994.
16. Feliciano DV, Bitondo CG, Cruse PA, et al: Liberal use of emergency center thoracotomy. *Am J Surg* 152:654–659, 1986.
17. Asensio JA, Wall M, Minei J, et al: Practice management guidelines for emergency department thoracotomy. *J Am Coll Surg* 193:303–309, 2001.
18. Feliciano DV, Rozycki GS: The management of penetrating abdominal trauma. In Cameron JL, et al., editors: *Adv Surg* 28:1–39, 1995.
19. Wiencek RG Jr, Wilson RF: Injuries to the abdominal vascular system: how much does aggressive resuscitation and prelaparotomy thoracotomy really help? *Surgery* 102:731–736, 1987.
20. Feliciano DV: Abdominal vascular injury. In Moore EE, Feliciano DV, Mattox KL, editors: *Trauma*, 5th ed. New York, McGraw-Hill, 2004, pp. 755–775.
21. Mattox KL, McCollum WB, Jordan GL Jr, et al: Management of upper abdominal vascular trauma. *Am J Surg* 128:823–828, 1974.
22. Fry WR, Fry RE, Fry WJ: Operative exposure of the abdominal arteries for trauma. *Arch Surg* 126:289–291, 1991.
23. Feliciano DV: Injuries to great vessels of the abdomen. In Souba WW, Fink MP, Jurkovich GJ, et al, editors: *ACS Surgery: Principles and Practice.* Web MD, 2006, pp. 1250–1261.
24. Illig KA, Green RM, Ouriel K, et al: Primary fibrinolysis during supraceliac aortic clamping. *J Vasc Surg* 25:244–251, 1997.
25. Asensio JA, Petrone P, Kimbrell B, Kuncir E: Lessons learned in the management of thirteen celiac axis injuries. *South Med J* 98(4):462–466, 2005.
26. Kavic SM, Atweh N, Ivy ME, et al: Celiac axis ligation after gunshot wound to the abdomen: case report and literature review. *J Trauma* 50:738–739, 2001.
27. Graham LM, Mattox KL, Beall AC Jr, et al: Injuries to the visceral arteries. *Surgery* 84:835–839, 1978.
28. Feliciano DV, Mattox KL: Thoracic and abdominal vascular trauma. In Hobson RW II, Wilson SE, Veith FJ, editors: *Vascular Surgery. Principles and Practice.* New York, Marcell Dekker Inc., 2004, pp. 1049–1070.
29. Fullen WD, Hunt J, Alexander WA: The clinical spectrum of penetrating injury to the superior mesenteric arterial circulation. *J Trauma* 12:656–664, 1972.
30. Accola KD, Feliciano DV, Mattox KL, et al: Management of injuries to the superior mesenteric artery. *J Trauma* 26:313–319, 1986.
31. Donahue TK, Strauch GO: Ligation as definitive management of injury to the superior mesenteric vein. *J Trauma* 28:541–543, 1988.
32. Stone HH, Fabian TC, Turkleson ML: Wounds of the portal venous system. *World J Surg* 6:335–341, 1982.
33. Nothmann A, Tung TC, Simon B: Aortoduodenal fistula in the acute trauma setting: case report. *J Trauma* 53:106–108, 2002.
34. Feliciano DV, Burch JM, Mattox KL, et al: Balloon catheter tamponade in cardiovascular wounds. *Am J Surg* 160:583–587, 1990.
35. Salam AA, Stewart MT: New approach to wounds of the aortic bifurcation and inferior vena cava. *Surgery* 98:105–108, 1985.
36. McAninch JW, Carrol PR: Renal trauma: kidney preservation through improved vascular control. *J Trauma* 22:285–290, 1985.
37. Gonzalez RP, Falimirski M, Holevar MR, et al: Surgical management of renal trauma: is vascular control necessary? *J Trauma* 47:1039–1042, 1999.
38. Barone GW, Kahn MB, Cook M, et al: Traumatic left renal artery stenosis managed with splenorenal bypass: case report. *J Trauma* 30:1594–1596, 1990.
39. Landreneau RJ, Mitchum P, Fry WJ: Iliac artery transposition. *Arch Surg* 124:978–981, 1989.
40. Mullins RJ, Lucas CE, Ledgerwood AM: The natural history following venous ligation for civilian injuries. *J Trauma* 20:737–743, 1980.
41. Moore EE, et al: Organ injury scaling. III: chest wall, abdominal vascular, ureter, bladder, and urethra. *J Trauma* 33(3):337–339, 1992.

COLON AND RECTAL INJURIES

David J. Ciesla and Jon M. Burch

Surgical management of colon and rectal injuries has evolved dramatically since World War II. Accepted treatment at that time generally consisted of resection and end colostomy based on experience with battlefield casualties. Although a difference between civilian and military injuries was recognized, the treatment by civilian trauma surgeons paralleled that of their military counterparts. In the ensuing decades following the Korean and Vietnam wars, primary repair began to replace the "colostomy only" approach in the nonmilitary setting. Numerous prospective randomized trials in civilian centers have since established primary repair as the preferred treatment for most colon and rectal injuries.

INCIDENCE AND MECHANISM

Mechanisms of colon and rectal injuries can be classified as direct penetration of the bowel wall by a foreign body as with stab or gunshot wounds, high-pressure blowout of the bowel wall as occurs in blunt trauma, or devascularization injury secondary to avulsion of the supporting mesentery. The vast majority of colon injuries are caused by penetrating trauma. Firearms account for 75%–90% of penetrating colon injuries. The colon is second only to the small bowel in the frequency of organs injured in penetrating trauma. The high incidence of colon injuries in penetrating trauma relative to other organs is a reflection of the size and distribution of the colon within the abdominal cavity. In contrast, blunt colon injuries are rare, occurring in less than 5% of patients with abdominal injuries. Most occur following high-energy motor vehicle crashes and present as blowout disruptions of colonic wall or mesenteric avulsions. Approximately 80% of rectal injuries are caused by firearms, 10% by blunt trauma, 6% by transanal or impalement injuries, and 3% by transabdominal stab wounds.

DIAGNOSIS

Colon injuries are most often diagnosed during operative exploration. Although it is rare to make an organ-specific diagnosis preoperatively, free intraperitoneal air may occasionally be seen on chest x-ray or abdominal CT scan. Blood or a positive occult hemoglobin test on digital rectal examination may also be seen. Suspicion of enteric injury should be raised in all patients with evidence of fever, tachycardia, peritonitis, and leukocytosis. Computed tomography (CT) scan evidence of intra-abdominal fluid in the absence of solid organ injury warrants further investigation, usually by diagnostic peritoneal lavage. A triple-contrast CT scan may be helpful in patients who have penetrating flank injuries with no clear evidence of intraperitoneal injury.

Blunt colonic injuries are evenly distributed around the colon and usually present as large blowout disruptions of the colon wall or avulsion injuries where the mesocolon is stripped from the adjacent colon. Although penetrating colon injuries are usually obvious, missed injuries are often the result of small-caliber gunshot wounds or stab wounds to areas that are difficult to examine, such as the splenic flexure and rectosigmoid junction. If a perforation is not obvious, feculent odor, hematoma, or mesenteric staining may

suggest an area that requires further evaluation. The suspicious area should be completely mobilized. Division of one or two terminal mesenteric vessels may be necessary to adequately evaluate potential injuries to the mesenteric border. A final diagnostic maneuver is to create a closed loop of colon by proximal and distal manual compression and gently milk the bowel contents toward the suspected injury. The extrusion of fecal material or gas is diagnostic, while its absence effectively rules out colonic injury.

All patients with truncal stab and gunshot wounds, or impalements of the lower abdomen, buttocks, perineum, or upper thighs, and any patient with a history of anal manipulation and lower abdominal or pelvic pain should be suspected of having a rectal injury. Evaluation begins with a digital rectal examination, where the presence of gross or occult blood should trigger further evaluation. However, it is important to note that a negative digital rectal examination does not rule out a rectal injury. Rigid proctoscopy should be performed in all patients with suspected rectal injury. Unstable patients who have undergone laparotomy for hemorrhage control, should have the abdomen temporarily closed and the patient should be repositioned for proctoscopy. Palpation or visualization of a perforation is definitive evidence of an injury. However, intraluminal blood or a submucosal hematoma is often the only evidence of rectal injury. In such cases with distal rectal injuries, transabdominal exploration and rectal mobilization does not improve the chance of definitive diagnosis and may increase the chance of iatrogenic vascular, urologic, or neurologic injury. Therefore, these patients should be treated in the same manner as patients with confirmed rectal injuries.

ANATOMIC LOCATION AND INJURY GRADING

The colon begins at the ileocecal valve and continues to the rectosigmoid junction. Blood is supplied via the ileocolic, right, and middle colic branches of the superior mesenteric artery and the left colic and sigmoidal branches of the inferior mesenteric artery. Venous drainage is via the mesenteric plexus to the superior and inferior mesenteric veins that empty into the portal vein. The rectum begins at the rectosigmoid junction and ends at the dentate line in the anal canal. Blood is supplied by the superior hemorrhoidal branch of the inferior mesenteric artery and the middle and inferior hemorrhoidal branches of the internal iliac or internal pudendal arteries. Venous drainage of the rectum follows the arteries with the superior hemorrhoidal vein draining into the portal system and the middle and inferior hemorrhoidal veins drain via the internal iliac veins.

The Organ Injury Scaling Committee of the American Association of the Surgery of Trauma has developed colon and rectal injury scales that facilitate comparison of injuries between patients and facilities and helps identify patients at high risk for postoperative complications (Tables 1 and 2).

SURGICAL MANAGEMENT

The current management strategies for colon and rectal injuries have been scientifically established in recent decades in civilian trauma centers where operations are generally performed shortly after injury in patients who have been resuscitated and treated with antibiotics. There are two generally accepted surgical options for contemporary management of colon injuries: primary repair or colostomy. Primary repair, whether direct closure of a defect or segmental resection and primary anastomosis, implies that the initial surgical intervention is definitive and no further treatment is necessary. Colostomy options include proximal end colostomy or ileostomy with distal mucous

Table 1: AAST Colon Injury Grading

	Grade	Injury Description
I	Hematoma	Contusion or hematoma without devascularization
	Laceration	Partial thickness, no perforation
II	Laceration	Laceration <50% of circumference
III	Laceration	Laceration >50% of circumference
IV	Laceration	Transection of colon
V	Laceration	Transection with segmental tissue loss

Note: Advance one grade for multiple injuries up to grade III.
Modified from Organ Injury Scaling Committee of the American Association of the Surgery of Trauma.

Table 2: AAST Rectal Injury Grading

	Grade	Injury Description
I	Hematoma	Contusion or hematoma without devascularization
	Laceration	Partial thickness, no perforation
II	Laceration	Laceration <50% of circumference
III	Laceration	Laceration >50% of circumference
IV	Laceration	Full-thickness laceration with extension into perineum
V	Vascular	Devascularized segment

Note: Advance one grade for multiple injuries to the same organ.
Modified from Organ Injury Scaling Committee of the American Association of the Surgery of Trauma.

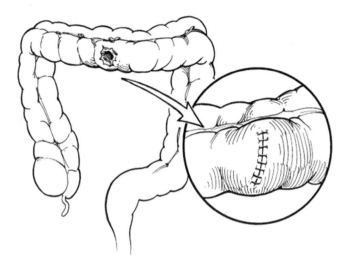

Figure 1 Primary repair of a nondestructive colon injury using a single-layer continuous suture. *(Baylor College of Medicine.)*

fistula or distal closure (Hartman's procedure), loop colostomy of the injured segment, and diverting colostomy proximal to suture repair.

Most authorities would agree that modern treatment of colon injuries is either by primary repair or colostomy. Although primary repair of all colon injuries in the nonmilitary setting is a desirable goal, it is not always possible. The key to successful management is patient selection based on the location and degree of injury and the physiologic state of the patient at the time of repair. For simple nondestructive injuries that do not require segmental resection (AAST CIS I–III), the treatment of choice is primary suture repair. Debridement is kept to a minimum except to remove grossly contaminated or ischemic tissue. We employ a single transverse closure using absorbable monofilament suture beginning a few millimeters from each end of the colostomy. Sutures are placed to gently oppose the seromuscular layer in a continuous Lembert fashion (Figure 1).

The choice between primary anastomosis and colostomy is more complex for destructive colon injuries. The first consideration is the physiologic state of the patient. A damage control approach should be strongly considered for patients with significant metabolic compromise. Critically injured patients with evidence of acidosis, coagulopathy, and hypothermia are at imminent risk of death. The damage control approach is founded on the principle that the metabolic status of the patient does not allow sufficient time to definitively repair all injuries.

The immediate priority is to control bleeding and abdominal contamination, temporarily close the abdomen, and transport the patient to the intensive care unit for vigorous metabolic resuscitation, correction of coagulopathy, and rewarming. The most expeditious method to control fecal contamination is to resect the injured segment of colon using a GIA stapler and close the abdomen with an adhesive plastic sheet. Definitive management of the injury is then performed once the patient has been adequately resuscitated, usually within 24 hours.

Primary repair has been established as the optimal treatment of destructive colon injuries. Destructive injuries proximal to the middle colic artery are generally treated with a right colectomy and ileocolostomy. Ileocolostomy has proven to be a robust anastomosis under emergent conditions and the low associated leak rate justifies its use for almost all injuries proximal to the middle colic artery. Primary repair by lateral suture or segmental resection and colocolostomy is also the procedure of choice for destructive injuries distal to the middle colic artery. Several contemporary retrospective and prospective randomized studies have demonstrated that the results following primary repair are as good as or better than routine colostomy with respect to postoperative complications. These studies have also identified a number of risk factors for suture line failure that include blood loss, concomitant solid organ injury, fecal contamination, mechanism of injury, delayed repair, and patient age. An additional consideration is the subjective evaluation of the degree of bowel edema present at the time of anastomosis. The visceral edema that occurs in the setting of large-volume resuscitation makes the placement and tension of anastomotic sutures uncertain and healing unpredictable. Therefore, colostomy should be considered for injuries distal to the middle colic artery in the presence of significant bowel edema.

Although several methods have been described for creation of ileocolostomy and colocolostomy, we prefer the end-to-end, single-layer technique using absorbable monofilament suture (Figure 2). The suture line is started at the mesenteric border using a double-armed 3-0 polydiaxone suture. Sutures are then placed 3–4 mm from the cut edge of the bowel to include all layers but the mucosa. Each arm is advanced around the bowel and tied at the antimesenteric border resembling a vascular anastomosis. Disparity in bowel caliber can be solved by extension of the enterotomy on the smaller end along the antimesenteric border. The mesenteric defect is then closed with a continuous absorbable suture.

Destructive colon injuries distal to the middle colic artery in patients with multiple risk factors for suture line failure should be treated with colostomy. The damaged section of the colon is resected using a GIA stapler and the proximal end of the colon used for the colostomy. The key technical aspects of colostomy are to ensure that

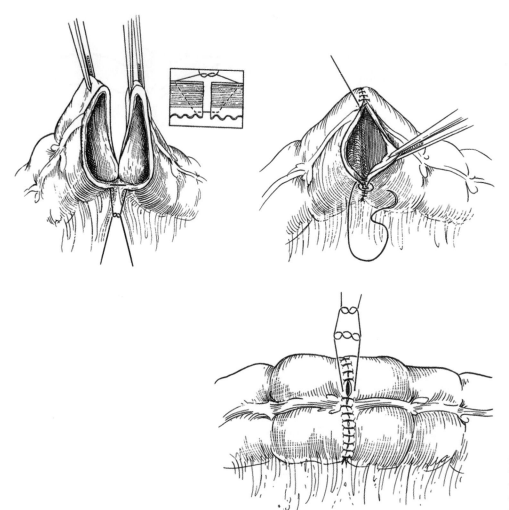

Figure 2   Resection and primary repair of a destructive colon injury using a single layer continuous suture to create an end-to-end anastomosis. *(Baylor College of Medicine.)*

the clamped end of the colon reaches the skin level with no tension, that the end of the colon has an adequate blood supply, and that the colostomy is immediately matured with sutures between the mucosa and the skin without tension. The distal end of the defunctionalized colon is left closed with staples. Treatment of the distal colon segment with mucous fistula is avoided because it is time consuming, is of no additional benefit, adds the potential complications of a second stoma, and adds difficulty to subsequent colostomy closure.

Rectal injuries identified either preoperatively or during abdominal exploration should be repaired. As noted previously, the only indication of a rectal injury may be the presence of intraluminal blood or a submucosal hematoma observed during rigid proctoscopy. Wounds to the extraperitoneal rectum with little or no loss of the rectal wall can be treated with colostomy and presacral drainage alone. Extensive dissection to definitively visualize distal rectal injuries should be avoided because of the potential for vascular, urologic, neurologic, or iatrogenic rectal injury. In such cases, the patient is treated as if a rectal injury is present with presacral drainage and proximal diversion (Figure 3). A curved incision is made posterior to the anus and the presacral space developed bluntly to the level of the sacrum. Ideally, Penrose drains are placed in proximity but not in contact with the injury. The drains are secured to the skin with silk sutures for better patient comfort and usually removed between 4 and 7 days postinjury. Although several methods for proximal diversion are described, it is essential that the chosen technique must completely divert the fecal stream from the rectal injury. We employ a loop colostomy located in the patient's left lower quadrant using the sigmoid colon. The critical technical elements to ensure complete diversion are creating a longitudinal

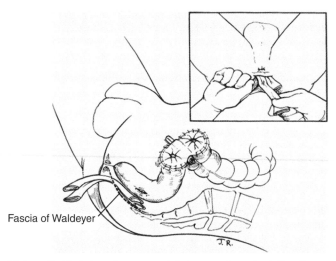

Fascia of Waldeyer

Figure 3   Technique for presacral drainage and proximal diversion for treatment of occult or unrepaired distal colon injuries. *(Baylor College of Medicine.)*

colotomy, maintaining the common wall or spur between the afferent and efferent limbs above the level of the skin, and maturing the stoma to the skin immediately. A loop colostomy created in this manner completely diverts the fecal stream.

Nondestructive rectal injuries that do not require resection based on intraoperative evaluation (AAST RIS I–III) are repaired primarily.

These injuries are generally lacerations with minimal surrounding tissue destruction that are easily exposed and sutured. The location may be intraperitoneal or extraperitoneal and exposed after mobilization of the proximal rectum. The technique used is the same as that for primary repair of colon injuries using a running single layer of 3-0 polydiaxone suture. Placement of drains in the pelvis is not necessary and may increase the risk of fistula.

Extensive loss of the rectal wall or devascularizing injuries (AAST RIS IV and V) are best treated by resection of the rectum distal to the injury and proximal end colostomy. The rectum can be divided within a few centimeters of the anal verge with the aid of a TA stapler after mobilization of the distal rectum. In addition, the advent of the end to end circular stapling device has facilitated elective colostomy closure. This has proved to be a much safer approach to destructive colon injuries than primary repair.

MORBIDITY AND COMPLICATIONS MANAGEMENT

Intra-abdominal abscess is the most frequent septic complication following colon repair, occurring in 5%–15% of patients. Small abscesses of less than 2 cm often respond to intravenous antibiotic therapy and do not require drainage. Many intra-abdominal abscesses can be managed by image guided percutaneous drainage. Occasionally, percutaneous drainage reveals an underlying fistula. In such cases when the patient has no evidence of sepsis, the percutaneous drain is left in place until serial fustulograms demonstrate obliteration of the abscess cavity. Once this occurs, the drain is slowly removed. Larger intra-abdominal abscess that are inaccessible to percutaneous drainage and those associated with sepsis require operative drainage.

Suture line failure and fecal fistula may occur regardless of the treatment method chosen and is observed in 1%–8% of patients. Fistulas that extend to the incision are often associated with intra-abdominal abscesses and evidence of sepsis. A fistulogram should also be performed to determine if there is diffuse leakage throughout the abdominal cavity and an abdominal CT obtained to look for intra-abdominal abscesses. Controlled fistula can be managed nonoperatively but the wound must be carefully inspected for evidence of necrotizing fasciitis. Uncontrolled fistulae require operative intervention and are usually treated by resection of the fistula and leaking segment of colon followed by proximal diversion with an end colostomy.

Stoma complications including stomal necrosis, obstruction, peristomal evisceration, and subcutaneous abscess occur in 3%–14% of patients. Most stomal complications require operative intervention.

Wound infections occur in up to 50% of patients with colon or rectal injuries but should not be considered a complication of the repair. Virtually all wound infections can be avoided by leaving the wound open at the time of abdominal closure. Closure of the wound during the initial operation should be reserved for patients with few associated injuries, minimal subcutaneous fat, little contamination, and who have not suffered prolonged shock.

Stab wound and missile tract infections occur frequently and must be considered in any patient with evidence of systemic sepsis. A reasonable effort should be made to remove missiles and material that have traversed the colon and lodged in the soft tissue to avoid soft tissue infection and possible necrotizing fasciitis.

MORTALITY

Early death in the multiply-injured patient with colon and rectal injuries is most often a result of exsanguination from associated injuries. The late mortality rate associated with colon injuries in contemporary studies ranges from 1%–4%, most often a result of sepsis or multiple organ failure. Death occurs more often in the patients treated with colostomy, but this may be a reflection of injury severity rather than treatment method.

CONCLUSIONS AND ALGORITHM

Despite the evolution in management of colon and rectal injuries in the recent past, the key elements to treatment have remained the same. Prompt recognition, hemorrhage control, and control of enteric spillage are the immediate management priorities followed by reconstruction or diversion. Although treatment must be individualized based on each injury, the constellation of associated injuries, and the physiologic state of the patient, it is important to have a generalized institutional approach to assess treatment outcomes.

With these considerations, we have adopted an institutional approach to colon and rectal injuries outlined in Figure 4. The critical decision-making points for colon injuries are the metabolic status of the patient, the need for segmental resection, the location of the

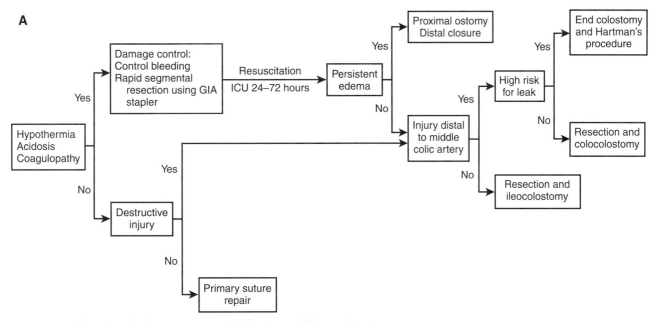

Figure 4   Algorithms for the management of **(A)** colon and **(B)** rectal injuries.

Continued

B

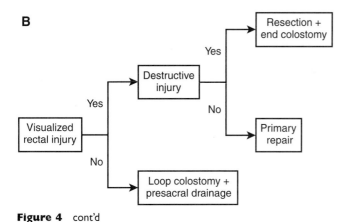

Figure 4 cont'd

injury, and the condition of the bowel at the time of repair. Adherence to this approach enables primary repair in 70%–90% of patients. The first consideration in rectal injuries is whether the injury is identified and repaired. Patients with suspected injuries that are not directly identified or not repaired because of anatomic location are treated with proximal diversion and presacral drainage. Rectal injuries requiring segmental resection are best treated with colostomy rather than primary anastomosis during the initial operation.

SUGGESTED READINGS

Burch JM, Brock JC, Gevirtzman L, et al: The injured colon. *Ann Surg* 203(6):701–711, 1986.

Burch JM, Feliciano DV, Mattox KL: Colostomy and drainage for civilian rectal injuries: is that all? *Ann Surg* 209(5):600–610, discussion 610–611, 1989.

Burch JM, Franciose RJ, Moore EE, et al: Single-layer continuous versus two-layer interrupted intestinal anastomosis: a prospective randomized trial. *Ann Surg* 231(6):832–837, 2000.

Burch JM, Ortiz VB, Richardson RJ, et al: Abbreviated laparotomy and planned reoperation for critically injured patients. *Ann Surg* 215(5):476–483, discussion 483–484, 1992.

Demetriades D, Murray JA, Chan L, et al: Penetrating colon injuries requiring resection: diversion or primary anastomosis? An AAST prospective multicenter study. *J Trauma* 50(5):765–775, 2001.

George SM Jr, Fabian TC, Voeller GR, et al: Primary repair of colon wounds. A prospective trial in nonselected patients. *Ann Surg* 209(6):728–733, 733–734, 1989.

Gonzalez RP, Merlotti GJ, Holevar MR: Colostomy in penetrating colon injury: is it necessary? *J Trauma* 41(2):271–275, 1996.

Ivatury RR, Licata J, Gunduz Y, et al: Management options in penetrating rectal injuries. *Am Surg* 57(1):50–55, 1991.

Maxwell RA, Fabian TC: Current management of colon trauma. *World J Surg* 27(6):632–639, 2003. (Epub 2003 May 2.)

Miller PR, Fabian TC, Croce MA, et al: Improving outcomes following penetrating colon wounds: application of a clinical pathway. *Ann Surg* 235(6):775–781, 2002.

Moore EE, Cogbill TH, Malangoni MA, et al: Organ injury scaling. II: pancreas, duodenum, small bowel, colon, and rectum. *J Trauma* 30(11):1427–1429, 1990.

Nelson R, Singer M: Primary repair for penetrating colon injuries. *Cochrane Database Syst Rev* (3):CD002247, 2003.

Renz BM, Feliciano DV, Sherman R: Same admission colostomy closure (SACC). A new approach to rectal wounds: a prospective study. *Ann Surg* 218(3):279–292, discussion 292–293, 1993.

Rombeau JL, Wilk PJ, Turnbull RB Jr, Fazio VW: Total fecal diversion by the temporary skin-level loop transverse colostomy. *Dis Colon Rectum* 21(4):223–226, 1978.

Vitale GC, Richardson JD, Flint LM: Successful management of injuries to the extraperitoneal rectum. *Am Surg* 49(3):159–162, 1983.

Williams MD, Watts D, Fakhry S: Colon injury after blunt abdominal trauma: results of the EAST Multi-Institutional Hollow Viscus Injury Study. *J Trauma* 55(5):906–912, 2003.

GENITOURINARY TRACT INJURY

Charles D. Best

KIDNEY INJURY

The most common indication of kidney injury on assessment in the emergency department is the presence of gross or microhematuria. Dipstick and urinalysis methods of determining the presence of hematuria have proved to be satisfactory for screening, with greater than 97.5% sensitivity and specificity,[1] and should initiate the process of staging by radiographic evaluation. The presence of hematuria does not correlate with the degree of injury, however.

There is ongoing evidence that adult patients sustaining blunt trauma can be selectively imaged on the basis of presence of hematuria and hemodynamic status. Based on the large experience of McAninch and colleagues,[1] as well as others, in working with patients with blunt trauma with microscopic hematuria and no evidence of shock, imaging is not required to assess urologic injury. Mee and colleagues[2] studied 1007 patients with blunt trauma and found that patients with gross hematuria or microscopic hematuria (>5 red blood cells per high-powered field [RBCs/hpf]) and shock (SBP <90 mm Hg) are most likely to have significant injuries, and radiographic imaging is mandatory. The selection criteria to determine need for imaging is based on blood pressure findings recorded at any time during the patient's initial evaluation, including paramedic assessment in the field.

These criteria do not apply to pediatric patients. The criteria for imaging in the pediatric population are different than for adults. This stems from the fact that there is not a well-established definition of shock in prepubertal children. Certainly, children with gross hematuria, regardless of hemodynamic stability, should be imaged. This will also allow for the detection of any congenital anomalies, such as ureteropelvic junction obstruction. Recent literature has been supportive of sparing imaging in stable children with only microhematuria. Brown et al.[3] revealed only a 4.6% significant renal injury rate in children with blunt trauma and microhematuria, defined as more than 3 rbc/hpf. Using more than 50 rbc/hpf as a criterion for imaging children with blunt trauma, Morey et al.[4] found only 1 in 147 patients with significant renal injury.

In addition, all patients with penetrating injuries and any degree of hematuria should be imaged or explored. At most major trauma centers, hemodynamically stable patients will undergo computed tomography (CT) scan of the abdomen and pelvis to rule out any abdominal injury. This incidentally allows visualization of the kidneys. The sensitivity and cost-effectiveness of the CT scan as a single imaging modality have for the most part replaced the routine use of IVP to exclude collecting system injury. Appropriate grading of renal injuries is crucial in determining management and expectant outcomes. The rate of urologic complications increases with increasing renal trauma grade. This can range from 0% complications with grade I injuries to 100% with grade V renal injuries. Performing follow-up CT scans in patients with grade III or higher injuries will detect 90% of delayed urologic complications.[5]

Blunt traumatic injuries as a result of automobile accidents, falls, or blows to the abdomen may cause significant damage to the kidney and represent at least 80% of all renal injuries seen in most urban hospitals. In rural hospitals, 90%–95% of kidney injuries are caused by blunt trauma. Bed rest and observation are successful in managing 95% of patients with blunt traumatic injuries. Santorelli et al.[6] showed that solid organ injuries secondary to blunt trauma, including renal injury, can be managed nonoperatively in hemodynamically stable patients with approximately a 90% success rate. Urologic complications occur in about 11% of patients managed expectantly.[7] These include delayed bleeding,[8] post renal hypertension, arteriovenous fistula, and urinary extravasation.[9] Similar findings are found in the pediatric population. Margenthaler et al.[10] reported an 87% success rate with nonoperative management in pediatric blunt renal injury, including 26% of patients with high-grade injury. Only two of the seven children requiring surgery had failed conservative management. No patient with follow-up developed hypertension. The patient should be maintained on strict bed rest until gross hematuria has cleared, at which point ambulation should be allowed to a limited extent. The patient must be carefully monitored for hematocrit and evidence of retroperitoneal bleeding. If gross hematuria returns after ambulation is allowed, reassessment of the injury is indicated.

Penetrating injuries account for approximately 20% of renal injuries in urban settings. These injuries generally occur from gunshot wounds and stab wounds. All penetrating renal injuries require operative exploration, unless the staging process indicates that the renal injury is minor. Indications for renal exploration in patients with renal injury are excessive and persistent retroperitoneal bleeding, pulsatile retroperitoneal hematoma, urinary extravasation in the presence of other significant injuries, significant amount of nonviable tissue, and vascular injury. Clinical judgment must be exercised in applying these indications for operation. The risk of late complications, such as hematuria, arteriovenous fistula, scarring or renal hypertension, after conservative management, has been cited as a reason for prompt exploration. Velmahoes et al.[11] evaluated the role of selective exploration of renal gunshot wounds and assessed the clinical and radiographic criteria of such a policy. Patients who underwent nephrectomy were more often hemodynamically unstable, had more severe kidney injuries, and had a higher Injury Severity Score (ISS) than patients who had renal reconstruction. In cases of renal exploration, proximal vascular control was practiced only in the presence of central injuries, provided that the patient was hemodynamically stable. This policy resulted in 38% of patients avoiding unnecessary renal exploration.

Grade IV renal injuries can be particularly challenging. Associated injuries are common, occurring in 80% of patients. These associated injuries are often the reason for laparotomy, with subsequent repair of the renal injury. In a patient who is hemodynamically stable after blunt injury, extravasation of urine would not necessitate renal exploration when additional indications for operation are not present. In fact, less than 10% of blunt traumatic renal injuries require exploration. A large retroperitoneal hematoma incidentally discovered during laparotomy calls for intraoperative excretory urography, which will give information regarding the injured kidney as well as whether the contralateral kidney is normal. If excretory urography reveals an abnormality, renal exploration is indicated. Carefully preoperative staging of the injury with use of CT (excretory urography optional) helps to identify patients who are candidates for nonoperative management. In the San Francisco experience of 113 grade IV renal injuries, 78% were explored, with only a 9% nephrectomy rate. Specific renal complications were rare (4%), with an overall complication rate of 23% in those patients managed conservatively. This was similar to those managed operatively, with a 4% renal complication rate, and an overall rate of 30%.[12]

The operative approach for exposure of an injured kidney is a transabdominal incision, which allows the surgeon to expose the renal vessels and control them with vessel loops. One of the main causes for total nephrectomy after trauma is uncontrollable renal bleeding. A retroperitoneal incision is made over the aorta just above the level of the inferior mesenteric artery. Dissection superiorly over the aorta should allow location of the left renal vein and both renal arteries. Applying vascular clamps to the individual vessel should control any massive bleeding if necessary. This method of control has been shown to significantly reduce nephrectomy.[13] Reflecting the colon off the hematoma should adequately expose the kidney, and the hematoma can be entered without fear of exsanguinating hemorrhage. Repair of the injured kidney is successful in 90% of cases. Total nephrectomy secondary to trauma is seldom necessary.

All nonviable tissue should be removed. Active bleeding at the margins indicates viability of the tissue. Hemostasis can be obtained by use of fine figure-of-8 chromic sutures on individual bleeding points. If the collecting system is violated, it should be closed with absorbable suture and made watertight. This can be confirmed by injecting methylene blue into the renal pelvis. The parenchymal defect should be covered with any preserved renal capsule, omental pedicle graft, or fibrin sealant. Partial nephrectomy may be appropriate in some cases. The presence of concomitant bowel injury should not change management of the renal injury.

Patients who undergo operative repair should be allowed to ambulate as soon as gross hematuria has cleared. The mean hospital stay for patients who have had renal injuries repaired surgically is less than 7 days. Patients who have gross hematuria and are managed nonoperatively should be hospitalized initially, and remain at bed rest until the gross hematuria is cleared. Once ambulation is allowed, the patient can be discharged if no further bleeding occurs, with restricted activity once at home. Patients with microscopic hematuria should be well staged and can be discharged home with restricted activity levels. Patients should be followed with periodic urinalysis and blood pressure determinations for several months. Follow-up excretory urography or CT scan will provide anatomic information on the healed renal unit, and/or diuretic renal scans will provide functional data. These should be done 2–3 months after injury.

URETERAL INJURY

The ureter or renal pelvis may be injured by a penetrating object (i.e., bullet or knife), surgical mishap, or blunt trauma. Blunt trauma is a rare cause, accounting for only 6% of ureteral injuries, and the other two types of injury occur approximately equally. Overall, ureteral injuries account for less than 1% of all genitourinary trauma. Patients with ureteral injuries from external trauma are often severely injured with multiple associated injuries. Diagnosis and management can often be challenging. Favorable outcomes are usually the result of early diagnosis and reconstruction. Failure to promptly recognize a ureteral injury frequently results in loss of functioning renal parenchyma, sepsis, and possibly death.[14]

In penetrating injuries of the ureter, microscopic hematuria is present in only 70%–80% of cases and should raise the suspicion for injury. On the other hand, there is a 30% false-negative rate.[14] Imaging should be performed on any patient with an abdominal injury and any degree of hematuria, or those patients where the trajectory may raise suspicion of ureteral, or renal injury. CT scan or intravenous pyelogram (IVP) approach 90% diagnostic accuracy in the acute setting.[15] Ureters that have been injured surgically and are unrecognized at the time, will often become obstructed and cause severe pain or prolonged ileus in the postoperative period. They may also present as excessive fluid drainage from surgical drain or wound. This fluid should be analyzed for creatinine. Excretory urography and retrograde ureterography can establish the diagnosis.

Penetrating injuries to the ureter require surgical reconstruction, in most cases by ureteroureterostomy, consisting of resection of the injured area and a primary repair. An exception of primary repair without debridement can be made in injuries resulting from blunt trauma or stab wounds. In all cases, internal stents using double-J catheters are recommended. In cases of surgical injury to the ureter that have been discovered within 2 weeks of operation, re-exploration and surgical management of the injury is recommended. Timing of diagnosis (early or late), location, grade of injury, and patient status should determine the type of management. Lower ureteral injuries may require ureteroneocystostomy, often with a psoas hitch. Mid- and upper-ureteral injuries can be managed by ureteroureterostomy or transureteroureterostomy. In all cases, adequate debridement of non-viable tissue, and a spatulated, mucosa-to-mucosa, tension-free anastomosis should be performed. Retroperitoneal drainage near the repair site is mandatory, and in some cases, use of omental flaps or other tissue should be used to further isolate the repair. Significant ureteral loss may require bowel interposition, autotransplantation, or nephrectomy.

Drains should be left in the retroperitoneum after reconstruction until output is minimal. Internal stents are generally left in place for 4–6 weeks and can be removed endoscopically through the bladder after excretory urography or retrograde pyelography. Excretory urography should be done again approximately 3 months after reconstruction to ascertain ureteral patency.

BLADDER INJURY

Approximately 10% of pelvic fractures are associated with bladder rupture. On the other hand, about 85% of traumatic bladder injuries are associated with pelvic fracture. Gross hematuria is present in most cases (94%),[16] and the remaining injuries will have microhematuria. The diagnosis is established by a traditional filling cystogram or CT cystogram. At least 400 ml of contrast medium should be used in either imaging study. Oblique and postvoid films should be performed with a fluoroscopic study. False-negative readings usually result from inadequate filling of the bladder with contrast. Injuries to the bladder are classified according to site of rupture. These sites, in decreasing order of frequency, are extraperitoneal (58%), intraperitoneal (~33%), and combined (~10%).

Patients who have intraperitoneal bladder rupture should undergo surgical exploration and repair of the bladder. A transabdominal mid-line incision in the lower abdomen can be used, and exposure of the bladder should be done at the mid-line. Lateral pelvic hematomas should be carefully avoided. The bladder should be opened at the mid-line and inspected from within. The length and number of lacerations cannot be assessed accurately by cystography. Any extraperitoneal lacerations are then closed from inside the bladder with a single layer of interrupted 2-0 or 3-0 absorbable suture. Intraperitoneal bladder rupture should be closed in two layers of running sutures. A suprapubic cystostomy tube may be left in place for 7–10 days, although modern experience has shown excellent success with urethral drainage alone. Parry et al. in a retrospective review, showed no difference in outcomes or complications in patients with bladder rupture treated with suprapubic tube and transurethral catheter versus transurethral catheter alone.[17] A drain should be placed in the region of the repair. The bladder nearly always returns to full function. During the early healing phases, the patient should be monitored carefully for potential urinary infection. Radiographic studies are seldom indicated unless the patient has complications.

URETHRAL INJURY

Approximately 5%–10% of pelvic fractures are associated with urethral injury, usually at the proximal bulbar urethra. In addition, straddle injuries occur to the deep bulbar urethra and pendulous

(anterior) urethra. These occur by forceful contact of the perineum with a blunt object such as handlebars or a fence. Another cause of blunt urethral trauma occurs in association with penile fracture. The incidence is about 20% in that situation. The most common indication of urethral injury is the finding of blood at the urethral meatus on initial examination, found in ~75% of patients. Other findings include hematuria, although nonspecific; inability to void; and perineal or penile hematoma. Passage of a urethral catheter is contraindicated when urethral injury is suspected. Urethrography is recommended as the first study done and the presence of extravasation will establish the diagnosis. This should ideally be performed with the patient in an oblique position. With widespread use of CT as the frontline imaging modality for the acutely traumatized patient, it may be essential to be familiar with CT findings suggestive of urethral injury. Extravasation of contrast above the urogenital diaphragm (UGD) is consistent with prostatic urethral disruption. Extravasation below the urogenital diaphragm is more consistent with bulbar urethral disruption. There may also be a combination above and below this muscle plane, indicting a more extensive injury of the posterior urethra. Other nonspecific findings include obscuring of the UGD fat plane, hematoma near the ischiocavernosus muscle, and distortion of the prostatic contour or bulbocavernosus muscle.[18]

Virtually all urethral injuries are the result of blunt trauma (motor vehicle accidents, falls, or blows) and occur in men. When penetrating injuries are seen, operative exploration and reconstruction of the specific injury are generally indicated. The urethral injury is often concomitant with injury of the corpora cavernosa. These injuries can be repaired simultaneously. Exceptions to this rule are when the following findings are associated with the urethral injury: hemodynamic instability, multiple associated injuries of nongenital organs, or a large urethral defect. In these situations, placement of a suprapubic cystostomy tube should be the initial management. Female urethral injuries are uncommon (0%–6.0% of female patients with pelvic fracture).[19]

The initial management of blunt traumatic anterior urethral disruption has traditionally been placement of suprapubic cystostomy tube. This is usually done percutaneously, or can be done by open exploration of the bladder if exploratory laparotomy is to be performed for other injuries. Only a small cystostomy incision is needed to permit inspection of the inside of the bladder for any potential associated rupture, as well as placement of the suprapubic catheter. Manipulation of the deep pelvis should be avoided, and no drains should be left in place; these measures can introduce infection in a perivesical hematoma. There is recent controversy with management by immediate urethral realignment. This is a reasonable option in patients with penetrating injuries to the urethra, or blunt injuries associated with pelvic fracture, that do not have the other findings described earlier. The stricture rate is significantly less with immediate realignment, and fewer subsequent procedures are required. When performed in select patients, the incidence of impotence and incontinence is also less than in patients undergoing delayed reconstruction.[20]

Patients with complete prostatomembranous urethral disruption invariably develop a stricture at the site of the disruption, but this can be repaired electively 2–3 months after injury. This repair can be accomplished by a combined transpubic perineal approach, by endoscopic urethrotomy, or more commonly, by perineal urethroplasty. Adequate planning of the reconstruction should include imaging by traditional retrograde urethrogram or urethral ultrasonography. Twenty to 30% of patients with pelvic fractures may become impotent. This is believed to be caused by nerve and vascular damage at the time of injury, which has been shown arteriographically.[21] Secondary stricture formation after urethroplasty may occur in 15%–20% of cases and often can be managed by endoscopic urethrotomy.

Patients with anterior urethral injury (bulbar and pendulous) who are managed by initial suprapubic cystostomy should have voiding cystourethrography approximately 2–3 weeks after injury; if no extravasation is noted, the patient should be allowed to continue voiding per urethra. Most of these patients develop relative strictures in the area of injury, but most do not require operative intervention or reconstruction. If operative correction is indicated, endoscopic urethrotomy is usually successful.

GENITAL INJURY

Penile fracture, although uncommon, demands immediate diagnosis and correction. The patient will have a history of a loud cracking sound while engaging in sexual activity, and in all cases an erection is present. A transverse tear in the tunica albuginea that surrounds the erectile bodies occurs as a result of the force applied to the area. Immediate detumescence occurs, and a hematoma develops on the penile shaft. This is often described as an "eggplant" deformity. In approximately 20% of cases, the urethra will be injured as well. These tunica injuries should be surgically corrected and involve degloving the penis, controlling the bleeding, and reapproximation of the tunica albuginea with interrupted polyglycolic acid sutures. Patients treated promptly in this manner almost always have a return of normal sexual function.

Blunt trauma to the scrotum may result in large hematoceles and testicular rupture. Testicular rupture is best diagnosed by ultrasonography, which will demonstrate areas of relative lucency of the echogenic patterns within the testicle parenchyma. Surgical correction of the ruptured testicle should be done by a trans-scrotal approach with evacuation of the hematoma and repair of the injury. The nonviable parenchyma that extrudes freely into the scrotal space should be removed, and the tunica albuginea of the testicle should be approximated with a running polyglycolic suture. These testicles heal after reconstruction and are useful for hormone production and cosmetic appearance. Return of spermatogenesis after such an injury is unpredictable. The need for complete orchiectomy is not often necessary when injury results from blunt trauma, particularly if diagnosed within 48 hours of injury.

Major skin loss to the penis and scrotum occurs from avulsion injuries, burns, gunshot wounds, and stab wounds. Urethrography should be done to determine whether concomitant urethral injury is present. Management should be aimed at reconstruction, using all attached salvageable skin. When local skin is not available, split-thickness skin grafts can be used to cover the testicles and penis. If the wound seems severely contaminated, testicles can be placed in subcutaneous pouches on the medial aspect of the thigh. More recent trends in management have involved wet-to-dry dressing changes to the exposed testicles, with grafting with split-thickness grafts once tissue bed is healthy. This has diminished the necessity of the thigh pouch technique, and delayed reconstruction. Third-degree burns of the penile shaft and scrotum should be corrected with total skin excision and immediate replacement with split-thickness skin grafts. With these methods, acceptable cosmetic and functional results can be expected.

REFERENCES

1. Chandhoke P, McAninch JW: Detection and significance of microscopic hematuria in patients with blunt renal trauma. *J Urol* 140:16–18, 1988.
2. Mee SL, McAninch JW, Robinson AL, et al: Radiographic assessment of renal trauma: a 10-year prospective study of patient selection. *J Urol* 141:1095–1098, 1989.
3. Brown SL, Haas CH, Dinchman KH, et al: Radiologic evaluation of pediatric blunt renal trauma in patients with microscopic hematuria. *World J Surg* 25:1557–1560, 2001.
4. Morey AF, Bruce JE, McAninch JW: Efficacy of radiographic imaging in pediatric blunt trauma. *J Urol* 156:2014–2018, 1996.
5. Blankenship JC, Gavant ML, Cox EC, et al: Importance of delayed imaging for blunt renal trauma. *World J Surg* 25:1561–1564, 2001.
6. Santorelli KH, Frumiento C, Rogers FB, et al: Nonoperative management of hepatic, splenic, and renal injuries in adults with multiple injuries. *J Trauma* 49:56–61, 2000.
7. Hershorn S, Radonski SB, Shoskes DA, et al: Evaluation and treatment of blunt renal trauma. *J Urol* 146:274–277, 1991.
8. Wein AJ, Murphy JJ, Mulholland SG, et al: A conservative approach to the management of blunt renal trauma. *J Urol* 117:425–427, 1977.
9. Carroll PR, Klosterman PW, McAninch JW: Surgical management of renal trauma: analysis of risk factors, technique and outcome. *J Trauma* 28:1071–1074, 1988.
10. Margenthaler JA, Weber TR, Keller MS: Blunt renal trauma in children: experience with conservative management at a pediatric trauma center. *J Trauma* 52:928–932, 2002.
11. Velmahoes GC, Demetriades D, Cornwell EE, et al: Selective management of renal gunshot wounds. *Br J Surg* 85:1121–1124, 1998.
12. Santucci RA, McAninch JW: Grade IV renal injuries: evaluation, treatment and outcome. *World J Surg* 25:1565–1572, 2001.
13. McAninch JW, Carroll PR: Renal trauma: kidney preservation through improved vascular control—a refined approach. *J Trauma* 22:285–288, 1982.
14. Presti JC, Carroll PR, McAninch JW: Ureteral and renal pelvic injuries from external trauma: diagnosis and management. *J Trauma* 29 370–374, 1989.
15. Carver BS, Bozeman CB, Venable DD: Ureteral injury due to penetrating trauma. *South Med J* 97:462–464, 2004.
16. Hsieh CH, Chen RJ, Fang JF, et al: Diagnosis and management of bladder injury by trauma surgeons. *Am J Surg* 184:143–147, 2002.
17. Parry NG, Rozycki GS, Feliciano DV, et al: Traumatic rupture of the urinary bladder: is the suprapubic tube necessary? *J Trauma* 54:431–436, 2003.
18. Ali M, Safried Y, Solafani S, Schulze R: CT signs of urethral injury. *Radiographics* 23:951–963, 2003.
19. Chapple C, Barbagli G, Mundy AR, et al: Consensus statement on urethral trauma. *BJU Int* 93:1195–1202, 2004.
20. Mouraview VB, Coburn M, Santucci RA: The treatment of posterior urethral disruption associated with pelvic fractures: comparative experience of early realignment versus delayed urethroplasty. *J Urol* 173:873–876, 2005.
21. Levine FJ, Greenfield AJ, Goldstein I: Arteriographically determined occlusive disease within hypogastric-cavernous bed in impotent patients following blunt perineal and pelvic trauma. *J Urol* 144:1147–1153, 1990.

GYNECOLOGIC INJURIES

Areti Tillou   and   Patrizio Petrone

TRAUMA IN PREGNANCY

Gynecologic trauma includes a large variety of relatively rare and challenging injuries from blunt and penetrating mechanisms. While motor vehicle crashes are the leading cause of major injury in pregnant women, penetrating trauma accounts for almost all injuries to the fallopian tubes, ovaries, and nongravid uterus. Pelvic fractures and straddle injuries often result in trauma to perineum, vagina, and less commonly the cervix and uterus. Injuries to the external genitalia are frequently associated with interpersonal violence and should be treated in that context.

In recent years, trauma has been recognized as the leading cause of death during pregnancy. As unsuspected pregnancy is relatively common in the reproductive years, this possibility must be considered when evaluating female trauma victims. Pregnancy produces significant physiologic and anatomic changes that must be recognized and understood by all health care providers treating pregnant trauma patients (Table 1).

Table 1: Changes in Maternal Physiology during Pregnancy

Change	Consequence
Cardiac output and blood volume increase	Shock after >40% of blood lost
Expansion of plasma volume	Physiologic anemia
Decline in arterial and venous pressure	Vital signs are not reflective of hemodynamic status
Increase of resting pulse	
Chest enlargement	Change in anatomic landmarks Caution during thoracic procedures (e.g., thoracostomy)
Diaphragm rise	
Substernal angle increase	
Decrease in functional residual capacity	Rapid decline in PO_2 during apnea or airway obstruction
Increase in oxygen consumption	
Airway closure when supine	
Increase in tidal volume and minute ventilation	Fall in PCO_2 and bicarbonates
Decrease in anesthetic requirements	Need for adjustment of sedative doses
Decreased gastric motility	Risk of aspiration
Relaxation of gastroesophageal sphincter	

Incidence

According to some authors, nearly 50% of maternal deaths are related to trauma. From 6%–7% of all pregnancies are complicated by trauma, and 0.4% of the patients require hospitalization for treatment of injuries. In 1995, Weiss reported an epidemiologic 1-year study in which all women of childbearing age who required hospitalization for injuries were screened for pregnancy; of 16,722 women, 761 were identified (4.6%) as being pregnant. The actual number of injured pregnant women is underestimated as many of them are unreported, especially with injuries resulting from domestic violence.

Mechanism of Injury

Motor vehicle collisions are the most common causes of injury during pregnancy. As the pregnancy progresses, the shift in the woman's center of gravity and diminished agility can result in falls and accidental injuries. Other common causes of injury include automobile–pedestrian collisions and firearm injuries. Younger women are at higher risk for injury during pregnancy, with a mean maternal age of 25 years.

Young pregnant women are also at high risk for injuries resulting from battery. It has been reported that 10%–30% of women are abused during pregnancy, and 5% of cases involving abuse result in fetal death. Of injured pregnant patients, 17% experience intentional trauma and 60% suffer repeated episodes of domestic violence. Physical abuse is suspected when the injuries are located proximally and in the midline, rather than distally, and trauma is evident to the neck, breast, face, upper arms, and lateral thighs, as well as with bizarre injuries such as cigarette burns or bites.

Diagnosis

Care is undertaken with attention to both mother and fetus. Uterine blood flow lacks autoregulation and is related directly to maternal blood pressure; consequently, treatment priorities are the same as for the nonpregnant trauma patient, as the best initial treatment for the fetus is the optimal resuscitation of the mother. A thorough physical exam complemented by imaging studies is necessary to identify some of the unique problems that might be present in any pregnant patient, including blunt or penetrating injury to the uterus, placental abruption, amniotic fluid embolism, isoimmunization, or premature rupture of membranes.

Prehospital Care

As a result of significant changes in maternal physiology (see Table 1), supplemental oxygen should be administered to prevent maternal and fetal hypoxia during transport and in the resuscitation room. Fluid resuscitation should be initiated even in the absence of signs of hypovolemia and shock. To avoid supine hypotension associated with the uterine compression of the inferior vena cava (IVC), patients in the second or third trimester of pregnancy should be transported on a backboard tilted to the left, with special attention to immobilization of the cervical spine. If the patient is kept in a supine position, the right hip should be elevated 4–6 inches, and the uterus should be displaced manually to the left. This maneuver increases cardiac output by 30% and restores circulating blood volume. Although only about 10% of pregnant patients at term develop symptoms of shock in the supine position, fetal distress may be present even in normotensive mothers; therefore, right hip elevation should be maintained at all times including during operative procedures.

Hospital Care

Primary survey includes assessment of airway, breathing, and circulation (ABCs), including volume replacement and hemorrhage control. Secondary survey includes the obstetrical history, physical examination, and evaluation and monitoring of the fetus. The history should include the date of the last menstrual cycle, expected date of delivery, and any problems or complications of the current and previous pregnancies such as preterm labor or placental abruption. Comorbidities such as pregnancy-induced hypertension and diabetes mellitus should also be documented.

The abdominal examination is critically important, as is a determination of uterine size, which provides an approximation of gestational age and fetal maturity. A discrepancy between dates and uterine size suggests uterine hemorrhage or rupture. Uterine rupture is suspected with peritoneal signs, abdominal palpation of fetal parts due to extrauterine location, and inability to palpate the uterine fundus. However, as the uterus enlarges, it displaces the intestines upward and laterally, stretching the peritoneum and making the abdominal physical examination unreliable.

Determination of gestational age is particularly important because this will guide the decision for a premature delivery if indicated. Most institutions will accept a 24–26 week pregnancy as viable, with a probability of survival ranging from 20%–70%. Radiographic estimation of gestational age is bound to an error of 1–2 weeks. Unless the date of the conception is known exactly, gestational age is particularly difficult to determine. A good rule of thumb is to consider patients with a uterus halfway between the umbilicus and the costal margin as having a viable pregnancy (Figure 1). An algorithm for initial maternal and fetal assessment is presented in Figure 2.

Physical evaluation of the pregnant patient must be directed to the detection of the following six pregnancy-related acute conditions.

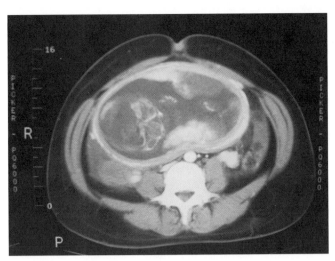

Figure 1 Computed tomography scan showing pregnant uterus above the level of umbilicus indicating a viable fetus.

Vaginal bleeding

This is an ominous sign that suggests premature cervical dilation, early labor, placental abruption, or placenta previa. Placental abruption after trauma occurs in 2%–4% of minor accidents and in up to 50% of major injuries. Maternal mortality from abruption is less than 1%, but fetal death ranges from 20% to 35%. Both fetal heart monitoring and sonographic evaluation should be used to investigate the possibility of abruption that most frequently becomes evident within several hours after trauma.

Ruptured membranes

In addition to increased risk of infection, prolapse of the umbilical cord can occur, resulting in compression of the umbilical vein and arteries.

Bulging perineum

This is caused most commonly by pressure from extrauterine location of fetal parts.

Presence and patterns of contractions

Direct or indirect trauma to the myometrium may result in release of arachidonic acid that can cause uterine contractions. Although most contractions will cease spontaneously, preparation for a premature delivery should be made.

Abnormal fetal heart rate and rhythm

An abnormal fetal heart rate may be the first indication of a major disruption in fetal homeostasis. During trauma resuscitation, evaluation of the fetus should begin with auscultation of heart tones and continuous electronic fetal heart rate monitoring (EFM). Any viable fetus of 24 or more weeks gestation requires monitoring after trauma. Cardiotocographic monitoring should be started in the resuscitation room and continued for a minimum of 4 hours; a

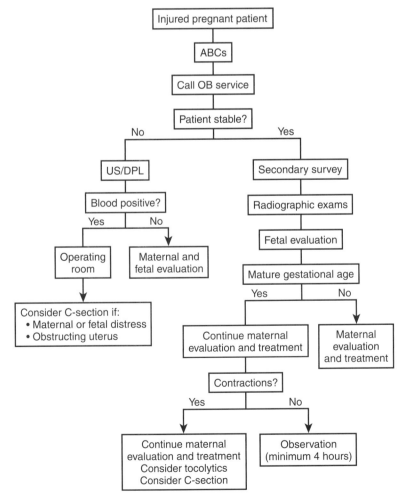

Figure 2 Algorithm for initial maternal and fetal assessment. *OB,* Obstetrics; *US,* ultrasound; *DPL,* diagnostic peritoneal lavage; *C-section,* cesarean section. *(Adapted from Knudson MM, Rozycki GS, Paquin MM: Reproductive system trauma. In Moore EE, Feliciano DV, Mattox KL, editors: Trauma, 5th ed. New York, McGraw-Hill, 2004, pp. 851–875.)*

minimum of 24 hours is recommended for patients with frequent uterine activity (more than six contractions per hour), abdominal or uterine tenderness, ruptured membranes, vaginal bleeding, or hypotension.

Fetomaternal hemorrhage

Fetomaternal hemorrhage (FMH) is the transplacental hemorrhage of fetal blood into the normally separate maternal circulation and occurs in 8%–30% of patients with trauma during pregnancy. The severity of injury and the gestational age have no correlation with the frequency and volume of FMH. The Kleihauer-Betke (KB) test is used after maternal injury to identify fetal blood in the maternal circulation. The ratio of fetal to maternal cells is recorded, allowing calculation of the volume of fetal blood leaked to the maternal circulation. Complications of FMH include Rh sensitization in the mother, fetal anemia, fetal paroxysmal atrial tachycardia, and fetal death from exsanguination. As the volume of FMH sufficient to sensitize most Rh-negative women is well below the 5-ml sensitivity level of the typical laboratory's KB test, all Rh-negative mothers who present with a history of abdominal trauma should receive one 300-mcg prophylactic dose of Rh immune globulin (anti-D immunoglobulin; Rhogam) within 72 hours of the traumatic event. An additional 300 mcg of Rh immune globulin should be given for every 30 ml of fetal blood found in maternal circulation. Only 3.1% of major trauma cases require more than one 300-mcg Rh immune globulin dose. The KB test is probably unnecessary before 16 weeks gestation because the fetal blood volume is below 30 ml at this gestational age.

Radiographic Examination

There are three phases of radiation damage related to gestational age of the fetus. Before 3 weeks of gestation, during preimplantation and early implantation, exposure to radiation can result in death of the embryo. Between 3 and 16 weeks of gestation, during organogenesis, radiation can damage the developing fetal tube, resulting in anomalies in the central nervous system. After 16 weeks, neurologic defects are the most common complication. Prenatal radiation exposure may be associated with certain childhood cancers.

Although there is existing concern about radiation exposure during pregnancy, in most instances the benefits outweigh the risks. It is generally believed that exposure of the fetus to less than 5–10 rad causes no significant increase in the risk of congenital malformations, intrauterine growth retardation, or miscarriage. Radiation doses from common imaging studies are shown in Table 2. All indicated radiographic studies should be performed, as for nonpregnant patients (Figure 3). It is obvious that unnecessary duplication of studies should be avoided.

Abdominal Evaluation

Evaluation of the abdomen in the pregnant patient may be challenging. Superior displacement of the viscera by the expanding uterus changes the anatomical relation of the intra-abdominal organs (Figure 4). Special attention is needed for patients with rib or pelvic fractures, unexplained hypotension, blood loss, hematuria, or altered sensorium caused by drugs, alcohol, or brain injury.

Table 2: Radiation Doses from Plain Radiographs and CT

Plain anteroposterior chest x-ray	<0.005 rad
Pelvic x-ray	<0.4 rad
CT scan of head (1-cm cuts)	0.05 rad
CT scan of upper abdomen (20 1-cm cuts)	3.0 rad
CT scan of lower abdomen (10 1-cm cuts)	3.0–9.0 rad

CT, Computed tomography.

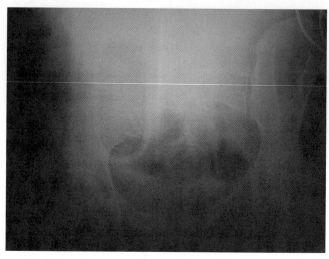

Figure 3 Pelvic x-ray of a pregnant patient after blunt trauma. Vertebrae and other parts of the fetus can be seen.

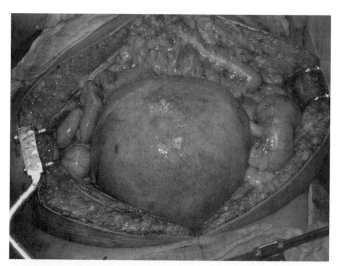

Figure 4 Exploratory laparotomy after motor vehicle collision. Gravid uterus displacing viscera.

Focused abdominal sonography for trauma (FAST) has a major role in the abdominal evaluation because it provides rapid detection of intra-abdominal and pericardial fluid in the mother as well as quick assessment of fetal condition. In the hemodynamically normal patient, abdominal CT scanning can also be done safely to evaluate both mother and fetus. If CT scan is necessary, both oral and intravenous contrast media should be administered as needed. The main drawback of a diagnostic peritoneal lavage (DPL) is its invasiveness, although the procedure can be done safely and has the same sensitivity as in the nonpregnant patient. DPL should be performed above the umbilicus using an open technique.

The American Association for the Surgery of Trauma (AAST) Organ Injury Scale for gravid uterus is shown in Table 3.

Surgical Treatment

Blunt Injury

Solid organ injuries may be managed nonoperatively in the hemodynamically stable pregnant patient. In contrast, unstable patients or those with intestinal injury clearly require early operation, as hypotension and infection can be harmful or even lethal for the fetus.

Table 3: AAST-OIS for Gravid Uterus

Grade	Injury Description	AIS-90 Score
I	Hematoma or contusion without placental abruption	2
II	Superficial laceration <1 cm in depth or partial placental abruption <25%	3
III	Deep laceration 1 cm in depth in second trimester or placental abruption 25% but <50%; deep laceration in third trimester	3–4
IV	Laceration extending to the uterine artery; deep laceration 1 cm with 50% placental abruption	4
V	Uterine rupture in second or third trimester; complete placental abruption	4–5

American Association for the Surgery of Trauma (AAST).
Modified from Moore EE, Jurkovich GJ, Knudson MM, et al: Organ injury scaling VI: extrahepatic biliary, esophagus, stomach, vulva, vagina, uterus (nonpregnant), uterus (pregnant), fallopian tube, and ovary. *J Trauma* 39(6):1069–1070, 1995.

Pelvic fractures represent the most challenging blunt injuries during pregnancy. Hemorrhage from dilated retroperitoneal veins can cause massive and fatal hemorrhagic shock. Maternal pelvic fracture is the most common cause of fetal death, with a fetal mortality approaching 25%. In nonpregnant patients, angioembolization is the usual treatment for pelvic hemorrhage, but the radiation dose for the procedure is considered excessive during pregnancy.

The abdominal wall, uterine myometrium, and amniotic fluid act as a cushion to direct forces from blunt trauma. Placental abruption is the most common cause of fetal death, resulting from anoxia, prematurity, or exsanguination. Manifestations include abdominal pain, vaginal bleeding, uterine tenderness, and contractions. One of the most serious complications associated with abruption is disseminated intravascular coagulation (DIC), caused when placental thromboplastin enters maternal circulation.

Penetrating Injury

As the uterus grows and expands out of the pelvis, it becomes an easier target for penetrating trauma. The thick density of its musculature allows the uterus to absorb energy from low-velocity penetrating injuries; maternal death is very uncommon except for injuries in the upper abdomen, which usually produce severe maternal damage. Gunshot wounds cause fetal injuries in 60%–70% of cases, with fetal death in 40%–65%. If the bullet has penetrated the uterus and the fetus is viable, cesarean section is indicated. Indications for C-section at celiotomy are summarized in Table 4.

Perimortem C-section is indicated in the case of maternal death if the fetus is viable (24 weeks). Timing is critical, as the probability of fetal survival is excellent when delivery occurs within 5 minutes or less of maternal demise. As the time increases, the chance of survival diminishes. In the rare situation where the mother is declared brain dead but maintains good vital signs, the fetus can be allowed to mature before delivery (Figure 5).

When performing an emergency C-section on a trauma patient, instead of the commonly used transverse incision, a vertical incision through all the layers into the uterus is safer and faster. This incision avoids injury to the uterine vessels, which enter the uterus from both sides.

Between gestational age 24–32 weeks, open cardiac massage (OCM) without aortic cross clamping should be seriously considered before an emergency C-section is performed. If OCM proves successful, the deliv-

Table 4: Indications for C-Section during Laparotomy for Trauma

Maternal shock
Threat to life from exsanguinations from any cause
Mechanical limitation for maternal repair
Irreparable uterine injury
Fetal distress in viable fetus
Unstable thoracolumbar spine injury
Pregnancy near term
Maternal death

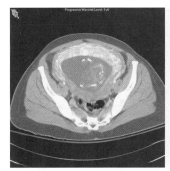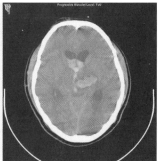

Figure 5 Intracranial hemorrhage (right panel) in an 18-week pregnant patient declared brain dead. As the fetus was not viable (*left panel*), the patient's family agreed to organ donation.

ery may be delayed so that chances of postnatal survival improve. A proposed algorithm for emergency C-section after trauma is presented in Figure 6.

Morbidity and Mortality

Trauma has become the most frequent cause of maternal death in the United States. Older reports attributed 80% maternal mortality to amniotic fluid embolism, which together with pulmonary thromboembolism was cited as the leading cause of maternal mortality. In contrast to declining maternal mortality from infection, hemorrhage, hypertension, and thromboembolism, accidental deaths during pregnancy have risen steadily. According to the latest statistics, as many as 36% of maternal deaths are caused by penetrating trauma. While overall maternal mortality from abdominal gunshot wounds is low (3.9%), fetal mortality ranges between 40% and 70%. Risk factors associated with poor fetal outcome are listed in Table 5.

Conclusions

Trauma has become the leading cause of death in women aged 34 and younger, including pregnant patients. Pathophysiologic changes in pregnancy affect all aspects of traumatic injury and require detailed assessment and meticulous management.

TRAUMA TO NONGRAVID UTERUS AND FEMALE GENITALIA

There is a relative abundance of information on trauma in pregnancy and a relative paucity regarding injuries to the female genitalia. Although these injuries are uncommon in the nonpregnant patient, they

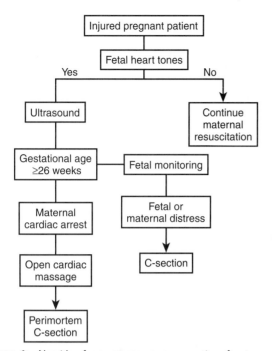

Figure 6 Algorithm for emergency cesarean section after trauma. *C-section,* Cesarean section; *CPR,* cardiopulmonary resuscitation. *(Adapted from Morris JA Jr, Rosenbower TJ, Jurkovich GJ, et al: Infant survival after cesarean section for trauma. Ann Surg 223:481–488, 1996.)*

Table 5: Predictors of Fetal Outcome

Maternal death

Maternal hypotension

Maternal traumatic brain injury

High Injury Severity Score (ISS)

Pelvic fracture

Ejection of pregnant woman from a vehicle

Severe abdominal injury to pregnant woman

are more often seen in cases where there is pathologic enlargement of the internal genitalia or in the early postpartum period. Missed or improperly treated female genital injuries can result in hemorrhage, sepsis, and loss of endocrine and reproductive function.

Incidence

The incidence of injuries to the female genitalia is largely unknown. Most information on the subject comes from isolated case reports or small series of patients. Vaginal lacerations complicate approximately 3.5% of pelvic fractures in female patients. Urethral and bladder injuries are also commonly present.

Mechanism of Injury

Blunt injuries involving the female genitalia are most frequently associated with pelvic fractures. Injuries to the external genitalia can also be the result of straddle injuries or accidental penetration. Water skiing, gymnastics, and bicycling accidents have been reported as the causes of blunt trauma to the lower genitalia. Penetrating injuries are almost exclusively responsible for injuries to the upper genital organs, although several reports of blunt trauma to normal ovaries and uterus have been reported.

Many of the injuries to the external genital organs are the result of violent acts in pregnant as well as nonpregnant women. This possibility should be always be considered, especially when the mechanism of injury is unclear. If sexual assault has occurred, informed consent for the remainder of the assessment must be obtained.

Domestic violence crosses lines of ethnicity/race, age, national origin, sexual orientation, religion, and/or socioeconomic status, although an overwhelming majority of the victims in heterosexual relationships are women. Typically, battery tends to occur as a pattern of violence rather than a one-time event. Physicians treating trauma victims should able to recognize the signs of domestic violence, refer patients to appropriate agencies, and provide social and other support.

Diagnosis

Initial assessment and resuscitation are performed as for any trauma patient. The secondary survey should include a detailed physical examination of the perineum. Examination under anesthesia may be needed for patients with severe pain or active bleeding. A complete examination should include bimanual palpation and speculum examinations of vagina and anorectum. Some authors recommend anesthesia for all patients with perineal trauma in order to evaluate the extent of the injury.

Intra-abdominal genital injuries are usually diagnosed at laparotomy for associated injuries. As blunt injury is more common with pathologically enlarged internal genitalia in the nongravid patient, CT scan of the abdomen or DPL may aid the diagnosis, although the latter is very rarely used. Detailed grading of gynecologic injuries is presented in Tables 6 through 10.

Table 6: AAST-OIS for Gynecologic Injuries: Vagina

Grade	Injury Description	AIS-90 Score
I	Contusion or hematoma	1
II	Superficial laceration involving mucosa	1
III	Deep laceration extending into submucosal fat or muscle	2
IV	Complex laceration extending into the cervix or peritoneum	3
V	Injury to adjacent organs	3

American Association for the Surgery of Trauma (AAST).
Modified from Moore EE, Jurkovich GJ, Knudson MM, et al: Organ injury scaling VI: extrahepatic biliary, esophagus, stomach, vulva, vagina, uterus (nonpregnant), uterus (pregnant), fallopian tube, and ovary. *J Trauma* 39(6):1069–1070, 1995.

Table 7: AAST-OIS for Gynecologic Injuries: Vulva

Grade	Injury Description	AIS-90 Score
I	Hematoma or contusion	1
II	Superficial laceration involving skin only	1
III	Deep laceration extending into subcutaneous fat or muscle	2
IV	Avulsion of skin, fat, or muscle	3
V	Injury to adjacent organs	3

American Association for the Surgery of Trauma (AAST).
Modified from Moore EE, Jurkovich GJ, Knudson MM, et al: Organ injury scaling VI: extrahepatic biliary, esophagus, stomach, vulva, vagina, uterus (nonpregnant), uterus (pregnant), fallopian tube, and ovary. *J Trauma* 39(6):1069–1070, 1995.

Table 8: AAST-OIS for Gynecologic Injuries: Nongravid Uterus

Grade	Injury Description	AIS-90 Score
I	Hematoma or contusion	2
II	Superficial laceration <1 cm in depth	2
III	Deep laceration 1 cm in depth	3
IV	Laceration extending to uterine artery	3
V	Devascularization or avulsion	3

American Association for the Surgery of Trauma (AAST).
Modified from Moore EE, Jurkovich GJ, Knudson MM, et al: Organ injury scaling VI: extrahepatic biliary, esophagus, stomach, vulva, vagina, uterus (nonpregnant), uterus (pregnant), fallopian tube, and ovary. *J Trauma* 39(6):1069–1070, 1995

Table 9: AAST-OIS for Gynecologic Injuries: Fallopian Tube

Grade	Injury Description	AIS-90 Score
I	Hematoma or contusion	2
II	Laceration involving <50% of circumference	2
III	Laceration involving 50% of circumference	2
IV	Complete transection	2
V	Devascularized segment	2

American Association for the Surgery of Trauma (AAST).
Modified from Moore EE, Jurkovich GJ, Knudson MM, et al: Organ injury scaling VI: extrahepatic biliary, esophagus, stomach, vulva, vagina, uterus (nonpregnant), uterus (pregnant), fallopian tube, and ovary. *J Trauma* 39(6):1069–1070, 1995

Table 10: AAST-OIS for Gynecologic Injuries: Ovary

Grade	Injury Description	AIS-90 Score
I	Contusion or hematoma	1
II	Superficial laceration <0.5 cm in depth	2
III	Deep laceration 0.5 cm in depth	3
IV	Partial disruption of blood supply	3
V	Complete parenchymal disruption or avulsion	3

American Association for the Surgery of Trauma (AAST).
Modified from Moore EE, Jurkovich GJ, Knudson MM, et al: Organ injury scaling VI: extrahepatic biliary, esophagus, stomach, vulva, vagina, uterus (nonpregnant), uterus (pregnant), fallopian tube, and ovary. *J Trauma* 39(6):1069–1070, 1995

Surgical Management

Isolated perineal lacerations should be repaired after appropriate irrigation and debridement with or without placement of drains. Large perineal hematomas require incision and drainage because of the high associated incidence of infection and sepsis. Vulvar lacerations may be closed primarily with absorbable sutures.

Repair of vaginal and cervical lacerations may be challenging because of the abundant blood supply. Absorbable sutures including the mucosal and submucosal layers are commonly used. These injuries must be diagnosed promptly in patients with pelvic fractures, as any delay can result in sepsis and death.

Injuries to the uterus are repaired in two layers using slowly absorbable running or interrupted figure-of-eight sutures. Hysterectomy for trauma is extremely rare and is only needed in extreme cases of massive destruction or exsanguinating hemorrhage. Injuries to the fallopian tubes and ovaries are also managed by either primary repair or excision according to injury severity. Vaginal packing with antibiotics is frequently used for 24 hours after procedures involving the vagina, cervix, or uterus.

Morbidity and Mortality

Morbidity is primarily determined by the associated injuries. Profuse bleeding from the perineal wounds as well as vagina, cervix, and uterus may be the cause of hemorrhagic shock. These wounds may be difficult to control. Missed perineal injuries in association with pelvic fracture may be fatal. Long-term complications include sexual dysfunction and infertility.

Conclusions

Injuries to the nongravid uterus as well as female genital organs are rare and should be suspected in all assault victims and all patients with direct perineal trauma, pelvic fractures, or penetrating injury to the pelvis. Thorough physical examination, preferably in the operating room, with prompt surgical treatment improves the outcome of these potentially challenging injuries.

SELECTED REFERENCES

1. Petrone P, Asensio JA: Trauma in pregnancy: assessment and treatment. *Scand J Surg* 95:4–10, 2006.
2. Desjardins G: Management of the injured pregnant patient. Resuscitation. http://www.trauma.org/archive/resus/pregnancytrauma.html.
3. Fildes J, Reed L, Jones N, et al: Trauma: the leading cause of maternal death. *J Trauma* 32:643–645, 1992.
4. Lavery JP, Staten-McCormick M: Management of moderate to severe trauma in pregnancy. *Obstet Gynecol Clin North Am* 22:69–90, 1995.
5. Weiss HB: Pregnancy-associated injury hospitalizations in Pennsylvania, 1995. *Ann Emerg Med* 34:626–636, 1999.
6. Weiss HB, Songer TJ, Fabio A: Fetal deaths related to maternal injury. *JAMA* 286:1863–1868, 2001.
7. Leggon RE, Wood GC, Indeck MC: Pelvic fractures in pregnancy: factors influencing maternal and fetal outcomes. *J Trauma* 53(4):796–804, 2002.
8. Guth AA, Patcher HL: Domestic violence and the trauma surgeon. *Am J Surg* 179:134–140, 2000.
9. McFarlane J, Parker B, Soeken K, Bullock L: Assessing for abuse during pregnancy. Severity and frequency of injuries and associated entry into prenatal care. *JAMA* 267:3176–3178, 1992.
10. ACS Committee on Trauma (ACS-COT): Trauma in women. In *Advanced Trauma Life Support Manual*, 6th ed. Chicago, American College of Surgeons, 1997.
11. Lavin JP Jr, Polsky SS: Abdominal trauma during pregnancy. *Clin Perinatol* 10:423–438, 1983.
12. Green JR: Placenta previa and abruption placentae. In Creasey RK, Resnik R, editors: *Maternal-Fetal Medicine: Principles and Practice*. Philadelphia, WB Saunders, 1994, p. 604.
13. Sandy EA Jr, Koerner M: Self inflicted gunshot wound to the pregnant abdomen: report of a case and review of the literature. *Am J Perinatol* 6:30–31, 1989.
14. Higgins SD: Trauma in pregnancy. *J Perinatol* 8:288–292, 1988.
15. Selden BS, Burke TJ: Complete maternal and fetal recovery after prolonged cardiac arrest. *Ann Emerg Med* 17:346–349, 1988.
16. Clark SL, Cotton DB, Pivarnik JM, Lee W, Hankins GD, Benedetti TJ, Phelan JP: Positional change and central hemodynamic profile during normal third trimester pregnancy and postpartum. *Am J Obstet Gynecol* 164:883–887, 1991.

17. Knudson MM, Rozycki GS, Paquin MM: Reproductive system trauma. In Moore EE, Feliciano DV, Mattox KL, editors: *Trauma*, 5th ed. New York, McGraw-Hill, 2004, pp. 851–875.
18. Eliot G, Rao D: Pregnancy and radiographic examination. In Haycock CE, editor: *Trauma and Pregnancy*. Littleton, MA, PSG Publishing, 1985, pp. 69–78.
19. Harvey EB, Boice JD Jr, Honeyman M, Flannery JT: Prenatal x-ray exposure and childhood cancer in twins. *N Engl J Med* 312:541–545, 1985.
20. Kaunitz AM, Hughes JM, Grimes DA, et al: Causes of maternal mortality in the United States. *Obstet Gynecol* 65:605–612, 1985.
21. Wessells H, Aninch J: Injuries to the urogenital tract. In American College of Surgeons: *ACS Surgery Principles and Practice*, pp. 1080–1085, New York, Web MD, 2005.

MULTIDISCIPLINARY MANAGEMENT OF PELVIC FRACTURES: OPERATIVE AND NONOPERATIVE HEMOSTASIS

Thomas M. Scalea

Very few injuries are as complicated as multisystem trauma and pelvic fracture. The pelvis is a complex anatomic region. The bony pelvis affords great protection to the structures it contains. Within the pelvis are important gastrointestinal, genitourinary, vascular, and neurologic structures. The force necessary to fracture a pelvis is extreme. Therefore, every pelvic fracture must be assumed to be a high-energy injury. The proximity of the pelvis to the abdomen makes combined injuries common. Patients with pelvic fracture often have other associated injuries as well. Over 50% will have either traumatic brain injury or associated long bone fracture.

Optimal management of multiply injured patients with pelvic fractures is perhaps the best example of true multidisciplinary care. This is especially true in patients who are hemodynamically unstable. Emergency physicians, trauma surgeons, orthopedic surgeons, and interventional radiologists all have key roles in managing these patients. A multiplicity of treatment options exists. The correct option for an individual patient is a function of the anatomy of the bony injury, the hemodynamic status of the patient, the presence or absence of other associated injuries, and local expertise within each individual institution. Very few centers have real expertise in every hemostatic technique.

It is vital to construct a plan before the patient arrives. Each institution should have an algorithm available that plays to that individual institution's strengths. Expertise and institutional resources must be instantly available 24 hours a day, 7 days a week, to care for these complicated patients. In this chapter, we will attempt to delineate all options available and discuss individual advantages and disadvantages. It is our hope that the reader will gain an understanding of this complex disease and that this work may serve as background for development for institutional guidelines.

PELVIC BLEEDING: MAKING THE DIAGNOSIS

There are four cavities into which a patient can exsanguinate—thorax, abdomen, retroperitoneum, muscle compartments, as well as externally. While bleeding into the mediastinum or into the brain may be life threatening, only a small volume is required to produce symptoms. Thus, exsanguination into these regions is not possible.

The diagnosis of intrathoracic bleeding can be made with a combination of physical exam and a chest x-ray or ultrasound exam. Tension pneumothorax and/or massive hemothorax can be identified rapidly. Muscle compartment bleeding should be identifiable on physical exam. Finally, external blood loss can generally be diagnosed by history. In addition, external blood loss may become apparent for the second time as the patients are resuscitated and blood pressure increases.

The distinction between intra-abdominal and retroperitoneal bleeding can be most difficult. Combined abdominal and pelvic injuries are common. Physical findings such as abdominal pain, distention, or tenderness do not differentiate between intra-abdominal or retroperitoneal bleeding. In addition, physical findings can be quite nonspecific. Patients can bleed a large volume of blood into the abdomen and/or retroperitoneum with minimal physical findings.

In the past, the diagnosis of intra-abdominal injury was generally made by diagnostic peritoneal lavage in patients who were hemodynamically labile. The advent of the focused ultrasound exam however, has revolutionized the early diagnosis of intra-abdominal injury. The focused assessment with sonography for trauma (FAST) is a rapid bedside technique that can make the diagnosis of intra-abdominal injury in several minutes. FAST is portable and can be repeated if results are equivocal.

While FAST is rapid, it is nonspecific. It can identify the presence of blood but is not an organ-specific test. Computed tomography (CT) scanning allows imaging of both the intra-abdominal as well as retroperitoneal structures. It can identify blood loss into both compartments. Unfortunately, this is not nearly as rapid as the FAST exam and is of limited utility in patients who are hemodynamically unstable.

The presence of retroperitoneal hemorrhage should be suspected in any patient with a pelvic fracture. A pelvic x-ray is a rapid screening test that should alert the clinician to the possibility of pelvic hemorrhage. This is usually performed as the screening radiograph with a chest x-ray. After blunt trauma, patients can bleed into the retroperitoneum without a pelvic fracture, but this is exceedingly rare. While a pelvic x-ray is a good screening test, it only describes pelvic anatomy in two dimensions and can vastly underestimate the degree of a pelvic bony injury posteriorly.

Initial physical exam of the pelvis can be helpful in determining skeletal stability even before an x-ray is taken. While some advocate rocking the pelvis vigorously, we believe that this is a potentially dangerous maneuver. In patients with skeletally unstable pelvic fractures, this produces excruciating pain. In addition, displacement of the fracture fragment may exacerbate bleeding that had stopped. Instead, we encourage clinicians to gently compress the pelvis inward at the level of the iliac crest. If the pelvis is skeletally stable, it will not give. If there is give in the pelvis, the patient almost certainly has a skeletally unstable pelvic fracture.

It is important to distinguish between patients with skeletally unstable pelvic fractures and patients who are hemodynamically unstable. Skeletal stability describes the bony architecture of the pelvic fracture. Hemodynamic stability describes the patient's physiologic

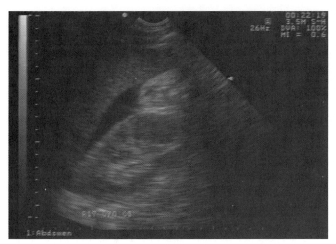

Figure 1 Fluid in the abdomen can signal a positive focused assessment with sonography for trauma (FAST), pelvic fracture, and hemodynamic instability. Such patients are almost certainly best served by an immediate laparotomy.

Table 1: Classification of Pelvic Fractures

Anteroposterior Compression	
Type I	Disruption of pubic symphysis of <2.5 cm of diastasis; no significant posterior pelvic injury
Type II	Disruption of pubic symphysis of >2.5 cm, with tearing of anterior sacroiliac and sacrospinous and sacrotuberous ligaments
Type III	Complete disruption of pubic symphysis and posterior ligament complexes, with hemipelvic displacement
Lateral Compression	
Type I	Posterior compression of sacroiliac joint without ligament disruption; oblique pubic ramus fracture
Type II	Rupture of posterior sacroiliac ligament; pivotal internal rotation of hemipelvis on anterior sacroiliac joint with a crush injury of sacrum and an oblique public ramus fracture
Type III	Findings in type II injury with evidence of an anteroposterior compression injury to contralateral hemipelvis

Data from Young JWR, Brumback RJ, Poka A: Pelvic fractures: value of plain radiography in early assessment and management. *Radiology* 160:445, 1986.

response. Not all patients with skeletally unstable pelvic fractures are hemodynamically unstable. In addition, patients who have skeletally stable fractures can still lose a substantial amount of blood into their retroperitoneum.

Patients with a pelvic fracture, a positive FAST, and hemodynamic instability are almost certainly best served by an immediate laparotomy. In most patients, the FAST turns positive with 200–300 cc of fluid in the abdomen (Figure 1). While free fluid could certainly be from a relatively minor intra-abdominal injury or a ruptured hollow viscus such as the bladder, diagnostic laparotomy is probably the most rapid and definitive test in patients who are hemodynamically unstable. If minor injury is found and bleeding is thought to be coming from the

pelvis, abbreviated laparotomy should be performed and other plans made to control the pelvic bleeding.

PELVIC FRACTURE CLASSIFICATIONS

A number of classification schemes are available that describe the bony architecture of pelvic fractures. Probably the most commonly used scheme was described by Young and Burgess in 1986 and classifies pelvic fractures by their vector of force (Table 1). Each classification is subdivided to describe the degree of pelvic instability. The authors originally thought that this classification scheme could predict the need for transfusions. While this may actually not be the

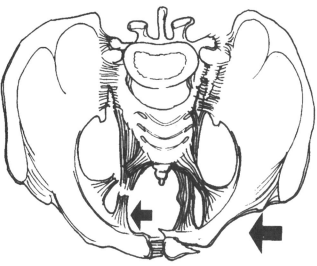

Lateral compression type III

Figure 2 Lateral compression pelvic fracture. *(From Moore EE, Feliciano DV, Mattox KL:* Trauma, *5th ed. New York, McGraw-Hill, 2003.)*

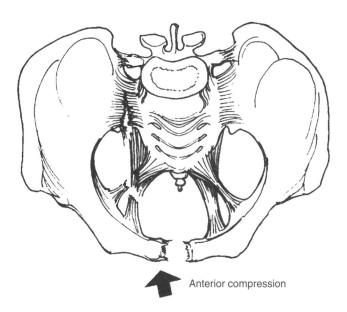

Anterior compression

Figure 3 Anterior/posterior compression fracture. *(From Moore EE, Feliciano DV, Mattox KL:* Trauma, *5th ed. New York, McGraw-Hill, 2003.)*

case, it is quite useful in describing fracture anatomy and guiding initial attempts at hemostasis.

Lateral compression (LC) pelvic fractures caused by side impact generally occur after T-bone vehicular crashes or car–pedestrian collisions (Figure 2). LC fractures cause an acute shortening of the pelvic diameter. The pelvis does not open but closes down. The pelvic ligaments generally stay intact. Thus, these fractures generally do not bleed. Hemodynamic instability after a lateral compression fracture more likely results from torso injuries such as intra-abdominal bleeding or intrathoracic bleeding. There is a known association with traumatic aortic injury and LC pelvic fractures.

Anteroposterior compression (AP) fractures generally occur after head-on vehicular crashes or may occur after equestrian injury, typically when patients are thrown from a horse or the horse lands on them (Figure 3). With this mechanism, pelvic diameter widens and the pelvis opens. The injuries can be purely ligamentous if the sacroiliac (SI) joints rupture, even in the absence of significant bony injury. Pelvic vascular injuries are quite common. AP compression fractures have the highest chance of bleeding, and transfusion requirements are the greatest in patients with these fractures.

Vertical shear (VS) injuries occur when patients land on an outstretched foot, which generally occurs after falling from a height (Figure 4). VS fractures can also occur in motorcycle crashes, particu-

larly if patients are riding with their legs outstretched. In vertical shear fractures, the force is transmitted up the axial skeleton through the posterior pelvis. Posterior fractures and/or ligamentous ruptures are quite common. If there is a complete disruption of both the anterior and posterior elements (Malgaigne fracture), the psoas muscle pulls the hemipelvis cephalad without opposition. This may be seen on a pelvic x-ray. Vertical shear injuries have an intermediate risk of bleeding.

Pelvic fractures do not always occur in pure form. For instance, a pedestrian may be struck obliquely, not truly from the front or side. Thus, a clear classification may not be obvious. The site of bleeding often correlates with pelvic fracture anatomy. AP compression fractures generally bleed from either the pudendal or obturator artery. Vertical shear fractures most often bleed from the superior gluteal artery. If lateral compression fractures bleed, they can bleed from virtually any vascular structure.

The notion that fracture anatomy could predict bleeding has been questioned recently. The group that Wake Forest reported on the use of angiography and embolization for pelvic hemostasis (Table 2). In their series, low grade AP compression fractures required angiography most often. Seventy percent of AP I injury were treated with embolization. This was substantially more common in AP II and about the same as AP III. In addition, the same was true for lateral compression fractures: nearly 70% of LC I fractures were treated without angiography and required embolization, about the same as LC II or LC III fractures.

It is also clear that pelvic fracture bleeding may be different by age group. In 2001, we demonstrated that lateral compression fractures occurred more common in patients over the age of 55. They were two times more likely to get blood than younger patients and required more blood transfusions (7.5 vs. 5 units). These lateral compression fractures were minor, yet still bled substantially. Not surprisingly, overall mortality was higher in the older patients.

While fracture anatomy may be able to predict both the likelihood and location of bleeding, clearly it is far from perfect. The wise clinician will recognize that any patient with a pelvic fracture can bleed. Patients with evidence of ongoing blood loss should obviously have a search for blood loss in other cavities. If none is found, the patient is probably bleeding from the pelvis. Regardless of the pelvic fracture anatomy, action should be taken to obtain hemostasis.

TREATING PELVIC FRACTURE BLEEDING

A number of techniques are available to stop bleeding from the bony pelvis. Bleeding from the pelvis can occur in a number of ways. The vast majority of bleeding is venous and tends to stop over time as the pelvic hematoma tamponades this low-pressure vascular injury. Patients can bleed from fracture fragments themselves as well as smaller pelvic arterial injuries. Larger arteries such as major branches of the hypogastric distribution (pudendal, obturator, or superior gluteal artery) can bleed. Major vascular structures, such as the proximal hypogastric artery or the external or common iliac artery, rarely bleed.

Hemostatic techniques for pelvic fracture bleeding can include external compressive devices, angiographic embolization, or intraoperative control. External compressive devices reduce the pelvic volume by reducing fracture fragments. This usually stops venous and bony bleeding by limiting pelvic volume. In addition, reducing the fracture fragments limits direct bony bleeding. External compression can help "stabilize the clot" that has formed. Stabilizing the fracture fragments limits recurrent fracture motion and should help prevent recurrent bleeding.

A number of devices are available to help achieve external compression. Perhaps the simplest is using a bed sheet. Ideally, the sheet is placed on the stretcher, even before the patient arrives. Alternatively, the patient can be gently lifted and the bed sheet placed underneath the patient. The bed sheet is then crisscrossed across the pelvis anteriorly and tied down (Figure 5). This low-tech technique has proven to be extraordinarily helpful. It can be especially helpful in

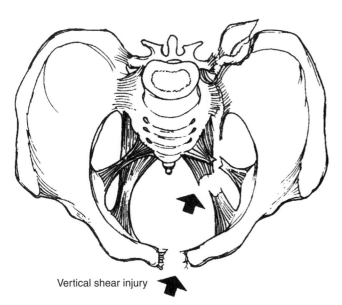

Vertical shear injury

Figure 4 Vertical shear fracture. *(From Moore EE, Feliciano DV, Mattox KL: Trauma, 5th ed. New York, McGraw-Hill, 2003.)*

Table 2: Pelvic Bleeding

		Angiography	Embolization
Anteroposterior compression	I	10	7
	II	4	1
	III	4	3
Lateral compression	I	8	5
	II	11	5
	III	5	3
Vertical shear		1	0

Data from Miller PR, Moore P, Meredith JW, Chang MC: External fixation or arteriogram in bleeding pelvic fracture: initial therapy guided by markers of arterial hemorrhage. *J Trauma* 54(3):437–443, 2003.

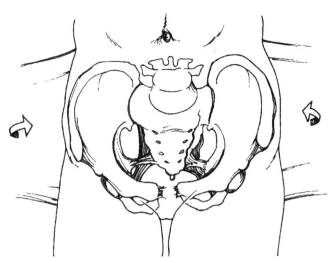

Figure 5   Achieving external compression by wrapping a bed sheet around the patient, crisscrossing anteriorly across the pelvis.   *(From Moore EE, Feliciano DV, Mattox KL: Trauma, 5th ed. New York, McGraw-Hill, 2003.)*

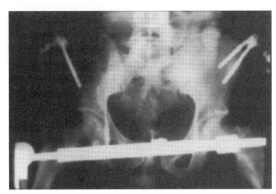

Figure 6   External fixation, commonly used in the past as a compressive device for pelvic hemostasis. External fixation is the most rigid of the external devices and closes the pelvis down definitively. *(From Moore EE, Feliciano DV, Mattox KL: Trauma, 5th ed. New York, McGraw-Hill, 2003.)*

small community emergency departments (EDs) that have limited resources and may not have sophisticated technology. We generally advise the emergency physician to tie the bed sheet down snugly but not excessively tightly. Patients can then be transported within the hospital or to a higher level of care.

The military antishock garment (MAST) was originally used as a resuscitative technique in the prehospital phase. The MAST was originally thought to autotransfuse blood from the capacitance vessels of the lower extremities. It is now clear that increases in blood pressure are caused by increases in systemic vascular resistance, not increases in cardiac preload. Use of the MAST has largely been abandoned. The MAST can, however, be an effective pelvic and lower extremity splint, and can keep pelvic fractures reduced similar to the bed sheet. The lower extremity portion must be inflated if the abdominal and pelvic portion is inflated. The MAST has the advantage of being able to set pressure, which obviously is not possible with the bed sheet. Increases in blood pressure may displace hemostatic clots and cause recurrent bleeding. If the pressure on the MAST is set too high, intra-abdominal pressure can go up, causing abdominal compartment syndrome. Patients must be carefully monitored for either potential complication.

The pelvic C clamp is inserted posteriorly to reduce the posterior fracture fragments. This is inserted percutaneously in the ED in many European trauma centers. In most American trauma centers, fluoroscopic guidance in the operating room is used, which limits its effectiveness as a resuscitation tool. The anterior portion of the C clamp can be rotated out of the way to provide access for angiography or laparotomy. Clearly, if the pin is poorly placed, complications can include gastrointestinal perforation or iatrogenic nerve injury.

In the past, external fixation was very commonly used as a compressive device for pelvic hemostasis. External fixation is the most rigid of the external devices and closes the pelvis down definitively (Figure 6). In centers with expertise, external fixators which can be rapidly applied in the ED. In other centers, this is often placed in the operating room similar to the C clamp. In some cases, external fixation may provide definitive fracture fixation. The anterior portion of the frame can be rotated similar to the C clamp to allow access for angiography and/or laparotomy.

Use of external fixation during the resuscitative phase requires that these resources be immediately available. External fixation degrades CT images and may interfere with patient motion through the CT gantry. The pins for external fixation are placed in the iliac crest

and the frame is then applied anteriorly. In patients with badly displaced posterior element pelvic fractures, the inward motion produced by tightening down the frame could cause further displacement of the posterior fracture fragments and increase blood loss.

Many American trauma centers have abandoned virtually all other external compressive devices and exclusively use a commercially available pelvic binder. The pelvic binder is a Velcro device that applies even direct pressure on the pelvis (Figure 7). The pressure is set by the Velcro and lace system on the anterior portion of the binder. The binders can be applied rapidly and require a minimum of expertise. The binder should be applied across the femoral trochanters, not across the lower abdomen. Correct placement of the binder can limit access to the groins for angiography. If angiography

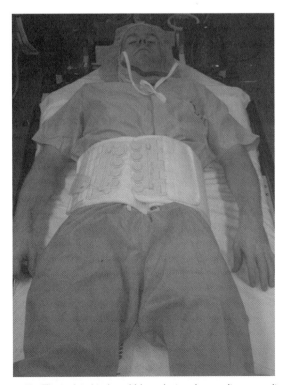

Figure 7   The pelvic binder, a Velcro device that applies even direct pressure on the pelvis, used exclusively by many American trauma centers.

is required, a hole can be cut in the binder or the binder must be placed slightly higher.

Deciding whether external compression would be helpful is a function of pelvic fracture anatomy. A wide open, AP III pelvic fracture is ideally treated with external compression. A lateral compression pelvic fracture where the pelvis has imploded—not exploded—is unlikely to be helped by external compression. Vertical shear injuries may respond in an intermittent manner. In the days of using external fixators, this discussion was quite germane. Was it wise to delay other hemostatic techniques, even for the 20 minutes it took to place an external fixator in the most sophisticated trauma center? The discussion would be even more important in centers where external fixation took a longer time.

The advent of the pelvic binder has obviated many of these discussions. While a pelvic binder is unlikely to help a lateral compression pelvic fracture, it can be applied quickly and almost certainly not exacerbate bleeding. The pelvic binder can act as a pelvic splint and limit fracture fragment motion during transport to the CT scanner, the operating room, or the angiography suite. Thus, we have become quite liberal in the use of pelvic binders, and place it on virtually any patient with a pelvic fracture who is hemodynamically unstable.

Angiographic embolization for pelvic hemostasis has been used for over 30 years. Diagnostic pelvic angiography should be able to identify all sites of pelvic arterial injury. Embolization with Gelfoam, stainless steel coils, or both can be quite effective in achieving pelvic hemostasis. The more liberal the use of angiography, the less the yield will be. Conversely, withholding angiography until a patient is in extremis, increases the yield of angiography but is probably not the wisest patient care. Our indications for angiography are in Table 3. These were developed nearly 20 years ago and are in current use.

A number of angiographic techniques are available. One would like to be as selective as possible with pelvic embolization to limit potential complications such as impotence or distal ischemia such as pelvic or buttock necrosis. The more selective technique, however, requires a greater amount of time and expertise to use. Another option is to use coil blockade. In this technique first described by Sclafani et al., the vascular injury is bridged and coils are placed distal to the injury. The catheter is then withdrawn and the area flooded with gel foam. This achieves hemostasis and prevents distal migration of the Gelfoam pledgets.

Another technique involves blind proximal hypogastric embolization with stainless steel coils. This is intended to reduce perfusion pressure within the hypogastric distribution and allow spontaneous hemostasis to occur. This could produce suboptimal hemostasis, as there is a rich collateral circulation within the pelvic vasculature. Vascular injuries could be fed by collaterals from the contralateral hypogastric or the circumflex vessels. With the proximal hypogastric artery embolized, the angiographic window to achieve hemostasis is now closed if recurrent bleeding occurs.

Despite this, we have had good success with proximal hypogastric embolization. We are not aware of any patient who has had significant ongoing pelvic hemorrhage from collateral flow. The concern

that bilateral proximal hypogastric embolization might cause an increase in problems also seems to be untrue even when bilateral embolization is used.

Operative approaches to achieve hemostasis have generally been discouraged. Laparotomy does not allow the surgeon to directly visualize the injured blood vessel. Opening the retroperitoneum releases tamponade and can restart bleeding that had been stopped, especially venous bleeding. The main hypogastric artery is a very short structure. In most patients, it is only several inches long. It then quickly branches into a large number of much smaller vessels that disappear deep into the pelvis. Identifying the injured blood vessel is extraordinarily difficult, and attempts to do this may only make a bad situation worse.

Hypogastric ligation is an option similar to proximal hypogastric embolization. It does carry risks of unroofing the pelvic hematoma, as well as risks of bleeding from collateral flow. In many centers, hypogastric embolization can be accomplished in approximately the same amount of time that it takes to achieve hypogastric ligation. However, if embolization is not available and patients are exsanguinating, hypogastric ligation remains an option.

Intraoperative hypogastric embolization is another option for patients in extremis. The proximal hypogastric artery is isolated with a vessel loop. The surgeon then mixes a slurry of hemostatic agents, which could include fresh frozen plasma and/or small-particulate Gelfoam. The hypogastric artery is accessed with a large Angiocath and blind embolization performed. There is limited experience in the literature with hypogastric embolization. This course should be avoided unless no other options exist.

Some patients almost certainly benefit from an attempt at operative hemostasis. Patients that present in hemorrhagic shock and have a unilateral absence of a femoral pulse likely have injury to either the common or external iliac artery. Typically, these patients have a traumatic hemipelvectomy (Figure 8). An extreme amount of force is necessary to produce this injury, and these patients usually are in refractory shock. A direct operative approach utilizing medial visceral rotation, combined with a direct approach to the iliac arteries is potentially life saving for these patients.

Early rigid fracture fixation is ideal, and definitive reduction of the fracture fragments can be quite helpful in achieving hemostasis. However, early open reduction and internal fixation risks torrential blood loss. Percutaneous SI screw fixation can reduce the posterior pelvis with minimal blood loss. These percutaneous screws are threaded under fluoroscopic guidance and rigidly reduce the pelvis. We typically use this technique with AP II or AP III fractures. The patients must be stable enough to undergo the operative procedure. This technique is not recommended for patients in profound shock. Percutaneous SI screws allow for good

Table 3: Indication for Angiography

4 units of blood in 24 hours
6 units of blood in 48 hours
Hypotension with negative focused assessment with sonography for trauma (FAST)/diagnostic peritoneal lavage
Large pelvic hematoma on computed tomography or in operating room
Pseudoaneurysm on computed tomography

Data from Moore EE, Feliciano DV, Mattox KL: *Trauma*, 5th ed. New York, McGraw-Hill, 2003.

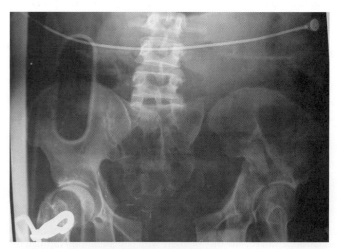

Figure 8 Traumatic internal hemipelvectomy.

reduction of the pelvic fracture, reduction of pelvic volume, and clot stabilization. Once the fracture is definitively fixed, patients can be mobilized out of bed, limiting pulmonary complications.

Anterior pelvic fixation can also be accomplished at the time of concomitant trauma laparotomy. In this scenario, patients undergo laparotomy and treatment for intra-abdominal injuries. When the abdominal portion is finished, the incision can be lengthened. The anterior fracture fragments are manually reduced and then an anterior pelvic plate placed. Again, this provides definitive anterior fracture fixation that obviates the need for other techniques such as external fixation or a binder. We have used this technique approximately 20 times, including in patients who have had gastrointestinal injuries and damage control procedures with an open abdomen. Our complication rate is low.

Pelvic hemostasis can also be achieved by pelvic packing. This technique should be reserved for patients in extremis who failed to respond to resuscitation and cannot be stabilized sufficiently for other techniques such as angioembolization.

Rather than approaching the pelvis via a laparotomy, it is wisest to pack via a retroperitoneal approach and approach the patient through a low midline incision. The pelvic hematoma has lifted the abdominal contents up out of the pelvis (Figure 9). The lower abdominal muscles are split in the midline and the pelvic hematoma entered directly. The pelvic hematoma must be completely evacuated and the pelvis then packed. It is important to stay extraperitoneal. When the packs are applied up against the peritoneum, the peritoneum increases the tamponade effect.

Virtually any material can be used for pelvic packing, such as towels, gauze, or laparotomy pack. We have favored the use of homemade fibrin bandages. These mesh packs can be constructed by using fibrin sealant and a Vicryl mesh. The mesh can be folded to the desired size (Figures 10 and 11). We generally pack these deep into the pelvis and supplement hemostasis with lap pads or towels.

Occasionally, this pelvic packing is used in concert with a laparotomy. In that case, we generally use a transverse incision to avoid having the abdominal and retroperitoneal incisions meet. The muscles can split and the pelvic packed in the same manner. We have used this technique in three patients over the past year. Thus, it is a technique that we apply only in desperate circumstances. However, it has been successful in all three cases.

MANAGEMENT OF OPEN PELVIC FRACTURES

Open pelvic fractures represent a distinct problem. They can be the source of torrential external blood loss. As the blood loss is external, there is often not a large component of retroperitoneal hemor-

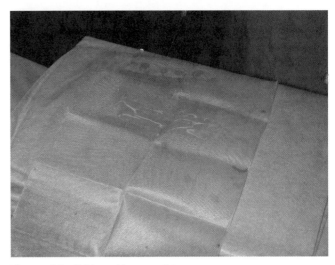

Figure 10   Pelvic packing material.

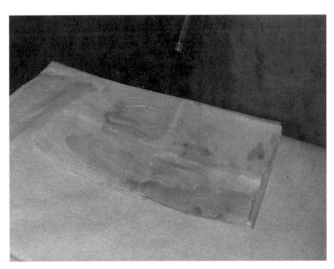

Figure 11   Folded pelvic packing material.

rhage. The clinician must first make the diagnosis and then control bleeding.

The diagnosis should be made on physical exam. As patients present supine, it is important to examine the perineum. It may be necessary to do a vaginal and/or rectal exam to appreciate the laceration. The abdomen should then be evaluated using a FAST. Patients with a positive FAST should proceed to laparotomy, and those with a negative FAST should undergo further diagnostic evaluations.

Bleeding can be controlled initially with packing. If the opening to the outside is small, it may be necessary to widen the external opening in order to get the packs up deep inside the pelvis. Definitive hemostasis can then be achieved later with either angiography or operative control. Once hemostasis is achieved, the patient should undergo debridement of nonviable soft tissue and muscle. Fecal diversion should be attempted later in any patient who has perirectal involvement.

It is important to characterize the anatomy of the pelvic fracture. It can generally be accomplished with a combination of physical exam and pelvic x-ray. The pelvic fracture should be reduced using any of the compressive devices discussed previously. The entire team should be alerted, including the operating room, the orthopedic service, and the

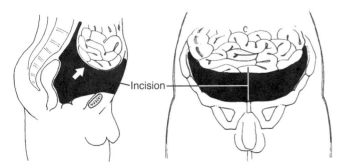

Figure 9   Low midline incision to approach pelvic hematoma.
(From Moore EE, Feliciano DV, Mattox KL: Trauma, 5th ed. New York, McGraw-Hill, 2003.)

angiography suite. Even if the bleeding looks venous and/or is controlled with packing, we advocate angiography for these patients.

The patient should go to the operating room for local exploration, repacking, and whatever hemostasis can be achieved via local control. This can be performed as the angiography team is setting up the angiography suite. If there is torrential bleeding when the patient is unpacked and explored, simply repacking the patient is the wisest course.

Exploring the wound in the ED is not recommended. There is neither adequate light nor appropriate instruments for adequate exploration. Patients almost always need to be placed in lithotomy position to get good access to the perineum. It is also unwise to unpack the patients in the ED. This only risks further blood loss.

Definitive hemostasis is generally achieved via a combination of operative exploration and angiography. There is virtxually no priority higher than achieving hemostasis. Early laparotomy is not necessary. Fecal diversion is not an emergency and can be accomplished later once the patient is hemodynamically stable and bleeding has been controlled.

SUMMARY

The multiply-injured patient with pelvic fractures represents one of the greatest challenges to the trauma service. Various techniques are available to evaluate the patient and help achieve hemostasis. Very few institutions in the United States have immediate access to all of these sophisticated techniques. It is important that an institutional algorithm be devised that will allow efficient, rapid, and effective care for these badly injured patients.

SELECTED REFERENCES

1. Burgess AR, Eastridge BJ, Young JWR: Pelvic ring disruptions: effective classification system and treatment protocols. *J Trauma* 30:848, 1990.
2. Ben-Menachem Y: Embolotherapy in pelvic trauma. In Neal MP, Tisnado J, Chu SR, editors: *Emergency Interventional Radiology*. Boston, Little & Brown, 1989.
3. Scalea TM, Burgess AR: Pelvic fractures. In Moore EE, Feliciano DV, Mattox KL, editors: *Trauma*, 5th ed. New York, McGraw-Hill Companies, 2004.
4. Miller PR, Moore PS, Mansell E, Meredith JW, Chang MC: External fixation or arteriogram in bleeding pelvic fracture: initial therapy guided by markers of arterial hemorrhage. *J Trauma* 54:437–443, 2003.

SPECIAL ISSUES IN MAJOR TORSO TRAUMA

CURRENT CONCEPTS IN THE DIAGNOSIS AND MANAGEMENT OF HEMORRHAGIC SHOCK

Juan Carlos Puyana, Samuel A. Tisherman, and Andrew B. Peitzman

The precipitating single common factor of hemorrhagic shock is severe acute blood loss, yet the clinical syndrome of hemorrhagic shock is heterogeneous. The diagnosis and management of this condition at first would appear to be simple. However, the very nature of how shock occurs and how the individual compensatory mechanisms respond to both the injury itself and the therapeutic interventions translate into a complex spectrum of diseases. This disease spectrum extends from immediate circulatory collapse to total body ischemia reperfusion injury with associated complex inflammatory and anti-inflammatory responses that in many instances evolve into multiple organ dysfunction. The purpose of this chapter is to provide a review of the current issues and a clinical perspective regarding the diagnosis and management of shock.

EPIDEMIOLOGY OF SEVERE HEMORRHAGIC SHOCK

Injury is the leading cause of death for individuals younger than age 44 years in the United States. Overall, trauma results in approximately 150,000 deaths per year, and severe hypovolemia caused by hemorrhage is a major factor in nearly half of those deaths. The leading causes of death remain head injury and hemorrhage. These findings have been reported both in the civilian literature[1] and military experiences—the Vietnam conflict,[2,3] and most recently in Baghdad.[4] Approximately one-third of trauma deaths occur out of hospital; exsanguination is a major cause of deaths occurring within 4 hours of injury. The distribution of battlefield injuries in the Vietnam War showed that 25% of the deaths occurred as a result of massive exsanguination and were not salvageable. An additional 19% of deaths were deemed salvageable, and these were the result of torso exsanguination (10%) and peripheral exsanguination (19%).[3]

CLINICAL PERSPECTIVE: LENGTH AND DEPTH OF HYPOTENSION

Severe hemorrhagic shock is characterized by cool, moist, pallid, or cyanotic skin. The patient is tachycardic and hypotensive, and the severity of these clinical manifestations may vary from patient to patient depending on age, underlying cardiovascular disease, and the presence of medications or associated toxic compounds such as drugs or alcohol. Hypotension is the hallmark of shock, is easily measured, and its presence is always a predictor of poor outcome.[5–7] The severity of shock, however, can only be partially quantified by the presence of hypotension. Obviously, patients with rapid and massive blood loss will manifest low blood pressure shortly after the injury. Sophisticated devices or monitoring techniques are not required to establish that such patients are close to dying. Prompt and efficient interventions must be instituted immediately, aimed at control of hemorrhage and replacement of the blood volume. Unfortunately, the absence of hypotension after injury does not rule out the presence of shock. In fact, it may mislead the inexperienced clinician to a false sense of security about the need for aggressive resuscitation.[8]

Injured patients arriving to the trauma center with hypotension or a history of transient hypotension comprise only 6%–9% of the total number of trauma patients.[5,6] From a practical viewpoint, patients with hemorrhagic shock can be stratified into three groups. Group 1 comprises patients with exsanguinating hemorrhage. They generally have significant chest injuries to the heart or great vessels, and/or massively disrupted abdominal visceral or significant retroperitoneal bleeding such as pelvic fractures. This group represents one-third of the total number of hypotensive patients or 2% of the total trauma patient population. They arrive alive to our trauma centers only as a direct result of well-organized prehospital and trauma systems. The response to fluid administration in this group is minimal or completely absent, and these patients are termed *nonresponders*.

Another one-third of hypotensive patients (2% of the total trauma population) constitute group 2 with moderate to severe hemorrhage, with bleeding at a slower rate than group 1. Group 2 patients can die within 6–12 hours if adequate and timely therapy and hemorrhage control are not provided. They respond to the initial resuscitation and may do so transiently. Even if managed appropriately, they may develop organ failure or infection.

The third group is also 2% of the total trauma population and comprises patients with transient hypotension whose compensatory response is sufficient to achieve spontaneous stabilization of their vital signs. The final outcome of these patients is better, but the onset of complications or organ dysfunction may result from the net time spent in a state of under-resuscitation, better described as unrecognized hypoperfusion or compensated shock.

Some clinicians suggest that most shock states can be reversed with more volume resuscitation, with correction of hypothermia, and with inotropic agents. Yet, many patients die, if not acutely from irreversible shock, then later from events initiated by severe, prolonged, or unrecognized shock. Clinically, however, circulatory collapse associated with shock is the common pathway of early progressive deterioration precipitated by trauma and hemorrhage. Patients suffering from severe penetrating trauma to the chest or abdomen, with major injuries to the thoracic or intra-abdominal vessels, who do not die at the scene, may undergo aggressive interventions that may include an emergency thoracotomy and massive transfusion. These patients usually require damage control interventions, and manifest severe hypothermia, coagulopathy, and circulatory failure, even after their hemorrhage has been controlled.[9] Much less common is the clinical scenario of combat casualty victims or civilian trauma patients from rural areas who may develop circulatory collapse and irreversible shock in a slow protracted fashion because of inadequate resuscitation as a result of lack of blood products, delayed evacuation, or prolonged hypotension before definitive care can be provided. Clearly these are two separate clinical scenarios that in the end may have similar outcomes. Because the spectrum of hypoperfusion, ischemia, and total body reperfusion may differ significantly from one clinical scenario to the next, future therapeutic interventions will need to be more sophisticated and targeted than what we offer today. Fluid resuscitation as currently prescribed represents a rather naive approach to therapy in a complicated pathophysiological process.[10]

The potential enhancement of early recognition of progressive or refractory shock and reducing the onset of circulatory collapse early in the management of the patient with hemorrhage offers the opportunity of redefining the "golden hour" (i.e., the window of opportunity for efficacious resuscitation).[11,12]

Discrepancies between Clinical Syndrome of Shock and Animal Models Used to Study Shock

When devising models of hemorrhagic shock, investigators in this field are challenged by two sometimes mutually incompatible goals. First, researchers desire to minimize animal-to-animal variability. Second, researchers seek to achieve a model with clinical relevance. Bleeding in the clinical environment is typically uncontrolled. As hemorrhage continues and arterial pressure decreases, the rate of bleeding tends to slow. Hemostatic mechanisms may come into play when blood pressure is low enough so that bleeding ceases entirely. Resuscitation can actually dislodge the nascent clot by raising blood pressure, and thereby precipitate recurrent hemorrhage.[13] Numerous animal models of uncontrolled bleeding have been described.[14] These models are generally useful for studying novel approaches to achieve hemostasis, for determining the optimal timing of resuscitation, or for determining the optimal parameters/endpoints for resuscitation.[15–17] However, uncontrolled hemorrhage models, while attractive because of their clinical relevance, suffer from a high degree of animal-to-animal variability. Therefore, the use of these models for preclinical efficacy studies of new therapeutic agents requires relatively large sample sizes to obtain statistically meaningful data.

On the other hand, controlled hypotension, as originally described by Wiggers, allows a more standardized grading of injury. When hemorrhagic shock is induced using the Wiggers model, it is initially necessary to periodically withdraw additional aliquots of blood to maintain the target blood pressure because of the body's normal compensatory responses to acute hypovolemia.[18] However, after the shock state has persisted for a period of time, it is no longer possible to withdraw blood to maintain the target blood pressure. On the contrary, it now becomes necessary to reinfuse aliquots of the shed blood to maintain the target blood pressure. This phase has little resemblance to what happens in clinical practice, but in the laboratory it is used to delineate what is known as the "decompensation endpoint," defined as the transition point from withdrawal

to reinfusion of blood. This transition point typically occurs after 90–120 minutes of shock depending on the species. This model is imperfect as well, because variability occurs as to the time of the decompensation endpoint from one animal to the next one. Obviously the Wiggers model allows for a more reproducible injury, one that has little resemblance to the clinical scenario but one that facilitates mechanistic or cause/effect studies and that has been used extensively to delineate many of the cellular and molecular events described after hemorrhage.[19,20]

Diagnosis of Shock

The phenomenon of ischemia and reperfusion has been extensively studied. Shock and resuscitation are functionally a total body ischemia/reperfusion injury. SIRS (systemic inflammatory response syndrome) and MODS (multiple organ dysfunction syndrome) are the expressions of a conglomerate of events associated with ischemia and reperfusion. Unfortunately, we rely on nonspecific global methods to provide indirect information regarding tissue perfusion. The current challenge is to identify innovative methods for quantifying the magnitude of shock. Some of the questions that should guide future research in this field include: how the interaction among the patient's physiological reserve, compensatory responses, and the individual organs endurance/response to ischemia may ultimately manifest, and identifying the best methods to accurately measure each of these components. Presently, we scarcely understand these issues and use rather crude methods to quantify the insult. The term *tissue perfusion* is used liberally to refer to an entity not readily quantifiable. In practical terms, we rely on base deficit and lactate as the global parameters used to gauge tissue perfusion. In the intensive care unit (ICU), we add to the interpretation of these values by hemodynamic parameters that are commonly obtained only after invasive monitoring techniques can be implemented, such as thermodilution cardiac output or continuous $S_V O_2$ from either the central or mixed venous circulation.[21,22]

Assessment of Tissue Perfusion

Base deficit (BD) and lactic acid provide information about the degree of anaerobic metabolism. Lactate is an indirect measure of oxygen debt. Base deficit is defined as the amount of buffer necessary to bring the pH back to 7.40 with pCO_2 of 40 torr. Davis et al.[23] stratified patients by BD as mild (2–5), moderate (6–14), and severe (>15). The magnitude of the initial BD was found to directly correlate with hypotension and further need for fluid resuscitation. In addition, 65% of patients who had a worsening BD despite resuscitation had ongoing hemorrhage. BD is considered a reliable marker for shock and the need for transfusion in multiple trauma patients.[24] Davis et al.[25] also demonstrated that BD could remain abnormal despite improvements in mean arterial pressure, cardiac output, mixed venous O_2 saturation, and oxygen extraction in an animal model of hemorrhagic shock. Rutherford et al.[26] found that BD, age, and head injury had an additive effect on the incidence of mortality. Base deficit is an expedient and sensitive measure of both the degree and the duration of inadequate perfusion. It is useful as a clinical tool and enhances the predictive ability of other trauma scores.

Lactate is the end product of anaerobic glycolysis. As a more direct measurement of tissue hypoxia induced acidosis, it has been shown to have strong prognostic value. Normalization of serum lactate below 2 mmol/l or less within the first 24 hours is associated with 100% survival. Only 78% of patients survived when lactate levels remained elevated during the period of 24–48 hours after shock. The mortality is greater than 85% if lactate remains elevated at 48 hours postshock.[27] Sauaia et al. demonstrated an association between an early (12 hours) rise in serum lactate above 2.5 mmol/l and multiorgan failure.[28] Manikis et al.[29] further found that initial and peak lactate levels, as well as the duration of hyperlactatemia, correlated with the development of MODS after trauma. In summary, the initial lactate level and time to normalization of lactate correlate with risk of MODS and death. However, improved survival using lactate or BD as endpoints for resuscitation has not been shown.[30]

Management of Shock

Shock may be managed by different strategies along the continuum of care from the moment of the insult to the time of stabilization in the ICU. Prehospital interventions may be life saving, but may be limited by the specific environment in the field, such as an urban inner city, a rural setting, the battlefield, or after a mass casualty scenario. During the hospital phase, more definitive therapies may be implemented with the level of care depending on the capabilities of the receiving hospital. When this is not the case, transfer to a Level I or II trauma center may be necessary. Therefore, the actual care that a patient may receive for a similar magnitude of injury may vary significantly depending on the variables listed above, the state of the regionalization of the trauma system, and the maturity of the trauma center. In this chapter, therapeutic strategies will be described according to the physiologic opportunities or therapeutic windows that may be available. These interventions may range from measures to control hemorrhage, enhancement of the compensatory response, replacement of volume lost, and support of the organs during the spectrum of hypoperfusion inherent to a particular clinical scenario. Prompt airway control and expedient control of bleeding are obviously fundamental tenets.

▮ HEMORRHAGE CONTROL

Local Hemorrhage Control

A number of agents are being used to achieve local hemostasis. Such agents may be used topically or systemically. Topical hemostatic agents include vasoconstrictive agents such as epinephrine and procoagulant agents such as thrombin, "hemostatic fibrin," gelatin, and cellulose material.

QuikClot is a new agent designed to induce local hemostasis of large wounds associated with vascular lesions. It is a zeolite mineral granular powder that increases the concentration of clotting factors in the wound. It has been used in models of extremity arterial injury and hepatic laceration with good results. QuikClot has been deployed with the U.S. military forces. Other local hemostatic dressings are currently being tested, such as Chitosan dressings and compressive dressings with a layer of fibrinogen thrombin and calcium chloride embedded in a Dexon mesh.[31,32]

Systemic Hemorrhage Control

Failure of coagulation in trauma is multifactorial and has been characterized by the combined presence of coagulation abnormalities resembling disseminated intravascular coagulation (DIC), caused by systemic activation of coagulation and fibrinolysis.[33] Fibrinolysis is probably caused by release of tissue plasminogen activator from injured tissues[33-35] and dilutional coagulopathy caused by aggressive fluid resuscitation.[36] This *massive transfusion syndrome* includes dilution of coagulation factors and impairment of platelet number and function.[37] Hypothermia may contribute to the coagulopathy by slowing of enzymatic activities of the coagulation cascade[38,39] and impeding platelet function.[40]

Ideally, the introduction of an effective hemostatic agent that would act *only* at the site of injury, without induction of systemic activation of coagulation, could improve hemorrhage control and

reduce hemorrhage-related mortality and morbidity in both military and civilian trauma victims.[41] Systemically administered hemostatic agents include coagulation factors in the form of cryoprecipitate and fresh frozen plasma. A general hemostatic agent may be one that enhances full thrombin generation, and thereby the formation of a stable, tight, fibrin hemostatic plug that is resistant to premature fibrinolysis.

Patients with profuse bleeding resulting from extensive surgery or trauma often develop a complex coagulation pattern that includes reduced plasma levels of fibrinogen, Factor VIII and Factor V, and decreased platelet counts. These patients may have an impaired capacity to generate thrombin. In addition, thrombocytopenia is common, as well as increased fibrinolysis as a result of massive tissue damage. Several of these factors are important for an adequate thrombin formation as well as for the formation of a tight fibrin plug. Thus, low levels of fibrinogen result in the formation of a loose fibrin structure and to decreased activation of Factor XIII, the fibrin-stabilizing factor.[42]

Factor VIIa

The use of recombinant-activated factor VII (rFVIIa) in otherwise normal patients with a trauma or surgery-induced coagulopathy may help in this situation. This is an innovative approach in cases for which there may not be other alternatives. Several case series continue to appear supporting the role of this drug in reversing the coagulopathy of trauma.

Trauma patients with massive bleeding thus may benefit from intravenous rFVIIa to help generate a thrombin peak, which may be enough to form a firm, stable fibrin hemostatic plug and thereby decrease the bleeding.[43] Because thrombin has such a crucial role in providing hemostasis, any agent that enhances thrombin generation in situations with impaired thrombin formation may be characterized as a "general hemostatic agent." Large animal studies with clinically relevant models have demonstrated the efficacy of rFactor VIIa in induction of clot and improved survival.[44-47]

An in vitro study reported by Meng et al.[48] indicated that rFVIIa may not be efficient in acidosis, but hypothermia has little effect on rFVIIa efficacy. These authors recommended that clinicians who may contemplate using FVIIa in trauma patients take note of the level of acidosis present and consider biochemical correction of acidosis before administration of FVIIa. Because of the profound effect of pH on the prothrombinase (FXa/FVa) complex, correction of acidosis may by itself improve hemostasis.

A preliminary study of FVIIa use reported three patients with high-velocity penetrating trauma, and four suffered blunt trauma. They had all received multiple transfusions and conventional interventions without achieving hemostasis. In all cases, the administration of rFVIIa caused a cessation of the diffuse bleeding and their coagulation parameters normalized.[44] Boffard and colleagues[49] published a larger multicenter trial demonstrating benefit from the use of rFVIIa. Both animal and human data indicate that there is a need for more research in the field using greater numbers of individuals both in human and animal research, as well as long-term follow-up to understand the issues regarding possible complications related to increased thrombosis.

Fluids

Management priorities in the bleeding trauma patient begin with airway control, ventilation, and oxygenation.[50] The goal of resuscitation is to stop the bleeding and replete intravascular blood volume to maximize tissue oxygen delivery. Cardiac output, blood pressure, and oxygenated blood flow to vital organs are important determinants of outcome. Measurement of blood pressure may not be feasible, and it is not a necessary requirement to initiate therapy during the primary survey. In fact, a quick global assessment of adequacy of perfusion can be obtained with examination of the characteristics of the pulse. Obvious signs of shock are sufficient to establish the diagnosis and determine the severity of blood volume deficit. Additional information such as blood pressure measurement, electrocardiographic monitoring, pulse oximetry, and capnography may be useful. Adequate intravenous (IV) access for infusion of normothermic fluids is the next priority while other causes of severe hypotension and shock are being sought, such as tension pneumothorax, pericardial tamponade, or neurogenic shock.

Ideally, any fluid therapy must be accompanied with control of bleeding. An estimate of blood volume deficit after blunt trauma may be obtained by calculating blood losses associated with specific injuries. A unilateral hemothorax may contain 3000 ml of blood, the abdomen can hold 2000–5000 ml, and abdominal distension may not be apparent. Other injuries that may precipitate massive hemorrhage include pelvic fracture, associated with blood losses of 1500–2000 ml in the retroperitoneum without any external signs of trauma. A femur fracture may bleed between 800–1200 ml, and a tibia fracture 350–650 ml.

Vascular Access for Patients with Severe Hemorrhage

Vascular access is essential to restore circulatory volume rapidly. The most important factor in considering the procedure for procuring vascular access is the anatomical location and magnitude of the injuries and the level of skill and expertise of the care provider. Venous access should be avoided in an injured limb. In patients with injuries below the diaphragm, at least one IV line should be placed in a tributary of the superior vena cava, as there may be vascular disruption of the inferior vena cava. For rapid administration of large amounts of intravenous fluids, short, large-bore catheters should be used. Doubling the internal diameter of the venous cannula increases the flow through the catheter 16-fold. A 14-gauge, 5-cm catheter in a peripheral vein will infuse fluid twice as fast as a 16-gauge, 20-cm catheter passed centrally. When using 8.5 French pulmonary catheter introducers, the side port should be removed, as this increases the resistance roughly four-fold.

ATLS™ (Advanced Trauma Life Support) guidelines recommend rapid placement of two large-bore (16-gauge or larger) IV catheters in the patient with serious injuries and hemorrhagic shock.[50] The first choice for IV insertion should be a peripheral extremity vein. The most suitable veins are at the wrist, the dorsum of the hand, the antecubital fossa in the arm, and the saphenous in the leg. These sites can be followed by the external jugular and femoral vein. The complication rate of properly placed intravenous catheters is low. Intravascular placement of a large-bore IV should be verified by checking for backflow of blood. An IV site should infuse easily without added pressure. Intravenous fluids can extravasate into soft tissues when pumped under pressure through an infiltrated IV line and may create a compartment syndrome. A patient in extremis who loses pulses in the trauma bay needs a cut-down in the femoral vein.

Subclavian and internal jugular catheterization should not be used routinely in hypovolemic trauma patients. The incidence of complications is higher and the rate of success is lower due to venous collapse. Rapid peripheral percutaneous IV access may be difficult to achieve in patients with hypovolemia and venous collapse, edema, obesity, scar tissue, history of IV drug abuse, or burns. Under such circumstances, central access with wide-bore catheters may be attempted by percutaneous femoral puncture or cut-down. Subclavian catheterization provides rapid venous access in experienced hands. The most frequent complication of subclavian venipuncture is pneumothorax. Pneumothorax is more likely to occur on the left side because the left pleural dome is anatomically higher. Subclavian and internal jugular catheters should be inserted on the side of injury in

patients with chest wounds, reducing the chances of collapse of the uninjured lung, especially if a thoracostomy tube is already in place. A simple pneumothorax may result in respiratory compromise in individuals with pulmonary contusions or a pneumothorax in the contralateral hemithorax. Venous air embolism is another complication of central line insertion.

Although percutaneous placement of internal jugular (IJ) catheters is an excellent means of attaining rapid large-bore catheter access, this is an unusual site for intravenous insertion in trauma patients because of the possibility of cervical trauma and the need for cervical collar immobilization.

Femoral vein cannulation is another alternative for line placement and is associated with fewer acute complications. Bowel perforation may occur, especially in patients with femoral hernia. Penetration of the hip may result in septic arthritis. Thrombophlebitis occurs more often with femoral than with IJ or subclavian catheters; however, this is most likely with prolonged use.

Venous cut-downs can be performed when rapid, secure, large-bore venous cannulation is desirable, and when percutaneous peripheral or central access is either contraindicated or impossible to achieve. Strict aseptic technique should be used. Surgical masks and caps should be worn. Venous cut-down has a low potential for anatomic damage. Cutaneous nerve injury is the most common problem. The infection rate is relatively low when used acutely but increases over time. Therefore, it is recommended that venous cut-down catheters be removed as soon as it is possible to achieve IV access through standard percutaneous IV catheters or a central venous catheter. In addition, any lines placed during resuscitation of a trauma patient without strict aseptic technique should be removed as soon as the patient's condition allows.

TIMING AND VOLUME OF RESUSCITATION FLUID THERAPY

The major controversy in intravenous fluid resuscitation relates to patients with uncontrolled hemorrhage. The optimal volume of intravenous fluid administered is a balance between improvement in tissue oxygen delivery against increase in the blood loss by raising blood pressure. Aggressive fluid resuscitation in an attempt to achieve normal systemic pressure before hemostasis and control of the bleeding may exacerbate blood loss and thereby potentially increase mortality. The knowledge regarding the best time to infuse fluids to patients with hemorrhagic shock dates from almost a century ago,[51] yet studies addressing the effects of massive resuscitation and best fluid management strategies during the prehospital phase have created controversy.[13,14] It is desirable that patients with penetrating injuries and without evidence of traumatic brain injury be resuscitated to a lower admissible blood pressure *(hypotensive resuscitation)* to prevent "popping the clot" until surgical or local control of the hemorrhage can be obtained. The effects of this strategy and the associated hypoperfusion on organs such an injured brain suggest that patients with central nervous system injuries should be managed with a higher blood pressure endpoint.

Type of Fluid

Crystalloids, the ATLS recommendation: Ringer's Lactate Solution

Shires' original studies of crystalloid volume replacement showed such an impressive improvement in survival compared with blood alone or plasma that these data were promptly translated into clinical practice. It is remarkable however that after having used Ringer's lactate as a volume expander and resuscitation fluid for more than half a century, only recently have investigators described the immunological and proinflammatory effects of this solution on neutrophils and other cells involved in host defense mechanisms.

Rhee et al.[52] described neutrophil activation caused by hemorrhagic shock and resuscitation. Using a swine model of shock, they compared the effects of fluid resuscitation in three separate groups: group I received Ringer's lactate solution; group II, shed blood; and group III, 7.5% hypertonic saline solution. Neutrophil activation was measured in whole blood using flow cytometry to detect intracellular superoxide burst activity. They found that neutrophil activation increased significantly immediately after hemorrhage, but it was greatest after resuscitation with Ringer's lactate solution. Animals that received shed blood or hypertonic saline had neutrophil activity return to baseline state after resuscitation. Furthermore, the same group later described that different resuscitative fluids may immediately affect the degree of apoptosis after hemorrhagic shock. In a study in rats, they described that resuscitation with Ringer's lactate solution resulted in a significant increase in small intestinal epithelial and smooth muscle cell and hepatocyte apoptosis.[53] These effects can be ameliorated by use of only the L-isomer of lactate or substitution of ketone for lactate.[54]

Colloids

Albumin

The use of albumin in critically ill patients has been analyzed in a Cochrane report.[55,56] The authors carried out a systematic review of randomized, controlled trials comparing administration of albumin or plasma protein fraction with no fluid or administration of crystalloid solution in critically ill patients with hypovolemia, burns, or hypoalbuminemia. A total of 1419 patients from 30 separate trials were studied. For each patient category, the risk of death in the albumin treated group was higher than in the comparison group. For hypovolemia, the relative risk of death after albumin administration was 1.46 (95% confidence interval 0.97–2.22), for burns the relative risk was 2.40 (1.11–5.19), and for hypoalbuminemia it was 1.69 (1.07–2.67). This review, however, was based on relatively small trials in which there were only a small number of deaths. Therefore, these results must be interpreted with caution. Interestingly, a recent abstract reported the results of a study comparing the safety and efficacy of 5% albumin solution and Ringer's lactate solution for resuscitation of adult ICU patients with shock.[57] This was an open-label randomized multicenter controlled trail. Nineteen patients were treated with albumin and 23 with Ringer's lactate solution. There were no statistically significant differences between groups with respect to days on mechanical ventilation, oxygenation failure, length of ICU stay, or 28-day mortality. The incidence of bacteremia was significantly lower in the albumin group. The authors requested access to the Cochrane database and added the results of this trial to the meta-analyses for the burn patients' subgroup. When the results from recent trials were added, the relative risk for death was no longer significant when comparing albumin versus crystalloids.[57] Finally, recently published results of the SAFE trial carried out in Australia and New Zealand (the Saline versus Albumin Fluid Evaluation [SAFE] Study is a collaboration of the Australian and New Zealand Intensive Care Society Clinical Trials Group) indicated that there is no difference in mortality or incidence of organ failure between albumin and saline in a double-blind randomized population of 7000 patients.[58] When treating patients with hypoalbuminemia, efforts must be centered on correction of the underlying disorder, rather than attempting to reverse primarily the hypoalbuminemia.[59]

Hextend

Hextend® (Abbott Laboratories, North Chicago, IL) is a modified, physiologically "balanced" first-generation, high-molecular-weight hydroxyethyl starch (HES) preparation (average molecular weight approximately 670 kDa; molecular weight 550 kDa). HES contains balanced electrolytes (Na, 143 mmol/l; Cl, 124 mmol/l; lactate, 28 mmol/l; Ca^{+2}, 2.5 mmol/l; K, 3 mmol/l; Mg^{+2}, 0.45 mmol/l; glucose, 5 mmol/l).[60] Hextend is currently being used as the fluid of choice for resuscitation in battlefield casualties because of its greater effect on intravascular volume compared with Ringer's lactate.[4] Unlike previously used preparations of starch such as Dextran or Hespan, Hextend may have less effect on coagulation parameters, but even this observation is debatable.[60–63] Animal studies have shown that Hextend is an efficient volume expander in models of hemorrhage and in models of combined hemorrhage and head injury. In addition, Hextend may be a more effective volume expander than smaller starches. A clinical study demonstrated that Hextend, with its novel buffered, balanced electrolyte formulation, is as effective as 6% hetastarch in saline for the treatment of hypovolemia.[60] There are no studies of the effect of Hextend in acute hemorrhage in humans.

Hypertonic Saline

Hypertonic saline is characterized by its osmotic properties that attract fluid into the intravascular compartment, where the addition of a dextran, or hetastarch, helps to prolong its effects through binding of the recruited water. The concept of resuscitation using hypertonic solutions entails rapid infusion of a 4 ml/kg of body weight dose of 7.2%–7.5% NaCl, which corresponds to a 250-ml bolus in an adult patient. This is given in combination with a colloid solution. This mode of therapy has been shown to have a rapid effect in the circulation. Studies suggest that hypertonic saline seems to be superior to conventional volume therapy with faster normalization of microvascular perfusion during shock phases and early resumption of organ function. Patients with head trauma in association with systemic hypotension particularly appear to benefit.[64,65]

The available literature suggests that there is no clear benefit of hypertonic saline solutions in terms of survival or reduced morbidity. However, recent reanalysis of individual studies of hypertonic saline/dextran found an improved survival in hypotensive patients with head injury.[65] A similar finding was reported in patients with penetrating injuries needing immediate surgery.[66] The prehospital use of hypertonic saline/colloid solutions is limited to a few countries, most of them in Europe and South America.

The Resuscitation Outcome Consortium (ROC) is a newly formed clinical trial network funded by the National Heart, Lung and Blood Institute, National Institute of Neurological Disorders and Stroke, the Canadian Institutes of Health Research, Defense Research and Development Canada, Heart and Stroke Foundation of Canada, and the U.S. Army Medical Research & Materiel Command. The ROC is focusing on research in the area of prehospital cardiopulmonary arrest and severe traumatic injury and is in the process of implementing a multicenter study in the United States and Canada to address the question of hypertonic saline resuscitation. This is a two-pronged study using two populations of trauma patients to be conducted simultaneously utilizing the same intervention and infrastructure. The objective of the first study is to determine the impact of hypertonic resuscitation on survival for blunt or penetrating trauma patients in hypovolemic shock. The second study aims to determine the impact of hypertonic resuscitation on long-term (6 months) neurologic outcome for blunt trauma patients with severe traumatic brain injury. Both studies will be three-arm, randomized, blinded intervention trials comparing hypertonic saline/dextran (7.5% saline/6% dextran 70, HSD), hypertonic saline alone (7.5% saline, HS), and normal saline (NS) as the initial resuscitation fluid administered to these patients prehospital.

Red Cell Transfusion

The decision to initiate blood transfusion during resuscitation is based on a clinical assessment which can be aided by estimating the mechanism of injury, the rate and magnitude of blood loss, the degree of cardiopulmonary reserve, and the overall oxygen consumption of the patient.[67] Any storage of blood products outside a blood bank is difficult and may not be possible in many institutions. Thus, blood products are ordered at the physician's discretion with the inherent risk of underestimating blood transfusion requirements. The options available are type O-negative, type-specific, typed and screened, or typed and cross-matched packed red blood cells (RBCs). (Fresh whole blood is generally not available, but has been used with success in wartime.) The initial choice will depend on the degree of hemodynamic instability. Type O-negative red cells have no major antigens and can be given reasonably safely to patients with any blood type. In patients with massive hemorrhage that require replacement of 50%–75% (e.g., ~10 units of red cells in an adult patient), of the patient's blood volume, it is recommended to continue to transfuse type O blood to avoid the risk of a major cross-match reaction. It is also advisable to have a massive transfusion protocol in place by which notification is given to the blood bank in anticipation for a major need for blood in the operating room. This will alert the blood bank personnel not only to have enough blood, but also to prepare the fresh frozen plasma and platelets that will be needed as a consequence of the ongoing massive hemorrhage.

The heart and brain are generally considered to be the organs most vulnerable to the effects of anemia. In normovolemic hemodilution, the heart begins to produce lactic acid at hematocrits between 15% and 20%,[68] and heart failure generally occurs at hematocrit of 10%.[69] One unit of packed RBCs will usually increase the hematocrit by ~3% and the hemoglobin by 1 g/dl in a 70-kg nonbleeding adult. Obtaining type-specific red cells requires 5–10 minutes in most institutions, and temporizing measures can sometimes be used to gain the necessary time. The use of type-specific red cells is preferred over O-negative and the risk of a hemolytic transfusion reaction is very low.[70] When blood is typed and screened, the patient's blood group is identified and the serum is screened for major blood group antibodies. A full cross-match generally requires 45 minutes and involves mixing donor cells with recipient serum to evaluate for any antigen/antibody reactions. In a recent prospective study of the use of blood transfusion in 104 patients with severe injuries, Beale et al.[71] found that 87% received a total of 324 transfusions; 6% were given in the emergency room, 60% after arrival to the ICU, and 30% in the operating room. The mean pretransfusion Hb level was 9.1 (±1.4) g/dl. This study showed that trauma patients received blood at a relatively high pretransfusion hemoglobin levels (mean of 9 g/dl). As shown previously, more than 4 units of blood was an independent risk factor for systemic inflammatory response.

Blood Substitutes

Attempts at developing artificial hemoglobin-based oxygen carriers (HBOCs) using hemoglobin derived from RBCs began in the 1930s. The greatest obstacle has been related to the toxic effect of stromal contamination. The hemoglobin molecule in HBOCs must be stabilized to prevent dissociation of the α2β2-hemoglobin tetramer. By doing so, intravascular retention is prolonged and nephrotoxicity is eliminated. Several products have been developed including diaspirin cross-linked hemoglobin (HemAssist), human recombinant hemoglobin (rHb1.1 and rHb2.0), polymerized bovine hemoglobin-based O_2 carrier (HBOC-201), human polymerized hemoglobin (PolyHeme®), hemoglobin raffimer (Hemolink™), and maleimide-activated polyethylene glycol-modified hemoglobin (MP4). The most advanced products are in clinical phase III trials, but no product has achieved market approval yet in the United States, Europe, or Canada.[72] Although the hemoglobin solutions may be considered as efficient resuscitative agents and good alternatives to RBC transfusion, their ability to improve microcirculation and to potentially restore metabolic parameters must be weighed against the excessive systemic vasoconstriction and oxidative damage described in some of these products. Diaspirin cross-linked hemoglobin looked promising in the laboratory, but the clinical trials were discontinued because of increased mortality.[73] Its vasopressor effects cannot be attributed to all hemoglobin solutions. Newer products have been developed to minimize the vasomotor effects of hemoglobin. The blood substitute product most studied in trauma patients currently awaiting FDA approval is human polymerized hemoglobin (PolyHeme, Northfield Laboratories, Evanston, IL). This is a

universally compatible, immediately available, disease-free, oxygen-carrying resuscitative fluid. The effect of treating patients with Poly-Heme has been assessed in massively bleeding patients with life-threatening hemorrhage.[74] In a more recent study, 171 patients received rapid infusion of up to 20 units (1000 g, 10 liters) of PolyHeme in lieu of red cells as initial oxygen-carrying fluid replacement in trauma patients and patients undergoing urgent surgery. Thirty-day mortality was compared with a historical control group of 300 surgical patients who refused red cells on religious grounds. Forty patients had RBC hemoglobin as low as 3 g/dl. Total plasma hemoglobin added by Poly-Heme was maintained at a mean of 6.8 (±1.2) g/dl. The 30-day mortality was 25.0% compared with 64.5% in historical control patients. In this study, PolyHeme increased survival from life-threatening acute anemia by maintaining an adequate level of total hemoglobin in the absence of red cell transfusion.[75] A large multicenter trial is in progress. HBOC-201 has been studied for perioperative use, with a trial in trauma patients planned as well. Use of HBOC, when blood is unavailable or perhaps instead of blood, seems promising. It seems likely that at least one product will be available in the near future.

PHARMACOTHERAPY

Vasopressin

Vasopressin is emerging as a potentially major advance in the treatment of a variety of shock states. Increasing interest in the clinical use of vasopressin has resulted from the recognition of its importance in the endogenous response to shock and from advances in understanding of its mechanism of action. Vasopressin has been shown to produce greater blood flow diversion from nonvital to vital organ beds when compared with epinephrine during vasodilatory shock.[76] Under normal conditions, the doses of vasopressin used have little or no pressor action, and significant elevation of plasma vasopressin resulting from the unregulated release of hormone (i.e., the syndrome of inappropriate secretion of antidiuretic hormone) does not cause hypertension.[77,78]

The likely effect of vasopressin in shock may be related to its effect on vascular smooth muscle. Vasopressin can inhibit both ATP-sensitive potassium (K^+ATP) channels[79] and nitric oxide (NO)–induced accumulation of cGMP.[80] Landry and colleagues[81] have shown that activation of the K^+ATP channels contributes to the hypotension of several types of shock, including hemorrhagic shock.[82] Furthermore, activation of NO synthesis also contributes to the hypotension of this condition.[83] Thus, vasopressin inhibits vasodilator mechanisms that contribute to both hypotension and vascular hyporeactivity in the late phase of hemorrhagic shock.[84–86] Arterial hypotension is the principal stimulus for vasopressin secretion via arterial baroreceptors located in the aortic arch and the carotid sinus. If central venous pressure diminishes, then these receptors first stimulate secretion of natriuretic factor, the sympathetic system, and renin secretion. Vasopressin is secreted when arterial pressure falls to the point that it can no longer be compensated for by the predominant action of the vascular baroreceptors.[87,88] Vasopressin potentiates the vasopressor efficacy of catecholamines. However, it has the further advantage of eliciting less pronounced vasoconstriction in the coronary and cerebral vascular regions. It benefits renal function, although these data should be confirmed. The effects on other regional circulations remain to be determined in humans.

New Therapeutic Possibilities

Ethyl Pyruvate

Pyruvate has been identified as an effective scavenger of reactive oxygen species (ROS). For this reason, it has been proposed as therapeutic agent for various pathological conditions that are thought to be mediated by redox dependent phenomena, such as myocardial, intestinal, or hepatic ischemia/reperfusion–induced injury. Ethyl pyruvate (EP) has been shown to be more effective and safer than equimolar doses of sodium pyruvate with significant anti-inflammatory effects.[89,90] The pharmacological basis for the anti-inflammatory effects of EP remains to be explained. It is plausible that EP mediates suppression of NF-KB activation and secretion of NO and of proinflammatory cytokines.[91] Because organ system injury after hemorrhage and resuscitation could be considered a total body ischemia and reperfusion injury, it has been proposed that EP may have a protective role in the management of shock. In an animal study of bleeding and hypotension to a MAP of 40mm Hg over a 60-minute period, Ringer's lactate resuscitation was compared with EP. Survival at 4 hours after resuscitation was 100% in the EP group versus 50% in the RL group.[92] In a similar study it was shown that EP had a protective effect on the shock associated permeability injury of the gut. Phase I and II studies on the effect of EP in humans are currently being undertaken in patients undergoing heart surgery and extracorporeal circulation.

HYPOTHERMIA AND HEMORRHAGIC SHOCK

Hypothermia during hemorrhagic shock appears to be a double-edged sword. Laboratory studies have consistently found that mild (33° C–36° C) to moderate (28° C–32° C) improves survival following hemorrhagic shock.[10,93–96] In contrast, retrospective clinical trials have suggested that trauma patients who become hypothermic are generally more severely injured,[97] with higher mortality than patients who remain normothermic.[98–100] Laboratory studies have demonstrated beneficial effects of hypothermia during hemorrhagic shock on individual organs and the entire organism. As an example, Mizushima et al.[93] found that mild hypothermia during hemorrhagic shock in rats with rewarming during resuscitation produced the best left ventricular performance and cardiac output, compared with normothermia throughout or prolonged hypothermia. Meyer and Horton[94,95] similarly found better cardiac performance with hypothermia compared with normothermia during hemorrhagic shock in dogs. They also demonstrated improved survival. Studies by Wu and associates[96,97] in rats have demonstrated benefit of continued hypothermia after cooling during hemorrhagic shock, mimicking exposure hypothermia as in patients, compared with active rewarming during resuscitation. Mild hypothermia is also beneficial during very prolonged hemorrhagic shock.

Clinically, retrospective studies by Luna et al.[98] and Jurkovich et al.[99] suggested that trauma patients who become hypothermic have increased mortality compared with those who remain normothermic. Because the more severely injured patients are more likely to become hypothermic, it has been difficult to separate the effects of hypothermia from those of confounding factors such as degree of shock, injury severity, volume of fluid and blood products infused, and need for operation. A more recent retrospective analysis from a large statewide database by Wang et al.[100] demonstrated that body temperature of 35° C or lower upon admission was independently associated with an increased risk of death (odds ratio 3).

The only prospective trial of temperature management in trauma patients was that of Gentilello et al.[101] Hypothermic trauma victims were randomized in the intensive care unit to standard rewarming versus more active rewarming via continuous arteriovenous rewarming (CAVR) using a countercurrent heat exchanger (Level I Technologies, Rockland, MA). The CAVR group rewarmed faster and required less fluids, but had similar hospital mortality compared with the standard treatment group.

To understand this dichotomy between the laboratory studies of hemorrhagic shock and the clinical findings with trauma victims, we must consider that uncontrolled, exposure hypothermia, which is common in trauma patients, is physiologically different from

controlled, therapeutic hypothermia, during which shivering and the sympathetic response are blocked. Another issue is potential coagulopathy from hypothermia, although clinically significant changes do not seem to occur unless the temperature is less than 34° C.[35,102]

SUMMARY

Shock after hemorrhage is a complex syndrome that may have a varied clinical manifestation associated with the magnitude of injury and the type of resuscitation or lack thereof. Innovative interventions targeting many of the therapeutic windows within the spectrum from injury to definitive resuscitation are available and were discussed. Active research in this area will bring new contributions and better understanding of this complex disease.

REFERENCES

1. Sauaia A, Moore FA, Moore EE, et al: Epidemiology of trauma deaths: a reassessment. *J Trauma* 38(2):185–193, 1995.
2. Bellamy RF: The causes of death in conventional land warfare: implications for combat casualty care research. *Mil Med* 149(2):55–62, 1984.
3. Blood CG, Puyana JC, Pitlyk PJ, et al: An assessment of the potential for reducing future combat deaths through medical technologies and training. *J Trauma* 53(6):1160–1165, 2002.
4. Holcomb JB: The 2004 Fitts Lecture: current perspective on combat casualty care. *J Trauma* 59(4):990–1002, 2005.
5. Hoyt DB: Fluid resuscitation: the target from an analysis of trauma systems and patient survival. *J Trauma* 54(5 Suppl):S31–35, 2003.
6. Heckbert SR, Vedder NB, Hoffman W, et al: Outcome after hemorrhagic shock in trauma patients. *J Trauma* 45(3):545–549, 1998.
7. Zenati MS, Billiar TR, Townsend RN, et al: A brief episode of hypotension increases mortality in critically ill trauma patients. *J Trauma* 53(2):232–236, discussion 236–237, 2002.
8. Porter JM, Ivatury RR: In search of the optimal end points of resuscitation in trauma patients: a review. *J Trauma* 44(5):908–914, 1998.
9. Hirshberg A, Mattox KL: Planned reoperation for severe trauma. *Ann Surg* 222(1):3–8, 1995.
10. Wu X, Stezoski J, Safar P, et al: After spontaneous hypothermia during hemorrhagic shock, continuing mild hypothermia (34 degrees C) improves early but not late survival in rats. *J Trauma* 55(2):308–316, 2003.
11. Trunkey DD: Prehospital fluid resuscitation of the trauma patient. An analysis and review. *Emerg Med Serv* 30(5):93–95, 2001.
12. Trunkey DD: In search of solutions. *J Trauma* 53(6):1189–1191, 2002.
13. Bickell WH, Wall MJ Jr, Pepe PE, et al: Immediate versus delayed fluid resuscitation for hypotensive patients with penetrating torso injuries. *N Engl J Med* 331(17):1105–1109, 1994.
14. Bickell WH, Shaftan GW, Mattox KL: Intravenous fluid administration and uncontrolled hemorrhage. *J Trauma* 29(3):409, 1989.
15. Capone A, Safar P, Stezoski SW, et al: Uncontrolled hemorrhagic shock outcome model in rats. *Resuscitation* 29(2):143–152, 1995.
16. Bar-Joseph G, Safar P, Saito R, et al: Monkey model of severe volume-controlled hemorrhagic shock with resuscitation to outcome. *Resuscitation* 22(1):27–43, 1991.
17. Abel FL. Animal models simulating human circulatory shock. *Prog Clin Biol Res* 299:287–290, 1989.
18. Peitzman AB, Billiar TR, Harbrecht BG, et al: Hemorrhagic shock. *Curr Probl Surg* 32(11):925–1002, 1995.
19. Hierholzer C, Harbrecht B, Menezes JM, et al: Essential role of induced nitric oxide in the initiation of the inflammatory response after hemorrhagic shock. *J Exp Med* 187(6):917–928, 1998.
20. Couch NP, Dmochowski JR, Van de Water JM, et al: Muscle surface pH as an index of peripheral perfusion in man. *Ann Surg* 173(2):173–183, 1971.
21. Chang MC, Meredith JW: Cardiac preload, splanchnic perfusion, and their relationship during resuscitation in trauma patients. *J Trauma* 42:577–584, 1997.
22. Chang MC, Mondy JS, Meredith JW, Holcroft JW: Redefining cardiovascular performance during resuscitation: ventricular stroke work, power and the pressure-volume diagram. *J Trauma* 45:470–478, 1998.
23. Davis JW, Parks SN, Kaups KL, et al: Admission base deficit predicts transfusion requirements and risk of complications. *J Trauma* 41(5):769–774, 1996.
24. Davis JW, Shackford SR, Mackersie RC, Hoyt DB: Base deficit as a guide to volume resuscitation. *J Trauma* 28(10):1464–1467, 1988.

25. Davis JW, Shackford SR, Holbrook TL: Base deficit as a sensitive indicator of compensated shock and tissue oxygen utilization. *Surg Gynecol Obstet* 173(6):473–476, 1991.

26. Rutherford EJ, Morris JA Jr, Reed GW, Hall KS: Base deficit stratifies mortality and determines therapy. *J Trauma* 33(3):417–423, 1992.

27. Abramson D, Scalea TM, Hitchcock R, et al: Lactate clearance and survival following injury. *J Trauma* 35(4):584–588, discussion 588–589, 1993.

28. Sauaia A, Moore FA, Moore EE, et al: Early predictors of postinjury multiple organ failure. *Arch Surg* 129(1):39–45, 1994.

29. Manikis P, Jankowski S, Zhang H, et al: Correlation of serial blood lactate levels to organ failure and mortality after trauma. *Am J Emerg Med* 13(6):619–622, 1995.

30. Tisherman SB, Barie P, Bokhari F, et al: Clinical practice guideline: endpoints of resuscitation. *J Trauma* 57(4):898–912, 2004.

31. Alam HB, Chen Z, Jaskilee A, et al: Application of a zeolite hemostatic agent achieves 100% survival in a lethal model of complex groin injury in swine. *J Trauma* 56:974–983, 2004.

32. Alam HB, Burris D, DaCorta JA, Rhee P: Hemorrhage control in the battlefield: role of new hemostatic agents. *Mil Med* 170:63–69, 2005.

33. Gando S, Tedo I, Kubota M: Posttrauma coagulation and fibrinolysis. *Crit Care Med* 20(5):594–600, 1992.

34. Kapsch DN, Metzler M, Harrington M, et al: Fibrinolytic response to trauma. *Surgery* 95(4):473–478, 1984.

35. Risberg B, Medegard A, Heideman M, et al: Early activation of humoral proteolytic systems in patients with multiple trauma. *Crit Care Med* 14(11):917–925, 1986.

36. Gubler KD, Gentilello LM, Hassantash SA, Maier RV: The impact of hypothermia on dilutional coagulopathy. *J Trauma* 36(6):847–851, 1994.

37. Reiss RF: Hemostatic defects in massive transfusion: rapid diagnosis and management. *Crit Care Am J Crit Care* 9(3):158–165, 2000.

38. Bergstein JM, Slakey DP, Wallace JR, Gottlieb M: Traumatic hypothermia is related to hypotension, not resuscitation. *Ann Emerg Med* 27(1):39–42, 1996.

39. Krause KR, Howells GA, Buhs CL, et al: Hypothermia-induced coagulopathy during hemorrhagic shock. *Am Surg* 66(4):348–354, 2000.

40. Valeri CR, Feingold H, Cassidy G, et al: Hypothermia-induced reversible platelet dysfunction. *Ann Surg* 205(2):175–181, 1987.

41. Hedner U: General haemostatic agents—fact or fiction? *Pathophysiol Haemost Thromb* 32(Suppl 1):33–36, 2002.

42. McDonagh J, Fukue H: Determinants of substrate specificity for factor XIII. *Semin Thromb Hemost* 22(5):369–376, 1996.

43. Hedner U: NovoSeven as a universal haemostatic agent. *Blood Coagul Fibrinolysis* 11(Suppl 1):107–111, 2000.

44. Martinowitz U, Holcomb JB, Pusateri AE, et al: Intravenous rFVIIa administered for hemorrhage control in hypothermic coagulopathic swine with grade V liver injuries. *J Trauma* 50(4):721–729, 2001.

45. Jeroukhimov I, Jewelewicz D, Zaias J, et al: Early injection of high-dose recombinant factor VIIa decreases blood loss and prolongs time from injury to death in experimental liver injury. *J Trauma* 53(6):1053–1057, 2002.

46. Schreiber MA, Holcomb JB, Hedner U, et al: The effect of recombinant factor VIIa on coagulopathic pigs with grade V liver injuries. *J Trauma* 53(2):252–257, 2002.

47. Sapsford KE, Watts S, Kenward C, Cooper GJ: Intravenous recombinant activated Factor VII improves survival in a pig model of uncontrolled hemorrhage from an aortotomy. St. Pete Beach, FL, 2003.

48. Meng ZH, Wolberg AS, Monroe DM 3rd, Hoffman M: The effect of temperature and pH on the activity of factor VIIa: implications for the efficacy of high-dose factor VIIa in hypothermic and acidotic patients. *J Trauma* 55(5):886–891, 2003.

49. Boffard KD, Riou B, Warren B, et al: Recombinant factor VIIa as adjunctive therapy for bleeding control in severely injured trauma patients: two parallel randomized, placebo-controlled, double blind clinical trials. *J Trauma* 59:8–15, 2005.

50. Carmont MR: The Advanced Trauma Life Support course: a history of its development and review of related literature. *Postgrad Med J* 81(952):87–91, 2005.

51. Cannon WF, Fraser J, Cowell E: The preventative treatment of wound shock. *JAMA* 70:618–621, 1918.

52. Rhee P, Burris D, Kaufmann C, et al: Lactated Ringer's solution resuscitation causes neutrophil activation after hemorrhagic shock. *J Trauma* 44(2):313–319, 1998.

53. Deb S, Martin B, Sun L, et al: Resuscitation with lactated Ringer's solution in rats with hemorrhagic shock induces immediate apoptosis. *J Trauma* 46(4):582–588, 1999.

54. Ayuste EC, Chen H, Koustova E, et al: Hepatic and pulmonary apoptosis after hemorrhagic shock in swine can be reduced through modifications of conventional Ringer's solution. *J Trauma* 60:52–63, 2006.

55. Cochrane Injuries Group Albumin Reviewers: Human albumin administration in critically ill patients: systematic review of randomised controlled trials. *BMJ* 317(7153):235–240, 1998.

56. Alderson P, Bunn F, et al: Human albumin solution for resuscitation and volume expansion in critically ill patients. *Cochrane Database Syst Rev* 4: CD001208, 2004.

57. Cooper A: Efficacy and safety of Plasbumin-5 for adult burn shock resuscitation. *Crit Care Med* 31(2 Suppl):abstract 71, 2003.

58. Finfer S, Bellomo R, Boyce N, et al: A comparison of albumin and saline for fluid resuscitation in the intensive care unit. *N Engl J Med* 350(22):2247–2256, 2004.

59. Pulimood TB, Park GR: Debate: albumin administration should be avoided in the critically ill. *Crit Care* 4(3):151–155, 2000.

60. Gan TJ, Bennett-Guerrero E, Phillips-Bute B, et al: Hextend, a physiologically balanced plasma expander for large volume use in major surgery: a randomized phase III clinical trial. Hextend Study Group. *Anesth Analg* 88(5):992–998, 1999.

61. Martin G, Bennett-Guerrero E, Wakeling H, et al: A prospective, randomized comparison of thromboelastographic coagulation profile in patients receiving lactated Ringer's solution, 6% hetastarch in a balanced-saline vehicle, or 6% hetastarch in saline during major surgery. *J Cardiothorac Vasc Anesth* 16(4):441–446, 2002.

62. Boldt J: New light on intravascular volume replacement regimens: what did we learn from the past three years? *Anesth Analg* 97(6):1595–1604, 2003.

63. Boldt J, Haisch G, Suttner S, et al: Effects of a new modified, balanced hydroxyethyl starch preparation (Hextend) on measures of coagulation. *Br J Anaesth* 89:722–728, 2002.

64. Kramer GC: Hypertonic resuscitation: physiologic mechanisms and recommendations for trauma care. *J Trauma* 54(5 Suppl):S89–S99, 2003.

65. Kreimeier U, Messmer K: Small-volume resuscitation: from experimental evidence to clinical routine. Advantages and disadvantages of hypertonic solutions. *Acta Anaesthesiol Scand* 46(6):625–638, 2002.

66. Younes RN, Aun F, Ching CT, et al: Prognostic factors to predict outcome following the administration of hypertonic/hyperoncotic solution in hypovolemic patients. *Shock* 7:79–83, 1997.

67. Ruchholtz S, Pehle B, Lewan U, et al: The emergency room transfusion score (ETS): prediction of blood transfusion requirement in initial resuscitation after severe trauma. *Transfus Med* 16(1):49–56, 2006.

68. Jan KM, Heldman J, Chien S: Coronary hemodynamics and oxygen utilization after hematocrit variations in hemorrhage. *Am J Physiol* 239(3):H326–H332, 1980.

69. Varat MA, Adolph RJ, Fowler NO: Cardiovascular effects of anemia. *Am Heart J* 83(3):415–426, 1972.

70. Gervin AS, Fischer RP: Resuscitation of trauma patients with type-specific uncrossmatched blood. *J Trauma* 24(4):327–331, 1984.

71. Beale E, Zhu J, Chan L, et al: Blood transfusion in critically injured patients: a prospective study. *Injury* 37:455–465, 2006.

72. Spahn DR, Kocian R: Artificial O_2 carriers: status in 2005. *Curr Pharm Des* 11(31):4099–4114, 2005.

73. Sloan EP, Koenigsberg M, Gens D, et al: Diaspirin cross-linked hemoglobin (DCLHb) in the treatment of severe traumatic hemorrhagic shock: a randomized controlled efficacy trial. *JAMA* 282(19):1857–1864, 1999.

74. Gould SA, Moore EE, Hoyt DB, et al: The first randomized trial of human polymerized hemoglobin as a blood substitute in acute trauma and emergent surgery. *J Am Coll Surg* 187(2):113–120, discussion 120–122, 1998.

75. Gould SA, Moore EE, Hoyt DB, et al: The life-sustaining capacity of human polymerized hemoglobin when red cells might be unavailable. *J Am Coll Surg* 195(4):445–452, discussion 452–455, 2002.

76. den Ouden DT, Meinders AE: Vasopressin: physiology and clinical use in patients with vasodilatory shock: a review. *Neth J Med* 63(1):4–13, 2005.

77. Padfield PL, Brown JJ, Lever AF, et al: Blood pressure in acute and chronic vasopressin excess: studies of malignant hypertension and the syndrome of inappropriate antidiuretic hormone secretion. *N Engl J Med* 304(18):1067–1070, 1981.

78. Tsai YT, Lee FY, Lin HC, et al: Hyposensitivity to vasopressin in patients with hepatitis B-related cirrhosis during acute variceal hemorrhage. *Hepatology* 13(3):407–412, 1991.

79. Wakatsuki T, Nakaya Y, Inoue I: Vasopressin modulates K(+)-channel activities of cultured smooth muscle cells from porcine coronary artery. *Am J Physiol* 263(2 Pt 2):H491–H496, 1992.

80. Kusano E, Tian S, Umino T, et al: Arginine vasopressin inhibits interleukin-1 beta-stimulated nitric oxide and cyclic guanosine monophosphate production via the V1 receptor in cultured rat vascular smooth muscle cells. *J Hypertens* 15(6):627–632, 1997.

81. Landry DW, Oliver JA: The ATP-sensitive K+ channel mediates hypotension in endotoxemia and hypoxic lactic acidosis in dog. *J Clin Invest* 89(6):2071–2074, 1992.

82. Salzman AL, Vromen A, Denenberg A, Szabo C: K(ATP)-channel inhibition improves hemodynamics and cellular energetics in hemorrhagic shock. *Am J Physiol* 272(2 Pt 2):H688–H694, 1997.

83. Thiemermann C, Szabo C, Mitchell JA, Vane JR: Vascular hyporeactivity to vasoconstrictor agents and hemodynamic decompensation in hemorrhagic shock is mediated by nitric oxide. *Proc Natl Acad Sci U S A* 90(1):267–271, 1993.

84. Voelckel WG, Raedler C, Wenzel V, et al: Arginine vasopressin, but not epinephrine, improves survival in uncontrolled hemorrhagic shock after liver trauma in pigs. *Crit Care Med* 31:1160–1165, 2003.

85. Krismer AC, Wenzel V, Voelckel WG, et al: Employing vasopressin as an adjunct vasopressor in uncontrolled traumatic hemorrhagic shock. *Anaesthesist* 54:220–224, 2005.

86. Morales D, Madigan J, Cullinane S, et al: Reversal by vasopressin of intractable hypotension in the late phase of hemorrhagic shock. *Circulation* 100:226–229, 1999.

87. Norsk P, Ellegaard P, Videbaek R, et al: Arterial pulse pressure and vasopressin release in humans during lower body negative pressure. *Am J Physiol* 264(5 Pt 2):R1024–R1030, 1993.

88. O'Donnell CP, Thompson CJ, Keil LC, Thrasher TN: Renin and vasopressin responses to graded reductions in atrial pressure in conscious dogs. *Am J Physiol* 266(3 Pt 2):R714–R721, 1994.

89. Sims CA, Wattanasirichaigoon S, Menconi MJ, et al: Ringer's ethyl pyruvate solution ameliorates ischemia/reperfusion-induced intestinal mucosal injury in rats. *Crit Care Med* 29(8):1513–1518, 2001.

90. Ulloa L, Fink MP, Tracey KJ: Ethyl pyruvate protects against lethal systemic inflammation by preventing HMGB1 release. *Ann N Y Acad Sci* 987:319–321, 2003.

91. Yang R, Gallo DJ, Baust JJ, et al: Ethyl pyruvate modulates inflammatory gene expression in mice subjected to hemorrhagic shock. *Am J Physiol Gastrointest Liver Physiol* 283(1):212–221, 2002.

92. Tawadrous ZS, Delude RL, Fink MP: Resuscitation from hemorrhagic shock with Ringer's ethyl pyruvate solution improves survival and ameliorates intestinal mucosal hyperpermeability in rats. *Shock* 17(6):473–477, 2002.

93. Mizushima Y, Wang P, Cioffi WG, et al: Should normothermia be restored and maintained during resuscitation after trauma and hemorrhage? *J Trauma* 48(1):58–65, 2000.

94. Meyer DM, Horton JW: Effect of different degrees of hypothermia on myocardium in treatment of hemorrhagic shock. *J Surg Res* 48(1):61–67, 1990.

95. Meyer DM, Horton JW: Prolonged survival times with induction of hypothermia after severe hemorrhagic shock. *Curr Surg* 45(4):295–298, 1988.

96. Wu X, Stezoski J, Safar P, et al: Mild hypothermia during hemorrhagic shock in rats improves survival without significant effects on inflammatory responses. *Crit Care Med* 31(1):195–202, 2003.

97. Gregory JS, Flancbaum L, Townsend MC, et al: Incidence and timing of hypothermia in trauma patients undergoing operations. *J Trauma* 31(6):795–798, discussion 798–800, 1991.

98. Luna GK, Maier RV, Pavlin EG, et al: Incidence and effect of hypothermia in seriously injured patients. *J Trauma* 27(9):1014–1048, 1987.

99. Jurkovich GJ, Greiser WB, Luterman A, Curreri PW: Hypothermia in trauma victims: an ominous predictor of survival. *J Trauma* 27(9):1019–1024, 1987.

100. Wang HE, Callaway CW, Peitzman AB, Tisherman SA: Admission hypothermia and outcome after major trauma. *Crit Care Med* 33(6):1296–1301, 2005.

101. Gentilello LM, Jurkovich GJ, Stark MS, et al: Is hypothermia in the victim of major trauma protective or harmful? A randomized, prospective study. *Ann Surg* 226(4):439–447, discussion 447–449, 1997.

102. Patt A, McCroskey BL, Moore EE: Hypothermia-induced coagulopathies in trauma. *Surg Clin North Am* 68(4):775–785, 1988.

EXSANGUINATION: RELIABLE MODELS TO INDICATE DAMAGE CONTROL

Alicia M. Mohr, Juan A. Asensio, Tamer Karsidag, Luis Manuel García-Núñez, Patrizio Petrone, Amanda J. Morehouse, Alexander D. Vara, John S. Weston, Donald Robinson, Edward Lineen, and Allan Capin

Exsanguination has been defined as an extreme form of hemorrhage with ongoing bleeding that, if not surgically controlled, will lead to death. Therefore, the speed by which the exsanguinating trauma patient moves from the prehospital, emergency department, operating room, and intensive care unit is important to survival. Certain conditions and complexes of injuries require damage control to prevent exsanguination. This chapter will describe validated indicators that can be used both preoperatively and intraoperatively to improve outcomes. This chapter will also outline current guidelines for the institution of damage control in trauma patients. Emphasis is placed on the current indications for damage control as defined by key studies. Awareness of these guidelines can improve outcomes after major intra-abdominal injuries and hemorrhage and also assist in the management of one of the well-known sequelae of damage control, the post-traumatic open abdomen.

HISTORY

Bailout/damage control surgery following trauma has developed as a major advance in surgical practice in the last 20 years. The principles of damage control surgery defied the traditional surgical teaching of definitive operative intervention and were slow to be adopted. Currently, techniques developed by trauma surgeons known as damage control surgery have been successfully used to manage traumatic thoracic, abdominal, extremity, and peripheral vascular injuries. In addition, damage control surgery has been extrapolated for use in general, vascular, cardiac, urologic, and orthopedic surgery.

In 1983, Stone was first to describe the "bailout" approach of staged surgical procedures for severely injured patients. This approach emerged after his observation that early death following trauma was associated with severe metabolic and physiologic derangements following severe exsanguinating injuries. Following massive transfusion exceeding two blood volumes in trauma and emergency surgery, severe physiologic derangement ensued and mortality was found to be greater than 60%. Profound shock along with major blood loss initiates the cycle of hypothermia, acidosis, and coagulopathy. It was at this time that hypothermia, acidosis, and coagulopathy were described as the "trauma triangle of death" or the "bloody vicious cycle." A fourth component, dysrhythmia, which usually heralded the patient's death, was later added by Asensio. Coagulopathy, acidosis, and hypothermia make the prolonged and definitive operative management of trauma patients dangerous. This approach, now called "damage control," describes it as multiphasic, where reoperation occurs after correcting physiologic abnormalities.

METABOLIC FAILURE

Hypothermia is a consequence of severe exsanguinating injury and subsequent resuscitative efforts. Severe hemorrhage leads to tissue hypoperfusion and diminished oxygen delivery, which leads to reduced heat generation. Clinically significant hypothermia is important if the body temperature drops to less than 36° C for more than 4 hours. Hypothermia can lead to cardiac arrhythmias, decreased cardiac output, increased systemic vascular resistance, and left shift of the oxygen–hemoglobin dissociation curve. Hypothermia exerts a negative inotropic effect on the myocardium with depression of left ventricular contractility. The initial ECG change seen with hypothermia is sinus tachycardia, but as the core temperature decreases, progressive bradycardia ensues. The cardiac response to catecholamines may also be blunted in hypothermic hearts, and cold cardiac tissue poorly tolerates hypervolemia and hypovolemia. Hypothermia can also induce coagulopathy by inhibition of the coagulation cascade. Low temperature also impairs the host's immunologic function. Hypothermia is aggravated by heat loss resulting from either environmental factors or surgical interventions. The multidisciplinary team caring for trauma patients must make every effort to prevent heat loss and help to correct hypothermia.

The causes of coagulopathy in patients with severe trauma are multifactorial, including consumption and dilution of platelets and coagulation factors, as well as dysfunction of platelets and the coagulation system. Clinical coagulopathy occurs because of hypothermia, platelet and coagulation factor dysfunction that occurs at low temperatures, activation of the fibrinolytic system, and hemodilution following massive resuscitation. Platelet dysfunction is secondary to the imbalance between thromboxane and prostacyclin that occurs in a hypothermic state. Hypothermia and hemodilution produce an additive effect on coagulopathy. After replacement of one blood volume (5000 ml or 15 units of packed red blood cells [pRBCs]), only 30%–40% of platelets remain in circulation. The prothrombin time (PT), partial prothrombin time (PTT), fibrinogen levels, and lactate levels are therefore not predictive of the severe coagulopathic state.

The predominant physiologic defect resulting from repetitive and persistent bouts of hypoperfusion is metabolic acidosis. Anaerobic metabolism starts when the shock stage of hypoperfusion is prolonged, leading to the production of lactate. Acidosis decreases myocardial contractility and cardiac output. Acidosis also worsens as a result of multiple transfusions, the use of vasopressors, aortic cross-clamping, and impaired myocardial performance. It is clear that a complex relationship exists among acidosis, hypothermia, and coagulopathy, and each factor compounds the other, leading to a high mortality rate once this cycle ensues and cannot be interrupted.

MODELS FOR DAMAGE CONTROL

Stone's original work in 1983 only provided the intraoperative observation of coagulopathy as an indication for "bailout." In this study, 17 patients underwent the "bailout" procedure, which included an initial laparotomy, followed by packing in patients with an observed clinical coagulopathy, and then completion of the surgical procedure once the coagulopathy was improved. This resulted in 11 survivors with a mortality rate of 35%. Subsequently, Rotondo et al. described the multiphase approach to the management of exsanguinating patients sustaining abdominal injury, but did not define any objective parameters during the intraoperative phase of damage control. The authors reported a survival rate of 77% in a very small subgroup of patients with major vascular injury and two or more physical injuries. Burch et al. proposed a model based on core temperature 32° C or less, pH 7.09 or less, and pRBC transfusion of more than 22 units that

could predict 48-hour survival; the authors also described the "lethal triad." In a study based on 39 patients, Sharp et al. defined a temperature 33° C or less, pH 7.18 or less, PT 16 seconds or higher, PTT 50 seconds or higher, and more than 10 units of pRBCs transfused as objective parameters to indicate the need for early packing.

Morris et al. described 107 patients who underwent staged laparotomy and abdominal packing. They proposed proceeding with damage control early in the course of operation based on patient's temperature of less than 35° C, a base deficit greater than 14, and the presence of coagulopathic bleeding. Similarly, Moore described a progressive coagulopathy as the most compelling reason for staged laparotomy. A severe coagulopathic state was described as PT and PTT greater than two times normal, massive and rapid blood transfusion exceeding 10 units in 4 hours, persistent shock defined as a oxygen consumption less than 110 ml/min/m², lactic acid level greater than 5 mmol/l, pH under 7.2, base deficit higher than 14, and core hypothermia less than 34° C. It was postulated that the ability to predict the onset of coagulopathy would have significant implications for instituting damage control. Another predictive model for life-threatening coagulopathy included systolic blood pressure less than 70 mm Hg, temperature higher than 34° C, pH less than 7.10, and Injury Severity Score (ISS) of 25 or higher.

No single model has been able to accurately predict the timing for institution of damage control. A pH less than 7.1 or a core temperature of less than 33° C may indicate that the "bloody vicious cycle" is too far advanced and cannot be interrupted. Similarly, it is difficult to obtain intraoperative results for PT, PTT, fibrinogen, and lactate levels at all hospitals, or to place a Swan-Ganz catheter in the operating room (OR).

To define the patient at greatest risk for exsanguination and death, one must determine the threshold levels of pH, temperature, and highest estimated level of blood loss. Therefore, in an attempt to institute the development of intraoperative guidelines for "damage control/bailout," Asensio et al. first retrospectively evaluated 548 patients over 6 years who were admitted to a large urban trauma center with the diagnosis of exsanguination. Inclusion criteria were intraoperative blood loss of 2000 ml or more, minimum transfusion requirement of 1500 ml pRBCs or greater during the initial resuscitation, and diagnosis of exsanguination. Data collected included demographics, prehospital and admission vital signs and physiologic predictors of outcome, Revised Trauma Score (RTS), Glasgow Coma Scale (GCS), Injury Severity Score (ISS), volume of resuscitative fluids, need for thoracotomy in the emergency department (EDT), volume of fluids in the operating room, need for thoracotomy in the operating room (ORT), and intraoperative complications. In this patient population, the Revised Trauma Score was 4.38 and the mean ISS was 32, denoting a physiologically compromised and severely injured patient population. There were 180 patients that underwent EDT with aortic cross-clamping, open CPR, 99 (55%) succumbed in the emergency department. In addition to the 81 patients that survived EDT, 117 required ORT for a total of 198 EDT and ORT, of which 56 (28%) survived to leave the operating room and the hospital. In this series, mean admission pH was 7.15, mean temperature was 34.3° C in the operating room, and these patients received an average of 14,165 ml of crystalloid, blood, and blood products. Overall, 449 patients survived to arrive in the OR with some signs of life and 281 patients died; 37% of these patients survived damage control. Table 1 shows the objective intraoperative parameters developed to predict outcome and provide guidelines on when to institute damage control based on these findings. This series also provided independent risk factors for survival, which included an injury severity score less than 20, spontaneous ventilation in the emergency room, no EDT or ORT, and the absence of abdominal vascular injury.

One of the natural sequelae in patients surviving damage control is an open abdomen. These guidelines were prospectively validated in a series of 139 patients who underwent damage control and had posttraumatic open abdomen. This study consisted of two groups of patients: 86 patients studied retrospectively prior to instituting the guidelines, and 53 patients studied prospectively after instituting the guidelines. The groups were comparable in all relevant parameters.

Table 1: Physiologic Guidelines That Predict Need for Damage Control

Hypothermia 34° C
Acidosis pH 7.2
Serum bicarbonate 15 mEq/l
Transfusion of 4000 ml blood
Transfusion of 5000 ml blood and blood products
Intraoperative volume replacement 12,000 ml
Clinical evidence of intraoperative coagulopathy

Although there was no difference in the mortality rate between the two groups (24% for each), there were statistically significant differences in the number of intraoperative transfusions, less hypothermia and bowel edema, less postoperative infections and gastrointestinal complications, and shorter intensive care unit and hospital length of stay for the prospective group. Another significant finding in this study was that 93% of patients were able to undergo definitive abdominal closure in their hospital stay as compared with the historic 22%.

Awareness of potential triggers to initiate damage control is vital. A study of 68 patients who underwent damage control surgery found that the inability to correct pH greater than 7.21 and PTT greater than 78.7 seconds was predictive of 100% mortality. Delayed recognition of the need for damage control as well as poor communication with the anesthesia and nursing team are deleterious to the care of the multiply injured patient.

PATIENT SELECTION

Not all trauma patients require damage control measures. In addition to the physiologic guidelines for the institution of damage control (see Table 1), certain conditions and complexes of injuries assessed both preoperatively and intraoperatively require damage control (Table 2). Multiple mass casualties and the need for EDT

Table 2: Preoperative and Intraoperative States That Suggest Need for Damage Control

Preoperative	Intraoperative
Multiple mass casualties	Need for intraoperative thoracotomy
Multisystem trauma with major abdominal injury	Major abdominal vascular injuries
Open pelvic fracture with major abdominal injury	Major thoracic vascular injuries
Major abdominal injury with need to evaluate extra-abdominal injury	Severe complex hepatic injuries
Traumatic amputation with major abdominal injury	Presence of sustained hypotension
Need for emergency department thoracotomy	Presence of coagulopathy
Presence of sustained hypotension	Presence of hypothermia
Presence of coagulopathy	
Presence of hypothermia	
Need for adjunctive use of angio-embolization	

predict the need for damage control. In the multiply injured trauma patient sustaining major abdominal injury, the need to evaluate for other extra-abdominal injuries in a timely fashion may also indicate damage control. The preoperative duration of hypotension (systolic blood pressure <90 mm Hg) was significantly different in those patients that exsanguinated as compared with survivors (45 minutes vs. 85 minutes). Therefore, in addition to other factors such as the preoperative assessment of hypothermia and coagulopathy, a period of sustained hypotension greater than 60 minutes would predict the need for damage control. Intraoperatively, certain complexes of injuries also predict the need for this technique. These injuries include major abdominal vascular, complex hepatic, major thoracic vascular injuries, and the need for intraoperative thoracotomy.

Patients with exsanguination are perhaps the best candidates to undergo damage control. Asensio has described an algorithm for the management of exsanguination that involves three phases (Figure 1). First, the patient is classified as exsanguinating; and second, resuscitation under the Advanced Trauma Life Support protocols is begun (see Figure 1). The third phase comprises rapid transport to the operating room (exsanguination from penetrating injuries is a dramatic ill-defined entity that requires leadership, fast thinking, aggressive surgical intervention, and a well-thought-out plan). Rapid damage control can lead to effective management of exsanguination and improve survival.

TECHNIQUE OF DAMAGE CONTROL

The most important goal of early institution of damage control is patient survival. A four-stage damage control approach has been recently defined by Johnson in a study of 24 patients who underwent damage control and were retrospectively compared with patients who underwent damage control a decade earlier (Figure 2). The "ground-zero" stage includes the prehospital phase as well as early resuscitation in the emergency room. This ground-zero phase includes short paramedic scene times and identification of injury

PHASE 1
  CLASSIFY PATIENT AS EXSANGUINATING
    Hemodynamic instability
    Initial blood loss >40%
    Massive ongoing blood loss
    Injuries prone to exsanguination

PHASE 2
  RESUSCITATE PER ATLS PROTOCOLS
    Crystalloids 2–3 L (Ringer's lactate)
    Blood (uncrossmatched, type specific, or crossmatched)
    Rapid infusion of warm fluids
    Determine need for ED thoracotomy and thoracic aortic cross-clamping

PHASE 3
  TO OR EXPEDIENTLY
    Determine need for OR thoracotomy and aortic cross-clamping
    Control bleeding source or sources
    Use adjunct techniques
      Rapid volume infusers
      Autotransfusion
      Packing
      Shunts
      Damage control
    Prevent hypothermia and coagulopathy
    Proper replacement of blood and blood products

Figure 1 Algorithm for the management of exsanguinations. *ATLS,* Advance Trauma Life Support; *ED,* emergency department; *OR,* operating room.

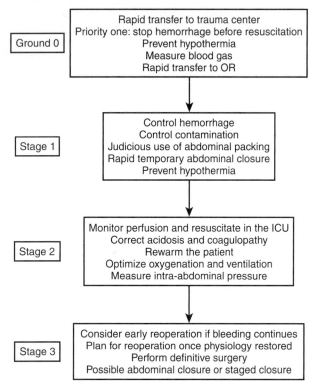

| Ground 0 | Rapid transfer to trauma center
Priority one: stop hemorrhage before resuscitation
Prevent hypothermia
Measure blood gas
Rapid transfer to OR |

| Stage 1 | Control hemorrhage
Control contamination
Judicious use of abdominal packing
Rapid temporary abdominal closure
Prevent hypothermia |

| Stage 2 | Monitor perfusion and resuscitate in the ICU
Correct acidosis and coagulopathy
Rewarm the patient
Optimize oxygenation and ventilation
Measure intra-abdominal pressure |

| Stage 3 | Consider early reoperation if bleeding continues
Plan for reoperation once physiology restored
Perform definitive surgery
Possible abdominal closure or staged closure |

Figure 2 Four stages of damage control. *ICU,* Intensive care unit; *OR,* operating room.

patterns in the ED that require damage control, as well as rewarming maneuvers that begin in the trauma bay.

Damage control implies immediate control of life-threatening hemorrhage, control of gastrointestinal contamination with rapid resections or closures, the use of intraluminal shunts, and judicious abdominal packing with temporary abdominal wall closures. Specifically, for chest injuries, one should repair cardiovascular injuries, perform stapled pulmonary tractotomy, pack if needed, place chest tubes, and close the skin. For abdominal injuries, damage control can involve control of major hemorrhage, hepatic packing, pancreatic drainage, temporary hollow viscus closures, rapid stapled resections, splenectomy, nephrectomy, vascular pedicle clamping in situ, and the use of intra-abdominal vascular shunts. Frequently, these patients experience abdominal compartment syndrome. Therefore, the posttraumatic open abdomen with temporary abdominal wall closure is used as an extension of damage control.

The second stage begins in the ICU where the metabolic disorder is corrected. Rewarming the patient is a high priority, as coagulopathy and acidosis can only be corrected and maintained once the body temperature returns to normal. Further inspections are then made to identify injuries that may have not been detected in the initial survey. Twenty-four to 72 hours may be needed to correct metabolic derangements.

The last stage of damage control involves the timing of reoperation when definitive procedures are performed. Reoperation is considered early if major blood losses continue. Usually, there is a window of 36–48 hours after the initial injury between the correction of the metabolic disorder and the onset of the systemic inflammatory response syndrome and/or multiple organ failure. In this phase,

definitive procedures are undertaken. Thorough re-exploration is made for any additional injuries and restoration of gastrointestinal continuity and vascular repair are done. Provisional feeding access may be placed, followed by washout of the abdominal cavity and attempts at definitive closure. The patient then returns to the intensive care unit for further care.

CONCLUSIONS

The management of exsanguination requires leadership, prompt thinking, aggressive surgical intervention, and a well-conceived plan. The exsanguinating trauma patient that requires massive transfusion incurs the greatest risk for the multifactorial interactions among acidosis, hypothermia, and coagulopathy. The ultimate goal is the prompt and effective control of the exsanguinating source; delays in the decision to perform damage control contribute to a higher morbidity and mortality. Therefore, damage control is a vital part of the management of the multiply injured patient and should be performed before metabolic exhaustion.

SUGGESTED READINGS

Aoki N, Wall M, Demsar J, et al: Predictive model for survival at the conclusion of damage control laparotomy. *Am J Surg* 180:540–545, 2001.

Asensio JA, Britt LD, Borzotta A, et al: Multiinstitutional experience with the management of superior mesenteric artery injuries. *J Am Coll Surg* 193:354–365, 2001.

Asensio JA, McDuffie L, Petrone P, et al: Reliable variables in the exsanguinated patient which indicate damage control and predict outcome. *Am J Surg* 182:743–751, 2001.

Asensio JA, Petrone P, O'Shanahan G, Kuncir EJ: Managing exsanguination: what we know about damage control/bailout is not enough. *BUMC Proc* 16:294–296, 2003.

Asensio JA, Petrone P, Roldan G, et al: Has evolution in awareness of guidelines for institution of damage control improved outcome in the management of the posttraumatic open abdomen? *Arch Surg* 139:209–214, 2004.

Burch JM, Ortiz VB, Richardson RJ, et al: Abbreviated laparotomy and planned reoperation for critically injured patients. *Ann Surg* 215:476–483, 1992.

Cosgriff N, Moore EE, Sauaia A, et al: Predicting life threatening coagulopathy in the massively transfused trauma patient: hypothermia and acidoses revisited. *J Trauma* 42:857–861, 1997.

Johnson JW, Gracias VH, Schwab CW, et al: Evolution in damage control for exsanguinating penetrating abdominal injury. *J Trauma* 51:261–269, 2001.

Moore EE: Staged laparotomy for the hypothermia, acidosis, and coagulopathy syndrome. *Am J Surg* 172:405–410, 1996.

Morris JA Jr, Eddy VA, Blinman TA, Rutherford EJ, Sharp KW: The staged celiotomy for trauma: issues in unpacking and reconstruction. *Ann Surg* 217:576–584, 1993.

Phillips TF, Soulier G, Wilson RF: Outcome of massive transfusion exceeding two blood volumes in trauma and emergency surgery. *J Trauma* 27:903–910, 1987.

Rotondo MF, Schwab CW, McGonigal MD, et al: "Damage control": an approach for improved survival in exsanguinating penetrating abdominal injury. *J Trauma* 35:375–382, 1993.

Stone HH, Strom PR, Mullins RJ: Management of the major coagulopathy with onset during laparotomy. *Ann Surg* 197:532–535, 1983.

Surgical Techniques for Thoracic, Abdominal, Pelvic, and Extremity Damage Control

Kimberly A. Davis   and   **Frederick A. Luchette**

Injury severity and spectrums of injury have continually evolved, resulting in greater and different challenges for the modern trauma surgeon. High energy blunt trauma, with resultant multisystem organ injury, as well as increasingly sophisticated firearms with greater wounding capacity, has resulted in greater severity of injury. Despite the fact that these injury patterns are more likely to result in the death of a patient, improvements in prehospital transport and trauma resuscitation have allowed more moribund patients to reach the hospital alive but in extremis. Damage control surgery, addressing the life-threatening injuries immediately but delaying definitive repair until the metabolic and physiologic perturbations have been corrected, has evolved to address this population of patients.

Damage control has three separate and distinct phases of management. The first phase includes aggressive volume expansion, rapid control of hemorrhage, and the minimization of contamination, often associated with placement of packing to tamponade bleeding. Next, contamination from hollow viscus injuries is quickly obtained. Temporary wound management strategies are implemented. The second phase, which occurs in the intensive care unit (ICU), involves the aggressive rewarming of the hypothermic patient, with correction of coagulopathy, and ongoing resuscitation with crystalloids and blood. Once normal physiology has been re-established, the third phase involves definitive operative management of the patient's injuries.

Indications for damage control strategy are multiple. The goal of the damage control procedure is to preserve life in the face of devastating injuries with profound hemorrhagic shock. As described by Moore et al., they include an inability to achieve hemostasis resulting from ongoing coagulopathy, a technically difficult or inaccessible major venous injury, a time-consuming procedure in the face of under-resuscitated shock, and a need to address other life-threatening injuries. These indications have been expanded to include hemodynamically unstable patients with high-energy blunt torso trauma or multiple penetrating injuries, or any trauma patient presenting in shock with hypothermia and coagulopathy (Table 1). Most commonly applied to the abdomen, damage control approaches have now been applied successfully to both devastating thoracic and orthopedic injuries.

PREDISPOSING FACTORS

The goal of damage control procedures is the early termination of surgical intervention before the development of irreversible physiologic derangement. Uncontrolled hemorrhage results in global ischemic injury, while resuscitation subjects the patient to further injury resulting from the period of reperfusion. Inevitably the lethal triad of hypothermia, coagulopathy, and acidosis develops. While each of these complications is potentially life threatening in and of them-

selves, the combination of the three together results in an exponential increase in morbidity, contributing to a downward spiral that eventually results in the patient's demise if not corrected. Damage control surgery, by abbreviating surgical intervention and returning the patient to the ICU for correction of the lethal triad, has resulted in improved mortality over time.

Hypothermia is defined as a core temperature of less than 35° C. The reasons for hypothermia after trauma include aggressive resuscitation with unwarmed fluids, exposure at the time of the primary and secondary survey with radiant heat loss to the environment, and evaporative loss from exposed peritoneal and pleural surfaces in the operating room. The incidence of clinical hypothermia after trauma laparotomy is 57%. Hypothermia has clearly been shown to increase mortality, increasing significantly in patients with a core temperature less than 34° C, and approaching 100% in patients with a core temperature less than 32° C.

Hypothermia has systemic effects, including negative impact on hemodynamics (decreased heart rate and cardiac output, increased systemic vascular resistance), renal function (decreased glomerular filtration rates), and central nervous system depression. Hypothermia also independently affects the coagulation cascade, as clot formation relies on a series of temperature-dependent enzymatic reactions. Studies have clearly demonstrated increases in prothrombin time (PT), thrombin time, and partial thromboplastin time (PTT). Hypothermia also affects platelet function, leading to sequestration in the portal circulation and prolonged bleeding times.

Metabolic acidosis occurs after hemorrhagic shock because of the switch from aerobic to anaerobic metabolism during periods of hypoperfusion. The detrimental effects of acidosis include depressed myocardial contractility and a diminished response to inotropic medications. Acidosis predisposes the myocardium to ventricular dysrhythmias and can worsen intracranial hypertension. Finally, acidosis has been shown to worsen coagulopathy by independently prolonging PTT and decreasing Factor V activity. Acidosis has been linked to the development of disseminated intravascular coagulation (DIC) and may exacerbate a consumptive coagulopathy.

Hypothermia, acidosis, and coagulopathy develop secondary to the dilutional effects when massive resuscitation initially is comprised of crystalloid and packed red blood cells without the addition of clotting factor replacement. Exposed tissue factor secondary to tissue injury also contributes to the development of coagulopathy through the activation of the clotting cascade and resultant consumption of clotting factors.

INITIAL RESUSCITATION CONCERNS

A systematic approach to the initial management of the injured patient has been promulgated by the Advanced Trauma Life Support course of the American College of Surgeons Committee on Trauma. The primary and secondary surveys as described in that course allow the rapid identification of life-threatening injuries and allow the surgeon to prioritize subsequent operative management of the unstable trauma patient. Patients with exsanguinating hemorrhage should be expeditiously transported to the operating room, where a decision regarding the initiation of damage control should be made early in the operative course, based on the patient's physiologic status, body temperature, and intravascular volume status (see Table 1). In patients with obvious ongoing resuscitation requirements, a central venous catheter should be placed for aggressive volume resuscitation. Given the multiple factors that predispose these patients to coagulopathy, early consideration should be given to the administration of coagulation factors (fresh frozen plasma and cryoprecipitate)

Table 1: Indications for Damage Control Procedures

Hemodynamic instability resulting from hemorrhagic shock
Presenting coagulopathy or hypothermia
Major abdominal vascular injury with or without associated visceral injury
Complex hepatic injuries with or without associated visceral injury
Multicavitary injuries with hemorrhagic shock
Multisystem trauma with competing management priorities
Metabolic acidosis with pH <7.3
Massive transfusion requirements

Adapted with permission from Rotondo MF, Zonies DH: The damage control sequence and underlying logic. *Surg Clin North Am* 77:761–777, 1997.

and platelets, in addition to the standard crystalloid and packed red blood cell resuscitation.

PHASE I: DAMAGE CONTROL OPERATION

Damage Control Laparotomy

Most damage control procedures are performed in the abdomen. In fact, the earliest descriptions of what subsequently became known as damage control surgery were in patients with major hepatic injuries, in whom the placement of perihepatic packing and staged operative management resulted in decreased morbidity and mortality. The most common injuries that trigger a damage control approach are major liver injuries and major vascular injuries.

The primary method of controlling hepatic hemorrhage is packing. The technique of pack placement is of the utmost importance and depends on the anatomic nature of the liver injury. Major hepatic lacerations require complete mobilization of the liver and inflow occlusion (the Pringle maneuver) to minimize blood loss. Direct ligation of bleeding vessels in the depth of the laceration is necessary to obtain surgical hemostasis. Once major vessel bleeding has been controlled, perihepatic packs should be placed anteriorly and posteriorly, compressing the liver between the two beds of packs and providing tamponade. In penetrating injuries, balloon tamponade of the missile tract, in conjunction with perihepatic packing, can be life saving.

There are several options available for the management of major vascular injuries. Some venous injuries will respond to packing. Ongoing bleeding, however, requires direct surgical intervention. Many abdominal vascular injuries can be managed with simple ligation of the bleeding vessel (Table 2). Ligation, however, is not tolerated in aortic or proximal superior mesenteric artery injuries, and is not technically feasible in retrohepatic caval injuries. These injuries are typically initially approached by an attempt at repair or the placement of a temporary intraluminal shunt, with planned repair at a second operation (phase 3). Commonly, Argyle carotid shunts and Javid shunts have been used for this purpose. Chest tubes may be used when larger conduits are necessary. The shunts should be secured using umbilical tapes, vessel loops, or suture, and do not require anticoagulation to maintain patency. Another technique for the management of exsanguinating vascular injury is the use of endoluminal balloon catheters to obtain proximal and distal control of hemorrhage. The catheters are inserted into the vessel at the site of injury, and the balloon inflated. This technique allows repair of the injured vessel in a relative dry operative field.

Table 2: Abdominal Vessel Ligation and Expected Complications

Vessel	Complication	Recommendations
Celiac axis	None	
Splenic artery	None if the short gastric vessels are intact	
Common hepatic artery	None if the portal vein is intact, possible gallbladder ischemia	Cholecystectomy (may be done at second look)
Superior mesenteric artery	Bowel ischemia	Second-look procedure
Superior mesenteric vein	Bowel ischemia	Second-look procedure
Portal vein	Bowel ischemia	Second-look procedure
Suprarenal inferior vena cava	Possible renal failure	Wrap and elevate legs, assess for compartment syndrome
Infrarenal inferior vena cava	Lower extremity edema	Wrap and elevate legs, assess for compartment syndrome
Left renal vein (proximal)	None	
Right renal vein	Renal ischemia	Nephrectomy
Common and external iliac artery	Lower extremity ischemia	Ipsilateral calf and sometimes thigh fasciotomies or extra-anatomic bypass
Common and external iliac vein	Lower extremity edema	Wrap and elevate legs
Internal iliac artery	None	
Internal iliac vein	None	

Adapted with permission from Shapiro MB, Jenkins DH, Schwab CW, Rotondo MF: Damage control: collective review. *J Trauma* 49:969–978, 2000.

Candidates for damage control surgery often have associated hollow viscus injury. The goal in management of these injuries is the control of contamination. Intestinal lacerations may be controlled by linear stapling or by stapled resection. After enterectomy, the gastrointestinal tract is left in discontinuity, and the decision to perform an anastomosis or stoma is postponed until the patient is stabilized and able to return to the operating room for definitive management (phase 3). Associated biliary or pancreatic injuries can often be managed with judicious placement of closed suction drains, with plans to address the injury at the second procedure (phase 3).

Hemodynamic instability caused by splenic lacerations should be managed with expeditious splenectomy. Similarly, hemorrhagic shock resulting from extensive renal lacerations or pedicle injuries should be managed by nephrectomy, especially if attempts at perinephric packing have failed. Ureteral injuries diagnosed during the damage control procedure should be ligated or drained with a percutaneous urostomy. Intraperitoneal bladder injuries should be rapidly oversewn with definitive management delayed until the second operation.

Given the volume of resuscitation after a damage control procedure, and the edema that results from reperfusion of previously ischemic tissue, formal closure of the abdomen is not an option. Forced closure of the abdomen is associated with a prohibitively high risk of subsequent abdominal compartment syndrome, adult respiratory distress syndrome (ARDS), and multisystem organ failure (MSOF). Multiple options exist for the temporary closure of the abdomen. The goals of temporary closure should be containment of the abdominal viscera, control of abdominal ascites, maintenance of tamponade on areas that have been packed, and optimization of later fascial closure.

Simple techniques involve closure of only the skin, with suture or towel clips. This technique will facilitate the tamponade of bleeding while coagulopathy, acidosis, and hypothermia are corrected. However, it does not expand abdominal volumes significantly and is often associated with development of secondary abdominal compartment syndrome. When this occurs, it can be managed in the ICU by simply reopening the skin. Techniques which expand the abdominal volume include coverage of the viscera with the Bogota bag, a 3-liter urologic bag that is stapled or sewn to the skin. The benefit of the Bogota bag over the vacuum-assisted techniques described below is that it allows visualization of the underlying viscera and assessment of viability, which may be important after the use of shunting or ligation for a major vascular injury.

Vacuum-assisted techniques for temporary abdominal closure have been well described. The vacuum-assisted wound coverage is constructed beginning with a nonadherent fenestrated drape placed over the viscera, followed by the application of a sterile surgical towel. Following placement of two closed suction drains, the wound is sealed with an adhesive plastic sheet applied to the skin. The benefits of this technique include maintenance of some tension on the abdominal wall fascia to minimize the risk of loss of domain and to facilitate subsequent delayed fascial closure at a later time. Commercial devices capable of similar functions are available. Another potential technique for temporary closure involves the use of Velcro, which is sutured to the fascia and sequentially tightened. In the acute setting, there is little role for prosthetic material for temporary closure of the abdomen. As there are no prospective trials comparing methods of temporary abdominal closure, the method used is at the discretion of the trauma surgeon and is often institution specific.

Damage Control Thoracotomy

Trauma patients with penetrating thoracic injuries who present in extremis should undergo emergency department (ED) thoracotomy. ED thoracotomy is rarely successful in patients with blunt trauma or with extrathoracic penetrating injury.

ED thoracotomy is classically performed through a left anterolateral thoracotomy at the level of the fifth intercostal space. This exposure permits rapid evacuation of the thoracic cavity as well as inspection of the pericardial sac to rule out tamponade. On entering the chest, any hemothorax is evacuated, and the pericardium inspected. If tamponade is present, a longitudinal pericardiotomy is performed from cephalad to caudad and avoiding the phrenic nerve. In the patient in extremis, the inferior pulmonary ligament is divided, allowing access to the posterior mediastinum, where aortic cross-clamping can be performed.

Cardiac lacerations may be temporarily controlled using a number of methods. Digital pressure over the hole is often quite effective, although the finger should not be inserted into the hole to avoid extending the laceration. A Foley catheter can be carefully passed through the injury into the ventricle and gentle traction applied after inflating the balloon to control hemorrhage. Finally, simple cardiac injuries can be repaired in the ED using a skin stapler to reapproximate the lacerated myocardium.

Exsanguination from pulmonary injuries may be controlled in several ways, including direct pressure, packing, hilar cross-clamping, or lung torsion at the hilar axis. Once in the operating room, penetrating pulmonary injuries are often amenable to a technique described by Asensio as stapled pulmonary tractotomy. A linear-cutting gastrointestinal stapler is placed within the injury tract and fired. With serial applications of the stapler, this will expose the base of the tract, permitting direct ligation of bleeding sites. Air leaks can be selectively oversewn. Patients undergoing tractotomy have a significantly lower mortality than patients undergoing formal resection.

Following damage control thoracotomy, it is not always possible to formally close the chest without prohibitive compromise of airway and ventilation mechanics. Temporary closure of the thoracic cavity can be accomplished should packing be necessary for control of medical bleeding. Following insertion of a chest tube, a skin-only closure may be fashioned to provide adequate tamponade. Routine closure of the incision can be accomplished in a delayed fashion at 48–72 hours (phase 3).

Damage Control Orthopedics

Damage control orthopedics is characterized by primary, rapid, temporary fracture stabilization. This concept applies particularly to femoral shaft fractures and pelvic fractures as these have an increased risk of adverse outcome. Both fractures are associated with significant soft tissue injury and blood loss. The impetus for the development of damage control orthopedics was the observation that patients with severe thoracic, abdominal, and head injuries had worse outcomes when subjected to extended operative procedures for fracture stabilization with ongoing evidence of hypothermia, coagulopathy, and acidosis.

The most common approach to fractures of the lower extremity is the application of an external fixator device to provide temporary fracture stabilization. External fixation is not a time-consuming procedure, and can safely be performed either in the operating room or ICU. The surgeon first obtains alignment of the extremity, and then places two pins above and two pins below the fracture site, avoiding neurovascular structures. The external fixator bars are then applied to the pins, spanning the fracture and providing stability. Although concerns have been raised over the increased risk for deep tissue infection caused by pin site sepsis, no significant increase in local infection has been reported.

Pelvic ring disruptions continue to be a significant source of both morbidity and mortality after trauma. Pelvic fractures account for 3%–8% of all skeletal fractures and most commonly result from high-energy trauma, with motor vehicle crashes being the predominant mechanism of injury. During the acute phase, the goal of treatment should be the control of hemorrhage. The retroperitoneum if intact can contain up to 4 liters of blood, and bleeding from the associated vascular injuries will continue until physiologic tamponade is obtained. However, if the retroperitoneal space is disrupted, pelvic fractures can lead to uncontrolled hemorrhage and increase the risk of exsanguination.

Decreasing the intrapelvic volume by restoring the normal pelvic anatomy remains the first step in the damage control management of the bleeding associated with pelvic fractures. This can be accomplished by multiple methods, including tying a bed sheet around the pelvis or using several commercially available pelvic slings and belts. External fixators and pelvic C clamps may also be used for this purpose and are ideal for "open-book" disruptions of the pelvic ring. The external fixator involves placement of two percutaneous pins per iliac crest. The pins are then connected with a frame that maintains reduction of the fracture and decreases pelvic volume. The C clamp consists of two pins applied on the posterior ilium in the region of the sacroiliac joints. The application of this device is relatively contraindicated in patients with fractures of the ilium and transiliac fracture dislocations.

If the patient remains hemodynamically labile after the application of an external stabilization device, ongoing bleeding from branches of the internal iliac arteries must be considered the source of hemorrhage. Arterial bleeding occurs in only 10% of patients with unstable pelvic fractures. In this patient population, pelvic arteriography with embolization of the bleeding vessel and collaterals is the optimal method of management. In situations where interventional radiology is not available, exploratory laparotomy with ligation of the ipsilateral internal iliac artery and pelvic packing is a viable alternative, although this procedure has a reported mortality rate of 25%.

PHASE 2: RESUSCITATION IN INTENSIVE CARE UNIT

After damage control procedures, patients are returned to the ICU for correction of their physiologic abnormalities, including hypothermia, acidosis, and coagulopathy. Aggressive correction of hypothermia is of paramount importance. External rewarming techniques include warming of the room and ventilator circuits, and application of a Bair Hugger. All fluids and blood products should be given through a Level I fluid rewarmer. In patients with severe hypothermia, defined as a temperature less than 32° C, consideration should be given to the use of continuous arteriovenous rewarming, as described by Gentilello et al. The technique involves the insertion of 8.5F femoral arterial and venous catheters, creating an AV fistula that then diverts a portion of the cardiac output through a heat exchanger, usually a Level 1 fluid warmer. The effectiveness of the technique is based on the patient's cardiac output, and is capable of raising a patient's core temperature approximately 4° C per hour. The patients who undergo continuous arteriovenous rewarming require less fluid during resuscitation and have significantly less early mortality than those warmed by conventional external methods.

Patients who are acidotic after damage control procedures are most likely under-resuscitated, and they require optimization of oxygen delivery for correction. Invasive monitoring, including central venous pressure monitoring or Swan-Ganz monitoring, may be necessary in the immediate postoperative period to guide resuscitative efforts. Persistent acidosis in a patient felt to be adequately resuscitated may be caused by a hypochloremic acidosis, which can follow aggressive resuscitation with normal saline. An anion gap can be used to differentiate lactic acidosis from hyperchloremic acidosis. Hyperchloremic acidosis results in a narrowed anion gap, while lactic acidosis results in a widened anion gap.

While correction of acidosis and hypothermia will aid in the correction of the coagulopathy seen after damage control procedures, these patients will require ongoing transfusion of fresh frozen plasma, cryoprecipitate, and platelets. All products should be delivered through a Level 1 fluid warmer to minimize the time to rewarming.

Recombinant human Factor VII has also been shown to be useful in this population, as it corrects coagulopathic defects rapidly.

PHASE 3: DEFINITIVE OPERATIVE MANAGEMENT

Following normalization of physiologic parameters, with particular attention to the correction of hypothermia, acidosis and coagulopathy, the patient should be returned to the operating room for definitive management of previously temporized injuries. The timing of reoperation has not been standardized, but most trauma surgeons will return to the operating room within 48–72 hours, as re-exploration prior to 72 hours is associated with decreased morbidity and mortality.

During re-exploration, a formal exploration is performed to identify any injuries that may have been missed. Previously placed packing is removed, and bleeding sites controlled. Intestinal continuity is re-established. Small bowel injures may be safely managed with primary repair or with anastomosis, while colon injuries may be primarily repaired, anastomosed, or exteriorized, depending on the extent of the injury and the surgeon's level of concern. Consideration should be given to delayed primary closure of the abdominal wall fascia, although this may not be feasible if significant edema persists. Most patients (80%) can have their fascia primarily closed within 5–7 days of injury. Those who cannot are candidates for split-thickness skin grafting of their open abdominal wound, with delayed closure of their planned ventral hernia at 6–12 months.

Following damage control thoracotomy, the patient may safely be returned to the operating room after correction of all physiologic derangements. Chest drainage (tube thoracostomy) and definitive thoracic closure are possible after removal of packing and control of bleeding or air leaks.

There are multiple data sets in the literature that suggest that the timing of definitive orthopedic stabilization should be delayed longer than 72 hours. It has been shown that days 2–4 after the initial damage control procedure are not optimal for definitive stabilization of orthopedic injuries, as this period is marked by ongoing systemic inflammatory response and generalized edema. A statistically significant increase in multisystem organ dysfunction has been reported in patients undergoing stabilization at 2–4 days compared with those patients whose fractures stabilized at 6–8 days.

COMPLICATIONS FOLLOWING DAMAGE CONTROL SURGERY

Immediate

The most common complication after damage control laparotomy is abdominal compartment syndrome (ACS). Despite liberal use of temporary abdominal closure methods, intra-abdominal hypertension may occur because of increased visceral swelling, ongoing bleeding, and the mechanical effects of intra-abdominal packing. Signs of ACS include a distended abdomen, increasing peak airway pressures, worsening acidosis, oliguria progressing to anuria, and decreased cardiac output with resultant systemic hypotension. The onset of ACS may be insidious or acute. Therefore, it is important to measure bladder pressures as a surrogate of intra-abdominal pressures. A pressure of greater than 25 mm Hg with evidence of physiologic compromise mandates abdominal decompression. Decompression should lead to immediate improvements in visceral perfusion, renal perfusion, cardiac function, and ventilatory mechanics.

Unplanned reoperation may be necessary in the patient with ongoing postoperative hemorrhage despite aggressive resuscitation and correction of the lethal triad. Indications for return to the operating room within the first 24 hours after a damage control procedure are listed in Table 3.

Table 3: Indications for Early Return to Operating Room

Continued bleeding and coagulopathy in face of normothermia (>6–10 units of packed red blood cells within 12 hours)
Abdominal compartment syndrome
Ischemic tissue causing metabolic derangement
Gastrointestinal soilage of the abdomen after failed repair, missed injury, or staple line disruption

Adapted with permission from Martin RR, Byrne M: Postoperative care and complications of damage control surgery. *Surg Clinics North Am* 77:929–942, 1997.

Delayed

Patients who undergo damage control procedures are at high risk of death or developing ARDS or MSOF. The presence of sepsis, transfusion requirements of greater than 15 units of packed red blood cells, pulmonary injury, and long bone fractures have been shown to be independent risk factors for post-traumatic ARDS. Shock, infections, multiple transfusions, and severe injury are all associated with late MSOF. Mortality following damage control surgery ranges from 20% to 67% depending on which series is read. When formal closure of the abdominal wound is not accomplished within the first week after injury, the presence of an open abdomen increases the risk of fistula formation. These patients will require re-establishment of abdominal wall continuity at the time of fistula takedown.

SUMMARY

Damage control procedures are life-saving in the critically injured patient with multiple injuries. Damage control allows life-threatening issues to be addressed expeditiously during truncated operative procedures. Normal physiology is then restored in the ICU. The ability to stage the definitive surgery allows correction of the lethal triad of hypothermia, coagulopathy, and acidosis, and has resulted in improved survival in patients who previously would have died of their injuries.

SUGGESTED READINGS

Asensio JA, Demetriades D, Berne JB, et al: Stapled pulmonary tractotomy: a rapid way to control hemorrhage in penetrating pulmonary injuries. *J Am Coll Surg* 185(5):486–487, 1997.

Asensio JA, McDuffie L, Petrone P, et al: Reliable variables in the exsanguinated patient which indicate damage control and predict outcome. *Am J Surg* 182:743–751, 2001.

Asensio JA, Petrone P, Roldan G: Has evolution in awareness of guidelines for institution of damage control improved outcome in the management of the post-traumatic open abdomen? *Arch Surg* 139:209–214, 2004.

Abikhaled JA, Granchi RS, Wall MJ, et al: Prolonged abdominal packing is associated with increased morbidity and mortality. *Am Surg* 63:1109–1113, 1997.

Barker DE, Kaufman HJ, Smith LA, et al: Vacuum pack technique of temporary abdominal closure: a 7-year experience with 112 patients. *J Trauma* 48:201–206, 2000.

Garner GB, Ware DN, Cocanour CS, et al: Vacuum-assisted wound closure provides early fascial reapproximation in trauma patients with open abdomens. *Am J Surg* 182:630–638, 2001.

Gentilello LM, Cobean RA, Offner PJ, et al: Continuous arteriovenous rewarming: rapid reversal of hypothermia in critically ill patients. *J Trauma* 32:316–327, 1992.

Gentilello LM, Jurkovich GJ, Stark MS, Hassantash SA, O'Keefe GE: Is hypothermia in the victim of major trauma protective or harmful? A randomized, prospective study. *Ann Surg* 226:439–449, 1997.

Giannoudis PV, Pape H-C: Damage control orthopaedics in unstable pelvic ring injuries. *Injury* 35:671–677, 2004.

Granchi T, Schmittling Z, Vasquez J, et al: Prolonged use of intraluminal arterial shunts without systemic anticoagulation. *Am J Surg* 180:493–497, 2000.

Gregory JS, Flancbaum L, Townsend MC, et al: Incidence and timing of hypothermia in trauma patients undergoing operations. *J Trauma* 31:795–800, 1991.

Jurkovich GJ, Greiser WB, Luterman A, et al: Hypothermia in trauma victims: an ominous predictor of survival. *J Trauma* 27:1019–1024, 1987.

Karmy-Jones R, Jurkovich GJ, Shatz DV, et al: Management of traumatic lung injury: a Western Trauma Association multi-center review. *J Trauma* 51:1049–1053, 2001.

Martin RR, Byrne M: Postoperative care and complications of damage control surgery. *Surg Clin North Am* 77:929–942, 1997.

Moore EE, Burch JM, Franciose RJ, et al: Staged physiologic restoration and damage control surgery. *World J Surg* 22:1184–1191, 1998.

Offner PJ, de Souza AL, Moore EE, et al: Avoidance of abdominal compartment syndrome in damage-control laparotomy after trauma. *Arch Surg* 136:676–681, 2001.

Pape H-C, Stalp M, Griensven M, Weiberg A, Dahlweit M, Tscherne H: Optimal timing for secondary surgery in polytrauma patients: an evaluation of 4314 serious-injury cases. *Chirurg* 70:1287–1293, 1999.

Raeburn CD, Moore EE, Biffl WL, et al: The abdominal compartment syndrome is a morbid complication of postinjury damage control surgery. *Am J Surg* 182:542–546, 2001.

Reed RL II, Bracey AW, Hudson JD, et al: Hypothermia and blood coagulation: dissociation between enzyme activity and clotting factor levels. *Circ Shock* 32:141–152, 1990.

Rotondo MF, Zonies DH: The damage control sequence and underlying logic. *Surg Clin North Am* 77:761–777, 1997.

Scalea TM, Boswell SA, Scott JD, Mitchell KA, Kramer ME, Pollak AN: External fixation as a bridge to intramedullary nailing for patients with multiple injuries and with femur fractures: damage control orthopedics. *J Trauma* 48:613–623, 2000.

Schreiber MA: Damage control surgery. *Crit Care Clin* 20:101–118, 2004.

Shapiro MB, Jenkins DH, Schwab CW, Rotondo MF: Damage control: collective review. *J Trauma* 49:969–978, 2000.

Wittmann DH, Aprahamian C, Gergstein JM: Etappenlavage: advanced diffuse peritonitis managed by planned multiple laparotomies using zippers, slide fastener and velcro analogue for temporary abdominal closure. *World J Surg* 14:218–226, 1990.

ABDOMINAL COMPARTMENT SYNDROME, DAMAGE CONTROL, AND THE POST-TRAUMATIC OPEN ABDOMEN

Richard S. Miller and **John A. Morris**

Major contributors to improved survival in the field of trauma and surgical critical care over the past decade include the early recognition and preventive strategies in the management of the abdominal compartment syndrome and the systematic, staged surgical approach to the trauma patient in extremis called damage control. However, in our efforts to cure one disease, we have created another: the post-traumatic open abdomen, defined as a large postoperative ventral hernia with the abdominal viscera covered by a temporary dressing or closure.

Many lessons have been learned in managing the complications associated with these critically ill patients and through these lessons, four essential principles in the management of the open abdomen have now evolved:

Protect the bowel.
Preserve the fascia and prevent its loss of domain.
Expedite early fascial closure primarily or with the use of biologic material.
Avoid committing the patient to a planned ventral hernia and delayed reconstruction unless absolutely necessary.

Before discussing these principles, both abdominal compartment syndrome and damage control deserve concomitant discussion regarding the initial management that then leads to the post-traumatic open abdomen.

ABDOMINAL COMPARTMENT SYNDROME

Generically, a compartment syndrome is a condition in which increased pressure in a confined space adversely effects the circulation and threatens the function and viability of the tissue within the space. This entity can occur in the extremities, orbital globe, intracranial cavity, and abdominal cavity.

The effects of increased intra-abdominal pressure were first described in 1863 by Marey and Burt, who reported the relationship between intrathoracic pressure and elevated intra-abdominal pressure. However, it was not until the 1980s that Kron and Richards coined the term "abdominal compartment syndrome" (ACS).[1,2] They reported a separate series of patients that developed a tense, distended abdomen with elevated pulmonary artery pressures and increased intra-abdominal pressures postoperatively despite normal mean arterial blood pressure and cardiac performance. All of these patients improved with re-exploration and abdominal decompression.

Intra-abdominal hypertension and the abdominal compartment syndrome are not synonymous. ACS is a late manifestation of uncontrolled intra-abdominal hypertension produced by ongoing ischemia and splanchnic hypoperfusion and the resuscitative measures to counteract the hemorrhagic shock state (Figure 1).

Table 1 lists the risk factors associated with ACS. Mortality from the fulminant abdominal compartment syndrome has been reported to be as high as 67%.

In addition to the accumulation of blood within the perineal cavity, other factors may contribute to occupying space within the abdominal cavity. This can occur by any shock-induced visceral ischemia and reperfusion edema including major injuries outside the abdominal cavity. Several recent reports have described this "secondary abdominal compartment syndrome," which occurs most frequently with major pelvic and long bone fractures, and hemorrhagic chest injuries. However, secondary ACS can occur in any setting associated with hemorrhagic shock.[3–5]

Balough and associates reviewed patients with major torso trauma and found that both primary and secondary abdominal compartment syndrome can be predicted early and are harbingers of multiorgan failure. Fourteen percent of these patients develop abdominal compartment syndrome, all of which require aggressive resuscitation using crystalloid, blood, and blood products early in their initial management in the emergency department. Therefore, the current emphasis in critical care management of the severely injured patients focuses on identification of predictive factors for the development of ACS and the recognition of intra-abdominal hypertension and treatment before full development of the syndrome.[7–12]

Intra-abdominal hypertension affects multiple organ systems in a graded fashion. The deleterious consequences appear gradually, and the adverse effects of elevated intra-abdominal pressure occur at lower levels than previously thought and manifest before the development of the fulminant syndrome (Table 2).

The classic picture of ACS includes a patient with a tense, distended abdomen and ventilatory insufficiency including hypoxia and hypercarbia, as well as increased peak inspiratory pressures. Progressive oliguria occurs despite adequate mean arterial pressure and cardiac output. This is followed by decreased cardiac performance and subsequent cardiovascular collapse unless treatment is instituted immediately (Table 3).

Figure 2 illustrates a high-risk patient for ACS: tense abdomen, respiratory failure, and progressive oliguria in a multitrauma patient requiring aggressive resuscitation for hemorrhagic shock.

Common computed tomography findings in this patient population include extraperitoneal hematoma and/or extravasation, intra- and retro-peritoneal edema, and "shock bowel" defined as an intense mucosal enhancement producing a prominent, feather-like appearance to the small intestines (Figure 3).

The most practical and reliable method of measuring intra-abdominal pressures is through the urinary bladder, which acts as a passive conduit. The urinary bladder transmits intra-abdominal pressures without imparting any additional pressures from its own musculature. Fifty to 100 ml of saline is injected into the fully drained bladder. A Foley catheter is clamped distal to the aspiration port and a 16-gauge needle is inserted into this port, which is then attached to a transducer system with the pubic symphysis used as the zero reference point. Commercial kits are available for measuring bladder pressures (AbVisor Intra-abdominal pressure monitor, Wolfe Tory Medical Inc., Salt Lake City, Utah).

The consensus at the World Congress on Abdominal Compartment Syndrome defines this disease entity as persistent bladder pressures over 20 mm of mercury with the new onset of organ failure. Figure 4 demonstrates the progression of organ dysfunction as intra-abdominal pressure increases over this level. Once defined, ACS mandates immediate decompressive celiotomy (Figure 5).

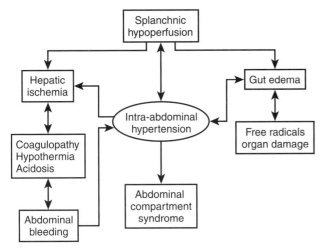

Figure 1 A cycle of ischemia producing intra-abdominal hypertension and the abdominal compartment syndrome. *(Reproduced with permission from Michael Rotondo, MD.)*

Table 1: Etiology of Abdominal Compartment Syndrome: Who Is at Risk?

Post-traumatic hemorrhage

Intraperitoneal bleeding

Retroperitoneal bleeding

Extraperitoneal bleeding

Any patient who requires vigorous fluid resuscitation from shock of any cause

Postresuscitative visceral edema

"Deadly triad"—hypothermia, acidosis, coagulopathy

Frequent prelude to abdominal compartment syndrome

This often rapidly reverses all the adverse affects of increased intra-abdominal pressure and dramatically improves oxygenation and pulmonary compliance, returning peak inspiratory pressures toward normal and promptly reversing the oliguria with a brisk diuresis of resuscitation fluids. Before decompression, all attempts to correct acid–base and electrolyte disturbances including potassium, magnesium, and calcium may avoid cardiac dysrhythmias after decompression. A respiratory therapist should also be immediately available to readjust ventilatory settings to prevent additional pulmonary barotrauma.

Decompression can be performed safely as a bedside procedure in the intensive care unit (ICU). However, with pressures greater the 35 mm Hg, decompression and re-exploration are required in the operating room to identify potential sources of ongoing hemorrhage.

DAMAGE CONTROL

An abbreviated celiotomy and intra-abdominal packing for hemorrhage control in the abdomen was first described by Stone[13] in 1983. However, the term "damage control" was first coined by Rotondo and Schwab at the University of Pennsylvania in 1993. The current management scheme has been revised to include four stages (Figure 6).[14–16]

During the initial trauma celiotomy (DC1), it is important to determine each patient's physiologic reserve in order to make appropriate operative decisions. Physiologic reserve is defined as an individual's unique ability to tolerate injury. It is a function of

Table 2: Effects of Intra-Abdominal Hypertension on Organ Systems

Head	↑ Intracranial pressure
	↓ Cerebral perfusion pressure
Heart	↓ CO
	↓ Venous return
	↑ Pulmonary artery occlusion pressure and central venous pressure
	↑ Systemic vascular resistance
Lungs	↑ Peak inspiratory pressure
	↑ Pulmonary artery wedge pressure
	↓ Dynamic compliance (Cdyn)
	↑ Arterial oxygen pressure (PaO$_2$)
	↑ Arterial carbon dioxide pressure (PaCO$_2$)
	↑ Intrapulmonary shunt (Qsp/Qt)
	↑ Fraction of dead space to total expired tidal volume (V$_D$/V$_T$)
Liver	↓ Portal flow
	↓ Mitochondria
	↑ Lactate
Kidney	↓ Urine output
	↓ Renal flow
	↓ Glomerular filtration rate (GFR)
Intestines	↓ Celiac flow
	↓ Superior mesenteric arterial (SMA) flow
	↓ Mucosal flow
Abdomen wall	↓ Compliance
	↓ Rectus flow

Table 3: Abdominal Compartment Syndrome: Classic Clinical Picture

Tense distended abdomen

Ventilator insufficiency

Hypoxia

Hypercarbia

Increased peak inspiratory pressure

Progressive oliguria despite adequate mean arterial pressure/carbon dioxide

↓ Cardiac performance

several host factors including age, gender, pre-existing disease, genetics, and immunocompetence (Figure 7). As physiologic reserve becomes depleted during hemorrhagic shock, regional and then global malperfusion occur, leading to physiologic exhaustion and subsequent death (Figure 8).[11]

Mortality associated with damage control procedures ranges between 25%–60%. Each patient responds and reacts differently to stress and injury, and each individual has a limited amount of compensatory reserve until physiologic exhaustion is reached.

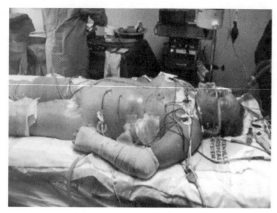

Figure 2   High-risk patient for abdominal compartment syndrome.

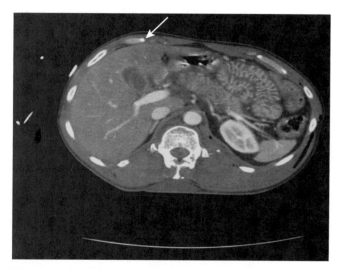

Figure 3   Shock bowel.

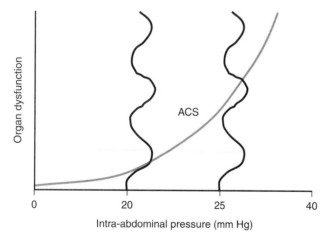

Figure 4   Progressive organ dysfunction with increasing intra-abdominal hypertension.

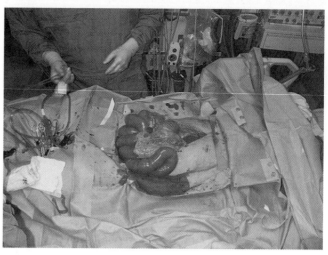

Figure 5   Bedside decompressive celiotomy for abdominal compartment syndrome (note massive small bowel edema).

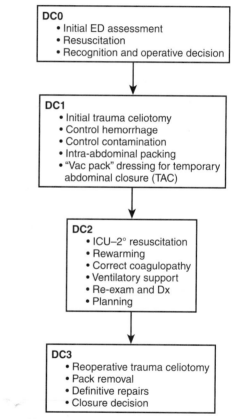

Figure 6   Algorithm for damage control.

Additionally, the extent of injury severity determines the slope leading to physiologic exhaustion (Figure 9).

Perioperative communication with the anesthesia team enhances survival and reduces complications. This communication includes maintaining the operating room as warm as possible, advising the anesthesia personnel of anticipated blood loss, and avoiding over resuscitation before surgical control of hemorrhage.

During the initial trauma celiotomy, the surgeon must recognize the need for immediate control of major hemorrhage and contamination with maximum replacement of coagulation factors including platelets, fresh frozen plasma, and cryoprecipitate, and in certain circumstances, factor VIIa for microvascular bleeding. Intraoperative monitoring of temperature, arterial blood gases, and volume of resuscitative fluids are important in determining whether a patient is descending down the physiologic curve toward physiologic exhaustion. In addition, for patients suffering hollow viscus injuries, contamination is controlled with linear staples to transect the bowel

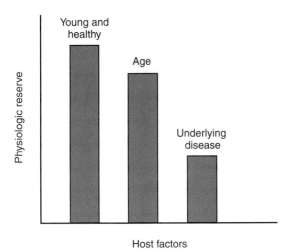

Figure 7   Host factors define physiologic reserve.

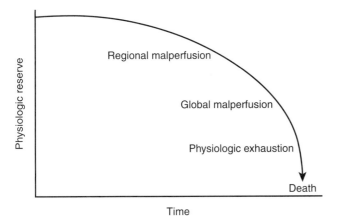

Figure 8   Depletion of physiologic reserve.

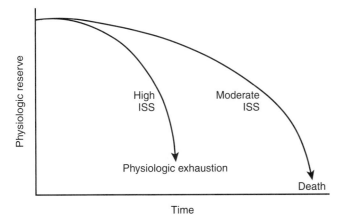

Figure 9   Physiologic reserve as related to Injury Severity Score (ISS).

ends and leave them in discontinuity until a later stage of damage control management.

Table 4 lists clinical parameters that should prompt the surgical team to initiate damage control maneuvers, abort the operation, and return to the ICU for resuscitation and restoration of reserve. Asensio[17,18] recommends instituting damage control early, well before reaching the upper limits of physiologic exhaustion, and describes statistically validated criteria. Using these statistically validated intraopera-

Table 4: Clinical Guidelines to Abort Initial Trauma Celiotomy and Initiate Damage Control Maneuvers

Hypothermia	<35° C
Acidosis	pH <7.2 Base deficit (BD) ≥−8 Lactate ≥4
Coagulopathy	Activated partial thromboplastic time (aPTT) >60 International normalized ratio (NR) >1.6
Ongoing resuscitation	Persistent shock systolic blood pressure <90 >10 liters crystalloid >10 units packed red blood cells
Operative time	>60–90 minutes with abdominal cavity opened

tive predictors of instituting damage control, patients with post-traumatic open abdomen incurred less hypothermia and fewer postoperative complications including intra-abdominal abscess and fistula formation. Patients with early damage control were also subjectively noted to have less bowel edema and were able to undergo definitive abdominal wall closure during their initial hospital stay.

Once a patient fulfills the requirements for DC or is decompressed for signs and symptoms of ACS, the surgeon must commit the patient to the post-traumatic open abdomen and a temporary abdominal closure.

Temporary Abdominal Closure

A TAC is defined as any technique that contains the abdominal viscera during the acute phase of care. Indications for creating a TAC are listed in Table 5.

Historically, a wide variety of techniques for TAC have been used to contain the abdominal viscera during the acute phase of care. However, the "vacuum pack" technique using the method described by Barker et al.[19] best fulfills the first two principles in the management of the post-traumatic open abdomen: protecting the bowel and preserving the fascia.

The bowel and abdominal viscera are protected by placing a perforated, nonadherent material such as a Steri-Drape (isolation bag 50 × 50 cm or 1010 large bowel bag 45 × 60 cm, 3M Health Care,

Table 5: Indications for Temporary Abdominal Closure

Depletion of physiologic reserve
Unable to close fascia without undue tension secondary to bowel edema
Avoid development of abdominal compartment syndrome after large fluid resuscitation
Planned return to operating room
Unpacking
Re-establish bowel continuity
Enteral access
Thorough exploration to re-evaluate known injuries and identify missed injuries
Associated need for management of extra-abdominal life-threatening injuries (e.g., major pelvic fracture, severe closed head injury)

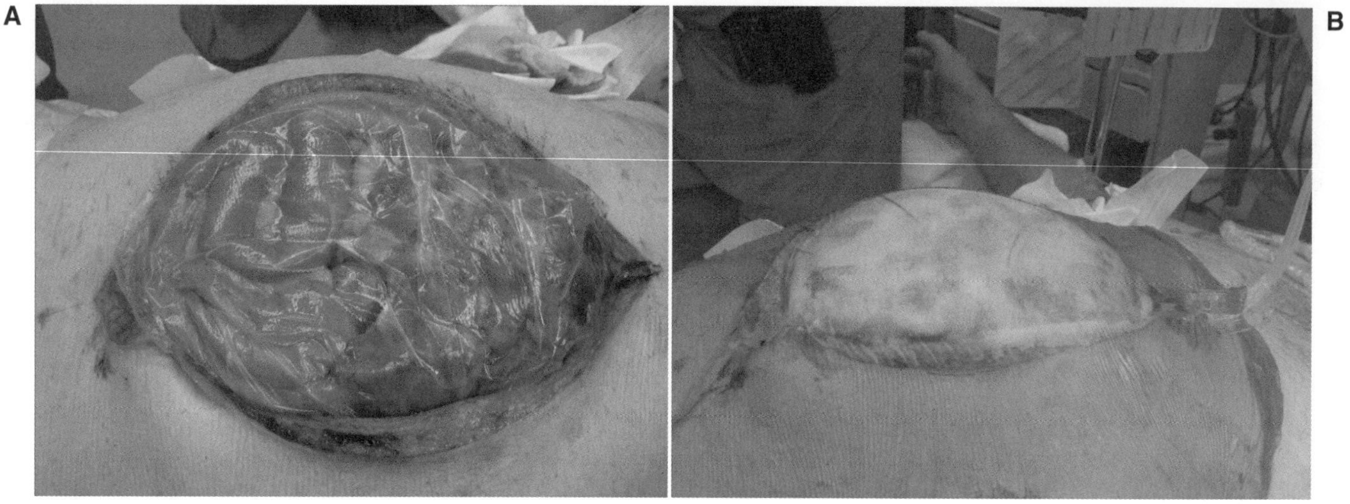

A   B

Figure 10   Vacuum pack temporary abdominal closure: **(A)** bowel bag, **(B)** sterile surgical towel/two large sump drains/large adhesive drape.

St. Paul, MN) over the intestines. This is followed by subfascial placement of a moist surgical towel with two large sump drains (Jackson-Pratt, Baxter Health Care Corp., Deerfield, IL) that are brought out through the superior portion of the wound. The entire abdominal defect is then covered with a large adhesive drape (Ioban, 3M Health Care, St. Paul, MN). The sump drains are attached to wall suction to create continuous negative pressure. This technique also counteracts the lateral retraction of the fascial edges and preserves the rectus musculofascial complex for subsequent closure (Figure 10).

Table 6: Advantages of Vacuum Pack Technique

Protects bowel and keeps it below fascia

Preserves fascia and prevents loss of domain

Readily available, rapidly applied, easily removed

Keeps patient dry and maintains sterility

Quantitates/qualitates fluid losses

Prevents intra-abdominal hypertension/abdominal compartment
  syndrome

Simple, atraumatic, and inexpensive

Advantages of the Vacuum Pack are listed in Table 6. Using this technique, the period before definitive fascia closure can be safely extended for up to a week after the initial celiotomy.[20]

Three potential stages (Figure 11) follow the placement of the vacuum pack for the post-traumatic open abdomen:

1. Resuscitation in the ICU (24 hours)
2. Restoration, or reoperation and attempts at early fascial closure (days to weeks)
3. Reconstruction, or planned ventral hernia and delayed fascia closure (6–12 months)

Resuscitation

The goals of the secondary resuscitation in the ICU after damage control or decompressive celiotomy for ACS are repayment of the oxygen debt sustained, restoration of adequate perfusion to meet metabolic needs, and reversal of hemorrhagic shock. This includes correction of the coagulopathy, clearing of the arterial lactic acidosis, correcting electrolyte disturbances, and rewarming the patient. A checklist of essential items necessary to perform this secondary resuscitation is listed in Table 7.

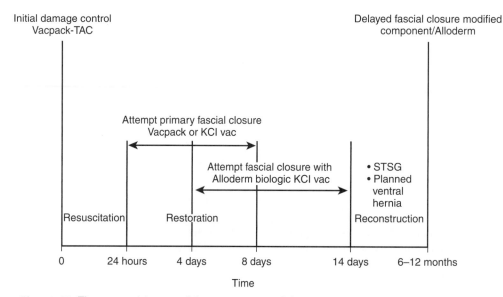

Figure 11   Three potential stages of the post-traumatic abdomen.

Table 7: Secondary Intensive Care Unit Resuscitation Checklist

Rewarming/Correct Hypothermia

Cordis introducer central line

Rapid infuser (Level I) with heat exchanger set at 40° C

  Infuse warm IV fluids, blood, blood products

Humidifier on vent set at 40° C

Convection air warmer (Bair Hugger)

  Placed over entire torso

Cover hands, feet, head

  Prevent insensible heat loss

Keep ambient temperature >85° F

Correct Coagulopathy, Acidosis, Electrolyte Imbalance

Measure hemoglobin and hematocrit, prothrombin time, partial prothrombin time, international normalized ratio (INR), platelet count, fibrinogen

  Replace with packed red blood cells, fresh frozen plasma, platelets, cryoprecipitate, ± FVIIa

Normalize arterial lactate, base deficit, correct K+, Mg+, Ca+ deficiency

Monitoring

Insert oximetric pulmonary artery catheter to maintain oxygen delivery and obtain endpoints of resuscitation.

  DO_2I (oxygen delivery index) 500 ml/minute

  Cardiac index (CI) >3 l/min

  End-diastolic volume index (EDVI) 120–140 ml

  Arterial oxygen saturation (SaO_2) >95%

  Venous oxygen saturation (SVO_2) >65%

  Temperature >36.5° C

  Hematocrit >21%

Check for adrenal insufficiency if not responding to resuscitation

  Random cortisol level

  Adrenocorticotropic hormone (ACTH) stimulation test

Medications

Peptic ulcer prophylaxis

  H_2 blockers or proton pump inhibitor

Deep venous thrombosis (DVT) prophylaxis

  Low molecular weight heparin   Sequential compression
                                                   devices or foot pumps

Insulin drip

  Maintain blood glucose 80–110 mg/dl

IV analgesia and sedation

  Continuous drips

Broad-spectrum antibiotics × 24 hours or until intra-abdominal packs out

  Cover Gram-negatives and anaerobes

Nursing

Elevate head of bed (HOB) 30 degrees

  Once TLS spine cleared

Frequent tracheal suctioning and oral hygiene

Functioning nasogastric tube

Wall suction for vacuum-pack sump drains

Foley catheter

  Check hourly urine output

  Check bladder pressures

Pad pressure points to reduce incidence decubiti

  Occiput, chin, scapulae, sacrum, heels

Additional resuscitative measures during ICU management also include the use of arteriography and embolization, especially for severe pelvic arterial hemorrhage and extensive hepatic vascular injuries. Complex lower extremity and pelvic fractures can also be temporarily realigned with the use of external fixators, deferring complex orthopedic reconstructive work until later stages in the patients' hospital course when the inflammatory response has dissipated.

Restoration

After the secondary resuscitation in the ICU and correction of physiologic and hemodynamic derangements that occurred during the initial trauma celiotomy or after decompression for ACS, patients with a temporary abdominal closure are returned to the operating room for further evaluation. During this re-exploration, the surgeon must once again make important clinical and technical decisions. All retained perihepatic and intra-abdominal lap pads are carefully removed, preventing dislodgment of clot over liver injuries and avoiding serosal tears from lap pads that are adherent to the bowel. Then a reevaluation of the known injuries and a thorough exploration to identify missed injuries are undertaken. If bowel resection was necessary during the initial damage control celiotomy, establishment of gastrointestinal (GI) continuity is performed and enteral access is established.

It is important to bury suture or staple lines deep within the abdomen and attempt to cover the anastomotic area with omentum. If creation of an ostomy is necessary, the stoma should be placed lateral to the rectus fascia to aid in future plans for colostomy takedown and abdominal wall reconstruction.

Nasoenteric feeding tubes or surgical placed enteral access procedures should be performed during the damage control reoperation stage. Either a nasoenteric feeding tube placed past the ligament of Treitz with nasogastric decompression or an open gastrojejunostomy feeding tube are options for long-term enteral access and supplemental nutrition.

Finally, extensive washout and evacuation of any further hematoma is performed and then a plan on definitive closure is made. If bowel edema is minimal or completely resolved and the fascial edges can be easily approximated without undue tension, then a primary fascial closure can be performed. Radiologic evaluation of the abdominal cavity on all patients must be obtained if the fascia is successfully closed at this stage to ensure that no retained foreign body remains.

If primary fascial closure is not possible because of ongoing physiologic insults or a prolonged inflammatory response with bowel edema and/or contamination, replacement of another vacuum pack is indicated. A good rule of thumb is that if the peak inspiratory pressures rise higher than 10 mm Hg from baseline during fascial approximation, attempts at primary fascial closure should be abandoned, as this can result in abdominal wall necrosis, recurrent abdominal compartment syndrome, serious infectious complications, and even death.

The complication rate associated with the post-traumatic open abdomen is between 25%–50%. The most common complications are listed in Table 8.

Figure 12 describes a recent study on complications after 344 post-traumatic open abdomen patients with TAC. The authors, Miller and colleagues,[21] reported a 65% success rate on early primary fascial closure. The remaining patients underwent delayed closures by either applying a split thickness skin graft (temporizing skin) to a granulating abdominal wound or using synthetic prosthetic mesh material (prosthetic fascial).

Primary fascial closure within the first week after the initial celiotomy was associated with a very low complication rate (9%). However, the complication rate increased significantly with three circumstances:

Attempts at closing the fascia primarily under too much tension
Awaiting the formation of granulation tissue before applying a STSG (8 days or more)
Using nonbiologic prosthetic material for closure

Table 8: Complications Associated with Post-Traumatic Open Abdomen

Abdominal	Extra-Abdominal
Wound infection	Ventilator-associated pneumonia
Wound dehiscence	Aspiration pneumonitis
Abdominal wall fasciitis/necrosis	Bloodstream infection
Intra-abdominal abscess/sepsis	Urinary tract infection
Enteroatmospheric fistula	Deep venous thrombosis/pulmonary embolism
	Pressure ulcers (occiput, scapulae, sacrum, heels)
	Multiple organ dysfunction syndrome/multiple organ system failure

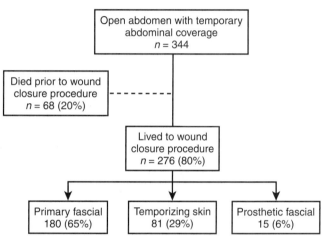

Figure 12 Outcome of 344 open abdomen patients with a temporary abdominal closure.

Figure 13 compares wound complications versus days to fascial closure. All three circumstances can potentially result in fistula formation, an expensive, labor-intensive, and morbid complication associated with the post-traumatic open abdomen. This occurred in 32 of 276 (8.6%) patients in this study (Figure 14).

In reviewing the literature, the incidence of fistula formation in this patient population is between 2%–25%. The etiology of fistulae formation is multifactorial and includes the presence of abdominal infection, bowel ischemia and/or obstruction, exposure of the bowel to atmospheric air for prolonged periods of time (causing desiccation), and the use of packs, dressings, or prosthetic materials that adhere to the serosa of the intestines.[22,23]

An enteroatmospheric fistula is defined as a postoperative complication with the open abdomen in which an enterotomy in the GI tract leaks succus or frank stool into the open wound. The absence of overlying soft tissue precludes closure (Figure 15).

Protecting the exposed abdominal viscera from injury and desiccation using the vacuum pack, limiting access to the wound to one or two senior surgeons, and early tension-free closure of the fascia are all good preventive measures. However, once a fistula forms, the adjacent viscera must be protected, and the effluent from the fistula controlled. Intubation of the fistula in the

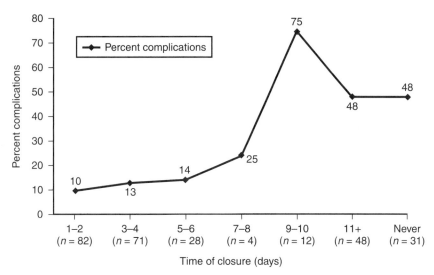

Figure 13 Percent of patients with wound complications versus days to fascial closure.

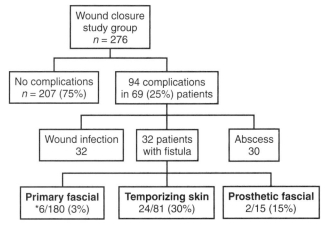

Figure 14 Wound closure complications associated with the post-traumatic open abdomen. *p=0.0001 when comparing fistula formation between primary and temporizing groups. *(From Miller et al[21].)*

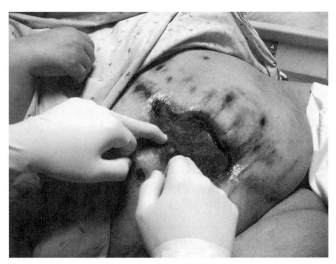

Figure 15 Enteroatmospheric fistula.

middle of the fixed visceral block is not recommended, and in this circumstance, repair of the fistula should not be performed until the patient is infection-free and in a stable physiologic state and has replenished protein and calorie stores. This usually occurs several months later. At that time the fistula can be resected in conjunction with delayed abdominal wall reconstruction.

Because all post-traumatic open abdomens are either colonized or chronically infected, it is now realized that use of synthetic prosthetic material is contraindicated. If the abdomen cannot be closed by the end of the first week, granulation tissue starts to develop, and a "frozen abdomen" is evident by the end of the second week. This creates a hostile environment for early fascial closure and thus necessitates a planned ventral hernia with a delayed reconstruction. A split-thickness skin graft (STSG) is applied over the granulation bed and the patient then requires a 6–12 month recovery period for protein and calorie stores to be replenished before successful abdominal wall reconstruction can be performed (Figure 16). This decision, although life-saving, is very costly and is associated with a loss of productive lifestyle and an inability to return to the workforce.

New solution

Because of the high complication rate under these circumstances, an aggressive approach to early fascial closure in the post-traumatic open abdomen is suggested, using a combination of the vacuum pack, vacuum-assisted closure technique (KCI VAC, KCI USA, Inc., San Antonio, TX), and a biologic material, human acellular tissue matrix (Alloderm, LifeCell Corp., Branchburg, NJ) to bridge the gap in the abdominal fascia.

Similar to the vacuum pack, the KCI VAC technique places a perforated, nonadherent plastic drape beneath the anterior abdominal wall to protect the bowel. However, the surgical towel in the middle layer is replaced with a polyurethane sponge cut to size to fit the facial defect. An 18 French suction tube is inserted into the sponge, which is then covered with an adherent occlusive drape, and constant application of negative pressure is obtained with wall suction (Figure 17).

This technique also protects the bowel and preserves the fascia and recaptures loss of abdominal domain. Additional advantages are listed in Table 9.

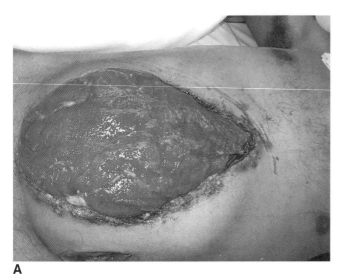

A

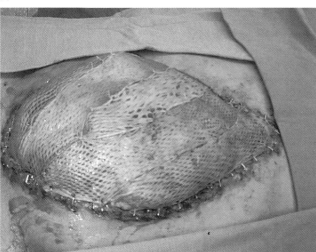

B

Figure 16 Mature granulation tissue in an open abdomen, which is then covered with a split-thickness skin graft.

Table 9: Additional Advantages of KCI VAC

Reduced need for frequent dressing changes
Removes excess interstitial fluid
Increases vascularity of wound
Decreased bacterial counts
Improves wound contraction
Delays onset of "frozen abdomen"—prevents granulation tissue adhering to fascia
Extends window of opportunity for definitive fascial closure

The KCI VAC allows for successful primary fascial closure or closure with the use of Alloderm in most post-traumatic open abdomen patients, even up to 3 weeks after initial damage control procedures or decompressive celiotomy.

Alloderm is a biologic material derived from partial thickness skin of tissue donors treated for removal of all cellular components so that only the native connective tissue matrix remains. Unlike synthetic prosthetic materials, which the body recognizes as foreign, causing encapsulation, Alloderm supports cellular growth and integration with rapid revascularization and transition to the patient's own tissue. This material serves as a bio-scaffold for the native autologous tissue (Figure 18).

Alloderm is also tolerant of contamination and can be used for closure in situations where synthetic material is contraindicated (Figure 19). It is best to underlay the Alloderm 4–5 cm lateral to the fascial edges using interrupted 0-prolene sutures and place this biologic material under moderate stretch to prevent future laxity of the abdominal wall.

Even though long-term results regarding recurrence rates and the development of abdominal wall laxity are not yet available, this method of fascial approximation certainly has significant advantages over the planned ventral hernia method of management with its inherent high risk of wound complications as mentioned previously.[24–30] The combination of using the KCI VAC and placement of Alloderm fulfills the final essential principle with post-traumatic open abdomen: expedite early fascial closure.

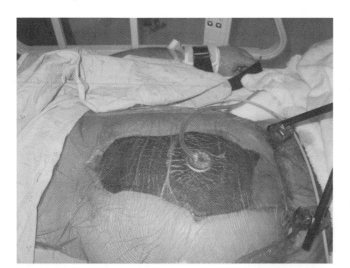

Figure 17 Vacuum-assisted closure—KCI VAC. Note external fixator for damage control orthopedics.

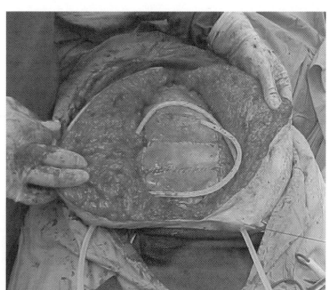

Figure 18 Alloderm with overlying skin flaps for early closure of abdominal fascia.

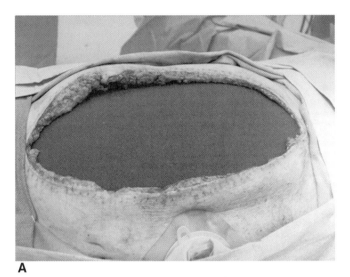

A

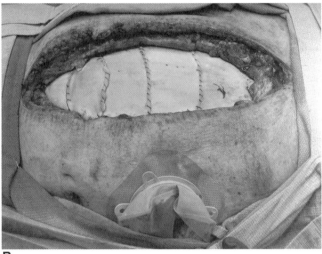

B

Figure 19   Alloderm used to bridge fascial gap in contaminated open abdomen wound with KCI VAC placed over the biologic fascial replacement.

Nutritional support for post-traumatic open abdomen

Ironically, after DC surgery, a large abdominal wound defect is created during the period of greatest physiologic stress with ongoing metabolic demands and catabolism. This can cause a tremendous barrier to primary fascial closure, wound healing, and overall rehabilitation. Therefore, close attention to nutritional support and caloric needs is essential to reduce both early and late complications.

During hemorrhagic shock and multitrauma, gut mucosal blood flow is decreased and remains below normal levels despite volume resuscitation. This decreased blood flow is associated with microbe translocation, ischemic bowel, and eventual multiorgan failure.

Basic science research has shown that enteral nutrition augments gut blood flow by locally mediated vasodilation. This enhances absorption of nutrients and preserves gut mucosal integrity and immunologic barrier functions. Additional research has studied the effects of enteral feeding during hemorrhagic shock, showing improved survival with no detrimental gut effects. The reduction in mesenteric blood flow caused by vasopressors is also inhibited and counteracted by the infusion of enteral nutrition. Thus, the gut is the preferred route for nutritional support during critical illness, and the initiation

of enteral nutrition within 36 hours of admission or surgery in critically ill patients results in fewer infections and reduced length of stay.

Nutritional support in the open abdomen should be initiated during the restoration phase, after intra-abdominal packing is removed, GI intestinal continuity re-established, and coagulopathy, acidosis, and hypothermia are corrected.

Immune-enhancing diets increase splanchnic blood flow to a greater degree than standard enteral diets. Head-injured and non-septic critically ill patients have been found to benefit from the use of immune enhancing diets. However, septic patients have a worse outcome with this diet and should be kept on standard formulas.

Although enteral feedings are the preferred route, it is not always possible in severely injured trauma patients with an open abdomen resulting from a prolonged inflammatory response with ongoing bowel wall edema, abdominal distention, high gastric output, and persistent adynamic ileus. In this circumstance, early enteral nutrition should be supplemented with parental nutrition to reach acceptable protein and calorie goals. In addition, enteral nutrition can continue safely during other extra-abdominal operations and procedures.[31,32]

Tsuei and colleagues[33] studied nasoenteric feeding in patients with an open abdomen and found it a safe effective method of nutritional support capable of meeting the nutritional goals in most patients. However, there have been no clinical studies to determine the exact percentage of caloric goals required to achieve maintenance of gut integrity and prevent bacterial translocation during the open abdomen. In animal models, over 50% of goal calories were needed to effectively reduce translocation and maintain adequate gut permeability.

Planned Ventral Hernia and Delayed Abdominal Wall Reconstruction

Once the window of opportunity for early fascial closure has passed secondary to an ongoing inflammatory response and bowel edema, a delayed staged closure of the abdominal wall is necessary. Because the open abdomen group remains at high risk for infectious complications, the use of synthetic prosthetic material for reconstruction is also not recommended.

Once the split thickness skin graft can be elevated from the underlying intestines (pinch sign–Figure 20), the inflammatory response has resolved and the underlying granulation tissue dissipated.

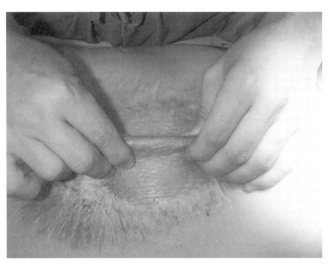

Figure 20   Pinch sign.

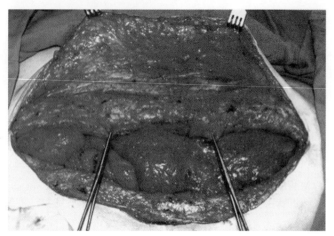

Figure 21 Fascial edges freed from surrounding tissue and skin flaps raised past edge of lateral rectus muscle.

This usually requires 6–12 months of recovery. Only then can reconstruction be performed safely.

The split thickness skin graft is removed and the fascia is mobilized from the surrounding tissue. The skin and subcutaneous tissue are then raised as lateral flaps circumferentially (Figure 21). Options for bridging the fascial gap at this point include the component separation technique and/or closure with Alloderm.

The component separation technique reconstructs the fascial defect with advancement flaps by transecting the external oblique just lateral to its insertion into the rectus sheath and separating it from the internal oblique. The rectus muscle can then be advanced medially and sutured in the midline to close the defect (Figure 22).[34]

This technique can approximate a 10-cm defect without undo tension. Using the modified component separation technique,[35,36] several more centimeters of mobility can be obtained by separating the rectus muscle from the posterior rectus sheath.

The recurrence rate with this method alone is 22%–32%.[37,38] Therefore, complementing or replacing this procedure with the use of Alloderm to bridge the fascial gap is an option.[39]

CONCLUSION

Damage control techniques and preventive measures to avoid the development of ACS are now the standards of care in the management of traumatic shock (Figure 23). Using a vacuum pack for temporary abdominal closure during the early stages of resuscitation protects the bowel and preserves the fascia.

Complications can then be avoided by not attempting to close the fascia under great tension and maintaining abdominal domain during the recovery phase with the use of the KCI VAC. Multiple attempts at fascial closure can then be safely performed either primarily or with the use of biologic material to bridge the fascial gap during initial hospitalization.

It is no longer acceptable to commit the post-trauma open abdomen patient to a large ventral hernia and delayed reconstruction except for unusual circumstances where a prolonged inflammatory response precludes early fascial approximation.

A

COMPONENT SEPARATION CLOSURE

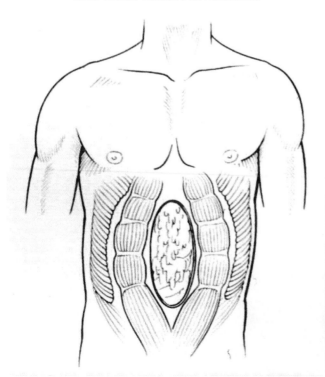

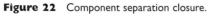

B

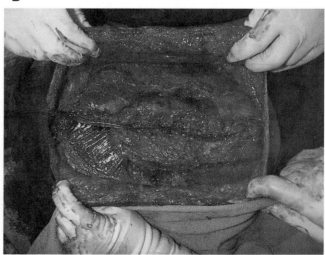

Figure 22 Component separation closure.

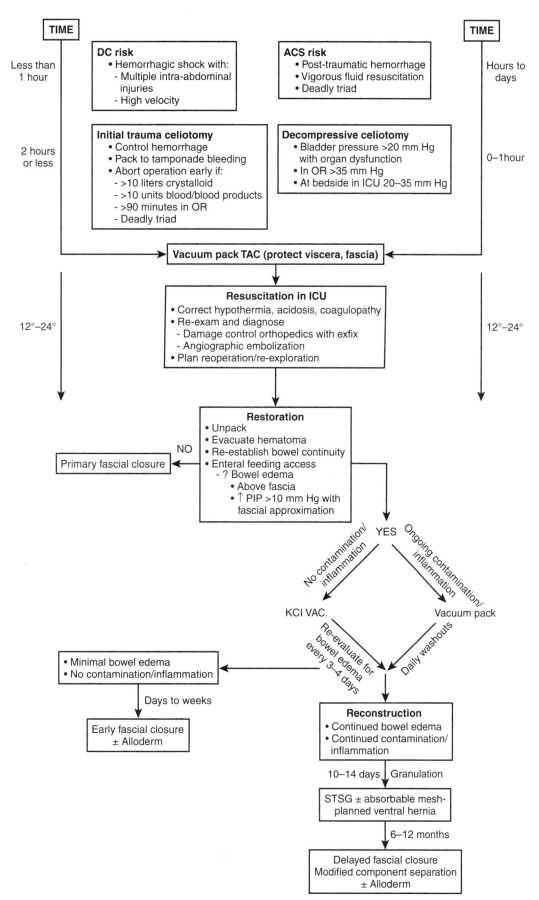

Figure 23 Algorithm for damage control and open abdomen management.

REFERENCES

1. Kron L, Harman PK, Nolan SP: The measurement of intra-abdominal pressure as a criterion for abdominal re-exploration. *Ann Surg* 199:28–30, 1984.
2. Richards WO, Scovill W, Shin B, Reed W: Acute renal failure associated with increased intra-abdominal pressure. *Ann Surg* 197:183–187, 1983.
3. Kopelman T, Harris C, Miller RS, Arrillaga A: Abdominal compartment syndrome in patients with isolated extraperitoneal injuries. *J Trauma* 49:744–749, 2000.
4. Biffl WL, Moore EE, Burch JM, et al: Secondary abdominal compartment syndrome is a highly lethal event. *Am J Surg* 182:645–648, 2001
5. Balough Z, McKinly BA, Cocanour CS, et al: Secondary abdominal compartment syndrome: an elusive complication of traumatic shock resuscitation. *Am J Surg* 184:538–544, 2002.
6. Balough Z, McKinley BA, Holcomb JB, Miller CC, Cocanour CS, Kozar RA: Both primary and secondary abdominal compartment syndrome can be predicted early and are harbingers of multiple organ failure. *J Trauma* 54:848–861, 2003.
7. Ertel W, Oberholzer A, Platz A, Stocker R, Trentz O: Incidence and clinical pattern of the abdominal compartment syndrome after "damage control" laparotomy in 311 patients with severe abdominal and/or pelvic trauma. *Crit Care Med* 28:1747–1753, 2000.
8. Saggi BH, Sugerman HJ, Ivatury RR, Bloomfield GL: Abdominal compartment syndrome. *J Trauma* 45:597–609, 1998.
9. McNelis J, Marini CP, Jurkiewicz A, Fields S, Caplin D, Stein D: Predictive factors associated with the development of abdominal compartment syndrome in the surgical intensive care unit. *Arch Surg* 137:133–136, 2002.
10. Morris JA Jr, Eddy VA, Blinman TA, Rutherford EJ, Sharp KWVA: The staged celiotomy for trauma issues in unpacking and reconstruction. *Ann Surg* 217:576–586, 1993.
11. Eddy VA, Nunn C, Morris JA Jr: Abdominal compartment syndrome: the Nashville experience. *Surg Clin North Am* 77:801–881, 1997.
12. Cheatham ML, Safcsak K, Block EFJ, Nelson LD: Predictors of mortality in patients with open abdomens. *Crit Care Med* 27(1 Suppl):170A, 1999.
13. Stone HH, Strom PR, Strom RJ, Mullins RJ: Management of the major coagulopathy with onset during laparotomy. *Ann Surg* 197:532–535, 1983.
14. Rotondo MF, Zonies DH: Damage control sequence and the underlying logic. *Surg Clin North Am* 77:761–777, 1997.
15. Shapiro MB, Jenkins DH, Schwab W, Rotondo MF: Damage control collective review. *J Trauma* 49:969–978, 2000.
16. Rotondo MF, Schwab CW, McGonigal MD, et al: "Damage control": an approach for improved survival in exsanguinating penetrating abdominal injury. *J Trauma* 35:375–382, 2003.
17. Asensio JA, McDuffie L, Petrone P, et al: Reliable variables in the exsanguinated patient which indicate damage control and predict outcome. *Am J Surg*. 182:743–751, 2001.
18. Asensio JA, Petrone P, Roldan G, et al: Has evolution in awareness of guidelines of institution of damage control improved outcome in the management of the posttraumatic open abdomen? *Arch Surg* 139:209–214, 2004.
19. Barker DE, Kaufman HJ, Smith LA, Ciraulo DL, Richart CL, Burns RP: Vacuum pack technique of temporary abdominal closure a 7-year experience with 112 patients. *J Trauma* 48:201–207, 2000.
20. Miller PR, Thompson JT, Faler BJ, Meredith JW, Chang MC: Late fascial closure in lieu of ventral hernia the next step in open abdomen management. *J Trauma* 53:843–849, 2002.
21. Miller RS, Morris JA Jr, Diaz JJ, et al: Complications after 344 damage-control open celiotomies. *J Trauma* 59:1365–1371, 2005.
22. Mayberry JC, Burgess EA, Goldman RK, et al: Enterocutaneous fistula and ventral hernia after absorbable mesh prosthesis closure for trauma: the plain truth. *J Trauma* 57:157–163, 2004.
23. Buechter KH, Leonvicz D, Hastings PR, Fonts C: Enterocutaneous fistulas following laparotomy for trauma. *Am Surg* 57:354–358, 1991.
24. Guy JS, Miller RS, Morris JA, Diaz J, May A: Early one-stage closure in patients with abdominal compartment syndrome: fascial replacement with human acellular dermis and bipedicle flaps. *Am Surg* 69:1025–1029, 2003.
25. Scott BG, Feanny MA, Hirshberg A: Early definitive closure of the open abdomen: a quiet revolution. *Scand J Surg* 94:9–14, 2005.
26. Holton LH III, Kim D, Silverman RP, Rodriguez ED, Singh N, Goldberg NH: Human acellular dermal matrix for repair of abdominal wall defects: review of clinical experience and experimental data. *J Long-Term Effects Med Implants* 15:547–558, 2005.
27. Kolker AR, Brown DJ, Redstone JS, Scarpinato VM, Wallack MK: Multi-layer reconstruction of abdominal wall defects with acellular dermal allograft (alloderm) and component separation. *Ann Plast Surg* 55:36–42, 2005.
28. Diaz JJ Jr, Guy J, Berkes MB, Guillamondegui O, Miller RS: Acellular dermal allograft for ventral hernia repair in the compromised surgical field. *Am Surg* 72(12):1181–1187, 2006.
29. Kim H, Bruen K, Vargo D: Acellular dermal matrix in the management of high-risk abdominal wall defects. *Am J Surg* 192(6):705–709, 2006.
30. Patton JH Jr, Berry S, Kralovich KA: Use of human acellular dermal matrix in complex and contaminated abdominal wall reconstructions. *Am J Surg* 193(3):360–363, 2007.
31. Cothren CC, Moore EE, Ciesla DJ, Johnson JL, Moore JB, Haenel JB, Burch JM: Postinjury abdominal compartment syndrome does not preclude early enteral feeding after definitive closure. *Am Surg* 188:653–658, 2004.
32. Blackburn GL, Jensen GL, Martindale RC: Nutrition support for the patient with an open abdomen after major abdominal trauma. *Nutrition* 19:563–566, 2003.
33. Tsuei BJ, Magnuson B, Swintosky M, Flynn J, Boulanger BR, Ochoa JB, Kearney PA: Enteral nutrition in patients with an open peritoneal cavity. *Nutr Clin Pract* 3:253–258, 2003.
34. Ramirez OM, Ruas E, Dellon AL: "Components separation" method for closure of abdominal-wall defects an anatomic and clinical study. *Plast Reconstr Surg*. 86:519–526, 1990.
35. Fabian TC, Croce MA, Pritchard FE, et al: Planned ventral hernia staged management for acute abdominal wall defects. *Ann Surg* 219:643–653, 1994.
36. Jernigan TW, Fabian TC, Croce MA, Moore N, Pritchard FE, Minard G: Staged management of giant abdominal wall defects acute and long-term results. *Ann Surg* 238:349–357, 2003.
37. Lowe JB 3rd, Lowe JB, Baty JD, Garza JR: Risks associated with "components separation" for closure of complex abdominal wall defects. *Plast Reconstr Surg* 111:1276–1283, 2003.
38. de Vries Reilingh TS, van Goor H, Rosman C, Bemelmans MH, de Jong D, van Nieuwenhoven EJ, van Engeland MI, Bleichrodt RP: "Components separation technique" for the repair of large abdominal wall hernias. *J Am Coll Surg* 196:32–37, 2003.
39. Espinosa-de-los-Menteros A, de la Torre JI, Marrero I, Andrades P, Davis MR, Vasconez LO: Utilization of human cadaveric acellular dermis for abdominal hernia reconstruction. *Ann Plast Surg* 58(3):264–267, 2007.

PERIPHERAL VASCULAR INJURY

VASCULAR ANATOMY OF THE EXTREMITIES

Enrique Ginzburg, Chee Kiong Chong, and Norman M. Rich

Extremity vascular injuries date as far back as the Greek and Roman civilization. Much of the knowledge regarding vascular trauma and the management of these injuries was gained from military conflicts. DeBakey and Simeone reported the amputation rate to be as high as 40% in World War II, when it was the main life-saving measure for soldiers who sustained extremity injuries. With the advance in surgical technologies and techniques, the rate of amputation dropped to as low as 15% during the Korean War. All this information provides modern surgeons with the ability to manage vascular trauma without the need to enter a combat zone.

DIAGNOSIS

Most patients that are admitted to a trauma center with extremity vascular injuries will be admitted from penetrating trauma. These are usually either stab wounds from knives or low velocity bullet wounds. In most cities, this is closely followed by patients who sustain blunt injuries as a result of motor vehicle crashes, and these are often associated with long bone fractures.

There are hard and soft clinical signs of vascular trauma. The hard signs include the following:

Pulsatile bleeding
Absence of pulses
Distal ischemia
Visible expanding or pulsatile hematoma
Presence of a thrill or bruit over the injured site

The soft signs of vascular injury include the following:

Bony injury
Proximity of penetrating wound
Presence of significant hemorrhage but stopped
Neurologic deficit
Well-contained hematoma
Swelling out of proportion to the injury

Patients with hard signs of vascular injury will undergo mandatory surgical exploration, as any delay will increase the risk of amputation, reperfusion injury, compartment syndrome, and infection. The management of patients with soft signs will usually include further diagnostic studies, close observation, and frequent re-examination. Diagnostic studies include Doppler ultrasound, computed tomography (CT) angiogram, or conventional angiography.

MANAGEMENT

The management of patients appearing with obvious peripheral vascular injuries should follow the protocols outlined by Advance Trauma Life Support (ATLS). Airway, breathing, and circulation will take priority. Injury to the brain, chest, and abdomen will also usually take precedence over extremity hemorrhage, which can usually be controlled by direct pressure.

Successful management of extremity vascular injury includes the following components:

Prompt resuscitation
Control of hemorrhage, usually with direct pressure
Timely diagnosis
Early surgical exploration
Minimized delay in transporting patient to operating room or extensive diagnostic studies when not indicated

A thorough knowledge of the relevant anatomy of the extremity is very important during surgical exploration. Destruction or distortion of tissue planes by hemorrhage is usually the rule rather than the exception, and when this is coupled with the retraction of the vessels into the surrounding tissue, it will increase the difficulty of achieving proximal and distal control of the bleeding vessel, which is the most important step in stopping the bleeding.

VASCULAR ANATOMY OF UPPER EXTREMITY

Axillary Artery

The axillary artery starts from the lateral border of the first rib, as a direct continuation of the subclavian artery. It enters the axilla at the apex and crosses the first intercostal space to run along the lateral wall of the axilla. As the artery emerges from beneath the costoclavicular passage, it becomes closely related to the brachial plexus, divisions, and cords. These nerves surround the artery and exchange fibers to eventually become the median, ulnar, and radial nerves at the distal portion of the axillary artery. This neurovascular bundle is enclosed in the axillary sheath, which separates it from the axillary vein. Distally, the axillary artery continues on as brachial artery at the lateral edge of the teres major muscle tendon.

Anteriorly, the axillary artery follows a course under the pectoralis minor muscle as it inserts into the coracoid process. The muscle divides the artery into three anatomical portions:

The first portion runs from lateral edge of the first rib to the upper border of the tendon pectoralis minor muscle, behind the clavipectoral fascia and the clavicular head of the pectoralis major muscle. It has only one branch in this portion, the supreme thoracic artery.

The second portion lies behind the pectoralis minor muscle. This is the shortest portion and it has two branches of clinical significance, the thoracoacromial artery and the lateral thoracic artery. The cords of the brachial plexus surround the axillary artery at this section.

The third portion starts from the lateral border of the pectoralis muscle to the lateral border of the teres major muscle. The axillary artery gives out three branches at the portion, the subscapular artery, the lateral humeral circumflex artery, and the medial circumflex artery. At this level, the brachial plexus becomes the medial nerve, which is anterior, the radial nerve, which is posterior, and the ulnar nerve, which is inferior to the axillary in the axillary sheath.

Axillary Vein

The basilic vein continues on at the lower edge of the teres major muscle as the axillary vein. Its main tributaries are brachial veins, which accompany the named arteries while they ascend in the axilla, and the cephalic vein, which courses through the deltopectoral groove, just below the clavicle. The axillary vein then becomes the subclavian vein above the lateral border of the first rib.

The axillary vein lies medial to the axillary artery. It is separated from artery by the medial pectoral nerve, medial cord of the brachial plexus, and the ulnar nerve. It is separated from the axillary sheath by a pad of fat. The close proximity of the vein to the artery often results in the occurrence of traumatic arteriovenous malformations. Penetrating injury to the upper part of axilla can cause profuse hemorrhage and risk of air embolism.

Surgical Exposure of Axillary Vessels

The axillary artery lies anterior to the capsule of the shoulder joint and might be injured when the shoulder is dislocated anteriorly. Fractures of the surgical neck of the humerus will also risk lacerating the vessel as it runs over the fusion of the subscapularis tendon and the joint capsule.

The axillary artery can be exposed through an infraclavicular incision placed 2 cm below and parallel to the mid-point of the clavicle, following a gentle curve along the anterior axillary line and then along the anterior border of the deltoid muscle. The first portion of the artery is the simplest to expose because it is medial to the pectoralis muscle and contains only one branch. Exposure of the second portion will require the detachment of the pectoralis minor tendon from the coracoid process. The cords of the brachial plexus surround this portion of the axillary artery, arranged medially, laterally, and posteriorly. From the posterior cord arises the axillary nerve, which follows a posterolateral course on the neck of the humerus. This nerve can be easily injured by dislocation of the humerus or fracture of the surgical neck, causing atrophy of the deltoid muscle and numbness of an area over the deltoid region. The third portion becomes superficial after emerging from under the pectoralis major muscle before becoming the brachial artery. Great care must be taken while exposing this portion because the nerves to the upper extremities run about it. The median nerve runs anterior to the artery and is frequently involved in axillary injuries resulting from its superficial position.

Brachial Artery

The brachial artery originates at the lower border of the teres major muscle as a direct continuation of the axillary artery. It takes a course toward the antecubital fossa, together with the median nerve, and bifurcates into radial and ulnar arteries opposite the neck of the radius. The medial bicipital sulcus, which separates the coracobrachialis and biceps muscle anteriorly from the triceps muscle posteriorly, marks the course of the basilic vein toward the axillary vein and provides the surface marking of the brachial vessels.

The proximal part of the brachial artery lies on the medial aspect of the arm, anterior to the long and median head of the triceps and bordered laterally by the coracobrachialis muscle. The median nerve lies between the coracobrachialis muscle and the brachial artery, whereas the ulnar nerve separates the artery from the basilic vein. The brachial artery gives rise to the profunda brachii artery posteriorly, which passes backward and accompanies the radial nerve in the radial groove to the lateral condyle of the humerus. This artery collateralizes about the shoulder with the circumflex humeral arteries arising from the axillary artery.

The brachial artery gradually inclines forward and outward and eventually comes to lie below the medial border of the biceps muscle. The median nerve crosses the artery obliquely at this part of the arm. The basilic vein and the medial cutaneous nerve are separated from the artery by the deep fascia sheath. The branches arising from this portion of the brachial artery include the nutrient artery to the humerus, muscular branches, and superior ulnar collateral artery, which accompanies the ulnar nerve to the groove on the posterior surface of the medial epicondyle. This artery subsequently takes part in the rich anastomosis around the elbow joint.

The distal part of the brachial artery is overlapped by the medial border of the biceps muscle and biceps tendon and eventually comes to lie medial to the biceps tendon before the bifurcation of the artery. The median nerve lies medial to the brachial artery. This inferior ulnar collateral artery arises near the elbow and forms a rich network of collaterals around the elbow joint. Brachial artery bifurcates opposite the neck of the radius bone to give rise to the ulnar artery medially and the radial artery laterally.

The artery is closely accompanied by a pair of venae comitantes that drain into the axillary vein.

Surgical Exposure of Brachial Artery

The brachial artery is the most commonly injured artery in the upper extremity, probably as a result of the superficial course that it takes. This artery accounts for 50% of all upper extremity injuries.

In the arm, exposure in any part of the artery can be achieved by a longitudinal incision along the course of the vessel just medial to the bicipital sulcus. This sulcus can be easily identified by grasping the head of the biceps and lifting it up to reveal the groove. The artery, along with the accompanying vein and nerves, is immediately visible after dividing the skin and subcutaneous tissue, investing the fascia, and splitting the biceps and triceps muscle. The basilic vein runs a superficial course along the bicipital sulcus. It can be identified and retracted laterally to prevent injury to the vein.

Just above the elbow, the brachial artery passes behind the bicipital aponeurosis, which may be divided to facilitate exposure of the vessel. The brachial artery is juxtaposed to the median nerve. Extension of incision across the antecubital fossa should be made with an S-shaped incision to reduce the risk of joint contracture. Care has to be exercised to prevent injury to the accompanying nerves and veins.

Radial Artery

The radial artery is usually the smaller branch that follows the general direction of the brachial artery. It is a fairly superficial vessel, covered mainly by skin, subcutaneous tissue, and fascia, save for the upper part, which is covered by the fleshy belly of brachioradialis muscle. The artery takes a course that travels laterally gradually, and after emerging from under the brachioradialis muscle, it comes to lie between the brachioradialis and the flexor carpi radialis muscles. The distal part, which is the most superficial part of the radial artery, travels between the tendon of flexor pollicis longus and the lateral border of the radius, until it passes behind the flexor retinaculum to enter the hand.

The radial artery gives rise to two major branches, the radial recurrent branch near the origin, and the superficial palmar branch, which takes part in the formation of the superficial palmar arch.

Ulnar Artery

The ulnar artery is the larger of the two terminal trunks of the brachial artery. It runs downward and medially to reach the medial aspect of the forearm from the bifurcation. During its course, the artery lies on the brachialis muscle in the upper part and then on the flexor digitorum profundus as it progresses distally. It is covered by the pronator teres muscle, flexor carpi radialis, and flexor digitorum superficialis. The medial nerve lies medial to the ulnar artery for the first 2.5 cm before it crosses in front of the artery to take up a lateral relationship. After the crossing over, the nerve is separated from the artery by the ulnar head of the pronator teres.

At the distal part, the ulnar artery emerges between the tendon of the flexor digitorum superficialis medially and flexor carpi ulnaris laterally to be covered by skin and fascia only. It subsequently passes behind the palmaris brevis to terminate in the superficial palmar arch. The branches that give out near the origin of the ulnar artery include the anterior and posterior ulnar recurrent arteries and the common interosseous artery.

Surgical Exposure of Ulnar and Radial Arteries

The incidence of ulnar and radial artery injuries ranges from 7%–35% of all upper extremity injuries. Ligation of a single vessel results in an amputation rate of 10%. Ligation of both vessels increases the rate to 39%.

Exposure of the ulnar artery is made through an incision over the medial volar aspect of the forearm, over the course of the vessel. The incision can be extended proximally to reach the antecubital fossa to gain control of the brachial artery. The skin incision is deepened to the subcutaneous, and the tissue between flexor carpi radialis and flexor digitorum superficialis can be split to facilitate exposure.

The radial artery can be exposed throughout its length via a longitudinal incision made on the medial aspect of the brachioradialis muscle. This will allow lateral retraction of the muscle to facilitate exposure. The artery runs superficially at the wrist, and exposure over the wrist will only require division of skin and subcutaneous tissue over the pulsation. However, this artery is very liable to spasm. Papaverine can be used to infiltrate the radial sheath, which is the deep fascia, before sharp dissection and mobilization.

VEINS OF UPPER EXTREMITY

The upper limb has deep and superficial sets of draining veins. The deep veins are the venae comitantes of the named arteries. The superficial vein runs in between the superficial fascia immediately beneath the skin. These two set of vessels have frequent anastomosis with each other.

In the forearm, the named arteries are accompanied by a pair of venae comitantes to provide venous drainage. These deep veins will drain into the two brachial veins. The brachial veins run with the brachial artery in the arm, draining blood proximally, until they join the axillary vein at the lower border of the subscapularis muscle.

The upper extremity also has a superficial venous network to provide drainage of the upper limb. These veins will eventually drain into the superficial veins, namely the basilic and cephalic veins.

Basilic Vein

The basilic vein receives tributaries from the ulnar component of the dorsal venous network. It runs up the posterior surface of the forearm and curves around the ulnar border below the elbow to the anterior surface of the forearm. In the elbow, it is joined by the vena mediana cubiti, a branch from the cephalic vein. The vein takes a medial and superficial relation to the brachial artery and the medial cutaneous nerve in this part of the course. It then runs upward along the medial border of the biceps brachii muscle, and perforates the deep fascia to run along the medial side of the brachial artery. At the lower border of the teres major muscles, the vein continues on as the axillary vein.

Cephalic Vein

The cephalic vein begins as the coalescence of the radial part of the dorsal venous network and winds upwards around the radial border. In the antecubital fossa just below the elbow, the cephalic vein gives off the vena mediana cubiti, which receives a perforating branch from the deep veins of the forearm and passes across to join the basilic vein. In the elbow, it crosses superficial to the musculocutaneous nerve and ascends along the lateral border of the biceps brachii muscle. In the upper part of the arm, the cephalic vein runs in the deltopectoral groove, where it is accompanied by the deltoid branch of the thoracoacromial artery. It then pierces the clavipectoral fascia to drain into the axillary vein just below the clavicle.

Axillary Vein

The basilic vein continues on at the lower edge of the teres major muscle as the axillary vein. Its main tributaries are brachial veins, tributaries that accompany the named arteries, while it ascends in the axilla, and the cephalic vein, which courses through the deltopectoral groove, just below the clavicle. The axillary vein then becomes the subclavian vein above the lateral border of the first rib.

The axillary vein lies medial to the axillary artery. It is separated from the artery by the medial pectoral nerve, medial cord of the brachial plexus, and the ulnar nerve. It is separated from the axillary sheath by a pad of fat. The close proximity of the vein to the artery often results in the occurrence of traumatic arteriovenous malformations. Penetrating injury to the upper part of axilla can cause profuse hemorrhage and risk of air embolism.

NERVES OF UPPER EXTREMITY

The nerves in the upper extremity have a close and important relationship to the major named artery. They can be easily injured along with the vessels in any trauma. However, iatrogenic injury to the nerve can also occur during surgical exploration if the relevant anatomy of the neurovascular bundle is not thoroughly understood.

Median Nerve

The median nerve originates from the lateral and medial cords of the brachial plexus at the distal part of the axillary artery. It accompanies the brachial artery throughout the whole course.

At first, the nerve lies laterally to the brachial artery. At the level of insertion of the coracobrachialis muscle, the median nerve crosses the artery superficially, occasionally deep to it, and descends along the medial side to the elbow. It traverses the cubital fossa together with the brachial artery in the same relationship, behind the aponeurosis of the biceps muscle and anterior to the brachialis muscle. It then passes into the forearm between the two heads of the pronator teres muscle, separated from the ulnar artery by the deep head of the muscle.

In the forearm, the median nerve runs between the flexor digitorum superficialis and flexor digitorum profundus, attaching firmly to the undersurface of the superficial flexor muscle of the fingers. There is no direct relationship between the median nerve and any of the major axial vessels in the forearm. At the wrist region, the median nerve lies superficially and thus prone to even minor laceration. It takes a course between the tendon of the palmaris longus and the tendon of flexor carpi radialis, and enters the wrist through the carpal tunnel along with tendons of flexor digitorum superficialis.

Ulnar Nerve

The ulnar nerve arises from the medial cord of the brachial plexus. It runs medial to the axillary artery in the axilla between the artery and the vein. In the arm, it accompanies the brachial artery on its medial side, anterior to the triceps muscle. At the distal half of the arm, the nerve deviates from the artery and pierces the medial intermuscular septum. It then runs downward and medially in the posterior compartment anterior to the medial head of the triceps muscle.

The nerve continues into the elbow between the medial epicondyle of the humerus and the olecranon. In the epicondyle groove, the nerve is just covered by skin and adipose tissue. It can be palpated as a cord-like structure and is prone to injury from any trauma to the medial epicondyle. Violent flexion of the elbow can also dislocate the nerve, and this will require surgical intervention. Through the ulnar groove on the medial epicondyle, the ulnar nerve enters the forearm between the two heads of flexor carpi ulnaris. It descends on top of the flexor digitorum profundus muscle and is overlapped by the flexor carpi ulnaris. In the upper half of the forearm, the ulnar nerve is still separated from the ulnar artery, but the two structures eventually come to travel together in the lower half of the forearm, with the nerve taking a medial relation to the artery throughout.

Radial Nerve

The radial nerve is the direct continuation of the posterior cord of the brachial plexus. It lies posterior to the axillary artery, and it is bigger in size when compared with the ulnar nerve. In the axilla, the radial nerve can be injured from prolonged exposure to pressure, such as falling asleep when the arm drapes across an arm rest and improper use of crutches. The nerve maintains the same relationship with the proximal part of the brachial artery, between the long head of the triceps and the shaft of the humerus. It then winds backward, accompanied by the profunda brachii artery, to run in the radial groove of the humerus laterally and distally across the back of the arm. The radial nerve is especially prone to injury in fracture of the midshaft of humerus resulting from its relation to the bone. Just distal to the midshaft, the nerve traverses the lateral muscular septum to enter the anterior brachii compartment, lying along the lateral margin of the brachialis muscle and deep to the brachioradialis and extensor carpi radialis longus muscle. The radial nerve may be injured in the fracture of the shaft of humerus or involved in the callus

formation when the bone heals. These might need surgical intervention for repair or release of the nerve. Anterior to the lateral epicondyle, the nerve gives rise to the posterior interosseous nerve.

In the forearm, the radial nerve descends deep to the brachioradialis, to take up a lateral relationship to the radial artery in the middle third of the forearm. The neurovascular bundles course further distally before separating prior to the styloid process of the radius to enter the dorsum of the hand. The posterior interosseous branch is a muscular branch that winds around the neck of the radius through the supinator muscle. It runs between the superficial and deep muscles of the back of the forearm to innervate them. As it is in close relation to the head of radius, the posterior interosseous nerve is prone to injury from fractures of the elbow or from exposure of the elbow during surgery.

VASCULAR ANATOMY OF LOWER EXTREMITY

Femoral Artery

The femoral artery, also known as the common femoral artery, is the direct continuation of the external iliac artery. It enters the femoral triangle behind the inguinal ligament, midway between the anterior superior iliac spine and the symphysis pubis.

The femoral triangle is bounded by the inguinal ligament superiorly, medial border of the sartorius muscle laterally, medial border of adductor longus, and pectineus muscle medially. The floor of the triangle is formed by the iliacus, psoas major, pectineus, and adductor longus muscles.

Within the triangle, the femoral artery is related laterally to the femoral nerve, medially to the femoral vein and femoral canal, and posteriorly to the psoas and pectineus muscles. Early in its course, the femoral artery gives rise to several branches—superficial epigastric, superficial circumflex iliac, superior geniculate, superficial, and deep external pudendal arteries. After traveling about 4 cm, the artery bifurcates within the femoral triangle into superficial femoral artery and profunda femoris artery.

Profunda Femoris Artery

The profunda femoris artery provides the main blood supply to the thigh. It usually arises from the posterolateral aspect of the femoral artery and descends first laterally, and then posterior to the superficial femoral artery. Subsequently, the artery runs down the thigh deep to the adductor longus muscle, in close relation to the linea aspera of the femur, and pierces the adductor magnus muscle to become the fourth perforating artery.

The medial and lateral circumflex femoral arteries arise soon after the origin of the profunda femoris artery, although they branch out from the common femoral artery at the level of bifurcation in 20% of patients. These important vessels can flow in either direction. They serve as collaterals via cruciate anastomosis around the hip when either the internal or external iliac artery is occluded. Three perforating arteries are also given out along the course of the profunda femoris artery to supply the muscle of the thigh. They are also connected by a rich anastomotic network.

Superficial Femoral Artery

This is usually the larger of the two terminating branches. It exits the femoral triangle at the apex and descends into the adductor canal. This canal is bordered by the sartorius muscle medially, vastus medialis anterolaterally, and the adductor longus and magnus muscles posteriorly. Within the canal, the artery is bound closely to the femoral vein by connective tissue. The saphenous nerve lies anterior to the vessel. The artery then pierces the adductor magnus at the adductor hiatus to become the popliteal artery. Near its termination, the superior geniculate artery branches from the femoral artery.

Surgical Exposure of Femoral Artery

In both wartime and peacetime, injuries to the femoral artery account for 20%–45% of all extremity injuries. Most of the injuries are penetrating in nature. Generally, penetrating injuries are most obvious and surgical intervention can be carried out without extensive diagnostic evaluation. However, blunt injuries are frequently obscured by concomitant injuries to the bone, nerve, and soft tissues. Angiography is known as the gold standard for diagnosing vascular injury. However, with the advance in technology, CT angiography is beginning to replace conventional angiography as the first line of investigation in some centers. It is noninvasive, and results can be obtained quickly. In the absence of pulses or with evidence of diminished perfusion, restoration of flow must be achieved as quickly as possible.

Exposure can be achieved by placing a longitudinal incision over the femoral pulse in the femoral triangle. In the absence of a pulse, the incision can be placed inferior to the midpoint between anterior superior iliac spine and pubic tubercle. Proximal control of the external iliac artery can be achieved through either a separate incision that runs parallel to the inguinal ligament or by extending the longitudinal incision superiorly and laterally through the inguinal ligament.

The incision is deepened to expose the deep fascia covering the femoral triangle. Incision of the fascia will allow the retraction of sartorius and adductor magnus to expose the femoral sheath. The sheath is then sharply incised to expose the femoral artery within. Exposure of the femoral vein is carried out in similar fashion.

The superficial femoral artery can be approached through an incision along the line joining the anterior superior iliac spine and medial femoral condyle. The incision is deepened through the superficial fascia, carefully retracting the greater saphenous vein. The fascia covering of the sartorius is divided and the muscle can be retracted medially to expose the superficial femoral vessels with the saphenous nerve on the anterior surface.

Popliteal Artery

The popliteal artery begins at the adductor hiatus as the direct continuation of the superficial femoral artery. It travels downward and slightly laterally to go behind the distal femur to enter the popliteal fossa.

The popliteal fossa is an important anatomical area because all neurovascular structures passing from the thigh to the leg traverse this space. It is filled with tissues that offer protection to the neurovascular structure and yet allow the movement at the knee joint. This is a diamond-shaped fossa located behind the knee. The floor consists of popliteal surface of the femur above, posterior surface of the joint capsule with overlying popliteus muscle. The superior border is made up of bicep femoris muscle and tendon laterally, and four muscles (namely, semimembranosus, semitendinosus, gracilis, and sartorius muscles) medially. The inferior boundaries are formed by the lateral and medial head of the gastrocnemius muscle, respectively. The roof consists of a strong sheet of deep investing fascia, which is pierced in the center by the short saphenous vein, subcutaneous tissue, and skin. This unites with the muscles and tendons forming the boundaries to form a well-enclosed space.

The popliteal artery runs on the floor of the popliteal fossa between the condyles of the femur until it reaches the distal border of the popliteus muscle and terminates by dividing into anterior tibial and tibioperoneal trunk. Throughout the course, it is in direct contact with the posterior ligament of the knee joint. Three pairs of branches are given out to supply the knee and these form important collaterals about the knee. No branches are given off at the upper portion of the popliteal artery, and this portion of the vessel is accessible for ligation if required.

Anterior Tibial Artery

The anterior tibial artery is the smaller terminating branch of the popliteal artery that arises from the lower border of the popliteus muscle. It passes forward through the interosseous membrane into the anterior compartment of the leg. At first, it lies close to the medial aspect of the neck of the fibula, but inclines medially and forward on the membrane as it descends and rests against the anterior surface of the shaft of tibia in the lower third of the leg. It lies deep between anterior tibialis and extensor digitorum longus muscle proximally and extensor hallucis longus muscle distally. In the final part of its course, it is covered only by skin, fascia, and extensor retinaculum. At the level of the ankle, the tendon of the extensor hallucis longus muscle crosses in front of the artery to become medially related. The artery then continues on as the dorsalis pedis.

Throughout the course, the anterior tibial artery is surrounded by two interlacing venae comitantes and the deep peroneal nerve. The deep peroneal nerve, after winding around the neck of the fibula, joins the anterior tibial artery soon after the artery enters the anterior compartment. Initially the nerve lies laterally to the artery, but from about the middle of the leg, the nerve takes up an anterolateral relationship with the artery for the rest of its course.

Tibioperoneal Trunk

The tibioperoneal trunk is the larger terminating branches of the popliteal artery. It originates and descends from just behind the soleal arch. The trunk lies on the tibialis posterior muscle and is covered by the gastrocnemius and soleus muscles. A network of complex and thin-walled venous vessels surrounds the artery and may bleed profusely during dissection of the tibioperoneal trunk. The tibial nerve accompanied the artery below the arch of the soleus muscle. It runs a variable length, ranging from 0 to 5 cm before bifurcating into posterior tibial and peroneal artery.

Posterior Tibial Artery

Posterior tibial artery is the direct continuation of the tibioperoneal trunk. It descends in the posterior compartment, lying on posterior tibialis for most of its course and covered by gastrocnemius and soleus muscles. In the upper two thirds, the posterior tibial artery lies deep to the covering muscles. For the rest of the course, the artery takes a superficial course. At its termination, the artery lies midway between the medial malleolus and the medial tubercle of the calcaneus, among the tendons of the deep leg muscles and under the cover of the flexor retinaculum. A pair of deep veins accompanies the artery as venae comitantes. Throughout the course, the posterior tibial nerve runs alongside the artery. The nerve takes a medial relationship initially and becomes posterior in the lower part of the leg. The posterior tibial artery terminates by dividing into medial and lateral plantar arteries.

Peroneal Artery

The peroneal artery descends laterally toward the fibula after branching off from the tibioperoneal trunk. It then follows the medial edge of the fibula, between flexor hallucis longus and tibialis posterior muscles, in close relation to the posterior aspect of the fibula and the interosseous membrane throughout the course. At the ankle, the artery gives off a branch that perforates the interosseous membrane.

This anterior malleolar branch of the peroneal artery descends in front of the lateral malleolus, and forms an anastomotic network around the malleolus with the lateral and posterior malleolar branches of the peroneal artery. A pair of deep veins accompanies the artery, but there is no major nerve that travels with the artery.

Surgical Exposure of Vessels in Leg

Most of these injuries are blunt injuries in peacetime, as opposed to most wartime injuries, which are penetrating in nature. Popliteal artery injury remains a serious affair. The amputation rate had been high with ligation, such as up to 73% in World War II. The rate of amputation has dropped significantly over the last decade, with the advance in arterial repair and liberal use of fasciotomy and intraoperative angiography. However, vascular insufficiency is a common sequelae when the limb survives.

The approach to the popliteal artery can be carried out in a posterior or a medial incision. A posterior S-shaped incision requires the patient to be placed in a prone position and have limited access to the anterior compartment of the leg; thus, it is seldom used for vascular injury. The medial approach tends to be more versatile, and lacks the disadvantages of the posterior approach. The incision is placed from the medial femoral condyle across the knee down to the leg. The incision of the superficial fascia will expose the underlying muscles. Anterior retraction of vastus medialis muscle and posterior retraction of sartorius muscle will expose the popliteal vessels and the saphenous nerve. This incision can also be extended distally behind the bony prominence of the tibia, to approach the origin of the anterior tibial artery and the tibioperoneal trunk. The exposure can be further enhanced by dividing the medial head of the gastrocnemius muscle, the tendon of the adductor magnus, sartorius, and the two medial hamstrings muscles.

The anterior tibial artery in the anterior compartment lies in front of the interosseous membrane. Exposure can be gained by a longitudinal lateral incision between the tibia and fibula. The incision is carried through the intermuscular septum between the tibialis anterior and extensor hallucis longus muscles, without disrupting the belly of the muscles. The extensor hallucis longus can be retracted laterally to facilitate exposure. Care must be taken to preserve the venae comitantes and the deep peroneal nerve. This approach, coupled with resection of fibula, will also facilitate exposure of the peroneal vessels that lie just behind the fibula in the posterior compartment. The anterior tibial artery in the lower part of the leg lies superficially. The incision placed over the pulse, dissection of the subcutaneous tissue, and investing fascia will allow exposure of vessel.

The posterior tibial artery is accessed through a medial approach. An incision is placed behind the posterior border of the tibia. The deep investing fascia is incised for the length of the wound and the intermuscular plane between the flexor digitorum longus anteriorly, and the medial head of gastrocnemius and soleus posteriorly. This will also allow exposure of the peroneal vessels, which lie in a more lateral position. Care must be taken to avoid injuring the tibial nerve, which lies adjacent to the posterior tibial artery. In the lower third of the calf, the posterior tibial artery takes a superficial course after emerging from under the soleus and gastrocnemius muscles. It is only covered by skin, subcutaneous tissue, and the deep investing fascia. The incision can be made directly over the pulse or about an inch anterior to the Achilles tendon and deepened to expose the vessel.

VEINS OF LOWER EXTREMITY

Like the upper extremity, the veins in the lower extremity are also divided into two sets—superficial and deep veins. The deep veins accompany the named arteries. In the thigh, they are usually single veins that run alongside the major arteries, namely, the common femoral vein, the superficial femoral vein, the deep femoral vein, and the popliteal veins. Those that accompany the smaller arteries usually consist of two smaller veins, the venae comitantes. These are the main capacitance vessels of the lower extremity.

The superficial veins, much like their counterparts in the upper limb, run below the skin in between the superficial fascia. In the lower extremity, the superficial veins are the long saphenous and the short saphenous veins with their tributaries. The deep and superficial systems are connected by perforating veins at various points in the lower extremity.

Long Saphenous Vein

The long saphenous vein is the longest vein in the body. It begins in the medial marginal vein of the dorsum of the foot. The vein runs in front of the medial malleolus and along the medial side of the leg, in relation with the saphenous nerve. It curves posteriorly at the level of the knee, and then sweeps upwards along the inner aspect of the thigh. The vein enters the femoral triangle, pierces the deep fascia, passes through the fossa ovalis, and finally gains entry into the common femoral vein. Near the fossa ovalis, it is joined by the superficial epigastric, the superficial iliac circumflex, the superficial external pudendal veins, and the accessory saphenous veins.

Short Saphenous Vein

The short saphenous begins behind the lateral malleolus as a continuation of the lateral marginal vein of the foot. It firsts ascends along the lateral border of the Achilles tendon, and then crosses the tendon to continue its ascent in the midline of the back of the leg. In the lower part of the popliteal fossa, the short saphenous vein perforates the deep fascia and ends in the popliteal vein between the heads of the gastrocnemius muscle. In the lower third of the leg, the vein is in close relation with the sural nerve, and in the upper two-thirds with the medial sural cutaneous nerve.

SUGGESTED READINGS

Lumley JSP: *Color Atlas of Vascular Surgery.* Baltimore, Williams & Wilkins, 1986.

Nyhus LM, Baker RJ, Fischer JE, editors: *Master of Surgery.* Boston, Little, Brown, 1997.

Rutherford RB, editor: *Vascular Surgery*, 3rd ed. Philadelphia, Saunders, 1989.

Stoney RJ, Effene DJ: *Comprehensive Vascular Exposures.* Philadelphia, Lippincott-Raven, 1998.

Zollinger RM Jr, Zollinger R: *Atlas of Surgical Operations.* New York, McGraw-Hill, 1993.

THE DIAGNOSIS OF VASCULAR TRAUMA

John T. Anderson   and   F. William Blaisdell

The diagnosis of vascular trauma is usually not a problem, as most injuries manifest overt blood loss, shock, or loss of critical pulses. However, in certain instances, the lesion may not be recognized initially, only to manifest itself later by sudden secondary hemorrhage or the development of critical organ or extremity ischemia.

Most of the vascular injuries of immediate concern to the clinician are those related to arteries. The reason for this is that venous hemorrhage is usually well controlled by the adjacent soft tissues, and excellent collateral flow compensates for occlusive lesions. Late progression of thrombosis and pulmonary embolism are the primary complications related to venous injury.

DIAGNOSIS

The first priority should be to identify and manage life-threatening injuries and treat shock. Except for head injuries, nearly all injuries associated with immediate fatality are related to the cardiovascular system.

Advanced Trauma Life Support (ATLS) guidelines should be followed while proceeding with evaluation and treatment simultaneously. Shock from internal hemorrhage can be differentiated from cardiac compression or injury by a quick glance at neck veins. If neck veins are full, the presumption is cardiac compression from tamponade, tension pneumothorax, or cardiac failure. Collapsed neck veins indicate hypovolemia, and failure of response to fluid therapy dictates immediate operative intervention involving the most likely body cavity. This is usually dictated by an emergency chest x-ray. External hemorrhage is usually obvious and immediate control is essential. Generally, direct pressure is effective for temporary control.

The presence of shock may lead to diminished pulses in the extremities and confusion about the location of vascular injury. Associated fractures and dislocations may compromise vascular patency and should be reduced before any decision about vascular injury is reached.

Prompt resuscitation and identification and management of vascular injuries should be the goals in order to minimize mortality and prevent permanent extremity ischemic damage.

History

Prehospital personnel should be questioned about bleeding at the scene and the presence or absence of shock. The need for resuscitation and the volume of fluid administered should be solicited. The use and duration of application of a tourniquet should be determined, and the amount and character of blood loss at the accident scene ascertained. A history of bright red pulsatile bleeding suggests arterial injury, while dark blood suggests venous origin. In many instances, bleeding may have ceased by the time the patient reaches the emergency room, leading to a false sense of security. In this type of patient, particularly one with an arterial injury, secondary hemorrhage is possible at any time.

Both the patient and prehospital personnel should be questioned about the mechanism of injury. Most civilian penetrating trauma results from low-velocity mechanisms such as knives or handguns. Arterial injuries in these cases are typically the result of direct injury, that is, from the knife or bullet. Information should be collected to aid in determining the trajectory of injury and potential structures injured. This could include the knife type and length, the number and direction of bullets, and the body position at the time of injury. Vascular injury from blunt mechanisms is often the result of stretching or compression from associated fractures or dislocations. Evidence of extremity fracture, dislocation, or altered perfusion should be elucidated. Additionally, specific mechanisms such as "car bumper" injuries or posterior knee dislocations are often associated with vascular injury and should be sought as appropriate.

Information about neurologic symptoms including sensory and motor deficits should be obtained. Potential confounding factors such as pre-existing peripheral vascular disease, diabetes, or neuropathies should be elicited.

Physical Examination

The patient should be undressed and thoroughly examined. The skin folds of the axilla or perineum and buttocks should not be neglected, as wounds resulting from penetrating trauma may be missed in these areas. Deformity resulting from fracture or dislocation should be identified. In the case of penetrating trauma, the location and number of wounds should be noted in an attempt to identify the trajectory of the wounding object (particularly with reference to major arteries).

Evidence of active bleeding or hematoma formation should be sought. The character of the bleeding, pulsatile bright red blood, or a steady ooze of dark blood should be noted. A tense or expanding hematoma indicates the presence of an arterial injury with bleeding contained by surrounding soft tissues. The opposite uninjured extremity should be evaluated as a comparison. Chronic peripheral vascular disease is generally symmetric. Absent pulses in the noninjured leg would support a diagnosis of pre-existing peripheral vascular disease.

The examination should include palpation of pulses proximal and distal to the injury. Perfusion and tissue viability can be further assessed with skin temperature and capillary refill distal to the injury and determination of motor function. Alterations in any of these parameters warrant further assessment. Conversely, an apparent "normal" pulse does not exclude the possibility of vascular injury. Pulses may be palpable and assessed as normal in up to $1/3$ of patients with later proven vascular injury. Again, the opposite noninjured extremity serves as a useful comparison.

Arteriovenous (AV) fistulas may occasionally be identified by auscultation of a bruit over the involved arterial segment. Generally the AV fistulas progress over time—often a bruit is not apparent early postinjury. A glove should be placed over the bell of the stethoscope to keep the stethoscope free of blood when there is an open injury.

A thorough neurologic examination should be documented. Anatomically, the blood vessels and nerves are located in close proximity to each other. A neurologic deficit may hint toward the presence of an associated vascular injury. Further, the examination is of prognostic importance, as functional outcome is very dependent on intact sensation and motor function. A "stocking glove" deficit frequently indicates neurologic dysfunction resulting from ischemia—peripheral nerves are susceptible to ischemia because of a high metabolic rate and low glycogen stores. Blood flow should promptly be re-established to prevent development of muscle death and gangrene.

HARD AND SOFT SIGNS OF VASCULAR INJURY

On the basis of history and physical examination, manifestations of vascular injury can be classified into two general prognostic categories, hard signs and soft signs (Table 1).

Hard signs are strong predictors of the presence of an arterial injury and the need for urgent operative intervention. Obvious examples include bright red pulsatile bleeding or a rapidly expanding hematoma. Evidence of extremity ischemia (manifested by the six P's—pulselessness, pallor, pain, paralysis, paresthesia, and poikilothermia) and a bruit or thrill are additional examples. For extremity trauma, we also consider an arterial pressure index (API), also known as the ankle-brachial index, of less than 0.90 to be a hard sign. The API is determined by dividing the systolic pressure of the injured limb by the systolic pressure of the noninjured limb. Johansen and colleagues[1] demonstrated 95% sensitivity and 97% specificity for identification of occult arterial injury with an API of less than 0.90. An API of more than 0.90 had a 99% negative predictive value for the presence of an arterial injury. The API is readily determined at bedside, and should be considered an extension of the physical examination. An important caveat is that the API may be normal in nonconduit vessels such as the profunda femoris.

Soft signs are those suggestive of an arterial injury, although with a much decreased likelihood than hard signs (see Table 1). These consist of mild pulse deficits, soft bruits, nonexpanding hematomas, and fractures or wounds in close proximity to major vessels. The actual incidence of arterial injury with these findings varies. For instance, patients with injury in proximity to a major vessel as the only finding are found to have an identifiable injury in less than 10% of cases; further, many of these injuries do not require additional treatment beyond simple observation. Most of the controversy of vascular trauma evaluation revolves around the assessment of patients with soft signs.

ADDITIONAL ANCILLARY TESTS

Ancillary imaging includes plain x-rays, duplex scanning, computed tomography (CT) angiography, and formal arteriography. A chest x-ray and plain x-ray imaging of the site of suspected vascular injury are warranted in essentially all patients. The utility of the remaining modalities are most beneficial when dealing with patients with soft signs, when the location of arterial injury is not obvious, or for assorted injuries, that is, thoracic aorta, where information gained may greatly impact subsequent management. In many patients, the presence of an arterial injury is obvious and the need for surgical intervention clear; these patients are generally best served by prompt operation without additional tests.

A chest x-ray and plain films are readily obtained in the emergency room and should be a part of the initial screening of the injured patient. Radio-opaque markers should be placed on all open wounds suspected to have resulted from a penetrating mechanism. Radiographs should completely cover the injured areas; often this requires imaging overlapping areas of the torso to ensure adequate coverage. Films should be scrutinized for foreign bodies, fractures, and dislocations. The trajectory of the injury is assessed as possible. The number of bullets identified and the number of wounds should sum to an even number. If not, the patient should be evaluated for additional unidentified wounds and films should be obtained to locate additional bullets. An important caveat is the possibility of a foreign body from a prior injury. At times, the bullet may travel as a missile embolism in the vascular system to a site distant from the site of entry. Occasionally, fluoroscopy (or the scout film of the CT scan) will assist in localizing additional bullets. A note should be made if the foreign body appears blurred, as this implies motion and the possibility of close contact with, or location within, a vascular structure.

Duplex ultrasonographic scanning combines two-dimensional imaging to assess anatomic detail and Doppler insonation to assess flow characteristics. Several investigators have demonstrated high sensitivity and specificity in the detection of vascular injury in various anatomic locations.[2–5] Duplex ultrasonography is more sensitive to the presence of vascular injury than the arterial pressure index (API). Importantly, duplex ultrasonography can identify arterial injuries in nonconduit vessels such as the profunda femoris (the API will remain normal). However, duplex ultrasonography is limited, as it is technician dependent and in most centers is not readily available after hours.

Recently, there has been a groundswell of interest in the use of CT angiography as a diagnostic modality for vascular injury in multiple anatomic locations.[6–11] Major advantages include almost universal availability and three-dimensional (3D) detail. Compared with formal angiography, an interventional radiologist does not need to be in attendance at the time of the examination. In general, the examination can be obtained more expeditiously than formal angiography, particularly after hours. Technological advancements in imaging resolution and software have been significant. Arterial anatomy can be reconstructed in 3D detail for easy evaluation. However, the modality is diagnostic only. A subsequent angiogram may be required for therapeutic embolization. Notably, the combined contrast load from both a CT angiogram and a subsequent angiogram can be significant. An additional technical limitation is that CT angiography is compromised by scatter from metallic fragments much more than formal angiography.[12] CT angiography is of particular value when thoracic vascular injury is suspected, and it has proven to be a highly sensitive screening test.[13] However, mediastinal hematoma alone, without evidence of arterial disruption, may still require arteriography to confirm large vessel injury.[14]

Arteriography has long been regarded the gold standard for assessment of arterial injury.[15] It is well tolerated and has a low complication rate. Major complications such as iatrogenic pseudoaneurysm or AV fistulas are very uncommon in the young population typical of most trauma centers. A major advantage of arteriography is the availability of therapeutic options (such as embolization). Further, compared with CT angiography, formal arteriography is not prone to scatter from the presence of metallic fragments. Even in centers that rely on CT imaging as the predominant diagnostic study, formal arteriography still has a diagnostic role in confirming or further delineating the presence of equivocal CT findings. This latter point is particularly applicable in the assessment of carotid injuries where even minor injuries may be of importance. An occasional patient requires urgent operation before availability of formal arteriography or CT angiography. In these patients, an on-table, surgeon-performed arteriogram can be obtained in the operating room. For instance, a

Table 1: Hard versus Soft Signs of Vascular Injury

Hard Signs	Soft Signs
Active arterial bleeding	Neurologic injury in proximity to vessel
Pulselessness/evidence of ischemia	Small- to moderate-sized hematoma
Expanding pulsatile hematoma	Unexplained hypotension
Bruit or thrill	Large blood loss at scene
Arterial pressure index <0.90 pulse deficit	Injury (due to penetrating mechanism, fracture, or dislocation) in proximity to major vessel

From Anderson JT, Blaisdell FW: Diagnosis of vascular trauma. In Rich N, Mattox KL, Hirshberg A, editors: *Vascular Trauma*, 2nd ed. Philadelphia, Elsevier/Saunders, 2004.

femoral artery can be cannulated with an arterial catheter, contrast injected, and images obtained either with plain films or fluoroscopy.[16–19] O'Gorman and colleagues[16,17] have demonstrated that the axillary artery can be visualized by injection of contrast into the brachial artery with distal outflow occlusion with a blood pressure cuff inflated to a level well beyond the systolic arterial blood pressure. A benefit of the recent popularity of endovascular techniques has been increased availability of formal arteriography in the operating room. In fact, some centers have the capability of embolization of pelvic or visceral vessels in the operating room, thereby precluding the need to transport an unstable patient to a radiology suite that may not have the resources of the operating room.

SPECIFIC AREAS OF INJURY

Each of the major anatomical areas presents some unique symptoms or requirements for diagnostic screening for vascular injury. These areas are the neck, chest, abdomen, and extremities.

Cervical vascular trauma may be manifested by initial signs of external hemorrhage, expanding hematoma[16] or ipsilateral hemispheric ischemic symptoms, including hemiplegia, hemiparesis, or monocular blindness. The latter neurologic symptoms must be assumed to result from carotid artery interruption or thrombosis until proven otherwise. Deficits resulting from cranial nerves IX, X, XI, and/or XII suggest the possibility of vascular injury because of their immediate proximity to the carotid artery and the jugular vein. Penetrating trauma is associated with hemorrhage or false aneurysms, whereas blunt trauma invariably produces symptoms through thrombosis. This can be either immediate or delayed. In cases of major neck trauma, duplex scanning has greatly facilitated screening for intimal disruption or dissection, and some institutions use it liberally. CT angiography has recently been established as a viable alternative to formal angiography in the screening of blunt carotid injury as well as in the assessment of penetrating neck injury.[8,9,11,] Formal angiography should still be considered the gold standard, and is required in equivocal cases as well as the occasional patient who requires embolization of a disrupted vertebral artery.

Thoracic great vessel injuries are those to the arteries at the base of the neck and the thoracic aorta. As is true of all penetrating trauma, massive hemorrhage is the usual manifestation of injury to any one or more of these vessels. In this instance, immediate operation is indicated, with location based on the presumed path of the missile, location of the stab wound, and/or chest x-ray. Because of the significance of delayed diagnosis, most patients who are stable and have penetrating injuries of the base of the neck should be evaluated with arteriography. CT angiography is an appropriate alternative in centers with late-generation multidetector/high-resolution CT scanners, and where appropriate radiologic expertise is readily available. Blunt trauma, particularly from deceleration injuries, is associated with traumatic rupture. As opposed to smaller vessels, subclavian, innominate, and aortic injuries are rarely associated with thrombotic symptoms, even though there has been intimal disruption. The primary problem relates to gross vessel disruption. Complete separation is rarely if ever a clinical problem, as death is usually instantaneous. Surviving patients manifest vascular injury by the presence of false aneurysms, mediastinal or cervical hematomas, or apical capping. CT scanning has been an excellent screening tool for these injuries. However, unless vessel disruption is demonstrated, arteriography should follow the demonstration of hematomas, as many of these are associated with small vessel disruption that does not require surgery.

Abdominal vascular injuries after penetrating trauma invariably are associated with hemorrhage. Because laparotomy is indicated for almost all gunshot wounds of the lower chest and abdomen and all stab wounds associated with blood loss, the diagnosis of arterial or venous injury is usually made at the time of operation. Because of the relatively protected nature of the abdominal great vessels, blunt traumatic injuries are quite rare, and when present are manifested by weak or absent femoral pulses. For the reasons given previously, special diagnostic studies are rarely necessary when dealing with abdominal vascular trauma. CT scanning is used frequently to assess the source of ongoing hemorrhage but is of greater value in identifying specific organ injury rather than major vascular injury. Notable exceptions that may require arteriography are unstable pelvic fractures with evidence of ongoing bleeding. Arteriography may be indicated to assess the internal iliac vessels and treat the bleeding embolically. There may be a role for CT angiography in patients with unstable pelvic fractures from blunt trauma to identify suspect areas to target for subsequent embolization; often the CT can be obtained while awaiting setup of the angiography suite. Further, additional intra-abdominal and pelvic injuries may be delineated and 3D information obtained regarding the pelvic fracture pattern.

Extremity vascular injuries lend themselves to the diagnostic and screening maneuvers described in the previous sections. These patients fall into three general categories: (1) patients with evidence of pulselessness/ischemia, active bleeding, or a pulsatile hematoma; (2) patients with hard signs and a palpable pulse; and (3) patients with soft signs or an injury known to be associated with vascular injury. Initially, all patients should be adequately resuscitated and undergo reduction and stabilization of associated dislocations and fractures. Perfusion should be reassessed after these initial measures. In some cases, perfusion normalizes, and subsequent workup can proceed more deliberately. Ongoing assessment of patients with suspected extremity vascular injuries is outlined in Figure 1 and in the following discussion.

In the first category, patients with evidence of pulselessness/ischemia, active bleeding, or a pulsatile hematoma, urgent attention is required to prevent exsanguination or tissue necrosis from ischemia. Generally, these patients should be taken promptly to the operating room. If ischemia is complete, such as with a tourniquet, muscle necrosis will result from 4 hours of ischemia; fortunately, there is often some collateral flow that extends this critical time period. In most cases, the location of injury is apparent from the history, physical, and preliminary plain films; operative intervention can proceed accordingly. In other situations, the exact location and degree of injury are not apparent (Table 2). To minimize the duration of warm ischemia, on-table angiography can be performed. In some centers, formal angiography is available in the operating room.

Patients in the second category manifest hard signs, but do not demonstrate evidence of active bleeding or absence of perfusion. These patients can undergo a more deliberate, albeit expedient, assessment. Often the location and extent of injury is delineated with formal angiography. More recently, enthusiasm for CT angiography has grown. An advantage of formal angiography is the ability to perform therapeutic endovascular interventions such as embolization of muscular bleeders, or to control pseudoaneurysms or AV fistulas. As mentioned, in some cases associated injuries warrant urgent operative intervention before angiography can be obtained. In these cases, on-table angiography or formal angiography in the operating room are viable alternatives.

The final category involves patients with suspected extremity vascular injuries who present with soft signs only. Much of the controversy regarding evaluation of vascular trauma concerns this category. In patients with an injury in proximity to a major artery (although without hard signs), radiologic abnormalities may be present in as many as 10% of patients who undergo arteriography. However, a much smaller proportion of patients require operative intervention—several series indicate a range of 0.6%–4.4% of patients. Dennis and colleagues have made a cogent argument in support of physical examination alone in this patient population.[20] They argue that patients requiring operative intervention will be identified from subsequent development of hard signs. Typically, patients are admitted for a short period of observation. Concerns regarding poor patient compliance for follow-up and a push to expeditiously identify significant injuries early (ideally, shortly after presentation to the emergency room to

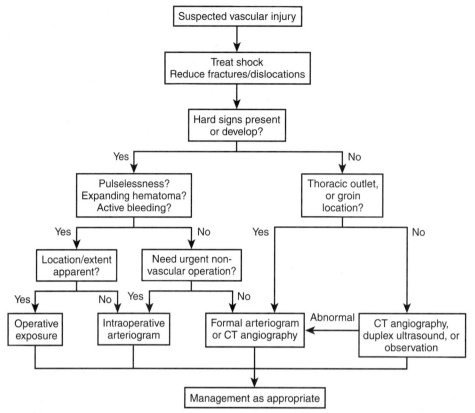

Figure 1 Algorithm: evaluation of extremity trauma. *(Modified from Anderson JT, Blaisdell FW: Diagnosis of vascular trauma. In Rich N, Mattox KL, Hirshberg A, editors: Vascular Trauma, 2nd ed. Philadelphia, Elsevier/Saunders, 2004.)*

Table 2: Indications for Arteriography: Extremity Trauma

Unclear location or extent of vascular injury
Extensive soft tissue injury
Fracture or dislocation
Trajectory parallel to an artery
Multiple wounds
Gunshot injuries
Peripheral vascular disease

From Anderson JT, Blaisdell FW: Diagnosis of vascular trauma. In Rich N, Mattox KL, Hirshberg A, editors: *Vascular Trauma*, 2nd ed. Philadelphia, Elsevier/Saunders, 2004.

guide appropriate disposition) have led many others to use alternative protocols involving ultrasonography or CT imaging. Ultimately, the choice is often determined by cost, availability of modalities, center volume/resources, and local expertise.

Although injuries to any of the two lower arm or three lower leg vessels can result in bleeding that requires treatment, for the most part, unless clinical symptoms point to the need for intervention, operation is rarely indicated and screening for injury is not indicated. These vessels have abundant collateral flow, so injury that results in occlusion to any one of them is rarely symptomatic, and hemorrhage from a disrupted vessel usually stops spontaneously.

Two scenarios that require mention are patients with a posterior knee dislocation and patients with an injury in the region of the groin or thoracic outlet. Unrecognized popliteal injuries can lead to delayed thrombosis and severe distal ischemia because of poor collateral flow about the knee. For this reason dislocations of the knee and major fractures of the supracondylar and proximal tibial areas should have vascular screening. The minimal comprises duplex assessment and/or vigilant observation/examination, and the more optimal, angiographic imaging. An additional critical area relates to the profunda femoral artery that is buried deep in the thigh, and may be responsible for deep hemorrhage and hematomas that require intervention. When there is any question regarding injury, femoral arteriography is the best screening method and lends itself to embolic treatment of distal bleeding (proximal injuries are best exposed and repaired). In the absence of hard signs of vascular injury, patients with injuries in the region of the groin, thoracic outlet, or neck generally should be evaluated with either formal angiography or CT angiography. Duplex ultrasonography of the subclavian and iliac vessels is generally limited. Prompt evaluation is mandatory, as missed vascular injuries in these regions may lead to exsanguination into the intrapleural or retroperitoneal space.

ACKNOWLEDGMENT

This chapter is adapted from Anderson JT, Blaisdell FW: Diagnosis of vascular trauma. In Rich N, Mattox KL, Hirshberg A, editors: *Vascular Trauma*, 2nd ed. Philadelphia, Elsevier/Saunders, 2004.

REFERENCES

1. Johansen K, Lynch K, Paun M, Copass M: Non-invasive vascular tests reliably exclude occult arterial trauma in injured extremities. *J Trauma* 31(4): 515–519, discussion 519–522, 1991.
2. Fry WR, Smith RS, Sayers DV, et al: The success of duplex ultrasonographic scanning in diagnosis of extremity vascular proximity trauma [see comments]. *Arch Surg* 128(12):1368–1372, 1993.

3. Ginzburg E, Montalvo B, LeBlang S, Nunez D, Martin L: The use of duplex ultrasonography in penetrating neck trauma. *Arch Surg* 131(7):691–693, 1996.
4. Knudson MM, Lewis FR, Atkinson K, Neuhaus A: The role of duplex ultrasound arterial imaging in patients with penetrating extremity trauma. *Arch Surg* 128(9):1033–1037, discussion 1037–1038, 1993.
5. Meissner M, Paun M, Johansen K: Duplex scanning for arterial trauma. *Am J Surg* 161(5):552–555, 1991.
6. Busquets AR, Acosta JA, Colon E, Alejandro KV, Rodriguez P: Helical computed tomographic angiography for the diagnosis of traumatic arterial injuries of the extremities. *J Trauma* 56:625–628, 2004.
7. Inaba K, Potzman J, Munera F, et al: Multi-slice CT angiography for arterial evaluation in the injured lower extremity. *J Trauma* 60:502–506, discussion 506–507, 2006.
8. Munera F, Soto JA, Palacio DM, et al: Penetrating neck injuries: helical CT angiography for initial evaluation. *Radiology* 224:366–372, 2002.
9. Nunez DB Jr, Torres-Leon M, Munera F: Vascular injuries of the neck and thoracic inlet: helical CT-angiographic correlation. *Radiographics* 24:1087–1098, discussion 1099–1100, 2004.
10. Soto JA, Munera F, Cardoso N, Guarin O, Medina S: Diagnostic performance of helical CT angiography in trauma to large arteries of the extremities. *J Comput Assist Tomogr* 23:188–196, 1999.
11. Utter GH, Hollingworth W, Hallam DK, Jarvik JG, Jurkovich GJ: Sixteen-slice CT angiography in patients with suspected blunt carotid and vertebral artery injuries. *J Am Coll Surg* 203:838–848, 2006.
12. Miller-Thomas MM, West OC, Cohen AM: Diagnosing traumatic arterial injury in the extremities with CT angiography: pearls and pitfalls. *Radiographics* 25(Suppl 1):S133–S142, 2005.
13. Melton SM, Kerby JD, McGiffin D, et al: The evolution of chest computed tomography for the definitive diagnosis of blunt aortic injury: a single-center experience. *J Trauma* 56:243–250, 2004.
14. Chen MY, Miller PR, McLaughlin CA, Kortesis BG, Kavanagh PV, Dyer RB: The trend of using computed tomography in the detection of acute thoracic aortic and branch vessel injury after blunt thoracic trauma: single-center experience over 13 years. *J Trauma* 56:783–785, 2004.
15. Snyder WH 3rd, Thal ER, Bridges RA, Gerlock AJ, Perry MO, Fry WJ: The validity of normal arteriography in penetrating trauma. *Arch Surg* 113(4):424–426, 1978.
16. O'Gorman RB, Feliciano DV: Arteriography performed in the emergency center. *Am J Surg* 152(3):323–325, 1986.
17. O'Gorman RB, Feliciano DV, Bitondo CG, Mattox KL, Burch JM, Jordan GL Jr: Emergency center arteriography in the evaluation of suspected peripheral vascular injuries. *Arch Surg* 119(5):568–573, 1984.
18. Pecunia RA, Raves JJ: A technique for evaluation of the injured extremity with single film exclusion arteriography. *Surg Gynecol Obstet* 170(5):448–450, 1990.
19. Ramanathan A, Perera DS, Sheriffdeen AH: Emergency femoral arteriography in lower limb vascular trauma. *Ceylon Med J* 40(3):105–106, 1995.
20. Dennis JW, Frykberg ER, Veldenz HC, Huffman S, Menawat SS: Validation of nonoperative management of occult vascular injuries and accuracy of physical examination alone in penetrating extremity trauma: 5- to 10-year follow-up. *J Trauma* 44(2):243–252, discussion 242–243, 1998.

UPPER EXTREMITY VASCULAR TRAUMA

Margaret M. Griffen   and   Eric R. Frykberg

Trauma to the upper extremities can have devastating results. The experience of wartime has taught many lessons about etiology, diagnosis, and treatment of upper extremity injury. Understanding the lessons learned from history provides the basis for treatment today.

Hemorrhage from injured blood vessels has been a well-known consequence of injury for several millennia. The diagnosis was made even in ancient times, but the treatment options were limited. Styptics were prepared from vegetable or mineral material and applied to bleeding vessels. Archigenes first advocated amputation of gangrenous extremities above the line of demarcation with linen ligatures placed on the vessels in the first century ACE.[1] Celsus records the first account of vessel ligation to establish hemostasis in 25 ACE[1]. These ancient recommendations were lost in later centuries, and mass cautery became the standard practice for extremity hemorrhage control until the late 1400s. Ambroise Pare reestablished the technique of amputation above the line of demarcation with linen ligatures of the injured vessels in 1552.[1] The tourniquet was introduced in 1674 by Morel. Direct vessel ligation was the treatment of choice by the 19th century, but the results were often disappointing. There was a 100% mortality associated with ligation of the aorta in 10 patients, a 77% mortality with ligation of the common iliac artery in 68 patients, and in 31 patients a 40% mortality when the femoral artery was ligated.[2]

The first known successful repair of an injured artery was performed in 1759 by Hallowell.[3] In 1889, Jassinowsky performed arterial reconstruction in animals and proved that interrupted silk sutures could successfully repair the carotid artery.[4] Murphy in Chicago was the first to successfully perform an end-to-end anastomosis on a femoral artery in 1897. He had firm beliefs that successful repair in vascular trauma required complete asepsis, atraumatic technique, temporary clamping of the vessel, accurate approximation, and meticulous hemostasis and cleansing of the wound.[2,3] Carrel and Guthrie described the basic techniques still used today for end-to-end anastomosis and lateral suture during the early 1900s. The use of veins as conduits for repair or bypass of arterial vessels was reported by Goyanes (1906) and Lexer (1907).[3,4] The unacceptably high thrombosis rate of these repair techniques precluded their widespread use.

World War I provided an opportunity to use the newly developed techniques for acute arterial repair. Over 100 successful repairs were documented, but the overall incidence of infection and secondary hemorrhage resulted in continued use of ligation as the preferred battlefield technique. Repair of pseudoaneurysms and arteriovenous fistulas identified after the acute period in wounded survivors of combat injuries had reasonable success at this time.

DeBakey and Simeone[5] published the management results of 2471 combat arterial injuries in World War II in 1946. Ligation continued to be the primary treatment during this conflict. However, 81 cases of suture repair were performed with an overall lower amputation rate, 35.8% versus 49%, when compared with ligation. This was perhaps the first indication that suture repair could be successful and improve outcome. Other factors stressed in the report included meticulous technique, wound debridement, delayed primary closure, and antibiotic use.

The Korean War began with a similar plan toward arterial injury. Patients were arriving at care facilities earlier than in any prior war because of improved evacuation techniques. An aggressive approach was then adopted, and surgical research teams were developed in both the Army and Navy to demonstrate the feasibility of acute arterial repair in wartime. Hughes (1958), Jahnke and Seeley (1953),

Shannon and Howard (1955), and Spencer and Grewe (1955) then presented successful data. The amputation rate dropped to 13% in Hughes's series after most patients had suture repair of their injuries.[6]

These wartime advances in vascular injury treatment crossed over into the civilian sector during the 1950s. Ferguson et al.[7] reported their success with suture repair of civilian arterial injuries from 1950 to 1959. Their amputation rate of 13.6% compared well with the military experience. Early diagnosis and treatment, debridement of devitalized vessel, intimal approximation, and achievement of distal pulses were considered vital to the success of arterial repair.

The Vietnam War provided further opportunity for advancement in the treatment of acute arterial injury. A vascular registry was established at Walter Reed hospital to track soldiers with arterial injuries. The patients were again evacuated quickly, and over 98% of 1000 patients reported by Rich et al.[8] underwent arterial repair. The amputation rate once again was 13.5% and consistent with the Korean War experience, despite more severe injuries encountered.

Since then, further advancement in the diagnosis and management of acute vascular injury has come from the civilian experience, and has been extrapolated to recent wars in the Middle East. Repair of the acute arterial injury is now the treatment of choice with several options to complete that plan. Newer techniques are now being developed to allow for endovascular repair of some upper extremity vascular injuries.

The focus of this chapter will be on vascular injury to the upper extremity. The anatomy of the upper extremity, the etiology of these injuries, their evaluation and diagnostic strategies, and finally treatment options will be discussed.

INCIDENCE

The overall incidence of vascular injury is quite low among all extremity injuries in both civilian and military settings. Beebe and DeBakey[9] reported a 0.25% incidence of arterial injury among all wounds in American troops in World War I. DeBakey and Simeone[5] reported a 0.96% incidence of arterial injury in World War II. The data on vascular trauma in the civilian population reported by Oller et al.[10] shows a 3.7% incidence of vascular trauma among 1148 injuries in over 26,000 patients in a state registry. The overall incidence of upper extremity vascular trauma is also low. Pillai et al. reported 21 (3.3%) arterial injuries in 643 cases of upper-extremity trauma.[11] However, the extremities are the most common site of vascular injury. Rich et al.[8] found that 93% of all vascular injuries occurred in the extremities of American casualties in the Vietnam War. The relative incidence of vascular injury in upper versus lower extremities varies according to the series reviewed. Civilian series demonstrate upper extremity vascular injury incidence between 17% and 53%, as compared with lower extremity involvement, but when series are combined the incidence is almost equal (Table 1).

Most upper extremity vascular injuries involve the arterial system, including the subclavian, axillary, brachial, ulnar, and radial arteries (Table 2). Associated bone, nerve, and soft tissue injuries also occur and substantially impact ultimate outcome. As in much of trauma, vascular injury to the upper extremity is mainly a disease of young males. Subclavian arterial injury accounts for 3%–9% of all vascular extremity injuries. The brachial artery is the most commonly injured vessel in the upper extremity. Brachial artery injury ranges from 12%–48% of all extremity vascular traumas and radial and ulnar artery injury among all upper extremity vascular traumas is 16%–17% (see Table 2).

MECHANISM OF INJURY

Penetrating trauma is the most common mechanism in upper extremity vascular injury. A penetrating mechanism of injury in military series is greater than 90% routinely, and consists of explosive shrapnel and high-velocity gunshot wounds. Civilian series demonstrate a penetrating mechanism for extremity vascular trauma in approximately 70%–85% of cases (Table 3). Blunt trauma comprises

Table 1: Location of Extremity Vascular Trauma

References	Extremity Injuries	Upper Extremity	Lower Extremity
Oller 1992[10]	632	361	271
Yupu 1993[33]	166	88	78
van Wijngaarden 1993[34]	106	20	86
Razmadze 1999[30]	157	62	95
Rozycki 2003[25]	93	16	77
Diamond 2003[29]	56	28	28
Total	1210	575	635

Table 2: Vessels Involved with Upper Extremity Vascular Trauma

References	Upper Extremity Injuries	Subclavian	Axillary	Brachial	Ulnar	Radial	Radial/Ulnar	Venous
Borman 1984[22]	298	0	59	126	48	65	0	0
Sitzmann 1984[15]	107	13	7	16	29	30	12	0
Orcutt 1986[16]	163	0	20	78	30	22	0	13
Cikrit 1990[21]	101	13	0	23	25	40	0	0
Myers 1990[24]	123	6	5	22	26	20	16	28
Fitridge 1994[28]	114	16	12	62	0	0	24	0
Sriussadaporn 1997[17]	28	6	10	12	0	0	0	0
Pillai 1997[11]	21	3	5	10	0	3	0	0
Manord 1998[32]	45	18	19	5	0	0	0	3
Wali 2002[23]	27	1	2	11	5	2	5	1
Total	1027	76	139	365	163	182	57	45

approximately 15%–30% of extremity vascular trauma seen in the civilian population (Table 4).

Of all penetrating extremity injuries, the most recent civilian data show stabbings to be the most common with gunshot wounds second. Other sources of penetrating trauma include glass, industrial/ farming incidence, and shotgun blasts (Table 5). Military series include high-velocity mechanisms of penetrating trauma from gunshots, bombs, and mine explosions. The high-velocity mechanism of military weapons may account for more extensive associated injuries, similar to blunt trauma.

McKinley et al.[12] collected data on 260 patients over a 19-year period with proximal axillary and subclavian artery injuries; only 11 patients had a blunt mechanism for their injury. In this study, stab wounds accounted for 82% of the penetrating trauma,[12] while Lin et al.[13] reviewed penetrating trauma to the subclavian artery and found gunshot wounds (85%) to be the most prevalent wounding agent. Demetriades et al.[14] reviewed their data for subclavian and axillary penetrating injuries and again gunshots were the most common mechanism.

DIAGNOSIS

All cases of extremity trauma should be fully examined to assess any immediate threats to life or limb. Airway, breathing, and circulation must be evaluated in each patient and all life-threatening

problems addressed. Specific examination of an injured upper extremity should first address the possibility of vascular injury, as this represents the greatest threat to limb salvage. This includes inspection for external bleeding, palpation for pain, temperature and instability, assessment of the pulses in each extremity, and a full sensory and motor examination with documentation of findings.

Patients with acute vascular injury to the upper extremity will present in a number of ways. The "hard signs" of vascular trauma include pulsatile bleeding; large, expanding, or pulsatile hematomas; palpable thrill; audible bruit; and/or evidence of regional ischemia (the 6 Ps of pain, pallor, pulselessness, paralysis, paresthesias, and poikilothermy, or coolness). Patients who present with one or more of these signs have a high risk of vascular injury requiring surgical repair, and vascular injury must be ruled out as a first priority. After uncomplicated penetrating trauma, the presence of one or more hard signs mandates immediate surgical exploration because of a probability of major vascular injury that approaches 100%. After blunt or complex penetrating limb trauma, when the presence or location of a vascular injury is not clear by physical examination, hard signs mandate immediate imaging to confirm injury, as these signs do not reliably predict vascular injury in this setting.

Ischemic changes were associated with absent pulses in over 70% of patients with upper extremity vascular trauma.[15–17] Hematomas

Table 3: Mechanism for Extremity Vascular Trauma

References	Extremity Injuries	Penetrating Mechanism	Blunt Mechanism
Borman 1984[22]	269	250	19
Orcutt 1986[16]	143	134	9
Cikrit 1990[21]	101	94	7
Myers 1990[24]	80	58	22
Oller 1992[10]	843	560	283
Yupu 1993[33]	148	107	41
Fitridge 1994[28]	114	62	52
Sriussadaporn 1997[17]	28	12	16
Manord 1998[32]	46	28	18
Demetriades 1999[14]	79	79	0
McKinley 2000[12]	260	249	11
Wali 2002[23]	27	16	11
Rozycki 2003[25]	93	0	93
Lin 2003[13]	54	54	0
Total	2285	1703	582

Table 4: Blunt Mechanisms for Extremity Vascular Trauma

References	Blunt Extremity Injuries	Motor Vehicle Collision	Motorcycle Collision	Industrial	Crush	Fall	Pedestrian	Elbow Dislocation	Humerus Fracture	Bike	Struck
Cikrit (1990[21]	7	2	0	1	0	1	0	2	1	0	0
Myers 1990[24]	22	13	0	7	0	2	0	0	0	0	0
Oller 1992[10]	270	139	17	43	10	18	24	0	0	3	16
Fitridge 1994[28]	47	47	0	0	0	0	0	0	0	0	0
Sriussadaporn 1997[17]	16	3	12	0	0	0	1	0	0	0	0
Wali 2002[23]	11	9	0	0	0	2	0	0	0	0	0
Rozycki 2003[25]	62	23	7	0	9	3	18	0	0	2	0
Total	435	236	36	51	19	26	43	2	1	5	16

Table 5: Penetrating Mechanisms for Extremity Vascular Trauma

References	Penetrating Extremity Injuries	Gunshot Wound	Stab	Shotgun	Glass	Machine	Angiogram	Laceration
Orcutt 1986[16]	134	47	69	0	7	0	11	0
Cikrit 1990[21]	94	12	15	8	15	0	0	44
Myers 1990[24]	54	7	7	4	29	0	6	1
Oller 1992[10]	432	135	203	56	0	38	0	0
Yupu 1993[33]	107	26	62	0	0	19	0	0
Fitridge 1994[28]	60	12	0	0	32	16	0	0
Sriussadaporn 1997[17]	12	4	8	0	0	0	0	0
Manord 1998[32]	28	17	7	4	0	0	0	0
Demetriades 1999[14]	58	58	0	0	0	0	0	0
McKinley 2000[12]	249	27	214	8	0	0	0	0
Wali 2002[23]	16	3	6	0	4	3	0	0
Lin 2003[13]	54	46	5	3	0	0	0	0
Total	1298	394	596	83	87	76	17	45

and bruits were less common than other hard signs. Neurologic deficits are common, but these should not always be attributed to nerve damage unless they persist after vascular repair, or a damaged nerve is directly visualized, as vascular insufficiency itself can give rise to these findings.

Noninvasive tests have been used to evaluate injured extremities for potential vascular injury, and include ankle:brachial pressure readings and duplex ultrasound. Limitations to this technology include the inability to provide the skilled individuals 24/7, and the lack of demonstrated reliability in complex injuries with large hematomas and bulky dressings. Johansen and colleagues[18] have found the ankle:brachial index (ABI) to have a high sensitivity and diagnostic accuracy for vascular injury. Duplex scanning combines B-mode ultrasound and Doppler technology to allow both visual and auditory evaluation of the blood vessel. Bynoe et al.[19] found duplex scanning to be both sensitive and specific when used to evaluate 198 injured extremities for vascular injury, with 20 documented cases of vascular trauma. This technique requires a highly skilled individual to perform and interpret, and limited availability of personnel and access to the extremity involved can limit its usefulness.

Conventional contrast arteriography remains the gold standard for the evaluation of injured extremities for vascular trauma, and should only be performed in hemodynamically stable patients as it requires transport of the patient to the radiology suite. With newer techniques for treatment of some vascular injuries, arteriography may also be therapeutic, allowing such interventional techniques as embolization and endovascular stenting to be performed. For many years, simple proximity of any asymptomatic injury to a major extremity artery mandated arteriography. Frykberg et al.[20] demonstrated a 10.5% incidence of injury in penetrating trauma when vessel proximity to an injury was the only indication for arteriography, although all injuries were nonocclusive with a largely benign natural history.[20] They concluded that in the absence of hard signs, proximity alone should not be an indication for arterial imaging or investigation. Certainly high-velocity penetrating mechanisms or complex blunt mechanisms may justify more liberal use of imaging.[11] Civilian studies currently demonstrate that 18%–57% of patients with extremity vascular trauma have arteriography performed preoperatively.[11,17,21–25] Complications from arteriography occur 2%–4% of the time, although major complications typically occur in far less than 1% of cases. Arteriography can also be performed more quickly, safely and cheaply in the emergency center or operating room by direct arterial injection of contrast by the surgeon.

Anatomic Location of Injury and Injury Grading

Knowledge of the anatomic structure of the upper extremity provides the clinician with the tools necessary to make informed decisions about treatment options. The arterial supply to the upper extremities includes multiple branches that provide excellent collateral circulation. The location of these branches in association to injury location can greatly affect the treatment options. The proximity of veins, nerves, and bone in the upper extremity explains the high incidence of associated injuries when arterial injury occurs.

The right subclavian artery originates from the innominate artery, while the left subclavian artery originates from the aortic arch. The subclavian vessel on both sides terminates at the lateral border of the first rib. The subclavian artery is typically divided into three portions according to the vessel location and the anterior scalene muscle location. The first portion is medial to the anterior scalene muscle and several branches originate from it. The vertebral artery arises first from the subclavian artery and travels cephalad to the transverse foramen of C6. The thyrocervical trunk is usually near the medial border of the anterior scalene and the inferior thyroid, transverse cervical, and transverse scapular branches arise from it. Inferiorly the internal mammary artery arises to course along the underside of the sternum. The second portion of the subclavian artery is located posterior to the anterior scalene, which separates it from the subclavian vein, and gives rise to the costocervical trunk. The third portion of the subclavian artery is lateral to the anterior scalene muscle and typically has no branches. The subclavian vein lies anterior to the anterior scalene muscle but in close proximity to the artery. The trunks of the brachial plexus lie posterior to the anterior scalene muscle and posterior to the subclavian artery but in close proximity.

The axillary artery begins lateral to the first rib and ends at the inferior border of the teres major muscle. The axillary artery is also divided into three portions. The first lies between the first rib and the upper border of the pectoralis minor muscle, and the supreme thoracic branch originates from the portion. The second part runs behind the pectoralis minor muscle and gives off the thoraco-acromial and the lateral thoracic branches. The final portion of the axillary artery extends from the inferior border of the pectoralis minor to lower border of the pectoralis major. Three branches arise from this final portion: subscapular, anterior circumflex humeral, and posterior circumflex humeral arteries. All the branches provide abundant circulation to the muscles of the shoulder and chest region, and to the bony structures of the shoulder and upper arm. The cords of the brachial plexus are in close proximity to the axillary artery. The axillary vein runs anterior to the axillary artery.

The brachial artery begins at the inferior border of the teres major and extends to just below the antecubital fossa. The first branch, the profunda, extends posteriorly through the medial and long heads of the triceps muscle along with the radial nerve to supply the posterior compartment. The superior ulnar collateral artery courses medially along with the ulnar nerve to supply a portion of the posterior compartment. A final branch, the inferior ulnar collateral, travels toward the medial epicondyle of the elbow. The median nerve follows the path of the brachial artery as it travels to the elbow. The brachial artery follows the inner border of the biceps muscle as it extends down the arm. Two brachial veins, venae comitantes, accompany the brachial artery. Extensive collateral circulation at the elbow is a result of the anastomosis of the branches of the brachial artery with inferior vessels.

The brachial artery terminates just below the elbow and divides into the radial and ulnar arteries. The ulnar artery is the larger of the two vessels. It branches into the anterior and posterior ulnar recurrent arteries and the common interosseous artery, which gives off the interosseous recurrent artery. These branches anastomose with the superior and inferior ulnar collaterals to provide extensive collateral blood flow. The ulnar nerve follows the path of the ulnar artery. The radial artery is smaller than the ulnar and is more superficial in the arm. Early in its course it gives off the radial recurrent branch, and later two branches arise along its course. The median runs down the center of the lower arm and is superficial in the lower third of the forearm. The superficial branch of the radial nerve, which is sensory only, runs along with the radial artery while the deep portion runs posteriorly. The palmar arch completes the arterial supply and is formed by the radial artery and the deep branch of the ulnar artery. This arch is an important anatomical consideration and is incomplete in 20% of people.

The innermost layer of the artery and vein is the intima, which consists of endothelial cells. Smooth muscle and elastic fibers make up the middle layer or media and the outer layer is the adventitia, which consists of connective tissue. Forces placed on the vessels will result in a variety of injury patterns. The particular injury will influence the way the patient presents with the injury and how a diagnosis may need to be made. The force of the wounding agent will also affect the extent of the injury and the options available for treatment. High-velocity gunshot wounds can cause significant soft tissue damage and disrupt more than the primary vessels but the collaterals as well. In fact, the blast effect from high velocity weapons can damage vessels even without directly hitting them.[3]

Lacerations and transections are the most common types of extremity vascular injury (Figure 1). A full-thickness tear in the wall

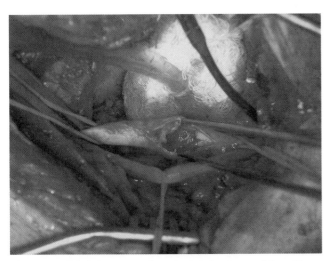

Figure 1 Subclavian artery thrombosis in intact vessel from blast effect after gunshot wound in right shoulder, showing the raised intimal flap causing the thrombosis.

with the vessel still intact is a laceration and can often be repaired by simple lateral suture. Hemorrhage is typically more pronounced with a laceration because the smooth muscle contracts and keeps the vessel open. These injuries may present a diagnostic dilemma because the pulse may be intact distal to the injury. A transection is a full-thickness cut through the vessel with disruption of the vessel. The ends of the vessel tend to constrict and bleeding will stop. Loss of the distal pulse with ischemia to the extremity is usually evident. The extent of the surrounding tissue destruction and or vessel loss will influence treatment strategies.

Contusions to blood vessels account for less than 10% of all vascular trauma. If the bruising with associated hematoma is in the adventitia it is of little consequence. Subintimal or intimal contusions can cause thrombosis of the vessel as they may partially occlude the vessel with a flap. Patients may present with a pulse and no immediate evidence of ischemia, and then have it develop over time. The index of suspicion for such injuries must be high, and aggressive observation should be applied. Contusion of vessels is more common in blunt trauma related to the stretching of the vessel.

Finally, if the surrounding soft tissues contain the bleeding from an injured vessel, a pseudoaneurysm or arteriovenous fistula may arise. Pulses may be intact, and so the diagnosis is sometimes hard to make. When found at the time of surgery these injuries are treated with resection and repair. The more chronic they become, the more complications may occur from direct pressure and erosion into surrounding structures, or delayed rupture and hemorrhage. Surgical repair of these chronic lesions is also more difficult than injuries found acutely. McKinley[12] reported transection and false aneurysm to be the two most common types of injury found in the subclavian and axillary arteries.

SURGICAL MANAGEMENT

The hemodynamically unstable patient with an injured extremity and hard signs of vascular trauma should be resuscitated and proceed to the operating room for surgical exploration. In this setting any doubt about the presence of a vascular injury can be clarified by immediate operating room arteriography by the surgeon. Active bleeding should be controlled with digital pressure as the patient is resuscitated, transported, prepped, and draped. The specific surgical incisions for exposure of the vessels will depend on the location of the wound. The hemodynamically stable patient with penetrating extremity trauma and hard signs should also proceed directly to surgery once life-threatening problems have been addressed. Those stable patients with blunt or complex penetrating extremity trauma may undergo arterial imaging to determine their treatment plan.

Nonoperative management of asymptomatic and nonocclusive extremity vascular injuries is feasible and safe. Dennis et al.[26] prospectively followed 43 patients with intimal flaps, arterial narrowing or small false aneurysms, and arteriovenous fistulas that fulfilled their criteria for nonoperative management, and were successful in avoiding surgery in 89%. To date, all published reports of this management have documented similar success rates, and not a single instance of limb loss or limb morbidity has yet been reported.

Endovascular techniques have proven efficacy and safety in the definitive treatment of upper extremity vascular injuries. The subclavian and axillary arteries are the vessels most amenable to this approach. The morbidity associated with an open repair of these vessels can be avoided with endovascular stenting. A guidewire must be able to traverse the lesion in order for a stent to be placed and repair the injury. Xenos et al.[27] presented their experience with five endovascular stents placed for subclavian and axillary artery injuries. The complication rate and long-term patency were comparable to open surgical repair. The small numbers and absence of long-term follow-up mandate further study before this approach can be widely applied.

Surgical repair is the standard treatment for upper extremity vascular trauma after several decades of published experience. General principles of vascular surgery apply to the exposure, preparation and repair of the injured vessel. The injured extremity can provide obstacles to exposure and identification of vasculature. Proximal and distal control of the injured vessel must be established. A detailed inspection of the wound and determination of vessel loss and surrounding soft tissue injury is done. The subclavian artery and proximal axillary artery can be difficult to surgically expose. Demetriades et al.[14] reported the use of an infraclavicular incision with extension into the deltopectoral groove to approach over 50% of these injuries. Another 48% were successfully exposed by adding a sternotomy or thoracotomy to the infraclavicular incision. Lin et al.[13] exposed most injuries using a supraclavicular incision on the left and a median sternotomy with infraclavicular extension, when necessary, on the right. McKinley et al.[12] exposed most vascular injuries with a supraclavicular or limited sternotomy incision with sternoclavicular dislocation.

Several methods can then be employed to repair the blood vessel (Table 6). Lateral suture repair can be performed if a simple laceration without tissue loss is found and the vessel is still intact, although this is rarely feasible for the relatively small brachial, radial, and ulnar arteries, which also tend to spasm after injury and manipulation. Mobilization of the vessel with debridement of the ends and a primary end-to-end anastomosis can be performed on transected vessels. Recent studies show this is performed in up to 69% of cases.[13,15,17,21–23,28] Uncomplicated penetrating injuries are more amenable to primary vascular repair than are blunt or complex injuries.[17,23,28] An interposition graft may be needed if extensive vessel loss occurs or mobilization for primary repair may cause undue tension or require ligation of collateral vessels. An autogenous vein is the recommended conduit for interposition grafting, and is used in up to 82% of cases requiring grafts. Prosthetic grafts are preferable when adequate vein is not available, or in unstable patients with multiple associated injuries when time is critical (Figure 2). In these circumstances, the risk of infection is outweighed by these considerations. In reviewing their treatment of subclavian and axillary injuries, Demetriades et al.[14] and McKinley et al.[12] found that over 20 prosthetic grafts were necessary for repair. Primary end-to-end anastomosis was performed in approximately one-third of these cases, as was interposition vein graft. Prosthetic graft was used as frequently as vein graft by Demetriades et al.[12–14] Extra-anatomic bypass may be necessary when the native vascular bed is contaminated or involved in extensive tissue destruction, in which setting it is recommended that the graft be tunneled through uninvolved clean tissue planes. Externally stented prosthetic grafts should be used for this approach. Finally,

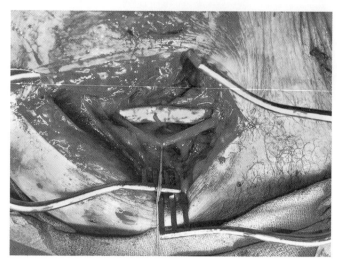

Figure 2 Subclavian artery repair after transection of injured area with interposition polytetrafluoroethylene (PTFE) graft.

ligation of the injured vessel may be a last-resort option in unstable patients with other life-threatening problems as a damage control measure. Temporary intraluminal arterial shunts are another option to allow limb salvage in these dire circumstances, as a means of maintaining extremity perfusion until the patient has been stabilized to the point that they may return to the operating room for definitive vascular repair. Ligation was used more frequently as management of radial and ulnar arterial injuries. Either artery may be ligated as long as the other is intact, and an intact palmar arch can be confirmed by performing an Allen test, or by observing brisk back-bleeding from the distal arterial segment.[13,15,20,28,29]

Fasciotomy may be necessary at the initial operation when prolonged ischemia or extensive soft tissue injury poses a high risk of compartment syndrome after reperfusion. The anatomy of the fascial compartments of the upper extremity must be understood to properly perform fasciotomy. In the postoperative period, serial clinical examinations, with compartment pressure measurements in suspicious cases, may demonstrate the need for fasciotomy.

Table 6: Surgical Procedures Performed to Repair Extremity Vascular Trauma

References	Extremity Injuries	Primary Repair	Vein Graft	Bypass Graft	Lateral Repair	Prosthetic Graft	Vein Patch	Ligation	Amputation	Endovascular
Borman 1984[22]	269	155	75	0	24	2	0	9	4	0
Sitzmann 1984[15]	107	62	19	0	8	0	0	18	0	0
Orcutt 1986[16]	158	76	33	0	16	1	1	31	0	0
Cikrit 1990[21]	100	54	26	0	0	0	3	17	0	0
Myers 1990[24]	123	74	44	0	0	5	0	0	0	0
Fitridge 1994[28]	107	26	50	0	0	0	13	14	4	0
Sruissadaporn 1997[17]	28	3	23	0	1	0	0	1	0	0
Pillai 1997[11]	20	2	16	0	0	0	0	2	0	0
Manord 1998[32]	45	19	25	0	0	0	0	1	0	0
Demetriades 1999[14]	100	33	18	0	0	22	0	26	0	1
McKinley 2000[12]	241	88	95	0	23	24	6	5	0	0
Wali 2002[23]	29	4	13	1	3	0	2	5	1	0
Lin 2003[13]	54	38	10	0	0	3	0	3	0	0
Total	1381	634	447	1	75	57	25	132	9	1

Primary amputation at the time of initial presentation may sometimes be an option to consider in patients with such severely injured upper extremities that prolonged and costly attempts at limb salvage are judged unlikely to succeed. The initial clinical examination is of major importance in this most difficult and challenging decision process, which should always involve the entire multidisciplinary team of trauma, vascular, plastic, and orthopedic surgeons. Most commonly a primary amputation is performed when the extremity is severely mangled without chance for recovery of limb function, and the potential for life-threatening complications related to attempted salvage are prohibitive. Primary amputation of the upper extremity is reported in up to 14% of cases of upper extremity trauma.[17,22,25,28,30] Secondary amputation is usually related to infectious complications from attempted salvage, and/or continued vascular, bony or soft tissue injury, or long-term disability from irreversible nerve injury and a nonfunctional extremity. Amputation of the upper extremity is less common than in lower extremity trauma, because of the more extensive collateral circulation, because problems with protective sensation, motor function and length discrepancy are easier to accommodate, and because limb prosthetics are not as advanced and useful.

MORBIDITY AND COMPLICATIONS MANAGEMENT

The loss of function of the upper extremity as a result of trauma is multifactorial. This multifactorial nature can influence recognition, evaluation, diagnosis, and treatment of upper extremity injury. Miller and Welch[31] specifically looked at limb loss as associated with ischemic times in canines with vascular disruption and reported a linear correlation between the time interval to revascularization and risk of limb loss. This correlation has since been confirmed in numerous experimental and clinical studies and emphasizes the essential importance of prompt diagnosis and treatment of vascular injuries. Associated subclavian vein and brachial plexus injury is high.[12,13] Associated nerve injury to the brachial plexus was identified in approximately 30% of patients in the previous series. Fitridge et al.[28] evaluated a patient population with a much higher blunt mechanism of injury to the subclavian and axillary vessels. Seventy-nine percent of their patients had associated major musculoskeletal trauma and only 32% of patients with subclavian/axillary vascular injuries had normal limb function after the 12-month follow-up. The extent of the nerve injury has a significant impact on the functional recovery of the extremity. Sitzmann et al.[15] had a lower incidence of associated nerve injury with brachial artery injury, whereas Cikrit et al.[21] reported a 65% incidence of associated nerve injury, which was the highest for all upper extremity vascular injuries in their series. Fitridge et al.[28] reported a 64% incidence of brachial plexus injury associated with subclavian/axillary arterial injuries, and only a 14% incidence of nerve injury associated with brachial artery injury. Associated nerve injury is found in as many as 58% of patients with radial and ulnar artery injury,[15] and the median nerve is most commonly injured. Late disability from upper extremity artery injury is related to the extent of nerve injury. Manord et al.[32] have shown that statistically significant recovery is possible, but continued disability is related to the extent of the initial nerve injury, which can be difficult to determine in the acute setting. Fracture of the distal humerus and proximal radius or ulna can be associated with brachial artery injury. Overall skeletal injury in association with an upper extremity vascular injury ranges from 11%–41%.[21,22,24,33]

MORTALITY

Experience from combat settings has shown that decreases in mortality correlate with decreased time from wounding to definitive care.[8] As time for evacuation went from 10 hours in World War II to 65 minutes in Vietnam, mortality among soldiers reaching medical care

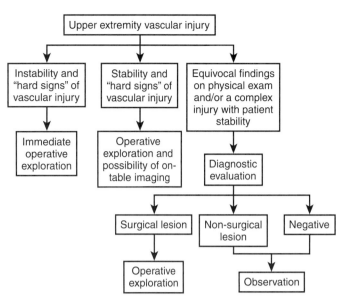

Figure 3 Algorithm for upper extremity vascular trauma.

alive dropped from 8% to 1.8%. Patients with injuries to the subclavian and axillary vessels presented in shock or with no signs of life in 23%–53% of cases.[12–15] Demetriades et al.[14] found isolated vein injuries in 20 patients, in whom the mortality was 50%, while isolated arterial injury resulted in a mortality rate of only 20%. In current civilian series, shock was seen in 15%–38% of patients with upper extremity vascular injury and is more commonly seen in patients with subclavian and axillary injuries.[14,15] Not surprisingly, patients presenting with shock had higher mortality.[13,14] Mortality associated with radial and ulnar vascular injury is low.

CONCLUSIONS AND ALGORITHM

Vascular injury to the upper extremity poses a variety of diagnostic and therapeutic challenges. Penetrating trauma is the most common mechanism. Diagnosis and most treatment decisions can often be made with clinical examination alone. Many diagnostic modalities are available for further evaluation of the extremity with equivocal findings. Nonoperative management is appropriate in certain situations but surgery remains the primary mode of treatment for upper extremity vascular trauma. Continued innovation in endovascular techniques will change the management strategies for certain extremity vascular injuries in the future. The functional recovery of a patient's upper extremity is related primarily to the associated neurologic injury and not the vascular injury. The algorithm in Figure 3 can be applied to upper extremity vascular trauma.

REFERENCES

1. Schwartz AM: The historical development of methods of hemostasis. *Surgery* 76:849–866, 1974.
2. Murphy JB: Resection of the arteries and veins injured in continuity—end-to-end suture—experimental clinical research. *Med Rec* 51:73–88, 1897.
3. Rich NM: Vascular trauma. *Surg Clin North Am* 53:1367–1392, 1973.
4. Dale WA: The beginnings of vascular surgery. *Surgery* 76:849–866, 1974.
5. DeBakey ME, Simeone FA: Battle injuries of the arteries in World War II: an analysis of 2,471 cases. *Ann Surg* 123:534–579, 1946.
6. Hughes CW: Arterial repair during the Korean War. *Ann Surg* 147:555–561, 1958.

7. Ferguson IA, Byrd WM, McAfee DK: Experiences in the management of arterial injuries. *Ann Surg* 153:980–986, 1961.
8. Rich NM, Baugh JH, Hughes CW: Acute arterial injuries in Vietnam: 1,000 cases. *J Trauma* 10:359–369, 1970.
9. Beebe GW, DeBakey ME: *Battle Casualties: Incidence, Mortality, and Logistic Considerations.* Charles C. Thomas, Springfield, IL, 1952.
10. Oller DW, Rutledge R, Clancy T, et al: Vascular injuries in a rural state: a review of 978 patients from a state trauma registry. *J Trauma* 32:740–746, 1992.
11. Pillai L, Luchette FA: Upper-extremity arterial injury. *Am Surg* 63:224–228, 1997.
12. McKinley AG, Carrim ATO, Robbs JV: Management of proximal axillary and subclavian artery injuries. *Br J Surg* 87:79–85, 2000.
13. Lin PH, Koffron AJ, Guske PJ, et al: Penetrating injuries of the subclavian artery. *Am J Surg* 185:580–584, 2003.
14. Demetriades D, Chahwan S, Gomez H, et al: Penetrating injuries to the subclavian and axillary vessels. *J Am Coll Surg.* 188:290–295, 1999.
15. Sitzmann JV, Ernst CB: Management of arm arterial injuries. *Surgery* 96:895–901, 1984.
16. Orcutt MB, Levine BA, Gaskill HV, et al: Civilian vascular trauma to the upper extremity. *J Trauma* 26:63–67, 1986.
17. Sriussadaporn S: Vascular injuries of the upper arm. *J Med Assoc Thai* 80:160–168, 1997.
18. Johansen K, Lynch K, Paun M et al: Non-invasive vascular tests reliably exclude occult arterial trauma in injured extremities. *J Trauma* 31:515–519, 1991.
19. Bynoe RP, Miles WAS, Bell RM, et al: Noninvasive diagnosis of vascular trauma by duplex ultrasonography. *J Vasc Surg* 14:346–352, 1991.
20. Frykberg ER, Crump JM, Vines FS, et al: A reassessment of the role of arteriography in penetrating proximity extremity trauma: a prospective study. *J Trauma* 29:1041–1050, 1989.
21. Cikrit DF, Dalsing MC, Bryant BJ, et al: An experience with upper-extremity vascular trauma. *Am J Surg* 160:229–233, 1990.
22. Borman KR, Snyder WH, Weigelt JA: Civilian arterial trauma of the upper extremity, an 11 year experience in 267 patients. *Am J Surg* 148:796–799, 1984.
23. Wali MA: Upper limb vascular trauma in the Asir region in Saudi Arabia. *Ann Thorac Cardiovasc Surg* 8:298–301, 2002.
24. Myers SI, Harward TRS, Maher DP, et al: Complex upper extremity vascular trauma in an urban population. *J Vasc Surg* 12:305–309, 1990.
25. Rozycki GS, Tremblay LN, Feliciano DV, et al: Blunt vascular trauma in the extremity: diagnosis, management and outcome. *J Trauma* 55: 814–824, 2003.
26. Dennis JW, Frykberg ER, Crump JM, et al: New perspectives on the management of penetrating trauma in proximity to major limb arteries. *J Vasc Surg.* 11:84–92, 1990.
27. Xenos ES, Freeman M, Steven S, et al: Covered stents for injuries of subclavian and axillary arteries. *J Vasc Surg.* 38:451–454, 2003.
28. Fitridge RA, Raptis S, Miller JH, et al: Upper extremity arterial injuries: experience at the Royal Adelaide Hospital, 1969 to 1991. *J Vasc Surg.* 20: 941–946, 1994.
29. Diamond S, Gaspard D, Katz S: Vascular injuries to the extremities in a suburban trauma center. *Am Surg.* 10:848–851, 2003.
30. Razmadze A: Vascular injuries of the limbs: a fifteen-year Georgian experience. *Eur J Vasc Endovasc Surg* 18:235–239, 1999.
31. Miller HH, Welch CS: Quantitative studies on the time factor in arterial injuries. *Ann Surg.* 130:428–438, 1949.
32. Manord JD, Garrard L, Kline DG, et al: Management of severe proximal vascular and neural injury of the upper extremity. *J Vasc Surg.* 27:43–49, 1998.
33. Yupu L, Yaotian H, Rensheng LL, et al: Management of major arterial injuries of limbs: a study of 166 cases. *Cardiovasc Surg* 1:486–488, 1993.
34. van Wijngaarden M, Omert L, Rodriguez A, et al: Management of blunt vascular trauma to the extremities. *Surg Gynecol Obstet.* 177:41–48.

LOWER EXTREMITY VASCULAR INJURIES: FEMORAL, POPLITEAL, AND SHANK VESSEL INJURY

Ziad C. Sifri,   Roxie Albrecht,   and   Juan A. Asensio

Lower extremity vascular injuries can be devastating and life threatening. The morbidity and mortality associated with these injuries are dependent on a multitude of factors, including the extent of injury, overall condition of the patient, and duration of ischemia. Deciding whether limb salvage is the optimal management for the injured patient requires good judgment. The initial decision to salvage the injured extremity depends on the ability of the patient to tolerate the procedure required to successfully repair the injury. It also depends on the likelihood of limb salvage as well as a satisfactory functional limb outcome. In the past, ligation of vascular injuries was often the approach taken to "save a life," and was favored because of a high amputation rate (up to 40%) reported when a surgical approach to repair the injuries was used.[1] Currently, the amputation rate in civilian trauma undergoing vascular repair is below 10% and this is not the preferred approach to manage extremity vascular injury. This reduction in the amputation rate over the past few decades has been attributed to a multitude of factors, including rapid transport time, improved prehospital care, soft tissue coverage, decreasing warm ischemia time (using the damage control approach and vascular shunt), low-velocity weapons, antibiotic utilization, and the early and aggressive use of fasciotomy.

This chapter's main focus is to illustrate a systematic approach to vascular injuries of the lower extremity, including diagnosis, indications for surgery, surgical approach and techniques for the repair of vascular injuries as well as common postoperative complications and outcomes after lower extremity vascular repairs.

INCIDENCE AND MECHANISM OF INJURY

Lower extremity vascular injuries occur most frequently in young men. In both the urban and rural setting, penetrating injuries to the extremity are the most common cause of peripheral vascular trauma. Penetrating injuries occur more commonly in the urban setting because of high levels of interpersonal violence and mostly result from gunshot wounds or stab wounds.[1] Blunt injuries occur more commonly in the rural setting because of a higher incidence of farming and industrial-type injuries. In part caused by a rise in urban violence and high-speed motor vehicles, the incidence of peripheral vascular trauma is increasing. Compared with other arterial injury, such as in the neck and chest, which may be rapidly fatal, most isolated peripheral vascular injuries are not immediately fatal and patients usually survive transportation to a medical center.[2] Extremity vascular injury accounts for up to 50% of all arterial injuries seen at civilian trauma centers. Although the exact incidence of peripheral vascular injuries is variable, upper and lower extremity vascular trauma has a similar incidence in an urban setting. Within the lower extremity, femoral arterial injuries are more common than popliteal injuries and account for up to 70% of all lower vascular injuries treated in urban trauma centers.[4–15]

DIAGNOSIS

The diagnosis of peripheral vascular trauma can usually be made based on a quick history and physical examination of the extremity, including a systematic and thorough neurovascular evaluation (Figure 1). There are a multitude of signs of vascular injury on examination. They are divided into hard and soft signs and reflect the likelihood that a significant vascular injury is present. Hard signs (Table 1) indicate a high likelihood that a significant vascular injury is present. Thus, patients with hard signs should be taken directly to the operating room to undergo immediate operative management.[2] Patients with soft signs of vascular injury (see Table 1) are less likely to have a significant vascular injury. This, however, must be confirmed using more invasive diagnostic modalities. Arteriography is currently the best available modality for the diagnosis of vascular injury in stable patients with soft signs of vascular injury but without evidence of peripheral ischemia. It can also be used in selected cases where the exact location of the injury is difficult to determine (e.g., pellet wounds or multiple gunshot wounds) and where the optimal incision and approach cannot be determined a priori. Arteriography can be performed in the angiography suite by an interventional radiologist or intraoperatively by the surgeon. It can be time consuming, but it is both sensitive and specific in the diagnosis of extremity vascular injury. Spiral computed tomographic angiography (CT-A) with the newest generation of high-speed scanner is an alternative diagnostic modality that has not yet been fully evaluated or widely accepted. It is rapid and does not require arterial catheterization. It does require contrast infusion, has no therapeutic potential, and can be limited by the artifacts generated if foreign bodies are present in the extremity.[2]

The types of arterial trauma that have been described include laceration, transection (complete or partial), contusion (with or without thrombosis), aneurysm (true or false), arteriovenous (AV) fistula, intimal disruption, and external compression by a hematoma.

Table 1: Signs of Vascular Injuries

Hard Signs

Signs of distal ischemia
Absent or diminished pulses
Expanding hematoma
Palpable thrill
Pulsatile bleeding
Bruit

Soft Signs

Cap refill >3 sec
Peripheral nerve deficit
Injury in proximity to major artery
Moderate bleeding (limited)
Diminished but palpable pulse

Lacerations and transections account for the great majority of arterial trauma.[1]

OPERATIVE MANAGEMENT FOR ALL PERIPHERAL VASCULAR INJURY

Preoperative Management

The initial objective in the management of peripheral vascular injury is to control bleeding to avoid exsanguination. This can immediately be accomplished using digital pressure, compressive bandages, or a tourniquet. Simultaneously, adequate fluid resuscitation is essential to limit the duration and extent of shock. Broad-spectrum antibiotics should also be administered in a timely fashion. Both groins, the lower abdomen, and both lower extremities should be prepped and draped. Prepping and draping the entire injured extremity including the distal aspect is important to assess for distal perfusion, assess the

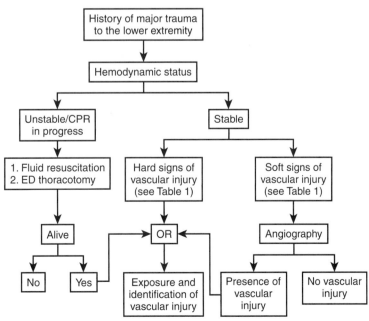

Figure 1 Algorithm for diagnosis of vascular injury in the lower extremity.

development of compartment syndrome, and perform fasciotomies if required. Prepping and draping the uninjured extremity allows for the harvesting of the greater saphenous vein if required to provide for a suitable replacement conduit. Vascular clamps, vessel loops, and fine monofilament sutures must be available before surgery begins.

Intraoperative Management

Controlling active bleeding before the start of the operation allows for sufficient time to obtain proximal and distal vascular control without further blood loss and prevents contamination of the surgical field by further bleeding. Approaching the hematoma directly may be useful in selected cases, but good judgment is required, as this can result in significant and potentially needless blood loss, which can further compromise the patient's hemodynamic and metabolic status, leading to a poor outcome. The cornerstone principle is to obtain proximal and distal control rapidly along with revascularization of the injured extremity. Surgical repair and temporary shunting are the main two options. The use of intraluminal shunt is advisable in patients who cannot tolerate surgical repair because of extreme systemic abnormalities such as acidosis, hypothermia, and coagulopathy. Also, when fracture stabilization may compromise the vascular repair, shunting should be performed before definitive vascular repair (Figure 2).

Surgical repair of arterial injury depends on the extent of vascular injury. Lateral arteriorrhaphy is recommended for management of small arterial lacerations that do not require debridement. Somewhat more extensive injuries requiring some debridement of the artery but without significant loss of the original length of the artery can be repaired via tension-free end-to-end anastomosis. Finally, for the most extensive injuries where free end-to-end anastomosis is not possible, the segmental defect can be bridged by autologous vein grafts (greater saphenous vein for lower extremity, cephalic vein for upper extremity) or synthetic conduits (PTFE, Dacron). Long-term patency rate and risk of infection should be taken into consideration when selecting between these two options. After surgical repair, adequate hemostasis must be insured, as well as distal limb perfusion. This can be evaluated using a continuous-wave Doppler device in the distal part of the affected extremity. If it is deemed unsatisfactory, a completion angiogram should be performed on the operating room table to look for technical problems with surgical repair, and the presence of common distal injury abnormalities such as thromboembolic complications or spasm or other traumatic injuries. When distal limb perfusion is deemed satisfactory, the wound should be assessed for adequate hemostasis, irrigated well, and debrided of necrotic and nonviable tissue before definitive wound closure. Complex wounds that involve large soft tissue defect may require live tissue flaps at a later time, which is beyond the scope of this chapter. Finally, patients with compartment syndrome or at a high risk for it, such as those with a combined arterial and venous injury, should undergo a therapeutic or prophylactic lower extremity fasciotomy.

Approach to Specific Vascular Injuries

Femoral Artery

The common femoral artery (CFA) is exposed via a longitudinal incision approximately 10 cm long placed over its course from the inguinal ligament inferiorly. If proximal control is needed, the external iliac artery must be explored and controlled. Using a similar incision, the profunda FA can be exposed and identified via a posterior lateral approach around the take-off of a superficial FA. Direct repair of the CFA is preferred; however, if a longitudinal injury or defect is identified, a vein patch may be necessary to preserve lumen diameter and avoid stenosis of the repair. An interposition graft is mandated when significant loss of artery has occurred, making it impossible to per-

form a tension free repair. Options for interposition grafts include the greater saphenous vein or synthetic grafts such as Dacron or PTFE with acceptable long-term patency rates. Profunda FA should be ligated when the patient is unstable or if serious associated injuries are present. It should be repaired if possible, but long-term complications are rare. The superficial FA courses deeper as it moves more distally. Because of their location, vascular injuries related to femur shaft fractures typically involve the superficial FA. The proximal portion is best exposed via a longitudinal groin incision as described previously; the middle and distal portion require an oblique incision in the thigh along the course of the sartorius muscle. Repair of this injury follows the same principles as those of the CFA described previously. However, patency rates using synthetic grafts are significantly lower than those for autologous vein graft, and therefore should be used in limited cases.[2]

Popliteal Artery

The most common presentation of a popliteal artery injury is thrombosis with limb ischemia. Because of its location, posterior knee dislocation can result in significant injury to the popliteal artery. The injury is best and most commonly approached through a medial incision extending from the posterior margin of the femur to the posterior margin of the tibia. The proximal artery is located as it exits from the adductor canal. Division of the medial head of the gastrocnemius, membranous, and semitendinous muscles is required to expose the area behind the knee. An incision along the posterior margin of the tibia helps expose the distal popliteal artery. A posterior approach, using an S-shaped incision, has also been described. It is faster and requires a less extensive dissection, but provides a more limited access to the proximal and distal popliteal vessel.

Tibial Arteries

The origin of the tibial arteries is identified by extending the incision used to locate the distal popliteal artery. The tibial arteries include the anterior tibial artery and the tibioperoneal trunk, which bifurcates into the peroneal and posterior tibial arteries. Division of the soleus muscle longitudinally helps expose the origin of the tibial arteries. Retracting on the popliteal vein posteriorly helps expose the anterior tibial artery. Retracting the popliteal vein anteriorly helps expose the peroneal and posterior tibial arteries. Exposure of the anterior tibial artery is done through an incision along the middle of the anterior compartment of the leg. The artery is located at the level of the interosseus membrane and can be reached by dissecting between the extension hallucis and the extensor digitorum muscle. Exposure to the distal aspect of peroneal and posterior tibial artery is via a medial incision along the posterior aspect of the tibia and posterior to the medial malleolus. Completion angiography is generally recommended after repair of popliteal and tibial artery injury so that any defects in the repair can be immediately addressed.

Venous Injuries

The management of venous injuries in the lower extremity is less complex than the management of arterial injury. The decision to ligate or primarily repair or reconstruct a venous injury depends on the patient's overall status, the extent and location of the venous injury, and the availability of collateral venous flow. Ligation is quick and definitive and more frequently performed. It can, however, result in significant postinjury edema of the lower extremity caused by venous thrombosis. This can result in acute complications such as compartment syndrome as well as late disability related to chronic venous insufficiency. Repair of venous injuries include most commonly a lateral venorrhaphy and rarely end-to-end repair or venous interposition grafts. The latter is often time consuming and may not be suitable for an unstable patient. Stenosis and thrombosis occur commonly after repair of venous injury and limit patency rates.

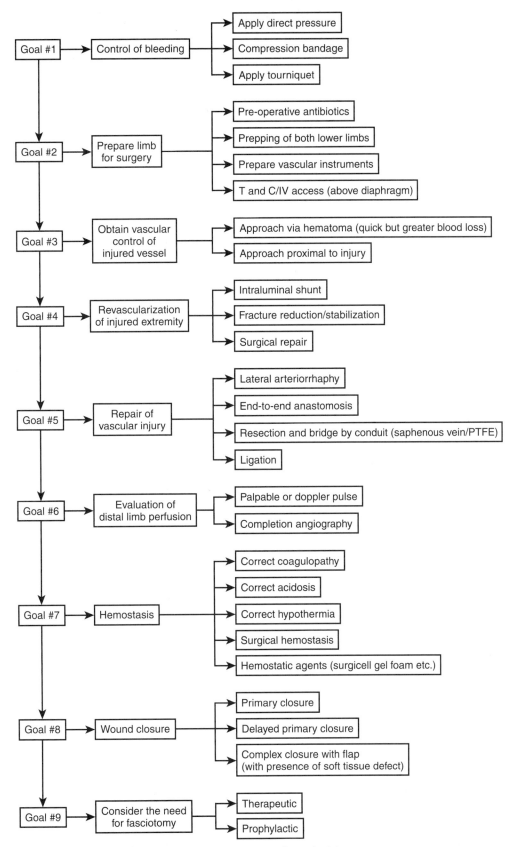

Figure 2 Algorithm for intra-operative management of vascular injury.

Postoperative Management

The goals of postoperative management are to rewarm the patient and replace blood and fluid losses in order to ensure adequate perfusion of the injured limb. Hypothermia and hypervolemia, which commonly occur after extensive surgery, can cause peripheral vasoconstrictions and compromise flow through the vascular repair. Elevation of the injured limb can reduce postoperative edema and is recommended after venous ligation. The use of anticoagulation (low-molecular-weight dextran or aspirin) can be helpful when small arteries and veins are repaired. On the other hand, the use of IV heparin is discouraged, especially in patients with multiple injuries. In addition, careful reassessment of the injured limb is essential for the early diagnosis of postoperative complications, as it may lead to immediate return to the operating room for re-exploration. Delays in the diagnosis of postoperative complication can lead to limb ischemia or necrosis.

MORBIDITY AND COMPLICATIONS

The most dangerous complications in the postoperative period are bleeding and thrombosis. Bleeding from the vascular repair may result in rapid swelling of the leg or external bleeding. This can be a life-threatening complication and mandates immediate return to the operating room for re-exploration and control of bleeding. At the same time, any coagulopathy should be corrected promptly. Arterial thrombosis at the site of the repair is suspected when the pulses are diminished or lost in the injured leg. Immediate return to the operating room to evaluate the vascular repair and to perform thrombectomy is essential to salvage the limb. The development of edema in the injured limb can result from thrombosis of the venous repair. Other complications include wound infection and deep infection at the site of the vascular repair. Delayed complications include stenosis and late thrombosis, pseudoaneurysm, and AV fistula. The surgical management of these complications is beyond the scope of this chapter. Chronic venous insufficiency has been associated with four-compartment fasciotomy.[1]

OUTCOME

There are three main outcomes after peripheral vascular trauma of the lower extremity: mortality rate, amputation rate, and functional outcome. The mortality rate after peripheral vascular injury has reached the lowest levels ever reported (<5%). This is attributable to rapid transport to a trauma center, adequate and prompt resuscitation, rapid diagnosis and treatment, and the use of damage control under the appropriate settings. In addition, the amputation rate has also dramatically improved (<2%), because of the institution of maneuvers resulting in abbreviated warm ischemia time. These include rapid transport from the scene to the operating room, better resuscitation, using intraluminal shunts, early stabilization of fractures, and liberal use of fasciotomy. The reported amputation rate after lower extremity vascular injury is highly variable.[1-3,16-19] Amputation rates for femoral artery injuries range from 0%–5%, and are much lower than those reported for popliteal injuries, which range from 0%–42%. Furthermore, any associated vein injury requiring ligation worsens the overall outcome and increases the amputation rate in the injured limb. A recently published study on blunt vascular trauma to the extremity reported that blunt vascular injuries reported an 18% amputation rate, which is considered to be three times the rate resulting from penetrating injuries. Higher amputation rates have been attributed to a delay in diagnosis as well as the presence of more significant injuries that delay the management of the extremity injury. Finally, the long-term functional outcomes

of limbs with vascular trauma remain under-reported because of poor follow-up in this patient population, warranting further investigation.[1] A recent study[20] dealing with lower extremity injury reported that in limbs at high risk for amputation, reconstruction versus amputation results in equivalent functional outcome at 2 years after injuries.

CONCLUSION

There has been a significant improvement in the management of lower extremity vascular injury, resulting in lower mortality and higher limb salvage rates. These improvements in management, including preoperative, intraoperative, and postoperative care, have been emphasized in this chapter. Trauma surgeons should be familiar with these advances so that they can improve on the current outcomes of lower extremity vascular injury.

REFERENCES

1. Shackford SR, Rich NM: Peripheral vascular injury. *Trauma*, 4th ed. McGraw-Hill, New York, 2000.
2. Sise MJ, Shackford SR: Extremity vascular trauma. In Rich N, Mattox KL, Hirshberg A, editors: *Vascular Trauma*, 2nd ed. Philadelphia, Elsevier Saunders, 2004, pp. 353–393.
3. Rich NM: Vascular trauma. *Surg Clin North Am* 53(6):1367–1392, 1973.
4. DeBakey ME, Simeone F: Battle injuries of the arteries in WWII: an analysis of 2471 cases. *Ann Surg* 123(4):534–579, 1946.
5. Jahnke EJ Jr, Seeley SF: Acute vascular injuries in the Korean War: an analysis of 77 consecutive cases. *Ann Surg* 138(2):158–177, 1953.
6. Hughes CW: Acute vascular trauma in Korean War casualties: an analysis of 180 cases. *Surg Gyne Obst* 99(20):91–100, 1954.
7. Rich NM, Baugh JH, Hughes CW: Acute arterial injuries Vietnam: 1000 cases. *J Trauma* 10(5):359–369, 1970.
8. Cargile JS, Hunt JL, Purdue GF: Acute trauma of the femoral artery and vein. *J Trauma* 32(3):364–370, 1992.
9. Degiannis E, Levy RD, Velmahos GC, Potokar R, Saadia R: Penetrating injuries to the femoral artery. *Br J Surg* 82(4):492–493, 1995.
10. Feliciano DV, Bitondo CG, Mattox KL: Civilian trauma in the 1980's: a one year experience with 456 vascular and cardiac injuries. *Ann Surg* 199: 717–724, 1984.
11. Carrillo EH, Spain DA, Miller FB, Richardson JD: Femoral vessel injuries in vascular trauma: complex and challenging injuries. *Surg Clin North Am* 82(1):49–65, 2002.
12. Richa NM, Hobson RW, Fedde CW, Collins GJ: Acute femoral arterial trauma. *J Trauma* 15(8):628–637, 1975.
13. Phifer TJ, Gerlock AJ, Vekovius WA, Rich NM, McDonald JC: Amputation risk factors in concomitant superficial femoral artery and vein injuries. *Ann Surg* 199(4):241–243, 1984.
14. Weaver FA, Rosenthal RE, Waterhouse G, Adkins RB: Combined skeletal and vascular injuries of the lower extremities. *Am Surg* 50:189–197, 1984.
15. Drost TF, Rosemurgy AS, Proctor D, Kearney RF: Outcome of treatment of combined orthopedic and arterial trauma to the lower extremity. *J Trauma* 29(10):1331–1334, 1989.
16. Reynolds R, McDowell HA, Diethelm AG: The surgical treatment of blunt and penetrating injuries of the popliteal artery. *Am Surg* 49(8):405–410, 1983.
17. Ashworth EM, Dalsing MC, Glover JL, Reilly MK: Lower extremity vascular trauma: a comprehensive aggressive approach. *J Trauma* 28(3):329–336, 1988.
18. Nanbashvili J, Kopadze T, Tvaladze M, Buachidze T, Nazvlishvili G: War injuries of major extremity arteries. *World J Surg* 27(2):134–139, 2003.
19. Feliciano DV, Herskowitz K, O'Gorman RB, Cruse PA, Brandt ML, Burch JM, Mattox KL: Management of vascular injuries in the lower extremities. *J Trauma* 28(3):319–328, 1988.
20. Bosse MJ, MacKenzie EJ, Kellam JF, Burgess AR, et al: An analysis of outcomes of reconstruction or amputation of leg-threatening injuries. *N Engl J Med* 347(24):1924–1931, 2002.
21. Asensio JA, Kuncir EV, Garcia-Nunez LM, Petrone P: Femoral vessel injuries: analysis of factors predictive of outcomes. *J Am Coll Surg* 203: 512–520, 2006.

COMPARTMENT SYNDROMES

Thomas S. Granchi

Compartment syndrome is a diagnosis that demands a decision. The diagnosis should be followed by immediate operation. Whether it occurs in a limb or the abdomen, compartment syndrome is a crisis that can be averted by surgical decompression. Fasciotomy treats compartment syndrome in limbs and laparotomy in the abdomen. Any alternative treatment should be compared with that standard.

Compartment syndrome occurs whenever pressure in a rigid compartment exceeds perfusion pressure. It can occur in any limb and in the abdomen. Despite advances in instruments for non-invasive measurements and the biology and chemistry of reperfusion injury, compartment syndrome stills threatens life and limb. The diagnosis is still missed or delayed resulting in avoidable death, limb loss, or crippling.

Common clinical presentations include reperfusion injury after vascular injury and repair, closed fractures, and electrical injuries. The astute clinician will suspect compartment syndrome early and act accordingly. Recognizing the potential for compartment syndrome should prompt serial examinations and pressure measurements. Inordinate pain and rapid loss of motor and sensory function in a limb are late clinical findings. Prophylactic fasciotomies should be considered in high-risk patients in whom serial examinations are not feasible.

Abdominal compartment syndrome (ACS) occurs in patients with massive intra-abdominal injuries and hemorrhagic shock. In the abdomen, elevated compartment pressure is manifested by oliguria and reduced cardiac output that do not improve with intravascular fluid replacement and increased airway pressures. Organ impairment and increased airway pressure can be detected at a pressure of 15 mm Hg. At 25–30 mm Hg, organ failure is evident and immediate laparotomy should be performed.[1] Measuring intra-abdominal pressures will confirm the diagnosis.

INCIDENCE

Trauma, vascular, and orthopedic surgeons will likely diagnose and treat compartment syndrome because of its association with vascular injury and fractures. The incidence is relatively low, even though the presentation and treatment are dramatic and memorable. In our Level 1 trauma center, the overall incidence of compartment syndrome was 0.004 among trauma admissions over a 2-year period.[2] This number includes compartment syndrome in the leg, arm, and abdomen.

The incidence varies according to anatomic site. Compartment syndrome in the leg occurred in 13 of 5226 trauma patients (i.e., incidence of 0.0025). Arm compartment syndrome occurred in six patients over the same period (i.e., incidence of 0.001). Abdominal compartment syndrome (ACS) occurred in four patients (i.e., incidence of 0.0008 among all trauma admissions and 0.008 among patients with trauma laparotomy).

Other published reports suggest that the incidence is much higher. A review of leg injuries reported an incidence of 30%–35% (up to 64%) of popliteal artery injuries with knee dislocations.[3] A large series of brachial artery injuries reported 12.1% incidence of fasciotomy.[4] Ivatury et al.[5] reported 100% incidence of ACS among patients with damage control laparotomy and primary fascial closure. The incidence was reduced to 38% with open abdomen techniques.[5] Improvements in open abdomen techniques and widespread appreciation of the syndrome have reduced the incidence of ACS even further. The low incidence of compartment syndrome among all trauma patients should not mitigate vigilance in patients with high-risk injuries.

MECHANISM OF INJURY

Arterial occlusion followed by reperfusion injury is a common presentation. Long bone fractures often precipitate compartment syndrome because of hematoma and tissue swelling at the site. Gulli and Templeton[6] report that it occurs in 3%–17% of closed tibia fractures. Compartment syndrome associated with femur injuries is rare if the fracture occurs at the shaft and absent associated vascular injuries.[7,8]

Venous pathology also causes compartment syndrome. There are several reports of compartment syndrome occurring with phlegmasia cerulea dolens.[9–11] The muscle compartments deserve attention in these patients.

In the upper arm and forearm, compartment syndrome can occur with supracondylar humerus fractures, IV drug abuse, electrical injuries, complications of IV sites, prolonged tourniquet use, and even weight lifting.[12] Many of these patients will present in ambulatory settings, where the index of suspicion may be low. Deep pain and tense swelling of the limb should prompt further investigation.

Abdominal compartment syndrome often develops in trauma patients who have had laparotomies and resuscitation for hemorrhagic shock. The abdominal cavity will stretch anteriorly and superiorly (along the diaphragm) to accommodate visceral edema or accumulating blood until it reaches the limits of its compliance. At this point, the abdomen becomes a rigid compartment, and pressure rises sharply, impairing organ function. Increased vascular resistance and reduced venous return impair cardiac output. Reduced renal perfusion pressure causes oliguria. Encroachment into the chest and tension on the diaphragm increase ventilator and airway pressures. Loss of functional residual capacity (FRC) and ventilation-perfusion mismatch (V/Q) cause hypoxia.[13]

Intoxications and systemic disease can cause compartment syndrome. Rutgers et al.[14] reported four cases of nontraumatic rhabdomyolysis and compartment syndrome in young male alcoholics receiving treatment with benzodiazepines. Ergotamine and cocaine intoxication have also been implicated in cases of compartment syndrome.[15,16] Patients with type I diabetes mellitus can suffer spontaneous compartment syndrome.[17–19]

Systemic diseases or drugs that cause vasoconstriction can induce muscle ischemia and subsequent compartment syndrome. Local factors that increase mass within the inelastic fascial compartments can also raise intracompartment pressure sufficiently to cause the feared syndrome. These include hematoma, fluid injection, infection, and even metastatic melanoma.[20] The careful clinician should remember the pathology, not only the common clinical settings, for compartment syndrome.

DIAGNOSIS

Physical Examination

The combination of inordinate muscle pain, pain on passive motion, muscle weakness or paralysis, hyperesthesia, and tense muscle compartments have been well described and repeated to generations of surgery residents.[21–23] Recognition of the symptom constellation should prompt immediate measurement of compartment pressure. If accurate measurements cannot be performed, or if the results are conflicting, then clinical diagnosis should supersede. Once the diagnosis has been made, the patient should not suffer delay in fasciotomy.

Abdominal compartment syndrome should be suspected in the patient with a tense, distended abdomen within a few hours after laparotomy for trauma or massive bleeding. Visceral swelling or continued bleeding push abdominal compliance beyond its limits. Oliguria that does not respond to fluid boluses is an early sign of intra-abdominal hypertension (IAH), and should prompt measurement of intra-abdominal pressure. This can be accomplished easily at the bedside by measuring the bladder pressure through a Foley catheter[1,9] (Figure 1). Frequent ventilator alarms from high airway pressures as the ventilator pushes against abdominal pressures of 60 cm H_2O or more herald the final stages of ACS. In this case, immediate abdominal decompression should be performed, even at the bedside, to permit ventilation and oxygenation.

Compartment Measurements

There are several techniques for measuring compartment pressures.[24–26] There are two variations—wick and slit—of the catheter technique. The catheters are inserted into the muscle through large-bore needles and then connected to a pressure transducer or manometer via saline-filled tubing. Because insertion and connection of the catheters are cumbersome, measuring several compartment pressures is difficult. The new electronic transducer-tipped catheter is promising, but shares many of the shortcomings with the other catheter techniques, such as need for tubes, catheter kinking, and poor placement beneath the fascia.[27] Other techniques for measuring compartments are readily available at the bedside and are easier to use.

Manufactured pressure monitors such as the Stryker (Stryker Instruments, Kalamazoo, MI) (Figure 2) employ modifications of the needle technique. They measure the pressure directly through a needle inserted into the muscle compartment. They are self-contained units requiring no assembly, which makes multiple measurements

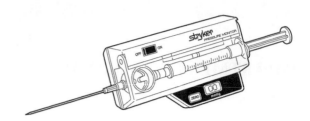

Figure 2   The Stryker pressure monitor is accurate, reliable, portable, and inexpensive. It can quickly and accurately measure compartment pressures at the bedside.   *(Stryker Instruments, Kalamazoo, MI.)*

easier at various sites or at different times. If a manufactured monitor is not available, a homemade version can be assembled using an 18-gauge needle, saline-filled pressure tubing, and a manometer or transducer.

Regardless of the device used, all compartments should be measured. Pressure may vary in different compartments. In the leg, the anterior and deep posterior compartments, at least, should be measured because they are most vulnerable to elevated pressure because of the neurovascular bundles they contain. The highest measurement should be used for clinical decisions.

Noninvasive Methods

There is a tenacious search for noninvasive diagnostics, and it extends to compartment syndrome. Several techniques that have clinical utility in other settings have been tried here. Near-infrared spectroscopy (NIRS) has been studied.[28–30] It measures muscle perfusion, not pressure, and can reliably diagnose ischemic tissue. Oxyhemoglobin saturation of less than 60% correlates with muscle compromise of compartment syndrome. Champions for its use argue that it directly identifies ischemic tissue rather than compartment pressure, which is a proxy for tissue compromise. If clinicians monitor for tissue ischemia rather than a rise in pressure, unnecessary fasciotomies might be prevented. Conversely, skeptics argue that waiting until ischemia is manifest may delay surgery. Also, the probe's range is limited to 2 cm or less below the skin surface. Therefore, it may miss deep muscle ischemia.

Digital pulse-oximetry is commonly available in the emergency room, operating room, and the intensive care unit. It is easy to use and inexpensive. It is not, however, sensitive in diagnosing compartment syndrome and muscle ischemia. It relies on pulsatile arterial flow to the distal digit to accurately measure the hemoglobin oxygen saturation. Because the arterial blood measured in the toe or finger bypasses the muscle compartments, measuring the former gives little useful information of the latter. A clinical series by Mars and Hadley[31] confirms this theoretical limitation.

Scintigraphy using 99mTc-methoxyisobutyl isonitrile (99mTc-MIBI) has been used to diagnose chronic exertional compartment syndrome.[32,33] The study requires a stable, ambulating patient, a trip to the nuclear medicine department, and a repeat study the next day with the patient at rest. With these limitations, nuclear medicine is no help with trauma patients.

Laboratory Studies

There are no laboratory tests to diagnose early compartment syndrome. Serum creatinine phosphokinase (CPK) is a marker for muscle cell injury, and is elevated in late or missed compartment syndrome.[12,34] The surgeon should not wait for a rise in serum CPK

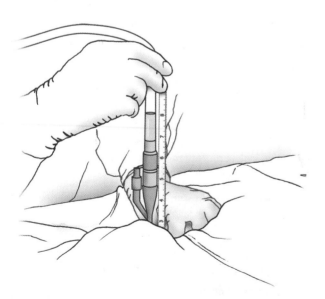

Figure 1   A simple method to measure intra-abdominal pressure via the Foley catheter. You may inject 50 mL of sterile saline into the bladder if there is insufficient urine in the tubing.

before operating. Postoperative levels may be useful in monitoring the response to treatment.

Similarly, myoglobinuria is a marker for muscle injury. It often occurs with crush or electrical injuries. These injuries frequently lead to compartment syndrome. The presence of myoglobinuria in such patients does not, per se, diagnose compartment syndrome. The muscle injury may follow from direct trauma rather than the ischemia from elevated compartment pressures. Therefore, myoglobinuria has little value in diagnosing acute early compartment syndrome.

Anatomic Location and Grading of Injury

Compartment syndrome usually occurs after injuries to peripheral arteries, especially the popliteal, superficial femoral, external iliac, hypogastric, and brachial arteries. These vessels provide the bulk of blood flow to their respective limbs, so relatively minor injuries to the vessel can cause devastating ischemia distally. Collateral arteries around the knee, hip, and elbow may be open, but are usually insufficient to perfuse the leg or arm.

Injuries to abdominal vessels can cause compartment syndromes in the abdomen and the legs. Massive bleeding from aortic, vena cava, or iliac injuries, and the massive transfusion required for resuscitation, can lead to ACS. Interruption of arterial inflow (or obstruction of venous outflow) and associated shock can cause compartment syndrome in the legs secondary to ischemia and reperfusion injury (or venous hypertension with venous injuries). Compartment syndrome in the legs and ACS can occur in the same patient.

Extensive abdominal visceral injuries can cause ACS. Liver injuries are especially prone to this complication because they bleed a lot and often require sponge packs. Multiple small bowel and mesentery injuries also lead to ACS because of blood loss and bowel edema. Any combination of solid and hollow organ injuries leading to damage control laparotomy increases the risk of ACS. Postoperative care should include provisions for measuring IAP.

Tables 1 through 3 show the visceral, abdominal vascular, and peripheral vascular injuries that may cause compartment syndromes. They also display the ICD-9 codes and Organ Injury Scores.[35]

Table 1: Peripheral Vascular Injuries Associated with Compartment Syndrome in Limbs

Abdominal Vascular Injury Scale			
Grade	Description of Injury	ICD-9	AIS-90
I	Non-named superior mesenteric artery or superior mesenteric vein branches	902.20/.39	NS
	Non-named inferior mesenteric artery or inferior mesenteric vein branches	902.27/.32	
	Phrenic artery or vein	902.89	
	Lumbar artery or vein	902.89	
	Gonadal artery or vein	902.89	
	Ovarian artery or vein	902.81/.82	
	Other non-named small arterial or venous structures requiring ligation	902.9	
II	Right, left, or common hepatic artery	902.22	3
	Splenic artery or vein	902.23/.34	
	Right or left gastric arteries	902.21	
	Gastroduodenal artery	902.24	
	Inferior mesenteric artery, or inferior mesenteric vein, trunk	902.27/.32	
	Primary named branches of mesenteric artery (e.g., ileocolic artery) or mesenteric vein	902.26/.31	
	Other named abdominal vessels requiring ligation or repair	902.89	
III	Superior mesenteric vein, trunk	902.31	3
	Renal artery or vein	902.41/.42	
	Iliac artery or vein	902.53/.54	
	Hypogastric artery or vein	902.51/.52	
	Vena cava, infrarenal	902.1	
IV	Superior mesenteric artery, trunk	902.25	3
	Celiac axis proper	902.24	
	Vena cava, suprarenal, and infrahepatic	902.1	
	Aorta, infrarenal	902.00	4
	Portal vein	902.33	3
V	Extraparenchymal hepatic vein	902.11	3/5
	Vena cava, retrohepatic, or suprahepatic	902.19	5
	Aorta suprarenal, subdiaphragmatic	902.0	4

Table 2: Abdominal Vascular Injuries Associated with Abdominal Compartment Syndrome

Grade	Type of Injury	Description of Injury	ICD-9	AIS-90
		Liver Injury Scale (1994 Revision)		
II	Hematoma	Subcapsular, 10%–50% surface area: intraparenchymal <10 cm in diameter	864.01	2
	Laceration	Capsular tear 1–3 cm parenchymal depth, <10 cm in length	864.11	
III	Hematoma	Subcapsular, >50% surface area of ruptured subcapsular or parenchymal hematoma; intraparenchymal hematoma >10 cm or expanding	864.03	3
	Laceration	3-cm parenchymal depth	864.03	
IV	Laceration	Parenchymal disruption involving 25%–75% hepatic lobe or 1–3 Couinaud's segments	864.04	4
V	Laceration	Parenchymal disruption involving >75% of hepatic lobe or more than three of Couinaud's segments within a single lobe	864.14	5
	Vascular	Juxtahepatic venous injuries; i.e., retrohepatic vena cava/central major hepatic veins	864.04	
	Vascular	Hepatic avulsion	864.14	
		Kidney Injury Scale		
III	Laceration	>1.0-cm parenchymal depth of renal cortex without collecting system rupture or urinary extravasation	866.02	3
IV	Laceration	Parenchymal laceration extending through renal cortex, medulla, and collecting system	866.12	4
	Vascular	Main renal artery or vein injury with contained hemorrhage	866.12	
V	Laceration	Completely shattered kidney	866.03	5
	Vascular	Avulsion of renal hilum that devascularizes kidney	866.13	
		Small Bowel Injury Scale		
II	Laceration	Laceration <50% of circumference	863.3	3
III	Laceration	Laceration >50% of circumference without transection	863.3	3
IV	Laceration	Transection of small bowel	863.3	4
V	Laceration	Transection of small bowel with segmental tissue loss	863.3	4
	Vascular	Devascularized segment	863.3	

Note: Aortic, vena cava, and iliac artery/vein injuries can also cause compartment syndrome in the legs.

Table 3: Abdominal Visceral Injuries Associated with Abdominal Compartment Syndrome

Grade	Description of Injury	ICD-9	AIS-90
	Peripheral Vascular Organ Injury Scale		
III	Superficial/deep femoral vein	903.02	2–3
	Popliteal vein	904.42	
	Brachial artery	903.1	
	Anterior tibial artery	904.51/904.52	1–3
	Posterior tibial artery	904.53/904.54	
	Peroneal artery	904.7	
IV	Tibioperoneal trunk	904.7	2–3
	Superficial/deep femoral artery	904.1/904.7	3–4
	Popliteal artery	904.41	2–3
V	Axillary artery	903.01	2–3
	Common femoral artery	904.0	3–4

SURGICAL MANAGEMENT

Surgery is the mainstay of treatment. Releasing the pressure through generous fascial incisions restores microvascular flow and rescues threatened tissue. For abdominal compartment syndrome, laparotomy accomplishes decompression. Medical therapies enjoy initial enthusiasm, but none so far have demonstrated adequate efficacy. Choices in operative treatment are choices of incision and wound closure. The necessity of fasciotomy for diagnosed compartment syndrome remains unassailable. Indications for prophylactic fasciotomies, however, have been questioned.[23,36,37]

The four muscle compartments in the calf are the anterior, lateral, superficial posterior, and deep posterior. The anterior compartment is bounded by the tibia medially, the interosseous membrane posteriorly anterior crural intermuscular septum laterally, and the crural fascia anteriorly. It contains the tibialis anterior, the extensor digitorum longus, and the extensor hallucis longus muscles. It also contains the anterior tibial artery and vein, and the deep peroneal nerve. The lateral compartment contains the peroneus longus and brevis muscles and the superficial peroneal nerve. The superficial posterior compartment contains the bulky soleus muscle. The deep posterior compartment encloses the tibialis posterior, flexor digitorum longus, and flexor hallucis longus muscles. The posterior tibial vessels and the tibial nerve run within this compartment. Note that the saphenous vein courses in the subcutaneous tissue along the medial border of the superficial compartment. It can be damaged during fasciotomy if care is not taken to protect it. Also, the sural nerve runs along the posterior lateral border of the superficial posterior compartment. Fasciotomies of the calf are usually performed through a medial incision, to open the posterior and deep posterior compartments, and a lateral incision for the anterior and lateral compartments (Figure 3).

Prophylactic fasciotomies in the calves have been advocated for combined popliteal artery and vein injuries and for ischemia for more than 6 hours. Advocates argue that delays in diagnosing compartment syndrome may lead to severe dysfunction or amputation, and therefore, waiting until compartment pressures reach threshold cannot be justified.[6] These authors recommend liberal fasciotomies, especially in the anesthetized or comatose patient.

The forearm contains three compartments, the volar, dorsal, and the mobile wad. The volar compartment contains the flexor and pronator muscles, the radial and ulnar arteries, and the median and ulnar nerves. The dorsal compartment contains the extensor muscles. The mobile wad is closely associated with the dorsal compartment and contains the radial nerve. Fasciotomies of all compartments can be performed through volar and radial incisions. The volar incision can be curved or straight. The radial incision is straight along the forearm axis (Figure 4).

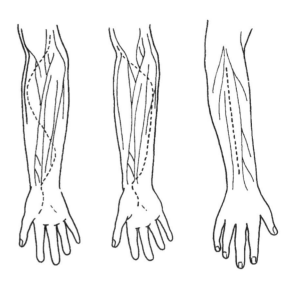

Figure 4 Incisions for forearm fasciotomies. Two possible volar incisions, curved (left), and straight (center). The radial incision is straight along forearm axis (right).

Hofmeister and Shin[38] recommend prophylactic fasciotomy of all muscle compartments of the arm after replantation. They reason that because the replantation requires 5–10 hours and the compromised muscle relies on tenuous arterial and venous anastomoses, fasciotomy should be performed before compartment syndrome develops. Under these circumstances, fasciotomy is prudent.

Advocates of liberal fasciotomies tend to discount the morbidity of the scars. Conversely, other experts hold that the complications from fasciotomies, including prophylactic ones, can be significant.[36,37,39] Wound complications include ulcers, skin tethering to the muscle, paresthesias, pruritus, muscle herniation, and disfigurement. Fitzgerald and colleagues[39] report that 28% of their patients changed hobbies, and 12% changed their occupations because of the unsightly scars. The authors recommend primary closure of the wounds whenever possible, and hope for less invasive methods for fascial release.

The feasibility of continuous compartment pressure or NIRS monitoring may influence the decision to refrain from fasciotomy. If the surgeon has continuous, reliable monitoring, he may choose to avoid the operation unless pressure exceeds the threshold. He must, however, recognize patients at risk for compartment syndrome and commit to frequent or continuous measurements and look for clear indications for fasciotomy.

The four compartments of the lower leg can be decompressed through a single lateral incision or through lateral and medial incisions. The two-incision technique is more common and the technique of choice because it is technically easier to reach the posterior compartments through the medial incision (see Figure 3). Fibulectomy has been described but has been abandoned because there are easier and less morbid operations that accomplish adequate decompression.[6,40]

Less invasive methods have been attempted. Ota et al.[41] described endoscopic release of the anterior leg compartment using an arthroscope and a transparent outer tube for chronic compartment syndrome in an athlete. The patient enjoyed relief of her symptoms postoperatively, and the compartment pressures diminished. Other authors have been less enthusiastic about endoscopic fasciotomies. Havig and colleagues[42] compared endoscopic and open forearm fasciotomies in cadavers. They found that the endoscopic procedure reduced compartment pressures, but not as dramatically as the open procedure. They caution against using the endoscopic forearm fasciotomy in the clinical setting.

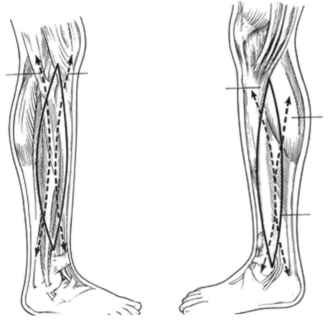

Figure 3 Medial and lateral incisions to open the calf compartments. The medial incision exposes the posterior and deep posterior compartments. The lateral incision exposes the lateral and anterior compartments.

Morbidity and Complication Management

After diagnosing compartment syndrome and performing fasciotomy, the surgeon faces a large, problematic wound. Primary closure is usually impossible because of exuberant muscle swelling. Delayed primary closure and later skin grafting are the most common methods of wound closure.

In the abdomen, primary closure of the fascia is usually impossible. Sometimes, a skin-only closure can be accomplished. The most common forms of closure after laparotomy for abdominal compartment syndrome involve some form of temporary prosthesis such as a "Bogota bag" or vacuum pack.[1,9] These maintain protection of the viscera while allowing loss of domain. They effectively increase the volume of the abdominal cavity. Removal of the prosthesis can be accomplished when the swelling recedes. If delayed primary closure cannot be performed, then skin grafting or component separation can cover the viscera.

Delayed primary closure of extremity wounds offers the benefit of a smaller scar, but is usually labor intensive. This method involves some daily manipulation of sutures, wires, or elastic bands. Steri-Strips® (3M Surgical Products, St. Paul, MN) have been used for gradual approximation of skin edges, closing the wound in 5–8 days.[43] Chiverton and Redden[44] used subcuticular Prolene suture to achieve skin closure. Harris[45] described using rubber vessel loops stretched between skin staples in shoelace fashion. A new device, the WoundBullet™ (Boehringer Laboratories, Norristown, PA) is promising. It uses a small internal ratchet to add tension to sutures for gradual wound closure.

We usually close the wounds with split thickness skin grafts in 5–7 days. This method requires little bedside wound manipulation and achieves closure of large wounds. It requires an additional general anesthetic for the patient and produces an uglier scar. Skin grafting, however, is a mainstay in this setting because of its simplicity and coverage of large wound areas.

Because of the morbidity of fasciotomy, medical treatments have been advanced. The results are equivocal. Most are used to ameliorate the damage from oxygen-free radicals.[38] They include deferoxamine to chelate iron, xanthine oxidase inhibitors, such as allopurinol, to block production of hypoxanthine, and superoxide dismutase, an enzyme to catalyze the superoxide radical to hydrogen peroxide. These antioxidants have been studied in many animal models, but not yet in human trials.

MORTALITY

Fortunately, death is rare after isolated limb compartment syndrome. When it occurs, it is usually from sepsis and systemic inflammatory response secondary to tissue necrosis. In these cases, the heroic attempts at limb salvage sacrifice the patient. Signs of distant organ failure or systemic inflammatory response syndrome should force the surgeon to abandon limb salvage and to proceed with amputation.

In patients with ACS, however, mortality is still high. Most series still report 25%–40% mortality in patients with damage control laparotomies. These patients still succumb to multiorgan failure and sepsis in the intensive care unit. With widespread appreciation of ACS, fewer die in the immediate postoperative period from untreated ACS. More of these patients are salvaged with decompression laparotomies.

CONCLUSIONS AND ALGORITHMS

Compartment syndrome is a threat to patients who suffer limb injuries. Abdominal compartment syndrome is well described and recognized in patients with massive injuries and hemorrhagic shock. It is a true compartment syndrome, with impaired organ perfusion.

Reperfusion injury after restoration of arterial inflow after prolonged ischemia is a common cause of compartment syndrome.

The tissue swelling and cell damage result from oxygen and lipid-free radicals produced during reperfusion. Although research has mapped the complex reactions in reperfusion injury, it has not produced a means for prevention or effective medical treatment. Effective treatment relies on early diagnosis through clinical examination and bedside measurements of compartment pressures. NIRS may have benefits as a noninvasive harbinger of muscle compromise.

Once the diagnosis is made, the surgeon should perform expeditious decompression. There are a variety of incisions described. In the lower leg, median and lateral longitudinal incisions are most commonly used. In the forearm, volar and radial incisions are preferred. For the abdomen, a midline laparotomy accomplishes decompression.

Prophylactic fasciotomies for high-risk patients are common, but may be unnecessary if reliable, frequent measurement is available. High rates of wound complications discourage some authors from unnecessary fasciotomies. Most experts do not hesitate to perform fasciotomy in the face of possible limb loss.

Wound coverage after fasciotomy and decompressing laparotomy remains problematic. The variety of techniques for delayed primary closure testify to the enthusiasm for it and the difficulty in achieving it. As a default method, split thickness skin grafting is an effective, but perhaps less attractive, means for closing these wounds. The surgeon must consider the trade-offs.

The following algorithms (Figures 5 and 6) show my approach to patients at risk for limb and abdominal compartment syndrome. They are not promoted as "the standard of care" nor to replace or supersede the judgment of a qualified surgeon. They have worked for me and my patients for many years, and I teach them to my residents.

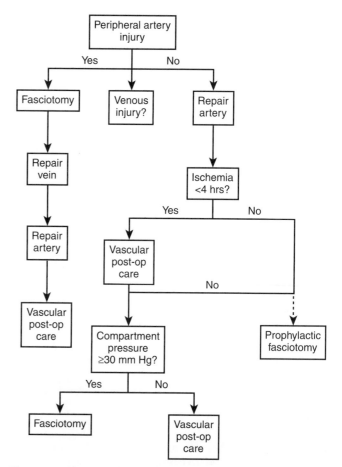

Figure 5 Algorithm for peripheral artery injuries. Note: Prophylactic fasciotomy is an option for select patients.

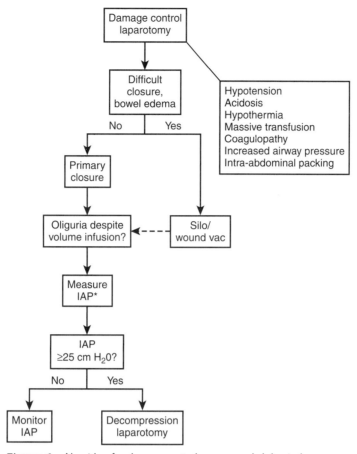

Figure 6 Algorithm for damage control surgery and abdominal compartment syndrome (ACS). Note: Even patients with silo closures can develop ACS.

REFERENCES

1. Burch JAM, Moore EE, Moore FA, Françoise R: The abdominal compartment syndrome in complex and challenging problems in trauma surgery. *Surge Clan North Am* 76(4):833–843, 1996.
2. Garza R: Trauma Registry. Ben Taub Trauma Center, Houston, TX, October 2005.
3. Heyse MS, Richardson MW, Miller MD: The dislocated knee. *Clan Sports Med* 19(3):519–543, 2000.
4. Zellweger R, Hess F, Nicol A, et al: An analysis of 124 surgically managed brachial artery injuries. *Am J Surge* 188:240–245, 2004.
5. Ivatury RR, Diebel L, Porter JM, Simon RJ: Intra-abdominal hypertension and the abdominal compartment syndrome. *Surg Clin North Am* 77(4):783–800, 1997.
6. Gulli B, Templeton D: Compartment syndrome of the lower extremity. *Orthop Clin North Am* 25(4):677–684, 1994.
7. Russel GV, Kregor PJ, Jarret CA, Zlowodowski M: Complicated femoral shaft fractures, in treatment of complex fractures. *Orthop Clin North Am* 33(1):1–17, 2002.
8. Schwartz JT Jr, Brumback RJ, Lakatos R, Poka A, Bathon GH, Burgess AR: Acute compartment syndrome of the thigh: a spectrum of injury. *J Bone Joint Surg [Am]* 71:392–400, 1989.
9. Dennis C: Disaster following femoral vein ligation for thrombophlebitis, relief by fasciotomy: clinical case of renal impairment following crush injury. *Surgery* 17:264–269, 1945.
10. Cywes S, Louw JH: Phlegmasia cerulea dolens: successful treatment by relieving fasciotomy. *Surgery* 51:169–172, 1962.
11. Wood KE, Reedy JS, Pozniak MA, Coursin DB: Phlegmasia cerulean dolens with compartment syndrome: a complication of femoral vein catheterization. *Crit Care Med* 28(5):1626–1630, 2000.
12. Moore RE III, Friedman RJ: Current concepts in pathophysiology and diagnosis of compartment syndromes. *J Emerg Med* 7:657–662, 1989.
13. Ivatury RR, Sugerman HJ, Peiztman AB: Abdominal compartment syndrome: recognition and management. *Adv Surg* 35:251–269, 2001.
14. Rutgers PH, van der Harst E, Koumans RKJ: Surgical implications of drug induced rhabdomyolysis. *Br J Surg* 78:490–492, 1991.
15. Gilman AG, Goodman LS, Murad F: *Goodman and Gilman's The Pharmacological Basis of Therapeutics*, 8th ed. New York, Macmillan, 1989.
16. Singhal P, Horowitz B, Quinones QC, et al: Acute renal failure following cocaine abuse. *Nephron* 52:76–78, 1989.
17. Lafforgue P, Janand-Delenne B, Lassman-Vague V, et al: *Diabetes Metab* 25(3):255–260, 1999.
18. Silberstein L, Britton KE, Marsh FP, et al: An unexpected cause of muscle pain in diabetes. *Ann Rheum Dis* 60(4):310–312, 2001.
19. Smith AL, Laing PW: Spontaneous tibial compartment syndrome in type I diabetes mellitus. *Diabetes Med* 16(2):168–169, 1999.
20. Simmons DJ: Compartment syndrome complicating metastatic malignant melanoma. *Br J Plast Surg* 53(3):255–257, 2000.
21. Matsen FA, Windquist RA, Krugmire RB: Diagnosis and management of compartment syndromes. *J Bone Joint Surg [Am]* 62:286, 1980.
22. Perry MO: Compartment syndromes and reperfusion injury: vascular trauma. *Surg Clin North Am* 68(4):853–864, 1988.
23. Velmahos GC, Toutouzas KG: Vascular trauma and compartment syndromes. *Surg Clin North Am* 82(1):125–141, 2002.
24. Matsen FA, Mayo KA, Sheridan GW, Krugmire RB: Monitoring of intramuscular pressure. *Surgery* 79(6):702–709, 1976.
25. Perron AD, Brady WJ, Keats TE: Orthopedic pitfalls in the ED: acute compartment syndrome. *Am J Emerg Med* 19(5):413–416, 2001.
26. Hargens AR, Mubarak SJ, Owen CA, et al: Interstitial fluid pressure in muscle and compartment syndromes in man. *Microvasc Res* 14:1–10, 1977.
27. Willy C, Gerngross H, Sterk J: Measurement of intracompartmental pressure with use of a new electronic transducer-tipped catheter system. *J Bone Joint Surg [Am]* 81(2):158–168, 1999.

28. Garr JL, Gentilello LM, Cole PA, et al: Monitoring for compartmental syndrome using near-infrared spectroscopy: a noninvasive, continuous, transcutaneous monitoring technique, *J Trauma* 46(4):613–618, 1999.

29. Giannotti G, Cohn SM, Brown M, et al: Utility of near-infrared spectroscopy in the diagnosis of lower extremity compartment syndrome, *J Trauma* 48(3):396–401, 2000.

30. Gentilello LM, Sanzone A, Wang L, et al: Near-infrared spectroscopy versus compartment pressure for the diagnosis of lower extremity compartmental syndrome using electromyography-determined measurements of neuromuscular function, *J Trauma* 51(1):1–9, 2001.

31. Mars M, Hadley GP: Failure of pulse oximetry in the assessment of raised limb intracompartmental pressure. *Injury* 25(6):379–381, 1994.

32. Edwards PD, Miles KA, Owens SJ, et al: A new non-invasive test for detection of compartment syndromes. *Nucl Med Commun* 20(3): 215–218, 1999.

33. Owens S, Edwards P, Miles K, et al: Chronic compartment syndrome affecting the lower limb: MIBI perfusion imaging as an alternative to pressure monitoring: two case reports. *Br J Sports Med* 33:49–51, 1999.

34. Robbs JV, Baker LW: Late revascularization of the lower limb following acute arterial occlusion. *Br J Surg* 78:490–493, 1979.

35. American Association for the Surgery of Trauma: October 26, 2005. http://www.aast.org/injury.

36. Field CK, Senkowsky J, Hollier LH, et al: Fasciotomy in vascular trauma: is it too much, too often? *Am Surg* 60(6):409–411, 1994.

37. Velmahos GC, Theodorou D, Demetriades D, et al: Complications and nonclosure rates of fasciotomy for trauma and related risk factors. *World J Surg* 21:247–253, 1997.

38. Hofmeister EP, Shin AY: The role of prophylactic fasciotomy and medical treatment in limb ischemia and revascularization, in compartment syndrome and Volkmann's ischemic contracture. *Hand Clin* 14(3):457–465, 1998.

39. Fitzgerald AM, Gaston P, Quaba A, McQueen MM: Long-term sequelae of fasciotomy wounds. *Br J Plast Surg* 53:690–693, 2000.

40. Mubarak SJ, Owen CA: Double-incision fasciotomy of the leg for decompression in compartment syndromes. *J Bone Joint Surg* 59A:184–187, 1977.

41. Ota Y, Senda M, Hashizume H, Inoue H: Chronic compartment syndrome of the lower leg: a new diagnostic method using near-infrared spectroscopy and a new endoscopic fasciotomy. *Arthroscopy* 15(4):439–443, 1999.

42. Havig MT, Leversedge FJ, Seiler JG 3rd: Forearm compartment pressure: an in vitro analysis of open and endoscopic assisted fasciotomy. *J Hand Surg (Am)* 24(6):1289–1297, 1999.

43. Harrah J, Gates R, Carl J, Harrah JD: A simpler, less expensive technique for delayed primary closure of fasciotomies. *Am J Surg* 180(1):55–57, 2000.

44. Chiverton N, Redden JF: A new technique for delayed primary closure of fasciotomy wounds. *Injury* 31(1):21–24, 2000.

45. Harris I: Gradual closure of fasciotomy wounds using a vessel loop shoelace. *Injury* 24(8):565–567, 1993.

MUSCULOSKELETAL AND PERIPHERAL CENTRAL NERVOUS SYSTEM INJURIES

UPPER EXTREMITY FRACTURES: ORTHOPEDIC MANAGEMENT

Robin M. Gehrmann, Virak Tan, and Alfred Behrens†

Fractures and dislocations of the upper extremity can vary from benign, requiring minimal intervention, to life and limb threatening. The treatment plan is based on the injury pattern including location, associated neurologic or vascular injury, status of the soft tissues, mechanism, and other associated injuries. In this chapter, several key issues in the decision-making process are discussed, followed by description and treatment of specific injuries.

OPEN FRACTURES

The associated soft tissue injuries add an element of urgency to the treatment of fractures. A fracture is classified as "open" if the fracture or fracture hematoma communicates with the air via a wound in the soft tissues. This can be caused from the bone protruding through the skin, "inside out," or if there is a penetrating mechanism causing an injury from the "outside in." Regardless, the implication is that environmental contamination can increase the incidence of infection and fracture healing complications. If there is a wound in the same limb segment as the fracture, it should be considered open until proven otherwise. A classification system for open fractures appears in Table 1. Infection rates are reported at 0%–2% for Type I, 2%–7% for Type II, and 10%–25% for Type III overall. Rates for type III are subclassified as follows: IIIA, 7%; IIIB, 10%–50%; and IIIC, 25%–50%.

Treatment of these fractures is therefore aimed at irrigation and debridement in the operating room within 8 hours. Preliminary or definitive stabilization of the fracture and appropriate antibiotic therapy should follow. It is apparent that short-course, high-dose antibiotic therapy is appropriate for open fractures and need not be continued over the course of the fracture healing process. Recommendations follow:

Grade I fractures: 2 g of cephalosporin on admission and 1 g every 6–8 hours for 48 hours.
Grade II and III fractures: therapy to cover both Gram-positive and -negative organisms is warranted. This includes recom-

mendations for grade I injuries plus 1.5 mg/kg on admission and 3–5 mg/kg/day in divided doses of an aminoglycoside. This may be adjusted for patients with renal failure or substituted with once/day dosing to minimize renal toxicity. Ten million units of penicillin are added for patients with farm injuries and tetanus prophylaxis is required as well in all cases.

Trauma to the arm involving a severe crush component such as that from a conveyer belt or injuries with prolonged vascular compromised are at risk for development of compartment syndrome. Prophylactic fasciotomy may be necessary.

DISLOCATIONS

This is another situation that requires more urgent assessment, diagnosis, and treatment. By definition a dislocation is present when the joint is disrupted such that the articular surfaces are no longer in contact. The diagnosis of a joint dislocation is often made from the history and physical examination. The limb will usually be held in a fixed position characteristic of the dislocation direction. A posterior hip dislocation, for example, is seen with the limb in flexion, adduction, and internal rotation. Loss of the normal contour of the joint can be seen as evidenced by a "sulcus" sign in an anterior shoulder dislocation.

Radiographic evaluation is essential in the management of these injuries because associated fractures will otherwise go unrecognized and can have significant effects on the prognosis if not taken into account before reduction.

Neurovascular compromise is the reason for emergent reduction of the joint. Sciatic nerve injury has been reported to occur in 8%–19% of hip dislocations. Osteonecrosis is a known complication of hip dislocations as well, occurring in up to 17% of these injuries. This is due to the interruption of capsular blood supply from the increased tension caused by the dislocation. Other associated neurologic injuries can be seen in Table 2.

Dislocations and fractures with neurologic or vascular compromise should therefore be reduced as quickly as possible in order to reduce potential irreversible injury to the affected structures. Following reduction a repeat examination is warranted to see if there has been a change in the neurovascular status of the limb.

GUNSHOT WOUNDS

Special attention is deserved here due to the need to make an important distinction for the treatment of these injuries. It is important to determine if the wound was inflicted by a "low-" or "high-velocity" weapon. The exact distinction is somewhat cloudy, but according to the *Wound Ballistics Manual* of the Office of the Surgeon General, muzzle velocity greater than 2500 ft/sec

†Deceased.

Table 1: Classification of Open Fractures

Grade I: Wound <1 cm, low-velocity trauma with minimal contamination or soft tissue damage. Fracture has little or no comminution.

Grade II: Wound >1 cm, without extensive soft tissue damage. Contamination and comminution are moderate.

Grade III: Characterized by extensive soft tissue damage including muscle, skin, and neurovascular structures with a high degree of contamination. Fractures are significantly comminuted.

Grade IIIA: Soft tissue coverage of the bone is adequate despite extensive laceration, flaps or high-energy trauma. This includes severely comminuted or segmental fractures regardless of the wound size.

Grade IIIB: Associated with extensive injury to the soft tissue with periosteal stripping, massive contamination, and severe comminution. After debridement a local or free flap is needed for coverage.

Grade IIIC: Includes any open fracture with an associated arterial injury that must be repaired.

Table 2: Neurologic Injuries Associated with Upper Extremity Fractures

Joint	Common Neurologic Injury	Deficit
Shoulder	Axillary nerve	Sensory deficit in deltoid region, weakness of deltoid and teres minor
Elbow	Posterior interosseous nerve	Weakness of wrist dorsiflexion
Knee	Peroneal nerve	Weakness of ankle and great toe dorsiflexion
Hip	Sciatic nerve	More frequently common peroneal portion giving dorsiflexion weakness

constitutes "high velocity." This is important because the kinetic energy of the bullet varies directly with the square of its velocity and only linearly with its mass.

Many low-velocity gunshot injuries can be treated to completion with closed methods, such as functional bracing or casting. If one chooses open management, it should be anticipated that the extent of the fracture is often more extensive than can be appreciated on plain radiographs. This should be taken into account in the preoperative planning.

There may also be associated neurologic deficits due to the "blast effect" of the initial injury that do not warrant immediate exploration, as many will often resolve. If persistent neurologic deficit occurs, an electromyograph (EMG) may be indicated at 3–6 weeks to assess the nerve for any evidence of fibrillation potential.

Gunshots to the forearm require special attention even if there is no associated fracture due to an increased risk for development of forearm compartment syndrome. During the past 4 years, we have treated five patients who developed forearm compartment syndrome from penetrating injuries. All were found to have arterial lacerations. Patients should be monitored for at least 8–12 hours for clinical evidence of increased pressure within the forearm, which include marked pain on passive digital extension, tense or swollen forearm,

and reduced hand sensibility or paresthesia. Intracompartmental pressure measurements may be helpful but the diagnosis is made on clinical grounds.

Once the diagnosis is established, an emergent forearm fasciotomy is required to prevent Volkmann's contracture.

IMAGING STUDIES

For fractures and dislocations, proper radiographic evaluation is essential before making any decisions regarding treatment of the injury. Ideally, two orthogonal views of the injured extremity should be obtained along with radiographs of the joints adjacent to the injured bone. Injuries to the shoulder girdle should have a minimum of three radiographic views in a standard trauma series, which includes anteroposterior (AP), scapular "Y," and axillary views. Subtle injuries can be missed if adequate radiographs are not obtained. This is seen in Figure 1 of this missed posterior dislocation that was not properly diagnosed until a magnetic resonance image was obtained 6 months after the initial injury.

INJURIES TO SHOULDER GIRDLE AND HUMERUS

Scapula Fractures

Fractures of the scapula are relatively uncommon, accounting for 3% of all shoulder girdle injuries. These generally occur as the result of high-energy trauma explaining the frequent association with other, often life-threatening, injuries that may be of greater significance than the fracture itself. It is not uncommon for scapular fractures to be overlooked in polytrauma patients and often noticed incidentally on a chest radiograph or CAT scan.

A classification system was developed by Ada and Miller (Table 3), which divided fractures into those involving the acromion, spine and coracoid, type 1, glenoid neck, type 2, intra-articular glenoid fractures, type 3, and isolated scapular body fractures, type 4.

Associated injuries are quite common due to the high-energy mechanisms in which they usually occur. In one study of 148 fractures in 116 scapulae, 96% had associated injuries with upper thoracic rib fractures being the most common. Pulmonary injuries were also common with an overall incidence of 37%, of which 29% were hemopneumothorax and 8% pulmonary contusion. Head injuries were observed in 34%, ipsilateral clavicle fractures were seen in 25%, and 12% of patients had cervical spine injuries, of which 4% had permanent cord injuries.

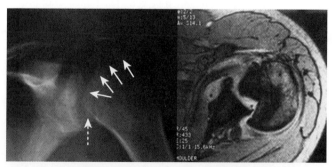

Figure 1 Anteroposterior radiograph on the left that depicts a missed posterior dislocation. There is overlap of the humerus and glenoid (*single dashed arrow*) and a large impaction fracture of the humeral head (*white arrow*). Magnetic resonance image on the right clearly shows the dislocation and associated humeral head impaction fracture.

Table 3: Scapular Fracture Classification System

Fracture Type	Anatomic Description/Location
1A	Fracture through acromion
1B	Fracture line through base of acromion or scapular spine
1C	Fracture through coracoid process
2A	Vertical glenoid neck fracture, lateral to base of acromion
2B	Vertical glenoid neck fracture that extends up through scapular spine and supraspinatus fossa
2C	Fracture line starts laterally at glenoid neck and propagates in transverse fashion through body exiting medially
3	Intra-articular glenoid fracture
4	Scapular body only

Data from Ada JR, Miller ME: Scapular fractures: analysis of 113 cases. *Clin Orthop* 269:174–180, 1991.

Management of these fractures is often nonsurgical as poor healing is an infrequent complication due to the rich blood supply from the investing rotator cuff musculature. Nonoperative management consists of admission for a period of 24 hours to assess pulmonary and cardiac status. A brief period of sling immobilization is initiated for comfort, followed by passive range of motion. Most fractures are united by 6 weeks such that active mobilization and strengthening can ensue safely. Maximal functional recovery can take 6–12 months.

Operative indications include intra-articular glenoid fractures with 5 mm of displacement, coracoid fractures with intra-articular extension and more than 5 mm of step-off, glenoid rim fractures with persistent or recurrent glenohumeral instability.

The injury pattern described as the "floating shoulder" deserves attention. This refers to a "double disruption" of the superior shoulder suspensory complex. This complex consists of a bone and soft tissue ring formed by the glenoid, coracoid process, coracoclavicular ligaments, distal clavicle, acromioclavicular joint, and acromion process. Isolated disruption of one of these components is generally tolerated well; however, when two or more structures are damaged, it is thought to produce an unstable situation. This is commonly seen with ipsilateral clavicle and glenoid neck fractures. The treatment of such injuries is somewhat controversial in that good results have been reported with fixation of both the glenoid and clavicle, clavicle alone, and more recently, nonoperative management. At this time, reasonable indications for operative intervention would include glenoid neck fractures with more than 3 cm of medial displacement in combination with injury to another structure. Each patient, however, must be evaluated individually.

Scapulothoracic Dissociation

Scapulothoracic dissociation is an infrequent injury that can be thought of as an internal forequarter amputation, which is almost always seen in conjunction with severe injuries to the brachial plexus and subclavian vessels. It is the result of a massive traction injury causing significant lateral displacement of the scapula relative to its thoracic articulation. According to the paper by Althausen et al., 88% have associated vascular lesions and 94% presented with severe neurologic injuries. A flail extremity resulted in approximately 52%, early amputation in 21%, and death in 10% of patients.

Diagnosis is made clinically by the presence of massive swelling, weakness, pain, tenderness, and absent or diminished pulses. It is crucial not to attribute pulselessness to a more distal injury when a more proximal, life threatening injury may be the underlying cause. Radiographically an AP film of the chest with the cassette oriented transversely may reveal lateral displacement of the scapula. Measurement from the medial border of the scapula to the spinous processes should alert the physician to the possibility of a scapulothoracic dissociation with a distance of more than 1 cm when compared to the opposite side. This may or may not be seen in conjunction with an acromioclavicular separation or clavicle fracture.

Management is controversial but arterial injuries may warrant immediate exploration and repair. As many as 10% of patients who survive the initial injury may die from exsanguination. Brachial plexus exploration may be carried out at the same time. Bony stabilization may be necessary to protect vascular repairs but the role of internal fixation is otherwise less clear.

Glenohumeral Dislocation

Due to its lack of bony constraint, the shoulder is the most commonly dislocated joint in the body. It is not a true ball and socket joint, but more like a golf ball resting on a golf tee. The static restraints to dislocation are composed of the glenoid labrum, capsule, and glenohumeral ligaments, while the rotator cuff musculature provides additional dynamic stability.

Anterior dislocations are by far the most common type. These are usually the result of an eccentric load applied to the arm while in an outstretched position as would be seen in a volleyball player while spiking the ball. Posterior dislocations occur with a posteriorly directed force on an adducted, flexed arm, and also have been noted to occur in patients who are seizing.

An anteriorly dislocated shoulder will present with the arm at the side or in slight abduction and external rotation. Normal loss of the shoulder contour may be seen with a prominent "sulcus" sign. Adduction and internal rotation are usually limited. A patient with a posterior dislocation will hold the arm in an adducted, internally rotated position.

Evaluation should include a thorough neurologic examination prior to any attempted reduction. Neurologic involvement is not infrequent with the axillary nerve being most commonly affected. Vascular status should likewise be documented, as vascular injuries can occur, although less commonly. Radiographic evaluation should also be completed prior to commencing treatment. A standard trauma series as described earlier is extremely helpful in delineating any associated glenoid rim or humeral head impaction fractures.

Reduction is most easily carried out with some form of sedation and or injection of lidocaine into the joint capsule. Gentle traction–counter traction will reduce most dislocations. Irreducible dislocations and fracture dislocations are best managed in the operating room with general anesthesia.

Postreduction, a period of immobilization in a sling from 10 days to 2 weeks is recommended followed by a supervised physical therapy program. In patients younger than 20 years, recurrence rates up to 90% have been reported most likely due to the violent nature of the dislocation and the very commonly associated anterior-inferior labral tear or "Bankart" lesion that occurs. In contrast, patients aged over 40 years commonly have associated rotator cuff tears. A high index of suspicion should be present at follow-up examination of these patients in the early recovery period.

Proximal Humerus Fractures

Proximal humerus fractures are common injuries, especially with our aging population. The majority of these injuries are minimally displaced or nondisplaced and can be treated conservatively. Factors to take into consideration in the treatment plan are age of the patient, hand dominance, bone quality, fracture type, and fracture displacement. Associated injuries in the multitrauma patient are also important in the decision-making process.

Assessment should consist of a thorough neurovascular examination along with a radiographic trauma series. The presence of an expanding axillary mass and absent distal pulses is concerning for a vascular injury. Nerve injuries occur in as many as one-third of patients and are more common with increasing age. In one study the incidence of nerve injury with proximal humeral fracture-dislocations was greater than 50% after age 50. If present, these injuries may take 9 months or more to recover neurologic function, which is often incomplete.

These fractures are classified according to the description by Neer. He described six variations of displaced proximal humerus fractures, and defined displacement as greater than 1 cm or 45 degrees of angulation. The anatomic "parts" consist of the anatomic neck, surgical neck, and greater and lesser tuberosities. Despite poor interobserver reliability, this is the most frequently used classification system. Figure 2 depicts various fracture patterns that are both considered "two-part fractures." The portion of the humerus that is displaced has clinical relevance due to the varying blood supply of the proximal humerus. Displacement of the anatomic neck for example, has a high chance of disrupting the blood supply and adversely affecting outcome, regardless of the treatment chosen.

Treatment varies from a period of immobilization in a sling followed by supervised physical therapy with close radiographic evaluation in nondisplaced or impacted fractures. Open reduction and internal fixation (ORIF) with aggressive therapy to reduce postoperative stiffness is preferable in fractures with greater displacement. The greater tuberosity fracture in Figure 2 was treated with suture fixation to the shaft, whereas the anatomic neck fracture underwent ORIF with a plate and screws as seen in Figure 3. In both cases, rapid aggressive physical therapy was possible postoperatively.

Humeral Shaft Fractures

There is a bimodal distribution of diaphyseal humeral shaft fractures, the first occurring in young males involved in high-energy motor vehicle accidents, falls from height, or gunshots. The second peak is seen in elderly women who sustain the fracture during a fall from a standing height. The reported incidence is approximately 14 per 100,000 per year.

Historically, treatment of these fractures has been successful with nonoperative management; initial splinting is followed by placement in a functional brace in the subacute phase. Gravity serves as an important factor in reduction and maintenance of alignment with this method of treatment. The complication rates of nerve injury and delayed union or nonunion have been lower than those reported for operative treatment. In one study of 922 patients treated with func-

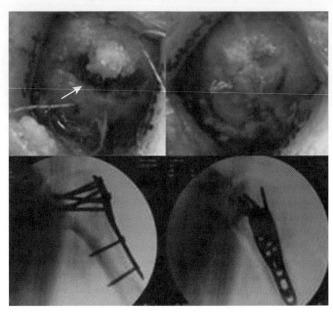

Figure 3 Intraoperative photos of greater tuberosity fracture being repaired with suture anchors *(above)*. Intraoperative fluoroscopy post–open reduction and internal fixation of anatomic neck fracture seen in Figure 2. *(Courtesy of Robin M. Gehrmann, MD.)*

tional bracing, only 3% of fractures failed to heal and 98% of patients regained near-full motion of the shoulder and elbow. Even in severely displaced or comminuted fractures such as the one seen in Figure 4, functional bracing may be the treatment of choice to minimize the risks associated with a major surgical procedure.

Treatment of fractures with associated nerve injury remains controversial. The reported incidence of radial nerve palsy varies from 1.8% to 24% with shaft fractures. The nerve is most commonly contused with a neuropraxia that recovers in greater than 70% of reported cases. Transverse fractures of the middle third are more likely to have a neuropraxia than spiral fractures of the distal third, which have a higher incidence of laceration or entrapment of the radial nerve as can be seen in Figure 5.

Low-velocity gunshot injuries to the humeral shaft have been shown to have similar infection and union rates when treated nonoperatively and given a 3-day course of oral ciprofloxacin versus 3 days of intravenous cephalosporin and amino glycoside.

The indications for operative intervention include open fractures, fractures with vascular injury, and injuries that cannot be acceptably aligned in a splint or functional brace as is most commonly seen in obese patients or severely comminuted fractures. Exploration for acute nerve injury cannot be universally recommended at this time.

ELBOW

Distal Humerus Fractures

Distal humerus fractures account for approximately 2% of all adult fractures. Both operative and nonoperative treatments have been reported to have poor outcomes due to pain, deformity, stiffness, nonunion, and ulnar neuropathy. The factors that appear to be most predictable of a good outcome are the ability to achieve an anatomic reduction of the joint surface and the ability to start early active motion.

When there is a displaced intra-articular component, operative treatment is the only way one can restore articular congruity.

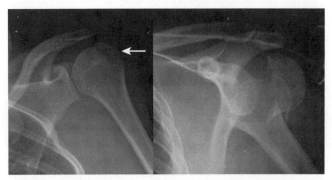

Figure 2 Displaced greater tuberosity fracture on left *(white arrow)*, and displaced anatomic neck fracture on right. Both are considered "two-part fractures" according to the Neer classification.

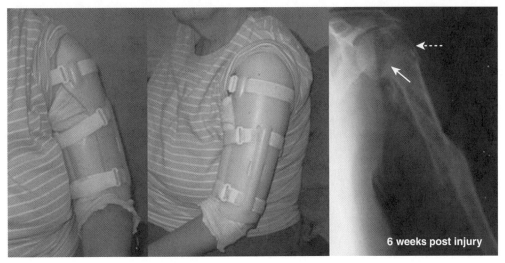

Figure 4 Clinical photos of a humeral fracture brace. Radiograph on right shows complex fracture being treated in this brace at 6 weeks with acceptable alignment of all components. Greater tuberosity component *(dotted arrow)*, surgical neck *(solid arrow)*, and comminuted shaft with early callus formation. *(Courtesy of Robin M. Gehrmann, MD.)*

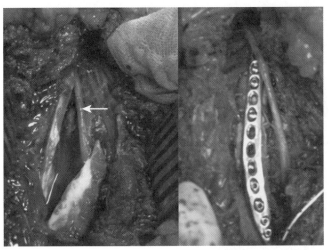

Figure 5 Intraoperative photograph of radial nerve. Incarcerated between bony spike of fracture fragments in a distal third humerus fracture *(left) (white arrow)*. Post–open reduction internal fixation (ORIF) with radial nerve crossing plate proximally *(right)*. *(Courtesy of Robin M. Gehrmann, MD.)*

maintenance of the reduction. Historically, this has led to the disastrous complications of Volkmann's ischemic contractures. It is therefore recommended that those fractures that are significantly displaced be closed reduced and pinned allowing the arm to be immobilized in 90 degrees or less, virtually eliminating this complication.

In adults the goals of reconstruction are aimed at re-creating the articular surface, and then re-establishing the medial and lateral columns of the humerus, Figure 6. An olecranon osteotomy is usually necessary in order to provide adequate exposure of the articular surface, after which the ulnar nerve is identified and retracted. Transposition of the nerve at the time of surgery is somewhat controversial at present.

Complications include ulnar neuropathy, heterotopic ossification, and painful impinging hardware, which can be removed once the fracture has healed, and if necessary ulnar nerve transposition can be carried out at the same time.

Nondisplaced or minimally displaced fractures can be treated nonoperatively if they are stable enough to allow for early range-of-motion (ROM) exercises. If the joint is not restored to its anatomic position, it will become painful as the high joint reactive forces lead to premature arthrosis.

In the case of a badly comminuted joint surface, in a low-demand elderly patient with poor bone quality other options would include early range-of-motion exercises to attempt to re-create some form of joint surface or primary total elbow arthroplasty. With modern fracture treatment principles and fixation devices good results can be achieved most of the time with ORIF.

Extra-articular fractures of the distal humerus occur more frequently in children than adults. They can be difficult to control in a splint or brace due to the muscle forces acting on the distal fragment, as well as the anatomy of the thin flat metaphyseal region, which makes it difficult to get any bony apposition for stability.

In children the more common "extension-type" fracture would require casting with the elbow in a greater-than-100 degrees flexion for

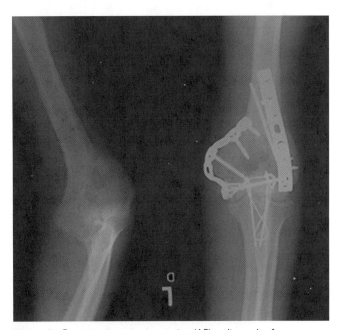

Figure 6 Preoperative anteroposterior (AP) radiograph of comminuted intra-articular distal humerus fracture *(left)*, and postoperative AP film *(right)* with restoration of the articular surface and the medial and lateral columns. *(Courtesy of Robin M. Gehrmann, MD.)*

In experienced hands, these fractures can be treated operatively with good to excellent results in most patients.

Elbow Dislocation

The elbow is the second most commonly dislocated joint (after the shoulder), accounting for 20% of all dislocations. Fifty percent of elbow stability is due to the highly congruent ulnohumeral joint, with the other 50% being provided by the collateral ligaments. The anterior band of the medial collateral ligament (also known as the anterior oblique ligament) is the primary stabilizer to valgus stress. The lateral collateral ligament complex (particularly the lateral ulnar collateral ligament) provides restraint to posterolateral rotatory subluxation and dislocation.

Elbow dislocation usually occurs in adolescents and young adults, frequently from a fall onto an outstretched arm with the shoulder abducted and elbow extended. Patients present with pain and inability to move the elbow. Gross deformity may be apparent, but can be under appreciated due to swelling. A thorough neurovascular exami-

nation and documentation is essential because 20% of cases have associated nerve injuries, usually neuropraxia of the ulnar or median nerves. The shoulder and wrist should be carefully evaluated to rule out concomitant injuries, which can occur in up to 15% of cases. Any forearm tenderness and instability of the distal radioulnar joint should be recognized as signs of disruption of the interosseous membrane (i.e., an Essex-Lopresti injury).

Radiographs of the elbow are used to confirm the clinical diagnosis of dislocation. An elbow dislocation that does not involve a fracture is known as a simple dislocation, and is classified according to the direction of the dislocation. Dislocation with associated fracture(s) of the radial head/neck and/or coronoid process (i.e., complex dislocation) must be determined on imaging studies because they have implications for definitive treatment (Figure 7).

An acute elbow dislocation should be initially managed by prompt closed reduction under adequate analgesia and muscle relaxation. This can usually be achieved in the emergency room with intramuscular or intravenous medication(s). Several reduction techniques have been described, but they all involve correcting the medial-lateral displacement, followed by longitudinal traction

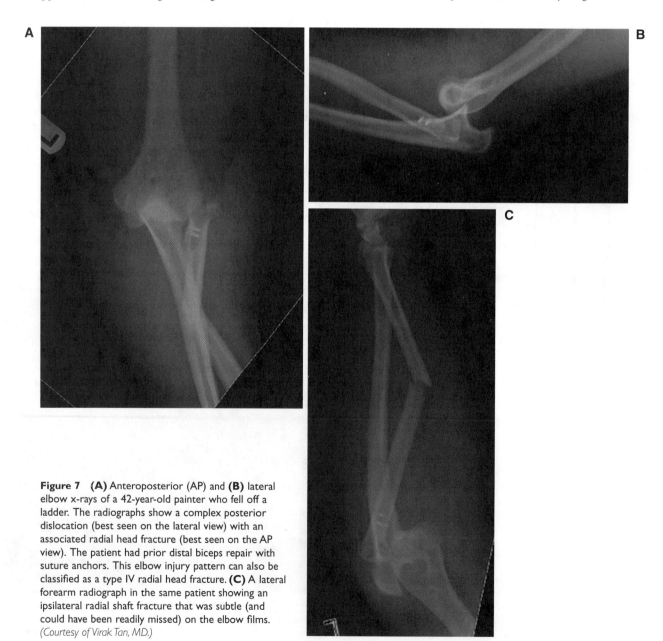

Figure 7 **(A)** Anteroposterior (AP) and **(B)** lateral elbow x-rays of a 42-year-old painter who fell off a ladder. The radiographs show a complex posterior dislocation (best seen on the lateral view) with an associated radial head fracture (best seen on the AP view). The patient had prior distal biceps repair with suture anchors. This elbow injury pattern can also be classified as a type IV radial head fracture. **(C)** A lateral forearm radiograph in the same patient showing an ipsilateral radial shaft fracture that was subtle (and could have been readily missed) on the elbow films. *(Courtesy of Virak Tan, MD.)*

and flexion of the forearm. A "clunk" is often felt with reduction of the joint.

After reduction, stability is assessed by checking range of motion with valgus-varus stress. Passive motion to within 30 degrees of full extension suggests a stable reduction and mobilization of the elbow can begin within a few days when the patient is more comfortable. If the elbow is unstable after reduction, then it should be immobilized in 90 degrees of flexion for approximately 3 weeks before beginning motion. Alternatively, an overhead rehabilitation protocol can be initiated with proper splinting and supervision. The overhead protocol takes advantage of gravity to maintain reduction during elbow motion.

Posterior elbow dislocation with associated fractures of the radial head and the coronoid process has been referred to as the "terrible triad of the elbow" because of the difficulties encountered in its management. Definitive treatment of these complex elbow dislocations usually involves surgery because they are highly unstable and are prone to numerous complications when inadequately treated. With operative treatment, the surgeon should attempt to restore elbow stability by (1) reestablishing radiocapitellar contact (by either repairing the radial head or replacing it with a prosthesis), (2) repairing the lateral collateral ligament, and (3) performing internal fixation of the coronoid fracture, as needed.

The outcome of nonoperative management of a simple elbow dislocation is highly successful. Poor results can occur with prolonged immobilization (usually greater than 3 weeks) and inadequate rehabilitation. Other complicating sequelae include heterotopic ossification and stiffness. Additionally, complex dislocations can also have recurrent instability, failure of fixation, post-traumatic arthritis, and tardy ulnar nerve palsy.

Radial Head Fractures

Radial head fractures are common injuries accounting for one-third of elbow fractures. Fifty percent to 60% of elbow dislocations have associated radial head and neck fractures. The mechanism of injury is usually an axial load on a pronated forearm. Patients with radial head fractures often present with lateral elbow pain upon extension or forearm rotation. Diagnosis and classification (modified Mason) of these injuries are based on radiographs. Type I is nondisplaced, type II is a displaced single fragment, and type III is a comminuted fracture. Type IV is a radial head fracture with an associated elbow dislocation.

Nondisplaced fractures are well managed with early mobilization. Operative indications for radial head fractures include displacement greater than 3 mm, bony block to elbow motion, Essex-Lopresti lesion (i.e., associated disruption of the interosseous membrane), and an unstable elbow. Surgery for radial head fracture may entail excision, internal fixation or prosthetic replacement. Isolated radial head fractures can be safely excised without compromising elbow stability or function, especially in the elderly patient. Ring et al. have shown that internal fixation is best reserved for radial head fractures with three or fewer fragments. Specialized precontoured radial head plates are available, and should be placed in the "safe zone" to prevent hardware impingement on the radial notch. Metallic prosthetic radial head replacement is performed when fixation of the head is not possible in the setting of an Essex-Lopresti lesion or a type IV fracture. At the time of this writing, there is no role for silicone radial head spacer due to silicone synovitis.

Coronoid Fractures

The coronoid process of the ulna serves as an anterior buttress of the greater sigmoid notch and is the attachment site for the anterior bundle of the medial collateral ligament and anterior capsule. Therefore it has an important role in providing stability to the elbow.

Coronoid fractures are common, and are associated with 10% of elbow dislocations. Classically, three types have been identified to occur in the coronal plane and are best seen on a lateral elbow x-ray: type I, tip avulsion; type II, less than 50%; and type II, greater than 50%. More recently, an oblique or vertical fracture line about the anteromedial coronoid is also recognized to cause instability of the ulnohumeral joint (Figure 8). This fragment is best seen on computed tomography scan. In general, types I and II coronoid fractures can be managed without fixation of the fragment itself. Because displaced type III or anteromedial fractures are associated with elbow instability, they should be treated with internal fixation and as part of the overall surgical management of elbow dislocation. Failure to stabilize these fractures will result in recurrent elbow subluxation or dislocation.

Olecranon Fractures

The greater sigmoid notch of the ulna is formed by the olecranon and coronoid processes. The olecranon makes up the proximal half of the notch, and by definition, isolated fractures involving this portion do not result in ulnohumeral instability. Olecranon fractures can result from direct force or from eccentric loading of the triceps. Minimally displaced fractures (<2-mm gap at 90 degrees of elbow flexion) are uncommon but can be treated with elbow splinting at 30 to 45 degrees of flexion. More commonly, the fractures are displaced and require operative fixation to restore active elbow extension. Several options exist for fixing olecranon fractures including tension band technique with supplemental Kirschner wires or screw(s), bicortical interfragmentary screw(s), and plating. Comminuted fractures are best managed with dorsal plate fixation. In cases of severe comminution, excision of the fragments, and reattachment of the triceps to the remaining portion of the proximal ulna may be required.

Complications of olecranon fixation most commonly involve hardware prominence, which can be managed by removal after the fracture has healed. In addition, elbow stiffness, malunion, nonunion, and post-traumatic arthritis can also occur.

FOREARM

Fractures of the forearm commonly result from high-energy trauma and are often associated with systemic and other musculoskeletal injuries. Clinical evaluation should include careful examination of the entire patient and not just the injured extremity. It is essential to determine if there is an open wound, neurovascular deficit, and/or impending forearm compartment syndrome. Radiographs should include AP and lateral views of the forearm, elbow, and wrist. All adult forearm fractures, except for the isolated nondisplaced or minimally displaced ulnar shaft fracture, require operative fixation. Surgical approach to the ulna is through the subcutaneous border between the flexor carpi ulnaris and extensor carpi ulnaris interval. The radial shaft is best approached from the volar side using the Henry approach. Alternatively, the Thompson dorsal approach may be used for middle and proximal third radial shaft fracture but puts the posterior interosseous nerve at risk for iatrogenic injury. The gold standard for fixation of forearm shaft fracture is 3.5-mm compression plating. In certain cases, intramedullary rodding or external fixation of ulnar or radial shaft may be done.

Monteggia Fracture

Monteggia fracture is a fracture of the proximal ulna with dislocation of the radial head. It occurs in 1%–2% of all forearm fractures. Bado described four types of injury patterns: type I, apex anterior ulnar fracture and anterior radial head dislocation; type II, apex posterior

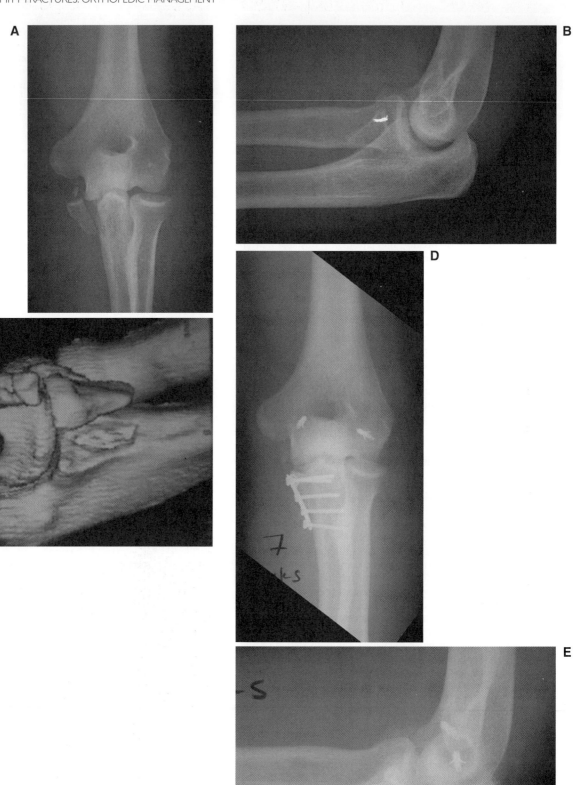

Figure 8 **(A)** Anteroposterior (AP) and **(B)** lateral elbow radiographs and **(C)** a three-dimensional computed tomography scan showing an anterior medial coronoid fracture. This patient had an elbow dislocation that was emergently reduced prior to these imaging studies. **(D)** and **(E)** The patient subsequently underwent operative fixation of his coronoid fracture and repair of both the lateral and medial collateral ligaments with suture anchors.   *(Courtesy of Virak Tan, MD.)*

ulnar fracture and posterior radial head dislocation; type III, proximal ulnar metaphyseal fracture and lateral radial head dislocation; and type IV, proximal ulnar and radial shaft fractures and anterior radial head dislocation (Figure 9). The key to successful outcome of Monteggia fracture is anatomic reduction and fixation of the ulna fracture. Upon reduction of the ulna, there is typically concomitant stable relocation of the radial head. Irreducible radial head dislocations can be associated with posterior interosseous nerve entrapment. In type IV lesions, open reduction and internal fixation of both the ulna and radius are required.

Complications of Monteggia fractures often result from nonanatomic or loss of fixation of the ulna fracture, leading to recurrent dislocation of the radial head. Poor outcomes can also be due to heterotopic ossification with proximal radioulnar synostosis.

Radial and/or Ulnar Shaft Fractures

Fractures of both the radial and ulnar shafts ("both-bone forearm" fractures) are operative injuries in the adult population. Most surgeons prefer compression plating of both bones using a separate incision for each. The anatomic bow of the radial shaft must be restored to prevent loss of forearm motion. In children, this injury may be treated with closed reduction and casting, provided that near-anatomic alignment of the shafts are established.

Isolated radial shaft fractures are uncommon but can occur from projectile injury such as a gunshot blast. A Galeazzi injury pattern must be ruled out by assessing the distal radioulnar joint (DRUJ) for instability. Even without DRUJ disruption, isolated radial shaft fractures are poorly controlled by casting, and therefore should generally have internal fixation.

Isolated ulnar shaft fractures are commonly referred to as "night stick fractures" because historically they occurred as a result of a direct blow to the ulnar aspect of the forearm from a night stick. In the modern era, motor vehicle accidents can also cause this injury. Fractures with less than 10 degrees of angulation and 50% shaft displacement can be treated by nonoperative means. Surgical treatment with compression plating is indicated for the more displaced fracture. Care should be taken to avoid injury to the dorsal sensory branch of the ulnar nerve during the approach for distal third fractures.

Galeazzi Fractures

A Galeazzi fracture is defined as a fracture of the middle to the distal radial shaft with subluxation or dislocation of the DRUJ. It is an uncommon injury, with incidence varying from 3% to 6% of all forearm fractures. The mechanism is a direct blow to the dorsoradial

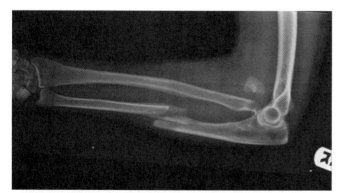

Figure 9 A single anteroposterior radiograph of the forearm showing a Monteggia type IV variant where there are fractures of the midshaft of the ulna and radial neck, and dislocation of the radial head. *(Courtesy of Virak Tan, MD.)*

wrist or a fall onto an outstretched hand with forced pronation of the forearm. Radiographic signs of a Galeazzi fracture include an ulnar styloid fracture, widened DRUJ on the AP view, dorsal dislocation of the distal ulna on the lateral view, and 5 mm or greater of radial shortening through the fracture site.

Operative treatment is essential in all Galeazzi fractures because closed treatment has resulted in a 92% failure rate due to loss of reduction of the radial shaft. After stable anatomic internal fixation of the radius, the distal radioulnar joint stability is assessed. If the joint is stable with forearm rotation, then immobilization is not necessary. However, if the DRUJ is reducible but is unstable, then either the arm must be immobilized in supination or the DRUJ pinned in the reduced position. Failure to reduce the DRJU by closed means necessitates open reduction of the joint.

The major concerns with treatment of Galeazzi fracture is loss of forearm rotation due to malalignment of the radius and incongruity of the DRUJ leading to painful motion.

WRIST

Distal Radius Fracture

Fractures of the distal radius are common, accounting for approximately 250,000 to 300,000 cases in the United States annually. This injury represents 20% of all fractures leading to emergency room visits and 75% of all forearm fractures. The mechanism is typically either a low-energy mechanism such as a fall onto an outstretched hand or a high-energy impact such as a motor vehicle accident or fall from height. Although in the past distal radius fractures were thought of as a homogeneous group of injuries, it is now widely recognized that there are different and often complex fracture patterns.

The diagnosis of a distal radius fracture is based on the history, examination, and imaging studies. Age, hand dominance, occupation/vocation, and mechanism of injury should be obtained in the history. Associated injuries in other areas of the body should be ruled out when there is a high-energy mechanism. Evaluation of the injured extremity should not just focus on the deformed wrist, but include examination of the elbow and forearm. Careful neurovascular examination must be performed with attention to the median nerve, since acute carpal tunnel syndrome can develop with displaced distal radius fractures.

Closed reduction and splinting of acute displaced fractures should be done in the emergency room to correct the wrist deformity and decrease the risk of traumatic carpal tunnel syndrome. In those cases in which there is minimal comminution and articular step-off, casting with close radiographic follow-up remains a good option. Loss of reduction is the main drawback of nonoperative treatment. Casting has also been associated with wrist/hand stiffness, compressive neuropathies, and complex regional pain syndrome.

For fractures that cannot be adequately reduced or maintained by closed methods, an external fixator with or without Kirschner wires may be indicated. Often times, overdistraction or flexion of the wrist is required to maintain reduction, which may lead to hand stiffness, median nerve compromise, and complex regional pain syndrome. Additionally, the risk of pin tract infection and soft tissue irritation is reported up to 60% of cases.

In light of the limitations of external fixation, open reduction and internal fixation have become a more widely used technique. Exposing the fracture through a dorsal or volar approach allows direct visualization and manipulation of the fracture fragments. A number of plate and screw constructs are available for both dorsal and volar fixation. Dorsally applied hardware has associated complications, such as tendon irritation or rupture and the possible need for removal of the hardware after fracture healing. Thus, the volar approach has recently become more popular. Newer fixed-angle plating systems allow early therapy to regain wrist and finger motion. However, the amount of soft tissue dissection and the extramedullary position of the implant still pose some disadvantages in treating wrist fractures.

Intramedullary devices such as the Micronail (Wright Medical Technology, Inc., Memphis, TN) attempt to counteract some of the disadvantages noted with open reduction and plating. By residing within the medullary canal, these devices minimize or eliminate soft tissue irritation and pin track infection, yet maintaining fracture reduction and alignment (Figure 10).

Perilunate Dislocations

Perilunate dislocations are relatively rare but complex injuries involving only 7% of all injuries of the carpus. They most often result from high energy mechanisms, including motor vehicle accidents, falls from height, or contact sports, and thus are often associated with other significant trauma. Mayfield et al. showed that an axial load with hyperextension and ulnar deviation of the wrist, coupled with intercarpal supination, reproduced a spectrum of "progressive perilunate instability." Four stages of perilunate injuries were described as the carpus is disrupted around the lunate. The pattern of sequential failure begins radially and is transmitted either through the body of the scaphoid (producing a trans-scaphoid fracture) or through the scapholunate (SL) interval (producing a SL dissociation). The force then propagates to the ulnodorsal aspects of the wrist. In stage I, there is disruption of the scapholunate and radioscaphocapitate ligaments. In stage II, the force disrupts the lunocapitate association. In stage III, there is failure of the lunotriquetral interosseous and ulnotriquetral ligaments, where the entire carpus separates from the lunate. Finally, stage IV involves palmar lunate dislocation into the carpal tunnel. Mayfield demonstrated that slower application of load produced fractures (radial styloid, scaphoid and/or capitate) prior to the lunate dislocation, termed "greater arc injuries." Conversely, a more rapidly applied force produced purely ligamentous disruptions, termed "lesser arc injuries."

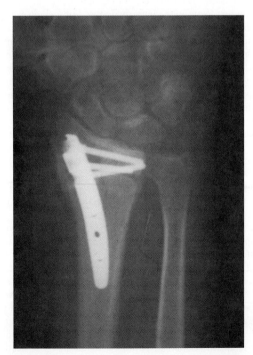

Figure 10 A single posteroanterior radiograph of the wrist in a patient who underwent distal radius fracture fixation with an intramedullary device. The fracture line is faintly visible just proximal to the distal screws. *(Courtesy of Virak Tan, MD.)*

Correct diagnosis and treatment of these injuries is imperative in order to restore wrist motion and function. The major pitfall in treating perilunate carpal injuries is delayed or missed diagnosis. The patient may have multiple (even life-threatening) injuries that preclude adequate workup and imaging of extremity injuries. Other times, the dislocation is missed because the radiographs are misread by inexperienced observers.

The typical presentation of an acute perilunate dislocation includes pain and swelling about the wrist. Deformity may be more subtle than expected. The carpus is usually displaced dorsally. In a lunate dislocation, the lunate can come to lie within the carpal tunnel; therefore, thorough neurovascular assessment of the upper extremity is important. A well-taken wrist series is the key to the diagnosis. Posterior-anterior view will show disruption of the normal carpal arcs (Figure 11A). Lateral radiograph will reveal loss of colinearity between the capitate, lunate, and the radius (Figure 11B). Traction radiographs may be indicated to further assess the injury pattern.

Once the diagnosis of a perilunate dislocation is made, treatment consists of immediate closed manipulation to achieve reduction and immobilization. Reduction is usually undertaken with the patient under intravenous sedation. The arm is first suspended in longitudinal traction. With the wrist extended and maintaining traction, a thumb is used to push the lunate back into its fossa as the wrist is then flexed to reduce the capitate over and into the concavity of the lunate. Failure to achieve a reduction via closed means often indicates interposed volar capsule and necessitates an urgent open procedure. A patient with an irreducible perilunate dislocation at minimum must undergo an urgent temporizing extended carpal tunnel release to decrease the pressure on the median nerve (Figure 11C). Failure to do so could result in permanent median nerve dysfunction.

Early definitive treatment of perilunate injuries is necessary to minimize the devastating complications of chronic carpal instability and traumatic arthritis associated from missed or inappropriately treated injuries. Despite the overall consensus that open reduction and internal fixation is the treatment of choice for restoring carpal alignment in acute perilunate dislocations, the ideal surgical approach is less explicit. There are three basic surgical approaches that can be used: volar, dorsal, and combined dorsal–volar approach.

The volar or palmar approach is typically used for reduction of the lunate and carpal tunnel release. Additionally, direct repair of the capsular rent at the space of Poirier can be done volarly. The dorsal approach provides exposure of the carpus for restoring alignment and repairing the scapholunate interosseous ligament (SLIL) which is thought to be the key to successful long-term results. Moreover, scaphoid and other carpal bone fractures can also be addressed dorsally. The combined dorsal–volar approach offers the advantages of both and is the preferred choice for the authors since it allows access to all the injured structures.

Carpal Fractures and Ligamentous Injuries

Trauma to the carpus can result in fractures or ligamentous disruptions. The scaphoid is the most common carpal fracture and can occur in isolation or in conjunction with distal radius or perilunate injuries. Emergency room management of isolated scaphoid fracture should include appropriate x-ray views, followed by a long-arm thumb-spica splint immobilization. Ninety percent to 95% of acute nondisplaced scaphoid fractures will heal with proper immobilization; however, it may take 8–12 weeks and several cast changes. Percutaneous headless screw fixation of acute scaphoid fractures has resulted in shorter healing time and less overall disability. Displaced scaphoid fractures require open reduction and fixation; there is no role for closed treatment under normal circumstances. Missed or inadequate treatment of a scaphoid fracture can result in malunion, nonunion, and/or avascular necrosis, which will lead to wrist arthritis in the long run.

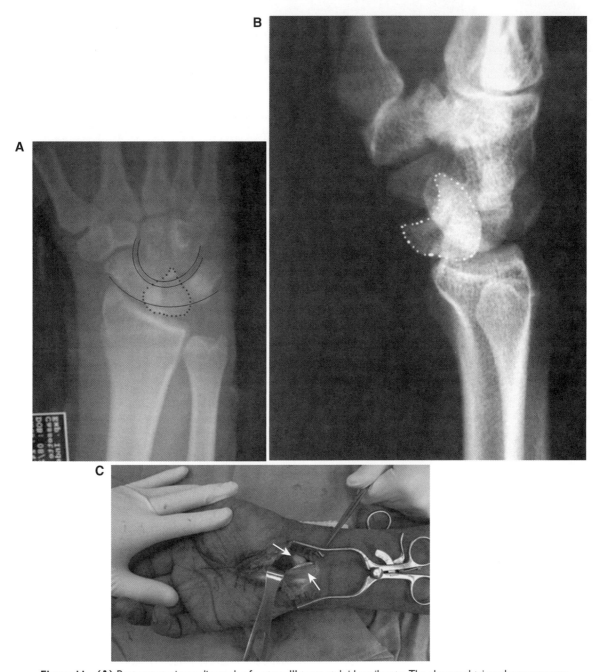

Figure 11 **(A)** Posteroanterior radiograph of a stage III trans-styloid perilunate. The abnormal triangular appearance of the lunate *(black dots)* has disrupted Gilula's arcs *(black lines)*. **(B)** Lateral radiograph of the same patient showing the lunate *(outlined)* is still articulating with the distal radius; however, there is dislocation of lunocapitate articulation. There is loss of colinearity among the radius, lunate, and capitate. **(C)** An emergent extended carpal tunnel release is required for irreducible perilunate dislocations. The transverse carpal ligament has been divided longitudinally, and the content of the carpal canal (including the median nerve, *bottom arrow*) is retracted ulnarly. The lunate *(top arrow)* is seen dislocated into the carpal canal.   *(Courtesy of Virak Tan, MD.)*

Fractures of the other carpal bones are uncommon and are usually a part of a larger injury spectrum. Kienbock's disease should be ruled out in patients with a lunate fracture but minimal trauma.

Scapholunate dissociation results from disruption of the scapholunate interosseous ligament. Dorsal wrist pain with tenderness over the scapholunate interval is the usual finding. The scaphoid shift test may also be positive. The space between the scaphoid and lunate will be widened on the AP radiograph. Early surgical treatment of this injury is simpler, and has better results than delayed reconstruction.

CONCLUSION

Trauma to the upper extremity can result in a variety of injury patterns, ranging from minor sprains to complex open fracture-dislocations. Often the injury can be treated or at least temporized by immobilization or splinting which will help with pain control and also minimize further damage to the extremity. Proper patient assessment and imaging studies are essential to initiating treatment. Although life-threatening injuries take precedence over the limb, a long-arm posterior splint can usually be applied expeditiously to the injured arm without interfering with the resuscitation effort.

There are several injury patterns that are orthopedic emergencies: dislocations, open fractures, acute trauma–related carpal tunnel syndrome, and compartment syndrome. Joint dislocations require prompt reduction in the emergency room or trauma bay. Failure to relocate the joint necessitates an emergent trip to the operating room for closed reduction under anesthesia or an open reduction. Open fractures are at risk for infection, and therefore need appropriate antibiotics and irrigation and debridement within 8 hours of the injury. Acute trauma–related median nerve compression often accompanies displaced distal radius fractures and perilunate dislocations. When the symptoms are progressive, an urgent surgical release of the transverse carpal ligament will prevent long-term sequelae. Compartment syndrome can occur after a crush or penetrating mechanism. These patients need close monitoring for sign and symptoms of increased compartment pressure. When compartment syndrome does occur, an immediate decompression of the compartments is warranted to prevent neurovascular compromise and eventual muscle necrosis and fibrosis.

SUGGESTED READINGS

Ada JR, Miller ME: Scapular fractures: analysis of 113 cases. *Clin Orthop* 269:174–180, 1991.

Althausen PL, Lee MA, Finkemeier CG: Scapulothoracic dissociation: diagnosis and treatment. *Clin Orthop Relat Res* 416:237–244, 2003.

Bado JL: The Monteggia lesion. *Clinical Orthopaedics & Related Research.* 50:71–86, 1967.

Blazar PE: Dislocations/instability. In Beredjiklian PK, Bozentka DJ, editors: *Review of Hand Surgery.* Philadelphia, Saunders, 2004, pp. 139–150.

Boyer MI, Galatz LM, Borrelli J Jr, et al: Intra-articular fractures of the upper extremity: new concepts in surgical treatment. *Instr Course Lect* 52: 591–605, 2003.

Egol KA, Connor PM, Karunakar MA, Sims SH, Bosse MJ, Kellam JF: The floating shoulder: clinical and functional results. *J Bone Joint Surg [Am]* 83:1188–1194, 2001.

Gustilo RB, Merkow RL, Tempelton D: Current concepts review: the management of open fracture. *J Bone Joint Surg* 72-A:299–304, 1990.

Hawkins RJ, Angelo RL: Displaced proximal humeral fractures: selecting treatment, avoiding pitfalls. *Orthop Clin North Am* 18:421–431, 1987.

Hughes SP: Antibiotics penetration into bone in relation to the immediate management of open fractures: a review. *Acta Orthopaed Belg* 58(1 Suppl): 217–221, 1992.

Jeon IH, Oh CW, Park BC, Ihn JC, Kim PT: Minimal invasive percutaneous Herbert screw fixation in acute unstable scaphoid fracture. *Hand Surg* 8(2):213–218, 2003.

Johansen K, Sangeorzan B, Copass MK: Traumatic scapulothoracic dissociation: case report. *J Trauma* 31:147–149, 1991.

Knapp TP, Patzakis MJ, Lee J, Seipel PR, Abdollahi K, Reisch RB: Comparison of intravenous and oral antibiotic therapy in the treatment of fractures caused by low-velocity gunshots. A prospective, randomized study of infection rates. *J Bone Joint Surg [Am]* 78:1167–1171, 1996.

Mayfield JK, Johnson RP, Kilcoyne RK: Carpal dislocations: pathomechanics and progressive perilunar instability. *J Hand Surg [Am]* 5(3):226–241, 1980.

Neer CS II: Displaced proximal humeral fractures: I. Classification and evaluation. *J Bone Joint Surg [Am]* 52:1077–1089, 1970.

O'Driscoll SW: Elbow dislocations. In: Morrey BF, editor: *The Elbow and Its Disorders.* Philadelphia, WB Saunders, 2000, pp. 409–420.

Orbay JL, Fernandez DL: Volar fixed-angle plate fixation for unstable distal radius fractures in the elderly patient. *J Hand Surg* 29(1):96–102, 2004.

Pugh DM, Wild LM, Schemitsch EH, King GJ, McKee MD: Standard surgical protocol to treat elbow dislocations with radial head and coronoid fractures. *J Bone Joint Surg [Am]* 86-A(6):1122–1130, 2004.

Regan WD, Morrey BF: Coronoid process and Monteggia fractures. In Morrey BF, editor: *The Elbow and Its Disorders.* Philadelphia, WB Saunders, 2000, pp. 396–408.

Ring D, Quintero J, Jupiter JB: Open reduction and internal fixation of fractures of the radial head. *Journal of Bone & Joint Surgery—American Volume.* 84-A(10):1811–1815, 2002.

Rozental TD, Beredjiklian PK, Bozentka DJ: Longitudinal radioulnar dissociation. *J Am Acad Orthop Surg* 11(1):68–73, 2003.

Sarmiento A, Zagorski JB, Zych GA, Latta LL, Capps CA: Functional bracing for the treatment of fractures of the humeral diaphysis. *J Bone Joint Surg [Am]* 82:478–486, 2000.

Simic PM, Weiland AJ: Fractures of the distal aspect of the radius: changes in treatment over the past two decades. *Instr Course Lect* 52:185–195, 2003.

Tan V, Capo J, Warburton M: Distal radius fixation with an intramedullary nail. *Tech Hand Upper Extrem Surg* 9(4):195–201, 2005.

LOWER EXTREMITY AND DEGLOVING INJURY

Peter G. Trafton, Herman P. Houin, and Donald D. Trunkey

Injuries of the lower extremity can be devastating (see Mangled Extremities section) and life-threatening or minimal and quickly healed. Advanced Trauma Life Support (ATLS) assessments should be made on all patients. The history, if obtainable, should include the mechanism of injury, initial physical examination by emergency medical services, and any pertinent medical information. Control of exsanguinating hemorrhage and splint immobilization should take priority.

The physical examination should include localization of pain and assessment of pulses, sensation, color, motor function, and angulated or rotational deformities. The entrance and exit of foreign objects that have caused penetration injuries and potentially embedded foreign objects should be noted.

RADIOLOGIC EVALUATION

Thorough evaluation of lower extremity injuries should include anteroposterior and lateral radiographs of the injured area and the joint above and below. Penetrating injuries are best evaluated with entrance and exit site markers. Careful clinical evaluations can minimize needless overuse of angiography (and subsequently its complications and expense); however, if one or more pulses distal to a penetrating injury are absent, the patient needs angiography, computed tomographic arteriography (CTA), or immediate surgery. If pulses are present, ankle brachial indices (ABIs) should be obtained. If the dorsalis pedis and posterior tibialis ABI are 1.0 or greater, the patient can be safely observed for other injuries and discharged with follow-up ABIs taken at 1 week. If the dorsalis pedis or posterior tibialis ABI is less than 1.0 with clinical ischemia, emergency angiography, CTA, or surgery (if distal perfusion is clearly inadequate) should be done if duplex scanning is not available or wounds are extensive, such as shotgun injuries. If distal perfusion is clinically adequate with an ABI less than 1.0, duplex ultrasonography can be done electively. If it is negative or shows only a minor injury (small intimal defect or small pseudoaneurysm), the patient can be observed with follow-up ABIs obtained in 1 week. If duplex scanning reveals a major injury, such as a large intimal defect, large pseudoaneurysm, or intraluminal clot, angiography or exploration should be performed.

FRACTURES

It is now generally accepted that aggressive, appropriate early management of the trauma patient's musculoskeletal injuries contributes substantially to overall care by reducing morbidity, mortality, and costs. Rehabilitation and ultimate function are also improved. This section is not a "how-to" discussion, but rather provides recommendations for immediate and knowledgeable collaboration with an experienced orthopedic traumatologist. Specific details of management for musculoskeletal injuries are treated only briefly (and thus arbitrarily) here. Several acceptable alternative treatments exist for many fractures. Differences of opinion are thus unavoidable.

Skeletal injuries cannot be managed safely in isolation. The treating physician must always think beyond the broken bone and assess associated soft tissue trauma, the status of the entire injured limb, and the whole patient. Other injuries, age and anticipated activity level, pre-existing musculoskeletal resources, and chances for meaningful participation in a rehabilitation program must also be considered. The choice of management for fractures and joint injuries may depend on whether an injury is isolated or is one of several problems in a patient with multiple injuries. Treatment is also affected by the resources available to the surgeon. In the absence of a well-equipped operating room, effective radiographic monitoring, and an experienced surgical team, modern techniques of internal fixation are likely to fail.

EARLY CARE OF MUSCULOSKELETAL INJURIES

Extremity injuries may be obvious or occult. Initial care of obvious injuries includes control of bleeding with pressure dressings, splinting unstable injuries in an acceptable position, and urgent identification and treatment of arterial occlusion.

Once resuscitation is proceeding satisfactorily, a thorough and systematic search must be made for more occult injuries. All skin surfaces, from digits to trunk, must be inspected for deformity, swelling, ecchymosis, and laceration. Skin abrasions are significant. If they are present in the region of a musculoskeletal injury, any needed operation must be done promptly or delayed until the abrasion heals. Palpate each bone and joint for swelling, deformity, and tenderness. Manually stress each bone to confirm stability. Move each joint to demonstrate normal passive range of motion and absence of abnormal motion (instability). When emergency surgery is a part of the resuscitation or early care of a trauma patient, examination of the extremities should always be completed before terminating the anesthetic. Confirm the presence of peripheral pulses. Obtain radiographs of all abnormal areas.

When the patient is conscious and able to cooperate, active voluntary motion of each joint must be assessed to check motor nerve and myotendinous integrity. Check sensation in the isolated sensory area of each major peripheral nerve. For critically ill patients who are unable to cooperate initially, completion of this evaluation may take several days. Such follow-through is mandatory to avoid missing injuries. Resuscitation of patients with multiple injuries necessarily places diagnosis and treatment of musculoskeletal conditions at a relatively low priority. Many injuries are not initially appreciated. Repeated examinations during the early recovery period are frequently rewarded by the discovery of additional injuries in time for effective treatment.

OPEN FRACTURES

Identification and Classification

Open fractures require special attention to minimize risk of clostridial and pyogenic infections. Treatment is guided by classification of the severity of the injury, primarily according to the extent of soft tissue trauma, and level of contamination (Table 1). It is important to consider the entire soft tissue wound and not just the skin opening. In severe crush injuries, small lacerations may overlie extensively contused or necrotic soft tissue.

Identification of an open fracture is the first step of early management. Although they are usually obvious, open fractures occasionally are missed because of an incomplete examination. Posterior surfaces must be checked. Seemingly superficial wounds may communicate with underlying injuries to bones or joints. Neurovascular status, myotendinous function, and the possibility of multiple injuries must be checked. If completely satisfactory examination and treatment of a wound near a fracture cannot be done in the emergency department (ED) assume that the fracture is open and proceed to the operating room (OR) where adequate anesthesia, assistance, hemostasis, and lighting usually confirm suspicions and facilitate treatment.

Once an injured limb has been examined, control of bleeding is achieved with sterile compression dressings, and a splint is applied before transportation to the radiology department or the OR. If a patient arrives with a well-described open fracture already covered, the dressing should optimally be removed only in the OR. Radiographs of injured or suspect areas are essential for evaluating the trauma patient. Unfortunately, the quality of emergency studies varies greatly, and it is risky for the patient to languish, poorly monitored, in the radiology department. The responsible surgeon must be prepared at any moment to conclude that the radiographs already obtained are the best possible and that the patient should proceed to surgery. Chest, pelvis, and cervical spine radiographs have the highest priority. Those of the extremities are necessary for a complete evaluation. Without adequate radiographs, the orthopedic surgeon may not be able to diagnose the extent of the fracture and whether it is an intra-articular injury. Of course, such radiographs may be obtained in the OR once the patient has been stabilized.

Management

It is strongly recommended that each open fracture be cared for in a well-prepared OR, with adequate anesthesia, as soon as is safely possible.

Table 1: Classification of Open Fractures

Grade I	Small wounds caused by low-velocity trauma, with minimal contamination and soft tissue damage (e.g., skin laceration by bone end or a low-velocity gunshot wound).
Grade II	Wounds more extensive in length and width, but that have little or no avascular or devitalized soft tissue and minimal contamination.
Grade IIIA	Significant wounds caused by high-energy trauma, often with extensive lacerations and soft tissue flaps, but such that after final debridement, adequate local soft tissue coverage is maintained and delayed primary closure is feasible.
Grade IIIB	Major wounds with considerable devitalized soft tissue, contamination, or both. Bone is exposed in the wound, and extensive periosteal avulsion may be present. Coverage of the soft tissue defect usually requires a local or free microvascular muscle pedicle graft.
Grade IIIC	Open fracture with an associated arterial injury that requires repair.

Immediate Wound Care

The basic aspects of surgical wound care have changed little since their description by Desault in the late 18th century. Effective medical adjuncts are more recent. Tetanus prophylaxis is administered immediately. The use of an appropriate IV antibiotic promptly after diagnosis of an open fracture is required. The value of this adjunct to surgical treatment has been shown by several comparative studies. A good requirement is the use 1 g of IV Cefazolin every 8 hours, beginning in the ED and continuing through the 48 hours after injury, regardless of whether the wound is left open. Depending on the source and extent of contamination, aminoglycosides for better Gram-negative coverage and/or penicillin for anaerobic organisms should be added to the initial antibiotic regimen, especially for grade III open fractures. Alternative antibiotics are required for allergic patients.

The properly evaluated patient is brought to the OR as soon as the team and equipment are assembled. Adequate anesthesia is induced, and definitive care of the open fracture is begun simultaneously with or following higher-priority surgical treatment.

Care of the open fracture starts with a thorough reassessment of the injured limb, which takes place under anesthesia. Is salvage warranted or must primary amputation be considered? If amputation seems to be a possibility, an effort to discuss this with the patient and/or the family preoperatively in the ED is optimal. It is also optimal to have another surgeon agree and write a note in the patient's chart that amputation is the best treatment alternative.

A pneumatic tourniquet is applied, but inflated only if necessary to control bleeding or to assess tissue viability with postischemic hyperemia. In principle, further contamination of the wound of an open fracture should be avoided during cleansing of an injured limb. However, in practice it is hard to scrub the limb adequately while a sterile occlusive dressing is kept over the wound. Most detergents and soaps are injurious to tissue; therefore, the wound itself should be avoided during use of a scrub solution. The scrub is done with the limb lying on a sterile waterproof disposable drape, which is replaced twice during the 10-minute wash. Detergent suds are rinsed, and the skin is dried with sterile towels. At that point, the entire limb, including the wound, is disinfected with iodophor antiseptic solution, and new waterproof sterile drapes are applied.

Irrigation and Debridement

Irrigation and debridement comprise the next step. It is often necessary to enlarge the wound to permit adequate inspection and cleansing. This should be carefully planned to avoid devitalizing skin flaps or interrupting superficial veins that might be essential for blood return. If possible, incisions should avoid contused skin and preserve a healthy flap of tissue to cover the fracture site and any internal fixation device that may be implanted. With sufficient exposure, all foreign matter and any dead or questionable tissue are removed. Nerves, major vessels, and as much bone as possible are not discarded. Grossly contaminated bone surfaces are removed with a rongeur or curet. All joints that have been penetrated are opened and inspected for debris, including osteochondral fragments. It is useful to leave questionably viable skin, which can readily be assessed during the days after injury. Subcutaneous fat, fascia, and injured muscle are aggressively removed if dead or dirty, although it is important not to excessively undermine a viable skin flap. Contractility, consistency, and especially the presence of bleeding from small intrinsic vessels are more helpful than color as indicators of muscle viability.

A pulsatile irrigation system enhances cleansing of injured tissue, although it should be used gently to minimize additional soft tissue injury. Pulsatile lavage pumps may permit use of less than the 10 or more liters of irrigant frequently recommended. Six liters of normal saline or Ringer's solution for the average grade II open fracture is recommended. Another adjunct, bacitracin solution (50,000 U in 1 liter of normal saline, with two ampules of sodium bicarbonate to alkalinize) as a final antibiotic rinse, can be applied with a bulb syringe.

During debridement, decisions must be made about two other aspects of care for the injured limb: fracture stabilization and wound closure. Complications arising from either of these areas can considerably increase the patient's period of disability and can jeopardize the eventual result. Avoidance of failure is best achieved by use of techniques with which the surgeon is thoroughly familiar and for which the proper equipment is available. Adequate fracture stabilization is important, and external or internal fixation may reduce the risk for infection and facilitate overall management. Meticulous wound toilet and delayed primary closure are essential if internal fixation is used, and in all grade II and III open wounds.

Reduction and Fixation

Although articular surface fractures should be reduced anatomically, extra-articular fractures generally require only adequate restoration of angular and rotational alignment with preservation of length. How to stabilize an open fracture is becoming less controversial. Traction, plaster cast, external skeletal fixation, and the several forms of internal fixation are all useful, individually and in combination. The problems that must be solved anew for each fracture patient follow: (1) How much stability is necessary, or even possible? and (2) What is the most beneficial and least hazardous way to obtain stability? Few direct comparative studies document the unequivocal superiority of one form of stabilization over another. We favor surgical fixation for all but the most minor open fractures, and prefer intramedullary nailing or external fixation to plate fixation in most cases because of the higher risk for infection and wound healing problems associated with plate fixation of open fractures.

Patients with severe soft tissue wounds over fractures that can be stabilized better with internal than external fixation (e.g., ankle fracture, some radius shaft fractures, and proximal femur fractures) are also more easily managed this way, despite the risk for infection. Primary internal fixation of fractures adjacent to arterial anastomoses is not necessary to protect the vascular repair.

External skeletal fixation must be carefully coordinated with wound management and bone grafting. It offers a powerful and adaptable technique for stabilizing open fractures without additional exposure or devascularization of bone and without the encumbrance of plaster casts or traction. External fixation can be applied rapidly and with minimal additional bleeding. An external fixator can span unstable joints and/or complex fracture. This provides stable provisional surgical fixation that can later be replaced with definitive internal and external fixation when the patient can better tolerate prolonged anesthesia and/or blood loss associated with complex fracture fixation procedures. This application of external fixation typically permits mobilization of a patient who might not tolerate recumbency. External skeletal fixation is especially applicable to unstable open fracture of the pelvis. Such fractures are associated with a mortality rate that approached 35% without modern treatment emphasizing aggressive resuscitation, pelvic stabilization, wound debridement, open wound management, and usually a diverting colostomy.

Larger-diameter threaded pins placed in predrilled holes are preferable for diaphyseal fixation. Ring fixators, fixed to the bone with tensioned wires, although somewhat more cumbersome, provide better control of many metaphyseal fractures. By temporarily spanning the injured joint with a simple half-pin fixator, placement of more complicated external fixation devices can be deferred until the patient is more stable.

Skeletal traction may provide an appropriate provisional or definitive means to stabilize open fractures for the patient with an isolated injury. However, compared with internal and external fixation, the poorer outcomes and increased systemic complications associated with skeletal traction with enforced recumbency have resulted in its being used only rarely and temporarily in modern trauma centers.

Wound Coverage

Whether, when, and how to close an open fracture wound are as controversial as the question of stabilization. Skin closure over a contaminated wound is dangerous. The risk for infection is increased when hardware is implanted, tension on skin flaps is excessive, or dead space is created by the closure. Nonetheless, an important early goal of open fracture care is to convert the initially contaminated open wound to a clean closed one. Several techniques are advocated for this, ranging from leaving the wound open until it heals secondarily to primary closure with any of several plastic surgical procedures if simple suture is not possible.

For all but the most trivial wounds and especially when open fractures are internally fixed, it is best to avoid primary wound closure. When wounds are left open, the use of antibiotic bead-pouch dressing technique developed by Seligson and colleagues[20] is still a good technique. Polymethylmethacrylate cement (one full sized batch) is mixed with 1.2 g of tobramycin powder. This is used to make beads of 5-mm diameter, which are molded onto twisted stainless steel wire, separated by 3–4 mm. Although this can be done by the surgical team in the OR, our pharmacy follows the procedures described by Seligson and colleagues[20] for prefabrication and gas sterilization of bead chains, which are made available to us in individual sterile peel-apart pouches. The beads are placed in the wound, and a large piece of Tegaderm or Opsite is used to cover and seal the opening and to keep the gentle traction of the wound flaps to prevent flap shrinkage.

Patients with more severe wounds should be returned to the OR in 1–2 days for a dressing change and further debridement as needed. As soon as all questionably viable tissues have been excised, the wound should be closed. Grades II and IIIA wounds can usually be sutured closed 5–7 days after injury but may require split-thickness skin grafts. More extensive wounds often benefit from closure with muscle pedicle flaps using local tissue or free microvascular transfers. Carefully chosen fasciocutaneous flaps are occasionally helpful, but other tissue flaps are not as effective in severely injured limbs. Split-thickness skin grafts can be used to cover healthy wound tissue at any time, although they are unsatisfactory over exposed blood vessels, tendons, and bare cortical bone. The multiple perforations produced by a meshing device minimize fluid accumulation under split thickness grafts.

It is entirely possible to manage most severe open fractures without the use of elaborate plastic surgical procedures. Open fractures heal successfully despite exposure of bone and hardware for several months or more.

COMPARTMENT SYNDROMES

Various injuries can cause progressive elevation of tissue pressure within the confines of "compartments" formed by the normal fascial envelopes around groups of skeletal muscles. Once compartment pressure is elevated sufficiently to obstruct microvascular perfusion, muscle and nerve ischemia leads to necrosis of the involved tissue. The pressure eventually recedes to normal levels, leaving behind dead muscle and nerve, the causes of Volkmann's contracture.

The key to effective treatment is early diagnosis. This requires suspicion of compartment syndrome whenever an extremity sustains a crushing or severely contusing injury, with or without a fracture. Conscious patients with compartment syndrome develop pain and firm swelling of the entire involved compartment and soon lose function of the muscles and nerves that lie within it. Pulses and skin perfusion are often normal. Compartment syndromes may occur in open fractures, which do not necessarily provide an adequate surgical incisions made for debridement alone.

For a minimum of every 2 hours, patients with significant extremity injuries must be monitored for inordinate pain and for loss of sensation or motor function distal to the area of injury. Release of any constricting bandage or cast is the essential first step in treatment of a suspected compartment syndrome to permit examination and to avoid external compression of the involved compartment. This may reduce pressure sufficiently to restore tissue perfusion and prevent necrosis. If the patient is unconscious, or has an associated nerve injury that prevents clinical assessment, compartment pressures are measured with a commercially available tissue pressure measuring device (e.g., Stryker STIC or a slit-wick catheter made from polyethylene tubing with the terminal end slit about 1 mm longitudinally in several places). The device is filled with sterile saline solution and connected to a strain gauge, as used for monitoring intra-arterial pressure. The catheter is then introduced through a large-bore needle into the compartment in question. A satisfactory measurement system elicits a prompt response to manual pressure on the compartment, and pressure will fall to a reproducible level soon after such external compression is released. It is important to measure the pressure in each compartment of the involved area. For the leg, this means anterior, lateral, deep posterior, and superficial posterior spaces. In the forearm, both flexor and extensor groups should be assessed at several sites. The pressure is typically highest close to the fracture.

If neuromuscular findings are normal, a patient with elevated compartment pressure may be monitored clinically or by repeated pressure measurements. If sensation of contractility is impaired or not accessible and compartmental pressure is within 30–40 mm Hg of mean arterial pressure, fasciotomy is required. All involved compartments must be released. For the leg, we use two incisions. One is lateral with identification and preservation of the superficial peroneal nerve, and is used for release of anterior and lateral compartments. The second is immediately posterior to the medial, tibial shaft for the deep and superficial posterior compartments. Skin incisions 8–10 cm long, with proximal and distal "blind" fasciotomies, may permit adequate decompression but are often insufficient in severely injured limbs. Such limbs are best treated with incisions that extend nearly the entire length of the compartment. The skin is left open for delayed closure by suture or split-thickness graft. If an associated fracture is present, fixing it at the time of fasciotomy simplifies wound management. Either external or internal skeletal fixation may be used, depending on the fracture configuration and the degree of additional soft tissue dissection required.

Forearm compartment syndromes may involve anterior (flexor) or posterior (extensor) muscles and may require releasing the intrinsic fascia of each involved muscle. An extensive surgical approach is required, such as McConnell's combined exposure of the median and ulnar nerves, as described by Henry in *Extensile Exposure*.[1]

For any open wound of the lower extremity that is to be treated open, vacuum-assisted wound closure (VAWC) is becoming a routine technique in mitral management of these wounds. After the wound is cleansed and irrigated, polyurethane foam is cut to fit the wound, and a Silastic sheet is placed over the polyurethane. An incision is made in the middle of the Silastic sheet, an adaptor fitted over this incision, and continuous suction is begun at 100–125 mm Hg. The dressing can be changed on the ward or in the OR if closing the wound is also planned. This is possible when the edema decreases and distention of the circumferential diameter of the extremity lessens. This is usually associated with a diuresis of the patient. Using this technique, it is often possible to eventually close the wound primarily. If the defect is too large after multiple dressing changes, a split-thickness graft is indicated.

Quantitative biopsies comprise another technique that may help the surgeon in determining when a wound can be closed. These biopsies help differentiate wound colonization or contamination from bacterial invasion of the wound bed. With a VAWC, there is also a salutary effect in keeping the wound dry, and typically there is less invasive bacterial into the wound.

Compartment syndromes that are recognized after necrosis is far advanced are probably best left closed rather than treated with fasciotomy because of the significant risk for infection and the lack of benefit from decompressing dead tissue.

DEGLOVING INJURIES

Treatment of degloving injuries requires careful assessment of the extent of the devitalized tissue, the layers of tissue in the flap, and the direction of the avulsion (whether proximally or distally based) and a thorough understanding of the blood supply to the affected tissues.

Degloved skin that remains attached to a pedicle will try to live as a flap and obtain its nutrients from the pedicle rather than the underlying bed. Thorough understanding of the muscular and fascial perforators to the skin will help to predict which flaps can be preserved. Extensive avulsions of the skin with narrow or distal pedicles with or without superficial subcutaneous tissue and without damage to the deeper tissues are best addressed by completely dividing the pedicle, defatting the skin, and replacing the avulsed skin as a full-thickness skin graft.

If the wound is too contaminated or too swollen, the avulsed tissue should be cleansed with pulsatile lavage, left with little or no tension, and addressed at a second exploration. Intraoperative fluorescein examination is a reliable predictor of tissue survival. If arterial in-flow is adequate, the soft tissues can be debrided and closed; tension should be minimal during closure.

Diminished venous return is a common cause for the ultimate death of tissue in degloving injuries. Pharmacologic manipulation with an antithromboxane treatment, such as Dermaid Aloe cream applied topically every 4 hours and 81 mg aspirin daily, coupled with the liberal use of leech therapy, has improved tissue survival with both delayed and immediate wound closures. Leeches are applied every 4 hours initially, and should remain on the wound until the cyanosis from venous congestion is relieved. Large flaps may require two leeches initially. Leeches can be stored on site with minimal tending or obtained within hours by calling a supplier (e.g., Leeches U.S.A., 1-800-645-3569). As venous re-canalization occurs, the frequency of leech application can be reduced and is usually unnecessary after 3 days.

MANGLED EXTREMITIES: DELAYED AMPUTATION

In a perfect world, it should be possible for a general or orthopedic surgeon to assess a patient with a mangled extremity and to make a perfect decision as to whether to do prompt amputation or to attempt reconstruction. Unfortunately, the literature does not help such surgeons in making these decisions, and most of the literature that addresses the mangled extremity focuses on the lower extremity. These fractures have been classified as 3C and are invariably open. Some have vascular injuries, and some do not. Some are insensate, and some are not.

Many scoring systems have been developed to predict those patients who should undergo immediate amputation and those who should have reconstruction. Our own bias is reflected by Bonanni et al.,[13] who state that predictive scoring is an exercise in futility. In their study, they could not show reliable sensitivity or specificity using the MESI, PSI, MESS, or the LSI. Surgical judgment based on experience is still the gold standard.

In a recent study by Bosse et al.,[17] of 569 patients with severe leg injuries who underwent reconstruction or amputation, the sickness impact profile (SIP) showed no difference in outcomes between these two groups. Their study did show that there was a poorer score for the SIP if the patient was rehospitalized or had a major complication, lower educational level, nonwhite ethnicity/race, poverty, lack of private health insurance, poor social support network, low self-efficiency, smoking, and involvement in disability-compensation litigation. Interestingly, patients who underwent reconstruction were more likely to be rehospitalized than those who underwent amputation. Return to work in the two groups was similar. The fact that the groups are similar reflects good decisions made by the surgeons.

Few other areas in trauma care are as controversial as whether amputations for mangled extremities should be done early or delayed. The most common reasons for delayed amputation are loss of wound cover in un-united fractures, infection in a nonunion fracture, an insensate limb, recurrent ulcerations, a dystrophic limb, sympathetic dystrophy, and phantom pain, to name a few. Some surgeons have argued that functional recovery is faster and less costly following amputation than with multiple procedures for salvage and reconstruction. In addition to the study by Bosse et al.[17] mentioned previously, Pozo et al.[18] studied 35 patients who had amputation following the failure of treatment for severe lower limb trauma. Seven of the amputations were for ischemia within 1 month of the injury; 13 were between 1 month and 1 year for infection, complicating loss of limb cover or un-united fractures; and 15 occurred later than 1 year postinjury mainly for infected nonunion. The latter group had an average of 12 operations and 50 months of treatments, including 8 months in hospital. Factors that contributed to salvage failure were vascular injuries, nerve damage, bone damage, muscle damage, skin cover, and sepsis. Overall, these authors concluded that if lower limb reconstruction is attempted, it should be assessed very early on by two specialists, one in trauma surgery and the other in orthopedic or plastic surgery, as to whether failure is inevitable. Obviously, this requires experience, and persistent attempts at salvage can be extremely difficult.

Another study that might influence surgeons on whether to salvage comes from Case Western Reserve.[16] Thirty-four patients were followed, of whom 16 had a successful limb salvage procedure, and 18 had an immediate below knee amputation (BKA). The patients who had a successful limb salvage procedure took significantly more time to achieve full weight bearing, were less willing or able to work, and had higher hospital charges than the patients who had been managed with an early BKA. Furthermore, patients who had limb salvage considered themselves severely disabled, and they had more problems than the amputation group with the performance of occupational and recreational activities. These quality-of-life evaluations, however, must be put into the perspective that Bosse and MacKenzie[17] have already outlined.

In a final study for consideration, Roessler and colleagues[19] reviewed 80 patients for a 4-year period and asked the question of when to amputate. They concluded that neurologic, bone, and tissue status influenced the decision regarding immediate amputation, but had little to do with delayed loss of limb or life. Somewhat surprisingly, they found that the circulation as determined by the presence or absence of a palpable or Doppler-detected pulse was critical. They concluded that in cases in which salvage is attempted, amputation should be performed at 24 hours if the patient's condition, including a markedly positive fluid balance, indicates systemic compromise. They also made the observation that in the absence of a distal pulse on presentation, the eventual amputation rate is high.

REFERENCES

1. Henry AK: *Extensile Exposure*, 2nd ed. Edinburgh, Churchill Livingstone, 1973.
2. Mackinnon SE, Dellon AL: *Surgery of the Peripheral Nerve.* New York, Thieme, 1988.
3. McCraw JB, Arnold PG: *McCraw and Arnold's Atlas of Muscle and Musculocutaneous Flaps.* Norfolk, Hampton Press, 1986.
4. Serafin D: *Atlas of Microsurgical Composite Tissue Transplantation.* Philadelphia, WB Saunders, 1996.
5. Caudle RJ, Stern PF: Severe open fractures of the tibia. *J Bone Joint Surg [Am]* 69:801–807, 1987.
6. Hansen ST Jr: The type-IIIC tibial fracture: salvage or amputation. *J Bone Joint Surg [Am]* 69:799–800, 1987.
7. Dagum AB, Best AK, Schemitsch EH, et al: Salvage after severe lower-extremity trauma: are the outcomes worth the means? *Plast Reconstr Surg* 103:1212–1220, 1999.
8. Fairhurst MJ: The function of below-knee amputee versus the patient with salvaged grade III tibial fracture. *Clin Orthop* 301:227–232, 1994.
9. Gustilo RB, Mendoza RM, Williams DN: Problems in the management of type III (severe) open fractures: a new classification of type III open fractures. *J Trauma* 24:742–746, 1984.
10. Swiontkowski MF, MacKenzie EJ, Bosse MJ, et al: Factors influencing the decision to amputate or reconstruct after high-energy lower extremity trauma. *J Trauma* 52:641–649, 2002.

11. Johansen K, Daines M, Howey T, et al: Objective criteria accurately predict amputation following lower extremity trauma. *J Trauma* 30:568–573.
12. Matsen SL, Malchow D, Matsen FA III: Correlations with patients' perspectives of the result of lower-extremity amputation. *J Bone Joint Surg [Am]* 82:1089–1095, 2000.
13. Bonanni F, Rhodes M, Lucke JF: The futility of predictive scoring of mangled lower extremities. *J Trauma* 34:99–104, 1993.
14. Bondurant FJ, Cotler HB, Buckle R, et al: The medical and economic impact of severely injured lower extremities. *J Trauma* 23:1270–1273, 1988.
15. Butcher JL, MacKenzie EJ, Cushing B, et al: Long-term outcomes after lower extremity trauma. *J Trauma* 41:4–9, 1996.
16. Georgiadis GM, Behrens FF, Joyce MJ, et al: Open tibial plateau fractures with severe soft-tissue loss. Limb salvage compared with

below-the-knee amputation. *J Bone Joint Surg [Am]* 75A:1431–1442, 1993.
17. MacKenzie EJ, Burgess AR, McAndrew MP, et al: Patient oriented functional outcome after unilateral lower extremity fracture. *J Orthop Trauma* 7:393–401, 1993.
18. Pozo JL, Powell B, Hutton PAN, Clarke J: The timing of amputation for lower limb trauma. *J Bone Joint Surg [Br]* 72B:288–292, 1990.
19. Roessler MS, Wisner DH, Holcroft JW: The mangled extremity: when to amputate? *Arch Surg* 126:1243–1249, 1991.
20. Henry SL, Ostermann PA, Seligson D: The antibiotic bead pouch technique: the management of severe compound fractures. *Clin Orthop* 295:54–62, 1993.

CERVICAL, THORACIC, AND LUMBAR FRACTURES

Robert L. Tatsumi and Robert A. Hart

Spinal column injuries in the United States occur at a rate of 4 to 5.3 injuries per 100,000 households. The most common causes of spinal column injuries include motor vehicle accidents (45%), falls (20%), sports-related accidents (15%), violence (15%), and miscellaneous causes (5%).

During the primary survey, as outlined by the American College of Surgeons guidelines, proper head mechanics should be employed for securing the airway. Manual in-line immobilization is preferred to avoid excessive head and neck movement. All patients with suspected spinal injuries should have proper immobilization of the neck and back to reduce the risk of spinal cord damage. Patients wearing a helmet at the time of injury should continue to wear the head apparatus during transport, but may have the face mask cut to provide ventilatory access.

Means of initial immobilization include a cervical collar, tape, or straps to secure the patient's neck/back and transportation on a firm spine board with lateral support devices. It is estimated that 3%–25% of spinal cord injuries may result from improper immobilization of the spinal column during the transport period.

The resuscitation period is a crucial time after airway management and provisional spinal stabilization have been performed. Maintaining a mean blood pressure greater than 95 mm Hg is recommended to provide adequate perfusion to the spinal cord, and has been shown to provide better neurologic outcomes. The treating physician must monitor for neurogenic shock, which presents as hypotension accompanied by bradycardia due to decreased sympathetic outflow as a result of a cervical or high thoracic spinal cord injury. Treatment consists of both volume replacement and the use of vasopressors if hypotension persists.

columns conduct ascending pain and temperature signals from the contralateral side of the body via the lateral spinothalamic tracts as well as descending voluntary motor signals from the ipsilateral side of the body via the lateral corticospinal tracts. Finally, the anterior column conducts ascending light touch signals from the contralateral side of the body via anterior spinothalamic tracts and descending fine motor control via anterior corticospinal tracts.

The end of the spinal cord (conus medullaris) is located at L1-L2 intervertebral disk. Below the level of the conus medullaris, the spinal canal is occupied by the lower motor roots called the cauda equina. As a lower motor neuron lesion, injury to the nerve roots has a much better prognosis for recovery than injury to the spinal cord (Figure 1).

Classification of Neurologic Injury

Determining the extent of a neurologic deficit in a patient with a spinal cord injury is paramount to understanding the overall prognosis. A complete injury is one in which "no motor or sensory function exists more than three segments below the level of the injury." Incomplete injuries retain some neurologic function further than three segments below the level of the injury with the caudal segment exhibiting greater than 60% motor strength and intact sensation.

Patients with complete injuries have less than a 3% chance of motor recovery in the first 24 hours. Patients with sacral sparing have partial continuity of the white matter long tracts and demonstrate an incomplete cord injury. The presence of the bulbocavernosus reflex, a spinal reflex mediated by the S3-S4 region of the conus medullaris, may be absent in the first 4–6 hours after injury while the patient is in "spinal shock," but usually returns within 24 hours. If the reflex does not return after 24 hours and distal neurological function remains absent, the injury is complete.

The secondary survey in patients with spinal cord injury includes a precise definition of neurologic deficits. Classification systems are useful to compare outcomes between different studies. While a variety of clinical grading systems exist, the American Spinal Injury Association (ASIA) scale has become the most widely accepted. The ASIA scale identifies motor, sensory, and general impairment deficits, and incorporates the functional independence measure (see page 163).

NEUROLOGIC INJURY

The spinal cord fills 35% of the canal at the level of the atlas and about 50% in the cervical and thoracolumbar regions. The spinal cord consists of white matter in the periphery and gray matter centrally. The gray, myelinated matter can be divided into three columns. The posterior columns conduct ascending proprioception, vibratory, and tactile signals from the ipsilateral side of the body. The lateral

Incomplete Spinal Cord Syndromes

Four incomplete spinal cord syndromes are defined based on the location of the trauma to the spinal cord. Central cord syndrome is the most common pattern of injury, resulting from gray matter destruction, which is worst in the central region of the spinal cord. This injury pattern often occurs due to hyperextension injury in a patient with degenerative cervical spinal stenosis. The patient experiences

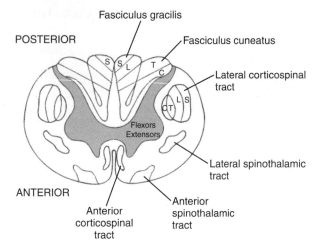

Figure 1 Spinal cord cross-section demonstrating the motor and sensory tracts.

motor and sensory deficits that are worse in the upper than in the lower extremities. The overall prognosis for central spinal cord injuries is good, with 75% of the patients experiencing at least partial motor recovery and most regaining the ability to ambulate.

Anterior cord syndrome is caused by vascular injury to the anterior portion of the spinal cord that causes motor/sensory deficits (lower greater than upper) with sparing of proprioception and position sense. This diagnosis carries the worst prognosis with only 10% of patients regaining substantial function.

Brown–Sequard syndrome is caused by isolated injury of one lateral half of the spinal cord and results in ipsilateral motor and contralateral sensory deficits. This syndrome has the best functional recovery.

Posterior cord syndrome is the rarest and causes decreased position and pressure sensation.

Spinal Cord Injury

Pharmacologic intervention for spinal cord injury continues to be a controversial topic. The recommended protocols based on the National Acute Spinal Cord Injury Study are a 30 mg/kg loading dose and 5.4 mg/kg/hr of methylprednisolone for 23 hours when delivered within 38 hours of injury, and a 47-hour infusion when started within 8 hours of injury. Despite the high acuity of these studies, the differences in the outcome are small, and bleeding and infectious complications were high in the steroid group compared to the control group. As a result, most spine societies do not regard these steroid protocols as an essential feature of initial spinal cord injury management.

CERVICAL SPINE TRAUMA

Evaluation

Cervical spine clearance for trauma patients continues to be a topic of debate. Class I evidence suggests that cervical spine radiographs are necessary for patients who present with neck pain or tenderness and have a decreased level of consciousness or are intoxicated, or who have distracting injuries. A cervical spine series consisting of anteroposterior (AP), lateral and open-mouth odontoid views has 85% sensitivity. The addition of flexion-extension views in the awake and alert patient to delineate spinal instability increases the negative predictive value to 99%.

It is important that radiographs include the C7-T1 interspace to identify any pathology around the cervicothoracic junction. The AP radiograph should be evaluated for symmetric disk height, lateral mass alignment, and spinous process orientation. The lateral radiograph should exhibit smooth anterior and posterior vertebral lines and spinolaminar lines as well as symmetric disk spaces and overlap of the lateral masses. Soft tissue planes should be evaluated and should be less than 6 mm at C2 and less than 2 cm at C6.

Computed tomography (CT) is useful to identify osseous pathology not seen on radiographs and is especially helpful at the craniocervical and cervicothoracic junctions. In some centers, CT scanning with sagittal and coronal plane reconstructions is replacing plain radiography as a screening study for high energy trauma admissions. Magnetic resonance imaging (MRI) may also be helpful in limited situations to diagnose soft tissue injury, such as the ligaments, disks, and facet capsules.

Anatomy

The cervical spine consists of seven vertebrae, and is subdivided into the atlas (C1), axis (C2), and subaxial spine (C3-C7). The atlas is ring-shaped, consisting of two articular lateral masses without a body or spinous process. The axis contains the odontoid process, which articulates with the anterior arch of the axis. The transverse ligament stabilizes this joint.

The subaxial spine consists of vertebral bodies with concave superior endplates. The facet joints are encapsulated synovial joints with overlying hyaline cartilage. The facet joint angle is 45 degrees in the sagittal plane.

Spinal stability primarily stems from ligament and disk integrity. Craniocervical stability involves intact anterior and posterior atlanto-occipital membranes and articular capsules. The atlantoaxial joint is stabilized by the transverse ligament primarily with the paired alar and apical ligaments provided secondary stabilization. The posterior ligamentum nuchae, interspinous ligaments, and ligamentum flavum acts as a "tension band" to provide resistance against flexion distraction injuries. The atlantoaxial joint provides 50% of the overall cervical rotation (Figure 2).

The vertebral artery passes through the vertebral foramina from C6 to C1 and then turns posteromedially around the superior articular process before entering the foramen magnum and joining the basilar artery. The vertebral artery follows a similar course, but enters at the C7 transverse foramina. Unilateral absence or hypoplasia of the vertebral artery is 5%–10%.

The vertebral canal sagittal diameter narrows from 23 mm at C1 to 15 mm at C7. Nerve roots exit the canal through the intervertebral foramen. The posterolateral uncovertebral joint and intervertebral disk forms the anterior border of the foramen while the posterior border is formed by the caudal superior articular facet. The C2 nerve root exits posterior to the C1-C2 facet joint, whereas the remaining cervical nerve roots exit anterior to the facet joints. The spinal nerves pass posterior to the vertebral artery at the middle of the corresponding lateral mass. The cervical plexus consists of the ventral rami of C1 through C4, whereas the brachial plexus is made up from the ventral rami of C5 through T1.

Cervical Spinal Ligamentous Instability

White and Panjabi defined instability as "the loss of ability of the spine under physiologic loads to maintain its pattern of displacement so that there is no initial or additional neurologic deficit, no major deformity, and no incapacitating pain." Acute radiographic instability criteria of the subaxial cervical spine include greater than 3.5 mm translation or greater than 11 degrees of angulation in the lateral plane. Because of the potential for late instability following the resolution of acute pain and muscle spasm, patients with significant axial neck ache but normal radiographs are indicated for follow-up flexion/extension films at around 2 weeks postinjury.

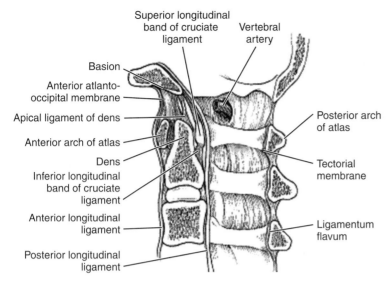

Figure 2 Sagittal cervical spine cross-section. *(Data from Heller J, Pedlow F: Anatomy of the cervical spine. In Clark CR, Dvorak J, Ducker TB, et al., editors: The Cervical Spine, 4th ed. Philadelphia, Lippincott-Raven, 2005, p. 9.)*

Occipital Condyle Fracture

Occipital condyle fracture should be considered a marker for potentially lethal trauma as patients experience an 11% mortality rate from associated injuries. Anderson and Montesano classified these fractures into the following types:

Type I: Impaction fractures due to an axial load (3%)

Type II: Extension of a basilar skull fracture into the condyle (22%)

Type III: Avulsion fractures (75%)

Types I and II fractures are caused by axial loading and have intact alar and tectoral membrane ligaments. Type III fractures are caused by skull distraction and have ligamentous disruption.

Stable type I, II, and III fractures can be managed in a cervical collar for 6–8 weeks. Displaced type II or III fractures are managed in a halo vest for 8–12 weeks. Grossly unstable type III fractures require occiput to C2 fusion and should raise the suspicion for an underlying occipitocervical dissociation. Cranial nerve palsies may develop days to weeks after the injury and most frequently involve cranial nerves IX, X, and XI (Figure 3).

Occipitocervical Dissociation

Occipitocervical dissociation (OCD) injuries have a high mortality rate. Patients who survive this injury demonstrate a wide variety of neurological sequelae ranging from cranial nerve palsies affecting VI, X, and XII, and cord lesions. OCDs are classified as I, anterior; II, longitudinal; and III, posterior.

Radiographic diagnosis of OCD can be evaluated by the Powers ratio, which divides the basion to posterior arch distance by the anterior arch to opisthion distance. A Power's ratio greater than 1.0 suggests anterior dissociation. Another radiographic measure known as Wachenheim's line can help evaluate for anterior or posterior subluxation. A line along the posterior surface of the clivus and extended caudally should just touch the posterior aspect of the tip of the dens. If this line runs anterior to the dens, anterior subluxation of the occipital condyles has occurred, while a position posterior to the dens indicates posterior subluxation.

The diagnosis can be difficult to make due to poor visualization of the osseous detail. The reported sensitivity for diagnosing OCD on plain radiographs is 57%, CT 84%, and MRI 87%. Treatment of OCD injuries requires instrumented occipitocervical fusion to at least C2, frequently augmented with halo vest placement.

Atlas Fractures

Atlas fractures comprise 7% of the cervical spine fractures. Fractures can involve the anterior or posterior arch, lateral masses, and transverse processes. Jefferson or burst fractures are bilateral, involving both the anterior and posterior arches resulting from axial load (Figure 4). Atlantoaxial stability depends on the integrity of the transverse ligament. Combined lateral mass displacement greater than 7 mm on AP radiographs (Figure 5).

Magnetic resonance imaging is a more sensitive means of detecting transverse ligament injury with mid-substance (type I) injuries having a poorer healing response than avulsion fractures (type II). Thus, type I injuries often require a C1-C2 arthrodesis, while type II injuries generally heal with halo vest immobilization. Most atlas fractures are stable and can be treated nonoperatively with 6–12 weeks of immobilization in a cervical collar.

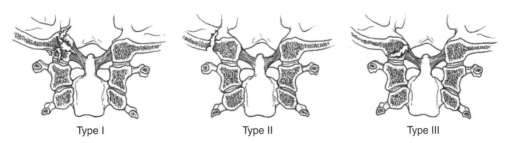

Type I   Type II   Type III

Figure 3 Types of occipital condyle fractures. *(From Anderson PA, Mirza SK, Chapman JR: Injuries to the Atlantooccipital articulation. In Clark CR, Dvorak J, Ducker TB, et al., editors: The Cervical Spine, 4th ed. Philadelphia, Lippincott-Raven, 2005, p. 594.)*

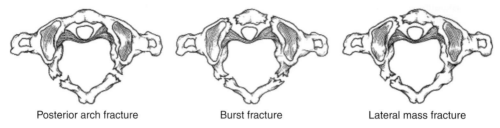

Posterior arch fracture   Burst fracture   Lateral mass fracture

Figure 4 Types of C1 arch fractures. *(From Hasharoni A, Errico TJ: Fracture of the first cervical vertebra. In Clark CR, Dvorak J, Ducker TB, et al., editors:* The Cervical Spine, *4th ed. Philadelphia, Lippincott-Raven, 2005, p. 610.)*

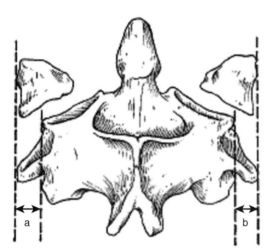

Figure 5 Radiographic assessment of transverse ligament instability. *(From Hasharoni A, Errico TJ: Fracture of the first cervical vertebra. In Clark CR, Dvorak J, Ducker TB, et al., editors:* The Cervical Spine, *4th ed. Philadelphia, Lippincott-Raven, 2005, p. 592.)*

Dens Fractures

Dens fractures have been classified by Anderson and D'Alonzo (Table 1; Figure 6). Type I and III fractures can generally be treated with an external orthosis. Management of type II fractures is more problematic and depends on patient age and associated injuries, as well as fracture displacement and stability. While nondisplaced fractures can sometimes be treated successfully with a halo vest, indications to operate include fracture comminution, displacement greater than 6 mm, posterior angulation, delay in diagnosis, and patient age greater than 50 years old. In general, elderly patients can be considered for C1-C2 fusion because of their decreased healing rates and poor tolerance of halo vest. Severely debilitated patients, on the other hand, can be treated with a cervical collar until comfortable, with the understanding that a successful fusion may not occur.

Surgical treatment can also be performed via anterior odontoid screw osteosynthesis, particularly for oblique fractures that run from anterosuperior to posteroinferior, patients with C1 ring fractures, and younger patients. C1-C2 arthrodesis can be performed via several techniques including wiring, transarticular screws, or rod and screw constructs.

Traumatic Spondylolisthesis of Axis

Bilateral fractures of the par interarticularis are called hangman's fractures. Most injuries are caused by motor vehicle accidents. Hangman's fractures are classified by Levine and Edwards (Table 2; Figure 7). Type I fractures require 6–12 weeks of halo vest immobilization. Surgical options for type II and III fractures include

Table 1: Classifications of Dens Fractures

Type I	Avulsion fractures of tip
Type II	Waist fractures
Type III	Fracture extends into C2 body

Source: Anderson LD, D'Alonzo RT: Fractures of the odontoid process of the axis. *J Bone Joint Surg* 56:1663–1674, 1974.

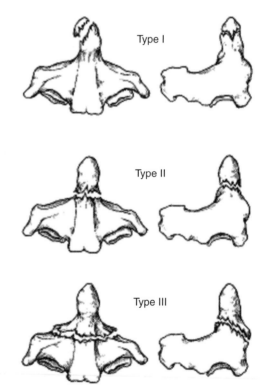

Type I

Type II

Type III

Figure 6 Types of odontoid fractures. *(From Anderson LD, D'Alonzo RT: Fractures of the odontoid process of the axis.* J Bone Joint Surg *56:1663–1674, 1974.)*

reduction followed by anterior C2-C3 interbody fusion, posterior C1-C3 fusion, or bilateral C2 pars screw osteosynthesis.

Subaxial Spine Fractures

Isolated fractures of the spinous process, lamina, and transverse processes occur frequently, and are most often stable as long as the facet articulations are competent and minimal vertebral translation has occurred.

Table 2: Classifications of Hangman's Fractures

Type I	Fractures with <3 mm of displacement and no angulation due to axial compression and hyperextension
Type IA	Asymmetric fracture line with minimal angulation or displacement due to hyperextension with lateral bending forces
Type II	Fractures with >3 mm of translation and angulation due to hyperextension and axial loading followed by rebound flexion
Type IIA	Fractures demonstrate angulation without translation due to a flexion-distraction injury
Type III	Fractures include C2-C3 facet dislocation due to hyperextension followed by flexion mechanism

Source: Levine AM, Edwards CC: The management of traumatic spondylolisthesis of the axis. *J Bone Joint Surg* 67:221–226, 1985.

Subaxial cervical spine fractures can be subclassified many ways. The most common injuries include compression, burst, and teardrop injuries.

Compression flexion injuries cause failure to the anterior half of the vertebral body without disruption of the posterior body cortex. The mechanism is a hyperflexion or axial loading injury. Patients are usually neurologically intact and in the absence of gross deformity or instability, most fractures heal with external immobilization in 6–12 weeks.

Burst fractures involve the anterior and middle columns and may extend into the posterior body cortex. Burst fractures that do not involve the posterior elements are more stable and can be treated in a halo for 12 weeks. Fractures that involve the posterior elements are unstable and can be associated with cord compromise. These types of fractures require anterior surgical decompression and stabilization via an anterior plate or added posterior fixation if necessary.

Extension tear drop injuries occur with hyperextension of the neck with an avulsion fracture of the anteroinferior vertebral body. This injury typically occurs at the C2-C3 interspace. Most of these injuries can be treated with a cervical collar for 6–8 weeks, even if the anterior longitudinal ligament has been disrupted. Flexion teardrop injuries are a more severe injury and may be associated with spinal cord injury. The teardrop fracture is located at the anteroinferior corner of the body, with the posteroinferior corner of the body rotating into the canal and possibly causing an anterior cord syndrome. Initial treatment consists of tong application for spinal reduction. Anterior decompression may be necessary to address cord compromise along with anterior and/or posterior stabilization.

Subaxial Spine Dislocations

Unilateral dislocations demonstrate 25% vertebral subluxation with associated monoradiculopathy that improves with traction. Bilateral dislocations demonstrate vertebral body subluxation greater than 50% without significant spinal cord injury. Awake and alert patients can safely undergo closed reduction with progressive application of traction as long as serial neurologic exams and radiographic assessments are taking place. A successful closed reduction without significant kyphotic deformity or radiculopathy can be managed with 6–12 weeks of external immobilization.

Patients who develop new or worsening neurologic deficits while having a closed reduction should proceed to have an MRI to identify a possible herniated disk. Overall, 25% of patients will fail a closed reduction will demonstrate signs of disk disruption on MRI. Patients who fail a closed reduction maneuver will require an open reduction and instrumented fusion. Additionally, patients with kyphotic deformity, significant subluxation, radiculopathy, bilateral facet fractures, and lateral mass dissociations may be treated with anterior or posterior instrumented fusions.

Special Considerations

Children less than 10 years of age frequently have spine injuries from the occiput to the third cervical spine due to the weight/size of the head being proportionally larger than the body. Children older than 10 years of age have spinal injuries similar to adults. Elderly patients frequently exhibit C1-C2 injuries that include transverse ligament disruption and dens fractures.

THORACIC AND LUMBAR SPINE TRAUMA

Anatomy

The thoracic spine is more rigid than the cervical or lumbar spine due to attachments of the ribs to the transverse processes and vertebral bodies. The thoracic spine also imparts its overall stability from the coronally orientated facets with shingled lamina, properties that limit extension. Because of the rigidity of the thoracic spine, the transition zones at T1 and T12 are highly susceptible to injury.

The thoracic spine has an overall kyphotic alignment with the apex centered around T6 through T8 with a range of 15–49 degrees. Maximal anterior column forces are generated and fractures within the rib cage usually occur at this location.

Motorcyclists have a high prevalence for blunt chest and thoracic spine trauma. Patients with lap belt echymosis are also at higher risk for flexion distraction T-L injuries.

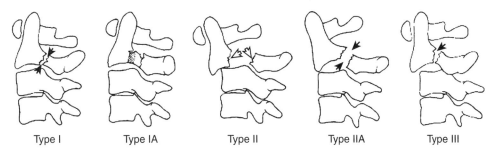

| Type I | Type IA | Type II | Type IIA | Type III |

Figure 7 Types of Hangman's fractures. *(From Levine AM, Edwards CC: The management of traumatic spondylolisthesis of the axis.* J Bone Joint Surg *67:221–226, 1985.)*

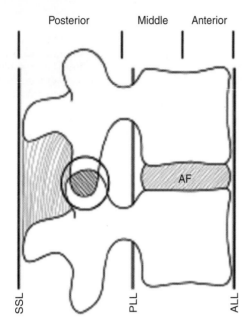

Posterior   Middle   Anterior

AF

SSL   PLL   ALL

Figure 8 Spinal columns. *SSL*, Supraspinal ligament; *PLL*, posterior longitudinal ligament; *ALL*, anterior longitudinal ligament; *AF*, annulus fibrosus. *(Adapted from McAfee PC, Yuan HA, Fredrickson BE, Lubicky JP: The value of computed tomography in thoracolumbar fractures: an analysis of one hundred consecutive cases and a new classification. J Bone Joint Surg 65: 461–473, 1983, with permission.)*

Fractures

Denis's three-column concept is frequently used because it includes the injury patterns most commonly seen and relates them to a specific mechanism of injury. The classification includes both minor and major injuries. Minor injuries include isolated fractures to the articular process, transverse process, and pars interarticularis. Major fracture types include compression, burst, flexion distraction, and fracture dislocations (Figure 8).

Compression Fractures

A compression fracture results from an axial load involves the anterior column of the spine. Radiographs show a wedge shaped defect in the vertebral body with varying degrees of kyphosis. Patients who are neurologically intact with less than 30 degrees of kyphosis and less than 50% vertebral body height loss can be managed in a hyperextension orthosis. Patients who do not meet these criteria need to be watched carefully for possible failure of the posterior ligamentous structures. Patients with fractures above T6 should wear a cervical extension for better spinal control (Figure 9).

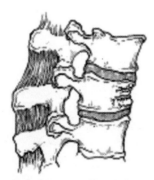

Figure 9 Compression fracture. *(From Holdsworth FW: Fractures, dislocations and fracture-dislocations of the spine. J Bone Joint Surg Br Dec 52(8):1534–1551, 1970).*

Burst Fractures

Burst fractures also occur from axial loads but involve the anterior and middle columns. Involvement of the posterior column equates to overall instability. Radiographically, burst fractures demonstrate widening of the pedicles and varying degrees of retropulsion into the canal. Patients without neurologic deficits, kyphosis less than 30 degrees, and less than 50% vertebral body height loss can be managed with a thoracolumbar orthosis for 3 months. Patients who do not meet these criteria should undergo a posterior instrumented fusion procedure (Figure 10).

Flexion Distraction

Flexion distraction injuries occur when the flexion moment occurs anterior to the vertebral column. This injury typically occurs in motor vehicle accidents where the lap belt acts as a fulcrum, and the anterior column fails in compression, whereas the middle and posterior columns fail in tension. Purely ligamentous injuries have a poor propensity to heal and usually require short-segment posterior procedures. Pure bony injuries have the potential to heal without surgical intervention as long as a nonunion or deformity does not occur (Figure 11).

Thoracolumbar Junction and Lumbar Spine Fractures

Injuries to the thoracolumbar junction (T11-L2) represent 50% of all the thoracic and lumbar fractures. The thoracolumbar junction is a transition area from the rigid thoracic spine to the more flexible lumbar spine. The thoracic spine is stiff due to rib articulations, alignment of facets, and disk alignment.

The thoracic spinal cord has poor vascularity as well as a constant medullary artery (artery of Adamkiewicz). This medullary artery originates from the intercostal artery on the left side between T10 and T12, and has an anastamoses with the anterior spinal artery.

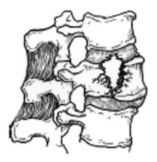

Figure 10 Burst fracture. *(From Holdsworth FW: Fractures, dislocations and fracture-dislocations of the spine. J Bone Joint Surg Br Dec 52(8):1534–1551, 1970.)*

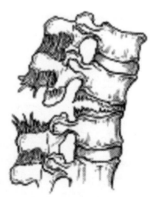

Figure 11 Flexion distraction. *(From Holdsworth FW: Fractures, dislocations and fracture-dislocations of the spine. J Bone Joint Surg Br Dec 52(8):1534–1551, 1970.)*

Injury to the artery of Adamkiewicz via trauma or iatrogenic can lead to frank paralysis.

Lumbar spine fractures occur predominantly to L3-S1. Normal lordosis is generally thought to be less than 60 degrees. The spinal cord usually terminates at L1. The conus can broaden to occupy as much as 50% of the canal diameter. Within the dural sac, the most lateral roots exit more proximally because they are tethered by the bony foramen anterolaterally. Fractures of the lower lumbar spine are less common (L3-L5). This region is intrinsically stable due to the lordotic nature of the lumbar spine, which places the weight-bearing axis in the middle and posterior columns, and the sagittal-oriented facets, which accommodate for greater flexion-extension moments.

Neurologic injuries are of two types in the lumbar spine. The first is a complete cauda equina syndrome, which is often seen with burst fractures with canal retropulsion. The second type is isolated nerve root injuries which may entail a root avulsion with associated transverse process avulsion or nerve impingement.

At the thoracolumbar junction, compression fractures are usually anterior but can be lateral. Typically the superior endplate is involved (68%), but both endplates may also be involved (16%). In the lumbar spine, compression fractures are quite infrequent because of the posteriorly oriented weight-bearing axis. The mechanism is predominantly a flexion type of injury that produces a fracture of the superior subchondral plate of the vertebral body. Compression fractures are more common in patients with osteopenia. Additionally, elderly patients may develop an ileus for a significant retroperitoneal hematoma due to the compression fracture.

Compression fractures with less than 50% height loss or less than 25 degrees of kyphosis are considered stable and can be managed in a thoracic lumbar sacral orthosis (TLSO) for 3 months, and are encouraged to lie in the prone position to minimize their deformity. L5 compression fractures can be accentuated by lumbar-only orthosis, and thus requires a single leg included in the orthosis to immobilize the lumbosacral junction. Patients should receive serial radiographs in the standing position at 1 week, 1 month, 2 months, and 3 months to be certain that healing has taken place.

Burst fractures usually occur with axial loading and usually involve the superior endplate in the thoracolumbar junction and the superior endplate in the lumbar spine. The presence of a longitudinal laminar fracture seems to be associated with traumatic dural tears with the potential of entrapping nerve roots within the lamina fracture.

Burst fractures that involve the anterior and middle columns are termed stable and are treated in a TLSO or total contact cast. Unstable burst fractures involve all three columns of the spine. Operative treatment should be considered for fractures with greater than 50% canal compromise, greater than 25 degrees of kyphosis, or the presence of a neurologic deficit. Anterior decompression and fusion should be considered for patients with significant neural compression and neurologic deficits with minimal kyphotic deformity. Cord decompression is best accomplished from an anterior approach when bony retropulsion exists into the canal. Posterior decompression, that is, laminectomy or laminotomy, can be performed below the cord level. Posterior instrumentation demonstrates the greatest rigidity because the hardware is closer to the center of the spinal axis.

Flexion distraction injuries typically occur from seat belts without shoulder harnesses where the fulcrum sits anterior to the spine. This fracture places the middle and posterior columns and anterior column in compression. The fracture can propagate purely through the ligaments (11%) or the bone (47%). Bony flexion-distraction injuries may be treated in a molded TLSO for 3–4 months, and then have serial standing radiographs to ensure that the deformity has not progressed. Ligamentous injuries require posterior instrumentation with compression techniques to provide stability and maintain alignment.

Flexion dislocation injuries involve all three columns of the spine. Three mechanisms have been described (1) flexion rotation, (2) shear fracture-dislocation, and (3) bilateral facet dislocation. In flexion rotation and bilateral facet dislocation, distraction is usually necessary to reduce the dislocation. After the reduction is performed, a neutralization plate may be used. Shear injuries are the most unstable because this is a three-column injury with ligamentous damage as well. These fractures require a combination of long distraction with short compression instrumented techniques.

IMPORTANT CONSIDERATIONS

Patients with ankylosing spondylitis or diffuse idiopathic skeletal hyperostosis represent a special subpopulation that requires extra attention. Ankylosing spondylitis can increase the risk of fracture, and patients with this condition should receive a CT scan when complaining of neck or back pain. Nondisplaced fractures in this patient population can be quite unstable and lead to spinal cord compromise.

SUGGESTED READINGS

Allen BL, Ferguson RL, Lehman TR, et al: A mechanistic classification of closed, indirect fractures and dislocations of the lower cervical spine. *Spine* 7:1–27, 1982.

An HS, Simpson JM, Ebranheim, NA, et al: Low lumbar burst fractures. *Orthopedics* 15:367–373, 1992.

Anderson LD, D'Alonzo RT: Fractures of the odontoid process of the axis. *JBGS* 56:1663–1674, 1974.

Anderson PA, Montesano PX: Orthology and treatment of occipital condyle fractures. *Spine* 13:731–736, 1988.

Bohlman HH: Acute fractures and dislocations of the cervical spine. An analysis of three hundred hospitalized patients and review of the literature. *J Bone Joint Surg [Am]* 61:1119–1142, 1979.

Bracken MB, Sheppard MJ, Collins WF, et al: A randomized, controlled trial of methylprednisolone or naloxone in the treatment of acute spinal cord injury: results of the Second National Acute Spinal Cord Injury Study. *N Engl J Med* 322:1405–1411, 1990.

Chapman JR, Anderson PA: Thoracolumbar spine fractures with neurologic deficit. *Orthop Clin North Am* 25:595–612, 1994.

Delamarter RB, Sherman JE, Carr JB: Cauda equine syndrome: neurologic recovery following immediate, early, or late decompression. *Spine* 16:1022–1029, 1991.

Denis F: Instability as defined by the three-column spine concept in acute spinal trauma. *Clin Orthop* 189:65–76, 1984.

Hoffman JR, Mower WR, Wolfson AB, et al: Validity of a set of clinical criteria to rule out injury to the cervical spine in patients with blunt trauma. *N Engl J Med* 343:94–99, 2000.

Hurlbert RJ: The role of steroids in acute spinal cord injury: an evidence-based analysis. *Spine* 26(Suppl 24):S39–S46.

Joint Section on Disorders of the Spine and Peripheral Nerves, American Association of Neurological Surgeons/Congress of Neurological Surgeons: management of vertebral artery injuries after nonpenetrating cervical trauma. Guidelines for management of acute cervical spinal injuries. *Neurosurgery* 50(Suppl 3):S1–179, 2002.

Levine AM, Edwards CC: The management of traumatic spondylolisthesis of the axis. *JBGS* 67:217–226, 1985.

Magerl F, Aebi M, Gertzbein SD, et al: A comprehensive classification of thoracic and lumbar injuries. *Eur Spine J* 3:184–201, 1994.

Peris MD, Donaldson WF, Towers J, et al: Helmet and shoulder pad removal in suspected cervical spine injury. *Spine* 27:995–999, 2002.

Nesathurai S: Steroids and spinal cord injury: revisiting the NASCIS II and NASCIS III trials. *J Trauma* 45:1088–1093, 1998.

White AA, Panjabi MM: Clinical Biomechanics of the Spine, 2nd ed. Philadelphia, JB Lippincott, 1990.

Wood K, Butterman G, Mehbod A, et al: Operative compared with nonoperative treatment of a thoracolumbar burst fracture without neurological deficit. *J Bone Joint Surg [Am]* 85:773–781, 2003.

Yue J, Sossan A, Selgrath C, et al: The treatment of unstable thoracic spine fractures with transpedicular screw instrumentation: a 3 year consecutive series. *Spine* 27:2782–2787.

PELVIC FRACTURES

Catherine A. Humphrey   and   Thomas J. Ellis

Pelvic fractures are a common injury among all trauma injuries (3%). They represent a spectrum of injuries from low-energy minimally displaced fractures in the elderly population to highly displaced fractures with major injury. While most low-energy fractures can be treated conservatively, higher-energy injuries are associated with significant multisystem morbidity. In Level I trauma centers, high-energy pelvic ring injuries are often seen in conjunction with severe head injury, chest and abdominal hemorrhage, genitourinary trauma, and severe peripheral neurologic injury (6%). This chapter will address diagnosis, early management and outcomes of pelvic ring injury. Prompt recognition of a displaced pelvic fractures aids trauma surgeons in the prediction and management of hemodynamic instability.

A multispecialty approach to the management of patients with hemodynamic instability and pelvic ring injuries is strongly supported throughout the literature. Early involvement of orthopedic traumatologists and interventional radiologists in addition to the primary trauma team improves morbidity and mortality from severe pelvic injuries. In the setting of hypotension, external fixation and angiography are beneficial but the treatment algorithm of such interventions should be individualized based on the resources available at each institution.

ANATOMY

The pelvic ring is comprised of three bones: the sacrum and the two innominate bones. There is no intrinsic bony stability to the ring itself. Integrity is maintained by a series of strong ligamentous complexes and the soft tissue envelope (Figure 1). Anatomic alignment is maintained primarily by a series of posterior ligaments. The strongest of these, the interosseous ligaments, connect the tuberosities of the ilium and sacrum. The posterior sacroiliac ligaments connect the superior and inferior posterior spines of the ilium to the lateral aspect of sacrum. Similarly, the anterior sacroiliac ligaments run from the anterior surface of the sacrum obliquely to the anterior surface of the ilium. The connecting ligaments are the sacrotuberous, which runs from the dorsum of the sacrum and posterior iliac spines to the ischial tuberosity; the sacrospinous, which courses from the lateral sacrum to the ischial spine; and the iliolumbar ligaments, which run from the transverse process of L5 to the iliac crest. This group of ligaments maintains the relationship between the sacrum and the sciatic buttress, which is the body's primary weight bearing axis. Under anatomic conditions, there is only microscopic motion at the sacroiliac joint.

The paired innominate bones meet anteriorly at the pubic symphysis, which is comprised of a hyaline cartilage interface reinforced by overlying fibrocartilage. The ligaments of pubic symphysis blend with the fibrocartilage to support the articulation superiorly and inferiorly. The anterior ring does not play an integral role in weight bearing but instead acts like a strut to maintain the posterior tension band.[1]

RADIOLOGY

A single anteroposterior (AP) radiograph of the pelvis provides valuable information about the unstable pelvic ring injuries. The anterior injury is readily apparent, and displaced/unstable posterior injuries should be apparent. Once the diagnosis of pelvic ring injury has been made, further imaging should include inlet and outlet views of the pelvis. These are obtained with the patient supine. The x-ray beam is then tilted approximately 45 degrees cephalad for the inlet view. This view elucidates displacement in the AP plane as well as rotation. The outlet view is obtained with the x-ray beam tilted 45 degrees caudad, and provides information regarding vertical displacement. Laboratory studies have demonstrated that static plain radiographs underestimate the injury displacement by 80%. CT scans provide additional valuable information regarding soft tissue injury and foraminal encroachment (Figures 2 and 3).[2]

CLASSIFICATION

Multiple classification systems have been described in an attempt to clarify mechanisms of injury, as well as predict treatment algorithms and outcomes. The Young and Burgess classification system is based on previous systems that divided pelvic injuries by the force vector (Figure 4). Injuries are grouped into lateral compression (LC), AP compression (APC), vertical shear (VS), and combined mechanical (CM) injuries. The Young system further subdivides LC and APC injuries by degree of force with increasing grade of injury correlating with an extension of the original vector to greater forces. For example, an APC-I injury describes symphyseal widening without widening of the sacroiliac joints, while an APC-III injury involves a complete hemipelvis disruption with complete injury to the symphysis as well as disruption of both the anterior and posterior sacroiliac ligaments (Table 1).[3]

This classification system has two major strengths. First, there is a reproducible association among the fracture classification, associated injuries, and mortality. Acute management and evaluation of the unstable patient may be guided by injury pattern. In addition, identification of the nature of the anterior ring lesion guides diagnosis of subtle posterior injuries often missed on screening imaging studies.[4]

ACUTE PATIENT MANAGEMENT

The initial evaluation of any trauma patient follows ATLS protocols. After completion of the primary survey examination proceeds to include plain radiographs of the chest and pelvis. The hemodynamic and respiratory status will direct further interventions. If possible, the injury mechanisms should be considered, as this will provide valuable insight into the nature and severity of the pelvic ring disruptions.

Initial examination must include assessment for open fractures. Despite advances in treatment and diagnosis, open pelvic fractures confer markedly increased risk for sepsis and overall mortality. A gentle but thorough rectal exam, careful inspection of perineum, and in the female patient, a vaginal exam, are critical to a complete initial evaluation.

Unstable anterior pelvic fractures are commonly associated with genitourinary injury particularly in male patients. Blood at the urethral meatus may signify a urologic injury including urethral tear or bladder rupture. Inability to pass a Foley catheter easily should prompt a retrograde urethrogram and consultation of a urologic surgeon.

A complete neurologic examination of the lower extremities with documentation of sensation and muscle grading is another critical component of the evaluation. Neurologic injuries increase in frequency and severity with increasing instability of the pelvic fracture. The nature of the nerve injury may help dictate the

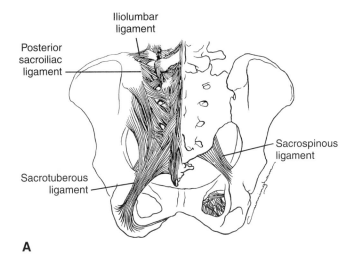

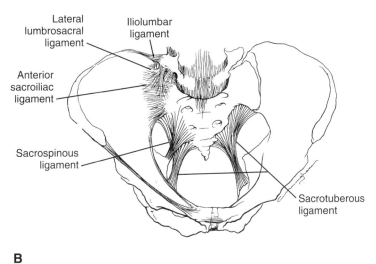

Figure 1   The bony pelvis and its major posterior ligaments.
(A) Posterior view. **(B)** Anterior view.   *(From Tile M, editor:* Fractures of
the Pelvis and Acetabulum, *3rd ed. Baltimore, Williams and Wilkins, 2003.)*

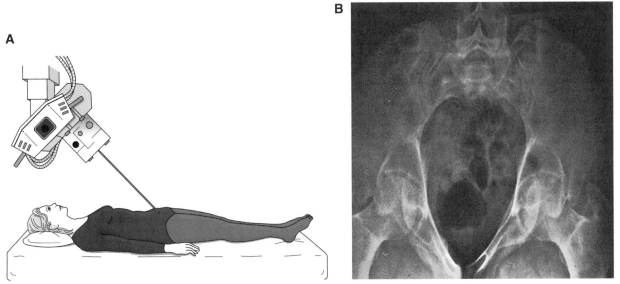

Figure 2   The inlet pelvic view. **(A)** Patient positioning. **(B)** Radiographic appearance.   *(From Kellam JF, Browner BD: Fractures of the
pelvic ring. In Browner BD, et al., editors:* Skeletal Trauma. *Philadelphia, WB Saunders, 1992, pp. 849–897.)*

A

B

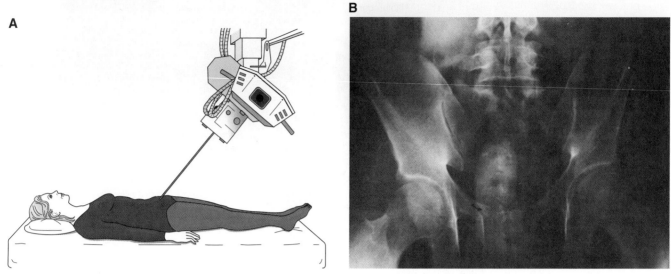

Figure 3   The outlet pelvic view. **(A)** Patient positioning. **(B)** Radiographic appearance.   *(From Kellam JF, Browner BD: Fractures of the pelvic ring. In Browner BD, et al., editors: Skeletal Trauma. Philadelphia, WB Saunders, 1992, pp. 849–897.)*

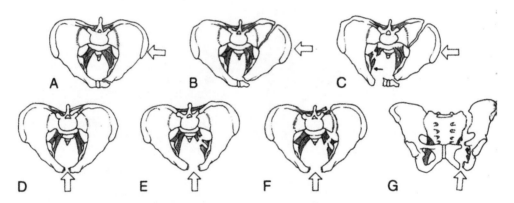

Figure 4   A diagrammatic depiction of the Young and Burgess classification system.   *(From Baumgaertner MR, Tornetta P, editors:* Orthopaedic Knowledge Update: Trauma 3. *Rosemont, IL, American Academy of Orthopaedic Surgeons, 2005, pp. 236–238, with permission.)*

Table 1: Pelvic Ring Fracture Classification System

Category	Primary Classifier	Secondary Classifier
LC-1	Anterior ring fracture	Ipsilateral sacral compression
LC-2	Anterior ring fracture	Crescent fracture
LC-3	Anterior ring fracture	Contralateral APC
APC-1	Symphysis diastasis	Intact anterior and posterior ligaments
APC-2	Symphysis diastasis or anterior ring fracture	Disrupted anterior and posterior ligaments
APC-3	Symphysis diastasis or anterior ring fracture	Disrupted anterior and posterior ligaments
VS	Symphysis diastasis or anterior ring fracture	Vertical displacement of posterior ring through sacroiliac joint, ilium, or sacrum
CM	Combination of previous patterns	Most common LC/VS or LC/APC

APC, Anteroposterior compression; *CM,* combined mechanical; *LC,* lateral compression; *VS,* vertical shear.
Adapted from Burgess AR, Eastridge BJ, Young JW, et al: Pelvic ring disruptions: effective classification system and treatment protocols. *J Trauma* 30(7):848–856, 1990.

appropriate surgical intervention, as well as provide useful prognostic information.

HEMODYNAMIC INSTABILITY

In the acute setting, the pelvic ring injury may be source of significant hemorrhage; however, biomechanically unstable pelvic ring injuries do not necessarily result in a hemodynamic compromise. Patients with pelvic ring injuries can be divided into two broad groups based on hemodynamic stability. While overall mortality rates for pelvic ring fractures are reported as 13%, the mortality rate among patients who present with a systolic blood pressure less than 90 mm Hg is as high as 52% in some series. Determining whether the pelvis is a contributor to a patient's hemodynamic status can be problematic.

Persistent hemodynamic instability should raise concern for arterial bleeding; however, this is uncommonly the source of blood loss in patients with pelvic fractures (approximately 15%). Large-volume hemorrhage from low-pressure sources, such as the pelvic venous plexus and cancellous bone, commonly accounts for the massive blood loss seen in unstable patients. The pelvic ring injury creates a disruption of the boundaries of the retroperitoneal space allowing for massive extravasation. Despite large-volume blood loss, the unconfined space is often inadequate to generate tamponade. Further manipulation through patient transfer and physical exam in the trauma bay contributes to clot disruption and further extravasation.

MODALITIES FOR INITIAL TREATMENT

Early interventions for management of pelvic hemorrhage have been the subject of extensive debate and study. Options include angiography/embolization, laparotomy with pelvic packing, and stabilization of pelvic fractures. The keys to early management are prompt recognition of the pelvis as the source of hemorrhage and rapid implementation of an institution specific protocol for systematic stepwise intervention (Figure 5). Each intervention may have a role depending on the nature of the injury and the availability of qualified personnel.[5]

Pelvic Binders

Circumferential wrapping of the pelvis is a quick and simple way to decrease gross fracture motion. First responders in the field can apply a sheet at the level of the greater trochanter to minimize fracture bleeding and stabilize hematoma formation. Currently several different binders are available commercially which can apply a controlled amount of force to the pelvis. These binders are designed to provide a reproducible amount of force which is evenly distributed around the pelvic ring. Circumferential wrapping is an invaluable component in early management of the unstable pelvic ring injury. The wrap is most valuable during the initial phases of evaluation and management but should not be left in place during the course of an extended, large-volume resuscitation.

Angiography

Bleeding from an arterial source occurs in less than 15% of unstable pelvic ring injuries. Although most commonly seen in APC II and III injuries, arterial bleeding may occur in any pelvic fracture pattern and thus should not be ruled out based on imaging alone. The most reliable predictor of pelvic arterial bleeding is persistent hemodynamic instability despite appropriate resuscitation. Patients who do not respond to an initial infusion of crystalloid and two units of packed red cells benefit from emergent angiography. Within the subgroup of patients with pelvic ring injuries presenting with hypotension, 70%–85% will have an arterial source of bleeding that can be successfully managed through angiographic embolization. Mortality rates in hemodynamically unstable patients who rapidly undergo embolization are markedly reduced. Complications related to embolization, including necrosis of the gluteus musculature, have been reported but are uncommon.

External Fixation

Anterior external fixation offers the advantage of a quick and reliable means of applying a fixation device to the pelvis without the added risk of an open surgical approach. Many types of anterior external fixation frames have been applied. Historically, the frame has been applied via pins in the iliac crest bilaterally, which are attached through anterior bars. Another more powerful approach involves placement of supracetabular pins. Both of these frames may provide enough stability to reduce bony motion and therefore allow clot formation. Application in the trauma bay, intensive care unit, or angiography suite may be readily accomplished in the hands of experienced surgeons with qualified staff.

Anterior external fixation may reduce bony motion in order to allow clot formation and early upright positioning. However, external fixation applied through the anterior ring can worsen the posterior ring injury. Frequently an anterior fixator reduces the anterior ring at the expense of the posterior injury and may aggravate bleeding from posterior sources.

C-Clamp

The pelvic c-clamp was designed with stabilization of the posterior injury as the primary goal. Two pins are applied to the posterior ilium and connected to a large C-shaped clamp anteriorly. It can be quickly applied in the resuscitation bay without interfering with definitive pelvic fixation. The dangers of poorly placed pins in the posterior pelvis due to distorted landmarks include pin perforation into the pelvis and further displacement of the fracture. Early experience with significant complications has limited the use of this technology in the United States.[6]

Surgical Management of Pelvic Bleeding

As noted earlier, the source of pelvic bleeding is largely venous. Thus the role of laparotomy alone for management of bleeding is limited. Some centers recommend pelvic packing in conjunction with application of a C-clamp and have demonstrated decreased mortality from this combined approach. If computed tomography scan shows no intraperitoneal bleeding or organ injury, and does show a significant pelvic hematoma, a suprapubic incision can be done, with packing of the space of Retzius and the lateral pelvic side wall.

TREATMENT AND OUTCOMES

Definitive reconstruction of unstable pelvic ring injuries is pursued once the acute inflammatory and resuscitation period has concluded. Stabilization of the ring allows early patient mobilization, improved pulmonary toilet, and decreased long-term morbidity. Many posterior ring injuries may be stabilized with percutaneous screw fixation following open or closed reduction. This avoids prominent hardware and decreases the risk of infection and soft tissue complication. The anterior injury pattern will dictate the need for and the type of operative stabilization. Anatomic restoration of the posterior ring injury is most

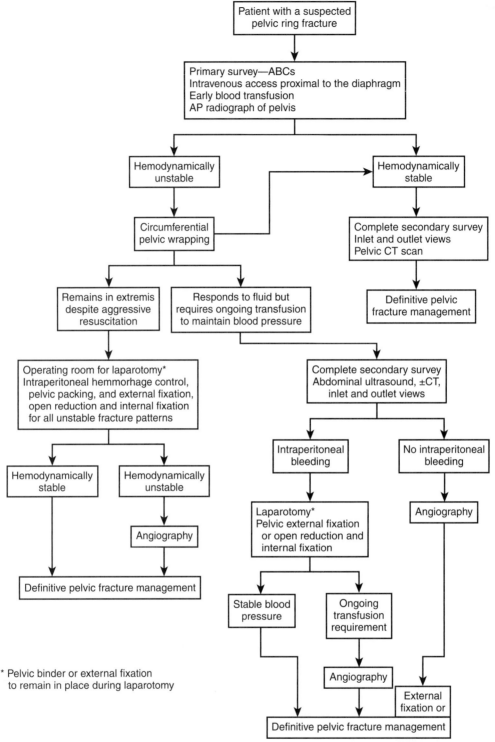

Figure 5 Acute management algorithm for unstable pelvic fractures. *(From Baumgaertner MR, Tornetta P, editors:* Orthopaedic Knowledge Update: Trauma 3. *Rosemont, IL, American Academy of Orthopaedic Surgeons, 2005, pp. 236–238, with permission.)*

critical for avoiding sitting imbalance and leg length discrepancy. In modern series, the majority of patients with anatomic fracture reductions maintained to union are able to return to their preinjury occupation, perform all activities of daily living, and walk without assistive devices. The minority of patients with good reductions who have suboptimal outcomes have one of several complications related to their initial injury complex.

The most significant factor in a patient's overall outcome score is the severity of the initial neurologic injury. Partial and complete injuries to the lumbosacral plexus result in muscle weakness, sensory deficits, and neurogenic pain. Reduction of the bony injury will not improve the neurologic prognosis. A large percentage of patients with significant nerve injury will not return to their preinjury occupation or functional status.

Genitourinary complications are a common complaint amongst patients with unstable pelvic fractures. Injuries to the urethra and perineum result in long-term complications such as stricture, incontinence, and erectile dysfunction. Female patients commonly develop incontinence and dyspareuenia. There is also an increased rate of cesarean section in female patients following pelvic injury.

Studies of overall outcomes in patients with pelvic fractures have documented small but significant impacts on mental and physical well-being over the long term. Although the vast majority of patients are able to return to work and ambulation, the residual effects of these devastating injuries continue to impact day-to-day life.[7]

SUMMARY

Unstable pelvic ring injuries are a relatively common problem in the trauma population. A multidisciplinary approach to initial management is effective at reducing both morbidity and mortality. Every institution should establish a specific pathway for the management of hemodynamic instability based on the availability of qualified personnel and facilities. Prompt recognition of the pelvic injury and its associated complications will guide appropriate therapeutic interventions.

REFERENCES

1. Tile M, editor: *Fractures of the Pelvis and Acetabulum*, 3rd ed. Baltimore, Williams and Wilkins, 2003.
2. Kellam JF, Browner BD: Fractures of the pelvic ring. In Browner BD, et al, editors: Skeletal Trauma. Philadelphia, WB Saunders, 1992, pp. 849–897.
3. O'Brien PJ, Dickson KF: Pelvic fractures: evaluation and acute management. In Baumgaertner MR, editor: *Orthopaedic Knowledge Update: Trauma 3.* Rosemont, IL, American Academy of Orthopaedic Surgeons, 2005, pp. 233–242.
4. Eastridge BJ, et al: The importance of fracture pattern in guiding therapeutic decision-making in patients with hemorrhagic shock and pelvic ring disruptions. *J Trauma* 53:446–451, 2002.
5. Biffi WL, et al: Evolution of a multidisciplinary pathway for the management of unstable patients with pelvic fractures. *Ann Surg* 233:843–850, 2001.
6. Ertel W, et al: Control of severe hemorrhage using c-clamp and pelvic packing in multiply injured patients with pelvic ring disruption. *J Orthop Trauma* 15:468–474, 2001.
7. Routt ML, Copeland C: Pelvic fractures: definitive treatment and expected outcomes. In Baumgaertner MR, editor: *Orthopaedic Knowledge Update: Trauma 3.* Rosemont, IL, American Academy of Orthopaedic Surgeons, 2005, pp. 243–258.

HAND FRACTURES

Roshini Gopinathan, Parham A. Ganchi,
and Mark S. Granick

The presence of an opposable thumb separates man from other primates. The hand serves many functions, ranging from precise prehension to power gripping. This requires finely coordinated interplay among the various components of the musculoskeletal architecture of the hand. A stable and well-aligned skeletal framework, stable joints, and balance between intrinsic and extrinsic muscles and tendinous systems are all necessary for good hand function.

Injuries to the hand can occur in isolation or may be one of many injuries in a multiply injured patient. Very often, injuries to the hand are overlooked initially, resulting in significant disability once the patient has recovered from life-threatening injuries. Particularly in the management of hand injuries, one should aim for optimal function rather than radiologic perfection.

Most hand fractures can be treated nonoperatively by means of closed manipulation, splinting, and protected motion. Certain fracture patterns, however, are best treated by operative intervention. The goals of treatment remain the same and include accurate reduction, stabilization, wound treatment, and early mobilization. Inability to achieve or maintain reduction in the so-called safe or functional position denotes that a fracture is unstable. The fracture pattern and integrity of the periosteal sleeve and surrounding soft tissues determine fracture stability. Unopposed pull of muscles can lead to instability. Fractures involving articular surfaces demand accurate reduction to achieve good motion. Severely comminuted fractures are often best treated closed, because open reduction can lead to devitalization of small bony fragments. These fractures are well suited for closed pinning. Open fractures with loss of bone, contamination, or poor soft tissue coverage are best treated with external fixation. This permits fixation and maintenance of length while allowing for soft tissue healing and dressing changes. Definitive procedures to achieve bony union and soft tissue coverage can be carried out in a delayed fashion. Indications for operative treatment are summarized in Table 1.

INCIDENCE

The most common upper extremity fractures are those of the metacarpals and phalanges. In a series of 4303 patients presenting to the emergency room with fractures, 19% had hand fractures.[1] The phalanges were most commonly fractured. Males between the ages of 15 and 35 were most commonly injured. Fractures of the little finger ray were most common.

Hove, in a series of 1000 consecutive patients, found that metacarpals, phalanges, and carpal bones accounted for 36%, 46%, and 18% of the fractures, respectively.[2] Chung and Spilson analyzed data from the 1998 National Hospital Ambulatory Medical Care Survey and estimated that in 1998, there were more than 600,000 metacarpal and phalangeal fractures in the United States.[3]

Fractures in children follow different patterns in various age groups because of differing mechanisms of injury. In a review of 242 hand fractures, Mahabir et al. found that 75% of injuries were in males, the mean age being 11 years.[4] The incidence of fractures was very low in the very young, rose sharply at age 9, and peaked at 12 years. Forty percent were epiphyseal fractures, predominantly Salter-Harris II. The fifth metacarpal was the most frequently fractured bone.

The incidence of hand injuries in polytrauma was studied by Schaller and Geldmacher.[5] They noted a 20% incidence of associated hand injuries, 75% of which were closed fractures. Ninety-three percent were involved in motor vehicle accidents.

MECHANISM OF INJURY

Chung and Spilson described the cause of injury in hand and forearm fractures.[3] Forty-seven percent of injuries were due to falls, while 15% were due to being struck by a person or object. Ten percent were due to vehicular accidents. Other causes included

Table 1: Indications for Operative Treatment in Hand Fractures

Displaced intra-articular fractures

Soft tissue interposition

Multiple fractures

Open fractures, to facilitate wound care

Tendinous or ligamentous avulsion

Segmental bone loss

Unstable fractures

being caught between objects, accidents involving machines or tools, injury due to another person, and nontraffic motor vehicle accidents.

De Jonge et al. studied the incidence and etiology of 6857 phalangeal fractures.[6] They found that falls were responsible for most injuries in patients 70 years or older, while sports were the main cause in the age group 10–29 years. The highest incidence was in males aged 40–70 years, and the cause was machinery. Over 45% of hand fractures in children occurred either during sports or in a fight.

DIAGNOSIS

Management of hand injuries requires a good understanding of hand anatomy and biomechanics. The individual needs of the patient need to be taken into account before devising a treatment plan. A detailed history needs to be obtained. Key points to be elicited are noted in Table 2.

Examination of the hand should assess deformity, tenderness, instability, sensation, and vascularity of the finger. The condition of the skin and soft tissues should be evaluated, including an assessment for injury to the tendons. It is particularly important to assess the finger cascade. On flexion of the fingers to make a fist, the tips of the fingers should converge toward the scaphoid. Scissoring of the fingers indicates rotational malalignment. Evaluation of stability is necessary to rule out ligamentous injury. This is done after administration of local anesthetic to prevent pain and reflex muscle spasm. The congruity of the joint is assessed during active motion and passive stress. Partial injuries can be treated by immobilization, while complete tears may require surgical repair.

Three views are necessary for adequate radiologic evaluation: anteroposterior, lateral (with the fingers fanned out), and an oblique view. The lateral view obtained in this manner, however, shows, at best, one finger in a true lateral position. Hence, it is better to get lateral views of individual fingers. Very rarely, special views of the hand are necessary to assess certain injuries. Occasionally, stress views of joints are used—for example, to evaluate collateral ligament injuries of the thumb metacarpophalangeal joint.

Table 2: History in Hand Injuries

Mechanism of injury

Associated injuries

Time delay in seeking treatment

Handedness of the individual

Occupation and hobbies

Pre-injury status

Medical conditions

Previous treatment

METACARPAL FRACTURES

The metacarpals are structurally divided into the head, neck, shaft, and base. The metacarpal head articulates with the base of the proximal phalanx. The collateral ligaments between the metacarpal and phalanx arise in an eccentric position. Hence, these ligaments are stretched in flexion and lax in extension, and the joint is stable in flexion (Figure 1). The thumb metacarpal and fourth and fifth metacarpals are mobile. Because of its unique anatomy, thumb fractures are dealt with separately. Common metacarpal fracture patterns are illustrated in Figure 2.

Metacarpal Shaft Fractures

Transverse fractures are caused by axial loading or direct blows. Because of the pull of the interossei, the fracture angulates dorsally. Patients can accept some angulation of the fourth and fifth metacarpals because of mobility. Greater than 30-degree angulations of the fifth metacarpal, 20 degrees in the fourth metacarpal, and any angulation in the second and third metacarpals require reduction. Oblique and spiral fractures, on the other hand, cause rotational malalignment. This is poorly tolerated, because the fingers overlap each other when the fingers are flexed. Transverse fractures are inherently stable, while spiral and oblique fractures are not.

Most metacarpal shaft fractures can be managed nonoperatively. The fracture is reduced if needed, and the hand is immobilized in the so-called safe position, with the wrist in 30–40 degrees of extension, the metacarpophalangeal joints in 80–90 degrees of flexion, and the interphalangeal joints in extension. Immobilization is maintained for 3–4 weeks and is followed by active mobilization.

Open reduction is indicated when the fracture is malaligned or unstable. Open fractures and those with associated soft tissue injuries are also best treated by open reduction. This permits earlier mobilization to prevent stiffness. With multiple metacarpal fractures, the stabilizing influence of the adjacent metacarpals is lost, and such fractures may need open reduction and internal fixation. Various techniques are available to stabilize fractures. Spiral or long oblique fractures can be stabilized by lag screws (Figure 3). The length of the fracture line should be at least twice the diameter of the bone. The proximal hole is over-drilled to a diameter wider than the thread of the screw. As the screw is tightened and the threads grip the distal fragment, interfragmentary compression is achieved.

Kirschner wires can be used to stabilize shaft fractures. Percutaneous insertion involves minimal soft tissue dissection; however, the stabilization is not rigid, and patients need to be splinted. Rarely, pin tract infec-

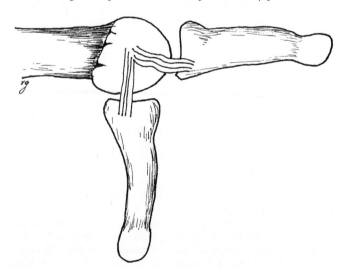

Figure 1 Metacarpophalangeal joint anatomy. The collateral ligaments arise in an eccentric fashion on the metacarpal head, resulting in a stable position in flexion.

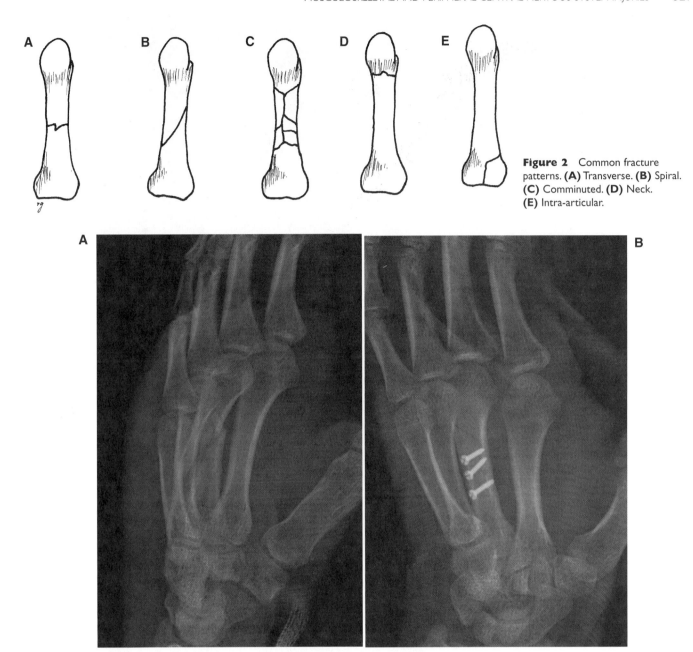

Figure 2 Common fracture patterns. **(A)** Transverse. **(B)** Spiral. **(C)** Comminuted. **(D)** Neck. **(E)** Intra-articular.

Figure 3 **(A)** Metacarpal shaft fracture sustained in a fist fight. **(B)** Fixation with three lag screws.

tions can complicate treatment. Multiple wires are usually placed to avoid rotation of fragments (Figure 4).

Fixation with plates and screws provides rigid fixation. This permits early mobilization, which can be critical to the successful rehabilitation of patients with concomitant tendon or other soft tissue injuries that are adversely affected by scar and adhesion formation. Plate fixation itself requires significant tissue dissection. This can result in adhesions, reduced tissue glide, and suboptimal functional outcomes. Again, early mobilization is essential to optimize functional outcomes. Plate fixation is particularly useful in the treatment of complications such as nonunion or malunion requiring corrective osteotomies.

Metacarpal Neck Fractures

The most commonly encountered fracture is that of the fifth metacarpal neck. These fractures are known as "boxer's fractures" and, as the name implies, are caused by impact of a clenched fist against a rigid surface, which is frequently the face of another individual or a wall. Impact of the closed fist against a tooth can lead to a serious human bite infection. The tooth can penetrate the joint space. As the finger is extended, the extensor tendon glides proximally and closes the joint space. This provides a good environment for growth of anaerobic bacteria. These bite injuries are commonly associated with metacarpal head fractures. If not treated or inadequately treated, these injuries can lead to severe infections and loss of function. Since these patients tend to be noncompliant and present late, they may need to be admitted to the hospital for debridement, open joint drainage, irrigation, and intravenous antibiotics. *Staphylococcus aureus* and *Streptococci* are the most common organisms cultured from these infections. Other organisms such as *Eikanella corrodens*, *Neisseria*, and *Clostridia* have also been cultured.

Metacarpal neck fractures angulate dorsally because of the pull of the intrinsic muscles. The fourth and fifth metacarpals have more mobility at the carpometacarpal joints, and hence angulation in the ulnar metacarpals is better tolerated from the functional standpoint. Patients

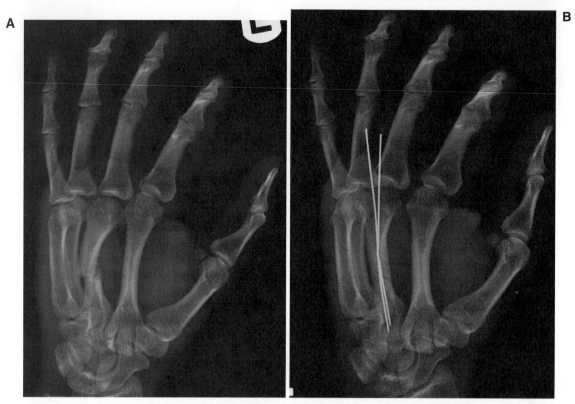

Figure 4 **(A)** Metacarpal shaft fracture sustained in a fist fight. **(B)** Fixation with Kirschner wires.

may complain about the resultant deformity—a loss of prominence of the knuckle—and also about feeling a mass in the clenched fist.

Closed reduction of metacarpal neck fractures is achieved by the Jahss maneuver[8] (Figure 5). Local anesthesia with a hematoma block is administered. Traction is applied and the fracture is disimpacted. The metacarpophalangeal and interphalangeal joints are flexed to 90 degrees. This relaxes the intrinsics and tightens the collateral ligaments. An upward push on the proximal phalanx transmits force to the distal fragment to achieve reduction. Reduction is confirmed by radiology. The hand is immobilized in an ulnar gutter splint. If the fracture is more than 7–10 days old, closed reduction is usually not possible.

Persistent dorsal angulation of more than 30–40 degrees of the ring and little finger metacarpals, more than 10–15 degrees in the index and long finger metacarpals, and any rotational malalignment require operative intervention. Percutaneous insertion of Kirschner pins usually suffices. On occasion, open reduction and pinning, or plate application is necessary.[6]

Metacarpal Head Fractures

Metacarpal head fractures are unusual and are usually intra-articular. Index metacarpal head fractures are the most common. These fractures usually result from direct trauma or axial loading. In addition to the standard three views, special views, such as the Brewerton view or skyline metacarpal view, are useful. Significant joint incongruity requires operative management.[6]

Thumb Metacarpal Fractures

Thumb metacarpal head, neck, and shaft fractures are treated as outlined previously (Figure 6). Fractures of the metacarpal base are important because loss of the carpometacarpal joint integrity can severely compromise hand function. Two patterns of injury are notable: Bennett's fracture and Rolando fracture.[6]

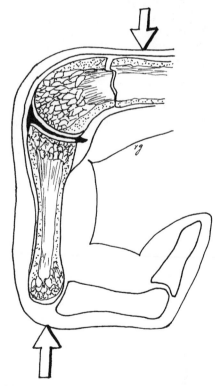

Figure 5 Jahss maneuver.

Bennett's Fracture

Bennett's fracture is an intra-articular fracture of the base of the thumb metacarpal (Figure 7). The smaller ulnar fragment remains attached to the trapezium by the volar oblique ligament, and the shaft is displaced

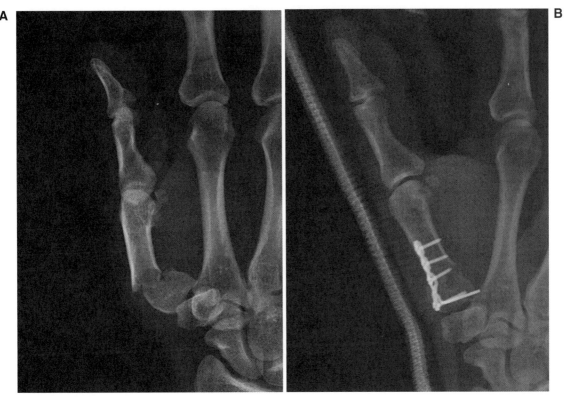

Figure 6 **(A)** Transverse fracture of thumb metacarpal base following a crush injury. **(B)** Fixation with a condylar plate.

by the pull of the adductor pollicis and abductor pollicis muscles. It is difficult to maintain reduction in a cast, so these fractures require operative intervention. Once reduced, the reduction is maintained by passing a Kirschner wire through the metacarpal shaft into the trapezium or the second metacarpal. It is not necessary to include the small fragment. If reduction is not possible by the closed technique, open reduction is necessary.

Rolando Fracture

This is a T- or Y-shaped fracture of the metacarpal base. The fracture results in joint incongruity and hence needs operative management. The fragments can be pinned together or plate and screws can be applied.

PHALANGEAL FRACTURES

Distal Phalangeal Fractures

These are divided into tuft fractures, shaft fractures, and articular fractures. Tuft fractures occur secondary to direct blows. These fractures are commonly associated with nail matrix injuries. Nail matrix injuries are treated by removal of the nail and careful repair of lacerations under loupe magnification using fine absorbable sutures. The nail is replaced to prevent adhesions of the nail fold. The finger is immobilized for 2–3 weeks using malleable aluminum splints.

Undisplaced shaft fractures are treated by splinting. If a fracture is not reducible, interposition of sterile matrix must be suspected and open reduction is necessary.

Epiphyseal injuries can be missed. Salter-Harris type I fractures are seen in young children, while type III fractures are seen in adolescents. Both injuries frequently require open reduction and pinning to maintain the reduction.

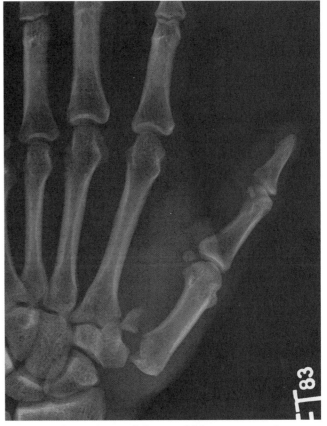

Figure 7   Bennet fracture following a fall from a motorcycle.

Proximal and Middle Phalangeal Fractures

Stable nondisplaced shaft fractures and those that are stable after reduction are immobilized with malleable aluminum splints and a short arm splint in the safe position. The finger can be "Buddy taped" to an adjacent noninjured finger to prevent rotational malalignment. Mobilization should be initiated early to prevent stiffness. Immobilization for more than 3 weeks is seldom necessary. Unstable fractures require pinning (Figure 8). Plate and screw application in the fingers can potentially compromise tendon function and soft tissue coverage.

Condylar fractures are serious injuries with poor outcomes. They require accurate reduction and fixation.

DISLOCATIONS

Proximal Interphalangeal Joint Dislocation

Dislocation of the proximal interphalangeal (PIP) joint is the most common ligamentous injury in the hand. These can be dorsal, volar, or lateral (Figure 9).

Dorsal dislocations are usually caused by hyperextension combined with longitudinal compression. Sometimes this can be associated with a fracture to the volar lip of the middle phalanx. Rarely, the volar plate can rupture and get interposed between the proximal and middle phalanges, producing an irreducible dislocation. Closed reduction is performed by traction and palmar flexion while applying pressure to the base of the middle phalanx. If after reduction of the dislocation, the joint is stable, the finger is splinted. Motion in a dorsal blocking splint is initiated in 1–2 weeks. Protected-range-of-motion exercises, by buddy taping the finger to an adjacent finger, are initiated at 3 weeks, and unprotected motion is started at 8 weeks. In fracture dislocations, if the fracture involves less than 40% of the articular surface, the joint is usually stable and can be treated as outlined previously. Larger fractures require pinning or dynamic skeletal traction, especially for pilon fractures.

Volar dislocations are unusual. These can be true volar dislocations or volar rotatory subluxations. Volar dislocations are usually associated with rupture of the central slip of the extensor tendon. After reduction, this should be treated with immobilization in full extension for 4–6 weeks. Failure to treat the central slip rupture results in a Boutonniere deformity. Volar rotatory dislocations are reduced by applying traction on the middle phalynx with the PIP flexed. Rotatory motion can reduce the dislocation. Open reduction is indicated if the dislocation is irreducible.

Lateral dislocations occur with rupture of a collateral ligament and a volar plate tear. Following reduction, the finger should be buddy taped and protected range of motion initiated.

Distal Interphalangeal Joint Dislocation

These are usually dorsal or lateral. Open dislocations are more common and require debridement, reduction, and splinting. Closed reduction is carried out by traction, flexion of the distal phalanx while maintaining pressure on the dorsum of the distal phalanx. The finger should be immobilized in slight flexion for 2–3 weeks.

METACARPOPHALANGEAL JOINTS

These are usually dorsal dislocations caused by hyperextension of the joint. They are divided into simple subluxations and complex dislocations. In simple subluxations, the volar plate is draped over the metacarpal head, and the proximal phalanx is in hyperextension over the metacarpal head. Simple dislocations are reduced by flexing the wrist while applying traction and flexing the MP joint. Following reduction, a dorsal extension block splint is applied (Figure 10).

In complex dislocations, the metacarpal head protrudes volarly between the lumbrical and flexor tendon. The volar plate is folded and entrapped between the two articular surfaces. Hyperextension of a simple subluxation can pull the volar plate further into the joint, entrapping it and converting it into a complex dislocation. Complex dislocations present with the MP joint in slight extension, palpable

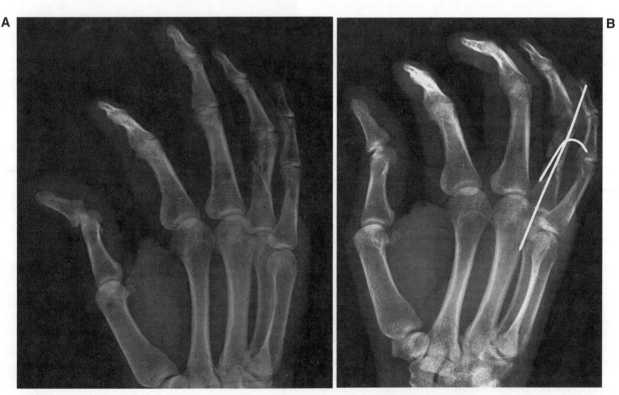

Figure 8 (A) Proximal phalanx fracture following a motorcycle accident, and **(B)** following pinning.

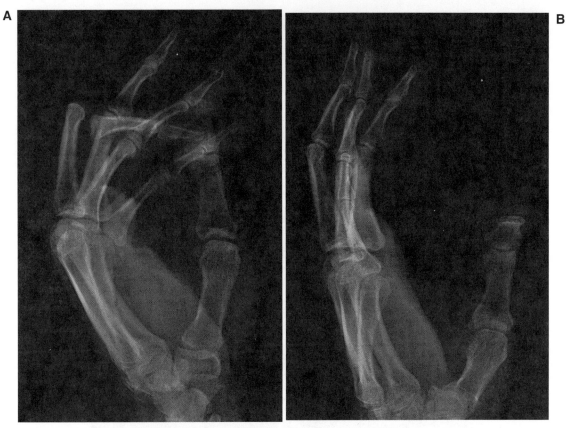

Figure 9 **(A)** Interphalangeal joint dislocation. **(B)** Post reduction.

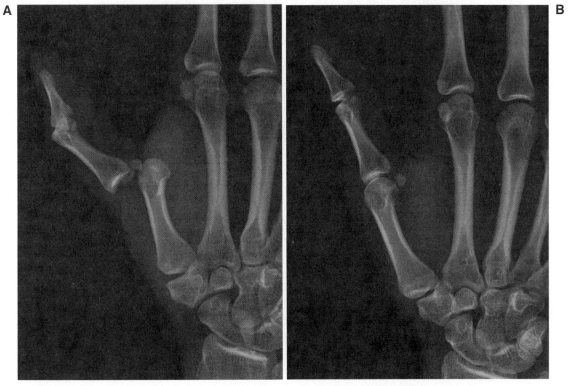

Figure 10 **(A)** Simple metacarpophalangeal joint dislocation following a fist fight. **(B)** Post reduction.

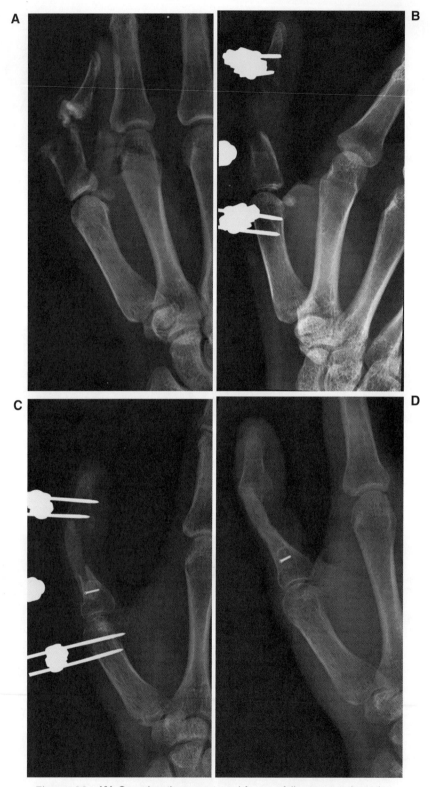

Figure 11   **(A)** Open, heavily contaminated fracture following an industrial accident, a crush injury with a plastic cutting device. **(B)** Following operative debridement and removal of devitalized bone, external fixator applied to maintain bone length and facilitate wound care. **(C)** Iliac crest bone graft applied following soft tissue healing. **(D)** Consolidated bone following removal of external fixator.

metacarpal head in the palm, and dimpling of the skin from pull on the periosteal dermal attachments. X-rays, especially of the first metacarpophalangeal joint, may show the sesamoid bones in the joint space, indicating volar plate entrapment. Complex dislocations require open reduction.

Forced lateral deviation of the fingers can lead to rupture of the collateral ligaments. Patients often present late. Tenderness along the collateral ligament and instability and pain on lateral stressing are noted on clinical examination. Immobilization followed by protected motion by buddy taping is used. In complete tears with significant instability, surgical repair is indicated.

Thumb Metacarpophalangeal Joints

Dislocation of the thumb metacarpophalangeal joint is treated similarly to that in the fingers. Collateral ligament injuries are quite common in athletes, especially injury to the ulnar collateral ligament.

Acute ulnar collateral ligament injury (skier's thumb) is caused by forced abduction of the thumb. This may be a partial or complete tear of the substance of the ligament, or it may be associated with an avulsion fracture at the site of insertion. Clinical examination under local anesthesia and stress x-rays are essential for diagnosis. Partial tears are treated by immobilization for 4–6 weeks in a thumb spica cast, followed by protected mobilization. Complete ruptures require surgical repair. Stener's lesion occurs when the adductor pollicis is interposed between the two ruptured ends of the collateral ligament, preventing healing.

Chronic instability of the ulnar collateral ligament caused by repetitive stress on the ligament is known as "game keeper's thumb." This may require ligament reconstruction.

COMPLICATIONS

Both undertreatment and overtreatment of hand fractures and dislocations can lead to complications. The most common complication is stiffness, and its prevention is of paramount importance in the restoration of hand function. Joint contractures can result from prolonged immobilization. The safe position must be utilized, whenever feasible. Scarring can result in tendon adhesions and entrapment of nerves, resulting in poor function. Stabilization of fractures and early protected motion are essential. Clinical healing precedes radiologic union. On the other hand, inadequate immobilization can lead to malunion, or nonunion. Malunion and nonunion may require operative intervention to correct. Corrective osteotomies and internal fixation are utilized to treat malunion. Nonunions may require bone grafting (Figure 11). Infection can be seen in open fractures and are more likely in human bite injuries. These injuries require antibiotic prophylaxis after adequate debridement.

Operative treatment of fractures can convert a previously closed fracture into an open fracture, hence risking infection. Injury to tendons, nerves, or vessels is also possible. Implants can fail with breakage of plates and screws.

REFERENCES

1. van Onselen EB, et al: Prevalence and distribution of hand fractures. *J Hand Surg [Br]* 28(5):491–495, 2003.
2. Hove LM: Fractures of the hand. Distribution and relative incidence. *Scand J Plast Reconstr Surg Hand Surg* 27(4):317–319, 1993.
3. Chung KC, Spilson SV: The frequency and epidemiology of hand and forearm fractures in the United States. *J Hand Surg [Am]* 26(5):908–915, 2001.
4. Mahabir RC, et al: Pediatric hand fractures: a review. *Pediatr Emerg Care* 17(3):153–156, 2001.
5. Schaller P, Geldmacher J: Hand injury in polytrauma. A retrospective study of 782 cases. *Handchir Mikrochir Plast Chir* 26(6):307–312, 1994.
6. De Jonge JJ, et al: Phalangeal fractures of the hand: an analysis of gender and age-related incidence and aetiology. *J Hand Surg* 19(2):168–170, 1994.
7. Jahss SA: Fractures of the metacarpals: a new method of reduction and immobilization. *J Bone Joint Surg* 20:178–186, 1938.

SCAPULOTHORACIC DISSOCIATION AND DEGLOVING INJURIES OF THE EXTREMITIES

Walter L. Biffl, Christopher Born, and William G. Cioffi

Scapulothoracic dissociation (STD) is the traumatic disruption of the shoulder from the chest wall. It is characterized by a complete loss of scapulothoracic articulation, typically with intact skin. Vascular and neurologic injuries are common, and when severe, the result is essentially a closed forequarter amputation.[1] Degloving injuries may occur to any extremity, with widely variable severity. The chapter will primarily address STD, with brief mention of the concepts associated with the management of degloving injuries.

INCIDENCE

The first report of STD was published in 1984 by Oreck and colleagues.[2] The literature on the topic consists mainly of case reports, small case series, and reviews.[1] One of the largest reported series consists of 25 patients, treated over a 24-year period.[3] Thus, one can expect to see a case of STD approximately once a year at a major trauma center. Extremity degloving injuries, on the other hand, are much more common.

MECHANISM OF INJURY

Scapulothoracic dissociation is typically the result of a massive traction force to the upper extremity, usually accompanied by a severe blunt force directed over the shoulder. Osseus and ligamentous injuries include clavicle fractures and acromioclavicular and sternoclavicular dislocations. Soft tissue destruction may involve the deltoid, latissimus dorsi, levator scapulae, pectoralis minor, rhomboids, and trapezius muscles. The skin is generally intact. Vascular injuries to the subclavian or axillary vessels and complete or partial avulsion of the brachial plexus are very common, and when severe result in a functional forequarter amputation.

DIAGNOSIS

The diagnosis of STD is made on the basis of clinical findings and radiographic studies. The diagnosis can be difficult, as patients often have severe associated injuries that impede the conduct of complete physical examination or distract the clinician from the involved extremity. Furthermore, intact skin and normal bony anatomy of the arm may be misleading as to the extent of the underlying injury.

Physical findings consistent with STD include massive soft tissue swelling, tenderness to palpation, and gross instability of the involved shoulder. The involved extremity may manifest vascular or neurologic compromise. Vascular injuries may be evidenced by the "Six P's": pain, pallor, pulselessness, paresthesias, paralysis, and poikilothermia. However, owing to the extensive collateral vascular network around the shoulder, a patient may have subclavian artery occlusion and still have a pulse in the distal extremity with a normal brachial-brachial index. On the other hand, a patient may have a cold, mottled extremity with diminished pulses due to shock or environmental conditions, in the absence of a vascular injury. The findings related to vascular and neurologic compromise may overlap. Diagnostic ambiguity calls for further vascular assessment.

The pathognomonic radiographic finding in STD is lateral displacement of the scapula on an anteroposterior (AP) chest x-ray.[4] The degree of displacement may be quantified by the scapula index. This is calculated by measuring the distance from the thoracic vertebral spinous processes to the medial border of the scapula, and dividing the distance on the injured side by that on the uninjured side (Figure 1). It requires an AP chest x-ray in a supine patient with nonrotated extremities, and an uninjured shoulder.[5] In the uninjured population, the scapula index averages 1.07 (±0.04).[6] Zelle and colleagues[3] reported an average index of 1.29 (±0.19) in a series of 25 patients with STD, but the diagnostic threshold is not well established. They noted that five of their patients had a scapula index within two standard deviations of the "normal" mean, and cautioned that it be used as a screen but not a definitive diagnostic test. Lange and Noel[7] suggested simply that a difference of greater than 1 cm suggests STD, while Ebraheim and colleagues[8] described alternative measurements from the sternal notch to the coracoid or glenoid margin. Because the accurate measurement of the scapula index requires a standardized x-ray and is affected by patient positioning, it is prudent to look for other clues such as distracted clavicle fractures and acromioclavicular or sternoclavicular joint disruptions, and to consider the overall clinical picture, in determining the possibility of STD.

Associated vascular injuries are very common. In a review of the literature, Damschen and colleagues[4] found that 88% of patients with STD had vascular injuries. More recently, in their large single-institution experience, Zelle and colleagues[3] reported vascular injuries in 16 (64%) of 25 patients. Duplex ultrasonography may be employed to document arterial flow, but arteriography is indicated in stable patients in whom STD is diagnosed or suspected, as it provides more definitive imaging. The subclavian, axillary, and brachial arteries should be interrogated.

Neurologic injury is also very common with STD. Damschen and colleagues[4] reported from their literature review that 94% of patients had a neurologic injury; in the series of Zelle and colleagues,[3] the incidence was 80%. The precise extent of injury can be difficult to determine initially. Complaints of severe pain in an anesthetic extremity are consistent with nerve root avulsion,[1] but a history and physical exam predict the site of injury in just 30%–50% of cases.[9] Evidence of concomitant spinal cord injury should be sought when there are any neurologic abnormalities. Computed tomography (CT) scanning and magnetic resonance imaging (MRI) may be complementary in the evaluation of these patients. A CT scan demonstrating paraspinous hematoma would be consistent with nerve root avulsion, and suggests that cervical myelography should be done.[6] In the case of incomplete motor deficits, MRI is preferred.[10] The T1-weighted images highlight the fat content of the spinal cord and nerve roots; the T2-weighted images highlight the water content and can demonstrate a pseudomeningocele that would suggest nerve root avulsion.[1] Electromyography (EMG) studies are useful in identifying the involved nerve roots and showing evidence of denervation.[9]

The diagnosis of an extremity degloving injury is usually obvious on inspection, although flap viability can be difficult to determine. It is important to ascertain the presence of concomitant bony fractures, ligamentous injuries, or joint dislocations, as well as the neurovascular integrity of the extremity. This is done by thorough physical examination. The Morel-Lavallee injury deserves special mention. This is a closed degloving, in which the skin is detached from subjacent layers by a shearing force but remains intact.[11] While it may not require any special treatment, it may result in skin necrosis or abscess. Additionally, if one makes an incision to operate in the area, it generally obligates open wound management.

INJURY GRADING

Damschen and colleagues[4] proposed a classification system for STD in 1997, on which to base clinical decision making. In their scheme, musculoskeletal injury alone was classified type I. Type II injuries included vascular (IIA) or neurologic (IIB) injuries. An STD with both vascular and neurologic injuries was called type III. Recently, Zelle and colleagues[3] examined the functional outcomes of 25 patients with STD. Their data demonstrated the pivotal importance of the neurologic injury in determining functional outcome. Consequently, they proposed a modified classification system that introduced a fourth category, type IV, which included all patients with complete brachial plexus avulsions (Table 1).

MANAGEMENT

Most patients with STD have significant associated injuries, and thus the first step in the management of these patients is initial evaluation and stabilization based on the principles of the Advanced Trauma Life Support course of the American College of Surgeons.[12] Management priorities are established with life-threatening injuries addressed first.

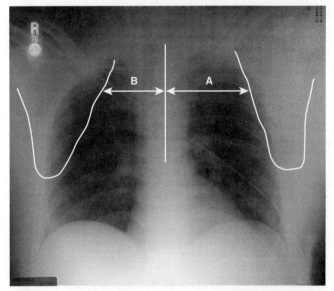

Figure 1   Anteroposterior chest x-ray demonstrating scapulothoracic dissociation. The scapula index is calculated by measuring the distance from the thoracic vertebral spinous processes to the medial border of the scapula, and dividing the distance on the injured side by that on the uninjured side (e.g., A/B in this image).

Table 1: Proposed Classification System for Severity of Scapulothoracic Dissociation

Type	Clinical Findings
I	Musculoskeletal injury alone
IIA	Musculoskeletal injury with vascular disruption
IIB	Musculoskeletal injury with incomplete neurologic impairment of the upper extremity
III	Musculoskeletal injury with vascular disruption and incomplete neurologic impairment of the upper extremity
IV	Musculoskeletal injury with complete brachial plexus avulsion

Adapted from Zelle BA, Pape HC, Gerich TG, et al: Functional outcome following scapulothoracic dissociation. *J Bone Joint Surg [Am]* 86:2–8, 2004.

Hemodynamically unstable patients who appear to be exsanguinating from subclavian vessels should proceed immediately to the operating room for control and repair. Left-sided injuries should be approached via a high anterolateral or "trapdoor" thoracotomy incision, while right-sided injuries are best managed via median sternotomy with supraclavicular extension.[13] Hemodynamically stable patients may undergo a more thorough diagnostic evaluation. If vascular injuries are identified by arteriography, management is dictated based on the presence of hemorrhage, location of the injury, perfusion of the distal extremity, and neurologic injury.[14] Active hemorrhage must be controlled surgically, unless a branch vessel injury is amenable to angioembolization. Venous injuries may be ligated without concern for significant upper extremity swelling.[15] The artery may be reconstructed with a saphenous vein graft or with a polytetrafluoroethylene graft. In the case of an exsanguinating patient, the vessel may be shunted temporarily, or ligated. If perfusion is inadequate, this may obligate amputation, but there is often sufficient collateral flow to sustain the extremity. The location of the injury dictates the approach for surgical exposure, proximal and distal control, and the appropriate level of graft interposition. An ischemic extremity must be vascularized within 4–6 hours to optimize functional outcome.[4] However, it is well recognized that an arm may be adequately perfused—and have a normal brachial-brachial index—even in the case of subclavian artery occlusion, due to the extensive collateral network around the shoulder.[16,17] In such a case, Sampson and colleagues[17] have suggested a nonoperative approach for hemodynamically stable patients with a viable, well-perfused upper extremity. Clearly, such a treatment course must be individualized. With the growing application of endovascular stents, there is likely a role in stable patients with amenable injuries, but they cannot be recommended as a standard at this time.

The neurologic injury is a major determinant of outcome and thus of treatment. In patients undergoing surgical exploration for vascular repair, the brachial plexus should be explored. If the brachial plexus is completely avulsed, a primary above-elbow amputation is the preferred initial management, as there is essentially no chance of functional recovery of the extremity.[1,3] If the brachial plexus is ruptured but not avulsed, repair is appropriate at the initial operation if the patient is a good physiologic candidate for the procedure. Nerve reconstruction does not need to be performed as an emergency but should be performed within 6 months to avoid muscle atrophy and fibrosis and as early as practically possible to minimize the scarring that will make the operation more challenging.[1,8,10] Treatment options for brachial plexus injuries include nerve repair, nerve grafting, neurotization, tendon transfers, or palliative pain-relieving procedures.[1] Treatment planning is facilitated by CT myelography and electromyography, done at 3 and 6 weeks after injury.[6] Clements and

Reisser[18] suggest that nerve repair is indicated if there are fewer than three pseudomeningoceles on CT myelography. On the other hand, the presence of three or more pseudomeningoceles indicates irreparable damage and warrants above-elbow amputation. Leffert[9] has suggested that the preoperative differentiation of preganglionic from postganglionic lesions facilitates planning and reduces operative time. The identification of a postganglionic lesion indicates that a proximal donor root will be available for repair or grafting. Identification of a preganglionic lesion allows the surgeon to proceed to neurotization without exploration of the brachial plexus. In this procedure, an uninjured, less important nerve is divided from its muscular insertion and attached (directly or via nerve grafts) to the distal stump of a nonfunctioning nerve.

The management of the bony injuries is a matter of some controversy. Open reduction and internal fixation may protect vascular repairs as well as facilitate early rehabilitation.[4,18] The concept of the shoulder suspensory complex helps determine the need for bony fixation.[19] The complex consists of the scapula, clavicle, and acromioclavicular joint, along with the ligamentous, tendinous, and supporting capsular structures. Injuries to individual components of the complex may be managed nonoperatively. However, injuries to two or more components usually result in instability and require repair. Definitive recommendations on this require further experience. If amputation is indicated, an above-elbow amputation is preferred. Early prosthetic application and rehabilitation are important in optimizing functional outcome.

In the case of open STD or degloving injuries, soft tissue coverage is important. Initial wound management consists of cleansing, with debridement of foreign material and necrotic tissue, and dressing changes. A vacuum-assisted wound dressing such as the VAC (Kinetic Concepts, Inc., San Antonio, TX) can be useful in facilitating wound care and hastening granulation of the wound bed. Skin grafts may be placed on a clean bed of granulation tissue, but myocutaneous flaps may be required.

MORBIDITY AND COMPLICATIONS

In the early postinjury period, the massive soft tissue injury can result in myoglobinuria, hyperkalemia, and vascular thrombosis. Hydration is important, but the surgeon should be mindful of this and prepared to perform amputation if the patient is compromised. Revascularization of the extremity may be associated with reperfusion injury and development of an extremity compartment syndrome. Thus, serial clinical evaluation of the extremity—with measurement of compartment pressures if there is uncertainty—is essential. These problems may be avoided by early amputation.

The major morbidity associated with STD is a flail upper extremity. Zelle and colleagues[3] reported that of the 62 well-documented cases of STD in the literature, of 40 patients who survived and did not undergo primary amputation, 24 (60%) were left with a flail extremity. In their experience, all complete brachial plexus avulsions resulted in a functionless extremity. Of seven patients with partial or no avulsion, shoulder function (as assessed by the Subjective Shoulder Rating System) was scored as poor in three, fair in two, and good in two. Long-term deficits were typically related to avulsed nerve roots. Zelle and colleagues[3] argue for early primary amputation in the setting of complete brachial plexus avulsion. It avoids the problems of myoglobinuria, hyperkalemia, and vascular thrombosis. The decision should be made initially. If early amputation is refused, later amputation should be considered within the first year to improve rehabilitation and functional outcome.[20] Unfortunately, patients and their families often refuse secondary amputation, despite a flail, anesthetic extremity.[7,8,18] This can lead to severe causalgia, pressure sores, and injury.[15,20] Furthermore, the longer the delay from injury to amputation to prosthetic fitting, the less likely the patient is to wear the prosthetic.[20]

MORTALITY

The STD-related mortality documented in the literature is 11%.[4] However, this may be underestimated, as patients may exsanguinate from uncontrolled subclavian vessel injuries, or die of associated injuries, without STD being definitively diagnosed.

CONCLUSIONS AND ALGORITHM

Scapulothoracic dissociation is a rare but devastating injury. Associated injuries are common. The timely diagnosis of vascular and neurologic injuries is critical. The rate of upper extremity loss is high, and many survivors are left with a flail upper extremity. Early amputation is indicated if there is a brachial plexus avulsion. A practical management algorithm, adapted from that proposed by Clements and Reisser,[18] is presented in Figure 2.

REFERENCES

1. Brucker PU, Gruen GS, Kaufmann RA: Scapulothoracic dissociation: evaluation and management. *Injury* 36:1147–1155, 2005.
2. Oreck SL, Burgess A, Levine AM: Traumatic lateral displacement of the scapula: a radiographic sign of neurovascular disruption. *J Bone Joint Surg [Am]* 66:758–763, 1984.
3. Zelle BA, Pape HC, Gerich TG, et al: Functional outcome following scapulothoracic dissociation. *J Bone Joint Surg [Am]* 86:2–8, 2004.
4. Damschen DD, Cogbill TH, Siegel MJ: Scapulothoracic dissociation caused by blunt trauma. *J Trauma* 42:537–540, 1997.
5. Rubenstein JD, Ebraheim NA, Kellam JF: Traumatic scapulothoracic dissociation. *Radiology* 157:297–298, 1985.
6. Kelbel JM, Jardon OM, Huurman WW: Scapulothoracic dissociation. A case report. *Clin Orthop* 209:210–214, 1986.
7. Lange RH, Noel SH: Traumatic lateral scapular displacement: an expanded spectrum of associated neurovascular injury. *J Orthop Trauma* 7:361–366, 1993.
8. Ebraheim NA, Pearlstein SR, Savolaine ER, et al: Scapulothoracic dissociation (closed avulsion of the scapula, subclavian artery and brachial plexus): a newly recognized variant, a new classification, and a review of the literature and treatment options. *J Orthop Trauma* 1:18–23, 1987.
9. Leffert RD: Clinical diagnosis, testing and electromyographic study in brachial plexus traction injuries. *Clin Orthop* 237:24–31, 1988.
10. Masmejean EH, Asfazadourian H, Alnot JY: Brachial plexus injuries in scapulothoracic dissociation. *J Hand Surg* 25B:336–340, 2000.
11. Kottmeier SA, Wilson SC, Born CT, et al: Surgical management of soft tissue lesions associated with pelvic ring injury. *Clin Orthop Relat Res* 329:46–53, 1996.
12. American College of Surgeons: *Advanced Trauma Life Support for Doctors.* Chicago, American College of Surgeons, 2004.
13. Biffl WL, Moore EE, Burch JM: Diagnosis and management of thoracic and abdominal vascular injuries. *Trauma* 4:105–115, 2002.
14. Katsamouris AN, Kafetzakis A, Kostas T, et al: The initial management of scapulothoracic dissociation: a challenging task for the vascular surgeon. *Eur J Endovasc Surg* 24:547–549, 2002.
15. Althausen PL, Lee MA, Finkemeier CG: Scapulothoracic dissociation: diagnosis and treatment. *Clin Orthop Relat Res* 416:237–244, 2003.
16. Levin PM, Rich NM, Hutton JE: Collateral circulation in arterial injuries. *Arch Surg* 102:392–398, 1971.
17. Sampson LN, Britton JC, Eldrup-Jorgensen J, et al: The neurovascular outcome of scapulothoracic dissociation. *J Vasc Surg* 17:1083–1089, 1993.
18. Clements RH, Reisser JR: Scapulothoracic dissociation: a devastating injury. *J Trauma* 40:146–149, 1996.
19. Goss TP: Scapular fractures and dislocations: diagnosis and treatment. *J Am Acad Orthop Surg* 3:22–33, 1995.
20. Rorabeck CH: The management of the flail upper extremity in brachial plexus injuries. *J Trauma* 198020:491–493, 1980.

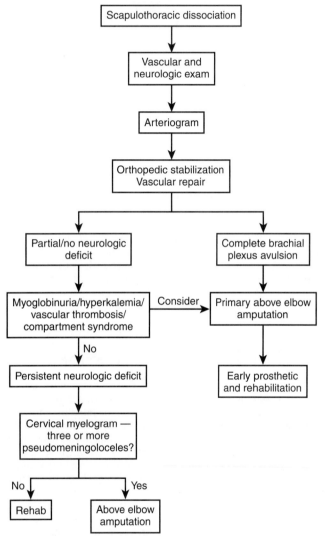

Figure 2 A management algorithm for scapulothoracic dissociation.

EXTREMITY REPLANTATION: INDICATIONS AND TIMING

Matthew Trovato, Boris Mordikovich, and Ramazi O. Datiashvili

The years since the first successful replantation of an arm in a 12-year-old boy by Malt and McKhann[1] in 1964 were marked by evident progress in the reconstructive surgery of limbs. That first revolutionary report was followed by the reports of revascularization of incompletely amputated fingers by Kleinert and colleagues in 1965[2] and the first successful thumb replantation by Komatsu and Tamai in 1968.[3,4] The evolution of microsurgical techniques and an accumulation of experience worldwide, along with the organization of specialized centers, has made replantation of completely or partially amputated extremities a generally accepted treatment of choice.

INCIDENCE

Traumatic amputation of the extremity is a devastating trauma, both physically and psychologically, leading to a lifelong disability of an individual.

According to the National Center for Health Statistics, the incidence of traumatic amputations is 38,500 per year. The exact number of replantations performed annually is unknown, although it seems to be on the decline, due to more conservative selection criteria and likely, as well, to improvements in safety protocols in the workplace.

Digital amputations comprise the group of the most common upper extremity amputations, followed by more proximal amputations.

The largest proportion of amputations occurs in the upper extremity distal to the elbow, accounting for 70%. Upper extremity amputations have the highest prevalence at ages 21–64 and account for 60% of the reported injuries. Fewer than 10% of all reported upper extremity amputations are sustained by persons less than 21 years of age.

Needless to say, the loss of an extremity or its parts has a great economic impact, accounting for billions of dollars lost every year.

CLASSIFICATION

All traumatic amputations of extremities are classified based on:

Type of amputation

Level of amputation

Mechanism and *character* of injury

This approach to classification serves both academic and clinical purposes and presents a foundation upon which the indications for replantation are predicated and functional outcomes assessed and compared.

Types of amputations are classified by anatomic criteria. The *complete* type is clearly defined by its term, that is, an amputation without any tissue connection between amputated and proximal parts of the extremity. An *incomplete,* or *partial* amputation is where most of vital anatomic structures are disrupted, and blood circulation in the amputated part of the extremity is absent; without replantation the amputated segment will neither survive nor be functional (Figure 1).

The *level* of traumatic amputation of the extremities is defined by the level of the skeletal rather than soft-tissue disruption. Based on these criteria, we divide all traumatic amputations (replantations) of the extremities into two main groups: *major* and *minor* amputations (replantations).

The necessity of differentiating the extremity amputations and replantations has been stressed by many authors for important clinical reasons, especially for indications and timing of surgery. This is due to the fact that major segments of the extremities contain large muscle mass, and anoxia of the muscles largely determines successful outcome of, and therefore indications for, replantation.

Minor segments are those amputated distal to the wrist or ankle level, and *major* segments are those amputated *at* and *proximal to* the level of the respective joints.

More precise classification of upper extremity amputations and replantations is based on the "zonal" principle, where the upper extremity is divided into six anatomic zones (Figure 2):

Zone I—distal to the insertion of the flexor digitorum superficialis (FDS) tendons

Zone II—at the level of the fibro-osseous canals of the flexor tendons, between anterior interosseous (AI) pulley and FDS tendon insertion

Zone III—the palm itself, between Zones II and IV

Zone IV—the level of carpal tunnel

Zone V—from the wrist to the musculotendinous junction

Zone VI—proximal to the musculotendinous junction

Based on the mechanism of trauma, we differentiate the following types of injury and various combinations of these in the same patient:

Guillotine: a very sharp wound with minimal skin and soft-tissue damage

Cutting: for instance, a guillotine with some zone of contusion

Crushing: the skin and soft-tissue injury zone is significant, often associated with comminuted fractures

Avulsion: dissociation in levels of amputation of bone and soft tissues, almost always requiring vessel grafts (Figure 3)

Patients with traumatic amputation of an extremity and associated significant injury to other organs, such as the head, chest or abdomen, usually represent a special challenge. These combined injuries are usually life-threatening and often preclude replantation.

INDICATIONS

We define replantation as a restorative surgery for the reestablishment of the anatomic integrity of major structures of an extremity in complete or partial amputation in order to regain the viability of the extremity and attain the acceptable functional outcome.

It appears from the review of the literature and our own experience that the indications for replantation have changed over the years.[5] Increasing experience has brought a clear understanding that, in evaluating the results of replantation, the only common denominator is functional outcome. We agree with Pederson that the indications for replantation should not be "based solely on potential viability but are predicated on the potential for long-term function."[6]

When considering replantation, one should take into account the status of the amputated part and the patient's general condition. In general, while any patient with complete or partial amputation can be considered as a candidate for replantation, an ideal candidate should have had not only a relatively benign local status, e.g., an

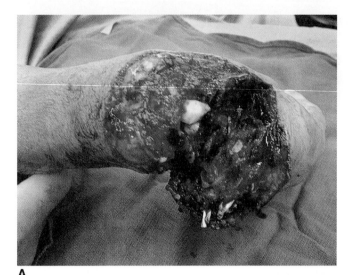

A

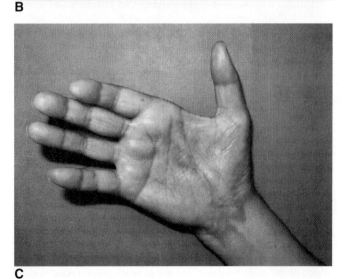

B

C

Figure I **(A)** Incomplete traumatic amputation of the hand at the level of carpus. **(B, C)** Functional result of replantation 1 year after replantation: **(B)** flexion; **(C)** extension.

amputation with minimal contamination and/or contusion but also, and maybe more importantly, a real determination for the continuous hard work later to attain and maintain the function of the replanted extremity or its part.

Assuming technical feasibility, the *indications* for replantation in traumatic amputations follow:

- The thumb provides 40%–50% of the hand's function. Usually replantation offers the best functional result as compared with other reconstructive options, including toe-to-hand transfer (Figure 4). Even with decreased motion and sensation, the replanted thumb provides such critical tasks of the hand as pinching and grasping. Therefore, all efforts should be made to replant the amputated thumb, unless the functional outcome is dismal.
- Multiple digital amputations always present a reconstructive puzzle. In general, all feasible replantations should be performed, aiming at the best possible functional result. If not all digits are replantable, the least damaged finger is usually replanted to the most functionally favorable position (heterotopic or transpositional).
- Amputations of a single digit in zone I—despite the recent conservative trend in replantations at the level distal to the flexor superficialis tendon insertion (e.g., Zone I), these usually have favorable functional outcome.
- All transmetacarpal amputations, or zone III, regardless of the thumb involvement—an absolute indication for replantation.
- Hand amputations at the level of the wrist and above, up to mid-humerus level—the risk of general complications increases with increasing anoxia time and muscle mass.
- Any amputation in a child where replantation is technically feasible.

General considerations, such as age, gender, occupation, and even a hobby, should be carefully considered every time replantation is contemplated. We recognize that any amputation in a selected group of patients with an extremely demanding occupation, such as musician or calligrapher, or with cosmetic demands in female patients, can be an indication for replantation.

Contraindications to replantation follow:

Relative

- Single digit in zone II (from AI pulley to FDS insertion)
- Prolonged warm ischemia
- Atherosclerotic vessels
- Mentally unstable patients

Absolute

- Multiple-level amputations
- Patients with severe combined trauma or systemic illness
- Significantly crushed or avulsed amputated part

TIMING

Anoxia of the amputated extremity is a critical factor for the success of replantation, especially of major segments. One should never underestimate the clinical implications of this fact, as it may lead to severe postoperative metabolic complications and potentially to death, especially in patients with prolonged warm anoxia of the replanted extremities. Most authors agree that after 6 hours of warm anoxia, the muscle undergoes irreversible changes. As the fingers devoid of muscles, their tolerance to ischemia, even warm anoxia, is relatively high. Adequate cooling of the amputated finger significantly prolongs its ischemic tolerance, thus increasing the time allowance between amputation and replantation.

The warm ischemic tolerance of amputated fingers is believed to be in the range of 812 hours, while cold anoxia can be tolerated for up to 40 hours and longer.

We performed successful replantation of three digits in one patient with a total period of warm anoxia of 28 hours. There have been reports of successful replantation of digits after 94 hours of cold anoxia.

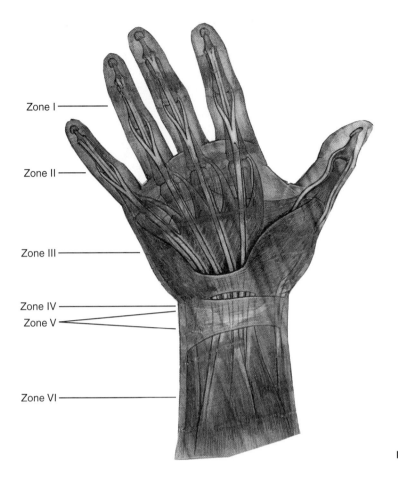

Zone I

Zone II

Zone III

Zone IV

Zone V

Zone VI

Figure 2 Flexor zones of the hand.

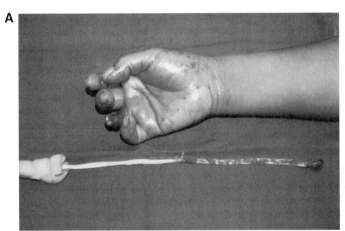

A

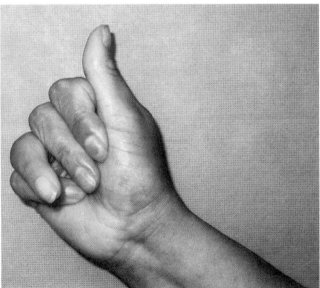

B

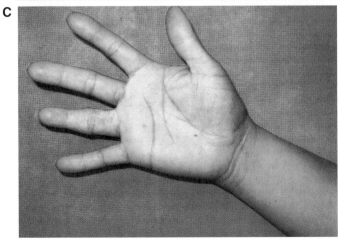

C

Figure 3 **(A)** Avulsion amputation of the ring finger. Note skeletal amputation at the level of distal interphalangeal joint, whereas soft tissues, vessels and nerves are avulsed from the base of the finger. **(B, C)** Functional result 6 months after replantation: **(B)** flexion; **(C)** extension.

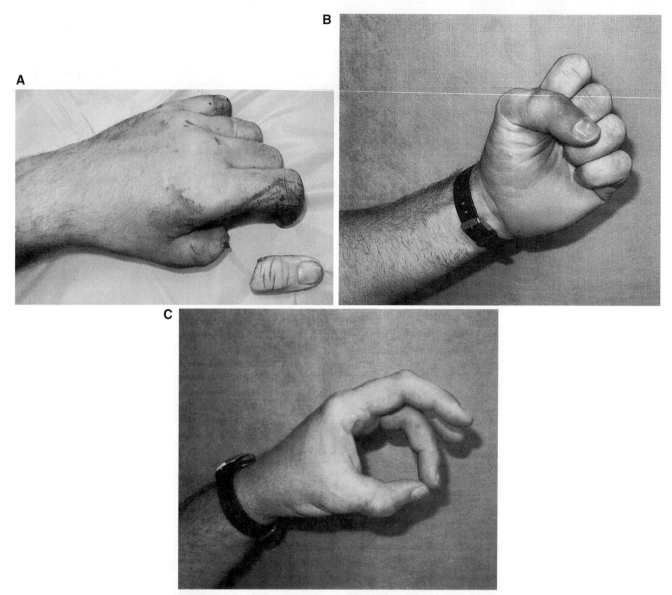

Figure 4 **(A)** Complete traumatic amputation of the thumb at the level of proximal phalanx. **(B, C)** Functional result 7 months after replantation: **(B)** flexion; **(C)** pinch.

CONCLUSION

Replantation is extremely challenging and, even when deemed successful, may involve long-term problems with infection, pain, difficult rehabilitation, and more reconstructive surgeries. The success of replantation is not defined as simply returning circulation. The goal of replantation is eventual restoration of function to an amputated part. Each type of amputation injury must warrant all treatment options to be considered. The location and extent of injury, the wishes of the patient, preservation of the amputated part, and the time elapsed since amputation all contribute to the final success.

REFERENCES

1. Malt RA, McKhann CF: Replantation of severed arms. *JAMA* 189:716, 1964.
2. Kleinert HE, Jablon M, Tsai T: An overview of replantation and results of 348 replants in 245 patients. *J Trauma* 20:390, 1980.
3. Komatsu S, Tamai S: Successful replantation of completely cut-off thumb. *Plast Reconstr Surg* 42:374, 1968.
4. Tamai S: Twenty years' experience of limb replantation: review of 293 upper extremity replants. *J Hand Surg* 7:549, 1982.
5. Datiashvili RO: *Limb Replantation.* Moscow, 1991.
6. Pederson WC: Replantation. *Plast Reconstr Surg* 107:3, 2001.

TECHNIQUES IN THE MANAGEMENT OF COMPLEX MUSCULOSKELETAL INJURY: ROLES OF MUSCLE, MUSCULOCUTANEOUS, AND FASCIOCUTANEOUS FLAPS

Matthew Trovato, Ramazi O. Datiashvili, and Mark S. Granick

Injuries involving skin and subcutaneous tissue loss require reconstructive solutions. In many cases, skin grafting alone may be sufficient. However, when skeletal fractures, tendons, viscera, or hardware is exposed, vascularized soft tissue coverage of the wound using muscle, musculocutaneous, and fasciocutaneous flaps is the preferred technique. The objective is to provide wound healing, optimal function, and the best possible aesthetic result.

DIAGNOSIS

Upon evaluation of a traumatic wound for reconstruction, many factors are considered. Assuming that the overall condition of the patient permits reconstructive surgery, the plastic surgeon must evaluate the nature and location of the wound. The wound bed needs to be clean and free of devitalized tissues. High-energy wounds and electrical burns produce extensive soft tissue damage, far beyond the zone of injury. All necrotic material needs to be aggressively debrided prior to embarking on reconstruction.

The concept of the "reconstructive ladder" recommends the use of the least invasive repair that will satisfactorily close a wound. The methods begin with secondary healing and progress through skin grafting to microvascular free-tissue transfer. This paradigm has been largely supplanted by the "reconstructive elevator" concept.[1] With this approach, the surgeon evaluates the wound and decides on the best option, not necessarily the least complicated one (Figure 1).

The ultimate goal for involvement of the plastic surgeon is to provide a reconstructive plan that gives special consideration to body symmetry and contouring and minimizes donor site defect and deformity.

ANATOMY

Split-thickness skin grafts (STSG) consist of the entire epidermis and a portion of the dermis, with an average thickness of 0.012–0.015 inches. STSGs require a vascularized wound bed, free of necrosis, with minimal bacterial burden. Healed grafts shrink considerably, bear abnormal pigmentation, and leave underlying tissues highly susceptible to trauma. Full-thickness grafts include the entire thickness of the skin, resist contraction, have potential for growth,

and have texture and pigment more similar to normal skin. However, they require an even better vascularized wound bed.

The most important anatomical aspect of muscle flaps is their vascularity. Because blood supply is usually the limiting factor in flap success, flaps are most often categorized by the vascular system on which they are based. McGregor proposed the concept of "random" and "axial" pattern flaps based on the importance of the presence or absence of a major vessel running along the axis of the flaps.[2] Random pattern flaps do not incorporate a dominant vascular supply, relying on the networks of small-diameter vessels to sustain the transferred tissue. They are limited in size and may require delay for successful transfer. Axial pattern flaps incorporate an anatomically recognized arteriovenous system running along the long axis of the tissue which permits successful transfer of vascularized flaps with high length-to-breadth ratios. They obtain their vascular supply from the musculocutaneous and fasciocutaneous systems, both of which rely on multiple "perforator" arteries. Knowledge of muscle vascular anatomy is helpful in predicting the viability of overlying skin territories based on such perforating vessels.

The now classic schema of Nahai and Mathes has divided muscles into groups according to their principal means of blood supply.[2] A type I muscle, such as the gastrocnemius or tensor fascia lata (TFL), is supplied by a single pedicle. A type II muscle, such as the trapezius or gracilis, has a dominant pedicle, with one or more minor pedicles. A type III, the serratus anterior (SA) or gluteus maximus (GM), for example, has dual dominant pedicles. A type IV, such as the tibialis anterior (TA) or sartorius, has segmental pedicles. The type V, such as the internal oblique muscle or latissimus dorsi (LD), has a dominant pedicle, with secondary segmental pedicles. Most muscles fall into the type II group. Types I, III, and V are the most reliable because complete muscle viability can be sustained by a single vessel. Sometimes the muscle territory of a minor pedicle is poorly captured by the dominant pedicle in a type II muscle. Owing to their segmental means of perfusion, type IV muscles would potentially only allow small flaps that have limited application.

Certain muscle flaps can be raised on a simple pedicle. Due to musculocutaneous vascular perforators, an island of skin can be carried with the muscle (myocutaneous/musculocutaneous flaps). When the perforator is traced through the muscle to the pedicle, thereby preserving the muscle, a cutaneous perforator flap results. Blood vessels also travel from major arteries and veins through intermuscular septae to the skin. When the skin and fascia are raised on septal perforators, a fasciocutaneous flap is created. Any flap with a dominant pedicle can become a free flap by division and subsequent reanastomosis of the vascular pedicle artery and vein into the recipient bed. Free flaps may be muscle only, musculocutaneous, fasciocutaneous, or osteomyocutaneous.

SURGICAL MANAGEMENT: PRIMARY FLAPS

Musculoskeletal trauma will be grouped into five soft tissue coverage regions: head and neck, upper extremity, chest and trunk, abdomen, and the lower extremity (Table 1).

Head and Neck

The pectoralis myocutaneous flap can be designed with a skin paddle centered over the lower portion of the muscle. It can be used to resurface the neck, cheek, oral cavity, palate, tonsillar area, and

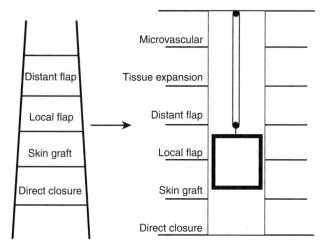

Figure 1 The "reconstructive elevator" evolved from the "reconstructive ladder" as the paradigm for approaching complex musculoskeletal reconstruction.

nasopharynx, tongue, floor of mouth, mandible, and cervical area. The flap has an upward arc of rotation of 180 degrees and may be raised as high as the orbits; however, in practicality, it is difficult to secure the closure without a significant downward pull on the muscle. The flap can be modified with an extended random skin component or with two separate skin paddles that can be divided. A rib may be harvested with the flap for bony reconstruction. Higher elevation of the flap can be performed with the division of the clavicle. The pectoralis was one of the early workhorse flaps, but it has largely been supplanted by free flaps.

The trapezius myocutaneous flap can be designed in several directions. The horizontal trapezius fasciocutaneous flap is an excellent choice for major coverage problems of the neck because of its proximity and favorable color match. As a transposition flap, it is more easily manipulated than either the pectoralis or latissimus myocutaneous flaps. A trapezius muscle or musculocutaneous flap provides unique coverage of the upper thoracic spine, and the donor site of the transposition of one or both muscles is inconsequential unless it is necessary to separate the trapezius muscle from the scapula.

Microvascular free-tissue transfer has gained a preeminent position as the reconstructive tool of choice in the head and neck for many of the complex defects facing the reconstructive surgeon. The technique offers a wide variety of potential donor tissues. Head and neck defects frequently require special considerations of form and function, such as preservation of a water-tight alimentary tract, a good match of skin color, texture, and hair-bearing qualities, composite tissue transfer requiring bone and soft tissue. These advantages permit a more critical appraisal of tissue requirements with the subsequent superior tissue match and greater latitude in tailoring the chosen flap to the defect.

Upper Extremity

Injuries involving the tactile surface of the hand with disruption of its sensory supply represent the most difficult reconstructive problems. The reconstructive goal must include restoration of sensibility if maximal function is to be achieved. A skin graft requires a suitable recipient bed such as muscle, fascia, paratenon, or periosteum. In the absence of structures capable of sustaining a graft, as in cases of exposed bone without periosteum or exposed tendon without paratendon, a well-vascularized flap is necessary to provide durable soft tissue coverage.

The groin flap (GF), reported by McGregor and Jackson in 1972, revolutionized the reconstruction of upper extremity wounds.[2] It is a versatile flap with a reliable vascular supply that is capable of covering large defects of the hand and wrist and provides an excellent tissue bed for subsequent procedures such as tendon reconstruction.

The radial forearm (RF) flap is designed to include the radial artery when raised as a pedicle fasciocutaneous flap. It can be raised proximally to cover defects involving the proximal forearm and elbow or distally (reversed) to cover defects involving the forearm, wrist, and hand. The main contraindication to its use is related to its dependence on the hand having adequate perfusion by the ulnar artery as demonstrated by a normal Allen's test.

Various situations preclude the use of local, regional, or distant pedicle flaps. Involvement of the hand and forearm in an injury may eliminate all potential local or regional flap options. Although distant pedicle flaps, such as the GF, are useful for coverage of large defects, defects resulting from circumferential injuries are extremely difficult to cover with such a flap. Occasionally, defects involving the volar and dorsal aspects of the hand or more proximal circumferential defects can be covered by a combined groin and epigastric flap. However, free flaps offer far greater versatility and availability of donor sites for coverage of extensive defects. Additionally, tailoring of the free flap to suit the reconstructive needs of the wound is more easily accomplished because of the diversity of available flaps. Limb elevation, early mobilization, and the ability to cover even extensive circumferential defects are additional advantages to the use of free-tissue transfer (Figure 2).

The most commonly used free flap in soft tissue coverage of the dorsum of the hand is the RF free flap. Thicker coverage for a palmar or forearm defect can be provided by a medial plantar, scapular, parascapular, or lateral arm flap. Coverage of an extensive circumferential defect can be provided by RA, SA, or LD flaps.

Chest Wall and Trunk

The principles of chest wall reconstruction follow: (1) adequate debridement and resection of all tumors, osteoradionecrotic tissue, infection, or crushed soft tissue or bone; (2) obliteration of intrathoracic dead space; (3) skeletal stabilization if more than four ribs or greater than 5 cm of chest wall are resected en bloc; (4) adequate soft

Table 1: Reconstructive Options for Soft Tissue Region

	Head and Neck	Upper Extremity	Chest and Trunk	Abdomen and Groin	Lower Extremity
Flap Selection	Pectoralis	Radial forearm	Pectoralis	Rectus abdominis	Gracilis
	Trapezius	Lateral arm	Rectus abdominis	Latissimus	Vastus lateralis
	Free	Island pedicle	Latissimus	Rectus femoris	Tensor fascia lata
		Groin flap	Free	Tensor fascia lata	Gastrocnemius
		Thoracoepigastric flap		Free	Soleus
		Free			Free

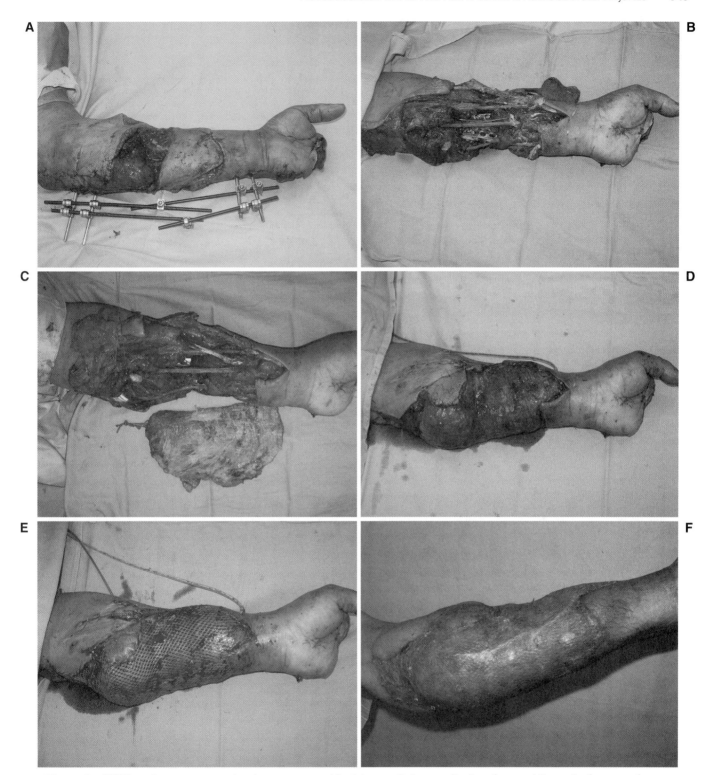

Figure 2 **(A)** View of an upper extremity after a severe crushing injury; preliminary application of external fixator for fractures of radius and ulna. **(B)** Appearance after serial debridements and internal fixation of fractures; note exposed vessels, nerves, and tendons. **(C)** Latissimus dorsi muscle free flap to be used for coverage of the wound. **(D)** Appearance after inset of flap. **(E)** Coverage of flap with meshed split-thickness skin graft. **(F)** Appearance at 3 months postoperative.

tissue coverage; and (5) aesthetic consideration. Muscle and musculocutaneous flaps are the tissues of choice for chest wall reconstruction. Local skin flaps, regional pedicle flaps, and thoracoabdominal tube flaps were used until the popularization of muscle and musculocutaneous flaps in the mid 1970s. The pectoralis major, LD, SA, and RA muscles are most frequently used.

In reconstruction of the posterior trunk, muscle coverage can be divided into thirds based on the location of the wound: the trapezius muscle for upper-third wounds, the latissimus dorsi for middle-third wounds, and the gluteus maximus for lower-third wounds. The scapular or parascapular fasciocutaneous flaps also may be used for small upper-third defects. Paraspinous muscle flaps may be advanced for relatively small vertical defects of the spine and paraspinal regions.[2]

Abdominal Wall and Groin

The objectives in abdominal wall reconstruction are to protect the intra-abdominal viscera, prevent herniation, and provide soft tissue coverage. It is critical that abdominal wounds not be closed under tension because of the risk of abdominal compartment syndrome. It is also best to avoid closure of acute injuries by elevation of local soft tissue flaps with the intention of later hernia repair. This approach merely opens new tissue planes that may spread infection and unnecessarily increases the operative time. Although exposed viscera can be directly skin-grafted, skin grafts lack the resilience to protect internal organs, promote adhesions, and provide unstable coverage. Moreover, the risk of early enteric fistulas is high. The treatment of choice in the acute setting is to use synthetic mesh for abdominal support.

The TFL is the ideal reconstructive option for abdominal wall defects. A dense, strong sheet of vascularized fascia and overlying skin can be transferred as a single unit in a single stage with minimal donor deficit. It is extremely useful in irradiated and contaminated fields. Protective sensation can be maintained by inclusion of the lateral femoral cutaneous nerve (T12), and voluntary control is provided by the descending branch of the superior gluteal nerve. Flaps wider than 8 cm usually require skin grafting of the donor site; narrower flaps can be closed primarily. There is tremendous disparity between the small size of the tensor muscle, originating from the greater trochanter, and the surrounding TFL flap. The flap is taken as distal as 10 cm from the knee so as to preserve lateral stability of the joint. The dominant pedicle—the lateral circumflex femoral vessels arising from the profunda femoris—pierces the medial aspect of the flap 8–10 cm below the anterosuperior iliac spine. The arc of rotation allows the tip of the flap to reach the ipsilateral lower chest wall and xiphoid, especially in a thin patient. The flap may be used to resurface the entire suprapubic region, lower abdominal quadrants, or ipsilateral abdomen.

Like the TFL, the rectus femoris (RFe) is an excellent flap choice for reconstruction of the ipsilateral or lower abdominal wall. For extensive defects, a larger cutaneous paddle may be incorporated with the adjacent fascia lata in the musculocutaneous flap. The tip of the flap reaches a point midway between the umbilicus and xiphoid. The flap is supplied by the lateral femoral circumflex vessels. It also can cover the entire suprapubic region and extend to the contralateral anterosuperior iliac spine. After transposition, the vastus lateralis and vastus medialis are approximated to prevent a functional deficit resulting in loss of the final 15 degrees of knee extension. Sacrifice of this muscle in ambulating patients causes minimal functional debility. The "mutton chop" or extended rectus femoris myocutaneous flap, described by Dibbell and colleagues, allows reconstruction of large full-thickness abdominal wall defects, including the epigastrium, without prosthetic material.[2]

Lower Extremity

Thigh

Lower extremity trauma wounds benefit from plastic surgical consultation and intervention because of large soft tissue defects and combined vascularized bone graft and soft tissue requirements. Common coverage methods for the thigh are: (1) flaps based on the thigh muscles, with or without skin grafts—in particular, the gracilis, sartorius, vastus lateralis, gluteal, and TFL flaps; (2) fasciocutaneous flaps such as the medial and posterior thigh; and

(3) more distant flaps such as the RA, based on the deep inferior epigastric pedicle.

Knee

The alternatives for soft tissue coverage of the knee are muscle flaps, fasciocutaneous flaps, and free-tissue transfer. The gastrocnemius muscle flap is readily available for knee coverage; however, it does not reliably cross the midline to the contralateral aspect of the knee or to the superior aspect of the knee. The distally based muscle flaps are unreliable. The saphenous fasciocutaneous flap, as described by Walton and Bunkis, is useful if available.[2] For extensive defects covering the entire surface of the knee, free-tissue transfer of a large fasciocutaneous flap or muscle flap is the most reliable.

Proximal Third

For soft tissue coverage of the proximal tibia, local muscle flap options include the medial and lateral gastrocnemius. The lateral is usually the shorter muscle and is compromised by the position of the peroneal nerve. Fasciocutaneous flaps include the saphenous flap, or a distally based medial or lateral fasciocutaneous flap. Free flaps are indicated when the local soft tissue injury contraindicates the use of local muscle or fasciocutaneous flaps or when the deficit is extensive (Figure 3).

Middle Third

Choices for coverage of the mid-tibial region include the soleus muscle, which is readily available and transposes well over this area. Fasciocutaneous flaps from the lateral or medial leg, based distally or proximally, are useful. Of course, free flaps are appropriate when local soft tissue coverage is not available or the defect is extensive.

Distal Third

The distal portion of the leg has poor skin elasticity, frequent severe edema, and osseous structures that lie in the subcutaneous tissue and are quite vulnerable. Such wounds also have a high rate of osteomyelitis, which often results in amputation. The distal third of the leg has significant tendinous structures that take skin grafts poorly. Finally, the foot and ankle require good flap durability because they are so frequently exposed to friction and shear by walking and footwear. Small ankle or distal tibial defects less than 4 cm[2] may be covered by the extensor brevis muscle flap, slightly larger defects by the supramalleolar flap, and somewhat larger defects by the dorsalis pedis fasciocutaneous flap. These flaps require a blood supply not compromised by the injury. The distally based muscle flaps are unreliable. Distally based fasciocutaneous flaps (based laterally or medially), including the sural neurocutaneous flap, may be safely used when perforators can be identified at the respective base of the flap.

Foot

Several small muscle flaps, such as the flexor hallucis, flexor digitorum brevis, and abductor hallucis brevis, are available for coverage of wounds of the foot but are rarely of practical use, given the frequent global injury to the foot and ankle area. The sural artery flap may be of benefit for small or moderate-sized wounds of the ankle and proximal foot as well as the heel area. Medial plantar flaps and dorsalis pedis flaps are examples of reliable local fasciocutaneous flaps. Island pedicle flaps of interdigital skin are useful for small defects. Most of these wounds, however, require some type of free-tissue transfer for satisfactory closure.

Indications for flap coverage of the foot are exposed bypass grafts, chronic osteomyelitis, open fractures, and tendon and nerve exposure. Indications for free-tissue transfer include large or circumferential defects exposing fractures, open joints, or the Achilles

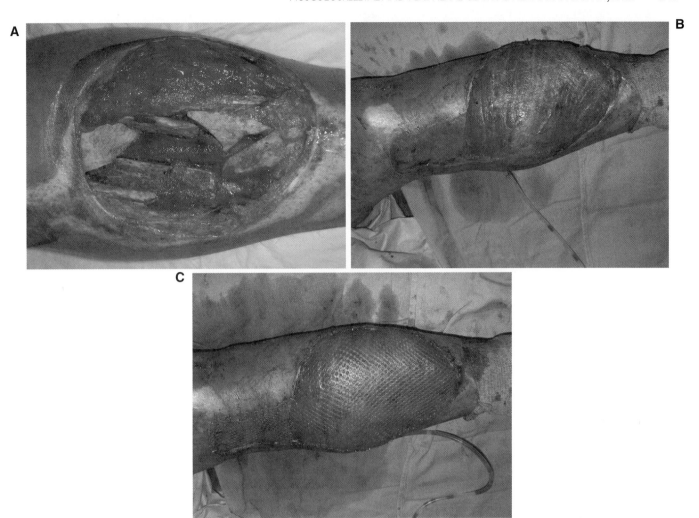

Figure 3 (A) View of a lower extremity after a severe crushing injury. Note fragments of fractured tibia and fibula exposed in the wound; preliminary appearance after debridement. **(B)** Appearance after inset of latissimus dorsi muscle free flap. **(C)** Coverage of flap with meshed split-thickness skin graft.

tendon; incisions or soft tissue trauma that compromise the lateral or medial fasciocutaneous areas; and compromise of the distal arterial flow, which may prevent the use of lateral supramalleolar or dorsalis pedis flaps.

COMPLICATIONS MANAGEMENT

In general, microvascular tissue transfers are a large metabolic challenge for patients; all of the complications common to major surgery are possible. Specifically, flap necrosis is the only serious complication. Loss of a few millimeters, or even 1–2 cm, at a margin of the flap usually has no deleterious effect. Loss of the major portion of the flap occurs in about 4% of the cases and is almost always explained by an obvious precipitating cause. A major flap loss may require the performance of a second flap, though most compromised free flaps can be salvaged. Venous congestion owing to insufficient venous outflow is the most common complication which, with early recognition, may

be rectified by flap revision or the use of medicinal leech therapy. Godina demonstrated the benefits of achieving healthy, soft tissue wound coverage over open lower extremity fracture within 5 days after injury.[2] This approach minimizes the risk of acute and chronic infection and maximizes flap survival.

REFERENCES

1. Bennet N, Choudary S: Why climb a ladder when you can take the elevator? *Plast Reconstr Surg* 105(6):2266, 2000.
2. Mathes SJ, Nahai F: *Reconstructive Surgery: Principles, Anatomy, and Technique.* New York, Churchill Livingstone, 1997.
3. Marsh JL: *Decision Making in Plastic Surgery.* St. Louis, MO, Mosby, 1993.
4. Strauch B, Vasconez LO, Hall-Findlay EJ: *Encyclopedia of Flaps.* Boston, Little, Brown, 1990.
5. Conley J, Patow C: *Flaps in Head and Neck Surgery.* New York, Thieme, 1989.
6. Aston SJ, Beasley RW, Thorne CHM: *Grabb and Smith's Plastic Surgery.* New York, Lippincott-Raven, 1997.

Special Issues and Situations in Trauma Management

Airway Management in the Trauma Patient: How to Intubate and Manage Neuromuscular Paralytic Agents

Ola Harrskog   and   Per-Olof Jarnberg

Injury is the leading cause of death in persons between the ages of 1 and 45 years in the United States and the third leading cause overall. Airway compromise is a common cause of death or severe morbidity in trauma victims. Management of the airway is a fundamental skill in trauma medicine. Obstruction of the airway has been reported in two-thirds of patients who die in the prehospital setting when death was not inevitable. Airway care is a cornerstone of resuscitation and is the first priority for patients both in the prehospital setting and in the emergency room (ER).

Over the last few decades, improvement in the management of trauma victims has helped to decrease mortality and morbidity. An organized systematic approach to treatment is particularly important and includes focus on the airway in the "primary survey," as outlined by the American College of Surgeons in their Advanced Trauma Life Support Course and Manual (ATLS). The ATLS emphasizes the importance of management during "the golden hour" after major trauma by stressing immediate attention to life-threatening conditions as soon as they are discovered. The development of new airway equipment as well as new techniques and algorithms for managing the difficult airway has significantly contributed to improved outcomes. The goal for emergency airway intervention is to make certain that the patient's ventilation is adequate to meet oxygen demands, thereby reducing the risk of ischemic injury to the brain, heart, and other organs as well as protecting the patient from the risks of aspiration and airway obstruction.

This review focuses on airway management of the adult traumatized patient. Specific aspects of pediatric airway management and the controversies of prehospital management of airways are not included.

AIRWAY CONSIDERATIONS IN THE TRAUMA PATIENT

Several circumstances make management of the trauma patient's airway unique. These include the frequent need for emergent intubation, the presence of complicating injuries, fixation in neck collars, and the risk of tracheopulmonary aspiration. There is no standard definition for a difficult airway, but it is often defined in the literature as an airway that requires more than two or three attempts for successful intubation. In the emergency department, difficult intubation conditions have been reported in at least 3% of cases. During the last few decades, we have seen a marked reduction in severe airway complications related to anesthesia for surgery in the operating room (OR). This, however, is not the case for airway management outside the OR. Management of the trauma airway is considered a task for the experienced physician.

Airway and breathing are the first two components of the ABCs (airway, breathing, and circulation) of initial evaluation of trauma patients. All seriously injured patients should receive supplemental oxygen, and many require intubation. Trauma victims are frequently either unconscious or combative as a result of head trauma or intoxication. The airway is vulnerable to mechanical obstruction from loss of muscle tone and airway reflexes. In addition, the airway is frequently contaminated with debris, blood, and secretions. Direct airway trauma and facial trauma may make the situation even more complex. The fully conscious, talking patient who maintains his/her own airway may not need airway intervention initially, but it must be kept in mind that the patient's status may change quickly. Continuous monitoring and frequent reevaluation of the airway is mandatory. Inhalation of oropharyngeal and gastric contents is always a risk in these individuals, but the actual frequency of aspiration is unknown. All trauma patients are presumed to have a full stomach and should be treated accordingly, using a technique to secure the airway that minimizes the risk of pulmonary aspiration.

The cervical spine is considered "unstable" in the trauma victim until proven otherwise. The evaluation of the spine and ruling out or diagnosing injury may be a prolonged procedure, especially in the patient with a decreased consciousness level. In the United States, 1.5%–3% of trauma victims suffer from spinal cord injury, and 55% of these injuries are located in the cervical spine. Complete spinal cord injury with loss of motor and sensory function distal to the lesion occurs in 43%–46% of cases. All trauma patients receive a rigid cervical collar to prevent secondary spine injury. However, this fixation usually makes an intubation more difficult and unpredictable.

There is an increased risk for awareness among trauma patients during airway manipulation and surgery. The incidence of awareness in the general adult patient population undergoing anesthesia is 0.1%–0.2%. Approximately 50% of these patients will have some psychological impact from their experience, and the most severe reaction is full-blown post-traumatic stress syndrome. The incidence of awareness is reported to be higher among trauma patients. These patients often have such hemodynamic instability that they tolerate only very light levels of anesthesia. It is, therefore, good practice to always consider giving amnesia-inducing drugs when neuromuscular blocking agents are used. To be paralyzed and unable to communicate is an extremely traumatic experience.

EVALUATION OF AIRWAY AND RESPIRATORY FUNCTION

Assessment of the airway as well as of the ventilatory and respiratory functions has the highest priority when a new trauma patient is encountered. Start by observing the patient's ventilatory pattern; and then auscultate the lungs. If time permits, obtain a chest film, and evaluate for the presence of hemothorax and/or pneumothorax. If there is an emergent need for airway intervention, the time for physical examination will be limited. The vital functions of a trauma patient can deteriorate rapidly, and constant monitoring with frequent reevaluation of the airway is crucial. The goal of the evaluation is to get as clear a picture as possible of the airway anatomy and the patient's ventilatory and respiratory functions, so that an appropriate plan for securing the airway can be established. The objective of the plan should always be a patient who is well oxygenated and ventilated and an airway that is protected after the intervention. The sophistication of the evaluation and the final plan are largely affected by the urgency of the needed intervention. It is not surprising that the incidence of difficult intubation is four to seven times higher in the emergency department than in the OR, largely due to challenging conditions in the trauma patient such as direct injury to the face and neck areas, fractures, hematomas, burns with edema, and secondary distortion of the airway.

In recent years, the development of classification systems to predict difficult intubations has reduced the incidence of airway complications in patients undergoing elective surgery. The Mallampati classification of the airway (see page 59) is commonly used and is based on assessment of tongue size in relation to other pharyngeal structures. The I to IV scoring scale predicts difficulty of intubation. The atlanto-occipital joint extension test measures the ability to extend the neck and, consequently, the ability to align pharyngeal and laryngeal axes to accommodate intubation. Measurements of the thyro-mental distance, sterno-mental distance, mandibulo-hyoid distance and inter-incisor distance are also helpful in evaluating the airway.

To provide high specificity and sensitivity for successful intubation and to assess the level of difficulty of an endotracheal intubation, several tests must be performed. These tests are usually correlated to the visualization of laryngeal structures and vocal cords. The gold standard for classifying the degree of exposure to the larynx entrance is the description by Cormac and Lehane (Figure 1). Grades III and IV are associated with difficult intubation. The dilemma is that all these tests are difficult to utilize in the trauma patient for many reasons, including an immobilized neck. Thus, alternative scoring systems such as the LEMON method have been proposed.

The LEMON method was developed by the U.S. National Emergency Airway Management Course and has a maximum score of 10 points, calculated by assigning 1 point for each criterion (Table 1). It has been demonstrated that an airway assessment score based on the LEMON criteria is helpful in predicting difficult intubation in the ER. The LEMON test is designed to be a quick and easy-to-use assessment tool. A poor laryngoscopic view is more common, for example, among patients with large incisors, a reduced inter-incisor distance, and a reduced thyroid-to-floor-of-mouth distance.

Another important component in an emergency evaluation is assessment of conditions that may compromise mask ventilation. Mask ventilation is usually used as an intermittent bridge until final airway control is established. Difficult mask ventilation is correlated to obesity, beards, facial trauma, upper airway obstruction, and absence of teeth and is reported in up to 5% of the normal adult population. It is a useful rule to make sure that mask ventilation is possible before paralytic drugs are administered to a patient. In the emergency situation, however, there are exceptions to this rule, and the pros and cons of using muscle blockade must be assessed in each case. Furthermore, the possibility of a "can't ventilate, can't intubate" situation is something that should be anticipated; therefore, it is essential that equipment and competence for creating a surgical airway are immediately available. In this circumstance, the team approach and communication among team members becomes crucial in establishing the final management plan, including rescue alternatives.

Planning an approach is the final step of the assessment (Figure 2). The team should then proceed with the airway management plan. When the patient can maintain adequate oxygenation and ventilation, and time permits, it may be beneficial to transport the patient to the OR which normally has better equipment and resources than the ER. In other situations, the right decision may be to immediately establish a surgical airway with the patient breathing spontaneously.

When reviewing the literature about airway management, it is remarkable how often the quality of professional competence/experience is mentioned. This is something that is very difficult to measure but is obviously critical to a successful outcome. All efforts should be made to have that experience accessible on short notice in a trauma organization that strives for excellence in airway management.

Original Cormack-Lehane system	I Full view of the glottis	II Partial view of the glottis or arytenoids	III Only epiglottis visible	IV Neither glottis nor epiglottis visible
View at laryngoscopy	E— —LI			
Modified system Cormack-Lehane	I As for original Cormack-Lehane above	IIa Partial view of the glottis	IIb Arytenoids or posterior part of the vocal cords only just visible	III As for original Cormack-Lehane above / IV As for original Cormack-Lehane above

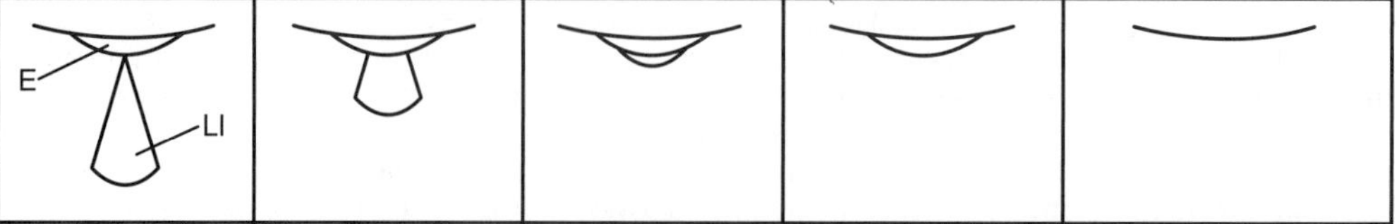

Figure 1 Cormack-Lehane original grading system compared with a modified Cormack-Lehane system (MCLS). *E*, Epiglottis; *LI*, laryngeal inlet. *(From Yentis SM, Lee DJH: Evaluation of an improved scoring system for the grading of direct laryngoscopy. Anesthesia 82:1197–1204, 1998.)*

Table 1: LEMON Criteria

Physical Sign	Less Difficult Airway	Indicators of Difficult Airway
Look at exterior	No face or neck pathology	Face or neck pathology, obesity, and so on
Evaluate the 3-3-2 rule	Mouth opening >3F Hyoid–chin distance >3F Thyroid cartilage–mouth floor distance >2F	Mouth opening <3F Hyoid–chin distance <3F Thyroid cartilage–mouth floor distance <2F
Mallampati	Classes I and II	Classes III and IV
Obstruction	None	Obstruction within or surrounding upper airway
Neck mobility	Normal extension and flexion	Limited range of motion

F, Finger-breadths.

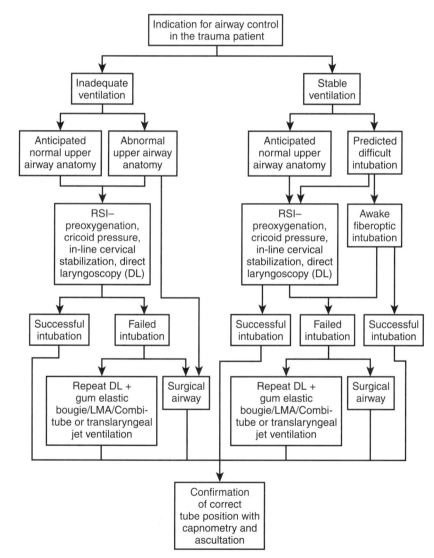

Figure 2 Airway management algorithm.

INDICATIONS FOR INTUBATION AND CONTROLLED VENTILATION

There are many indications for intubation and controlled ventilation in trauma patients. The decision to intubate is not always easy, but for the severely injured patient, the threshold should be low. The decision to intubate the trauma patient is usually made after a rapid assessment of injuries and identification of an indication to control the airway. Indications for intubation are:

Airway obstruction
Hypoventilation

Hypoxemia
Severe cognitive impairment
Cardiac arrest
Severe hemorrhagic shock
Smoke inhalation

Airway obstruction in the trauma patient can result from many conditions. Direct trauma to the larynx and trachea or maxillofacial injuries can result in severe obstruction, sometimes with delayed onset. These injuries are associated with high risk of aspiration. Cervical spine injury can be associated with hematoma formation and obstruction and also with direct paralysis of respiratory muscles. Patients with cognitive impairment, resulting from brain injury or intoxication, are prone to obstruction and secondary hypoxemia. Smoke inhalation and burns frequently result in edema formation and obstruction, which can have a delayed onset and require preventive intubation.

Hypoventilating patients need tracheal intubation. Patients with cervical spine fractures frequently hypoventilate, as do patients with cognitive impairment.

Persistent hypoxemia, despite supplemental oxygen, is also an indication for airway intervention. This condition can result from airway obstruction, hypoventilation, and lung injury, including aspiration and lung contusion. Low consciousness levels frequently result in hypoxemia that affects neurologic outcome. However, prevention of hypoxemia is associated with reduced mortality and morbidity in trauma victims.

The patient with severe cognitive impairment (Glasgow Coma Score <8) frequently has airway obstruction, is hypoventilating, and has hypoxemia. Usually, these patients have brain injury, and early intubation reduces mortality and morbidity. Other reasons for low consciousness levels include intoxication and smoke inhalation.

Trauma victims with cardiac arrest have a higher survival rate if early intubation is performed.

Patients with severe hemorrhagic shock should be intubated emergently to improve oxygenation. Immediate surgical intervention is almost inevitable.

Smoke inhalation is associated with burn injuries and inhalation of toxic products, such as carbon monoxide and cyanide. When cognitive impairment from inhalation is suspected, or airway obstruction from thermal injury is present, immediate intubation is necessary. If the patient is not intubated, close observation is required. Edema formation and airway obstruction can develop quickly, and many authors recommend routine intubation. Measurement of blood concentrations of carbon monoxide and cyanide is fundamental. Toxic carbon monoxide concentrations are indication for intubation and ventilation with 100% oxygen.

INDUCTION AGENTS AND MUSCLE RELAXANTS

A number of pharmacological agents are used to facilitate intubation of the trauma patient. Most patients will benefit from anesthesia prior to paralysis and intubation, with the exception of profoundly hypotensive and unconscious patients. Intubation of the brain-injured patient without the use of anesthesia can produce a severe increase in intracranial pressure and cause herniation.

Many anesthesia induction agents have qualities that limit their usefulness in the trauma setting. The ideal induction agent should have a quick onset, provide deep hypnosis, have a short duration, and render hemodynamic stability. Intracranial and intraocular pressures should be minimally affected, and a reduction of cerebral metabolic rate is ideal. If the potential for increased blood pressure and heart rate is a concern, pretreatment with an opioid usually diminishes this response.

Many of these properties are also desirable for muscle relaxants. For example, when intubation and mask ventilation are not accom-

plished, the duration of neuromuscular blocking agents should ideally be so short that spontaneous ventilation is reestablished before severe desaturation occurs.

Currently, we do not have agents that satisfy all of these criteria. However, the most commonly used induction agents and muscle relaxants are discussed below.

Sodium thiopental has been one of the most commonly used induction agents for many years. Maximum concentration at the receptor site occurs within a minute, and the patient is usually unconscious within 30–45 seconds. Rapid redistribution results in a short duration after a single dose. Barbiturates act at the GABA receptor site and depress the reticular activating system. The respiratory center is depressed, and the response to carbon dioxide is reduced. In the hypovolemic patient, sodium thiopental may cause a dangerous decrease in blood pressure due to depression of the medullary vasomotor center and reduced activity of the sympathetic nervous system, causing vasodilatation and decreased venous return. If thiopental is used, it must be dosed cautiously, using a lower dose in the circulatory-compromised patient. Thiopental causes cerebral vasoconstriction as well as decreased intracranial blood volume and intracranial pressure. Therefore, it is often an excellent choice in a patient with an isolated brain injury and stable circulation, when elevated intracranial pressure is a concern. Thiopental may induce acute intermittent porphyria in susceptible patients.

Propofol is a relatively new agent which can be used for sedation and induction and maintenance of anesthesia. It is an alkylphenol with high lipid solubility. It causes marked vasodilatation, making it less suitable for induction of trauma patients. If propofol is used, the induction dose must be drastically reduced. It is attractive for continuous sedation in the circulatory-stable patient because of its short half-life and its properties that reduce cerebral metabolism and blood flow. Propofol depresses pharyngeal and laryngeal reflexes and muscle tone more than other induction agents.

Etomidate is a carboxylated imidazole that produces unconsciousness within 30 seconds after intravenous (IV) administration. The duration is short, and etomidate has very favorable circulatory properties. Its direct cardiovascular effects are minimal, but it can cause hypotension by affecting sympathetic output. Etomidate also reduces cerebral blood flow, cerebral oxygen consumption, and intracranial pressure. These traits make it very attractive for the unstable trauma patient with head injuries; and it is, therefore, considered by many to be the induction agent of choice for trauma patients. Although the circulatory properties are beneficial, careful dose reduction should be considered in the hypovolemic patient, as even etomidate may drop the cardiac output. There is also some concern that it causes adrenocortical suppression for a few hours after administration, and it may theoretically cause instability in the catecholamine-depleted patient and potentially modify the humoral stress response.

Ketamine is another choice for induction of anesthesia. It is derived from phenylcyclidine and induces a condition called dissociative anesthesia. Onset occurs within a minute after IV administration. Ketamine stimulates the cardiovascular system via endogenous release of catecholamines, which often results in tachycardia and hypertension. However, it has direct negative inotropic properties and can produce further hypotension in patients with long-standing shock and depleted endogenous catecholamine stores. This drug should probably be avoided in victims with head injuries because of its properties to increase cerebral metabolism, blood flow, and intracranial pressure. It is often the preferred induction agent in hypotensive, hypovolemic patients; and with ketamine, ventilation is preserved and airway reflexes are more or less intact. Ketamine is also a potent analgesic. All these qualities make ketamine a useful drug under field conditions. However, it is well known for its potential to produce unpleasant hallucinations and psychomimetic reactions during emergence. This risk can be reduced by pretreatment with benzodiazepines.

Muscle relaxants are used to create conditions that facilitate the intubation procedure. The larynx, for example, must be visualized as optimally as possible, and muscle tone suppression is integral to creating this condition. To help prevent hypoxemia and hypercapnia, a short onset time for muscle paralysis is important. Today, succinylcholine and rocuronium are the two drugs available that fulfill this criterion. Succinylcholine has some undesirable side effects, and substantial research has been underway to find an alternative drug. So far, however, no superior replacement has been introduced on the market, although promising drugs are under investigation. The current alternative to succinylcholine is rocuronium, but it does not match the short onset and short duration of succinylcholine.

Techniques that shorten the onset of alternative drugs have been studied. One such technique is known as "priming" and results when approximately one-tenth of the intubating dose is given 60 seconds prior to the remainder of the full dose. This partially preoccupies the receptor sites, thereby shortening the time required to achieve adequate intubation conditions. Another method, called "timing," requires that the administration of the muscle relaxant be carefully timed before the induction agent so that the patient does not experience the unpleasant sensation of being conscious while paralyzed. Each of these techniques is unreliable, and all alternatives to succinylcholine render a prolonged duration of muscle relaxation that can be detrimental in the "can't intubate, can't ventilate" situation.

Succinylcholine is a depolarizing muscle relaxant. Its onset is 30–45 seconds, and its offset is about 6–12 minutes. Shortly after administration of succinylcholine, muscle fasciculations occur. Observation of these fasciculations can help to predict when the patient is sufficiently paralyzed to commence the intubation process.

A brief increase in intracranial and intraocular pressure will follow administration of succinylcholine. The increase in intracranial pressure is small and not considered important enough to avoid succinylcholine in the brain-injured patient. Furthermore, it has never been proven that this increase in intracranial and intraocular pressure is of clinical importance. After all, laryngoscopy alone increases intracranial and intraocular pressure.

An increase in intragastric pressure after succinylcholine injection has also been documented. However, this does not likely increase the risk for aspiration of stomach contents because succinylcholine increases the tone of the lower esophageal sphincter.

A transient elevation of plasma potassium concentration of up to 1 mmol/l is seen in conjunction with administration of succinylcholine. This can be more pronounced in victims of burns, spinal cord trauma, and severe soft tissue injuries and can lead to cardiac dysrhythmias or asystole. The resulting massive release of potassium is an effect of extrajunctional receptor proliferation. This is not a relevant problem in the acute situation but must be considered later during hospital treatment of these patients.

Finally, succinylcholine also triggers malignant hyperthermia and can produce severe anaphylactic reactions.

Rocuronium is a nondepolarizing muscle relaxant. It does not trigger malignant hyperthermia or other side effects associated with succinylcholine. However, allergic reactions are still a possibility. To obtain good intubation conditions, rocuronium usually requires up to 60 seconds, and its duration after an intubation dose is approximately 45 minutes. These time factors are the primary reasons that succinylcholine is still considered the muscle relaxant of choice.

INTUBATION TECHNIQUES

During all advanced airway management procedures, the patient should be monitored adequately. The standard is electrocardiogram (ECG), pulse oximetry, end tidal CO_2 monitoring, and an automated blood pressure cuff. The choice of intubation technique depends on the severity of respiratory compromise, the expected difficulty of intubation, and the skills of the practitioner.

In most cases when the airway must be controlled immediately, the best technique is the modified rapid sequence approach, using preoxygenation and cricothyroid pressure to block esophageal passage of gastric contents. This technique has an acceptable success rate of 95%–97%, but is inherently risky.

For this approach, drugs are injected at predetermined doses. Taking into consideration that the decisions regarding medications must often be made within seconds of the patient's arrival, it is fundamental to have a thorough knowledge about drug actions in order to tailor the choice and dose and to avoid causing harm and circulatory instability (Table 2).

During the intubation process, the potential risk of spinal cord injury is always a concern if cervical fractures are present. In the past, because of this risk, blind nasal intubation of the conscious patient was frequently advocated. Today, we know more about spinal movements and different intubation techniques; and the nasal route is used mainly if the jaw is locked and the patient's condition is relatively stable. As long as manual in-line neck stabilization is applied and axial traction is avoided to prevent distraction, rapid sequence intubation, followed by direct laryngoscopy and oral intubation, appears to be safe, even if it produces more motion in the spine compared with the use of the nasal route. Ideally, when a spine injury is present, and spine motion is the primary concern, intubation should be executed using a fiberoptic bronchoscope. This is rarely possible in an emergency situation. Preintubation maneuvers, such as jaw trust, insertion of Combitubes, and positioning of laryngeal masks, cause as much motion as some of the intubation techniques. There are no data that suggest better outcome with any particular technique, and the most immediate threat to patients with spinal cord injury is hypoxemia from hypoventilation or aspiration of gastric contents. The most severe injury to the spinal cord probably occurs at the time of the trauma; and if rapid sequence intubation is performed with care and in-line stabilization, the risk for secondary neurological injury is minimal. The most common complication of rapid sequence intubation is probably hypotension.

The rapid sequence intubation procedure can be divided into a predetermined sequence of four phases: preoxygenation, drug administration, endotracheal tube positioning, and confirmation of endotracheal tube position. Usually, the patient will present with the neck immobilized in neutral position by a cervical collar. This position should be retained throughout the intubation sequence. The patient is preoxygenated with a high flow of 100% oxygen using a non-rebreathing system before the induction agent is injected. The mask should have a tight seal. The preoxygenation process will significantly increase the time lapse until desaturation begins after apnea.

Table 2: Dosages of Induction and Muscle Relaxant Drugs

Drug	Dose	Onset Time	Duration
Etomidate	0.15–0.3 mg/kg	30–60 sec	3–5 min
Ketamine	2 mg/kg	1–2 min	5–15 min
Propofol	0.5–2 mg/kg	30–60 sec	3–10 min
Thiopental	1–3 mg/kg	30–60 sec	5–10 min
Succinylcholine	1.5 mg/kg	30–60 sec	5–10 min
Rocuronium	1 mg/kg	45–60 sec	45–60 min

The induction agent is injected as a bolus and is immediately followed by the muscle relaxant. When the patient starts to lose consciousness, one assistant will hold the patient's neck in in-line stabilization, and a second assistant will apply cricoid pressure using Sellick's maneuver to compress the esophagus between the cricoid cartilage and C6, prohibiting the regurgitation of stomach contents during airway manipulation. It is permissible to open the cervical collar to facilitate intubation as long as strict attention is maintained to prevent cervical movements.

When the patient is paralyzed, intubation should proceed in a gentle and nontraumatic fashion. After the cuff is insufflated, the correct position of the tube should be verified by direct visual inspection during the intubation process, end tidal CO_2 monitoring, and auscultation in both flanks and over the stomach. Indirect signs, such as chest movements and condensation in the tube, are helpful when verifying tube positioning. If the breath sounds are not bilateral and equal, an explanation must be determined. The most common explanations for this situation include mainstem intubation, pneumothorax, hemothorax, and obstruction of the airway. Since the right mainstem bronchus leaves the trachea at a steeper angle than the left, foreign bodies and endotracheal tubes that have been placed too deeply frequently end up on the right side. Absence of breath sounds and a gurgling sound over the epigastrium indicate esophageal intubation. After correct placement, the tube should be taped securely. Note the distance from the upper sixth molar. When the tube is correctly positioned, the average distance from the tip of the endotracheal tube is 21 cm in an adult female and 23 cm in an adult male.

The in-line stabilization of the patient's head, which is required, is not optimal for visualization of the larynx during direct laryngoscopy; and it is not uncommon that suboptimal conditions are encountered during the intubation procedure and the larynx is not fully exposed. The gum elastic bougie is an excellent tool that allows tracheal intubation in most cases when the laryngeal inlet is not optimally exposed. After the bougie is inserted into the trachea, vibrations can usually be felt when its tip is sliding against tracheal cartilages. Then, the endotracheal tube is advanced over the bougie and into the trachea. Frequently, a twisting motion must be applied if the tip of the tube is trapped against the anterior larynx wall.

If intubation of the patient fails, a surgical airway usually needs to be created. Multiple intubation attempts increase the risk for edema, bleeding, and diminished visualization of the glottic opening. The incidence of hypoxemia, regurgitation of gastric contents, and cardiovascular complications are significantly increased after more than two attempts. An alternative technique should be selected before entering into the vicious cycle of multiple attempts and complications. Under some circumstances, rescue devices, such as the laryngeal mask or an esophagotracheal airway (Combitube), can be used to bridge the gap until definite control of the airway is established. Correct placement of these devices usually requires release of the cricoid pressure; and although the risk of aspiration is increased, ventilation is generally much more effective than with a face mask.

Several methods are used to create a surgical airway. Cricothyroidotomy is performed by penetrating the cricothyroid membrane to create an airway and can be executed as an open or percutaneous procedure. Tracheostomy may be selected as the primary technique under some conditions, especially if the larynx is fractured. Translaryngeal jet-ventilation can be life saving and is particularly useful if the knowledge to establish other surgical airways is not immediately present. This method is executed by inserting a catheter percutaneously into the trachea and insufflating it with oxygen. There are several potential complications, and the risk for barotraumas must be kept in mind. Once the airway is secured, it is important to keep the patient pain free and adequately sedated, especially if the patient has received long-term muscle relaxants.

SUMMARY

Although we have many choices of techniques and equipment to manage the airway today, the gold standard is still rapid sequence intubation, with creation of a surgical airway as a backup technique. The critical component of teamwork underlies the entire process. In fact, the whole trauma team should remain focused on their interdependence in order to create the most effective outcome for the patient, and this mutual cooperation must not be forgotten. A better understanding of the effects of induction agents and muscle relaxants as well as knowledge about alternative airway management techniques allow the team to work more effectively and improve patient care.

SUGGESTED READINGS

Arne J, et al: Preoperative assessment for difficult intubation in general and ENT surgery: predictive value of a clinical multivariate risk index. *Br J Anaesth* 80(2):140–146, 1998.

Barash PG, Cullen BF, Stoelting RK: *Clinical Anesthesia*, 4th ed. Philadelphia, Lippincott, Williams and Wilkins, 2001.

Bell RM, Krantz BE, Weigelt JA: ATLS: a foundation for trauma training. *Ann Emerg Med* 34(2):233–237, 1999.

Caplan RA, et al: Adverse respiratory events in anesthesia: a closed claims analysis. *Anesthesiology* 72(5):828–833, 1990.

Copass MK, et al: Prehospital cardiopulmonary resuscitation of the critically injured patient. *Am J Surg* 148(1):20–26, 1984.

Cormack RS, Lehane J: Difficult tracheal intubation in obstetrics. *Anaesthesia* 39(11):1105–1111, 1984.

Cormack RS, et al: Laryngoscopy grades and percentage glottic opening. *Anaesthesia* 55(2):184, 2000.

Crosby ET, et al: The unanticipated difficult airway with recommendations for management. *Can J Anaesth* 45(8):757–776, 1998.

Eastern Association for the Surgery of Trauma (EAST): *Guidelines for Emergency Tracheal Intubation Immediately Following Traumatic Injury*. Allentown, PA, Eastern Association for the Surgery of Trauma, 2002.

Foley LJ, Ochroch EA: Bridges to establish an emergency airway and alternate intubating techniques. *Crit Care Clin* 16(3):429–444, vi, 2000.

Ghoneim MM: Awareness during anesthesia. *Anesthesiology* 92(2):597–602, 2000.

Hussain LM, Redmond AD: Are pre-hospital deaths from accidental injury preventable? *BMJ* 308(6936):1077–1080, 1994.

Ivy ME, Cohn SM: Addressing the myths of cervical spine injury management. *Am J Emerg Med* 15(6):591–595, 1994.

Langeron O, et al: Prediction of difficult mask ventilation. *Anesthesiology* 92(5):1229–1236, 2000.

Mallampati SR, et al: A clinical sign to predict difficult tracheal intubation: a prospective study. *Can Anaesth Soc J* 32(4):429–434, 1985.

Mort TC: Emergency tracheal intubation: complications associated with repeated laryngoscopic attempts. *Anesth Analg* 99(2):607–613, 2004.

Morton T, Brady S, Clancy M: Difficult airway equipment in English emergency departments. *Anaesthesia* 55(5):485–488, 2000.

O'Callaghan-Enrigh S, Finucane BT: Anesthetizing the airway. *Anesthesiol Clin North Am* 13(2):325–336, 1995.

Osterman JE, et al: Awareness under anesthesia and the development of post-traumatic stress disorder. *Gen Hosp Psychiatry* 23(4):198–204, 2001.

Peterson GN, et al: Management of the difficult airway: a closed claims analysis. *Anesthesiology* 103(1):33–39, 2005.

Practice guidelines for management of the difficult airway. A report by the American Society of Anesthesiologists Task Force on Management of the Difficult Airway. *Anesthesiology* 78(3):597–602, 1993.

Practice guidelines for management of the difficult airway: an updated report by the American Society of Anesthesiologists Task Force on Management of the Difficult Airway. *Anesthesiology* 98(5):1269–1277, 2003.

Reed MJ, Dunn MJ, McKeown DW: Can an airway assessment score predict difficulty at intubation in the emergency department? *Emerg Med J* 22(2):99–102, 2005.

Rose DK, Cohen MM: The airway: problems and predictions in 18,500 patients. *Can J Anaesth* 41(5 Pt 1):372–383, 1994.

Sakles JC, et al: Airway management in the emergency department: a one-year study of 610 tracheal intubations. *Ann Emerg Med* 31(3):325–332, 1998.

Sebel PS, et al: The incidence of awareness during anesthesia: a multicenter United States study. *Anesth Analg* 99(3):833–839, 2004.

Sekhon LH, Fehlings MG: Epidemiology, demographics, and pathophysiology of acute spinal cord injury. *Spine* 26(24 Suppl):S2–S12, 2001.

Tayal VS, et al: Rapid-sequence intubation at an emergency medicine residency: success rate and adverse events during a two-year period. *Acad Emerg Med* 6(1):31–37, 1999.

Trunkey DD: Trauma: accidental and intentional injuries account for more years of life lost in the U.S. than cancer and heart disease. Among the

prescribed remedies are improved preventive efforts, speedier surgery and further research. *Sci Am* 249(2):28–35, 1983.

Walls RM: Management of the difficult airway in the trauma patient. *Emerg Med Clin North Am* 16(1):45–61, 1998.

Winchell RJ, Hoyt DB: Endotracheal intubation in the field improves survival in patients with severe head injury. Trauma Research and Education Foundation of San Diego. *Arch Surg* 132(6):592–597, 1997.

PEDIATRIC TRAUMA

David W. Tuggle   and   L. R. Tres Scherer

Pediatric trauma is the number one killer of children. It is also the number one cause of permanent disability in this population. It has often been said that children are not merely small adults, and this is never more accurate than in pediatric trauma. Although the principles of trauma care are the same for children as for adults, the differences in care required to optimally treat the injured child do require special knowledge, careful management, and attention to the unique physiology and psychology of the growing child or adolescent.

INCIDENCE OF PEDIATRIC TRAUMA

While medical science has made vast strides in the surgical care of the neonate and child, injury and homicide remain the leading causes of death in patients under 19 years of age. When combined, they account for more than 50% of all deaths in this age group. For children ages 1–4, motor vehicle injuries are the leading cause of death. Nearly half of children 4 and younger who died in motor vehicle crashes were riding unrestrained. Drowning is the second leading cause of injury-related death for children ages 1–4. In 1999, children under 5 accounted for more than half of all poison exposures. Children under 5 are among those most at risk for injuries from residential fires. Head trauma is the leading cause of death and disability among abused infants and children. For children ages 5–14, motor vehicle injuries are the leading cause of death. Drowning is the second leading cause of injury-related death among children 5–14. For children ages 10–14, suicide is the third leading cause of death. Between 1980 and 1997, the suicide rate for children 10–14 years old increased 109%. Nearly one-third of bicyclists killed in traffic crashes are children ages 5–14. An estimated 140,000 children are treated each year in emergency departments for traumatic brain injuries sustained while bicycling. Children 15 and younger accounted for 11% of pedestrian fatalities and 30% of nonfatal pedestrian injuries in 1998. Children are at increased risk for dog bites; 2.5% of children are bitten each year compared with 1.6% of adults. Nearly 30% of rapes occur before age 12. Despite these gloomy facts, there has been a 45.3% reduction in unintentional injury mortality rates in children in the United States between 1979 and 1996.

MECHANISMS OF PEDIATRIC TRAUMA

The mechanism of injury and mortality in children has remained remarkably consistent. In children over 1 year and under 14 years, motor vehicle–related mortality remains the greatest killer of children, at 46.5% of all causes (2002).[1] Drowning is the second cause,

followed by burns. A detailed view of mortality statistics reveals the home as an area of continuing concern. Other areas of concern include falls and bicycle-related injuries; a growing area of death and disability now includes all-terrain vehicle (ATV) crashes.[2]

Childhood injuries most commonly occur as energy is transferred abruptly either by rapid acceleration or deceleration, or a combination of both. The body of a child is very elastic, and energy can be transferred in a way that creates internal injuries without significant external signs. Due to the closer proximity of vital organs, children can have multiple injuries from a single exchange of energy, more so than older patients. Penetrating trauma is a much less common form of injury in small children, ranging from 1% to 10% in pediatric trauma centers. No matter the type of injury, the health care professional evaluating the injured child should keep in mind these significant differences during evaluation and management.

INITIAL ASSESSMENT, STABILIZATION, AND MANAGEMENT OF INJURED CHILD

Airway Management

Most children do not have pre-existing pulmonary disease; therefore, an oxygen saturation of greater than 90% on room air is often proof of adequate pulmonary function. If oxygenation is difficult, then a lung injury, pneumothorax, or aspiration should be considered. Hypoventilation is common in the presence of a head injury or shock. If any of these conditions exist, intubation is appropriate. Respiratory compromise requiring intubation commonly indicates a very severe injury. While no criteria have been validated to determine what constitutes a "major resuscitation" in children, intubation and airway compromise have been shown to suggest a population that has a higher incidence of mortality compared with injured children who do not have airway issues.[3] As with all patients, care should be taken to avoid cervical spine motion during intubation. It should be noted that nasotracheal intubation is generally not used in small children in the emergency setting.

Intubation also facilitates evaluation and resuscitation in many circumstances. The combative child should be evaluated for hypoxia in the acute setting, although an alert, uncooperative child may also indicate the presence of minimal injuries. The use of the Broselow Pediatric Resuscitation Measuring Tape has become the standard for determining the height, weight, and appropriate size for resuscitative equipment in a child. The Broselow cart has been found to be more useful than older "standard" carts for children. In addition, this device has been useful in determining drug doses and drip concentrations during the entire hospitalization.

The need for emergency airway access for acute pediatric airway obstruction is a very uncommon event. If needed, a 14- or 16-gauge angiocatheter may be placed through the cricothyroid membrane, or even the tracheal wall. Care should be taken to avoid penetrating the posterior tracheal membrane. Oxygen can then be administered through the catheter, allowing time for attempts at intubation. This technique, although rarely required, may be followed by tracheotomy or cricothyroidotomy. It should be noted that a cricothyroidotomy in a child may lead to subglottic stenosis and should be avoided.

Postintubation management includes gastric decompression and performing a chest x-ray for pneumothorax and endotracheal tube positioning. Gastric decompression with a nasogastric or orogastric tube should be employed in every case, since gastric distention will impair diaphragmatic excursion, with resulting respiratory compromise in the small child. If a pneumothorax is present, needle decompression can be employed, but this should be followed by immediate tube thoracostomy.

Vascular Access

The ideal initial sites for vascular access in children are the peripheral veins in the upper extremities, especially the antecubital fossa. If access cannot be achieved in these vessels, central venous access may be employed (Figure 1). A percutaneous femoral venous catheter is the next best choice and the most commonly used route for emergency venous access in the child. This should be done without attempting a cut-down, preferably using the Seldinger technique. Surgeons familiar with subclavian catheterization in the child may utilize this route as the next choice.[4] For surgeons comfortable with this technique in children, complications are rare. Intraosseous access is acceptable in injured children. Contraindications include proximal fractures and sites of infection nearby. The anteromedial surface of the proximal tibia is used, 2–4 cm distal to the tibial tuberosity. For insertion in the proximal tibia, the needle is directed inferiorly at a 45-degree angle from the perpendicular. If the insertion site is the distal tibia, the needle should be angled 45 degrees superiorly. In both instances, the

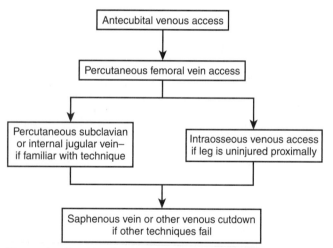

Figure 1 Algorithm for venous access in children.

goal is to angle away from the region of the growth plate and/or joint. There are specialized needles readily available to use with this technique, but if these are not available, a spinal needle with a trochar may be employed. Multiple entries into the medullary cavity should be avoided, as the leakage that occurs with multiple attempts may cause a compartment syndrome. For surgeons not familiar with peripheral, central, or intraosseous access in children, a cut-down of the saphenous vein may be employed,[5] although intravenous (IV) access by cut-down is no easier or faster than any of the abovementioned methods.

Circulatory Management

Age-specific hypotension is an indication for designating the necessity for major resuscitation in an injured child. In an analysis of the National Pediatric Trauma Registry, 38% of recorded deaths occurred in children whose systolic blood pressure was less than 90 mm Hg. This group represented 2.4% of the study population. To determine if a child has "age-specific hypotension" requires knowledge of normal blood pressures in children.[6] New national guidelines for the ranges of normal childhood blood pressures based on age were published in 2004 (Table 1). A child with an injury that produces significant blood loss may present with a normal blood pressure. The otherwise healthy child can readily compensate for blood loss by mounting a significant tachycardia coupled with peripheral vasoconstriction. Therefore, a normal blood pressure in a child does not mean that circulating blood volume is at normal levels. A more accurate determination includes a blood pressure evaluation along with monitoring heart rate and assessing peripheral perfusion. Clinical signs of poor perfusion in conjunction with altered mentation are classic findings in pediatric hypovolemic shock. If these are present, then an immediate bolus of 20 cc/kg of isotonic crystalloid is in order. If a second bolus of this amount is needed, and there is little improvement, blood should be started immediately (Figure 2). Caution must be taken, as over-resuscitation may be as problematic as under-resuscitation, especially in the presence of a head injury. Enthusiastic administration of crystalloid solutions may exacerbate cerebral edema in certain circumstances. Overtreatment with crystalloid infusions may result in poor clot formation, worsening the compromised hemorrhagic state, and may have no impact on survival. Supranormal trauma resuscitation increases the likelihood of the abdominal compartment syndrome in adult trauma victims, and there are reports of the same problem in children.[7] Typically, a bolus of 20 cc/kg of isotonic crystalloid in the presence of hypotension is the first treatment. If there is evidence of continuing instability, a second bolus of this amount may be given. If after two boluses of crystalloid the child does not have stable vital signs, blood should be started immediately. Type-specific packed red blood cells should be given, or O negative blood if necessary, in certain circumstances. Fresh frozen plasma and platelets should be considered early in the resuscitation period if large amounts of blood are needed for resuscitation. If there is a decreased level of consciousness without signs

Table 1: Normal Vital Signs and Weights for Various Age Groups in Pediatric Population

Age	Respiratory Rate	Pulse	Systolic Blood Pressure	Weight (kg)	Weight (lb)
Newborn	30–50	120–160	50–70	2–4	4–7
1–12 months	20–30	80–140	70–100	4–10	10–22
1–3 years	20–30	80–130	80–110	10–15	22–33
3–5 years	20–30	80–120	80–110	15–20	33–44
6–13 years	20–30	70–110	80–120	20–45	44–99
14 years and up	12–20	55–90	90–120	45 and up	99 and up

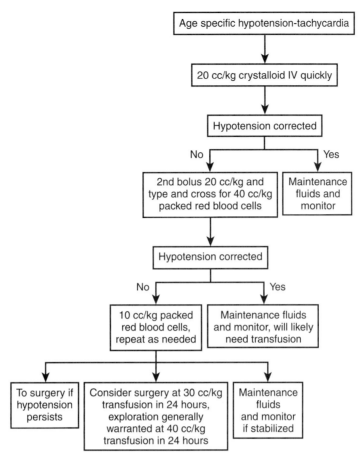

Figure 2 Algorithm for fluid and blood resuscitation in children.

of hypovolemia, then modest fluid resuscitation is in order. Hypothermia is an extremely common occurrence in injured children. Hypothermia in the injured child may occur at any time of the year, even during the extremes of summer. The response to hypothermia includes catecholamine release and shivering, with an increase in oxygen consumption and metabolic acidosis. Hypothermia as well as acidosis contribute to a post-traumatic coagulopathy. Prevention and treatment of hypothermia require attention to this serious complication during the initial evaluation of the injured child. A warm room, warmed fluids, heated air-warming blankets, or externally warmed blankets should be utilized during the initial resuscitation. An aggressive approach to rewarming should begin in the emergency department and should be continued in the radiology suite during evaluation. There is some evidence to suggest that early, carefully controlled hypothermia in the severely head-injured child who has no other injuries may be beneficial, but this treatment option is still experimental.

Diagnostic Assessment

The diagnostic assessment of the injured child begins with the initial evaluation and resuscitation phase of trauma management. The physical exam is a crucial first step, as it will direct all other forms of assessment. The initial physical examination also becomes the baseline for serial physical examinations by the trauma team performed later in the hospitalization. After the physical examination, other adjuncts may be employed.

While the patient is undergoing resuscitation in the emergency department, the diagnosis of injuries begins with standard radiographs. The most frequently ordered imaging studies in the emer-

gency department include plain radiographs of the chest, abdomen, pelvis, cervical spine, and extremities. Thoracic and lumbar spinal x-rays are commonly ordered when neurological injuries are suspected, or when the physical examination reveals point tenderness over the spine. Detecting a pneumothorax, pneumoperitoneum, pelvic fracture, or long bone fracture is an important component of the initial care of an injured child. Plain x-rays of the skull may document fractures, but they have little value in directing management of the head-injured child, except for penetrating injury and suspected child abuse.

Several recent studies by adult and pediatric trauma surgeons have attempted to determine the role of focused acute sonography for trauma (FAST) in the evaluation of the injured child.[8,9] The most common FAST evaluation examines the heart, right and left upper quadrants, and the pelvis for fluid (Figure 3). Some surgeons include an evaluation of the thorax for fluid in the pleural space and for pneumothorax.

Currently, non–radiologist-directed ultrasound evaluation in children should be coupled with the physical examination and should not be considered a conclusive diagnostic study. Although its sensitivity, specificity, and accuracy are high, it is used mostly as a screening tool to determine the need for more in-depth imaging studies or invasive evaluation. The relative lack of subcutaneous tissue in most children makes this an easy study to perform on children, compared with adolescents and adults. Obvious benefits of the FAST evaluation include its portability, eliminating the need to transport the child to the radiology suite, and the child's decreased radiation exposure.

Computerized tomography (CT) is the accepted diagnostic radiologic tool of choice for the vast majority of injured children suspected of having a potentially life-threatening injury.[10] CT scans of

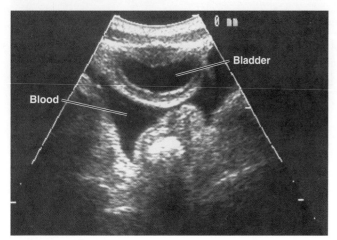

Figure 3 A positive focused acute sonography for trauma (FAST) in a 4-year-old. Blood in the pelvis.

the head, abdomen, and chest are considered the standard of care for the evaluation of an internal injury in a stable, traumatized child. The majority of children with suspected intra-abdominal injuries, providing they are stable, should have a CT scan performed prior to instituting operative or nonoperative management, unless an absolute indication for surgery is present. Physiologically unstable children in the emergency department are evaluated by other modalities, such as diagnostic peritoneal lavage or ultrasound. While CT scanning is the imaging modality of choice for evaluating a stable injured child, it is generally accepted that a high percentage of those scans will reveal no injuries. Abnormal abdominal CT scans are seen in only one-fourth of patients (Figure 4). A CT scan affects the decision to operate on children with a solid organ injury in a very small number of cases. Despite the liberal use of head CT scans, it is possible for the child with a severe neurologic injury to have a normal initial scan, or for a child to develop late manifestation of a neurologic injury or cerebral edema despite an initial normal study.

Evidence, on a CT scan, of intra-abdominal injuries requiring operative correction may be subtle. Findings of free intraperitoneal or retroperitoneal air, extraluminal gastrointestinal contrast me-

dium, bowel wall defects, and active hemorrhage are often obvious and have a high correlation with intestinal injury requiring operative intervention. There are, however, potentially life-threatening intestinal injuries that may be manifest only by focal bowel wall thickening or peritoneal fluid accumulation without solid organ injury. Other less specific findings associated with intestinal injuries include mesenteric stranding, fluid at the mesenteric root, focal hematomas, mesenteric pseudoaneurysm, and the hypoperfusion complex. Other adjuncts to the management of the injured child may include interventional radiologic techniques, magnetic resonance imaging, and invasive and noninvasive vascular studies.

The routine use of laboratory studies in the emergency department, in general, has not been shown to be of significant value in the pediatric trauma population. Some specific clinical laboratory testing, such as base deficit tests, urinalysis, and arterial blood gas tests, may be of limited benefit in selected circumstances. Most often, laboratory testing has lagged behind the clinical decision-making process occurring in the emergency department during evaluation and resuscitation. Point-of-care testing has not altered this concept. In the presence of a head injury, testing for a coagulopathy, thrombocytopenia, or hyperglycemia may be of benefit to establish a baseline for later determinations or to assist in assessing morbidity or mortality risks. During hospitalization, routine laboratory testing is appropriate as long as specific indications exist for monitoring, such as nonoperative management of a spleen or pancreatic injury, blood gases for patients receiving mechanical ventilation and patients with head injuries.

MANAGEMENT OF SPECIFIC INJURIES

It should be noted that the scale used for every injured organ—namely, the American Association for the Surgery of Trauma's Organ Injury Scale—is the same for adults and children. The management of specific injuries in children is virtually identical to that used for adults, except where indicated.

Head and Central Nervous System Injury

Acute traumatic brain injury is the most common cause of death and disability in the pediatric population. In those who survive, minor injuries can be associated with reversible defects, while major injuries can result in severe disabilities. The mechanisms of head injury in children are related to age. Infants typically suffer more from falls, such as from a table or the arms of a care giver. Intentional injury is a common cause of death in children under 2 years. Injury with intention, independent of severity, raises the mortality in brain-injured children. In older children, the usual cause of head injuries is from vehicle-related accidents or recreational activities.[11] While children have a better survival rate with head injury than adults do, this does not mean they have less morbidity with similar injuries. Children have a plasticity of the neuron related to the myelination and establishment of neuron interconnections. This allows a given focal injury to produce a less severe deficit as compared with a mature brain. But this same lack of maturity may also make the child more susceptible to a diffuse injury and subject to greater cognitive impairment.

During the initial evaluation and resuscitation of the brain-injured child, care should be taken to avoid secondary brain injury due to causes such as hypotension and hypoxia.[12] Control of the cervical spine is also mandatory during this period. Clinical and radiologic evaluation of the c-spine is important to rule out injury. The Glasgow Coma Scale (GCS) can be used for children over the age of 5, while some modification of the GCS is often used for children under 5. If a score of less than 9 is determined, that patient typically requires airway management, and intracranial pressure (ICP) measurement and treatment options should be considered. A score of less

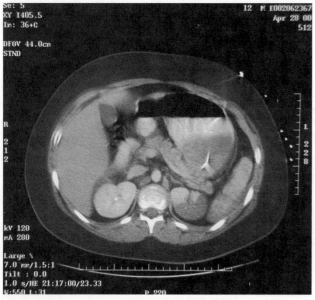

Figure 4 A positive computed tomography scan for a renal and spleen injury in an 8-year-old.

than 8 indicates the patient is comatose. Maintaining good oxygenation and perfusion is crucial during the entire resuscitation period, and this often mandates endotracheal intubation, taking care to protect the cervical spine, as injury may not be known.

Once the patient is initially evaluated and causes of secondary brain injury are managed, a head CT should be obtained. If there is evidence of brain swelling, monitoring of ICP is indicated. This is best done with a system that allows drainage of cerebrospinal fluid, such as a ventriculostomy. Avoiding hyperthermia is important, as this may cause secondary brain injury.[13] Other management techniques include hyperosmolar therapy with mannitol or hypertonic saline. Sedation is used as needed to maintain a low ICP. Hyperventilation as prophylaxis should generally be avoided. High-dose barbiturate therapy to create a coma has been suggested to be of some benefit. Decompressive craniectomy is now considered an alternative for the surgical management of head-injured children in specific circumstances. It should be considered in head-injured children with cerebral edema and medically uncontrolled intracranial hypertension. It may be of some benefit in children with a potentially recoverable head injury. It is not likely to be useful in children who have suffered an extensive secondary brain injury, or those who have a GCS of 3, with no improvement. Nutritional support, avoidance of steroid use, and treatment of postinjury seizures when indicated are also important aspects of the care of the head-injured patient.

Thoracic Injuries

Thoracic trauma is an important cause of morbidity and mortality in children. It accounts for 4%–25% of pediatric trauma injuries, but these chest injuries are associated with a greater mortality rate when compared with other system injuries. Thoracic trauma can be anticipated in children who present with a low systolic blood pressure, an elevated respiratory rate, abnormalities on thoracic physical examination including abnormal chest auscultation, and femur fractures.[14]

In general, the pediatric airway is more susceptible to mucus plugging and small amounts of airway edema. The chest wall is more compliant in children, with less muscle mass for soft tissue protection. This allows a greater transmission of energy to underlying organs when injury occurs. In children, the mediastinum is more mobile than in older patients, particularly in young children. Unilateral changes in thoracic pressure, such as with a tension pneumothorax, can lead to a shift of the mediastinum to the extent that venous return is markedly reduced. The pathophysiologic effect is similar to hypovolemic shock. This response is more pronounced in children than is typically in the case in an adult.

Rib fractures are relatively uncommon in young children and occur more frequently in adolescents. Even though rib fractures are uncommon, internal injuries of the organs lying underneath the ribs, such as liver or spleen injuries, and pulmonary contusion, are quite common. Flail chest is seen less commonly in children than in adults. One of the most common thoracic injuries in children is a pulmonary contusion. The flexible chest wall of the child allows contusion of the lung without rib fracture. The presence of a pulmonary contusion contributes to decreased pulmonary compliance, hypoxia, hypoventilation, and a ventilation perfusion mismatch. A chest radiograph taken during the initial assessment may demonstrate a pulmonary contusion; however, a chest CT scan can show areas of pulmonary contusion not appreciated on the radiograph. Treatment includes appropriate fluid resuscitation, supplemental oxygen, pain management, and strategies to prevent atelectasis and pneumonia. Children with pulmonary contusions may have prolonged changes in respiratory function and radiographic abnormalities.

Pneumothorax and hemothorax are not uncommon injuries in children. A pneumothorax is typically treated with a chest tube appropriately sized for the patient. A hemothorax is also treated with a tube thoracostomy, typically with the largest tube that can be inserted. Intrathoracic blood loss of 15 ml/kg immediately or ongoing losses of 2–3 ml/kg/hour for 3 or more hours suggest the need for thoracic exploration to control bleeding in children. Cardiac injuries are extremely rare, as are tracheobronchial injuries and esophageal injuries. Injuries to the great vessels occur in children with rapid deceleration injuries, and these types of injuries should be considered, with the appropriate mechanism, in any injured child.[15]

Abdominal Injuries

Due to the relative thinness of the pediatric abdominal wall, a modest amount of force may cause a greater injury to one or more organs in the abdomen. Multiple organs may be injured from a single blow due to closer proximity. The assessment for abdominal injury begins with the physical examination. Inspection may reveal bruising, a lap belt mark, or abdominal distention. Tenderness on physical examination should prompt a higher level of evaluation with CT scanning. A nasogastric or orogastric tube should be placed to decompress the stomach.

During the course of routine nonoperative management of abdominal injuries, injuries requiring operative management may be overlooked for quite some time. It has been noted that a delay in diagnosis, although not uncommon, is not associated with increased mortality.[16] However, an increase in septic complications has been seen when operative intervention occurred more than 24 hours after injury. Therefore, in-hospital observation with serial examinations should be employed in all children with abdominal examinations that are not perfectly normal. When abdominal injuries occur under suspicious circumstances, the diagnosis of child abuse should be entertained.

Blunt diaphragmatic rupture is an uncommon occurrence. The left diaphragm is involved more often than the right; however, bilateral injury can occur. The frequency of associated injuries, especially of liver and spleen, is very high. Blunt injury to the diaphragm may have several manifestations. An abnormal diaphragm contour, a high riding diaphragm, or a questionable overlap of abdominal visceral shadows may indicate injury. Visceral herniation, the abnormal placement of a nasogastric tube into the hemithorax, or intestinal obstruction should be considered diagnostic. Computerized tomography has been used to establish this diagnosis, but the CT may appear normal in some patients. Many diaphragmatic ruptures are not identified in the first few days after injury and may not be detected for a considerable period of time. Repair of an acute diaphragmatic rupture is often best accomplished with an abdominal approach. If a late diagnosis of a diaphragmatic injury is made, a thoracic approach to repair should be considered.

Blunt injuries to the stomach are likely the third most common intestinal perforation in the child. Gastric perforations occur relatively more frequently in children than adults. The site of perforation is most often the greater curve of the stomach. The diagnosis is usually made quickly, due to free air seen on initial radiographs in the emergency department or bloody nasogastric aspirate. Pneumoperitoneum and peritonitis occur early in this injury. The liver and spleen are often injured along with the stomach. Operative repair is required. The use of a decompressive gastrostomy can be considered when massive injury is present. Every effort should be made to salvage the spleen during repair of the stomach injury.

The child with a duodenal injury that requires surgery more often presents with abdominal distention, bilious vomiting, pneumoperitoneum, and peritonitis.[17] A duodenal hematoma is usually treated nonoperatively with nasogastric decompression and total parenteral nutrition. This management is associated with a high rate of success, but may take as long as 3 weeks for the obstruction to resolve. A late diagnosis of duodenal perforation can occur with this injury and is usually associated with an increase in complications, but not mortality.

The small bowel, both jejunum and ileum, is the most common part of the intestinal tract to be injured in a child. The mechanism of injury to the small bowel is the result of its being trapped between the delivered force and the vertebral column. Adult-sized seatbelts are often used to secure children in a car, and as a result the risk of small bowel injury rises. If a seatbelt bruise is present, the risk of an intra-abdominal injury is much more likely, and therefore a higher index of suspicion should be employed. Children with small bowel injury due to blunt trauma invariably have an abnormal physical examination. Free fluid seen on an ultrasound or CT scan, coupled with a tender abdomen, and no solid organ injury, almost mandates an abdominal exploration for bowel injury. Even if no perforation is identified in surgery, care should be taken to evaluate for mesenteric rents, hematomas, and possibly retroperitoneal injuries. In this same setting, compression injury of the lumbar vertebrae (chance fracture) is also common; and when present, the patient usually requires a longer hospital stay due to pain management.

Injuries to the colon and rectum are not common in children.[18] Accidental causes of colon and rectal injuries include motor vehicle collisions involving pelvic fractures and rectal wall penetration by bone shards. Nonaccidental injuries caused by child abuse, typically from blunt instrumentation, are also seen. If the mucosa is injured or the injury is superficial, observation is appropriate. Full thickness injuries of the distal rectum can be managed with primary repair in many cases. Devastating colon injuries above the peritoneal reflection often need a temporary colostomy. Penetrating injuries often can be managed by primary repair, but in the face of complicating features may also need diversion at the time of repair.

The injured spleen in a child will almost always stop bleeding without any intervention. Nonoperative management is the standard of care, and the incidence of any potential operative intervention is very small.[19] The rate of operative intervention is likely cut in half when a trained pediatric surgeon is managing the patient. Children who require surgery are those who have received or are likely to receive half their blood volume in transfusions within 24 hours of injury (40 cc/kg). The physiologic response to splenic injury correlates with the grade of splenic injury. Most often children who need operative intervention will need splenectomy. If splenectomy must be performed, post-splenectomy immunization is appropriate. Many children are given penicillin on a daily basis if the splenectomy is performed before age 5 years of age. If immunosuppression is suspected, hepatitis B vaccine should also be administered.

When only the liver is injured, without major vascular or bile duct involvement, then observation will almost always succeed. This is especially true in patients with isolated solid organ injuries. However, it is possible that hepatic injuries may be associated with a slightly higher mortality rate than splenic injuries. The combination of hepatic and splenic injury is clearly associated with a higher mortality rate, which goes up as the severity of injury rises. The concept of operation when half of the blood volume has been transfused, as noted for splenic injury, is valid for liver injury as well. If a blush is seen on CT, angioembolization may be of benefit prior to operation. Early operative damage-control laparotomy, coupled with embolization and early reoperation as a means to improve survival, has seen some success. The physiologic and hematologic effects of a massive transfusion in the child often make the operative management of liver injury very difficult.

Pediatric pancreatic injuries are uncommon and are most often due to blunt trauma. Bicycle-related injuries should be included in this category. The majority of pancreatic injuries in children may be treated successfully with nonoperative management, including gut rest, intravenous nutrition, and occasionally pancreatic antisecretory medication. Conservative management of children with a pancreatic transection may be more controversial. The beneficial effects of a spleen-sparing distal pancreatectomy, even in the face of a delayed diagnosis, have been noted.[20] When the capabilities for pediatric endoscopic retrograde cholangiopancreatography (ERCP) are available, ductal stenting may be of significant benefit. Other surgeons, as well as our group, have been able to employ laparoscopic

distal pancreatectomy with splenic salvage for pancreatic transection when stenting could not be accomplished.

Blunt trauma is the most common mechanism of renal injury in children. Contusion is the most common injury seen. Renal injury can occur in the absence of hematuria. Nonoperative management of most pediatric renal injuries (grades I–III) can be accomplished safely. Nonoperative management for renal salvage appears to be successful in most cases, even with grade IV injuries, but operative renal salvage for grade V injuries appears to be uncommon. Ureteral stenting for urine leaks may be needed in patients with injuries of the collecting system. Rarely, nephrectomy for exsanguinating injury may be needed. This would typically be initiated when 40 cc/kg of blood transfusion had been necessary and administered. Angioembolism may be considered in some cases; however, the majority of patients will not require emergency procedural intervention. Since most injured children now undergo abdominal CT scanning, CT cystography should be considered on every child to evaluate for bladder injury. The majority of bladder injuries can be treated successfully with urethral catheters, without the need for additional suprapubic drainage.

Vascular injuries in children are uncommon. Children can tolerate complete vascular occlusion to arms and legs to a greater degree than adults. Extremity vascular injuries are equally divided between blunt and penetrating mechanisms. Limb salvage is typically greater than 95%. Abdominal aortic injuries can occur due to seat-belt injuries, bicycle injuries, and ATV-related injuries. Immediate direct vessel repair is an optimal management plan, due to related internal injuries. Endovascular stents have not been evaluated for long-term use in children, and especially in the growing child.

Orthopedic injuries are the greatest cause of required operative intervention in injured children. These injuries are often of such magnitude that they distract the child from complaining of other, more serious injuries. Thus orthopedic injuries are also a significant source of missed injury in the injured child. Missed injuries are the most important reason that a tertiary examination should be considered for all children admitted to the hospital. Cervical spine injuries are often misdiagnosed, and most of the missed injuries are due to normal variants.

ACKNOWLEDGMENT

Supported in part by the Paula Milburn Miller/Children's Medical Research Institute, Chair in Pediatric Surgery, Oklahoma City, Oklahoma.

REFERENCES

1. Kissoon N, Dreyer J, Walia M: Pediatric trauma: differences in pathophysiology, injury patterns and treatment compared with adult trauma. *CMAJ* 142:27, 1990.
2. Killingsworth JB, Tilford JM, Parker JG, Graham JJ, Dick RM, Aitken ME: National hospitalization impact of pediatric all-terrain vehicle injuries. *Pediatrics* 115(3):e316–321, 2005.
3. Edil BH, Tuggle DW, Jones S, Albrecht R, Kuhn A, Mantor PC, Puffinbarger NK: Pediatric major resuscitation—respiratory compromise as a criterion for mandatory surgeon presence. *J Pediatr Surg* 40(6): 926–928, 2005.
4. Chiang VW, Baskin MN: Uses and complications of central venous catheters inserted in a pediatric emergency department. *Pediatr Emerg Care* 16(4):230–232, 2000.
5. Rogers FB: Technical note: a quick and simple method of obtaining venous access in traumatic exsanguination. *J Trauma* 34(1):142–143, 1993.
6. National High Blood Pressure Education Program Working Group on High Blood Pressure in Children and Adolescents: the fourth report on the diagnosis, evaluation, and treatment of high blood pressure in children and adolescents. *Pediatrics* 114(2 Suppl):555–576, 2004.
7. Balogh Z, McKinley BA, Cocanour CS, Kozar RA, Valdivia A, Sailors RM, Moore FA: Supranormal trauma resuscitation causes more cases of abdominal compartment syndrome. *Arch Surg* 138(6):637–642, 2003.
8. Mutabagani KH, Coley BD, Zumberge N, McCarthy DW, Besner GE, Caniano DA, Cooney DR: Preliminary experience with focused

abdominal sonography for trauma (FAST) in children: is it useful? *J Pediatr Surg* 34(1):48–52, 1999.

9. Suthers SE, Albrecht R, Foley D, Mantor PC, Puffinbarger NK, Jones SK, Tuggle DW: Surgeon-directed ultrasound for trauma is a predictor of intra-abdominal injury in children. *Am Surg* 70(2):164–167, 2004.

10. Ruess L, Sivit CJ, Eichelberger MR, Gotschall CS, Taylor GA: Blunt abdominal trauma in children: impact of CT on operative and nonoperative management. *AJR* 169:1011–1014, 1997.

11. Kriel RL, Krach LE, Panser LA: Closed head injury: comparison of children younger and older than 6 years of age. *Pediatr Neurol* 5(5):296–300, 1989.

12. Selden PD, Bratton SL, Carney NA, et al: Guidelines for the acute medical management of severe traumatic brain injury in infants, children, and adolescents following severe pediatric traumatic brain injury. *Pediatr Crit Care Med* 4(3 Suppl):S53–S55, 2003.

13. Adelson PD, Ragheb J, Kanev P, Brockmeyer D, Beers SR, Brown SD, Cassidy LD, Chang Y, Levin H: Phase II clinical trial of moderate hypothermia after severe traumatic brain injury in children. *Neurosurgery* 56(4):740–754, 2005.

14. Holmes JF, Sokolove PE, Brant WE, et al: A clinical decision rule for identifying children with thoracic injuries after blunt torso trauma. *Ann Emerg Med* 39:492–499, 2002.

15. Tiao GM, Griffith PM, Szmuszkovicz JR, et al: Cardiac and great vessel injuries in children after blunt trauma. An institutional review. *J Pediatr Surg* 35:1656–1660, 2002.

16. Canty TG Sr, Canty TG Jr, Brown C: Injuries of the gastrointestinal tract from blunt trauma in children: a 12-year experience at a designated pediatric trauma center. *J Trauma* 46:234–240, 1999.

17. Clendenon JN, Meyers RL, Nance ML, Scaife ER: Management of duodenal injuries in children. *J Pediatr Surg* 39(6):964–968, 2004.

18. Haut ER, Nance ML, Keller MS, Groner JI, Ford HR, Kuhn A, Tuchfarber B, Garcia V, Schwab CW, Stafford PW: Management of penetrating colon and rectal injuries in the pediatric patient. *Dis Colon Rectum* 47(9):1526–1532, 2004.

19. Mooney DP, Forbes PW: Variation in the management of pediatric splenic injuries in New England. *J Trauma* 56(2):328–333, 2004.

20. Meier DE, Coln CD, Hicks BA, Guzzetta PC: Early operation in children with pancreas transection. *J Pediatr Surg* 36(2):341–344, 2001.

TRAUMA IN PREGNANCY

Amy C. Sisley and William C. Chiu

The pregnant trauma patient presents significant challenges to the trauma surgeon. The physiologic changes in the mother during pregnancy represent both diagnostic and treatment dilemmas, while the need to treat two patients simultaneously may represent both clinical and emotional challenges for the trauma team.

INCIDENCE

Trauma complicates 7%–8% of pregnancies and is the leading cause of maternal death.[1] The incidence of significant maternal and fetal injury increases with gestational age, with slightly over 50% of injuries occurring in the third trimester.[2]

The most common mechanisms of injury for maternal trauma are motor vehicle collisions (MVCs) at 55%–70%, followed by assault at 12%–22%. In contrast, fetal death is a consequence of motor vehicle collisions in 82% of cases, followed by gunshot wounds (GSWs) in 6%, and falls in 3%.[3]

MECHANISM OF INJURY

Blunt Trauma

Blunt trauma is the leading cause of both maternal and fetal death and is usually a consequence of MVCs, assaults, or falls. Although mortality rates are similar for pregnant versus nonpregnant blunt trauma patients, with equivalent Injury Severity Scores (ISS), their patterns of injury are notably different. Pregnant patients injured in MVCs are more likely to sustain significant abdominal injuries and less likely to sustain head injuries than their nonpregnant counterparts. Splenic, hepatic, and retroperitoneal injuries occur more frequently in gravid trauma patients, due in part to the increased vascularity associated with pregnancy as well as to the displacement of the abdominal contents by the uterus. Up to 25% of pregnant blunt trauma patients sustain significant splenic or hepatic lacerations.[4]

Direct injury to the fetus from blunt trauma is rare (<1%). The leading cause of fetal mortality after blunt trauma is maternal mortality followed by placental abruption. Since the uterus is elastic and the placenta is not, sheering forces can result in placental abruption, even in otherwise minor blunt abdominal trauma. The estimated incidence of abruption is 2%–3% for minor trauma and up to 40% for severe blunt abdominal trauma. Uterine rupture occurs less commonly than placental abruption but increases in incidence with gestational age.[3] Although uterine rupture is life-threatening to both the mother and the fetus, its diagnosis is often difficult, given the variable and sometimes subtle clinical presentation. The clinician must maintain a high index of suspicion for both placental abruption and uterine rupture in any patient with blunt abdominal trauma, especially in late gestation.

Penetrating Trauma

Penetrating trauma is usually the result of either GSWs or stabbing. This type of injury in pregnant patients is most often sustained at the hands of a spouse or intimate partner. Death rates for these injuries are actually decreased in pregnant patients compared with nonpregnant patients, owing to the protective effect for the mother of the gravid uterus. Unfortunately, the consequence to the fetus is a mortality rate of 71% for abdominal GSWs and 42% for abdominal stab wounds. It should also be noted that due to the upward displacement of intra-abdominal content by the uterus in pregnancy, upper quadrant abdominal stab wounds carry a high risk for small bowel injury in pregnant patients.[1,3]

Intimate Partner Violence

Intimate partner violence (IPV) is not uncommon in pregnancy. Between 7.4% and 21% of pregnant patients reported physical abuse at the hands of an intimate partner and fully two-thirds reported an escalation of violence during pregnancy. Physically abused women have higher rates of miscarriage and low birthweight infants than nonabused women. Battering during pregnancy is not only associated with an increase in the frequency of abuse but also with a threefold increase in risk of homicide compared with physically abused women who are not pregnant.[5] Hence, intrapartum battering is a marker for a particularly violent and potentially lethal relationship.

PHYSIOLOGIC ALTERATIONS OF PREGNANCY

The extent of the anatomic and physiologic changes that occur during normal pregnancy is dependent on gestational age. During the first trimester, early changes are easily adapted to, so there is minimal functional alteration. By the third trimester, virtually every organ system has undergone change to compensate for the enlarged uterus and growing fetus. It is most important to remember that the presence of a fetus and the physical size of the abdomen are not the only aspects to consider when caring for the injured pregnant patient.

During the entire first trimester, the uterine size is small enough so that it remains relatively well protected by the bony pelvis. The earliest physiologic changes result from the presence of the placenta. Hormones released from the placenta include human chorionic gonadotropin (hCG), human placental lactogen (hPL), progesterone, estrogen, adrenocorticotropic hormone (ACTH), and thyroid stimulating hormone (TSH). These hormones increase maternal insulin resistance and promote hyperglycemia. The subsequent increase in insulin and glucose levels translate into enhanced protein synthesis for the fetus. The reproductive hormones also inhibit gastrointestinal motility, which increases the potential for aspiration as early as 8–12 weeks gestation.

Increased levels of estrogen and progesterone, as well as of renin and aldosterone, lead to increased sodium resorption and plasma volume expansion beginning at about 10 weeks gestation. While heart rate, mean arterial pressure, and central venous pressure are not yet altered, the cardiac output may start to increase by 1–1.5 l/min (Table 1). Progesterone also promotes hypertrophy of the kidneys from 10 weeks gestation and leads to impaired gallbladder contraction and bile stasis. Beginning at the end of the first trimester, there may be an increase in gallstone formation.

Second Trimester

During the second trimester, the uterus begins to rise out of the pelvis, and by 20 weeks, it may reach the umbilicus (Figure 1). Blood pressure falls by about 5–15 mm Hg and reaches its lowest level of the pregnancy. In traumatic maternal hemorrhage, placental blood flow is preferentially reduced, and 30% of maternal blood volume may be lost prior to signs of shock.[6] The "supine hypotensive syndrome" is caused by compression of the inferior vena cava by the gravid uterus, decreasing venous blood return and thereby decreasing preload and cardiac output. Turning the mother left side down increases cardiac output by about 30% after 20 weeks gestation.[7]

Table 1: Cardiovascular Alterations during Pregnancy

Parameter	Trimester		
	1st	2nd	3rd
Cardiac output	Increased	Increased	Increased
Stroke volume	Increased	Increased	Increased
Heart rate	Normal	Normal	Increased
MAP	Normal	Decreased	Normal
SVR	Normal	Decreased	Decreased

MAP, Mean arterial pressure; *SVR*, systemic vascular resistance.

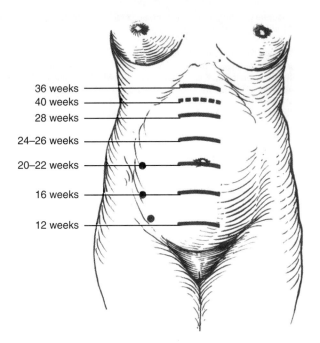

Figure 1   The height of the uterine fundus relative to the abdominal wall.   *(Courtesy of David Gens, MD.)*

Third Trimester

By the 7th month, the pubic symphysis and sacroiliac joints widen. At approximately 36 weeks gestation, the uterus reaches its maximal height near the costal margins. Intraperitoneal structures are displaced cephalad and laterally.

During the third trimester, blood pressure returns to more normal levels and heart rate increases up to 20 beats per minute relative to the nonpregnant state. This physiologic tachycardia must be considered when evaluating the pregnant trauma patient. Pulmonary capillary wedge pressure and left ventricular function remain normal, while systemic and pulmonary vascular resistances are decreased.[8]

After 30 weeks gestation, plasma volume has increased 40%, accompanied by a 15% increase in red blood cell mass. This discrepancy leads to the "physiologic anemia of pregnancy."[9] Serum albumin declines by up to 30% because of this volume expansion. Benign physiologic pericardial effusion is more prevalent and may complicate the Focused Assessment with Sonography for Trauma (FAST). The decrease in colloid oncotic pressure may increase the risk for pulmonary edema. A hypercoagulable state is also induced because of an increase in nearly all coagulation factors, procoagulants and fibrinogen, and a reduction in fibrinolytic activity.[10]

Anatomic changes in the thorax include the diaphragm rising about 4 cm and the chest diameter increasing by 2 cm.[11] The most significant changes in respiratory function include an increase in minute ventilation by as much as 50%, mostly by an increase in tidal volume. Functional residual capacity decreases largely due to elevation of the diaphragm. A state of compensated respiratory alkalosis results in a chronic reduced $PaCO_2$ to approximately 30 mm Hg and reduced plasma bicarbonate level.[12]

The movement of gastrointestinal viscera cephalad is associated with a displacement of the gastroesophageal sphincter into the thorax. Placental release of gastrin augments the acid production of the stomach, making the risk for aspiration greatest at this time.

Uterine compression of the bladder and ureters results in a compensated hydronephrosis. The increase in blood volume and cardiac output is associated with increased renal blood flow of up to 80% and increased glomerular filtration rate of 50%. Blood urea nitrogen and serum creatinine are commonly reduced, but urine output volume does not significantly change.

DIAGNOSIS

Primary Survey

The initial evaluation of the pregnant trauma patient should include early consultation with the obstetrics service as well as neonatology if appropriate (>24 weeks gestation). The general principles of evaluation of trauma patients are similar to those of the nonpregnant patient and include initial focus on assessing and stabilizing maternal vital signs. These include the standard Advanced Trauma Life Support (ATLS) primary survey, which is then followed by a rapid and brief assessment of the fetus for viability. Because pressure from the pregnant uterus on the inferior vena cava can result in a decrease in cardiac return, an effort should be made to displace the uterus laterally in pregnant patients. This may be accomplished by tilting the backboard to the side or by manually displacing the uterus to the left side.

Indications for intubation in the pregnant trauma patient are similar to those in the nonpregnant patient, although aspiration risk is higher during pregnancy. It should be kept in mind, however, that the fetus will not tolerate hypoxemia as well as the mother, so supplemental oxygen should always be applied and oxygen saturation monitored in all pregnant patients.

Accurate assessment of maternal volume status may be complicated by the physiologic changes of pregnancy. Since the fetus will be compromised by even minor maternal hypovolemia, aggressive volume replacement should be undertaken. Vasopressors and inotropes may actually reduce maternal blood flow to the fetus and should not be used as a substitute for volume resuscitation in alleviating maternal hypotension. Immediate jeopardy of the mother's life may occasionally necessitate the use of vasopressors or inotropes for circulatory support, but they should be used sparingly and discontinued as rapidly as possible.

Secondary Survey

The secondary survey is then performed in accordance with ATLS guidelines, with the caveat that examination of the perineum must include a formal examination of the vagina and cervix to evaluate for bleeding. The pelvic examination should be performed by an obstetrician if possible.

The physical examination of the abdomen is difficult in pregnancy due to displacement of abdominal contents from their normal position. Additionally, stretching of the abdominal wall by the uterus in late pregnancy may result in a relative insensitivity to peritoneal irritation, resulting in difficulty in detecting peritonitis on clinical examination alone. The FAST examination represents a rapid and noninvasive means of evaluating the patient for the presence of intra-abdominal fluid. The sensitivity of the FAST examination in pregnant patients, at 83%, is slightly lower than in the nonpregnant population,; however, the specificity is similar at 96%.[13] Although it does not replace formal fetal ultrasonography, the FAST examination may be used to get a rapid picture of the fetal status during the initial resuscitation by detecting the fetal heart rate. The FAST has also been reported to detect unsuspected pregnancies in some trauma patients, thus influencing subsequent management.[14] The use of ultrasonography does not involve ionizing radiation and poses no known risk to the developing fetus.

Initial Evaluation of the Fetus

The initial evaluation of the fetus is part of the secondary survey and potentially includes ultrasonography, fetal monitoring, and obstetric consultation if not previously obtained. Formal pelvic ultrasonography can determine if the fetus is still viable and can calculate gestational age. It should be noted that ultrasonography is unreliable in predicting placental abruption.

Cardiotrophic monitoring is the mainstay of fetal assessment in the third trimester. The practice management guidelines of the Eastern Association for the Surgery of Trauma (EAST) include a recommendation that all pregnancies greater than 20 weeks gestation should undergo fetal monitoring for a minimum of 6 hours.[15] More prolonged monitoring has been recommended in cases of uterine contractions, abnormal fetal heart rate patterns, and in cases of severe maternal trauma.[3] Fetal monitoring is used to evaluate both the state of the fetus as well as the presence and frequency of uterine contractions. It is the single most reliable tool available for the assessment of placental abruption. The use of fetal monitoring routinely, even in cases of apparently minor maternal trauma, must be emphasized. A recent multi-institutional study of 13 Level I and Level II trauma centers revealed that fetal monitoring was obtained on only 61% of trauma patients with third trimester pregnancies.[16]

Exposure to Radiation from Diagnostic Radiographs

Invariably, the necessity of obtaining radiographs in the evaluation of the pregnant patient raises concern about radiation exposure and subsequent damage to the fetus. Since the most important predictor of fetal outcome is maternal outcome, the clinician caring for the injured pregnant patient should not hesitate to obtain diagnostic radiographs that are necessary for the evaluation of the mother. These diagnostic tests should be limited to those that will have impact on maternal outcome and for which there is no alternative test. Redundancy should be eliminated. Hence, if it is known that the patient will require computed tomography (CT) scans of the chest and abdomen, plain films of the chest and thoracolumbar spine need not be obtained. The dose of ionizing radiation to the fetus can be further reduced by the use of lead shielding whenever possible.

Predicting teratogenicity as a consequence of fetal radiation exposure is difficult; however, no study has shown an increase above baseline for exposures of 10 rad (100 mGy).[15] According to the recommendations on radiation exposure during pregnancy made by the American College of Obstetrics and Gynecology (ACOG), exposure of 5 rad (50 mGy) is not associated with any increase in risk of fetal loss or of birth defects.[17] Other than teratogenicity, the principal concern in exposing a fetus to radiation is that of increasing the risk of childhood cancers. The National Radiation Protection Board of Britain cites a 6% excess risk per 100 rad exposure.[18]

Most of the common radiographic tests employed in the evaluation of trauma patients are associated with fetal radiation doses of 1/100 rad or less (Table 2). The exception to this is the abdominal CT, with a radiation dose of 2.60 rad for 10-mm slices. This is still only about half of the 5-rad dose cited by ACOG as safe. However, it should be kept in mind that the newer multiplanar scanners may have a higher radiation exposure. Consultation with the radiology department is strongly recommended in planning a diagnostic workup that will minimize the risk of radiation exposure.

SURGICAL MANAGEMENT

The majority of traumatic injuries to the pregnant patient are treated similarly to those in nonpregnant patients. In general, injuries requiring operative intervention would be the same in the pregnant patient and in the nonpregnant patient. The additional considerations necessary in pregnancy are that general anesthesia and abdominal surgery may precipitate premature labor. Direct injury to the uterus, maternal shock, or fetal distress may require emergency cesarean section.

Table 2: Estimated Fetal Exposure from Radiographs

Procedure	Approximate Fetal Dose[a] (rad)
Plain Films	
Chest (two views)	0.00002–0.00007
Abdomen	0.1
Cervical spine	0.002
Pelvis	0.040
Thoracolumbar spine	0.370
CT Scans[b]	
Head CT	<0.05
Chest CT	<0.100
Abdominal CT	2.60

[a]Dose varies depending on exact procedure used and on body habits.
[b]Estimate based on 10-mm slices.
Adapted from Barraco RD, Chiu WC, Clancy, et al: Practice management guidelines for the diagnosis and management of injury in the pregnant patient: the EAST practice management guidelines work group, Eastern Association for the Surgery of Trauma World Wide Web site, http://www.east.org/tpg/pregnancy.pdf; and Wakeford R, Little MP: Risk coefficients for childhood cancer after intrauterine irradiation: a review. *Int J Rad Biol* 79(5):293–299, 2003.

Blunt Trauma

Uterine rupture occurs in only 0.6% of instances of blunt trauma during pregnancy.[19] Direct fetal injury is also very rare and complicates <1% of cases. As it is in the nonpregnant patient, nonoperative management of abdominal solid organ injuries should be the treatment of choice in hemodynamically stable pregnant patients. The greatest difference in nonoperative management of abdominal injuries is that angiographic therapeutic adjuncts are not advisable because of the potential for large radiation exposure. In unstable patients, operative management may best limit maternal and fetal shock, and the indications for laparotomy are similar to those in nonpregnant patients. Hemodynamic instability in patients with blunt abdominal trauma and free intraperitoneal fluid found by ultrasonography are indications for urgent laparotomy (Figure 2). At laparotomy, the uterus should be left intact unless there is direct uterine injury.

Pelvic fractures have several serious implications in the pregnant patient and may be associated with fetal demise in up to 25% of cases. Engorgement of pelvic and retroperitoneal vasculature renders any pelvic fracture at increased risk for significant hemorrhage. Fetal injury or death may result from direct placental injury or from maternal shock (Figure 3). Pelvic angiography for embolization should be an adjunct used for life-threatening pelvic hemorrhage, as the radiation required for the procedure exceeds safe levels for the fetus.

Penetrating Trauma

As the uterus enlarges and rises out of the bony pelvis, the risk of injury from penetrating trauma increases. The muscular uterine wall is somewhat resilient to low-velocity stab wounds to the abdomen but is not an adequate barrier to GSWs. Patients who should have urgent laparotomy are those who are hemodynamically unstable, those with obvious transperitoneal penetration, and those with free intraperitoneal fluid found on ultrasonography. While the diagnostic options available are similar to those of nonpregnant patients, the main concern would be the exposure of ionizing radiation. It may be prudent to use local wound exploration to evaluate superficial stab wounds whenever possible. Diagnostic peritoneal lavage (DPL) has relative contraindications in pregnancy, and there is the special consideration for the need of a supraumbilical location for access.

The use of CT scanning in penetrating torso trauma in the pregnant patient is an area that has not yet been well studied. In blunt trauma, the judicious use of abdominopelvic CT scanning to evaluate for abdominal injury is recommended. In penetrating trauma, the benefits and risks of the options must be considered. In penetrating torso trauma in nonpregnant patients, triple contrast abdominopelvic CT reliably excludes peritoneal penetration to prevent unnecessary laparotomy.[20] The risks of CT scanning include the fetal exposure to ionizing radiation. The risks of general anesthesia and unnecessary laparotomy must be considered in balance. Without clear evidence and recommendations on the utility of CT in penetrating torso trauma, careful individual decision making and judgment are required between immediate laparotomy and diagnostic CT scanning.

Cesarean Section

While the importance of emergency cesarean section for fetal salvage is evident, the indications for perimortem cesarean section remain controversial (Table 3). Morris et al. showed that emer-

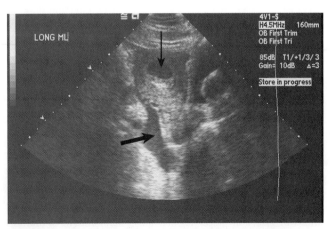

Figure 2 Ultrasound of a car crash victim showing an early intrauterine pregnancy (*small arrow*) and free fluid in the abdomen (*large arrow*).

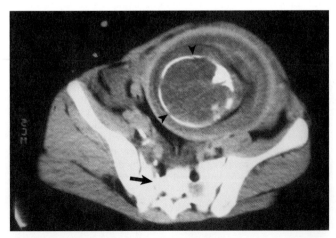

Figure 3 Computed tomography scan demonstrating fracture of the maternal pelvis (*long arrow*) with concomitant fracture of the fetal skull (*short arrows*).

Table 3: Indications for Emergency and Perimortem Cesarean Section

Fetal hypoxia or distress
Premature rupture of membranes
Uterine injury or rupture
Amniotic fluid embolism
Disseminated intravascular coagulation
Gravid uterus complicating management at laparotomy
Maternal refractory shock or cardiac arrest

gency cesarean section for patients at greater than 25 weeks gestation was associated with a 45% fetal survival and that 60% of infant deaths resulted from delay in recognition of fetal distress.[21] In this multicenter study, infant survival was independent of maternal injury, and no fetus delivered without fetal heart tones survived.

Perimortem cesarean section refers to those cases of emergency cesarean section performed surrounding maternal death, whether fetal delivery is performed prior to or after actual maternal death, and should be considered in any moribund pregnant patient of at least 24 weeks gestational age if fetal heart tones are still present.[15] When performed following maternal death, fetal neurological outcome and survival are closely dependent upon the time interval between maternal death and fetal delivery. Fetal delivery must occur within 20 minutes of maternal death, but should ideally start within 4 minutes of maternal cardiac arrest. The anticipated fetal survival rate is up to 70% when delivery is performed within 5 minutes of maternal death.

MORBIDITY AND COMPLICATIONS MANAGEMENT

The pregnant trauma patient is at risk for complications specifically associated with the pregnancy and fetus. Changes in the anatomy and physiology of pregnancy may also place the pregnant patient at increased risk for some potential complications that are not directly related to the pregnancy.

Fetomaternal Hemorrhage

Fetomaternal hemorrhage occurs in up to 28% of pregnancies after trauma.[22] The amount of Rh-positive fetal blood required to sensitize the Rh-negative mother is variable, but most patients are sensitized by as little as 0.01 ml of blood. The extent of fetomaternal hemorrhage and Rh alloimmunization is evaluated with the Kleihauer-Betke (KB) test. The test utilizes a stain that identifies fetal red blood cells with hemoglobin F in maternal blood. The ratio of fetal:maternal red blood cells can be assessed. Treatment with Rh immunoglobulin should be given early, along with obstetric consultation, but definitely within 72 hours of injury.

Premature Labor

Many cases of mild uterine contractions after trauma resolve spontaneously. Instances of true premature labor involve both preterm contractions and evidence of cervical dilation and may need to be treated with pharmacologic tocolytics. Several agents are available for tocolysis, including terbutaline and magnesium sulfate, and should only be administered with obstetric consultation. Traumatic injury, surgery, and general anesthesia may increase the risk of premature

labor. Drost et al. reported an 80% efficacy using tocolysis in a study of major trauma in pregnancy.[23] Blunt abdominal trauma may cause premature rupture of membranes leading to premature labor.

Pre-eclampsia and Eclampsia

Systemic blood pressure is normally decreased beginning in the second trimester. Any hypertension in these patients may be a sign of pre-eclampsia. Control of pregnancy-induced hypertension is important to prevent uterine vasoconstriction and placental ischemia. The initial treatment includes fluid resuscitation to expand intravascular volume. These patients may also require vasodilator therapy or inotropic support to improve perfusion. Pre-eclampsia typically resolves following fetal delivery.

Pregnant trauma patients with altered sensorium, coma, or seizures may have eclampsia. Associated signs may include hypertension, oliguria, proteinuria, pulmonary edema, and disseminated intravascular coagulation (DIC). As in the treatment of pre-eclampsia, fluid resuscitation and hemodynamic support is necessary. Intravenous magnesium sulfate should be administered, and cesarean section should be considered in those patients at 28 weeks gestation or greater.

Placental Abruption

In surviving pregnant trauma patients, placental abruption is the most common cause for fetal death, and occurs in 30%–70% of severely injured patients. The mechanisms for abruption in blunt trauma may be either from uteroplacental ischemia from maternal shock or from mechanical shearing as a result of deceleration forces. Later in pregnancy, relatively minor blunt trauma may result in abruption.

In the setting of trauma, the signs of abruption may be as subtle as occult vaginal bleeding and abdominal pain, or may be severe enough to result in shock or DIC. The absence of vaginal bleeding does not exclude abruption. Uteroplacental separation of up to 25% may result in vaginal bleeding and premature labor. Separation of greater than 50% usually results in fetal demise.

Amniotic Fluid Embolization

Amniotic fluid embolism refers to the entrance of amniotic fluid into the maternal circulation. It more commonly presents during labor or the immediate postpartum period, and the risk of maternal mortality is up to 80%. Pregnant trauma patients suffering from premature labor may be at risk. The diagnosis is mostly made on clinical signs, and the manifestations include severe dyspnea, hypoxia, hypotension, altered sensorium or seizures, and possible cardiac arrest. Respiratory failure mimics that seen in the acute respiratory distress syndrome. Patients may develop thrombocytopenia or DIC. Following fetal delivery, the maternal treatment for this condition is largely supportive. These supportive measures include supplemental oxygen or mechanical ventilation, fluid resuscitation, inotropes, vasopressors, and blood product replacement.[24]

Venous Thromboembolism

The hypercoagulable state associated with pregnancy is caused by an increase in coagulation factors and inhibition of fibrinolysis. The hypercoagulable state exacerbates conditions of prolonged immobilization in trauma patients with neurologic injury, pelvic or lower extremity fractures, and critical illness. Prophylaxis with subcutaneous low-molecular-weight heparin or low-dose unfractionated heparin, in combination with lower extremity intermittent pneumatic venous compression devices, is recommended. Heparin products do not cross the placental barrier and are considered safe during pregnancy. While warfarin products are contraindicated during pregnancy, patients may be transitioned to warfarin postpartum.

Acute deep venous thrombosis (DVT) should be treated with full anticoagulation doses of heparin. While both unfractionated heparin and low-molecular-weight heparin are considered safe and effective during pregnancy, the ability to titrate continuous infusion heparin has advantages with acute traumatic injury and the potential need for unplanned delivery.

The method of radiological diagnosis for pulmonary embolism (PE) remains controversial.[24] Winer-Muram et al. showed that the average fetal dose of ionizing radiation from a helical thoracic CT scan for PE is less than that with ventilation-perfusion lung scanning and was safe in all three trimesters.[25] The utility of inferior vena caval filters for PE prophylaxis and the safety of thrombolytic agents for severe cases of PE have not been well studied.

Intra-Abdominal Infection

While unnecessary laparotomy may have a risk for maternal and fetal morbidity, missed gastrointestinal injury may result in greater complications. Intra-abdominal infection is particularly harmful to the fetus, and aggressive surgical or interventional therapy should be considered. Antibiotic therapy should be administered with infectious diseases and pharmacy consultation, since many agents may have adverse effects on the fetus. Empiric antibiotic selection should consider both the likely etiologic organisms and the safety for the fetus.

Mortality

Reported fetal mortality rates due to trauma vary, but are as high as 61% for major trauma and 80% for maternal shock. Even minor trauma is associated with a 1%–5% fetal mortality. The incidence of significant maternal and fetal injury increases with gestational age, with slightly over 50% of injuries occurring in the third trimester. The most common cause of fetal death is maternal death followed by placental abruption. The most common mechanism associated with mortality for both mother and fetus is the MVC. This mechanism alone accounts for 82% of fetal deaths. It should be noted that the fetal death rate is affected by maternal age, with peak fetal death rates in mothers aged 15–19.[26] This may reflect the greater propensity for patients in that age group to participate in risk-taking behavior such as alcohol and substance abuse, with an increased incidence of both MVCs and interpersonal violence.

The single most important measure to be taken to reduce mortality among pregnant women is the promotion of seatbelt use. The use of seatbelts results in a significant decrease in maternal (and hence fetal) mortality. It has been shown that along with crash severity, the use of seatbelts is the best predictor of maternal and fetal outcome.[27] Three-point restraints should be used with the belt low on the pelvis, below the uterine fundus, with the shoulder belt placed between the breasts.

CONCLUSIONS

The evaluation and treatment of the pregnant trauma patient represents a significant challenge to the trauma team. Optimization of the outcome depends on an understanding of the physiologic changes that occur in pregnancy as well as a firm grasp of the strategies that are necessary to assess both the mother and the fetus. Care must be maternally directed at the outset, since the best way to save the fetus is to save the mother. Fetal monitoring of third trimester pregnancies is essential in the early detection of both premature labor and fetal

distress. Finally, a multidisciplinary approach, with early involvement of consultants from obstetrics, is an essential element of successful care.

References

1. Lavery JP, Staten-McCormick M: Management of moderate to severe trauma in pregnancy. *Obstet Gynecol Clin North Am* 22:69–90, 1995.
2. Baerga-Varela Y, Zietlow SP, Bannon MP, et al: Trauma in pregnancy. *Mayo Clinic Proc* 75(12):1243–1248, 2000.
3. Van Hook JW: Trauma in pregnancy. *Clin Obstet Gynecol* 45(2):414–424, 2002.
4. Shah KH, Simons RK, Holbrook T, et al: Trauma in pregnancy: maternal and fetal outcomes. *J Trauma* 45(1):83–86, 1998.
5. McFarlane J, Campbell JC, Sharps P, et al: Abuse during pregnancy and femicide: urgent implications for women's health. *Obstet Gynecol* 100(1): 27–36, 2002.
6. American College of Surgeons: *Advanced Trauma Life Support Course for Physicians*, 5th ed. Chicago, American College of Surgeons, 1993.
7. Metcalfe J, McAnulty JH, Ueland K: Cardiovascular physiology. *Clin Obstet Gynecol* 24:693–710, 1981.
8. Clark SL, Cotton DB, Lee W, et al: Central hemodynamic assessment of normal term pregnancy. *Am Obstet Gynecol* 161:1439–1442, 1989.
9. Knudson MM, Rozycki GS, Strear CM: Reproductive system trauma. In Mattox KL, Feliciano DV, Moore EE, editors: *Trauma*, 4th ed. New York, McGraw-Hill, 2000, pp. 879–906.
10. Yeomans ER, Gilstrap LC III: Physiologic changes in pregnancy and their impact on critical care. *Crit Care Med* 33:S256–S258, 2005.
11. Elkus R, Popovich J Jr: Respiratory physiology in pregnancy. *Clin Chest Med* 13:555–565, 1992.
12. Awe RJ, Nicotra MB, Newsom TD, et al: Arterial oxygenation and alveolar-arterial gradients in term pregnancy. *Obstet Gynecol* 197953: 182–186, 1979.
13. Goodwin H, Holmes JF, Wisner DH: Abdominal ultrasound examination in pregnant blunt trauma patients. *J Trauma* 50(4):689–694, 2001.
14. Bochicchio GV, Haan J, Scalea TM: Surgeon-performed focused assessment with sonography for trauma as an early screening tool for pregnancy after trauma. *J Trauma* 52(6):1125–1128, 2002.
15. Barraco RD, Chiu WC, Clancy, et al: Practice management guidelines for the diagnosis and management of injury in the pregnant patient. The EAST Practice Management Guidelines Work Group, Eastern Association for the Surgery of Trauma World Wide Web site. http://www.east.org/tpg/pregnancy.pdf.
16. American College of Obstetricians and Gynecologists Committee: Opinion #299: guidelines for diagnostic imaging during pregnancy. *Obstet Gynecol* 104:647, 2004.
17. Wakeford R, Little MP: Risk coefficients for childhood cancer after intrauterine irradiation: a review. *Int J Rad Biol* 79(5):293–299, 2003.
18. Rogers FB, Rozycki GS, Osler TM, et al: A multi-institutional study of factors associated with fetal death in injured pregnant patients. *Arch Surg* 134(11):1274–1277, 1999.
19. Mattox KL, Goetzl L: Trauma in pregnancy. *Criti Care Med* 33(10): S385–S389, 2005.
20. Chiu WC, Shanmuganathan K, Mirvis SE, et al: Determining the need for laparotomy in penetrating torso trauma: a prospective study using triple-contrast enhanced abdominopelvic computed tomography. *J Trauma* 51:860–869, 2001.
21. Morris JA Jr, Rosenbower TJ, Jurkovich GJ, et al: Infant survival after cesarean section for trauma. *Ann Surg* 223:481–491, 1996.
22. Rose PG, Strohm PL, Zuspan FP: Fetomaternal hemorrhage following trauma. *Am Obstet Gynecol* 153:844–847, 1985.
23. Drost TF, Rosemurgy AS, Sherman HF, et al: Major trauma in pregnant women: maternal/fetal outcome. *J Trauma* 30:574–578, 1990.
24. Moore J, Baldisseri MR: Amniotic fluid embolism. *Crit Care Med* 33: S279–S285, 2005.
25. Winer-Muram HT, Boone JM, Brown HL, et al: Pulmonary embolism in pregnant patients: fetal radiation dose with helical CT. *Radiology* 224: 487–492, 2002.
26. Weiss HB, Songer TJ, Fabio A: Fetal deaths related to maternal injury. *JAMA* 286(15):1863–1868, 2001.
27. Pearlman MD, Klinich KD, Schneider LW, et al: A comprehensive program to improve safety for pregnant women and fetuses in motor vehicle crashes: a preliminary report. *Am Obstet Gynecol* 182:1554–1564, 2000.

Trauma in the Elderly

Benjamin Braslow, Donald R. Kauder, and C. William Schwab

The age at which a person becomes elderly has not been resolved by a clear consensus in the literature, but most agree that it falls in the span between ages 55 and 75. According to the 2000 census, 35 million (12.4%) Americans were over age 65, and by 2050, this age cohort is projected to reach 86 million (20.7%). The elderly constitute the most rapidly growing segment of the U.S. population. Today's elderly enjoy a level of physical freedom unmatched by prior generations. Improved access to health care and assisted living communities allow many older Americans to function relatively independently well into their ninth decade. Traumatic injuries very often compromise this autonomy, creating dependence on relatives or caregivers for assistance with activities of daily living. Unfortunately, a number of physical factors predispose the elderly to injury, including diminished postural stability, motor strength, coordination, visual acuity, and hearing. These common changes often lead to an inability to recognize and avoid many environmental hazards, thus converting normal daily activities into treacherous and frequently lethal events. In direct correlation with this rapid expansion of this sector of the population, hospitals are treating increased numbers of geriatric trauma patients. In 2001, over 3.2 million elderly patients who sustained unintentional injuries were evaluated in U.S. emergency departments; 2.2 million (68.7%) were admitted. These patients have been shown to have more adverse outcomes, including case fatality rates and complications. In 2002, unintentional injury was the fifth leading cause of death in the United States overall and the ninth leading cause of death in those aged 65 and older, accounting for over 33,000 victims. Survivors exhibit a higher prevalence of functional impairment, often requiring longer hospital stays and complex discharge arrangements. Not surprisingly, the elderly, comprising just over one-tenth of the population, account for nearly one-third of health care resources expended on trauma.

PHYSIOLOGY

There are numerous physiologic changes that influence the treatment of injury in elderly patients. With advancing age there is a normal, unavoidable, progressive loss of functional reserve in each organ system. The degree of loss is subject to individual variations and is distinct from the pathologic loss of function associated with comorbid diseases prevalent in senescence. Such conditions include but are not limited to hypertension, pulmonary disease, cardiovascular disease, diabetes, and renal failure. This combination of diminished reserve and concomitant disease significantly limits the ability of the elderly trauma patient to absorb physical insult and subsequently recover. It also impacts the care rendered to such patients at every level of intervention, from prehospital provider to trauma surgeon to surgical intensivist to physical therapist.

Most significantly, the cardiovascular system demonstrates age-related changes that affect the elderly patient's response to severe trauma. With age there is a progressive loss of myocytes and a compensatory increase in myocyte volume in both ventricles along with fat cell infiltration in the interstitial space of the ventricular walls and septum. The myocardium progressively stiffens, resulting in decreased diastolic relaxation and slowed ventricular filling. The heart becomes less efficient, with a progressive decrease in its ejection fraction. Stroke volume is diminished, leading to an increased reliance on the atrial contribution to increase end-diastolic volume in order to maintain cardiac output. The heart can be extremely sensitive to both hypovolemia and hypervolemia, resulting in a very narrow therapeutic window. Further, there is a decreased inotropic and chronotropic response to both endogenous and exogenous beta-adrenergic stimulation and progressive deterioration of the conducting system by cell atrophy, fibrosis, and calcification. This ultimately leads to a lowering of the maximal achievable heart rate and of the ability to adequately increase cardiac output during stress. Structural changes in the arterial tree also affect cardiac function in the elderly. Arterial intimal hyperplasia with concomitant atherosclerosis produces stiffness of the arterial walls, resulting in a reduction of diastolic pressure despite systolic hypertension and limiting coronary blood flow. This becomes most clinically important during stress, when myocardial oxygen demand increases but coronary blood flow is restricted. Prescription antihypertensive medications such as beta-blockers, calcium channel blockers, and diuretics—all very commonly prescribed for the elderly population—can also play a major role in the impairment of the cardiovascular response to stress and injury. The multifaceted age-related decline in cardiovascular function makes it incumbent upon the treating trauma physician to carefully plan treatment regimens and closely monitor this patient population during resuscitation.

The aging process significantly affects pulmonary physiology as well. With age, costal cartilage becomes calcified and the chest wall becomes more rigid, decreasing lung compliance. Respiratory muscles atrophy, and an increased reliance on diaphragm function and abdominal musculature for breathing develops. Forced vital capacity is decreased, as is forced expiratory volume in one second (FEV_1). Lung parenchymal changes are noted with aging as well. Fusion of adjacent alveoli occurs, which decreases surface tension forces and reduces pulmonary elastic recoil. Thickening of the alveolar basement membrane decreases gas-diffusing capability, resulting in V/Q mismatch and higher alveolar-arterial oxygen gradients. There is also decreased airway sensitivity and efficiency of the mucociliary clearance mechanism. A history of smoking compounds the deleterious affects of aging on pulmonary anatomy and function. Clinically, these changes manifest as decreased cough effectiveness, predisposition to aspiration and pneumonia, and decreased compensatory responses to hypoxia and hypercarbia. Aggressive pulmonary toilet, adequate pain control, judicious use of mechanical ventilation, and careful monitoring of fluid status become imperative in preventing pulmonary complications in the elderly trauma population.

Anatomic changes evident in the elderly kidney include cortical mass loss secondary to glomerulosclerosis (acellular obliteration of glomerular capillary architecture) and tubular senescence. Hypertension, diabetes mellitus, and atherosclerosis accelerate these processes. Physiologically, these changes manifest as a reduced glomerular filtration rate (GFR). After the age of 40 years, the GFR decreases 1 ml/min/year. Tubular senescence blunts the reabsorption and secretion of solutes. Most significant is the decreased capacity to reabsorb sodium and to secrete potassium and hydrogen ions. The juxtaglomerular apparatus in elderly patients produces less renin and limits the response to aldosterone. The response to antidiuretic hormone is also attenuated. All of these changes mandate hypervigilant monitoring of fluid, electrolyte, and acid base balance in the injured elderly patient, especially those requiring surgery, during which massive fluid shifts are expected. Yet another factor leading to hypovolemia is a decreased thirst response, which often predisposes them to hypovolemia. Predicting decreased renal function in the acute setting can be difficult. A reduction in muscle mass with age often results in a normal serum creatinine despite a reduced creatinine clearance. Age-adjusted formulas for creatinine clearance are much better estimates of renal function in the elderly patient than serum creatinine levels. Potentially nephrotoxic agents, such as intravenous radiographic contrast, should be used with extreme caution even if serum creatinine levels appear within normal limits.

Significant age-related changes also occur in the central nervous system. Cortical atrophy progresses with age, resulting in an increased volume of the subdural space. This allows for greater movement of the brain during traumatic impact, which can result in serious parenchymal damage. Relatively minor mechanisms of injury may result in more frequent subdural and subarachnoid hemorrhage secondary to greater shearing forces on parasagittal bridging veins. Large volumes of blood may accumulate intracranially before symptoms of intracranial hypertension develop. This process is compounded by the frequent use of anticoagulant and/or antiplatelet medications in this population for a variety of prophylactic and therapeutic indications. Likewise, a greater degree of brain swelling may occur before symptoms appear. Vision, auditory function, vibrotactile sensation, reflex timing, and pain perception are all blunted with age. These changes, in combination with age-related deterioration in cognitive ability, memory, and information processing, not only contribute to an increased predisposition to injury in the elderly, but also may obscure their post-traumatic evaluation.

Changes in the musculoskeletal system have significant impact on the elderly patient's predisposition to injury. There is a progressive loss of muscle mass and strength with age. Loss of motor neurons, collagen and adipocyte infiltration, and diminished myosin-ATP activity are also contributing factors. Progressive erosion of cartilage and ligamentous stiffening, especially in weight-bearing joints, affects mobility and can be a source of chronic pain. Attempts at postural compensation can alter weight-bearing mechanics and cause injury to other musculoskeletal structures. Age-related bone loss secondary to osteoporosis causes further loss of strength and greater susceptibility to fracture, most commonly seen in the hip, pelvis, wrist, and ribs. Vertebral collapse is associated with progressive kyphosis, which alters the center of gravity and contributes to balance disturbances. This process is more pronounced in women but is relevant to both sexes. Women lose up to 35% of cortical bone mass and 50% of trabecular bone mass over their lifetime; men lose about one-third less. These changes in strength and flexibility contribute to progressive limitation of movement, making the elderly patient more vulnerable to injury and complicating the recovery process.

Neurohumoral senescence is also quite common. There is a global decreased sympathetic response to stress in the elderly. This is multifactorial, related to neurologic, musculoskeletal, and endocrine alterations associated with age. Thermoregulation is impaired secondary to a decreased cutaneous vasoconstriction response to cold environments, which renders the elderly trauma patient more susceptible to hypothermia. Immune function also shows an age-related decline, specifically related to T-lymphocyte-mediated immunity. The response of T lymphocytes to interleukin 2 is impaired, as is the stress-related increase in natural killer-cell activity. These changes increase the elderly trauma patient's susceptibility to infection. Furthermore, markers of the systemic response to surgical stress (tumor necrosis factor α, interleukin 6, and CD11b/CD18 expression) have been shown to be more elevated after surgical stress in older (compared with younger) patients. This increase in cytokine response to surgical stress has been postulated to increase the incidence of systemic inflammatory response syndrome in the elderly and may explain an increased incidence of postoperative morbidity.

MECHANISM OF INJURY

Blunt trauma accounts for the overwhelming majority of geriatric injuries, with falls being the most common mechanism. The Center for Disease Control reported over 3.6 million geriatric fall-related injuries in 2003. Although multilevel falls do occur in the elderly population, same-level falls predominate. Interestingly, the associated morbidity of these low-level falls in the elderly is significant, producing a spectrum of injuries similar to those seen in falls from a height. It is estimated that 28%–45% of elderly people residing in the community and 45%–61% of elderly nursing home residents will fall each year. Falls are the leading cause of injury-related death in people over 75 years of age and are second only to motor vehicle crashes in those between 65 and 74 years. Although elderly men and women seem to fall with the same frequency, serious injuries are twice as common among women. This is likely because of their more extensive osteoporosis and decreased muscle mass. When compared with a younger population, elderly fall victims sustain more severe injuries over multiple body regions for similar mechanisms of injury. Most concerning is the fact that half of all hospitalized elderly fall victims who fall at home are subsequently discharged to a nursing home. Common risk factors for falls include inappropriate use of assist devices, alterations in gait, declines in proprioceptive and vestibular function, peripheral neuropathies, and overall loss of strength and coordination. Many medications may be implicated as well, especially those that may induce hypotension (beta-blockers, calcium channel blockers, etc.) or sedation (sleeping pills, anxiolytics, etc.). Approximately 25% of falls in the elderly are caused by an underlying medical problem, mandating medical investigation beyond simply treating the injuries sustained in the fall. Implementation of fall-intervention programs, modification of environmental hazards (repair of loose carpets, improved lighting, appropriate placement of grip bars), modification of medicine doses and schedules, use of mobility aids (walkers, wheelchairs, canes), and participation in physical strength and conditioning programs were shown to reduce fall incidence rates at participating elderly residence facilities from 2.9 to 1.7 per person year for active seniors.

Motor vehicle crashes are the second most common mechanism of injury leading to death following geriatric trauma, totaling over 7200 deaths in 2001. In 2003, there were 19.8 million older licensed drivers in the United States (10% of all licensed drivers compared with 9% in 1993), an increase of 27% since 1993. According to the National Highway Traffic Safety Administration, drivers aged 65–74 years old have the second highest rate of vehicular crash fatalities, falling just behind drivers aged 16–20. Despite driving less frequently and over shorter distances, drivers older than 75 years have the highest incidence of traffic fatalities per mile driven. The elderly are more likely to be involved in crashes in good weather and at a location close to home. Most traffic fatalities involving older drivers occur in daylight, on a weekday, and involve at least one other vehicle. Age-related impairment of driving skills, including diminished visual acuity and delayed reaction times, no doubt contributes to this increased crash rate. Luckily, this is countered by the relative absence of other significant causative factors such as speeding and intoxication. Older drivers involved in fatal crashes have the lowest proportion of intoxication of all adult drivers. Geriatric drivers involved in a motor vehicle crash should be evaluated as to their physical and cognitive abilities and counseled on driving restrictions and the need for frequent ongoing assessment.

Declines in peripheral vision, hearing, judgment, gait speed, and reaction time put older pedestrians at considerable risk for being struck by moving vehicles; they account for 18% of all pedestrian fatalities. The pedestrian struck death rate for this age group (3.17 per 100,000) is higher than for any other age group. Recent studies show that regarding injuries to a pedestrian struck, age plays a critical role in the anatomic distribution and severity of injuries. Older victims are significantly more likely to suffer severe injuries, especially to the head and chest. Severe abdominal trauma, spinal injuries, and fractures of the pelvis and tibia also increase significantly with age. One causative mediator of elderly pedestrian injury might be that the standard time allotted for most crosswalks in the United States assumes a walking speed of 4 feet per second, which is often unobtainable in this population. This correlates with the observation that one-third of all pedestrian fatalities in individuals over 65 years occurred within a crosswalk, double that of other pedestrians. Municipal identification of particularly dangerous intersections can result in crosswalk modification to provide better visibility, longer crossing times, and more appropriate danger notification to both drivers and pedestrians.

The elderly population is especially vulnerable to violent crime, both in and out of the home. Violent assaults account for approximately 10% of all geriatric trauma admissions. Although the elderly comprise only about 6% of all assault victims in this country, they are five times more likely to die as a result of their attack as compared with their younger counterparts. Decreased mobility and strength and impaired cognition and judgment are major factors that contribute to the inability of the elderly to adequately defend themselves. Attacks on the elderly primarily involve blunt instruments. Penetrating injuries via knife or firearm are increasing in frequency in the United States and were recently reported by the Center for Disease Control and Prevention to account for over 50% of assault related fatal injuries in the elderly.

Domestic abuse is unfortunately a growing source of nonaccidental trauma in the elderly. The true magnitude of this problem is clouded by variances in legal definitions and reporting accuracy. The National Aging Resource Center on Elder Abuse estimated in 1998 that only 1 in 15 cases of geriatric abuse is reported. Often this is a result of denial on the part of the victim as well as the abuser. Over 2 million cases of elder abuse and/or neglect are thought to occur annually in the United States, involving up to 6% of the elderly population. Longer life expectancy coupled with altered family dynamics and financial difficulties are frequent reasons for such mistreatment. Elderly females experience abuse more often than males, and persons older than 80 are abused two to three times more often than those between 65 and 80. Similar to child abuse, detection mandates a high degree of suspicion, especially when there are signs of physical injury or neglect that are inconsistent with the mechanism described.

Sadly, self-inflicted injury in the elderly is not a rare event. Depression secondary to the death of a loved one, chronic illness, and unmitigated pain are common reasons given for self-inflicted injury in the elderly population. Of the more than 11,000 geriatric self-inflicted injuries reported in this country in 2001, 48% resulted in mortality. In over half of these self-inflicted deaths, a firearm was used.

Burns account for approximately 8% of traumatic deaths in the elderly. Geriatric patients often have decreased cutaneous sensation and diminished reaction times. They are more likely to experience prolonged thermal exposure and to sustain more extensive and more severe burns than younger patients at the same scene. Scalding is the most common form of burn injury in the elderly, typically from bath water. Not surprisingly, elderly burn victims have a higher mortality rate for the same extent of burn than do younger patients. Burns exceeding 50% of total body surface area are almost uniformly fatal in elderly victims. Inhalation injury is poorly tolerated in the geriatric burn population secondary to limited pulmonary reserve and, if present, can increase the already prominent mortality rate. The same is true of the cardiovascular system with respect to the massive volume resuscitation that is required for optimal burn management. Cardiac intolerance is frequently implicated in early post-burn death in the elderly.

OUTCOMES

Both short- and long-term outcomes after trauma are worse in geriatric patients when compared with their younger counterparts. A higher prevalence of pre-existing medical conditions in the elderly patient as well as a reduced physiologic reserve are thought to account for these poor outcomes. Elderly trauma victims poorly tolerate hemodynamic instability or the increased physiologic demands that often accompany even minor trauma or its complications. Geriatric patients have been shown to have increased rates of cardiac, respiratory, renal, and infectious complications during hospitalization when compared with younger patients. As expected, the most severely injured patients and the patients with the most significant pre-existing conditions manifest the most nosocomial complications, which negatively impact survival. More than 33% of patients over 65 years of age have at least one chronic medical condition. Gubler et al. showed that the increased risk of death in elderly trauma patients persists for up to 5 years from the time of hospitalization for injury. In this study of over 9400 elderly patients, the presence of any pre-existing comorbidity was shown to increase the risk of mortality within those 5 years following hospitalization for an injury between 2 and 8.4 times, depending on the number of comorbid diagnoses. Pre-existing conditions such as liver disease, renal disease, malignancy, congestive heart failure, and a prior spinal cord injury have been shown in multiple studies to increase the risk of death in elderly trauma patients with minor injury severity scores (ISS). This relationship does not appear to hold for more severely injured patients. As a patient's ISS rises above 15, chronic medical conditions cease to have a significant effect on outcomes; and above 25, survival becomes a primary function of the severity of injury. Grossman et al. identified an ISS of 30 as "LD_{50}" (50% of the geriatric population that sustained this magnitude of injury died) for blunt geriatric trauma independent of mechanism or comorbidities. Interestingly, Perdue et al. found that despite controlling for ISS, Revised Trauma Score (RTS), pre-existing disease, and the development of complications, elderly patients were almost five times more likely to die after trauma than younger patients.

The high morbidity and mortality rates seen in geriatric trauma have led some authors to advocate routine admission to the intensive care unit and invasive hemodynamic monitoring (pulmonary artery catheters, arterial lines, central venous pressure monitors) for elderly patients with predicted ISS of over 9, any evidence of hypoperfusion, or significant pre-existing disease. Scalea et al. compared elderly, multiply injured trauma patients who appeared clinically stable after initial evaluation and underwent early invasive monitoring and goal-directed resuscitation with historical controls. Forty-three percent of patients were found to be in cardiogenic shock and showed further evidence of a systemic low flow state despite initial "normal" vital signs. With early intervention, mortality was reduced by half. Schultz et al. showed this benefit in a randomized trial of elderly patients with isolated hip fractures. Patients who received perioperative invasive monitoring had a tenfold reduction in postoperative mortality when compared with controls.

Despite their initially higher mortality rate, and the increased likelihood of dying within the 5-year period following injury, a significant number of elderly patients who survive their acute injury are able to eventually return to levels of reasonable function and resume independent living. In an analysis of nearly 39,000 elderly trauma patients in Pennsylvania, Richmond et al. showed that overall, more than half (52%) of those discharged from the hospital went directly home. Twenty-five percent were discharged to a skilled nursing facility (SNF), and 20% went to a rehabilitation facility. Grossman et al. showed a predisposition for those patients aged more than 80 years to require SNF placement (37%), whereas patients aged 65–79 more frequently returned home (53%). It is estimated that 50% of geriatric trauma patients discharged to a SNF eventually return home, and on average about 63% of patients discharged home with assistance will eventually return to some reasonable level of independent living. Often, home care agencies, spouses, and family members play an integral role in allowing patients to remain living at home.

MANAGEMENT OF SPECIFIC ORGAN INJURIES

The nonoperative management of splenic injuries has become a well-established practice in hemodynamically stable patients. Splenectomy has been all but eliminated in the pediatric trauma population, and its incidence is quite low in young adults. However, this strategy remains controversial in patients older than 55 years. This reluctance dates back to early reports by Smith and Godley demonstrating high failure rates in this population. Anatomic explanations of this have indicated that older spleens have a weakened capsule and fragile vasculature secondary to a decrease in the amount of smooth muscle and elastin fibers. This prevents older spleens from adequately contracting and retracting damaged vessels within the injured parenchyma. More recent published results of nonoperative management of splenic injury in older patients have challenged age 55 and older as an exclusion criterion, with reported success rates up to 80%. Despite these published successes, a recent large, multicenter study sponsored by the Eastern Association for the Surgery of Trauma concluded that older patients fail this nonoperative approach more often than their younger counterparts, and those who do so suffer increased mortality and morbidity. Factors associated with an increased risk of failure of nonoperative management of splenic injury include higher grade injuries (grades IV and V), a contrast blush or pseudoaneurysm seen on computed tomography (CT) scans, combined liver and splenic injuries, and the need for multiple blood transfusions. Although the optimal management of geriatric blunt splenic injuries is still a matter of debate, the limited physical reserve of the elderly patient must be carefully considered when determining an individualized plan of care. Knowing that hypotension is poorly tolerated in this population has led many surgeons to consider splenectomy as the more conservative approach.

Blunt chest injury and rib fractures are commonly encountered in the geriatric trauma patient and can account for a significant amount of morbidity and even mortality. Aside from treating the inherent complications associated with pneumothorax, hemothorax, and pulmonary contusion, managing chest wall pain is imperative in this population, the goal being to minimize chest wall splinting and maximize pulmonary effort. Inadequate pain control in the setting of decreased pulmonary reserve or underlying intrinsic lung disease can have devastating clinical consequences. Older trauma patients with isolated thoracic trauma suffer increased rates of acute respiratory distress syndrome and symptomatic pleural effusions, and have three times the risk of developing pneumonia when compared with their younger counterparts. For the elderly, in-hospital mortality increases in a linear fashion, with the number of rib fractures present starting at about 10% for one to two ribs fractured and approaching 40% when seven or more ribs are involved. Providing adequate analgesia to support deep breathing and coughing so as to limit atelectasis and hypoxia and to clear secretions is the mainstay of care but can be very difficult to achieve. Use of parenteral narcotics, while usually effective, can be dangerous if not closely titrated and monitored. Oversedation can result in hypoventilation, leading to hypercarbia and hypoxia. In a population already predisposed to coronary ischemia, hypoxia, even for brief periods, can be lethal. Oversedation also interferes with pulmonary toilet efforts and can lead to aspiration complicated by chemical pneumonitis or pneumonia. Ileus is also a common untoward effect of systemic narcotic analgesia. Many recent reports show significant decreases in pulmonary complications and mortality with the use of epidural analgesia compared with parenteral analgesia. Bulger et al. found that when comparing elderly patients with rib fractures who did not receive epidural analgesia with those who did, the mortality rate decreased from 25% to 11%. A randomized study by Ullman et al. showed a statistically significant decrease in length of intensive care unit stay, duration of mechanical ventilatory assistance, and hospital length of stay with epidural analgesia use. These benefits were achieved with few complications and lower overall hospital costs.

Elderly patients receiving oral anticoagulant therapy, including warfarin, clopidogrel, and aspirin, present a particularly difficult clinical challenge to the trauma surgeon. These medications are most commonly prescribed for a variety of prophylactic and therapeutic indications, including atrial fibrillation, prosthetic mechanical heart valves, pulmonary thromboembolism, previous deep venous thrombosis, and atherosclerotic coronary and/or peripheral vascular disease.

Common sense would dictate that patients taking the medications would suffer more severe bleeding and worse outcomes than patients with a normal coagulation profile, but this has not been consistently supported in the literature. However, the subset of anticoagulated older patients who have sustained traumatic intracranial bleeding clearly fare worse. A recent analysis by Mina et al. of patients on anticoagulation medications with intracranial injury found a near 40% mortality rate as compared with less than 10% for matched controls not receiving any anticoagulation. Anticoagulated patients presenting with suspected closed head injury should undergo expedient head CT scanning and reversal of their anticoagulation if bleeding pathology is identified. The ideal strategy for when and how to reverse anticoagulation after injury remains ill defined and is fraught with complex decisions regarding the risks and benefits of such therapy. Usually fresh frozen plasma and/or vitamin K is used in Coumadin reversal and for correction of the International Normalized Ratio (INR), whereas platelet transfusion and desmopressin serve to counter the antiplatelet effect of clopidogrel. Recently recombinant coagulation factors (i.e., Factor VIIa) and prothrombin complex concentrates have also demonstrated efficacy in the reversal of oral anticoagulant therapy, but their use in the elderly population is limited by the high risk of thrombotic complications.

The evaluation of spinal injury in the geriatric patient can also be clinically challenging. Pre-existing organic brain syndrome or pre-existing neurological deficits can further confound the diagnosis. Radiographic clearance can be equally difficult because of degenerative changes commonly present. Upper cervical injuries are predominant in the elderly population, with odontoid fractures being the most common. Age-related cervical spinal stenosis and increased osteophyte formation put older patients at especially high risk of central cord syndrome. This is seen most often following a forward fall with the chin striking an object or the floor, resulting in cervical hyperextension and acute pinching of the spinal cord. This results in bleeding in the more central regions of the spinal cord, producing preferential neurologic deficits in the upper extremities. Because there is often no concomitant bony injury, CT scanning can miss this diagnosis. In this clinical setting, magnetic resonance imaging becomes the imaging modality of choice to elucidate the injury. Prognosis for complete recovery following central cord syndrome is poor for older patients. In those over 70, bladder control and ambulatory function are restored only 20% and 40% of the time, respectively, and mortality can be in excess of 50%.

CONCLUSIONS

While geriatric patients have many physical and psychological factors predisposing them to injury and complicating their recovery, many have good outcomes and maintain a high quality of life after injury. Health care providers must pay careful attention to comorbidities and the potential impact of reduced physiologic reserve. Although the morbidity and mortality observed in the injured elderly population may be higher when viewed in the aggregate, each patient must be aggressively evaluated and managed with the goal of expedient return to the highest possible quality of life and level of functioning. When caring for the injured elderly, one must maintain a high index of suspicion for injury and a low threshold for aggressive invasive monitoring in an intensive care setting.

SUGGESTED READINGS

Aalami OO, Fang TD, Song HM, et al: Physiological features of aging persons. *Arch Surg* 138:1068–1076, 2003.

Bergeron E, Lavoie A, Clas D, et al: Elderly trauma patients, with rib fractures are at greater risk of death and pneumonia. *J Trauma* 54(3):478–485, 2003.

Bulger EM, Arneson MA, Mock CN, et al: Rib fractures in the elderly. *J Trauma* 48(6):1040–1047, 2000.

Grossman M, Scaff DW, Miller D, et al: Functional outcomes in octogenarian trauma. *J Trauma* 55(1):26–32, 2003.

Inaba K, Goecke M, Sharkey P, et al: Long-term outcomes after injury in the elderly. *J Trauma* 54(3):486–491, 2003.

Jacobs DG: Special considerations in geriatric injury. *Curr Opin Crit Care* 9:535–539, 2003.

Jacobs DG, Plaisier BR, et al: *Practice Management Guidelines for Geriatric Trauma.* east.org, Eastern Association for the Surgery of Trauma, 2001.

McGwin G, MacLennan PA, Fife JB, et al: Preexisting conditions and mortality in older trauma patients. *J Trauma* 56(6):1291–1296, 2004.

Perdue PW, Watts DD, Kaufmann CR, et al: Differences in mortality between elderly and younger adult trauma patients: geriatric status increases risk of delayed death. *J Trauma* 45(4):805–810, 1998.

Richmond TS, Kauder DR, et al: Characteristics and outcomes of serious traumatic injury in older adults. *J Am Geriatr Soc* 50:215–222, 2002.

Victorino GP, Chong TJ, Pal JD: Trauma in the elderly patient. *Arch Surg* 138:1093–1098, 2003.

Vyrostek SB, Annest JL, Ryan GW: Surveillance for fatal and non fatal injuries—United States, 2001. *MMWR Morb Mort Wkly Rep*53(SS07), 2004.

BURNS

Kimberly A. Davis   and   Richard L. Gamelli

The frequency of burn injury and its subsequent multisystem effects make the treatment of burn patients a commonly encountered management challenge for the trauma/critical care surgeon. The emergency surgery components of initial burn care include fluid resuscitation and ventilatory support, as well as preservation and restoration of remote organ function. Following appropriate resuscitation, burn patient management is focused on wound care and provision of the necessary metabolic support. The involvement of the emergency/trauma surgeon in burn wound management is dependent on the extent and depth of the wound and the rapid identification of those patients who are best cared for at a burn center.

INCIDENCE

The precise number of burns that occur in the United States each year is unknown because only 21 of 50 states mandate the reporting of burn injury. An estimated total number of burns has been obtained by extrapolation of those data. At present, 1.25 million is regarded as a realistic estimate of the annual incidence of burns in the United States, 80% of which involve less than 20% of the total body surface. Approximately 190–263 patients per million population are estimated to require admission to a hospital for burn care each year. In the population of burn patients requiring hospital care, there is a smaller subset of approximately 20,000 burn patients who, as defined by the American Burn Association (Table 1), are best cared for in a burn center each year. This subset consists of 42 patients per million population with major burns, and 40 patients per million population having lesser burns but a complicating cofactor.

MECHANISM OF INJURY

Certain populations are at high risk for specific types of injuries that require treatment by the trauma/critical care surgeon. Scald burns are the most frequent form of burn injury overall, causing 58% of burn injuries and over 100,000 emergency department visits annually. Sixty-five percent of children age 4 and under who require hospitalization for burn care have scald burns, the majority of which are due to contact with hot foods and liquids. The occurrence of accidental tap water scalds can be minimized by adjusting the temperature settings on hot water heaters or by installing special faucet valves that prevent delivery of water at unsafe temperatures. Scald burns with injury typically involving the feet, posterior legs, buttocks, and sometimes the hands are most often caused by immersion in scalding

water by an abusive caretaker. It is important that the trauma/critical care surgeon identify and report child abuse, because when abuse is undetected and the child is returned to the abusive environment, repeated abuse is associated with a high risk of fatality.

Fire and flame sources cause 34% of burn injuries and are the most common causes of burns in adults. One-fifth to one-quarter of all serious burns are related to employment. Kitchen workers are at relatively high risk for scald injury, and roofers and paving workers are at greatest risk for burns due to hot tar. Workers involved in plating processes and the manufacture of fertilizer are at greatest risk for injury due to strong acids, and those involved with soap manufacturing and the use of oven cleaners are at greatest risk of injury due to strong alkalis.

Electric current causes approximately 1000 deaths per year. Young children have the highest incidence of electric injury caused by household current as a consequence of inserting objects into an electrical receptacle or biting or sucking on electric cords and sockets. Adults at greatest risk of high-voltage electric injury are the employees of utility companies, electricians, construction workers (particularly those manning cranes), farm workers moving irrigation pipes, oil field workers, truck drivers, and individuals installing antennae. Lightning strikes result in an average of 107 deaths annually. The vast majority (92%) of lightning-associated deaths occur during the summer months among people engaged in outdoor activities such as golfing or fishing.

Abuse is a special form of burn injury, affecting the extremes of age. Child abuse is typically inflicted by parents but also perpetrated by siblings and child care personnel. The most common form of thermal injury abuse in children is caused by intentional application of a lighted cigarette. Burning the dorsum of a hand by application of a hot clothing iron is another common form of child abuse. Scald burns, as previously discussed, are also common. In recent years, elder abuse by caretakers or family members has become more common, and it too should be reported and the victim protected.

PATHOPHYSIOLOGY

Local Effects

The cutaneous injury caused by a burn is related to the temperature of the energy source, the duration of the exposure, and the tissue surface involved. At temperatures less than 45° C, tissue damage is unlikely to occur even with an extended period of exposure. In the adult, exposure for 30 seconds when the temperature is 54° C will cause a burn injury, while an identical burn will occur with only a 10-second exposure in a child. When the temperature is elevated to 60° C, a common setting for home water heaters, tissue destruction can occur in less than 5 seconds in children. It is not surprising, therefore, that significant injury can occur when patients come in contact with boiling liquids or live flames.

Table 1: Burn Center Referral Criteria

Partial-thickness burns involving more than 10% of the total body surface area

Full-thickness in any age group

Burns involving face, hands, feet, genitalia, perineum, or major joints

Significant electric burns, including lightning injury

Chemical burns

Inhalation injury

Burns in patients with pre-existing medical conditions that can complicate management, prolong recovery, or affect mortality

Lesser burns in association with concomitant trauma sufficient to influence outcome[a]

Any size burn in a child in a hospital without qualified personnel or the equipment needed for the care of children

Any size burn in a patient who will require special social or psychiatric intervention or long-term rehabilitation

[a]If the mechanical trauma poses the greater immediate risk, the patient may be stabilized and receive initial care at a trauma center before transfer to a burn center.
Adapted with permission from Stabilization, Transfer and Transport, Chapter 8. In *Advanced Life Burn Support Course Instructors Manual.* Chicago, American Burn Association, 2001, pp. 73–78.

Burn injury causes three zones of damage. Centrally located is the zone of coagulation. In a full-thickness burn, the zone of coagulation involves all layers of the skin, extending down through the dermis and into the subcutaneous tissue. In partial-thickness injuries, this zone extends down only into the dermis, and there are surviving epithelial elements capable of ultimately resurfacing the wound. Surrounding the zone of coagulation is an area of lesser cell injury, the zone of stasis. In this area, blood flow is altered but is restored with time as resuscitation proceeds. If patients are inadequately resuscitated, thrombosis can occur and the zone of stasis can be converted to a zone of coagulation. The most peripheral zone is an area of minimally damaged tissue, the zone of hyperemia, which abuts undamaged tissue. The zone of hyperemia is best seen in patients with superficial partial-thickness injuries as occur with severe sun exposure.

Along with the changes in wound blood supply, there is significant formation of edema in the burn-injured tissues. Factors elaborated in the damaged tissues and released as local mediators include histamine, serotonin, bradykinin, prostaglandins, leukotrienes, and interleukin-1, all of which cause alterations in local tissue homeostasis and increases in vascular permeability. Complement is also activated which can further modify transcapillary fluid flux. The net effect of these various changes is significant movement of fluid into the extravascular fluid compartment. Maximum accumulation of both water and protein in the burn wound occurs at 24 hours post injury and can persist beyond the first week post-burn. Additionally, patients who have greater than a 20%–25% body surface burn have similar fluid movement in undamaged tissue beds. This may be related in part to the changes in transcapillary fluid flux and also may be in response to the volume of resuscitation fluids administered.

Systemic Response

The physiologic response to a major burn injury results in some of the most profound changes that a patient is capable of enduring. The magnitude of the response is proportional to the burn size, reaching a maximum at about a 50% body surface area burn. The duration of the changes is related to the persistence of the burn wound and

therefore resolves with wound closure. The organ-specific response follows the pattern that occurs with other forms of trauma, with an initial level of hypofunction, the "ebb phase," followed by a hyperdynamic "flow" phase.

Changes in the cardiovascular response are critical and directly impact the initial care and management of the burn patient. Immediately following burn injury, there is a transient period of decreased cardiac performance and elevated peripheral vascular resistance, which can be exacerbated by inadequate volume replacement. Systemic hypoperfusion can result in further increases in systemic vascular resistances and reprioritization of regional blood flow. Failure to adequately resuscitate a burn patient worsens myocardial performance. Conversely, adequate resuscitation restores normal cardiac performance values within 24 hours of injury, and by the second 24 hours those values further increase to supranormal levels, resulting in a hyperdynamic state, which will revert back to more normal levels with wound closure.

Pulmonary changes following burn injury are the consequences of direct parenchymal damage that occurs with inhalation injury. In patients without inhalation injury, pulmonary changes following burn injury are reflective of the generalized hyperdynamic state of the patient. Lung ventilation increases in proportion to the total body surface area of the burn, with increases in both respiratory rate and tidal volume. Worsening of the burned patient's respiratory status should indicate a supervening process, including sepsis, pneumonia, occult pneumothorax, pulmonary embolism, congestive heart failure, or an acute intra-abdominal process. In patients without these events, pulmonary gas exchange is relatively preserved, and there is little change in pulmonary mechanics.

The renal response to burn injuries is largely dependent on the cardiovascular response. Initially there is a reduction in renal blood flow, which is restored with resuscitation. If a patient is underresuscitated, renal hypoperfusion will persist, with early onset renal dysfunction secondary to renal ischemia. This can be exacerbated if the patient exhibits myoglobinuria or hemoglobinuria, either of which is capable of causing direct tubular damage.

Burn injury is capable of affecting both gastrointestinal motility and mucosal integrity, usually as a result of underresuscitation leading to intestinal hypoperfusion. Conversely, patients who are massively resuscitated will have significant edema of the retroperitoneum, bowel mesentery, and bowel wall contributing to a paralytic ileus. With near-immediate initiation of enteral feedings, gastrointestinal motility can be preserved, mucosal integrity protected, and effective nutrient delivery achieved. Delay in the initiation of enteral feeding is associated with the onset of ileus, which can also occur when the burn resuscitation has been complicated.

From a neuroendocrine standpoint, burn injury results in an elevated hormonal and neurotransmitter response similar in magnitude to that of the "fight or flight" response. The duration of the neurohumoral response is prolonged and is exacerbated by surgical stress. The increases in glucocorticoids and catecholamines are necessary to support the stress response of the injured patient. When there is an insufficient stress hormone response, an otherwise survivable insult can become fatal. Many of the multisystem changes occurring post-burn can be related in part to the alterations in catecholamine secretion, particularly the changes in resting metabolic expenditures, substrate utilization, and cardiac performance. As wound closure is accomplished, the increased neurohumoral response abates and anabolic hormones become predominant.

Burn injury affects the hematopoietic system, resulting in the loss of balance in both leukocyte and erythrocyte production and function. Burns of greater than 20% of total body surface area are associated with both alterations in red cell production and increases in red cell destruction at the level of the cutaneous circulation, resulting in anemia. Such anemia can be further compounded by frequent phlebotomy, surgical blood loss, hemodilution due to resuscitation, and transient alterations in erythrocyte membrane integrity. Longer-term changes appear to be related to hyporesponsiveness of the erythroid progenitor cells in the bone marrow to erythropoietin. During the early stages of resuscitation, reductions in platelet number, depressed fibrinogen levels, and alterations in coagulation factors return to normal or near normal values with appropriate resuscitation. Changes in white cell number occur early, with an increase in neutrophils due to demargination and accelerated bone marrow release. With uncomplicated burn injury, bone marrow myelopoiesis is preserved.

In addition to the changes occurring in the bone marrow, there are significant further depressions in the immune response. Burn injury causes a global impairment in host defense. Alterations of the humoral immune response include reductions in IgG and IgM secretion, decreased fibronectin levels, and increases in complement activation. Cellular changes include alterations in T-cell responsiveness and cell populations, leading to alterations in antigen presentation and impairment of delayed-type hypersensitivity reactions. Leukocyte function is adversely affected. Granulocytes have been noted to have impaired chemotaxis, decreased phagocytic activity, decreased antibody-dependent cell cytotoxicity, and a relative impairment in their capacity to respond to a second challenge. The clinical significance of these observations is that the burn patient is at significant risk for post-burn infectious complications.

GRADING OF BURN WOUND DEPTH

The injuries that will be apparent on examination are the consequences of the level of tissue destruction. Wounds that are superficial are associated with hyperemia, fine blistering, increased sensation, and exquisite pain upon palpation. The wounds are hyperemic, warm, and readily blanch. These types of injuries represent first-degree burns or are alternatively termed superficial partial-thickness injuries. With a second degree or deeper partial-thickness burn, the wound presents with intact or ruptured blisters or is covered by a thin coagulum termed "pseudoeschar." The key physical finding is

preservation of sensation in the burned tissue, although it is reduced (Table 2). With proper care, superficial and even deeper partial-thickness injuries are capable of spontaneous healing without grafting. The risk of infection in deep partial-thickness wounds is significant, and if an infection develops it can lead to a greater depth of skin loss. A full-thickness wound occurs when the injury penetrates all layers of the skin or extends into the subcutaneous or deeper tissues. These wounds will appear pale or waxy, be anesthetic, dry, and inelastic, and contain thrombosed vessels. Occasionally in children or young women, the initial appearance of a wound may be more that of a brick red coloration. Such wounds will have significant edema and are inelastic and insensate. Full-thickness wounds are infection-prone wounds, as they no longer provide any viable barrier to invading organisms and if left untreated become rapidly colonized and a portal for invasive burn wound sepsis.

RESUSCITATION PRIORITIES

Fluid Administration

Immediately following burn injury, the changes induced in the cardiovascular system must receive therapeutic priority. In all patients with burns of more than 20% of the total body surface area and those with lesser burns in whom physiologic indices indicate a need for fluid infusion, a large-caliber intravenous cannula should be placed in an appropriately sized peripheral vein, preferably underlying unburned skin. If there are no peripheral veins available, central venous access is indicated. Lactated Ringer's solution should be infused at an initial rate of 1 liter/hr in the adult and 20 ml/kg/hr for children who weigh 50 kg or less. That infusion rate is adjusted following estimation of the fluid needed for the first 24 hours following the burn.

Resuscitation fluid needs are proportional to the extent of the burn (combined extent of partial- and full-thickness burns expressed

Table 2: Clinical Characteristics of Burn Injuries

	Partial-Thickness Burns		Full-Thickness Burns
	First Degree	**Second Degree**	**Third Degree**
Cause	Sun or minor flash	Higher intensity or longer exposure to flash Relatively brief exposure to hot liquids, flames	Higher intensity or longer exposure to flash Longer exposure to flames or "hot" liquids Contact with steam or hot metal High-voltage electricity Chemicals
Color	Bright red	Mottled red	Pearly white Translucent and parchment-like Charred
Surface	Dry No bullae	Moist Bullae present	Dry, leathery, and stiff Remnants of burned skin present Liquefaction of tissue
Sensation	Hyperesthetic	Pain to pin prick inversely proportional to depth of injury	Surface insensate Deep pressure sense retained
Healing	3–6 days	Time proportional to depth of burns, 10–35 days	Requires grafting

Source: Pruitt BA Jr, Gamelli RL: Burns. In Britt LD, Trunkey DD, Organ CH, Feliciano DV, editors: *Acute Care Surgery.* New York, Springer, 2007, pp. 128, with permission.

as a percentage of total body surface area) and are related to body size (most readily expressed as body weight) and age (the surface area per unit of body mass is greater in children than in adults). The patient should be weighed on admission and the extent of partial- and full-thickness burns estimated according to standard nomograms (Figure 1). The fluid needs for the first 24 hours can be estimated on the basis of the Advanced Burn Life Support and Advanced Trauma Life Support consensus formula (Table 3).

Because of the greater surface area per unit of body mass in children, the volume of fluid required for the first 24 hours is relatively greater than that for an adult. In all patients, one-half of the estimated volume should be administered in the first 8 hours after the burn. If the initiation of fluid therapy is delayed, the initial half of the volume estimated for the first 24 hours should be administered in the hours remaining before the 8th post-burn hour. The remaining half of the fluid is administered over the subsequent 16 hours.

The limited glycogen stores in a child may be rapidly exhausted by the marked stress hormone response to burn injury. Serum glucose levels in the burned child should be monitored, and 5% dextrose in lactated Ringer's administered if serum glucose decreases to

BURN ESTIMATE AND DIAGRAM
Age vs. area

Area	Birth–1 yr	1–4 yr	5–9 yr	10–14 yr	15 yr	Adult	2*	3*	Total	Donor areas
Head	19	17	13	11	9	7				
Neck	2	2	2	2	2	2				
Ant. trunk	13	13	13	13	13	13				
Post. trunk	13	13	13	13	13	13				
R. buttock	2½	2½	2½	2½	2½	2½				
L. buttock	2½	2½	2½	2½	2½	2½				
Genitalia	1	1	1	1	1	1				
R.U. arm	4	4	4	4	4	4				
L.U. arm	4	4	4	4	4	4				
R.L. arm	3	3	3	3	3	3				
L.L. arm	3	3	3	3	3	3				
R. hand	2½	2½	2½	2½	2½	2½				
L. hand	2½	2½	2½	2½	2½	2½				
R. thigh	5½	6½	8	8½	9	9½				
L. thigh	5½	6½	8	8½	9	9½				
R. leg	5	5	5½	6	6½	7				
L. leg	5	5	5½	6	6½	7				
R. foot	3½	3½	3½	3½	3½	3½				
L. foot	3½	3½	3½	3½	3½	3½				
						Total				

BURN DIAGRAM

Age_____

Sex_____

Weight_____

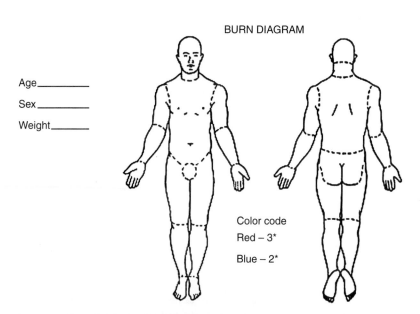

Color code
Red – 3*
Blue – 2*

Figure 1 Example of a form used for documenting extent of burn. Figure outlines are filled in with a blue pencil and a red pencil to indicate distribution of partial-thickness and full-thickness burns, respectively. Note the columns indicating how the percentage of total body-surface area represented by body-part surface changes with time. *(Used with permission from Martin RR, Becker WK, Cioffi WG, and Pruitt BP Jr: Thermal Injuries. In Wilson RF and Walt AJ, editors: Mangement of Trauma: Pitfalls and Practice, 2nd ed. Baltimore, Williams and Wilkins, 1996, p. 765.)*

Table 3: Fluid Required for the First 24 Hours Post-Burn

Adults = 2–4 ml LR/%TBSAB/Kg, BW
Children = 3–4 ml LR/%/TBSAB/Kg, BW + maintenance in children <30 kg

BW, Body weight; *LR,* lactated Ringer's; *TBSAB,* total body surface area burned.

hypoglycemic levels. In the case of small children with small burns, the resuscitation fluid volume as estimated on the basis of burn size may not meet normal daily metabolic requirements. In such patients, maintenance fluids should be added to the resuscitation regimen.

The infusion rate is adjusted according to the individual patient's response to the injury and the resuscitation regimen. The progressive edema formation in burned and even unburned limbs commonly make measurements of pulse rate, pulse quality, and even blood pressure difficult and unreliable as indices of resuscitation adequacy. Therefore, hourly urine output should be used as a measure of the adequacy of resuscitation. The fluid infusion rate is adjusted to obtain 30 ml of urine per hour in the adult and 1 mg/kg of body weight per hour in children weighing less than 30 kg. The administration of fluid is increased or decreased only if the hourly urinary output is one-third or more below, or 25% or more above, the target level for 2 successive hours. If in either adults or children the resuscitation volume infused in the first 12 hours will result in administration of 6 ml or more per percent of body surface area burned per kilogram of body weight in the first 24 hours, human albumin diluted to a physiologic concentration in normal saline should be infused and the volume of crystalloid solution reduced by a comparable amount.

Restoration of functional capillary integrity occurs at or near 24 hours after burn injury. Consequently, the volume of fluid needed for the second 24 hours post-burn is less, and colloid-containing fluids can be infused to reduce further volume and salt loading. Human albumin diluted to physiologic concentration in normal saline is the colloid-containing solution of choice, infused in a dosage of 0.3 ml per percent of burn per kilogram of body weight for patients with 30%–50% burns, 0.4 ml per percent of burn per kilogram of body weight for patients with 50%–70% burns, and 0.5 ml per percent of burn per kilogram of body weight for patients whose burns exceed 70% of the total body surface area. Water containing 5% dextrose is also given in the amount necessary to maintain an adequate urinary output. The colloid-containing fluids for children are estimated according to the same formula, but half normal saline is infused to maintain urinary output and avoid inducing physiologically significant hyponatremia by infusion of large volumes of electrolyte-free fluid into the relatively small intravascular and interstitial volume of the child. Fluid infusion "weaning" should also be initiated during this time period, to further minimize volume loading. In a patient who is assessed to be adequately resuscitated, the volume of fluid infused per hour should be arbitrarily decreased by 25%–50%. If urinary output falls below target level, the prior infusion rate should be resumed. If urinary output remains adequate, the reduced infusion rate should be maintained over the next 3 hours, at which time another similar fractional reduction of fluid infusion rate should be made. This decremental process will establish the minimum infusion rate that maintains resuscitation adequacy in the second post-burn day.

Fluid management after the first 48 hours post-burn should permit excretion of the retained fraction of the water and salt loads infused to achieve resuscitation, prevent dehydration, and electrolyte abnormalities, and allow the patient to return to pre-burn weight by post-burn day 8–10. Infusion of the large volumes of lactated Ringer's required for resuscitation commonly produces a weight gain of 20% or more and a reduction of serum sodium concentration to approximate that of lactated Ringer's—that is, 130 mEq/l. Correction of that relative hyponatremia is facilitated by the prodigious evaporative water loss from the surface of the burn wound, which is the major component of the markedly increased insensible water loss that is present following resuscitation. Inadequate replacement of insensible water loss makes hypernatremia the most commonly encountered electrolyte disturbance in the extensively burned patient following resuscitation. Such hypernatremia should be managed by provision of sufficient electrolyte-free water to allow excretion of the increased total body sodium mass and replace insensible water loss to the extent needed to prevent hypovolemia.

Electrolyte abnormalities are frequently encountered in the immediate post-burn period. Hyperkalemia is frequently encountered and is typically a laboratory sign of hemolysis but may also be a sign of muscle destruction by high-voltage electric injury or a particularly deep thermal burn. Hyperkalemia may also occur in association with acidosis in patients who are grossly under-resuscitated. In the case of patients with high-voltage electric injury, emergency debridement of nonviable tissue and even amputation may be necessary to remove the source of the potassium. Hypophosphatemia is also extremely common after burn resuscitation due to either prolonged administration of parenteral nutrition or failure to supply sufficient phosphate to meet the needs of tissue anabolism following wound closure. Hypophosphatemia can be prevented and treated by appropriate dietary phosphate supplementation.

Ventilatory Support

The most critical factor in the initial assessment of a burn patient is the patency of the airway and the ability of the patient to maintain and protect the airway. Standard criteria should be used to determine the need for mechanical stabilization of the airway, also keeping in mind the systemic response to a major burn and the local response to an airway injury which may combine to cause progressive airway swelling and edema that will impair air flow. Circumferential torso burns will further impair the ability of the patient to respire. Allowing airway compromise to proceed to a critical state before intubating the patient and stabilizing the airway is not appropriate care. The safest approach when there is concern about the airway, particularly in a patient needing transport for definitive care, is to perform early intubation.

Patients suffering both inhalation injuries and thermal burns have a significantly increased incidence of complications and probability of death. While an inhalation injury alone carries a mortality of 5%–8%, a combination of a thermal injury plus inhalation injury can easily result in a mortality 20% above that predicted on the basis of age and burn size. Injuries to the airway are due to the direct damage by the inhaled products of combustion that cause inflammation and edema. Damage to the oropharynx and upper airway is related to the heat content of the inhaled material. In the distal airways, however, injury is principally related to the particulate material contained within the smoke and the chemical composition of inhaled materials. Moist heat, which occurs with steam, has 4000 times the heat-carrying capacity of dry smoke and is capable of causing more extensive thermal damage of the tracheobronchial tree.

Presenting signs and symptoms of an inhalation injury are stridor, hypoxia, and respiratory distress. The probability that a patient has suffered an inhalation injury is highly correlated with being burned in an enclosed space, having burns of the head and neck, and having elevated carbon monoxide levels. The extent and severity of the inhalation injury are directly related to the duration of exposure and the types of toxins contained within the smoke, and exacerbates the ensuing host inflammatory response. Activation of the inflammatory cascade results in the recruitment of neutrophils and macrophages which propagate the injury. Altered surfactant release causes obstruction and collapse of distal airway segments. As part of the response to injury, there is a marked and near-immediate increase in bronchial artery blood flow, which is associated with marked alterations in vascular permeability within the lung. The net effect is that extensive destruction and inflammation reduce pulmonary compliance and impair gas exchange, resulting in altered pulmonary blood flow patterns and ventilation perfusion mismatches.

Part of the initial management of the patient with inhalation injury should include a thorough evaluation of the airway, including bronchoscopy. The clinical findings of an inhalation injury on bronchoscopy include airway edema, inflammation, increased bronchial secretions, presence of carbonaceous material which can diffusely carpet the airway, mucosal ulcerations and even endoluminal obliteration due to sloughing mucosa, mucous plugging, and cast formation. Signs of gastric aspiration may also be evident. Repeat bronchoscopy can be performed for removal of debris and casts as well as surveillance for infection.

Carbon monoxide and cyanide gases are present in smoke and when inhaled are rapidly absorbed and cause systemic toxicity as well as impaired oxygen utilization and delivery. Carbon monoxide is an odorless, nonirritating gas that rapidly diffuses into the bloodstream and has a 240-fold greater affinity for hemoglobin than does oxygen, thus easily displacing oxygen. The diagnosis of carbon monoxide poisoning is made in a burn patient on the basis of circumstances of injury, physical findings, and the measurement of blood carboxyhemoglobin level. It is important to note that pulse oximetry values do not differentiate between carboxyhemoglobin and oxyhemoglobin. Patients with significant carbon monoxide intoxication can have normal oxygen saturations but will not have satisfactory blood oxygen content. Signs and symptoms of carbon monoxide poisoning are typically mild to absent when carbon monoxide-hemoglobin (carboxyhemoglobin) levels are 10% or less. When carboxyhemoglobin levels are between 10% and 30%, symptoms are present and often manifested by headache and dizziness. Severe poisoning is seen in patients with carboxyhemoglobin levels of greater than 50%, which may be associated with syncope, seizures, and coma. The primary treatment modality for carbon monoxide intoxication is the administration of increased levels of inspired oxygen.

Cyanide poisoning, which can occur in combination with carbon monoxide intoxication, disrupts normal cellular utilization of oxygen by binding to the cytochrome oxidase and resulting in cellular lactic acid production and greater cellular dysfunction due to uncoupling of the oxidative phosphorylation system. Blood concentrations of cyanide greater than 0.5 mg/l are toxic. Treatment of cyanide poisoning includes the administration of oxygen as well as decontaminating agents such as amyl and sodium nitrates. These compounds induce the formation of methemoglobin, which can act as a scavenger of cyanide. Hydroxycobalamin is the antidote of choice.

The goal of mechanical ventilation following inhalation injury is to minimize further damage to the airway and lung parenchyma while providing adequate gas exchange. This is best achieved through careful control of airway pressures, thereby limiting ventilation-induced barotrauma. Lung damage following burn injury is not homogeneous but patchy in distribution and requires that the level of positive end expiratory pressure (PEEP) used to maximize airway recruitment be limited to avoid ventilator-induced lung injury. In severe lung injury, mechanical ventilation can lead to increases in alveolar sheer forces and changes in pulmonary blood flow. This, in association with reductions in elasticity and alterations in lung compliance, results in further lung injury and ventilation perfusion abnormalities.

For patients who have signs of inhalation injury on bronchoscopy, it is beneficial to initiate aggressive management of retained secretions with the use of bronchodilators and mucolytic agents. Meticulous control of airway pressure should be practiced, with the early performance of torso escharotomies and prompt treatment of abdominal compartment syndrome. Mean airway pressures should be maintained at less than 32–34 cm of water and chemical paralysis liberally used, with a low threshold for conversion to pressure-controlled ventilation with titration of tidal volumes to lessen further the risk of ventilator-induced barotrauma. This may require the acceptance of smaller than usual tidal volumes and permissive hypercapnia, which is acceptable as long as arterial blood pH is above 7.26 and the patient is hemodynamically stable.

Initial Wound Care

Initial wound care is focused on preventing further injury. Burning clothing should be removed, contact disrupted with metal objects that may retain heat, and only molten materials adherent to the skin surface should be cooled. Attempted cooling of burn wounds should not be done, as local vasoconstriction can impair wound blood flow and extend the depth of the injury, as well as exacerbate systemic hypothermia. Patients being prepared for transport or admitted for definitive care should be placed in sterile or clean, dry dressings and be kept warm. Items of clothing or jewelry should be removed prior to the onset of burn wound edema to prevent further compromise of the circulation. In cases of chemical injury, the removal of contaminated clothing with copious water lavage of liquid chemicals and removal by brushing of powdered materials at the scene can limit the extent of the resultant burn injury. No attempt should be made at chemical neutralization, as such treatment would result in an exothermic reaction and cause additional tissue damage. The care provider must exercise extreme caution when working with victims of chemical injury to prevent self-contamination and personal injury.

After admission to the hospital and as soon as resuscitative measures have been instituted, the burn wounds should cleansed with warm fluids and a detergent disinfectant like chlorhexidine gluconate, which has an excellent antimicrobial spectrum. During cleansing, hypothermia must be avoided. Materials that are densely adherent to the wound, such as wax, tar, plastic, and metal, should be gently removed or allowed to separate during the course of subsequent dressing changes. Sloughing skin, devitalized tissue, and ruptured blisters should be gently trimmed from the wound. Careful wound cleansing should be done at each dressing change, with serial debridement of devitalized tissue performed as necessary. The wound should be monitored for signs of infection and change in depth from the initial assessment.

The damaged skin surface can serve as the portal for microbial invasion if it becomes progressively colonized. As microbial numbers increase within the wound to levels of 100,000 organisms per gram of tissue, an invasive wound infection and ultimately systemic sepsis may occur. Topically applied antimicrobial agents, which penetrate the burn eschar, are capable of achieving sufficient levels to control microbial proliferation within the wound. Systemic antibiotics are not indicated, as they do not adequately penetrate eschar. Topical antimicrobial agents are used in the prophylactic treatment of the burn wound and as a part of the management of burn wound infections. Topical agents do not heal the wound but prevent local burn wound infection from destroying viable tissue in wounds capable of spontaneous healing.

Silver sulfadiazine, the most widely used agent, is available as a 1% suspension in a water-soluble micronized cream base. The cream is easily applied and causes little or no pain on application. The cream can be directly applied to the wound as a continuous layer and covered over with a dressing. At each dressing change, the cream should be totally removed and not allowed to form a caseous layer that will obscure the wound bed. The most common toxic side effect of silver sulfadiazine is a transient leukopenia which, when it does occur in up to 15% of treated patients, resolves spontaneously without discontinuation of the drug. Silver sulfadiazine is active against a wide range of microbes, including *Staphylococcus aureus*, *Escherichia coli*, *Klebsiella* sp., many but not all *Pseudomonas aeruginosa*, *Proteus* sp., and *Candida albicans*.

Mafenide acetate was one of the first effective topical agents introduced for the management of the burn wound. It was initially available as Sulfamylon® Burn Cream, which is highly effective against

Gram-positive and Gram-negative organisms but provides little antifungal activity. Mafenide acetate readily diffuses into the eschar and is the agent of choice for significant burns of the ears because it is also capable of penetrating cartilage. Drawbacks with the use of mafenide acetate include pain on application to partial-thickness burns, and limited activity against methicillin-resistant *S. aureus.* Mafenide acetate also inhibits carbonic anhydrase and may cause a self-limiting hyperchloremic acidosis. Mafenide acetate has more recently become available as a 5% aqueous solution and is an excellent agent to use on freshly grafted wounds and is not associated with the problems found with the cream formulation.

Silver nitrate as a 0.5% solution is effective against Gram-positive and Gram-negative organisms but does not penetrate the eschar. Silver nitrate solution leaches sodium, potassium, chloride, and calcium from the wound, in association with transeschar water absorption which can result in mineral deficits, alkalosis, and water loading. Those side effects can be minimized by giving sodium and other mineral supplements and modifying fluid therapy. These problems and the labor required to use silver nitrate effectively limit its routine use, and most see silver sulfadiazine as a highly acceptable alternative.

Silver-impregnated dressings have recently become available for clinical use. When the fabric base is in contact with wound fluids, the silver is released continuously and serves as the antimicrobial agent deposited onto the wound. The treatment interval with such a composite may extend up to several days depending on the fabrication design, with dressing changes needed only once or twice per week. The effectiveness of this membrane in treating extensive full-thickness burns is unconfirmed, and at present it is used to treat partial-thickness burns.

In superficial partial-thickness burns, the use of bacitracin ointment represents a satisfactory alternative, particularly in patients with a known sulfa allergy. It may be used open, especially with superficial facial burns or as a component of a closed dressing. Other topical agents include antibiotic combinations such as triple antibiotic ointment (neomycin, bacitracin zinc, and polymyxin B) and Polysporin (bacitracin zinc and polymyxin B). In the case of methicillin-resistant staphylococci, mupirocin is a useful agent.

The application of topical antimicrobial agents to the burns of patients who will be transferred to a burn center may preclude the use of biological membrane dressings that must adhere to the wound surface to be effective. Additionally, as soon as a patient is admitted to a burn center, any previously placed dressing must be removed to permit the burn team to make a precise assessment of the extent of the burn and the depth of injury. Unless there will be an extended period of time before the patient is transferred to a burn center, the preferred initial management entails placing the patient in a dry dressing, particularly one with a nonadherent lining, and keeping the patient warm.

Burn Wound Excision and Grafting

Excision of the burned tissue and grafting are required for wounds that are full thickness in depth; this treatment is also now considered the optimum management of wounds with a mixed depth of injury. Wounds that are capable of spontaneous closure within 2–3 weeks post-injury can be managed expectantly, provided the cosmetic and functional outcomes will be acceptable. Wounds needing excision and closure should undergo excision as soon as possible, as this reduces the period of disability and the overall cost of the injury. In patients with a large burn wound, the timing and extent of the surgery are based on the patient's relative physiologic stability and his or her capacity to undergo a major operative procedure. Early burn wound excision and closure in patients with large wounds shortens the length of hospitalization, reduces cost, and favorably impacts overall burn mortality.

Wounds that are small or linear in shape can be managed by excision of the burn and primary wound closure. This is useful in burns

of the upper inner arm in the elderly, localized burns of a pendulous breast, abdominal burns, buttock injuries, and thigh burns. This approach works quite well when these wounds are excised early, before significant microbial colonization of the wound occurs.

In selected cases, the injury may be such that amputation of the burned part is most appropriate. In the patient with significant multisystem trauma, the expeditious removal of the burn injury might be the best option for the patient's overall survival. A mangled extremity, which has also suffered a severe burn that is deemed nonsalvageable, should undergo early amputation. It is not necessary to extend the amputation to a level that allows closure with unburned tissue. If viable muscle is available to close the amputation site, that wound bed can be resurfaced with an autogenous skin graft. A grafted amputation site can, with a modern prosthesis, function as a durable stump. In a patient who is paraplegic and suffers an extensive, deep lower extremity burn injury, amputation can be a viable alternative to excision and grafting. A similar option may need to be considered for the patient in whom significant pre-existing peripheral vascular disease makes the likelihood of a healed and functional extremity very low.

Excision and grafting will be required for wounds not amenable to primary closure. The extent of the procedure that a patient can undergo is related to the patient's age and physiologic status. Implicit in this approach is the use of experienced operating teams, an anesthesiologist who thoroughly understands the unique problems of the patient with a major body surface-area burn, and an operating room fully equipped to treat such a patient, as well as ready availability of blood products and the capacity to care for the patient postoperatively. A patient having this extent of surgery in essence undergoes a doubling of the surface area of "injury"—the now excised and grafted wound along with the partial-thickness wound produced by the donor site. In patients with wounds of a larger size (>30% total body surface area) or those who cannot tolerate a single procedure to achieve closure, staged excision of burned tissue is performed and the resulting wounds are closed with available cutaneous autografts or a biologic dressing.

The technique of burn wound excision is based on the depth of the wound and anatomic site to be excised. The most common method of excision is tangential. Excision of deep partial-thickness wounds to the level of a uniformly viable bed of deep dermis by tangential technique and immediate coverage with cutaneous autograft results in rapid wound closure with a typically excellent result. Optimally, the desired wound bed is achieved in one pass of the Weck blade as evidenced by diffuse bleeding. A frequent error is attempting this technique in wounds of an inappropriate depth and assuming that punctuate bleeding indicates a viable bed. Such wounds will heal with a poor take, as the bed contains marginally viable tissue incapable of supporting the cutaneous autograft. During the performance of this procedure, the amount of blood loss can be minimized with the use of a tourniquet on extremity burns or subeschar clysis containing epinephrine. An alternative to tangential excision is fascial excision, which involves excision of the burn wound to fascia or deep subcutaneous tissue. Viability of the fascia should be carefully assessed, and if the viability is questionable, the excision should be carried down to the underlying muscle prior to grafting.

The blood loss occurring with burn wound excision is related to the time of excision post-burn, the area to be excised, the presence of infection, and the type of excision. Donor sites can also represent a significant portion of the blood loss. The quantity of blood loss has been estimated to range from 0.45 to 1.25 ml/cm^2 of burn area excised. Adjunctive measures that can be used to control blood loss include elevation of limbs undergoing excision, applications of topical thrombin and/or vasoconstrictive agents in solutions to the excised wound and donor site, clysis of skin graft harvest sites and/or the eschar prior to removal, and application of tourniquets. Spray application of fibrin sealant can also reduce bleeding from the excised wound after release of the tourniquet. Blood loss will be compounded if the patient becomes coagulopathic, hypothermic, or acidotic during the procedure, a triad that can be avoided by partnership with an experienced anesthesiologist.

Grafting of the burn wound is usually done at the time of excision. However, there are instances where it advisable to stage the skin grafting procedure. The surgeon must be aware of the patient's status throughout the surgical procedure and, if necessary, truncate the procedure. It may be best to perform only the excision, and stage the timing of the grafting. Additionally, if the viability of the wound bed is suspect, only excision should be performed. The wound can be dressed with a 5% Sulfamylon solution dressing or covered with a skin substitute and subsequently re-evaluated.

Several skin substitutes exist. The two most commonly used naturally occurring biologic dressings are human cutaneous allograft and porcine cutaneous xenograft. Both of these preparations are capable of becoming vascularized. Allograft skin can provide wound coverage for 3–4 weeks before rejection. Xenograft tissue is available as reconstituted sheets of meshed porcine dermis or as fresh or prepared split-thickness skin. Xenograft skin can be used to cover partial-thickness injuries or donor sites, which re-epithelialize beneath the xenograft. Additionally, various synthetic membranes have been developed that provide wound protection and possess vapor and bacterial barrier properties. Either Biobrane™ (Dow-Hickham, Sugarland, TX) or Integra™ (Integra LifeScience Corporation, Plainsboro, NJ) can be placed over freshly excised full-thickness wounds, and once fully vascularized, the epidermal analog is removed and the vascularized "neodermis" covered with a thin split-thickness cutaneous autograft. A permanent skin substitute for burn care victims continues to represent the holy grail. Presently, cultured epithelial autografts are commercially available but are limited in their use because of suboptimal graft take, fragility of the skin surface, and high cost. Use of any biologic dressing requires that the excised wound and the dressing that has been applied be meticulously examined on at least a daily basis. Submembrane suppuration or the development of infection necessitates removal of the dressing, cleansing of the wound with a surgical detergent disinfectant solution, and even re-excision of the wound if residual nonviable or infected tissue is present.

The proper management of the patient's burn wounds is critical to achieve the optimum cosmetic and functional outcome and the timely return of the patient to full activity. In patients with major burns, the wound must be properly cared for and closure achieved expeditiously to lessen the level of physiologic disruption that accompanies a major burn. Failure to do so can result in invasive wound infection, chronic inflammation, erosion of lean body mass, progressive functional deficits, and even death.

Specialized Injuries: Electrical Burns

The principal mechanism by which electricity damages tissue is by conversion to thermal energy. Currents of 1000 volts and above are classified as high voltage. Upon contact with such currents, the body acts as a volume conductor. The electric current may induce cardiac and/or respiratory arrest, necessitating cardiopulmonary resuscitation at any time after injury. Arrhythmias may also occur, necessitating electrocardiogram monitoring for at least 24 hours after the last recorded episode of arrhythmia.

Two characteristics of high-voltage electric injury increase the incidence of acute renal failure in patients. First, there is often extensive unapparent subcutaneous tissue injury in a limb underlying unburned skin. The limited cutaneous injury may lead to gross underestimation of resuscitation fluid needs. Second, the mass of muscle injured by the electric current may cause rhabdomyolysis, resulting in direct damage to the renal tubules. Resuscitation fluids should be based on the extent of burn visible plus the estimated daily needs of the patient, adjusted according to the patient's response. If the urine contains hemochromogens (dark red pigments), fluid should be administered to obtain 75–100 ml of urine per hour, with

sodium bicarbonate added to the fluids to alkalinize the urine. If the hemochromogens do not clear promptly, or the patient remains oliguric, 25 g of mannitol should be given as a bolus and 12.5 g of mannitol added to each liter of lactated Ringer's until the pigment clears. The addition of mannitol, an osmotic diuretic, makes measurements of urine output unreliable as a monitor of the adequacy of resuscitation, and central venous monitoring is indicated.

When the body functions as a volume conductor, current flow is proportional to the cross-sectional area of the body part involved. Consequently, severe tissue destruction may occur in a limb with a relatively small cross-section area, whereas relatively little tissue damage may occur as current flows through the trunk. Damage to the muscle in a limb is often associated with marked increase in the pressure within the compartment containing the damaged muscle, which, if unrelieved, may cause further tissue necrosis. A limb compartment, which is hard to palpation, should alert one to the need for immediate surgical exploration. Operative intervention and extensive fasciotomy are mandated by extensive deep tissue necrosis, compartment syndrome, or persistent or progressively severe hyperkalemia. The extent of destruction may necessitate amputation at the time of exploration, particularly if the nonviable muscle is the source of persistent hyperkalemia. Following debridement or amputation, the wound should be dressed open. The patient is returned to the operating room in 24–36 hours for reinspection and further debridement of nonviable tissue if necessary. When all tissue in the wound is viable, it may be closed definitively.

Tissue damage can also be caused by low-voltage or house current. Burns of the oral commissure occur in young children who bite electric cords or suck on the end of a live extension cord or an electric outlet. The lesion may have the characteristics of full-thickness tissue damage, but early surgical debridement may only accentuate the defect and should be avoided. These injuries will usually heal with minimal cosmetic sequelae, which can be addressed electively if needed.

Specialized Injuries: Chemical Injuries

A variety of chemical agents can cause tissue injury as a consequence of an exothermic chemical reaction, protein coagulation, desiccation, and delipidation. The severity of a chemical injury is related to the concentration and amount of chemical agent and the duration with which it is in contact with tissue. Consequently, initial wound care to remove or dilute the offending agent takes priority in the management of patients with chemical injuries, brushing away dry material and instituting immediate, copious water lavage. For patients in whom extensive surface injury has occurred, the irrigation fluid should be warmed to prevent the induction of hypothermia.

The appearance of skin damaged by chemical agents can be misleading. In the case of patients injured by strong acids, the involved skin surface may have a silky texture and a light brown appearance, which may be mistaken for a sunburn rather than the full-thickness injury that it is. Skin injured by delipidation caused by petroleum distillates may be dry, show little if any inflammation, and appear to be undamaged but yet found to be a full-thickness injury on histologic examination.

Specialized Injuries: Cold Injuries

Injuries occurring secondary to environmental exposure can result in local injuries, frostbite, or systemic hypothermia. The pathophysiology of frostbite is crystal formation due to freezing of both extracellular and intracellular fluids. Patients presenting with frostbite will have coldness of the injured body part, with loss of sensation and proprioception. On initial examination, the limb may well appear pale, cyanotic, or have a yellow-white discoloration. During rapid rewarming at 40°–42° C in water for 15–30 minutes, hyperemia will occur followed by pain, paresthesias, and sensory deficits. Greater than 1 week may pass before a true determination of the depth and extent of the injury can be obtained. The injured extremity should be elevated in an attempt to control edema and padded to avoid pressure-induced ischemia as a secondary insult. Frostbite wounds are tetanus-prone wounds, and therefore tetanus toxoid should be administered based on the patient's immunization status.

MORBIDITY AND COMPLICATIONS MANAGEMENT

Early Complications

As resuscitation proceeds and edema forms beneath the inelastic eschar of encircling full-thickness burns of a limb, blood flow to underlying and distal unburned tissue may be compromised. Cyanosis of distal unburned skin and progressive paresthesias, particularly unrelenting deep tissue pain, which are the most reliable clinical signs of impaired circulation, may become evident only after relatively long periods of relative or absolute ischemia. Since the full-thickness eschar is insensate, the escharotomy can be performed as a bedside procedure without anesthesia, using a scalpel or an electrocautery device. On an extremity, the escharotomy incision, which is carried only through the eschar and the immediately subjacent superficial fascia, is placed in the mid-lateral line and must extend from the upper to the lower limit of the burn wound (Figure 2). The circulatory status of the limb should then be

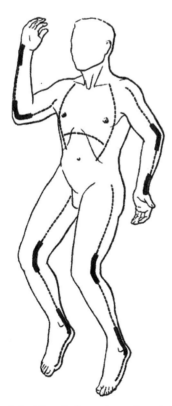

Figure 2 The dashed lines indicate the preferred sites of escharotomy incisions for the limbs (mid-lateral and mid-medial lines), thorax (anterior axillary lines and costal margin), and neck (lateral aspect). The thickened areas of the lines on the limbs emphasize the importance of carrying the incisions across involved joints. *(Used with permission from Martin RR, Becker WK, Cioffi WG, and Pruitt BP Jr: Thermal Injuries. In Wilson RF and Walt AJ, editors: Management of Trauma: Pitfalls and Practice, 2nd ed. Baltimore, Williams and Wilkins, 1996, p. 765.)*

reassessed. If that escharotomy has not restored distal flow, another escharotomy should be placed in the mid-medial line of the involved limb. A fasciotomy may be needed when there has been a delay in restoring the patient's limb circulation and in particular if the patient is receiving a massive fluid load.

Edema formation beneath encircling full-thickness truncal burns can restrict the respiratory excursion of the chest wall. If the limitation of chest wall motion is associated with hypoxia and elevated peak inspiratory pressure, chest escharotomy is indicated to restore chest wall motion and improve ventilation. These escharotomy incisions are placed in the anterior axillary line bilaterally, and if the eschar extends onto the abdominal wall, the anterior axillary line incisions are joined by a costal margin escharotomy incision (see Figure 2).

The timely administration of adequate fluid as detailed previously has essentially eliminated acute renal failure after burn injury. Far more common today are the complications of excessive resuscitation—that is, compartment syndromes and pulmonary compromise. Compartment syndromes can be produced in the calvarium, muscle compartments beneath the investing fascia, and the abdominal cavity.

Excessive fluid administration may also cause formation of enough ascitic fluid and edema of the abdominal contents resulting in intra-abdominal hypertension. The abdominal compartment syndrome represents progression of intra-abdominal hypertension to the point of organ dysfunction, including decreased cardiac output with resultant hypotension, increased peak airway pressures, oliguria, and worsening metabolic acidosis due to hypoperfusion. Bladder pressure measurements serve as an indirect measurement of intra-abdominal pressures. Elevation of the bladder pressure above 25 mm Hg should prompt therapeutic intervention, beginning with adequate sedation, reduction of fluid infusion rate, diuresis, and paracentesis. If organ failure becomes evident, decompressive laparotomy is indicated.

Compartment syndromes may also occur in the muscle compartments underlying the investing fascia of the limbs of burn patients, even in limbs that are unburned. To assess compartment pressure, the turgor of the muscle compartments should be assessed on a scheduled basis by simple palpation. A stony hard compartment is an ominous finding which should prompt direct measurement of intracompartmental pressure. A muscle compartment pressure of 25 mm of mercury or more necessitates performing a fasciotomy of the involved compartment in the operating room using general anesthesia.

Metabolic and Nutritional Support

Burn injury alters the distribution and utilization of nutrients as well as the metabolic rate. All of these post-burn metabolic changes must be considered in planning nutritional support of the hypermetabolic burn patient. This is necessary to minimize loss of lean body mass, accelerate convalescence, and restore physical abilities. Bedside indirect calorimetry is the most accurate means of determining metabolic rate and nutritional requirements, but bedside metabolic care may not always be available. A rule of thumb estimate for nutritional needs of patients whose burns exceed 30% of the body surface area is 2000–2200 kcal and 12–18 g of nitrogen per square meter of body surface per day.

At the time of admission, patients should have a nasogastric or nasoduodenal tube placed. It is preferable to start enteral feedings as soon as possible after the patient is admitted. When feedings are initiated early, the desired rate of administration can typically be reached within 24–48 hours after admission. If the patient is intolerant to gastric feedings, the administration of metoclopramide will often resolve the problem. If a patient fails to respond to metoclopramide, an attempt should be made to pass a feeding tube distal to the ligament of Treitz. In patients who become intolerant of enteral feedings, or who develop gastrointestinal complications that prevent enteral feeding, total parenteral nutrition will be required.

Burn injury induces insulin resistance, which may lead to hyperglycemia. The maintenance of blood glucose values below 120 mg/dl with aggressive insulin infusion has been demonstrated to have a favorable impact on the outcome of critically ill patients. Potassium and phosphorous must also be given to meet the patient's needs, which often exceed initial estimates, particularly when large loads of glucose are being given with exogenous insulin. Over the course of the patient's care, as the open wound area decreases and the hypermetabolic state slowly resolves, the nutrient load should be adjusted so that balance is maintained between metabolic needs and substrate delivery, preventing overfeeding.

TRANSPORTATION AND TRANSFER

Many important advances have been made in the care and management of burn-injured victims during the past 50 years. One of the more significant advances has been the recognition of the benefits of a team approach in the care of critically injured burn patients. The American College of Surgeons and the American Burn Association have developed optimal standards for providing burn care and a burn center verification program that identifies those units that have undergone peer review of their performance and outcomes. Patients with burns and/or associated injuries and conditions listed in Table 1 should be referred to a burn center.

Once the decision has been made to transfer a patient to a burn center, there should be physician-to-physician communication regarding the patient's status and need for transfer. It is critical that the patient be properly stabilized in preparation for the transfer. During transport the need to perform life-saving interventions such as endotracheal intubation or re-establishing vascular access may be very difficult to accomplish in the relatively unstable and limited space of a moving ambulance or a helicopter in flight. That difficulty makes it important to institute hemodynamic and pulmonary resuscitation and to achieve "stability" prior to undertaking transfer by either aeromedical or ground transport. A secure large-bore intravenous cannula must be in place to permit continuous fluid resuscitation. Patients should be placed on 100% oxygen. If there is any question about airway adequacy, an endotracheal tube should be placed and mechanical ventilation instituted. The hourly urinary output should also be monitored, with fluid infusion adjusted as necessary. All patients should be placed NPO, and those with a greater than 20% body surface area burn require placement of a nasogastric tube. The burn wound should be covered with a clean and/or sterile dry sheet. The application of topical antimicrobial agents is contraindicated prior to transfer, since they will have to be removed on admission to the burn center. Maintenance of the patient's body temperature is vital. The patient should be covered with a heat-reflective space blanket to minimize heat loss. Burn wounds, as tetanus-prone wounds, mandate immunization in accordance with the recommendations of the American College of Surgeons.

MORTALITY

Early post-burn renal failure as a consequence of delayed and/or inadequate resuscitation has been eliminated, and inhalation injury as a comorbid factor has been tamed. Invasive burn wound sepsis has been controlled, and early excision with prompt skin grafting and general improvements in critical care have reduced the incidence of infection, eliminated many previously life-threatening complications, and accelerated the convalescence of burn patients. Mortality for various ages and burn sizes is reported in Table 4. Not only has

Table 4: Changes in Burn Patient Mortality at U.S. Army Burn Center, 1945–1991

Age Group	Percentage of Body Surface Burn Causing 50% Mortality (LA$_{50}$)	
	1945–1957	1987–1991
Children (0–14)	51	72 [a]
Young adults (15–40)	43	82 [b]
		73 [c]
Older adults	23	46 [d]

[a]5 years
[b]21 years
[c]40 years
[d]60 years

Source: Pruitt BA Jr, Gamelli RL: Burns. In Britt LD, Trunkey DD, Organ CH, Feliciano DV, editors: *Acute Care Surgery.* New York, Springer, 2006, p. 155, with permission.

survival improved, but the elimination of many life-threatening complications and advances in wound care have improved the quality of life of even those patients who have survived extensive, severe thermal injuries.

SUGGESTED READINGS

American Burn Association: *Advanced Life Burn Support Course Instructors Manual.* Chicago, American Burn Association, 2001.

American Burn Association: *Burn Care Resources in North America.* Chicago, American Burn Association, 2004.

Asch MJ, Fellman RJ, Walker HL, Foley FD, Popp RL, Mason AD Jr, Pruitt BA Jr: Systemic and pulmonary hemodynamic changes accompanying thermal injury. *Ann Surg* 178:218–221, 1973.

Bennett B, Gamelli RL: Profile of an abused child. *J Burn Care Rehabil* 19:88–94, 1998.

Ernst A, Zibrak JD: Carbon monoxide poisoning. *N Engl J Med* 339: 1603–1608, 1998.

Heinrich JJ, Brand DA, Cuono CB: The role of topical treatment as a determinant of an infection in outpatient burns. *J Burn Care Rehabil* 9: 253–257, 1988.

Kowal-Vern A, McGill V, Gamelli R: Ischemic necrotic bowel disease in thermal injury. *Arch Surg* 132:440–443, 1997.

Martin RR. Becker WK, Cioffi WG, Pruitt BP Jr: Thermal injuries. In Wilson RF, Walt AJ, editors: *Mangement of Trauma: Pitfalls and Practice,* 2nd ed. Baltimore, Williams and Wilkins, 1996, pp. 760–771.

McManus WF, Mason AD Jr, Pruitt BA Jr: Excision of the burn wound in patients with large burns. *Arch Surg* 124:718–720, 1989.

Mochizuki H, Trocki O, Dominion L, Brackett KA, Joffe SN, Alexander JW: Mechanism of prevention of postburn hypermetabolism and catabolism by early enteral feeding. *Ann Surg* 200:297–300, 1984.

Peck M: Practice guidelines for burn care: nutritional support. *J Burn Care Rehabil* 12:59S–66S, 2001.

Pruitt BA Jr, Gamelli RL: Burns. In Britt LD, Trunkey DD, Organ CH, Feliciano DV, editors: *Acute Care Surgery: Principles and Practice.* New York, Springer, 2007, pp. 125–160.

Pruitt BA Jr, Goodwin CW Jr: Critical care management of the severely burned patient. In Parrillo JE, Dellinger RP, editors: *Critical Care Medicine,* 2nd ed. St. Louis, Mosby, 2001, pp. 1475–1500.

Rico RM, Ripamonti R, Burns AL, Gamelli RL, DiPietro LA: The effect of sepsis on wound healing. *J Surg Res* 102(2):193–197, 2002.

Tasaki O, Goodwin CW, Saitoh D, Mozingo DW, Ishihara S, Brinkley WW, Cioffi WG Jr, Pruitt BA Jr: Effects of burns on inhalation injury. *J Trauma* 43:603–607, 1997.

SOFT TISSUE INFECTIONS

Sharon Henry

Soft tissue infections occur frequently and account for approximately 48.3 in 1000 outpatient visits. The severity of these infections varies from trivial to life-threatening.

Severe soft tissue infections have been described throughout the medical literature since ancient times. Necrotizing fasciitis was described in the fifth century BC by Hippocrates, though Wilson coined the term in 1952.

Much of our knowledge regarding the treatment of soft tissue infection has been based on the experience gained during military conflicts. For instance, hospital gangrene was described first by Joseph Jones, a Confederate surgeon during the Civil War. The treatment of battlefield infections has influenced civilian practice. This review will begin with a description of the anatomically more superficial infections and progress to the deeper, life-threatening infections (Figure 1).

SUPERFICIAL INFECTIONS

Superficial infections are limited anatomically to the epidermis and the dermis. These infections can occur spontaneously or secondary to minor trauma. Impetigo usually presents with vesicles that leak, producing a thick yellow crust. These lesions are typically located on the face, neck, and extremities. *Staphylococcus aureus* and *Streptococcus pyogenes* are the most common causative agents. Bullous impetigo, like impetigo, is most commonly caused by *S. aureus*. It is characterized by small vesicles that coalesce to form large bullae.

Folliculitis develops as an infection of the hair follicle. The lesions appear as pustules or papules, commonly on the extremities, scalp, or beard. Whirlpool folliculitis is associated with immersion in inadequately chlorinated pools, whirlpools, or hot tubs. Diffuse pustules are seen. *Pseudomonas aeruginosa* is the classic causative agent. Swimmer's itch is a folliculitis that develops after freshwater exposure.

Furuncles, deeper inflammatory nodules, can develop from folliculitis. *S. aureus* is often the causative agent. Carbuncles are coalescing furuncles formed by connecting sinuses. The nape of the neck is the most common anatomic location. *S. aureus* is most often isolated. Patients often have comorbidities such as diabetes mellitus, alcoholism, immunosuppression, or malnutrition. Systemic infection may result from these lesions.

Cellulitis is an inflammation of the subcutaneous tissue. There is erythema, pain, and edema of varying severity. A portal of entry for the bacteria is usually present. It may be as mundane as a crack in the skin from dryness or athlete's foot. More substantial trauma may be involved, such as shotgun or shrapnel penetrations. Systemic symptoms may manifest and include fever, chills, malaise, and (infrequently) organ failure. Streptococcus (Groups A, B, C, and G) as well as staphylococcus are frequent culprits. Areas of compromised venous or lymphatic drainage are prone to this infection, and recurrence is common. Pelvic radiation or having had lymphadenectomy, mastectomy, or venectomy makes the development of cellulitis more likely.

DEEP INFECTION

Deeper infections are more frequently life- and limb-threatening. The literature concerning the potentially life-threatening infections is confusing. Multiple terms are used to describe the same disease, depending on the clinical setting in which it arises. The treatment is the same regardless of the term used to describe it. It therefore seems that anatomic classification is more logical and easily remembered. This review uses anatomic characterizations and relate them to older terminology as necessary.

In the medical literature, deep structure infection has masqueraded under a variety of pseudonyms. The term "necrotizing soft tissue infection" (NSTI) is used here. Table 1 lists a variety of terms that may appear in the medical literature to describe this infective process.

All the terms describe an infection involving the subcutaneous fat and fascia, with variable skin involvement. The incidence of this infection is not known. A recent report quotes World Health Organization statistics of 500–1500 cases of necrotizing fasciitis annually. Though uncommon, it is not rare. The Centers for Disease Control has monitored Group A streptococcal infections and estimated 10–20 cases per 100,000 population. In Ontario, Canada, a population study estimated an incidence of 0.6 per 100,000.

CLINICAL PRESENTATION

Signs and symptoms of NSTI can be quite nonspecific (Table 2). Pain, erythema, and swelling of the affected area are most frequently present. This same constellation of symptoms may be seen in pathologic processes that have a much more benign course and respond effectively to antibiotic therapy alone. "Hard signs" of necrotizing infection include tense erythema, bullae, skin discoloration, and crepitus, pain out of proportion to examination, or anesthesia of the affected area. Unfortunately, many of these are late signs and indicate that the infective process is well established or they occur only in a small percentage of patients.

Signs of systemic toxicity may also be present. These may include pyrexia, tachycardia, hypotension, and organ dysfunction. The progression of symptoms may be rapid over the course of hours to days or more indolent over the course of days to weeks. The rate of progression of symptoms may be ameliorated by partial treatment. Some suggest classifying the disease by its clinical course. Fulminant disease presents in patients with acute onset and rapid progression over the course of hours with shock. Acute disease presents with large surface area involvement and over the course of days. Subacute disease presents for weeks and is usually localized. Differentiating this process from cellulitis or simple abscess can be a challenge. Clinically, failure to improve with appropriate antibiotics or worsening systemic toxicity portends this diagnosis (Table 3).

Laboratory data are equally nonspecific. Leukocytosis, hyponatremia, and elevated creatinine phosphokinase have been evaluated in clinical studies and may be markers of the disease. Wall et al. matched 21 patients with necrotizing fasciitis with controls and attempted to identify parameters that would distinguish the groups. White blood cell count (WBC) $> 15.4 \times 10^9/l$, serum sodium (Na) less than 135 mmol/l, or both, were the best factors to distinguish necrotizing fasciitis from non-necrotizing fasciitis. The sensitivity was 90%, and the specificity was 76%. In this study, 40% of the patients with necrotizing fasciitis lacked "hard signs." Wong and colleagues developed the Laboratory Risk Indicator for Necrotizing Fasciitis (LRINEC) score. The score was developed retrospectively based on WBC, hemoglobin (Hgb), serum Na, C-reactive protein, creatinine, and glucose in patients with necrotizing fasciitis and patients with other severe soft tissue infections. A score of ≥6 had a positive predictive value of 92% and a negative predictive value of 96%. In a cohort of prospectively evaluated patients, the model was found to have a positive predictive value of 40% and a negative predictive value of 95%. Creatinine phosphokinase (CPK) elevation was found by one group to distinguish patients with group

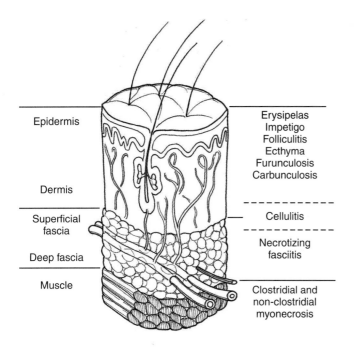

Figure 1   Skin structures with corresponding infection.

Epidermis
Dermis
Superficial fascia
Deep fascia
Muscle

Erysipelas
Impetigo
Folliculitis
Ecthyma
Furunculosis
Carbunculosis

Cellulitis

Necrotizing fasciitis

Clostridial and non-clostridial myonecrosis

Table 1: Terms Used to Describe NSTI

Meleney's synergistic gangrene	Hospital gangrene
Streptococcal gangrene	Fournier's gangrene
Gas gangrene	Acute dermal gangrene
Suppurativa fasciitis	Necrotizing erysipelas
Phagedena	Phagedena gangrenosum
"Flesh-eating disease"	Necrotizing fasciitis
Clostridial cellulitis	

A streptococcal necrotizing fasciitis (GAS) from non–group A streptococcal necrotizing fasciitis. CPK elevations were >600 IU/l in the GAS group.

DIAGNOSTIC IMAGING

Diagnostic imaging may be useful in diagnosis or in defining the extent of disease. The hallmark of necrotizing, air in subcutaneous tissues, can be seen with a variety of imaging techniques. Plain radiographs will demonstrate subcutaneous air in only 16% of patients. Plain films may also demonstrate foreign bodies. This is especially

important when treating intravenous drug users. Ultrasonography, computed tomography (CT scan), and magnetic resonance imaging (MRI) are more sensitive than plain radiography in demonstrating air in the tissues. These modalities may additionally identify fluid collections in the subcutaneous tissues or within the muscle. They may be very helpful in cases without significant skin changes in planning incisions. MRI has the advantage of not requiring the administration of intravenous contrast material which may be toxic to the kidneys. This is especially helpful in patients who already have compromised renal function. However, systemically compromised patients are often logistically poor candidates for MRI scanning. In most cases, diagnostic imaging is only confirmatory, as patients with nonspecific findings on evaluation, such as edema, may still harbor the disease. Failure to improve with appropriate antibiotics, development of systemic toxicity, or profound elevation of the WBC should markedly raise the index of suspicion.

PATHOPHYSIOLOGY

The ability of an organism to cause infection is dependent on the virility of the organism and the resistance of the host. This disease is unique in that it affects both the compromised and the uncompromised host. Multiple reviews identify multiple risk factors associated with increased susceptibility; however, exceptionally virulent bacteria such as GAS are able to affect otherwise uncompromised hosts. These bacteria produce exotoxins that activate cytokines, leading to a robust systemic response. At the cellular level, the toxins and enzymes (hyaluronidases and lipases) facilitate the spread of bacteria along fascial planes and through the subcutaneous tissue. Necrosis of the superficial fascia and fat often produce a thin, watery, foul-smelling fluid (dishwater pus). The skin necrosis that may accompany this infection results when thrombosis of the skin's nutrient vessels occurs. Microscopic findings are usually severe subcutaneous fat necrosis, severe inflammation of the dermis and subcutaneous fat, vasculitis, endarteritis, and local hemorrhage. The fascia may be edematous and suppurative, and thrombosis of vessels may be seen. Myonecrosis may also be seen in advanced cases.

SURGICAL TREATMENT

Necrotizing fasciitis is a surgical emergency. The mainstay of treatment is surgical debridement. These procedures can be quite deforming, requiring the removal of large amounts of skin, subcutaneous fat, fascia, and possibly muscle or bone. Explorations on the extremities are usually begun by making generous vertical incisions. When involvement is diffuse, fasciotomy incisions on the extremities are often a useful starting place. The dissection must extend down to the level of the deep fascia. The muscle should also be inspected to confirm its viability (Figure 2). Formal fasciotomies may be necessary in cases with very intense edema in order to prevent myonecrosis (Figure 3).

Table 2: Frequency of Clinical Signs

Author	Erythema (%)	Crepitans (%)	Edema (%)	Year Published	# Patients in Study
Callahan	77	3	20	1988	30
McHenry	72	12	75	1995	65
Brook	89	39	77	1995	83
Elliot	66	45	75	1996	197
Tang	50		58	2001	24
Theis	54			2002	13
Wong	100	13	92	2002	89

Table 3: Bacteriology

Rapid progression:

Incubation <24 hours following inciting event
Streptococcus pyogenes (GAS)
Clostridia perfringens (gas gangrene)
Pasteurella multocida (animal bite)
Aeromonas hydrophilia (freshwater exposure)
Vibrio vulnificus (shellfish exposure)

Slower progression:

Staphylococcus aureus
Enterobacteria
Escherichia coli
Klebsiella pneumonia
Pseudomonas aeruginosa
In immunocompromised host
Coagulase negative staphylococci
Diphtheroids
Bacillus sp.

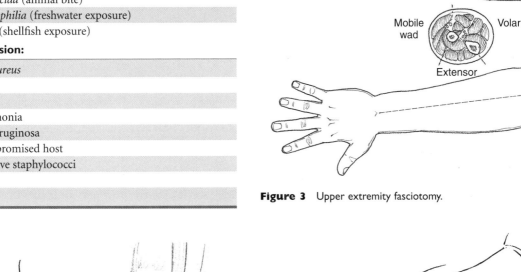

Figure 3 Upper extremity fasciotomy.

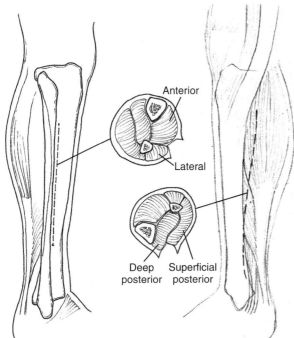

Figure 2 Lower extremity fasciotomy.

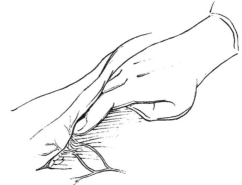

Figure 4 Loss of tissue plane integrity.

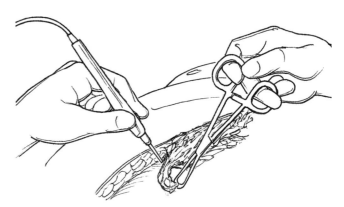

Figure 5 Thorough debridement.

The integrity of the tissue plane between the subcutaneous fat or superficial fascia and the deep fascia is tested with either a finger or clamp (Figure 4). Lack of resistance to this probing is the hallmark of the diagnosis in early cases. "Dishwater pus" may be encountered as this plane is opened. In more advanced cases, frankly necrotic or purulent material is encountered. Cultures for stat Gram stain and aerobic and anaerobic cultures should be obtained. If the patient is immunosuppressed, cultures for *Mycobacterium* and fungus should also be sent. It is imperative to widely open all affected tissue planes and debride all obviously devitalized tissue (Figure 5).

When the presentation is more focal, incisions can be placed over the area of maximal skin abnormality and the incision extended as abnormalities of the deeper tissue are encountered. A colostomy may be helpful in cases with extensive perianal involvement to prevent ongoing stool contamination. Surgical feeding tube placement should be considered in critically ill patients or in patients with large surface area wounds that are likely to remain open for some time.

Plans should be made at the end of the case for return to the operating room for re-evaluation of the wounds within 48 hours. Adequate evaluation of these deep and often painful wounds is not possible at the bedside. A variety of wound dressings can be applied. Negative pressure wound therapy (NPWT) is optimally suited for this purpose. It allows removal of exudate, which may further decrease bacterial counts. It prevents maceration of the surrounding tissue and keeps the patient and their bed linens dry. It is often helpful to be able to quantify the fluid losses that are occurring. Replacement of these losses may be necessary. The skin surrounding the wound can be evaluated for advancing cellulitis or edema. The character of the fluid can also be assessed.

It is imperative if this type of wound care is to be used that hemostasis is meticulous and coagulopathy corrected. Parameters must be given to the nursing staff regarding volume and character of the fluid loss that is acceptable. When this type of dressing is not available or prudent, the wounds may be packed with Kerlix (Kendall Kerlix AMD) or gauze impregnated with antimicrobial material. Although some of these materials may be cytotoxic, the antimicrobial properties may outweigh the negative effect of the cytotoxicity on normal tissues. Once the infection is controlled, non-cytotoxic products should be used. Silver ion–based products are a good choice.

BACTERIOLOGY

Necrotizing fasciitis is usually divided into two categories. Type I is a polymicrobial infection and is the most common variety. Typically this infection is seen in patients with comorbidities. Gram-negative enteric bacteria are seen in combination with Gram positives and anaerobes. Type II is GAS either alone or in combination with *S. aureus*. This type takes a more virulent course and occurs in younger, healthier patients. Clostridial infections classically produce air in the soft tissues, although the polymicrobial type I infections may also produce GAS. *Vibrio vulnificus* and *Aeromonas hydrophilia* should be suspected when the patient has been exposed to shellfish or freshwater.

PHARMACOLOGIC THERAPY

Initial treatment of the patient in shock should be aimed at resuscitation. Fluids and blood products are given as needed to replace deficits. Coagulation abnormalities should be corrected. It must be stressed that resuscitation is begun, but all abnormalities will not and need not be fully corrected before proceeding to surgery. Resuscitation must continue throughout the preoperative, operative, and postoperative phases. Many abnormalities will not fully correct until there is adequate source control. Pressors and steroids may be necessary in severe cases. When GAS is involved, intravenous immunoglobulin (IVIG) may also be given. Broad spectrum antibiotic therapy is initiated to cover the most likely causative organisms. Extended spectrum penicillins are a good first-line choice. Clindamycin should be added in cases that may involve GAS. Methicillin resistance is emerging in the community, and this must be considered in choosing antibiotics. Vancomycin or daptomycin should be considered when resistance is suspected or in cases where the patient is severely compromised. Patients with penicillin allergies can be treated with fluoroquinolones in combination with Gram-negative and anaerobic therapy or carbapenems.

HYPERBARIC OXYGEN

Hyperbaric oxygen (HBO) is an adjunct to resuscitation, surgical debridement, and broad spectrum antibiotics. A variety of salutary affects have been attributed to HBO therapy (Table 4). There are no

Table 4: Beneficial Effects of HBO

Inhibits growth of anaerobic organisms
Reduces the production of clostridial toxin
Improves leukocyte bacterial killing
Bacteriocidal and bacteriostatic effects on a variety of organisms
Enhances efficacy of certain antibiotics
Modulates cytokine levels
Decreases tissue edema
Increases collagen formation

prospective randomized studies to scientifically validate the efficacy of hyperbaric oxygen therapy. There are a number of retrospective studies that seem to support its use in severe necrotizing infections. Several studies demonstrated decrease mortality in patients treated with HBO compared with historic controls. Other studies demonstrated improved preservation of tissue as evidenced by a decrease in the number of debridements to achieve control of the infection. Some studies, however, have questioned the efficacy of HBO. These studies showed no statistically significant difference in mortality between patients treated with HBO and those who received only surgical debridement. HBO therapy is not uniformly available throughout the country, so it is not an option for every patient who presents with this problem. When available, given the relatively high mortality and morbidity, use of this modality as an adjunct makes sense.

MORTALITY, MORBIDITY, AND COMPLICATIONS MANAGEMENT

The morbidity following the treatment of severe necrotizing soft tissue infections can be severe. Most of the morbidity results from the tissue destruction brought about by the infection. The extent of morbidity depends on the area involved and the extent of the necessary debridement. During debridement, iatrogenic injury to nerves and blood supply can compound dysfunction. This is most common in the management of extremity infections. Tissues may be distorted by the inflammation and necrosis or scarred by prior surgery, making the identification of vital structures a challenge. It is vitally important to be familiar with the anatomy of the area. Patients may be left with significant deficits in function solely related to the magnitude of the surgical debridement. Amputation rates from 17%–33% have been documented in patients with extremity severe soft tissue infections.

Patients with abdominal sites of infection, who require debridement of their abdominal wall, are subject to the development of enterocutaneous fistulae. Management of the output of the fistula and providing for adequate nutrition are the primary management issues in the early management of this problem.

Mortality rates as high as 76% have been recorded, although contemporary studies report overall mortality in the range of 20%. Multiple factors affect mortality. Clinical presentation and speed to surgery appear to be the two most important determinants. Patients who suffer delays in obtaining surgical treatment had higher mortalities. Patients who present with organ failure or increased serum lactates also have higher mortalities. Comorbidities such as diabetes mellitus, renal failure, and advanced age, and the need for large surface area debridements have also been noted to increase mortality.

CONCLUSIONS

NSTI can occur under a variety of clinical conditions. It should be considered in postsurgical, post-traumatic wounds as well as in wounds from insect or animal bites. Differentiation from superficial infection is mandatory to assure appropriate surgical therapy is performed. Patients who fail to respond to appropriate medical therapy or who present with evidence of shock or organ dysfunction often harbor deeper infections. Patients with leukocytosis, hyponatremia, hyperglycemia, elevated creatinine, C-reactive protein, or CPK on laboratory evaluation should elicit an aggressive evaluation. This may include radiographic workup or surgical exploration. Progression of physical findings, including worsening edema, blistering, and crepitans or skin necrosis, mandates surgical exploration. Delays in treatment result in increased mortality and morbidity.

SUGGESTED READINGS

Bosshardt TL, Henderson VJ, Organ CH: Necrotizing soft-tissue infections. *Arch Surg* 131:846–854, 1996.

Brook I, Fraxier EH: Clinical and microbiological features of necrotizing fasciitis. *J Clin Microbiol* 33:2382–2387, 1995.

Callahan TE, Schecter WP, Horn JK: Necrotizing soft tissue infection masquerading as cutaneous abscess following illicit drug injection. *Arch Surg* 133:812–818, 1998.

Elliott DC, Kufera FA, Meyers RA: Necrotizing soft tissue infections: risk factors for mortality and strategies for management. *Ann Surg* 224:672–683, 1996.

Simonart T, Nakafusa J, Narisawa Y: The importance of serum creatinine phosphokinase level in the early diagnosis and microbiological evaluation of necrotizing fasciitis. *Eur Acad Dermatol Venereol* 18:687–690, 2004.

Tang WM, Ho PL, Fung KK, Yuen KY, Leong JC: Necrotizing fasciitis of a limb. *J Bone Joint Surg* 83:709–714, 2001.

Theis FC, Rietveld J, Danesh-Clough T: Severe necrotising soft tissue infections in orthopaedic surgery. *J Orthop Surg* 10:108–113, 2002.

Wall DB, de Virgilio C, Black S, Klein S: Objective criteria may assist in distinguishing necrotizing fasciitis from nonnecrotizing soft tissue infection. *Am J Surg* 179:17–21, 2000.

Wall DB, Klein SR, Black S, de Virgilio C: A simple model to help distinguish necrotizing fasciitis for nonnecrotizing soft tissue infection. *J Am Coll Surg* 191:227–300, 2000.

Wilkinson D, Doolette D: Hyperbaric oxygen treatment and survival from necrotizing soft tissue infections. *Arch Surg* 139:1339–1345, 2004.

Wong CH, Chang HC, Pasupathy S, Khin LW, Tan JL, Low CO: Necrotizing fasciitis: clinical presentation, microbiology, and determinants of mortality. *J Bone Joint Surg* 85A:1454–1460, 2003.

Wong CH, Khin LW, Heng KS, Tan KC, Low CO: The LRINEC (Laboratory Risk Indicator for Necrotizing Fasciitis) score: a tool for distinguishing necrotizing fasciitis from other soft tissue infections. *Crit Care Med* 32:1535–1541, 2004.

Wu W, Scannell C, Lieber MJ, Huang W: Hyperbaric oxygen therapy: current status in the management of severe nonclostridial necrotizing soft tissue infections. *Curr Treat Opin Infect Dis* 3:217–225, 2001.

COMMON ERRORS IN TRAUMA CARE

R. Stephen Smith,   R. Joseph Nold,
and   Jonathan M. Dort

Errors in management occur frequently in medicine. A recent Institute of Medicine report estimated that 44,000–98,000 deaths each year were caused by medical errors. This represents more deaths in the United States each year than are caused by breast cancer or AIDS. Most of these errors occur in low-intensity, nonemergent scenarios. Obviously, trauma care is a much more difficult setting to perform in an errorless fashion. Care of injured patients must occur in an emergent fashion. Decisions must be made rapidly, based on limited information. In many instances, interventions must be initiated before a complete evaluation is performed. Frequently, the history of the mechanism of injury is obscure, or injured patients involved with criminal activities may mislead the trauma team. Moreover, injured patients are frequently unresponsive, have a decreased level of consciousness, or are uncooperative due to intoxication. Seriously injured patients frequently present with multiple injuries that require the involvement of multiple providers. Routinely, numerous surgeons, surgical subspecialists, emergency medicine physicians, and residents must accurately communicate and coordinate care for an optimal outcome. The list of potential causes for errors in trauma care is infinite. Because of these many difficulties, the surgeon who cares for trauma must pay particular attention to the factors that cause errors in management and should make every effort to prevent these errors. In this chapter, a number of common errors in the management of injured patients are discussed. This discussion includes missed diaphragmatic injury, failure to recognize extremity compartment syndrome, failure to prevent or treat abdominal compartment syndrome, delayed damage-control laparotomy, missed hollow viscus injuries, failure to perform a tertiary survey, futile or emergency department thoracotomy, and the dogma of mandatory colostomy.

MISSED DIAPHRAGMATIC INJURY

Injuries to the diaphragm are common. Approximately 5% of patients injured in motor vehicle crashes have injuries to the diaphragm. A more frequently encountered scenario involves penetrating thoracoabdominal wounds. Approximately 15% of patients with this history will have injury to the diaphragm. Unfortunately, the diagnostic modalities used routinely for evaluation of injured patients have low sensitivity and a high rate of false negatives for diaphragmatic injury. Delayed diagnosis is the usual situation with diaphragmatic injury and may occur in up to 62% of patients. Cases of delayed recognition and treatment of up to 50 years have been reported in the literature. Diaphragmatic injuries should be recognized and treated as soon as possible to prevent complications. The most serious complications of diaphragmatic injury include herniation, incarceration, and strangulation of hollow viscera. The true incidence of this devastating complication is unknown but has historically resulted in mortality rates of 20%–36%.

Optimal diagnosis of diaphragmatic injury requires a high index of suspicion. It is virtually impossible to evaluate the diaphragm with 100% certainty without operative evaluation. Direct visualization, either through laparotomy, thoracotomy, laparoscopy, or thoracoscopy, is required to make this diagnosis with certainty. Conversely, not every patient with a history of injury should be explored, as this would lead to an unacceptable rate of negative and nontherapeutic operations.

A number of physical findings should increase the surgeon's suspicion for diaphragmatic injury. These include penetrating thoracoabdominal injury or blunt trauma involving injuries to the abdomen or chest. Unfortunately, physical examination is unreliable in patients with diaphragmatic injury. In fact, 20%–40% of patients with isolated diaphragmatic injury have an initially normal physical examination. A number of noninvasive diagnostic adjuncts are routinely used in the evaluation of trauma patients. These include chest x-ray, focused assessment with sonography for trauma (FAST), and computed tomography (CT). Unfortunately, all of these diagnostic modalities used either alone or in combination are unreliable for the diagnosis of diaphragmatic injury. Additionally, diagnostic peritoneal lavage is nonspecific and fails to diagnose isolated diaphragmatic injury in a large percentage of cases. The only methods that evaluate the diaphragm with certainty are invasive operative procedures that directly visualize the diaphragm.

Isolated diaphragmatic lacerations are rarely life-threatening immediately following the injury. Direct evaluation of the diaphragm frequently holds a lower priority than treatment of other potentially life-threatening injuries. However, it must be emphasized that eventual evaluation of the diaphragm is indicated in at-risk patients. Once identified, diaphragmatic injury should be expeditiously repaired.

FAILURE TO RECOGNIZE EXTREMITY COMPARTMENT SYNDROME

Development of a compartment syndrome occurs commonly in patients with injuries to the upper and lower extremities. Compartment syndrome may also occur in any muscular compartment encased by fascia. This includes the hand, shoulder, arm, buttocks, thigh, and foot. A commonly held misconception is that patients with open fractures are protected from the development of compartment syndrome. Approximately 10% of patients with open fractures develop a limb-threatening compartment syndrome. Compartment syndrome is diagnosed on history and physical findings as well as a few adjunctive evaluations. Physical findings suggestive of compartment syndrome include a tense extremity with increased pain. Paresthesia indicates advanced ischemia involving nerves. It is an error to assume that a compartment syndrome is not present if a distal pulse is palpable. In fact, pulselessness is a late sign of compartment syndrome and may only occur after irreversible nerve and muscular injury have taken place.

Compartment syndrome develops in injured extremities secondary to a number of factors. Hemorrhage and muscle edema within a compartment may occur secondary to fracture. As pressure within the compartment increases and compartment pressure exceeds perfusion pressures, muscle and nerve ischemia will occur. Additionally, venous outflow obstruction results when compartment pressures rise. Compartment syndrome is a well-recognized complication of electrical burns. Ischemia with reperfusion is also a well-known cause of compartment syndrome. Iatrogenic causes of compartment syndrome include misplaced intravenous catheters into a muscle compartment followed by infusion of fluids into the compartment. Prolonged utilization of military antishock trousers (MAST) has also been associated with the development of compartment syndrome.

The diagnosis of compartment syndrome is based on clinical assessment and invasive evaluation of compartment pressure. Measurement of compartment pressure is easily accomplished using a number of techniques. If pressures within a muscular compartment are greater than 30 mm Hg, then compartment syndrome must be considered. A more elegant approach to determining compartment syndrome is measurement of the compartment perfusion pressure. The compartment perfusion pressure is calculated by subtracting the compartment pressure from the mean arterial blood pressure. If the compartment perfusion pressure is less than 40 mm Hg, then compartment syndrome must be considered.

Definitive therapy for compartment syndrome exists in the form of fasciotomy. Techniques of fasciotomy for both the upper and lower extremities are well known and involve decompression of all compartments of the involved extremity.

ABDOMINAL COMPARTMENT SYNDROME

The abdominal compartment syndrome (ACS) is defined as the pathophysiology and organ dysfunction that occurs as a result of intra-abdominal hypertension (IAH). The renal, cardiovascular, and pulmonary systems are most affected. Treatment of the syndrome is early decompression. However, even when treated appropriately, mortality approaches 50%.

Appreciation of the adverse affects of intra-abdominal hypertension began in the nineteenth century. Marey (1863) and Burt (1870) demonstrated the affects of IAH on respiratory function. In 1890, Heinricius observed increased mortality in cats and guinea pigs when intra-abdominal pressure (IAP) increased from 27–46 cm H_2O.

Emerson showed the relationship between IAH and adverse cardiovascular affects in 1911. In 1913, Wendt demonstrated the relationship between IAH and renal dysfunction. Later in the century, pediatric surgeons became aware of the adverse physiologic affects of IAH and developed techniques to allow expansion of the abdominal contents. In 1984, Kron described a technique to measure intra-abdominal pressure and first used the phrase "abdominal compartment syndrome."

The cardiovascular effects of IAH are consistent and well defined. Cardiac output is reduced as a result of decreased venous return secondary to increased intrathoracic pressure. This phenomenon occurs at IAP greater than 20 mm Hg, although venous return has been shown to be impaired at pressures as low as 15 mm Hg. Elevated intrathoracic pressure also contributes to a reduction in ventricular compliance, which reduces cardiac contractility. The diminished cardiac output seen with IAH has been shown to be exacerbated by hypovolemia and inhalational anesthetics.

The respiratory effects of IAH are mechanical. As the diaphragm is displaced cephalad, increased airway pressures are required to maintain adequate ventilation. Ultimately, this leads to ventilation/perfusion mismatch with resultant hypoxia and hypercarbia.

The mechanism of renal failure with ACS is multifactorial. Inadequate renal perfusion secondary to poor cardiac output, decreased perfusion, obstruction of renal venous outflow, and compression of the kidney all contribute to the renal failure associated with increasing IAP. Numerous studies have demonstrated that the oliguria and anuria seen with ACS are reversible with abdominal decompression.

Very little evidence exists on the effects of ACS on other organ systems. However, decreased blood flow in all abdominal organs occurs when IAP is more than 40 mm Hg. Hepatic artery, portal vein, and microcirculatory perfusion decrease when IAP surpasses 20 mm Hg. Intracranial hypertension and decreased cerebral perfusion pressure consistently improve with abdominal decompression when IAH is present.

Many etiologies exist for the development of ACS. Massive fluid resuscitation with crystalloid solutions plays a prominent and potentially preventable role in the development of this syndrome. Any condition associated with intra-abdominal hemorrhage places the patient at risk for ACS. This includes abdominal trauma, ruptured abdominal aortic aneurysm, retroperitoneal hemorrhage, elective abdominal operations, complications of pregnancy, and hepatic transplantation. In addition to blood, other intraperitoneal fluid collections may contribute to the development of ACS. Edema of the bowel and retroperitoneum, abdominal packing, ileus, ascites, massive volume resuscitation for shock, and inadvisable closure of abdominal fascia, all increase the risk of IAH and ACS.

The diagnosis of ACS is based on clinical parameters and the measurement of IAP. Findings of oliguria (<0.5 ml/kg/hr), hypoxia (oxygen delivery <600 ml/min/m²) with increasing airway pressures (peak >45 cm H_2O), SVR greater than 1000, and a distended abdomen, are all suggestive of ACS. Two methods of IAP measurement are clinically useful: intragastric and intravesicular. The latter is the most widely employed. First described by Kron et al., the technique involves clamping the bladder catheter, followed by the injection of

50–100 ml of sterile saline into the bladder. The catheter is then connected to a pressure manometer.

Based on the adverse physiologic changes at different IAP levels, most experienced surgeons suggest that the abdomen be decompressed with IAP above 25 mm Hg and that all patients be decompressed above 35 mm Hg. Early decompression, which may be performed in the intensive care unit (ICU), can reverse the pathophysiology of ACS. To avoid hypotension upon decompression, it is important to ensure that adequate intravascular volume resuscitation has been accomplished. Complications of abdominal decompression include hyperkalemia, respiratory alkalosis, hemorrhage, and reperfusion injury. The final step in decompressive laparotomy is to provide temporary abdominal closure that prevents recurrent IAH. Additional concerns include infection, fluid loss, evisceration, enterocutaneous fistula formation, and exposure of the abdominal viscera. Many methods of closure are available, including absorbable mesh, plastic intravenous (IV) (Bogota) bags, and vacuum-assisted closure. The large ventral hernia which results from temporary closure frequently requires delayed repair with nonabsorbable mesh. The mortality rate of ACS, despite decompression, still approaches 50%. Left untreated, it is routinely fatal. Early clinical suspicion in patients at risk, combined with aggressive measurement of IAP, can lead to life-saving decompression.

THE MYTH OF MANDATORY COLOSTOMY

Interpersonal violence remains prevalent in North America. The colon is the second most commonly injured abdominal organ in penetrating trauma (Table 1). Multiple associated injuries and infectious complications are common. When these patients present, the trauma surgeon must decide to primarily repair the colon, resect and perform an anastomosis, or create a colostomy. There is continuing debate as to the optimal treatment for penetrating colon injuries. During World War I, many patients underwent primary repair. Colostomy was reserved for extensive injuries or left colon injuries. No matter what treatment was employed, there was a high mortality rate. These dismal survival statistics occurred in an era of delayed treatment, inadequate volume resuscitation, no blood transfusions or antibiotics, and the absence of critical care. The dogma of mandatory colostomy began after the U.S. Army Surgeon General W. H. Ogilvie published a letter in 1943 that required the performance of colostomy for colon injuries:

> The treatment of colon injuries is based on the known insecurity of suture and the dangers of leakage. Simple closure of a wound of the colon, however small, is unwarranted; men have survived such an operation, but others have died who would still be alive had they fallen into the hands of a surgeon with less optimism and more sense. Injured segments must either be exteriorized, or functionally excluded by a proximal colostomy.

This mandate was based on scant evidence but was issued in response to a mortality rate of greater than 50%. From Ogilvie's own data, 50% of patients primarily repaired died, while 59% of

patients treated with colostomy died. As military surgeons returned home, they continued to treat colon injuries with colostomy. But, as early as 1951, Woodhall and Ochsner reported decreased mortality with primary repair compared to colostomy in civilian practice (8.3% vs. 35%). In recent decades, surgeons have become more comfortable with primary repair of colon injuries that previously would have been diverted. More surgeons accept repair or resection and anastomosis of right colon injury, but treatment of left colon injuries are increasingly treated without colostomy. In previous decades, surgeons had to justify primary repair of a colon injury, but now the tide has turned. In 1991, Chappuis et al. reported the first prospective, randomized study of primary repair versus diversion in penetrating colon injuries. Patients were randomized irrespective of injury, contamination, transfusions, or shock. There was no difference in morbidity between the groups (17.9% vs. 21.4%). Length of hospitalization was 6 days longer in the colostomy group.

A 1996 prospective, randomized study by Gonzalez evaluated patients with penetrating colon injuries. These patients were randomized to either primary repair with or without resection versus mandatory colostomy. Randomization occurred irrespective of concomitant injuries or other risk factors. Septic complications were lower in the primary repair group (20% vs. 25%,) although this was not statistically significant. In severely injured patients with a PATI (penetrating abdominal trauma index) score higher than 25, there was a lower complication rate in the primary repair group as compared with the diversion group. Although these differences were not statistically significant, this experience demonstrated that primary repair was at least equal to, if not superior to, mandatory colostomy.

Subsequently, Gonzalez et al. reported their 6-year experience with 181 patients with penetrating colon injury. These patients were again randomized to primary repair or colostomy, regardless of other injuries, heavy fecal contamination, or hypotension. Septic complications were lower in the primary repair group (18% vs. 21%, $p = 0.05$). In hemodynamically unstable patients, the complication rate was also lower in the primary repair group (26% vs. 50%). Complications declined over time in both groups, which can be explained by improvement in the overall care of trauma victims.

Sasaki et al. published a prospective randomized study of 71 patients with penetrating colon injuries. There were no exclusionary criteria used in the randomization. Sixty percent of patients were treated with primary repair or resection and anastomosis. There was no significant difference in the grade of injury. There was a 19% complication rate (colon and non-colon related) in the primary repair group as compared with a 36% complication rate in the diversion group. In patients with a PATI greater than 25, the complication rate was 33% in primarily repaired patients and 93% in diverted patients. The PATI score has been used as an argument for mandatory colostomy in the past, but in this and other studies, the complication rate is higher in patients with higher PATI scores regardless of the choice of treatment. The authors also report a 7% complication rate at the time of colostomy reversal. Berne et al. performed a retrospective review of 40 patients who underwent colostomy reversal after trauma. They found a morbidity rate of 55% in patients initially treated with colostomy for colon injury.

The decision to perform a diverting colostomy may seem inherently sound. But contemporary trauma care must be based on evidence and not intuition. Diverting colostomy condemns patients to a subsequent operation for reanatomosis and exposes them to stoma-specific complications, including peristomal hernia, stenosis of the ostomy, ostomy retraction, necrosis and skin damage at the ostomy site. Based on current evidence, mandatory colostomy for penetrating colon injury should be abandoned. Consideration of colostomy for any colon injury, regardless of the coexisting injuries or comorbidities, must be justified based on current evidence and the status of the individual patient.

Table 1: American Association for the Surgery of Trauma (AAST) Colon Injury Scale

Grade I	Hematoma or contusion without devascularization
Grade I	Laceration: partial thickness without perforation
Grade II	Laceration <50% of circumference
Grade III	Laceration >50% of circumference
Grade IV	Transection of colon
Grade V	Transection of colon with segmental tissue loss

DELAYED DAMAGE-CONTROL LAPAROTOMY

"Damage control," a term originating from the U.S. Navy definition of a ship's ability to absorb damage and maintain mission integrity, is now a phrase that describes a surgical strategy utilized in many body regions. It describes a modified operative sequence in which the immediate repair of injuries is abandoned in favor of a staged approach. This is done in recognition of the physiologic insult suffered by the critically injured patient, and the continued deterioration during the operation which may render that insult irreversible. The concept of abbreviated laparotomy dates to 1908, when Pringle described the principles of compression and hepatic packing for control of portal venous hemorrhage. This practice fell out of favor after World War II, but reports emerged in the 1960s and 1970s that suggested improved outcomes with this technique. In 1983, Stone et al. introduced the modern concept of the abbreviated laparotomy with subsequent resuscitation and interval completion laparotomy after physiologic restoration. In 1993, Rotondo and associates popularized the term "damage control," and it has rapidly become a standard in the treatment of critically injured patients with deteriorating physiologic parameters.

Three stages of damage-control laparotomy were originally described. The first stage is the truncated laparotomy in the face of life-threatening physiologic circumstances. It involves the control of hemorrhage with intra-abdominal packing and control of contamination from bowel, pancreatic, or biliary tract injuries. Lengthy vascular repairs are not pursued, but temporary shunting is used liberally. Enteric contamination is controlled by rapid suture, stapling, or resection. No attempt at definitive reconstruction of bowel continuity is required. Most authors describe the use of laparotomy pads for packing; however, the use of Kerlex gauze has also been described. Overpacking can lead to increased intra-abdominal pressure and abdominal compartment syndrome. Underpacking may fail to stop hemorrhage. Packing should provide pressure in vectors that recreate the disrupted tissue planes. It is difficult to obtain hemostasis of arterial injuries with packing. If rapid repair, ligation, or stenting cannot be accomplished, then other methods, such as angiographic embolization, should be employed. Biliary tract and pancreatic injuries can be managed with external tube drainage. Rarely, a pancreatoduodenectomy without reconstruction may be required. Once the abbreviated laparotomy is completed, the abdomen is closed by temporary methods. Many techniques for temporary closure have been described, including penetrating towel clamp closure, running skin sutures, use of an IV bag (Bogota bag) and vacuum closure device. Whichever method is used, the goals are identical: prevent evisceration, protect the bowel, and minimize the risk of intra-abdominal hypertension and abdominal compartment syndrome.

The second phase of damage control involves ongoing resuscitation in the ICU with the reversal of the lethal triad: hypothermia, acidosis, and coagulopathy. Each of these devastating physiologic complications has a compounding effect on the others. Hypothermia, defined as a core temperature less than 35° C, is exacerbated by prolonged exposure, inadequate perfusion, and inadequate warming in the emergency department or operating room. Hypothermia exists in as many as half of injured patients following trauma laparotomy. Hypothermia increases the requirement for fluid resuscitation, vasopressors, inotropes, and transfusions. It is associated with increased morbidity, organ dysfunction, coagulopathy, and mortality. In the ICU, the ambient temperature, airway circuit, intravenous fluids, and blood products should all be warmed. Warm blankets and a forced-air heater should be used aggressively. Acidosis results from inadequate oxygen delivery secondary to hemorrhage which results in anaerobic metabolism and the release of lactic acid. Acidosis worsens coagulopathy, depresses myocardial contractility, diminishes inotropic response to catecholamines, and predisposes to ventricular dysrhythmias. Correction of acidosis is directed at improvement of oxygen delivery and optimizing cardiac output. Failure to correct

elevated lactic acid levels or base deficit within 48 hours is associated with rates of mortality approaching 100%. Coagulopathy is worsened by the combined effects of hypothermia, acidosis, and dilution of clotting factors by massive crystalloid resuscitation. Correction of coagulopathy is achieved by the reversal of hypothermia and acidosis, as well as the aggressive replacement of clotting factors with fresh frozen plasma, cryoprecipitate, and platelets. Recombinant factor VIIa may be beneficial in reversing recalcitrant coagulopathy in trauma.

The third phase of damage control refers to definitive operative repair of injuries after reversal of physiologic impairments. The timing of definitive repair is based on clinical parameters rather than the clock. It may be necessary to perform more than one subsequent laparotomy to repair all injuries. The decision to employ damage control techniques is ultimately made by the surgeon. The decision should be made early if the benefits of the technique are to be fully realized. Indications for the damage control approach include the inability to achieve hemostasis, inaccessible source of hemorrhage, multiple severe injuries, poor response to resuscitation, and as dictated by the direct measurement of physiologic parameters of temperature, pH, and the vital signs. Complications of damage control include wound infection, abscess formation, enterocutaneous fistula formation, dehiscence, bile leak, pancreatic pseudocyst formation, intestinal necrosis, abdominal compartment syndrome, multisystem organ failure, acute respiratory distress syndrome (ARDS), and death.

Damage control represents a unique surgical philosophy which can be life-saving in a select population of critically injured patients. Success is dependent on timing, patient selection, rapid operative control of hemorrhage and contamination, aggressive resuscitation, and the reversal of the lethal triad of hypothermia, acidosis, and coagulopathy.

MISSED HOLLOW VISCUS INJURY

With the increasing utilization of nonoperative management of solid organ injuries in blunt trauma, the incidence of missed hollow viscus must be considered. Hollow viscus injury affects about 1% of all trauma patients and 15% of patients with blunt abdominal trauma. Motor vehicle collisions are the most common mechanism of injury. Even as diagnostic imaging has evolved, it is still inferior to laparotomy in establishing the diagnosis of hollow viscus injury. Some of these injuries are evident on close examination of initial computed tomography (CT) scans, but others become apparent after hours or days. The FAST exam has proven useful to diagnose hemoperitoneum, but it is not capable of reliably identifying hollow viscus injury. Physical examination, diagnostic peritoneal lavage (DPL), and laboratory tests are similarly unreliable.

The use of CT has dramatically increased over recent years. The ability to identify solid organ injuries with CT scans is far superior to the ability to diagnose hollow viscus injury. Killeen et al. examined 150 CT scans of blunt trauma victims and compared these to operative findings. Helical CT scan showed a sensitivity of 94% for bowel injuries and 96% for mesenteric injuries. The number of solid organ injuries influences the diagnosis of hollow viscus injuries. With a single solid organ injury, a hollow viscus injury was found in 7.3% of patients. The incidence doubled (15.4%) with two solid organ injuries and was 34.4% with three solid organ injuries. Malhotra et al. also found that the following findings on CT were predictive of hollow viscus injury: unexplained intraperitoneal fluid, pneumoperitoneum, bowel wall thickening, mesenteric fat streaking, mesenteric hematoma, extravasation of luminal contrast, and extravasation of vascular contrast. They recommend that patients with a single positive finding undergo confirmatory DPL, and those with more than one finding should undergo urgent exploration.

In 1999, Fang et al. examined patients with a delayed diagnosis of small bowel injury. Their retrospective review of 111 blunt trauma victims with small bowel injury showed no difference in mortality if the injury was treated within 24 hours. But patients with a delay in diagnosis of greater than 4 hours had an increased incidence of wound infection, abscess formation, enterocutaneous fistula, wound dehiscence, and sepsis. Those whose injury was repaired after 24 hours averaged a 20-day increase in hospital stay and a 6-day delay in initiation of oral intake when compared with those whose injury was repaired between 12 and 24 hours. Fakhry et al. found an increase in mortality and morbidity with diagnostic delays in small bowel injuries. Mortality was 2% when the injury was treated within 8 hours, 9.1% when treated between 8 and 16 hours, 16.7% when treated between 16 and 24 hours, and 30.8% when delayed more than 24 hours.

Missed injuries are not isolated to blunt mechanism of injury. Sung et al. found, in a retrospective review of 607 patients with penetrating trauma, a missed injury rate of 2%. These injuries were missed at the initial operation. These injuries included two gastric perforations, two retroperitoneal rectal injuries, one pancreatic transection, and one duodenal injury. Forty-two percent of patients with missed injuries developed sepsis, and 17% developed renal failure. Mortality was significantly higher in patients with missed injuries (17% vs. 6.4%, $p = 0.007$). This study highlights the need for a standard, systematic approach to trauma laparotomy. In our institution, after a physical exam, all patients undergo a surgeon-performed FAST exam. In the stable patient with free fluid, we then obtain a contrast-enhanced CT. If the patient's physical findings change or a hollow viscus injury is still suspected, but unproven, a repeat CT scan and/or diagnostic laparoscopy is then considered. The increased mortality and morbidity associated with diagnostic delays mandates an aggressive search for suspected hollow viscus injuries.

FAILURE TO PERFORM TERTIARY SURVEY

Missed injuries plague all trauma centers. The Advanced Trauma Life Support Course (ATLS) has become the gold standard for initial recognition and treatment of life-threatening injuries in the initial evaluation period through the use of a primary and secondary survey. However, it is clear from published reports that this approach allows injuries to go undetected. While there is no consensus on the specific criteria to define a missed injury, it refers to any injury not appreciated in the initial evaluation. The reported rates of missed injuries vary from 2%–50%. The majority of these may not be clinically significant, but some are potentially fatal. Even less severe injuries can cause prolonged disability, expense, pain, and deterioration in the relationship between the trauma team and the patient. Factors that contribute to the prevalence of missed injuries include the attention focused on more urgent treatment priorities, altered patient sensorium, poorly appreciated physical findings, and radiologic studies that are not appropriately performed, are misinterpreted, or are omitted. Missed injuries are more common in patients involved in motor vehicle crashes, those with higher injury severity scores (ISS), and those with a greater number of injuries. One other factor reported to increase the frequency of missed injuries is the level of experience of the treating physician.

There are a number of reports that recommend the use of a tertiary survey as a mechanism to address this issue. The tertiary survey is a thorough re-examination of the trauma patient within the first 24 hours of admission and after all contributing sources of examination difficulty have resolved. This exam includes symptom review, physical examination, and review or ordering of appropriate radiologic or laboratory studies. Since factors of hemodynamic instability and altered sensorium may still exist after 24 hours of treatment, it is important to complete the tertiary survey again when a patient is stabilized and neurologically competent. Many surgeons have suggested formal radiology rounds as a standard part of the tertiary survey, since over 25% of missed injuries can be correctly identified on the original x-ray studies. Enderson et al. reported identifying additional injuries in 9% of blunt trauma patients with the routine use of a tertiary survey. Janjua et al. detected 56% of early missed injuries and 90% of clinically significant missed injuries with the performance of a tertiary survey within 24 hours of admission. Biffl et al. were able to reduce the incidence of missed injuries from 2.4%–1.5% after implementation of a tertiary survey policy. Soundappan et al. reported similar results in a pediatric population.

The distribution of missed injuries involves almost every anatomic region. The most commonly missed injuries are fractures. These include fractures of the extremities, spine, and pelvis. Missed skull and facial fractures are reported routinely. Strategies to avoid delayed diagnosis include a thorough physical examination of all extremities and the back to search for deformity, swelling, ecchymosis, and decreased range of motion. In neurologically intact patients, a meticulous interrogation of symptoms is warranted. Radiologic evaluation of any questionable area should be performed and reviewed in a timely fashion. Delays in the diagnosis of abdominal injuries, including both solid organ, intestinal, and diaphragm injuries, can cause preventable trauma deaths. Inability to perform a meaningful abdominal exam, hemodynamic instability precluding the ability to perform a CT scan, and the immediacy of an operative procedure for other serious injuries, can all contribute to a delay in diagnosis. Useful measures to reduce these delays include repeat physical examination, the use of serial sonography, and repeat CT scan to improve the diagnosis of a hollow viscus injury. Frequently missed injuries in the thorax include aortic rupture, rib fractures, pneumothorax, and hemothorax. Careful physical examination and radiologic evaluation can reduce the rate of diagnostic delays.

Missed injuries occur with significant frequency and with the potential for significant morbidity and mortality. The tertiary survey is a comprehensive patient evaluation that occurs after the initial resuscitation period. Tertiary survey should become a standard and necessary feature of the care of every trauma patient.

FUTILE RESUSCITATIVE THORACOTOMY

One of the most dramatic procedures performed is the emergency department (ED) thoracotomy. It is performed in a hectic environment, but when carried out in the proper patient, can be life saving. Unfortunately, it is frequently performed in poorly selected patients without valid indications, with predictably dismal results. There is little doubt that a patient with cardiac tamponade secondary to a small stab wound to the right ventricle who loses vital signs in the trauma bay may be salvaged. But in many instances, indications for resuscitative thoracotomy are less clear. Futile thoracotomy performed for patients with lethal injuries is distressingly common.

Rhee et al. recently retrospectively reviewed a 25-year multicenter experience with resuscitative thoracotomy. Blunt trauma victims undergoing ED thoracotomy had a survival rate of 1.4%. Survival of blunt trauma victims ranged from 0%–12.5% for the various trauma centers. If the 12.5% rate of survival from one center is excluded, most survival rates are less than 2%. Many blunt trauma "survivors" of ED thoracotomy were not neurologically intact. In 2004, Powell et al. evaluated their experience with ED thoracotomy for victims of penetrating and blunt trauma who required prehospital cardiopulmonary resuscitation (CPR). They documented four blunt trauma survivors, all of whom had a severe neurologic deficit. Even in blunt trauma patients with cardiac tamponade, the outcome after ED thoracotomy is routinely fatal. In a retrospective review of ED thoracotomy patients, Grove et al. reported four blunt trauma victims with cardiac tamponade who survived ED thoracotomy and were admitted to the ICU; all died within 9 days. Clearly, blunt trauma victims without signs of life in the field or upon arrival in the trauma bay should be declared dead. The blunt trauma patient who loses vital signs shortly after arrival in the ED will have a dismal outcome with any therapy, and we believe that thoracotomy should not be performed.

Some victims of penetrating trauma clearly may benefit from ED thoracotomy. Proper selection of potentially salvageable patients is key. Powell found that the duration of CPR was critical. All survivors of ED thoracotomy had CPR for 15 minutes or less. Any penetrating trauma patient with prolonged CPR (>15 minutes) should be pronounced dead upon arrival.

Few patients will survive if the duration of prehospital CPR is greater than 5 minutes. ED thoracotomy is a potentially life-saving procedure, but there are few survivors. Utilization of this intervention should be limited to patients with penetrating mechanisms of injury. Those with noncardiac injuries have a poor prognosis. The FAST exam may help to delineate treatable intrathoracic injury and decrease the number of futile ED thoracotomies in the future.

SUMMARY

The circumstances involved in the evaluation and treatment of injured patients makes errors likely. It is inevitable that delays in diagnosis and intervention will occur in multiply injured patients. However, it is incumbent upon all those who care for trauma patients to have a high index of suspicion for common errors so that the frequency of these may be minimized. A low threshold of suspicion for difficult to diagnose injuries must be maintained if optimal care is to be delivered to injured patients. Futile attempts to salvage lethally injured patients are costly and time consuming and should be minimized.

Suggested Readings

Biffl WL, Harrington DT, Cioffi WG: Implementation of a trauma survey decreases missed injuries. *J Trauma* 54(1):38–43, 2003.

Burch JM, Moore EE, Moore FA, Franciose R: The abdominal compartment syndrome. *Surg Clin North Am* 76:833–842, 1996.

Chappuis CW, Frey DJ, Dietzen CD, et al: Management of penetrating colon injuries: a randomized controlled trial. *Ann Surg* 213:492–498, 1991.

Eddy V, Nunn C, Morris JA Jr: Abdominal compartment syndrome: the Nashville experience. *Surg Clin North Am* 77:801–812, 1997.

Enderson BL, Reath DB, Meadors J, et al: The tertiary survey: a prospective study of missed injury. *J Trauma* 30:666–669, 1990.

Grove L, et al: Emergency thoracotomy: appropriate use in the resuscitation of trauma patients. *Am Surg* 68:313–317, 2002.

Hirshberg A, Walden R: Damage control for abdominal trauma. *Surg Clin North Am* 77(4):813–820, 1997.

Houshian S, Larsen MS, Holm C: Missed injuries in a level I trauma center. *J Trauma* 52:715–719, 2002.

Janjua KJ, Sugrue M, Deane SA: Prospective evaluation of early missed injuries and the role of tertiary trauma survey. *J Trauma* 44:1000–1006, 1998.

Moore AFK, Hargest R, Martin M, Delicata RJ: Intra-abdominal hypertension and the abdominal compartment syndrome. *Br J Surg* 91:1102–1110, 2004.

Ogilvie WH: Abdominal wounds in the Western Desert. *Surg Gynecol Obstet* 78:225, 1944.

Powell DW, et al: Is emergency department resuscitative thoracotomy futile care for the critically injured patient requiring prehospital cardiopulmonary resuscitation? *J Am Coll Surg* 199(2):211–215, 2004.

Rhee P, et al: Survival after emergency department thoracotomy: review of published data from the past 25 years. *J Am Coll Surg* 190(3):288–298, 2000.

Rotondo M, Schwab C, McGonigal M, et al: Damage control: an approach for improved survival in exsanguinating penetrating abdominal injury. *J Trauma* 35(3):375–382, 1993.

Saggi BH, Sugerman HJ, Ivatury RR, Bloomfield GL: Abdominal compartment syndrome. *J Trauma* 45(3):597–609, 1998.

Schreiber M: Damage control surgery. *Crit Care Clin* 20:101–118, 2004.

Shapiro MB, Jenkins DH, Schwab CW, et al: Damage control: collective review. *J Trauma* 49(5):969–978, 2000.

Stone H, Strom P, Mullins R: Management of the major coagulopathy with onset during laparotomy. *Ann Surg* 197:532–535, 1983.

Sugrue M, D'Amours SK, Joshipura M: Damage control surgery and the abdomen. *Injury* 35:642–648, 2004.

Woodall JP, Oschner A: The management of perforating injuries of the colon and rectum in civilian practice. *Surgery* 29:305, 1951.

Working Group, Ad Hoc Subcommittee on Outcomes, American College of Surgeons, Committee on Trauma: Practice management guidelines for emergency department thoracotomy. *J Am Coll Surg* 193(3):303–309, 2001.

CARDIAC HEMODYNAMICS: THE PULMONARY ARTERY CATHETER AND THE MEANING OF ITS READINGS

Mitchell J. Cohen and **Robert C. Mackersie**

The pulmonary artery catheter (PAC) is a physical object creating a conundrum. Since its introduction in the 1970s, the PAC has been simultaneously hailed for its ability to provide physiological data not easily obtainable by other means, and condemned as a useless and potentially harmful invasive monitor. Very little hard data support continued use of the PAC, and some data support avoiding it altogether. Despite considerable controversy over the clinical utility and safety of the PAC, which has intermittently led to confusion and conjecture regarding its use and future, the PAC remains a mainstay of invasive intensive care unit (ICU) monitoring. In this chapter, we aim to provide a concise history of right-heart catheterization. We will then examine the basis of insertion, data collection, interpretation, and troubleshooting. Finally, we will reexamine the clinical data for and against the use of PA catheterization and determination of resuscitation in critically ill surgical patients.

HISTORY OF CONTROVERSY

The PAC was introduced in the late 1960s, approved for clinical use in 1970 and quickly became the de facto tool of the critical care physician. By 1999, 1.5 million catheters were sold, and presumably used, each year in the United States. Due to its introduction prior to a 1976 policy change, which mandated the testing of medical devices, the PAC was grandfathered by the Food and Drug Administration (FDA), and has to date never been required to undergo safety testing. Even as considerable controversy and political debate over its utility continues, the catheter has never been considered a life-saving device and, as a result, is exempt from licensing and required study.[1]

Since its invention, the PAC has enjoyed growing use and acceptance as a monitoring tool. Indeed, its popularity has followed closely the advent of critical care as a specialty, and thus is considered by many a primary tool of the critical care physician. After years of use with little data supporting benefits, concerns about the overall utility and safety of the PAC first appeared in several papers written in the late 1980s.[1] Gore et al. examined 3000 patients with acute myo-

cardial infarction (MI) and the relationship of outcome to PA catheterization.[2] This study of over 3000 patients with acute MI reported higher mortality in patients with hypotension who received a PAC (42% vs. 32%). Higher mortality was also reported in the subgroup or patients with CHF who received a PAC (44% vs. 25%). In addition, patients who received a PAC had longer hospital stay. Several observational and retrospective studies quickly followed with similar concerning results.[3] Many in the critical care community discounted these trials, believing that PAC placement was more common in patients with greater illness, which would explain the higher mortality rates. A 1990 Canadian trial was the first to attempt to prospectively study the use of PAC in critically ill patients. In what was to become a recurring theme, however, the study failed due to a 35% exclusion rate as many clinicians refused to randomize their patients, arguing instead that it was unethical not to use a PAC (which had become the de facto tool of the ICU physician). A lack of clinical agreement regarding PAC use or perhaps just a lack of interest in the problem followed, and the PAC enjoyed continued widespread use until the debate was reignited by Connors et al., who studied PAC use in 5735 critically ill ICU patients. The Connors group was careful to attempt to match illness severity and other confounding variables between the PAC and control groups. Ultimately, his group found that patients treated with PAC had increased 30-day mortality, mean cost, and ICU stay. Subgroup analysis identified no groups of patients who benefited from PAC.[4]

As a result of these and similar data, in the same issue of the *Journal of the American Medical Association*, Bone and Drhen called for a National Heart, Lung, and Blood Institute (NHLBI) randomized prospective clinical trail to test the efficacy and safety of the PAC. They went on to spark considerable controversy by suggesting that the FDA issue a moratorium on the use of the pulmonary catheter until such time that the safety and use be measured in an appropriate clinical trial. In response to this call for a moratorium, both a National Heart, Lung, and Blood Institute (NHLBI) and a Society of Critical Care Medicine (SCCM) consensus conference were convened in 1997. The Pulmonary Artery Catheter Consensus Conference Consensus Statement was published that same year. According to the statement, there was no need of a moratorium on PACs, given adequate level-IV evidence to support the possibility of benefit of PAC in patient groups including MI and trauma, but conceded that appropriate clinical trials should be undertaken to measure its use and safety.[5,6] The NHLBI conference came to similar findings.[7] Many trials followed, all with limited numbers of patients or low randomization rates.

In 2003, a Canadian group published the first prospective randomized study with sufficient patient enrollment to have statistical power and authority.[8] In this study, 1994 patients were randomized to surgery without a pulmonary catheter versus with a PAC. The authors found that there were no differences in hospital survival, and in 6- and 12-month survival. There was however, an increase in the number of pulmonary embolism (PE) events with eight reported in the catheter group versus 0 in the observation group. The authors concluded that no benefit from PA catheterization could be found in elderly high-risk surgical patients. While this study was important in that it was the first to randomize a significant cohort of patients, the randomization rate remained a low 52%. Furthermore, it represented a subset of older critically ill patients, while excluding younger trauma or septic patients. Other trials have followed and shown mixed results.[9–12] More recently Shah et al. performed a meta-analysis of 13 randomized clinical trials between 1985 and 2005.[13] This study totaling 5051 patients was performed using a random effects model to estimate the odds ratio for death, hospital days, and pressors and found no difference between patients with and without a PAC.

No randomized prospective trial to date, however, has shown a definite benefit to PA catheterization in critically injured patients. In data limited to trauma patients, there is some recent evidence to show a benefit for PAC use in the injured. A database study of over 53,000 patients drawn from the National Trauma Data Bank showed a reduction in mortality in older patients and patients with higher injury severity scores. Overall, PAC use was shown to be beneficial in patients with severe shock with a base deficit of 11 or more, injury severity scores higher than 25, and age over 61. This large cohort database study is the first and only study to show a clear benefit from PAC use in the severely injured patient.[14]

One bias confounding PAC use and study are disparate factors that affect which patients are treated with the PAC. In 2000, Rapoport et al. reported a comprehensive look at the characteristics of PAC use.[15] This group retrospectively examined 10,217 patients in 34 ICUs in the United States and showed that full-time ICU staffing was associated with a decreased likelihood of PAC use. Catheter use was associated with white race/ethnicity and private insurance. Patients admitted to a surgical ICU were two times more likely to have a PAC. This study is revealing in that it is indicative of the lack of an established protocol and the presence of an established bias in PAC placement.

PULMONARY ARTERY CATHETER USE AND INSERTION: WHAT IT IS AND HOW IT WORKS

Pulmonary artery catheters are commonly 100 cm long with an exterior French diameter of 7.5. Available with or without a heparin or antibiotic coating, they commonly contain latex rubber, an important consideration in latex-allergic patients. The 7.5–French diameter is further separated into three lumens. At the far distal end of the catheter is the PA port, which is used to transduce PA pressure and draw mixed venous blood. Just proximal to this port is a 1.5-cc balloon, which facilitates both the "floating" of the catheter and is also used to distally occlude the PA to measure pulmonary artery occlusion pressure (PAOP). Another side infusion port, used for instillation of fluid, vasoactive agents, and medications, is located 15 cm proximal to the end of the catheter. Proximal to the side infusion port is the right atrial (RA)/central venous pressure (CVP) port, which is designed to be positioned at the vena cava/right atrial junction. This RA/CVP port is transduced to measure the CVP. Like the proximal infusion port, it can also be used as an infusion port for medication and fluids.

Along with ports that allow for pressure transduction and fluid infusion, the PAC also incorporates a thermal coil and proximal and distal thermistor for the measurement of cardiac output. Cardiac output is calculated by measurement of the change in temperature of blood between a proximal and distally placed thermistor. Traditionally, a cooled fluid bolus was injected proximally and the temperature of this bolus (now slightly warmed by blood flow) was measured by the thermistor at the tip of the catheter. Using formulas discussed later in the chapter, the cardiac output could be calculated. Most modern catheters now utilize a proximally placed thermal coil incorporated

into the catheter which gently warms blood proximally extrapolation from the temperature difference proximally and distally gives a continuous calculation of cardiac output. (A more detailed discussion of cardiac output monitoring appears later in the chapter.)

Insertion Tips and Guidelines

Insertion of the catheter is done through the gasketed introducer port of a Cordis™ catheter. Full sterile technique is paramount in order to reduce infection rates. We commonly place the introducer catheter and the PAC sequentially with one sterile prep and setup, which prevents contamination at the introducer gasket as well as the necessity of reprepping of a previously placed introducer. At times, however, this cannot be avoided, or a PAC will be placed through a previously located introducer line. In this instance, the introducer catheter and surrounding skin should be prepped widely with chlorohexidine preparation. In all cases, wide sterile prep with chlorohexidine, full sterile precautions including gown, hat, mask, and sterile gloves are essential. Any break in sterile technique has been shown in many studies to significantly increase the infection rate and implementation of the above precautions has been reported to reduce the infection rate to near zero.[16–21] Another tip is to prep widely. We cannot stress this seemingly trivial point too strongly. Opening, preparing, and inserting a PAC results in an often-unwieldy octopus of catheter, tubing, and transducers that have to cross through a sterile to unsterile transition zone. Wide prep of all or most of the bed with a sterile half-sheet facilitates easy handling and reduced risk of contamination. Once an introducer catheter is in place, the PAC is removed from the packaging and the proximal end is passed to an assistant who will connect and flush the catheter ports. At this time, the transducer is connected, zeroed, and tested. The balloon is also tested. Placement of the catheter sheath allows future adjustments without additional sterile prep.

Constant verbal communication between the floater and the assistant is essential. Once the tip of the catheter is passed through the introducer and into the blood vessel, it must be advanced only when the balloon is inflated (up), and conversely it must never be withdrawn unless the balloon is deflated (down). The slang "floating" a swan refers to the fact that the catheter advances by floating along with the blood flow. Direct advancement can cause vascular injury or perforation. A constant communicative banter—"balloon up?," "balloon up," "balloon down?," "balloon down"—can prevent injuries such as arterial, cardiac, and PA rupture.

Initially the catheter is inserted to the 10–15-cm mark, allowing the balloon to pass through the introducer. Once the catheter tip is safely past the introducer, the balloon is inflated and the catheter slowly advanced by feeding slack catheter and allowing the catheter to be pulled downstream by the blood flow. A combination of clinical experience, length of catheter inserted, and careful attention to the monitored transducer tracing allow successful placement. As the catheter tip enters the vessel, the initial pressure reading will be the CVP, which first transduced at ~15–25 cm depending on patient size and insertion site. With another 5–10 cm of advancement, the catheter passes into the right atrium and the transducer will register a distinct right arterial waveform. Another few centimeters of advancement passes the catheter tip through the tricuspid valve (around 30 cm) and the easily recognizable spike of RV pressure will register on the monitor. Slow careful advancement of another 5–10 cm will pass the catheter into the PA (tracing), and will soon wedge the catheter to produce a flattening of the waveform and characteristic wedge tracing.

Often several attempts to ensure proper wedging are required. When a RV waveform is not evident after 35–45 cm or no wedge tracing occurs after the catheter has advanced 10–15 cm past the RV tracing, the balloon should be deflated, and the catheter pulled back to the RA or RV. Once a distinct tracing identifies the catheter location, another careful attempt at reinsertion and wedging can begin. When the catheter is inserted and wedged, the pulmonary capillary wedge pressure (PCWP) is noted and the balloon deflated. The catheter is locked into place and the sterile covering advanced to cover the full length of the catheter. Placement of the catheter is confirmed by a chest x-ray.

INTERPRETATION: WHAT DOES IT MEASURE AND WHAT DOES IT MEAN?

Initial Warnings and Potential Measurement Problems

While the PAC provides a lot of otherwise unobtainable data, only diligent attention and educated interpretation make PA catheterization worth the risk, time, and cost. Without proper placement, all obtained data are erroneous and will lead to false interpretation and incorrect (and possibly harmful) intervention. Careful attention to the PAC waveform helps confirm catheter placement. Entry into the pulmonary artery is evidenced by a decrease in mean pressure and characteristic wave form. Upon entering the PA, a triphasic waveform is seen, which reflects atrial and ventricular contraction. From the PA careful advancement of the catheter will "wedge" the catheter.[22]

From the PAOP and CVP, we begin the pressure-volume measures. Once wedged or occluded, the inflated balloon prevents forward blood flow from the right ventricle or proximal pulmonary artery and allows only back-pressure to be transduced at the catheter tip. This transduced "wedge" pressure reflects a contiguous fluid column from the PA through the pulmonary vasculature to the left atrium (LA). The unobstructed column continues through the mitral valve into the (when open) left ventricle (LV), and hence,

$$PA \sim LA \sim LV \sim LVEDP,$$

where LVEDP is left ventricle end-diastolic pressure. It is crucial to note that this relationship holds true only when there is a contiguous fluid column between the PA and LV. A common reason for improper interpretation of PAOP occurs when this contiguous fluid column is interrupted or affected. Examples of interrupted fluid column include mitral valve disease (stenosis or insufficiency) and pulmonary venous obstruction. Also affecting the relationship between PAOP and left ventricular end-diastolic volume (LVEDV) is the ability to extrapolate volume from pressure measurements. Since PCWP is ultimately used as a measure of ventricular filling (volume), this necessitates the ability to predictably extrapolate volume from pressure, which is only possible with normal compliance. Indeed, LVEDP is analogous to left ventricular end-diastolic volume (LVEDV) only in a normally compliant heart and thorax. Many factors influence the ability to use PCWP as an accurate measure of left heart–filling pressures. As described previously, the analogous relationship between LVEDP and LVEDV is accurate only insofar as the ventricle is normally compliant. In cases where left heart compliance is reduced such as ventricular hypertrophy or ischemic myocardial damage, the PCWP will be elevated for a corresponding left ventricular pressure/volume and cannot be considered an accurate measure. While trend analysis can be used to monitor fluid resuscitation in these patients, injured or septic patients often manifest rapidly changing cardiac compliance making interpretation difficult and suspect. Indeed multiple animal models have shown a rapid flux of cardiac edema resulting from injury, resuscitation, and inflammation, all of which can rapidly change ventricular compliance and render the PAC an unreliable measure of cardiac filling.[22]

Along with proper wedging in the pulmonary artery and a normally compliant heart, the pulmonary catheter must be placed in the proper lung zone. In order for PCWP to reflect a vascular rather than alveolar pressure, the catheter must be placed in West zone 3 of the lung. Here Pa > PV > PA, so the measured pulmonary venous pressure reflects vascular pressure instead of pulmonary alveolar pressure. If the catheter is in zone 1, PA > Pa > PV, or 2 Pa > PA > PV, the catheter will reflect alveolar pressure rather than the PA pressure.

Constantly changing thoracic pressures from ventilation (spontaneous or mechanical) are reflected in the PAC tracing. In a positive pressure–ventilated patient, the PCWP should be measured at expiration when the pleural pressures are closest to zero. This is reversed if the patient is spontaneously breathing. In a spontaneously breathing patient the pressure normalizes somewhere between expansion and inhalation and by convention, the pressure is measured at end inspiration. Direct monitoring and examination of the tracing rather than reliance on automatically collected single number display is always better. In an extreme situation, brief paralysis might be necessary to get a useful PAWP tracing in an agitated or ventilatory dyssynchronous patient.

Positive end-expiratory pressure (PEEP) also affects the PAC tracing, and interpretation of the PCWP in a patient affected by intrinsic or intrinsic PEEP is the subject of much conjecture and misinformation. PEEP (both intrinsic and extrinsic) causes transmural thoracic pressure, which positively effects PAWP measurements. To correctly determine the PAWP, the PEEP can be temporally disconnected (for a few seconds or breath cycles). Alternatively, the effect of intrinsic or extrinsic PEEP can be estimated by adding 2–3 cm H_2O to each 5 cm of PEEP >10.[22]

Cardiac output (CO) is measured by thermodilution. Traditionally, a cooled saline bolus was injected proximally, and the temperature of the bolus was measured by a thermistor at the catheter tip. CO is calculated by determining the area under the curve and plotting the integral. An average of three to five injections were used to minimize variability. Newer catheters measure CO continuously by integrating a thermal coil, which gently heats the proximal blood, measures the temperature drop at the catheter tip and uses a similar method to calculate CO. In either method, intracardiac shunt and tricuspid regurgitation will lead to unpredictable error in cardiac output measurement. At least one set of authors suggest that greater reliability can be had by calculating CO through plotting of the Fick curve and extrapolating CO.

Pressure, Volume, and Work Measures

While modern PAC monitoring units or ICU nurses provide continuous data readouts of hemodynamic parameters, it remains essential to have a grounded understanding of the physiologic principles and calculations involved in PAC monitoring. Actual measured parameters begin with CVP. CVP is directly transduced from the proximal or CVP port of the catheter. Without obstruction between the right atrium and the vena cava, CVP is analogous to right atrial pressure (RAP), which is again analogous to right ventricle end-diastolic pressure (RVEDP) and right ventricle end-diastolic volume (RVEDV). Hence,

$$CVP \sim RAP \sim RVEDP \sim RVEDV.$$

CVP is a direct measured extrapolation of RVEDV or cardiac preload. Just as CVP is a measure of right heart filling, PCWP measures left-sided pressure and volume. As described previously when the catheter is "wedged" in the pulmonary artery, there is a continuous fluid column between the PA and LV. Hence,

$$PCWP \sim LAP \sim LVEDP \sim LVEDV.$$

Cardiac output is also measured directly through the previously mentioned thermodilution. CO is converted to a more normalized cardiac index (CI) by dividing CO by body surface area (BSA). BSA is derived from height and weight normograms, but can also be easily calculated as follows:

$$BSA\ (m^2) = \{Ht\ (cm) + wt\ (kg) - 60\}/100\ (IB).$$

Once CO is known, stroke volume (SV) can be calculated:

$$SV = CO / HR,$$

where HR is heart rate.

Right-sided ejection fraction (RVEF) is then calculated as follows:

$$RVEF = SV / RVEDV.$$

Calculation of RVEDV requires a continuous thermistor, which is callable of dividing CI into systolic and diastolic components. Knowing RVEF allows RVEDV to be calculated:

$$RVEDV = SV / RVEF.$$

Right-sided heart work estimates the work of the right heart as it pumps blood through the lungs back to the left ventricle. The right ventricle stroke work index (RVSWI) is estimated as follows:

$$RVSWI = (PAP - CVP) \times SVI \times 0.0136,$$

where PAP is pulmonary artery pressure, and SVI is stroke volume index.

The left heart volume and work are calculated similarly to the right. The left ventricular work is the work of the blood circulating through the systemic circulation. This is estimated by

$$LVSWI = (MAP - PCWP) \times SVI \times 0.0136,$$

where LVSWI is left ventricle stroke work index, and MAP is mean arterial pressure.

Among the most useful calculated measures provided by the PAC is the pulmonary and systemic vascular resistance. Each estimates the resistance across the pulmonary or systemic circulation and is an extrapolation of vascular tone. Systemic vascular resistance (SVR) is the drop in pressure across the systemic circulation times the flow and is calculated as

$$SVR = (MAP - RAP) \times 80 / CI,$$

where RAP is renal arterial pressure.

Pulmonary vascular resistance (PVR) is the drop in pressure across the pulmonary circulation multiplied by right-sided flow:

$$PVR = (PAP - PCWP) \times 80 / CI.$$

Goal-Directed Therapy Using Pulmonary Artery Catheter

There is little disagreement regarding the large amount of data provided by a properly placed and interpreted PA catheter. Whether the data provided result in better patient outcome is the source of considerable debate. Much clinical research has been done in an attempt to determine which PAC-derived physiologic parameters should be measured and which are predictive of outcome. Shoemaker and his group provided the initial work toward defining and grouping patient physiologic response to trauma.[23] As early as 1973 Shoemaker and colleagues showed in several studies that PAWP measured reduced cardiac output. They further showed that decreased oxygen delivery along with increased peripheral vascular resistance characterized non-survivors after trauma.[24] Based on these and other similar study results, many groups targeted resuscitation of severely injured trauma patients to achieve physiologic values retrospectively associated with survival. Ten years after his initial studies, Shoemaker and colleagues showed an overall survival benefit in patients who achieved normal physiologic values.[25,26] Finally, this group showed that there was less oxygen debt as measured by VO_2 in surviving patients.[27] Interestingly, there was no difference in oxygen consumption between the groups. In similar research, Bishop et al. examined physiologic parameters in 90 trauma patients and found that patients who achieved higher levels of CI, oxygen delivery, and oxygen consumption within the first 24 hours after admission had a lower incidence of ARDS and reduced overall mortality.[28] Based on these and similar findings, several groups then randomized patients to supernormal resuscitation versus traditional resuscitation with the intent of proving that invasive monitoring of aggressive resuscitation would allow achievement of supranor-

mal physiology and better outcome. These studies showed mixed results. Bishop's group randomized patients to be supranormally resuscitated to a cardiac index of more than 4.5, DO_2I greater than 670, and a VO_2I greater than 166, versus traditional resuscitation as defined by achievement of normal urine output and CVP.[29] The supranormally resuscitated group showed significantly lower mortality and decreased organ failure. Interestingly, optimal parameters were reached in 70% of the study group and 29% of the control group. Similarly, Flemming et al. randomized trauma patients with blood loss of more than 2000 cc to supernormal CI, DO_2, and VO_2, and found that attainment of these goals resulted in statistically significant decreases in organ failure, ICU stay, and ventilator days, and a trend toward decreased mortality.[30]

Other studies, however, pointed out that attainment of resuscitation was more important than the means by which it was achieved and many more recent studies have been unable to show similar benefit to monitoring or goal-directed resuscitation. Velmahos et al. randomized severely injured patients to supranormal resuscitation versus traditional hemodynamic monitoring. While there was no difference in mortality, organ failure, sepsis, ICU days, or hospital stay between the two groups, they found that 70% of the supranormal group and 40% of the traditional group achieved supranormal physiologic parameters, and that attainment of these optimal values was associated with better outcome independent of treatment protocol. There were no outcome differences between the two groups. What was perhaps most interesting in this study, however, was the finding that nonresponders (those who failed to reach the set goals despite volume and ionotropic manipulation) fared significantly worse than the control group. This suggests the likelihood that aggressive resuscitation toward supranormal physiology will be harmful in those whose physiology cannot attain it, and is in fact exhausted such attempts. Other groups have reported similar results, which indicate that that the ability to achieve normal parameters is associated with the mortality benefit, and is ultimately more important than whatever treatment was designed to achieve them.[31] Taken together, these results cast doubt regarding the usefulness of interventional monitoring and resuscitation. Indeed, many believe that aggressive resuscitation should be instituted in all patients without any need for invasive monitoring. Others argue for limited supraphysiologic resuscitation. Some data points to poorer outcome from PAC use. Indeed, deleterious consequences of aggressive resuscitation and the PAC have been reported. Hayes et al. reported that increasing oxygen delivery with ionotropic augmentation with dobutamine was associated with increased mortality.[32] Others have reported similar increased mortality in supranormally resuscitated patients. At least one group has purported to show that the PAC is itself a predictor of morbidity independent of protocol-driven resuscitation. Rhodes et al. performed a prospective randomized trial of 200 patients where no protocol-driven resuscitation was instituted.[33] In this study, patients were randomized to PAC placement versus no PAC where patients were resuscitated based up the clinical judgment of the ICU staff. Data were obtained prospectively and examined retrospectively, and revealed that the PAC group received significantly more fluid in the first 24 hours and exhibited increased morbidity. Evidence for the deleterious effects of PAC protocol–driven resuscitation were seen in a study by Hayes et al. that showed an increased mortality in PAC-treated patients (54% vs. 34%).[32] In this study there was a rigorous goal-directed attempt to achieve supranormal physiologic parameters. To achieve these goals, aggressive fluid resuscitation and ionotropic support were used.

In an attempt to make sense of the huge amount of data regarding PACs and endpoints of resuscitation, Kern and Shoemaker performed a meta-analysis on 21 randomized clinical trials and found that early hemodynamic optimization achieved significant mortality reduction only if optimized parameters were achieved prior to the onset of sepsis or organ dysfunction.[34] Heyland and associates analyzed seven studies and found no significant reductions in mortality achieved with optimization.[35] Lastly, an analysis by Poeze et al.

showed that physiologic optimization resulted in decreased mortality. In this analysis the entire benefit was from patients who hemodynamically optimized perioperatively. Patients with established sepsis or organ failure prior to treatment were unlikely to benefit from "optimization."[36]

Others have questioned the accuracy of the actual PAC measurements. Epstein et al. studied the accuracy of VO_2 measurements by the calculated reverse Fick method versus direct measurement by indirect calorimetry in an attempt to determine the accuracy of PAC determined oxygen consumption measures. Their study showed a bias of 41 ml/min/m^2, indicative of an undermeasurement of VO_2 by PAC measures.[37] Finally, Luchette and colleagues studied the accuracy of continuous cardiac output measurements and found that there was higher signal-to-noise ratio and degraded accuracy when patient temperature was above 38.5° C, resulting in further questioning of the accuracy and usefulness of PAC measurements in severely injured or septic patients.[38]

Mixed Venous Saturation: Monitoring Tissue Metabolism

While the results of supranormal resuscitation are mixed, many believe that the best use of a PAC is as a measure of tissue perfusion. PAC sampling of mixed venous saturation should serve as an adjunctive measure of tissue-level perfusion. Even if supranormal resuscitation remains controversial with mixed data, surely SVO_2 should provide useful data. Unfortunately, this measure of tissue perfusion, while seemingly useful as a measure of tissue oxygenation and subsequent outcome has also not ultimately been shown useful as the targeted endpoint of resuscitation. Gattinoini and associates published a randomized prospective trial involving 762 patients across 56 ICUs who were randomized to either traditional resuscitation or targeting of CI > 4.5 or SvO_2 > 70%. There was no difference in mortality or organ dysfunction among the three groups. Like the studies discussed above, subgroup analysis showed that patients who achieved hemodynamic targets had similar mortality rates independent of the group to which they were randomized.

Right Ventricle End-Diastolic Pressure as Measure of Cardiac Index and Cardiac Function

As predicted by the Starling curve, end-diastolic volume is the best predictor of preload. Unfortunately, PAC pressure measurements as discussed previously are confounded in the setting of changing intrinsic ventricular compliance and extrinsic PEEP. RVEDV monitoring provides the first actual measurement of preload. Rather than being a pressure surrogate for volume, RVEDV utilizes a PAC with a fast thermistor to give a directly measured volume measure. In an attempt to find an alternative to PAOP as a measure of cardiac function, Chetham et al. showed that CI correlated better with RVEDVI than PAOP.[39] The same group then studied 64 patients with respiratory failure and high PEEP requirements, and suggested that RVEDVI was a better measure of CI than PAOP at all levels of PEEP. CI was inversely correlated with PCWP at PEEP levels over 15. Taken together, these findings caused this group to conclude that RVEDVI should be used in lieu of PAOP as a measure of cardiac function.

Despite initial reservations that mathematical coupling was responsible for the close correlation between RVEDV and CI, several groups have shown that the directly measured volume measures are superior to extrapolations from pressure (CVP and PAWP) measures. Chang and colleagues showed that splanchnic malperfusion was better predicted by RVEDV than PCWP, which was in turn associated with MODS and mortality.[40] Other correlations among RVEDV, tissue perfusion, and outcome have been similarly reported by several groups.[42] Lastly Kincaid et al.[41] presented data to show that optimal RVEDV could be calculated for each individual patient.

Taken together, these data support the use of RVEDV as a superior measure of cardiac function and goal-directed resuscitation.

CONCLUSIONS: USE THE PULMONARY ARTERY CATHETER WISELY

Since its inception, the PAC has been a data tool of the critical care physician. As can be seen from a careful review of the literature, little prospective, conclusive data exist to support its continued use. At the same time, however, there is a recent literature and clinical support for early goal-driven resuscitation of critically ill patients. Trauma patients are often hyper-protocolized based on their mechanism and injuries. The PAC is also subject to extreme difficulties in proper measurement and interpretation of collected data, and it is impossible to know the precise accuracy of collected data and how well they were interpreted in the many PAC and resuscitation trials. In the midst of controversy, however, it is important to remember that the PAC is not a drug or intervention, and its utility therefore cannot be directly assessed. The potential effectiveness of the PAC depends on a number of other factors, many of which are not measured or assessed in clinical studies. These include proper indications and risk assessment, proper placement and risk reduction measures, knowledgeable use and interpretation, and the contextual relevance and utility of the data obtained from the PAC.

Because of these confounders and the powerful data that can be procured from measurement, we advocate continued selected and diligent use of the PAC as a tool for proper resuscitation in the critically injured and ill patient. While the proper resuscitative parameters and goals may not be absolutely known, and may change from minute to minute in our patients, more frequent and better data collection properly filtered through clinical judgment should only benefit patient care. To be used correctly, however, perfect attention to proper and safe placement and use must be assumed. From there, continued data collection and monitoring corroborated with patient state is also essential. It is not enough to intermittently examine a few select physiologic variables. Indeed, at any given moment a patient's physiology and subsequent predicted outcome are the sum of a huge number of measured and unmeasured variables and the interactions between these patterns of variables. As technology becomes sufficiently advanced to allow for pattern recognition of more than a few variables, the utility of each measure should increase and be revealed. To discount the important measures derived from the PAC based on studies that failed to find utility of these independent measures is probably shortsighted, and ignores the utility of these otherwise unobtainable data. Indeed, the continued use of the PAC despite multiple studies reflects the clinician's belief that the PAC data combined with other monitoring and clinical acumen will be beneficial on a patient-to-patient basis, which might not be measured in a large trial. That said, use of the PAC requires continual attention, monitoring, and intervention, and we believe that much of the confusion and negative data regarding PA catheterization results from a once-a-day glance at the Swan numbers (usually without regard to their accuracy) without careful perusal of the ongoing flux of the patient's state. Discounting the PAC is foolish. It is a tool that can only be made useful and better through physician education and diligence.

REFERENCES

1. Williams G, Grounds M, Rhodes A: Pulmonary artery catheter. *Curr Opin Crit Care* 8, 251–256, 2002.
2. Gore JM, Goldberg RJ, Spodick DH, Alpert JS, Dalen JE: A community-wide assessment of the use of pulmonary artery catheters in patients with acute myocardial infarction. *Chest* 92:721–727, 1987.
3. Zion MM, et al: Use of pulmonary artery catheters in patients with acute myocardial infarction. Analysis of experience in 5,841 patients in the SPRINT Registry. SPRINT Study Group. *Chest* 98:1331–1335, 1990.
4. Connors AF Jr, et al: The effectiveness of right heart catheterization in the initial care of critically ill patients. SUPPORT Investigators. *JAMA* 276: 889–897, 1996.

5. Pulmonary Artery Catheter Consensus Conference: Consensus statement. *N Horiz* 5:175–194, 1997.
6. Sibbald WJ, Keenan SP: Show me the evidence: a critical appraisal of the Pulmonary Artery Catheter Consensus Conference and other musings on how critical care practitioners need to improve the way we conduct business. *Crit Care Med* 25:2060–2063, 1997.
7. Bernard GR, et al: Pulmonary artery catheterization and clinical outcomes: National Heart, Lung, and Blood Institute and Food and Drug Administration Workshop Report. Consensus statement. *JAMA* 283:2568–2572, 2000.
8. Sandham JD, et al: A randomized, controlled trial of the use of pulmonary-artery catheters in high-risk surgical patients. *N Engl J Med* 348:5–14, 2003.
9. Polanczyk CA, et al: Right heart catheterization and cardiac complications in patients undergoing noncardiac surgery: an observational study. *JAMA* 286:309–314, 2001.
10. Guyatt G: A randomized control trial of right-heart catheterization in critically ill patients. Ontario Intensive Care Study Group. *Intensive Care Med J Intensive Care Med* 6:91–95, 1991.
11. Wilson J, et al: Reducing the risk of major elective surgery: randomised controlled trial of preoperative optimisation of oxygen delivery. *BMJ* 318:1099–1103, 1999.
12. Afessa B, et al: Association of pulmonary artery catheter use with in-hospital mortality. *Crit Care Med* 29:1145–1148, 2001.
13. Shah MR, et al: Impact of the pulmonary artery catheter in critically ill patients: meta-analysis of randomized clinical trials. *JAMA* 294:1664–1670, 2005.
14. Friese RS, Shafi S, Gentilello LM: Pulmonary artery catheter use is associated with reduced mortality in severely injured patients: a National Trauma Data Bank analysis of 53,312 patients. *Crit Care Med* 34:1597–1601, 2006.
15. Rapoport J, et al: Patient characteristics and ICU organizational factors that influence frequency of pulmonary artery catheterization. *JAMA* 283:2559–2567, 2000.
16. Chen YY, et al: Comparison between replacement at 4 days and 7 days of the infection rate for pulmonary artery catheters in an intensive care unit. *Crit Care Med* 31:1353–1358, 2003.
17. Blot F, et al: Mechanisms and risk factors for infection of pulmonary artery catheters and introducer sheaths in cancer patients admitted to an intensive care unit. *J Hosp Infect* 48:289–297, 2001.
18. Kac G, et al: Colonization and infection of pulmonary artery catheter in cardiac surgery patients: epidemiology and multivariate analysis of risk factors. *Crit Care Med* 29:971–975, 2001.
19. Rello J, Coll P, Net A, Prats G: Infection of pulmonary artery catheters. Epidemiologic characteristics and multivariate analysis of risk factors. *Chest* 103:132–136, 1993.
20. Horowitz HW, Dworkin BM, Savino JA, Byrne DW, Pecora NA: Central catheter-related infections: comparison of pulmonary artery catheters and triple lumen catheters for the delivery of hyperalimentation in a critical care setting. *J Parenter Enteral Nutr* 14:588–592, 1990.
21. Eyer S, Brummitt C, Crossley K, Siegel R, Cerra F: Catheter-related sepsis: prospective, randomized study of three methods of long-term catheter maintenance. *Crit Care Med* 18:1073–1079, 1990.
22. Marino PL: *The ICU Book.* Baltimore, Williams and Wilkins, 1998.
23. Shoemaker WC, Reinhard JM: Tissue perfusion defects in shock and trauma states. *Surg Gynecol Obstet* 137:980–986, 1973.
24. Shoemaker WC, Montgomery ES, Kaplan E, Elwyn DH: Physiologic patterns in surviving and nonsurviving shock patients. Use of sequential cardiorespiratory variables in defining criteria for therapeutic goals and early warning of death. *Arch Surg* 106:630–636, 1973.
25. Shoemaker WC, Hopkins JA: Clinical aspects of resuscitation with and without an algorithm: relative importance of various decisions. *Crit Care Med* 11:630–639, 1983.
26. Shoemaker WC, Appel P, Bland R: Use of physiologic monitoring to predict outcome and to assist in clinical decisions in critically ill postoperative patients. *Am J Surg* 146:43–50, 1983.
27. Shoemaker WC, Appel PL, Kram HB, Waxman K, Lee TS: Prospective trial of supranormal values of survivors as therapeutic goals in high-risk surgical patients. *Chest* 94:1176–1186, 1988.
28. Bishop MH, et al: Relationship between supranormal circulatory values, time delays, and outcome in severely traumatized patients. *Crit Care Med* 21:56–63, 1993.
29. Bishop MH, et al: Prospective, randomized trial of survivor values of cardiac index, oxygen delivery, and oxygen consumption as resuscitation endpoints in severe trauma. *J Trauma* 38:780–787, 1995.
30. Fleming A, et al: Prospective trial of supranormal values as goals of resuscitation in severe trauma. *Arch Surg* 127:1175–1179, discussion 1179–1181, 1992.
31. McKinley BA, et al: Normal versus supranormal oxygen delivery goals in shock resuscitation: the response is the same. *J Trauma* 53:825–832, 2002.
32. Hayes MA, et al: Elevation of systemic oxygen delivery in the treatment of critically ill patients. *N Engl J Med* 330:1717–1722, 1994.
33. Rhodes A, Cusack RJ, Newman PJ, Grounds RM, Bennett ED: A randomised, controlled trial of the pulmonary artery catheter in critically ill patients. *Intensive Care Med* 28:256–264, 2002.
34. Kern JW, Shoemaker WC: Meta-analysis of hemodynamic optimization in high-risk patients. *Crit Care Med* 30:1686–1692, 2002.
35. Heyland DK, Cook DJ, King D, Kernerman P, Brun-Buisson C: Maximizing oxygen delivery in critically ill patients: a methodologic appraisal of the evidence. *Crit Care Med* 24:517–524, 1996.
36. Poeze M, Solberg BC, Greve JW, Ramsay G: Monitoring global volume-related hemodynamic or regional variables after initial resuscitation: What is a better predictor of outcome in critically ill septic patients? *Crit Care Med* 33:2494–2500, 2005.
37. Epstein CD, Peerless JR, Martin JE, Malangoni MA: Comparison of methods of measurements of oxygen consumption in mechanically ventilated patients with multiple trauma: the Fick method versus indirect calorimetry. *Crit Care Med* 28:1363–1369, 2000.
38. Luchette FA, et al: Effects of body temperature on accuracy of continuous cardiac output measurements. *J Invest Surg* 13:147–152, 2000.
39. Cheatham ML, Nelson LD, Chang MC, Safcsak K: Right ventricular end-diastolic volume index as a predictor of preload status in patients on positive end-expiratory pressure. *Crit Care Med* 26:1801–1806, 1998.
40. Chang MC, Meredith JW: Cardiac preload, splanchnic perfusion, and their relationship during resuscitation in trauma patients. *J Trauma* 42:577–582, discussion 582–584, 1997.
41. Kincaid EH, Meredith JW, Chang MC: Determining optimal cardiac preload during resuscitation using measurements of ventricular compliance. *J Trauma* 50:665–669, 2001.
42. Miller PR, Meredith JW, Chang MC: Randomized, prospective comparison of increased preload versus inotropes in the resuscitation of trauma patients: effects on cardiopulmonary function and visceral perfusion. *J Trauma* 44:107–113, 1998.

OXYGEN TRANSPORT

**Patricio M. Polanco,   Mitchell P. Fink,   Juan Carlos Puyana,
and   Juan B. Ochoa**

Unicellular organisms evolved to efficiently harness large amounts of energy from organic molecules (especially glucose) through the utilization of oxygen as an electron acceptor. In this process, CO_2 is generated and chemical energy is transferred to high-energy containing molecules of ATP. Oxygen cannot be stored in our cells; therefore, the generation of energy through aerobic (oxygen consuming) processes is completely dependent on its supply. Without oxygen, death rapidly ensues.

In unicellular organisms, the oxygen consumed and the CO_2 produced easily diffuses across the cell membrane. This cannot occur in multicellular organisms such as humans. Instead, complex mechanisms of oxygen delivery and CO_2 removal had to evolve in order to maintain aerobic metabolism. We are therefore totally reliant on the coordinated function of respiratory, cardiovascular, and hematologic systems to maintain energy production.[1]

At a molecular-cellular level, *shock* is defined as the pathologic state that occurs when oxygen supply becomes the rate-limiting step in the generation of energy.[2] We can now measure the degree of failure in the supply and utilization of oxygen during shock, and in fact using these variables, can monitor the effectiveness of therapy.[3] This chapter intimately explains how we can quantify the delivery and consumption of oxygen.

ENERGY GENERATION IN THE CELL

The process of glucose breakdown to CO_2, water, and energy make up the metabolic backbone of the energy production of the cell, although other molecules such as amino acids and fatty acids can also enter at different steps of this process.

Glycolysis (the first step in the process of glucose metabolism) requires the breakdown of glucose to two molecules of pyruvate. This first step occurs universally in the cytoplasm of all mammalian cells, yielding two molecules of ATP. This constitutes only 5.2% of the total potential energy that can be released from glucose. In the absence of oxygen, pyruvate is metabolized by lactic dehydrogenase to lactate. Under anaerobic conditions, such as that seen in intense physical activity or during shock, lactate rapidly accumulates in the circulation. Lactate uptake with regeneration of glucose occurs in the liver. Lactate concentrations in blood of less than 2 mmol/l are considered normal. Increased lactate production, poor lactate clearance, and accumulation in plasma reflect increased anaerobic metabolism and a state of shock. The degree of increase in plasma lactate is a reliable prognostic sign.[4] Lactate levels can also be used as an endpoint of therapy in trauma resuscitation so that successful treatments of shock should be followed by normalization of lactate in plasma.[5]

In the presence of oxygen, pyruvate is oxidized to and ultimately metabolized to CO_2 and water. This aerobic phase of glucose metabolism is called respiration, and occurs entirely in the mitochondria. The generation of energy from pyruvate involves three stages. The first stage generates acetyl-coenzyme A (acetyl CoA), an irreversible process. In the second stage, acetyl-CoA is metabolized in an eight-step process (the citric acid cycle) through enzymatic oxidation generating CO_2, and energy that is conserved in NADH and $FADH_2$. In the final stage (called the electron transfer chain), NADH and $FADH_2$ are oxidized through an electron-carrying process that uses oxygen as the final electron acceptor.

In the aerobic portion of glucose metabolism, 36 molecules of ATP are generated. Thus, cellular respiration yields 18 times more energy than anaerobic glycolysis. Most of the cells in our body are dependent on cellular respiration for the generation of energy and ultimate survival. Organic molecules that generate pyruvate are not limited to glucose since other molecules such as certain amino acids and fatty acids can be utilized. It is therefore oxygen, not pyruvate, which becomes the rate-limiting step in the generation of energy in our bodies.[6]

Pathologic states that involve abnormal mitochondrial utilization of oxygen are observed in various clinical processes. For example, cyanide poisoning of the electron transfer chain results in a rapid development of a severe energy deficit, accumulation of lactate, and death. More commonly, states of septic shock are thought to cause "mitochondrial disease" that renders these organelles incapable of efficiently utilizing oxygen for the generation of energy.[7] To date, physicians can do little to correct mitochondrial dysfunction.

MICROCIRCULATION AND OXYGEN DELIVERY

The diffusion of oxygen into the cell is limited by the distance between the cell itself and the source of oxygen, and is limited to only 100–200 micrometers. A highly complex capillary network (microcirculation) exists to distribute the oxygen to cells and tissues. The surface area in the microcirculation far exceeds the circulating blood volume. Thus, a hypovolemic state would occur if all capillary beds were open at any given time. To avoid this, blood flow is selectively distributed to various vascular beds as needed to meet oxygen demands.

A breakdown in the regulation of oxygen distribution (dysoxia) across the microcirculation occurs in septic shock; thus, septic shock is a form of distributive shock. Excessive amounts of nitric oxide, a potent vasodilator, are thought to be a central aspect of sepsis dysoxia. In addition, the resultant tissue edema increases the distance between the cells and the capillaries, which also contributes to poor oxygen diffusion. Thus, sepsis is characterized by poor oxygen extraction.[8]

Hemoglobin, the Ultimate Oxygen Carrier

Hemoglobin (Hb) serves as a unique oxygen carrier capturing oxygen in the alveoli, distributing it through the microcirculation, and ultimately discharging it in the pericellular environment. Each gram of hemoglobin binds 1.34 ml of O_2. Since Hb concentration is easily measured, the content of O_2 carried per 100 ml of blood can be calculated as follows[7,9]:

$$1.34 \text{ (ml/g)} \times \text{Hb (g/dl)} \times O_2 \text{ saturation (SaO}_2\text{, fraction of 1)}$$
$$= \text{Hb oxygen content} / 100 \text{ ml.}$$

Example:

$$1.34 \times 15 \times 0.98 = 19.7 \text{ ml} / 100 \text{ ml.}$$

The degree of oxygen saturation in Hb through spectrophotometric absorption of light (pulse oximeter) is a widely used tool in intensive care. The saturation of hemoglobin is highly nonlinear, roughly following an S curve (Figure 1). This determines that Hb can easily upload or download O_2 under physiologic conditions. It also determines that minor drops in SaO_2 at saturations of less than 90% reflect higher degrees in the change of the partial pressures of

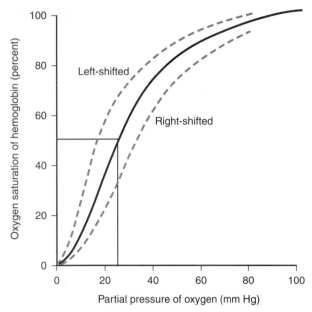

Figure 1 Oxyhemoglobin dissociation curve. The solid line represents the oxyhemoglobin dissociation curve for normal adult hemoglobin. The right or left shifted curves represent increase or decrease capacity of hemoglobin to delivery of oxygen at a define partial pressure of oxygen (pO$_2$).

O_2 (PO$_2$) than drops at a lower SaO$_2$. Roughly, a 90% SaO$_2$ reflects a PO$_2$ of 60 mm Hg. Pathologic alterations of the Hb-oxygen saturation curve are observed with alterations in pH, temperature, and the concentration of 2-3 diphosphoglycerate (2-3 DPG).

A small percentage of O_2 is also carried by the plasma and is a function of the PO$_2$. This concentration is approximately

$$0.003 \text{ ml} / 100 \text{ ml (of plasma)} / (PO_2) \text{ mm Hg.}$$

Thus, we can calculate the total amount of O_2 contained in a given amount of blood (CaO$_2$) as

$$(1.34 \text{ [Hb]} \times SaO_2) + 0.003 \text{ (PO}_2) = CaO_2.$$

Based on this formula, we could assume that increasing levels of serum hemoglobin through blood transfusion will increase CaO$_2$ and therefore oxygen delivery. This is theoretically true; however, attempts aimed at achieving normal levels of serum Hb in all critically ill patients are not uniformly beneficial. Hebert et al. in a randomized, controlled clinical study showed increased mortality in patients who were treated with a liberal transfusion strategy (transfused when Hb falls below 10.0 g/dl) versus those with a restrictive transfusion therapy (Hb maintained at 7.0–9.0 g/dl). However, oxygen consumption and delivery were not measured in this study.[10]

Heart as Oxygen Delivery Pump

How much oxygen is ultimately delivered (DO$_2$) to the cells is determined by the amount of blood pumped by the heart, making cardiac performance an essential aspect in analyzing oxygen-dependent cellular energy production. Cardiac output (Q) is calculated at the bedside through several methods. Although the utility of the Swan-Ganz catheter has been questioned, it is still the most practical tool to provide the following measurement[11–14]:

$$Q \times CaO_2 = DO_2 \text{ (ml/min/m}^2).$$

Cardiac output is determined by preload (intravascular volume), contractility, afterload (vascular resistance), and heart rate. Inappro-

priate cardiac performance rapidly leads to shock. Thus, inadequate contractility observed after myocardial infarction leads to inadequate oxygen delivery, a state known as cardiogenic shock.

PUTTING IT ALL TOGETHER: MEASURING CELLULAR OXYGEN CONSUMPTION AND EXTRACTION IN PATIENTS

We can easily quantify the amount of oxygen consumed in whole organisms using the functions developed previously. The amount of oxygen taken up by the cells (VO$_2$) is a function of measuring Q and the difference in arterial (CaO$_2$) and venous oxygen content (CVO$_2$). CVO$_2$ is calculated using the same variables as in arterial content with the exception that venous oxygen saturation (SvO$_2$) is measured in the central circulation (right atrium or ventricle):

$$Q (CaO_2 - CVO_2) = VO_2.$$

Not all oxygen delivered to the periphery is consumed or extracted in the periphery. In fact, only approximately 25% of the oxygen delivered is normally extracted, although there are significant variations by organ. Oxygen extraction ratio (O$_2$ER) is calculated as a percentage of the oxygen consumed divided by the oxygen delivered:

$$(VO_2 / DO_2) = O_2ER.$$

The amount of oxygen extracted by the tissues can be increased significantly under physiologic conditions to satisfy cellular needs. This provides a very important buffer that allows the maintenance of adequate oxygen consumption during times of increased demand. In addition, oxygen extraction allows tissues to maintain adequate oxygen consumption when delivery is decreased.

Several authors have described the use of oxygen delivery and S$_V$O$_2$ as a valid endpoint of resuscitation in what has been defined as early goal-directed therapy (EGDT). Despite its widespread use, the validity of S$_V$O$_2$ as a tool for monitoring resuscitation remains controversial. Shoemaker reported that mortality was decreased when high-risk surgical patients were treated to supranormal values for cardiac index ($\geq$4.5 l/min/m^2) and oxygen delivery ($\geq$600 ml/min/m^2).[15] Gattinoni et al.[16] and Hayes et al.[17] found no improvement in outcome using cardiac index, oxygen delivery, and S$_V$O$_2$ compared with traditional treatments of resuscitation. In contrast, Rivers et al. showed that EGDT using a constant measurement of central venous oxygen saturation using a central line instead a Swan-Ganz catheter (defined as S$_V$CO$_2$) was associated with mortality improvement from 30.5% compared to 46.5% in patients receiving standard therapy.[18]

Relationship of Oxygen Consumption and Oxygen Delivery during Pathologic States

During physiologic states, oxygen delivery exceeds oxygen consumption; it is therefore said that oxygen consumption is independent of the delivery (Figure 2). In experimental models, a gradual decrease in oxygen delivery is associated with an increase in O$_2$ER and maintenance of normal aerobic metabolism. A critical point in DO$_2$ is reached (cDO$_2$) where oxygen consumption becomes dependent on oxygen delivery and aerobic energy generation fails. As a result, lactate accumulates in the blood. Not surprisingly, variables that measure the state of oxygen delivery and consumption are excellent biomarkers of clinical outcome.

Serum levels of lactate and base deficit have been described as indirect indicators of tissue perfusion and cellular oxygen utilization. Several authors have determined a strong correlation of serum lactate and/or base deficit with outcome in hemorrhagic shock. Broder and Weil in 1964,[19] and later on Vincent et al.[20] and Dunham et al.[21]

OXYGEN DELIVERY AND CONSUMPTION

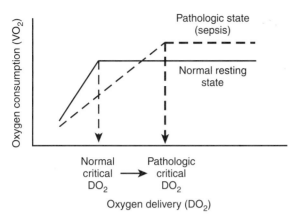

Figure 2 Oxygen delivery (DO$_2$) and consumption (VO$_2$). Solid line represents the normal state in which VO$_2$ stays constant over a decrease of DO$_2$ until it falls below a critical DO$_2$ (cDCO$_2$). The dashed line represents a pathologic state (sepsis) with an increase of VO$_2$ and cDO$_2$ due to impaired oxygen utilization.

confirmed the previous findings, both in clinical studies and animal models.

Determining the cDO$_2$ in a given patient would give clinicians the advantage of determining when shock is present. However, cDO$_2$ is not easily determined using conventional technology. For one, the cDO$_2$ varies from patient to patient, and differs according to pathologic state. In addition, VO$_2$ and DO$_2$ share several variables including Hb and cardiac performance. Varying one or more of these shared variables will alter both VO$_2$ and DO$_2$, a phenomenon known as "mathematical coupling."

Despite these limitations, measuring oxygen transport and consumption remains an essential tool for clinicians treating shock states. Careful measurements of oxygen variables allow the "fine-tuning" of resuscitation-optimizing oxygen transport and cardiac performance while minimizing physiologic costs. An array of variables are routinely manipulated by the clinician, including increasing oxygen saturation, hemoglobin concentrations, optimizing preload and myocardial contractility, altering afterload, and decreasing cellular oxygen consumption. How these variables are changed in a given patient depends in great part on the type of shock present.

Characteristic Oxygen Transport Variables in States of Shock

Hemorrhagic Shock

Hemorrhagic shock is characterized by the loss of Hb, thereby decreasing oxygen carrying capacity and by loss of intravascular volume to negatively affect preload. Thus, in hemorrhagic shock, there is a decrease in DO$_2$ due to decreased hemoglobin and cardiac output, associated with an increase in O$_2$ER. Hemorrhagic shock is best treated by controlling the site of bleeding and restoring intravascular volume and hemoglobin levels. Whole fresh blood, although not normally available, should ideally be used in cases of severe hemorrhagic shock. Provision of adequate volumes restores cardiac output and hemoglobin levels.

Cardiogenic Shock

Cardiogenic shock is characterized by decreased myocardial contractility most often as a result of myocardial infarction. Cardiogenic shock is characterized by very low cardiac output associated with normal or elevated preload and increased O$_2$ER.

Septic Shock

Septic shock is characterized by increased cardiac output associated with decreased afterload. O$_2$ER is decreased, and therefore characteristically elevated SvO$_2$ is observed.

Neurogenic Shock

Neurogenic shock observed after traumatic high spinal cord injuries are associated with a normal cardiac output, an absence of reactive tachycardia and decreased afterload.

CONCLUSIONS

Utilization of oxygen in mammalian cells is necessary for the production of adequate amounts of energy. Oxygen has to be transported to the pericellular environment, as it only diffuses through small distances in tissues. A complex network of capillaries is designed so that adequate delivery of oxygen transported by hemoglobin can occur. Systemic assessment of oxygen delivery and consumption can be readily performed to provide important prognostic information that also allows optimization of therapeutic approaches to the treatment of various forms of shock.

REFERENCES

1. Wells RM: Evolution of haemoglobin function: molecular adaptations to environment. *Clin Exp Pharmacol Physiol* 26:591–595, 1999.
2. Gutierrez G, Reines HD, Wulf-Gutierrez ME: Clinical review: hemorrhagic shock. *Crit Care* 8:373–381, 2004.
3. Bilkovski RN, Rivers EP, Horst HM: Targeted resuscitation strategies after injury. *Curr Opin Crit Care* 10:529–538, 2004.
4. Shah NS, Kelly E, Billiar TR, Marshall HM, Harbrecht BG, Udekwu AO, Peitzman AB: Utility of clinical parameters of tissue oxygenation in a quantitative model of irreversible hemorrhagic shock. *Shock* 10:343–346, 1998.
5. McNelis J, Marini CP, Jurkiewicz A, Szomstein S, Simms HH, Ritter G, Nathan IM: Prolonged lactate clearance is associated with increased mortality in the surgical intensive care unit. *Am J Surg* 182:481–485, 2001.
6. Gutierrez G: Cellular energy metabolism during hypoxia. *Crit Care Med* 19:619–626, 1991.
7. Fink MP: Cytopathic hypoxia. Mitochondrial dysfunction as mechanism contributing to organ dysfunction in sepsis. *Crit Care Clin* 17:219–237, 2001.
8. Spronk PE, Zandstra DF, Ince C: Bench-to-bedside review: sepsis is a disease of the microcirculation. *Crit Care* 8:462–468, 2004.
9. Peruzzi WT, Martin M: Oxygen transport. *Respir Care Clin North Am* 1:23–34, 1995.
10. Hebert PC, Wells G, Blajchman MA, Marshall J, Martin C, Pagliarello G, Tweeddale M, Schweitzer I, Yetisir E: A multicenter, randomized, controlled clinical trial of transfusion requirements in critical care. Transfusion Requirements in Critical Care Investigators, Canadian Critical Care Trials Group. *N Engl J Med* 340(6):409–417, 1999.
11. Connors AF Jr, Speroff T, Dawson NV, Thomas C, Harrell FE Jr, Wagner D, Desbiens N, Goldman L, Wu AW, Califf RM, Fulkerson WJ Jr, Vidaillet H, Broste S, Bellamy P, Lynn J, Knaus WA: The effectiveness of right heart catheterization in the initial care of critically ill patients. *JAMA* 276(11):889–897, 1996.
12. Sandham JD, Hull RD, Brant RF, Knox L, Pineo GF, Doig CJ, Laporta DP, Viner S, Passerini L, Devitt H, Kirby A, Jacka M: A randomized, controlled trial of the use of pulmonary-artery catheters in high-risk surgical patients. *N Engl J Med* 348(1):5–14, 2003.
13. Richard C, Warszawski J, Anguel N, Deye N, Combes A, Barnoud D, Boulain T, Lefort Y, Fartoukh M, Baud F, Boyer A, Brochard L, Teboul JL: Early use of the pulmonary artery catheter and outcomes in patients with shock and acute respiratory distress syndrome: a randomized controlled trial. *JAMA* 290(20):2713–2720, 2003.
14. Harvey S, Harrison DA, Singer M, Ashcroft J, Jones CM, Elbourne D, Brampton W, Williams D, Young D, Rowan K: Assessment of the clinical effectiveness of pulmonary artery catheters in management of patients in intensive care (PAC-Man): a randomised controlled trial. *Lancet* 366(9484):472–477, 2005.

15. Shoemaker WC, Appel PL, Kram HB, et al: Comparison of hemodynamic and oxygen transport effects of dopamine and dobutamine in critically ill surgical patients. *Chest* 96:120, 1989.
16. Gattinoni L, Brazzi L, Pelosi P, et al: A trial of goal-oriented hemodynamic therapy in critically ill patients. *N Engl J Med* 333:1025–1032, 1995.
17. Hayes MA, Timmins AC, Yau EH, et al: Elevation of systemic oxygen delivery in the treatment of critically ill patients. *N Engl J Med* 330:1717, 1994.
18. Rivers E, Nguyen B, Havstad S, Ressler J, Muzzin A, Knoblich B, Peterson E, Tomlanovich M: The Early Goal-Directed Therapy Collaborative Group: early goal-directed therapy in the treatment of severe sepsis and septic shock. *N Engl J Med* 345:1368–1377, 2001.
19. Broder G, Weil MH: Excess lactate: an index of reversibility of shock in human patients. *Science* 143:1457, 1964.
20. Vincent JL, DuFaye P, Bere J, et al: Serial lactate determinations during circulatory shock. *Crit Care Med* 11:449, 1983.
21. Dunham CM, Siegel JH, Weireter L, et al: Oxygen debt and metabolic acidemia as quantitative predictors of mortality and the severity of the ischemic insult in hemorrhagic shock. *Crit Care Med* 19:231–243, 1991.

PHARMACOLOGIC SUPPORT OF CARDIAC FAILURE

John W. Mah   and   **Orlando C. Kirton**

Cardiovascular disease affects more than 70 million people, according to statistics from the American Heart Association in 2002. Congestive heart failure affects approximately 4.9 million of these Americans, resulting in about 1 million admissions and costs of about $27.9 billion annually.[1] Admission for acute decompensated heart failure (ADHF) often results from exacerbation of pre-existing disease or following any number of events, including acute myocardial infarction, valvular disease, and arrhythmias. Additionally, patients today are older and sicker and may be undergoing cardiac and noncardiac surgery as well as developing other causes of acute heart failure such as from sepsis or pulmonary embolus. Patients with ADHF are often triaged to the medical intensive care unit (ICU); however, these patients are also presenting for urgent exploratory and elective surgery. Whether presenting with acute or chronic heart disease, this sicker population represents an increasingly difficult challenge for the surgical intensivist. Diagnosing and treating the initiating cause is imperative; the mainstay of therapy is optimal pharmacologic hemodynamic management.

PATHOPHYSIOLOGY

The pathophysiologic mechanisms leading to ADHF, as well as the goals of pharmacologic treatment, must be identified in order to successfully treat patients with ADHF. Understanding the complex nature of each specific disease process and its physiologic response is crucial for improving function and outcome. Cardiac failure is usually a result of derangement in any number of physiologic factors, including preload, afterload, contractility, heart rate, and heart rhythm.[2]

Increased preload is common in ADHF and is usually secondary to volume overload but can also occur with myocardial ischemia and valvular dysfunction. The body's natural compensatory response is to increase filling pressures to improve myocardial contractility by increasing wall stress on the ventricle (moving up on the Frank-Starling curve).[3] Heart failure generally causes a decrease in renal blood flow and subsequently activates the renin-angiotensin-aldosterone axis (RAAA). The end results of these compensatory mechanisms are vasoconstriction by angiotensin II with increased renal blood flow, release of aldosterone, which increases sodium absorption in exchange for potassium, and promotion of ventricular

hypertrophy, fibrosis, and remodeling that ultimately leads to increased ventricular stiffness.[4]

Increased cardiac afterload is common in the perioperative setting due to multiple causes such as pre-existing hypertension, catecholamine surge, postoperative hypertension, and release of cytokines and inflammatory mediators. Moreover, pulmonary artery hypertension is increased due to similar causes, but can be exacerbated as well by relative hypoxic vasoconstriction and acidosis. In the failing heart, the sympathetic nervous system (SNS) is stimulated as the body acts to increase systemic vascular resistance to maintain normal perfusion to vital organs. The failing heart is further strained as it attempts to increase cardiac output against higher outflow pressures.[3] The increased sympathetic tone also stimulates the release of renin, further activating the RAAA and its inherent problems in heart failure. Subsequently, there is an increase in myocardial oxygen demand, worsening sodium and water retention and a heightened potential to exacerbate lethal cardiac arrhythmias.[3] Furthermore, higher plasma levels of circulating catecholamine have been correlated with worse prognosis.

Myocardial contractility is largely affected by stimulation of the SNS. Adrenergic agents increase intracellular adenosine monophosphate (cAMP), which in turn, increases calcium influx and strengthens the contraction. However, with chronically increased sympathetic tone, the failing heart becomes less responsive to circulating catecholamines, seemingly protecting the myocytes from the excessive catecholamines and their resulting inotropic and chronotropic drive. This dampened response is due to decreased sensitivity and down regulation of the β-receptors from the chronically elevated catecholamine levels that persist in congestive heart failure.[2] Contractility becomes impaired and is less responsive to physiologic needs as well as to pharmacologic agents that act at the β-receptors. In addition, the failing heart responds inadequately to volume overload. The Frank-Starling mechanism is blunted, and significant increases in preload are poorly tolerated, further exacerbating congestive symptoms.

Right ventricular (RV) failure is becoming increasingly recognized as a significant cause of morbidity and mortality in the ICU.[5,6] The RV is thin-walled and compliant relative to the left ventricle (LV) and is designed to function in a low-pressure, low-resistance environment. Contraction occurs in three stages: papillary muscle contraction, RV movement toward the interventricular septum, and LV contraction with twisting of the RV. There is minimal time spent in isovolemic contraction and relaxation, resulting in almost continuous flow to the lungs.[5] The RV is vulnerable to elevation in pulmonary vascular resistance, which will increase the time spent in isovolemic contraction and relaxation, decreasing overall forward blood flow. The RV is perfused primarily from the right coronary artery (RCA), with perfusion occurring in systole and diastole as long as the low-pressure system remains intact. Both ventricles are dependent on movement of the interventricular septum, which can shift toward either the RV or LV, both of which can impair adequate filling and increase end diastolic pressures.

Following cardiac surgery, ventricular function is transiently impaired even in patients with normal preoperative ventricular function. This is due to several factors, including aortic cross clamping, inadequate myocardial protection, hypothermia and cardioplegia, reperfusion injury, as well as excessive levels of inotropes in the perioperative setting. There is a biphasic pattern, with initial recovery following weaning from cardiopulmonary bypass, a nadir at about 3–6 hours, and then full recovery at 8–24 hours. This pattern can obviously be delayed by poor preoperative ventricular function.[7] Pharmacologic support is frequently necessary until adequate function returns.

TREATMENT

The general pharmacologic goals of supporting the acutely decompensated heart are to ameliorate afterload, optimize preload and myocardial performance while modulating myocardial oxygen consumption, and minimizing further activation of the neurohormonal cascade. Additional support is often needed to maintain an adequate mean arterial blood pressure to ensure sufficient coronary blood flow.

Diuretics

Diuretics are the mainstay and building block in treating patients with ADHF, as volume overload is a common occurrence. However, there are no randomized clinical trials demonstrating the efficacy of diuretics on mortality in ADHF. Nonetheless, diuretics remain an effective therapy for the volume-overloaded patient; they act by decreasing preload and intravascular volume and relieving the symptoms of dyspnea and pulmonary congestion.[3] Also, hypervolemia is common in the surgical patient who has pre-existing congestive heart failure due to volume resuscitation from trauma, sepsis, major surgery, or perioperative fluid management. Loop diuretics such as furosemide are commonly used; more potent alternatives such as bumetanide or torasemide are useful in the diuretic-resistant patient. Intravenous boluses can be used, but continuous drips have been shown to be as effective and produce a more "gentle" diuresis. Continuous infusions have been shown to be less toxic and even more efficacious in patients with renal insufficiency.[8] Volume status should be addressed clinically or with invasive monitoring if needed, as overdiuresis or diuresis of the normovolemic patient can cause hypotension or hypoperfusion of end organs. Diuretics may be detrimental in the face of an acute myocardial infarction or other organ dysfunction, as well as in the early postoperative setting in the presence of capillary leak and third space fluid sequestration. Other concerns include the use of high-dose diuretics, which can activate the RAAA and the SNS, and which have their own adverse long-term effects.

Vasodilators

Nitroglycerin can be an effective agent for the rapid treatment of cardiogenic pulmonary edema and ADHF and provides rapid relief of symptoms. The primary effect of nitroglycerin (NTG) is venodilation, with vasodilation occurring at higher dosing (>30 mcg/min). Nitroglycerin has minimal effects on cardiac and skeletal muscle and causes smooth muscle relaxation mainly in the venous system, allowing for increased venous capacitance. It effectively and rapidly reduces ventricular filling pressures (preload), relieving unwanted ventricular wall stress and, more importantly, reduces myocardial oxygen demand. In addition, NTG can improve coronary blood flow by reducing coronary artery resistance and prolonging diastole. The half-life of NTG is short, allowing for rapid escalation and discontinuation of the drug, but tachyphylaxis occurs and often requires persistently increasing dosage. Other unwanted side effects include headache and abdominal pain related to the powerful vasodilation.[3] Volume status must be determined, and diuretics can be helpful in negating the increasing resistance to nitrates.

Nitroprusside induces a more balanced dilation of arterial and venous systems independent of dosing. Venous tone is reduced, producing benefits of decreased preload. In addition, nitroprusside causes a dramatic reduction in afterload, allowing for improvement in cardiac output, stroke volume, and reduced LV filling pressures and ventricular wall stress and ultimately decreased myocardial oxygen demand. It can be especially useful in ADHF for rapid afterload reduction in conditions such as acute mitral or acute aortic regurgitation. Nitroprusside also causes coronary vasodilation and can improve myocardial perfusion if ventricular diastolic pressure reduction exceeds aortic diastolic pressure reduction. Patients with coronary artery disease, however, have the potential to develop a "coronary steal," redirecting blood flow away from ischemic to nonischemic myocardium. Specific cautions include precipitous drops in blood pressure and cyanide and thiocyanate toxicity.

Nesiritide is a recombinant form of a human brain type natriuretic peptide (hBNP) that binds to vascular and endothelial receptors to increase the intracellular levels of cyclic guanosine monophosphate (cGMP). This results in smooth muscle relaxation with predominant vasodilation and some venodilation. Although considered a "natriuretic," diuresis has not been shown to be a major effect. It may, however, potentiate the effects of other diuretics.[9] Nesiritide has been shown to be effective in controlling the symptoms of congestive heart failure and lowering pulmonary capillary wedge pressures (PCWP), with a better safety profile in studies comparing it with dobutamine-based treatments. Symptomatic hypotension can occur, so nesiritide should not be used in patients who are volume depleted, hypotensive, or underperfused. At best, nesiritide appears to be better than placebo, safer than dobutamine, and equal to noninotropic regimens using diuretics and vasodilators. Furthermore, investigators have recently brought to light nesiritide's increased incidence of renal failure and overall increased short-term risk of death in a pooled analysis of randomized controlled trials (RCT) and suggest that its use be limited to failure of traditional therapy with combination of diuresis and nitroglycerin.[10]

Inotropes and Vasopressors

The ideal inotropic agent would increase contractility without increasing heart rate, afterload, preload, or myocardial consumption.[2] The receptor-based agonists exert their effects through α_1, α_2, β_1, β_2, or dopaminergic receptor agonism, while the phosphodiesterase III inhibitors increase intracellular cAMP concentrations to enhance the contractile force in cardiac muscle (Table 1). Vasopressors, although having some intrinsic inotropic activity, are most useful in treating hypotension and maintaining an appropriate mean arterial blood pressure to ensure adequate coronary flow.

Table 1: Catecholamine Activity at Adrenergic Receptor Sites

	Dopamine	β_1	β_2	α
Dopamine	+++	++	+	+++
Dobutamine	0	+++	++	+
Norepinephrine	0	+++	0	++
Epinephrine	0	+++	++	+++

0, No activity; +, minimal activity; ++, moderate activity; +++, predominant activity.

Inotropic Agents

Dobutamine is a synthetic catecholamine with predominant β_1 and weak β_2 agonist effects as well as weak α_1 activity; its main effect is enhanced contractility and heart rate, augmenting cardiac output and stroke volume (Table 2). Systemic vasodilation occurs secondary to dobutamine's β_2 activity, affecting peripheral circulation as well as the pulmonary circulation. Although dobutamine increases myocardial oxygen consumption, this is balanced with improvement in myocardial oxygen supply by coronary vascular dilation. However, this beneficial effect only occurs if the deleterious increase in heart rate can be avoided.[11] Dobutamine is contraindicated in idiopathic hypertrophic subaortic stenosis due to an increasing pressure gradient between the LV and aorta. Dobutamine should be used with caution in patients with atrial fibrillation or flutter because of its pro-arrhythmic pharmacologic effect. Its use may also be limited in the patient already taking doses of long-term beta-blockers or those with pre-existing chronic heart failure, because of the need for higher levels of medication to achieve effect. In these circumstances, combination therapy with phosphodiesterase inhibitors has been shown to be useful.

Epinephrine acts predominantly at the α_1, β_1, and β_2 receptors, and its cardiac effects are most beneficial when used at lower doses (up to 0.02 mcg/kg/min) where the β effects predominate. Contractility is improved along with peripheral vasodilatation and increase in heart rate. The end result in the normovolemic patient is increased cardiac output and systolic pressure with decreased diastolic pressure, systemic vascular resistance (SVR), and pulmonary vascular resistance (PVR). In fact, following cardiac bypass, epinephrine produces equal increases in stroke volume as dobutamine or dopamine, with less significant tachycardia at lower dosing.[2,6] At higher dosing, arrhythmias become more frequent and α activity significantly increases, which tends to encourage alternative inotropic support.

Phosphodiesterase (PDE) inhibitors are a unique class of drugs that inhibit the phosphodiesterase III isoenzyme found in myocardial and vascular smooth muscle cells, leading to increased levels of cAMP. This higher level of intracellular cAMP results in increased myocardial contractility and myocardial and vascular smooth muscle relaxation. Systemic vasodilation is also enhanced, with significant reduction in both PVR and SVR. Mean arterial blood pressure can decrease, but there is usually minimal effect on myocardial oxygen consumption and heart rate.[6] This unique mechanism of action improves contractility in these situations when desensitization secondary to down regulation of β receptors has occurred. PDE inhibitors may in fact work synergistically with the β agonists, thereby decreasing the necessary concentrations of these agents and reducing their

harmful side effects. The addition of even small doses of PDE inhibitor can have a large impact on cardiac index without augmenting systolic blood pressure. PDE inhibitors have been found to be beneficial for RV failure due to its inotropic ability and pulmonary vasodilatory properties (decreased RV afterload). The PDE inhibitors have a longer half-life than most inotropes but have a fairly quick onset of action. Milrinone has essentially replaced amrinone due to its improved safety profile and potency. It is 20 times as potent as amrinone and reaches peak concentration in 2 minutes, with a half-life of approximately 2–4 hours. The half-life is significantly longer than the adrenergic agents, and the risk of systemic hypotension must be taken under consideration prior to its use. It causes significantly more vasodilation compared with dobutamine at similar increases in cardiac output.[12] Also, the half-life is further prolonged by its decreased elimination in patients with congestive heart failure or renal insufficiency. Other cautions of its use include ventricular and supraventricular arrhythmias, hypotension, headache, and rare occurrences of thrombocytopenia.

Vasopressors

Dopamine is a naturally occurring agent and stimulates different receptors based on serum concentration. At least part of its effect is due to release of norepinephrine from nerve terminals in myocardial cells. Dopamine is usually the drug of choice for acute heart failure with associated hypotension, also deemed cardiogenic shock. At lower doses (up to 3 mcg/kg/min), it is mainly a dopaminergic agonist. As the rate increases to 5–10 mcg/kg/min, it acts at the β_1 receptor. It is in this range that cardiac contractility is stimulated, with minimal increase in heart rate, blood pressure, or SVR. Higher doses result in increasing α_1 receptor stimulation.[6] Because dopamine has no β_2 effects, the overwhelming result is strong systemic as well as coronary vasoconstriction. At higher dosing, dopamine usually becomes limited by its profound tachycardia, arrhythmias, and coronary vasoconstriction. Hence, its use in cardiac failure is best utilized at low to moderate dosing.

Norepinephrine is of little value in the treatment of acute heart failure and remains in use only after other drugs have failed. Its predominant activity is at the α receptor, with only mild β_1 agonist activity. Any β activity is usually countered by the strong vasoconstriction and increase in afterload, further offsetting the myocardial oxygen supply and demand ratio. It is, however, one of the first-line agents useful in septic shock or other causes of marked vasodilatory shock. Its use in cardiac failure is supportive to keep arterial blood pressure adequate for coronary artery perfusion, such as in cardiogenic shock.

Table 2: Hemodynamic Actions and Infusion Rates

	CO	Inotropy	HR	SVR	Infusion Rate
Dobutamine	↑↑	↑↑	↑↑	↑↓	2–40 mcg/kg/min
Epinephrine	↑↑	↑↑	↑	↑	1–4 mcg/min
	↑	↑↑	↑↑	↑↑	4–7 mcg/min
	↑↓	↑↑	↑↑	↑↑↑	>7 mcg/min
Milrinone	↑↑	↑↑↑	↑↓	↑↓	50 mcg/kg bolus, then
					0.375–0.75 mcg/kg/min
Norepinephrine	↑↓	↑	↓	↑↑↑	0.01–0.1 mcg/kg/min
Dopamine	↑↓			↑↓	0.5–2 mcg/kg/min
	↑			↑↓	2–5 mcg/kg/min
	↑↓	↑↑	↑↑↑	↑↑	5–10 mcg/kg/min
Phenylephrine	↓		↓	↑↑	20–400 mcg/min

Arginine vasopressin (AVP) is an endogenous hormone released from the posterior pituitary gland usually in response to changes in volume as well as blood pressure and osmolality. Its role is limited in treatment of acute heart failure but has recently been found to be useful in refractory septic shock. In early septic shock, AVP levels are high, followed by a relative depletion in circulating AVP and a relative vasoplegic state by 36 hours. Replacement of low-dose AVP to physiologic levels has been shown to restore normal vascular tone while providing paradoxical vasodilation and increased blood flow to other organs. AVP binds to motor (V_1) and renal (V_2) receptors, allowing some potential for renal protection, and may have pulmonary vasodilatory or rather minimal pulmonary vasoconstricting effects. Regardless, administration of low-dose AVP (0.01–0.04 unit/min) can potentially restore a catecholamine-resistant state while reducing the high dosage of additional first-line vasopressors and their added harmful effects.[13]

Other Agents

Thyroid hormone has been used in transplant organ donors to improve cardiac function. Sick euthyroid syndrome is being frequently diagnosed, and other nonthyroidal illnesses are relatively common in the critically ill patient. Replacement of thyroid hormone has been suggested to improve cardiac performance and enhance recovery of ventricular function after an ischemic event. In the cardiac patient, T_3 hormone levels have been shown to be significantly decreased following cardiopulmonary bypass (CPB), unrelated to dilution or heparin administration. These levels then return to normal after 12–24 hours.[2] Although there is some evidence that administration of T_3 improves cardiac function, studies are conflicting for using T_3 in the perioperative setting to wean patients from CPB.[14,15] Although no adverse effects have been reported with the use of thyroid hormone in the T_3-deficient patient, its use has not been clearly supported and remains relatively controversial.

Methylene blue is mentioned for its potential use in refractory shock but obviously lacks strong evidence-based studies. It is mentioned for its unique and untapped potential as a mechanism of action in sepsis or other systemic inflammatory responses (SIRS) resulting in shock. The SIRS state results in increased production of nitric oxide (NO) and subsequently smooth muscle cGMP leading to hypotension, decreased response to catecholamines, and myocardial depression. Methylene blue inhibits the production of NO and cGMP, increasing arterial blood pressure, improving myocardial function, and maintaining oxygen transport, and has been shown in a few small studies to be effective in refractory septic shock, reducing the requirement of adrenergic agents.[16] There have been some reports of worsening hypoxia in those patients with acute lung injury who have been administered methylene blue, due to apparent pulmonary vasoconstriction. This appears to be lessened by lower dosing and continuous infusions.

SPECIAL CIRCUMSTANCES

Heart Failure in Septic Shock

Multiple factors contribute to the hypotensive state and relative cardiac failure associated with septic shock. Although sepsis usually results in a high output cardiac state, there is, nevertheless, a reduction in the contractile performance that is often unable to meet the metabolic demands of the tissues. RV and LV contractility is directly impaired. Preload is reduced due to a marked drop in the SVR and a loss of fluid from capillary leakage and thus poor venous return.[17] Endogenous vasopressin, although initially enhanced, is quickly exhausted from prolonged intense stimulation of neurohypophyseal stores. Although dopamine, epinephrine, norepinephrine, phenylephrine, and vasopressin have been shown to increase blood pressure in septic shock,

there appears to be a survival advantage specifically with norepinephrine. Both dopamine and norepinephrine are acceptable first-line agents for maintenance of normal blood pressure after adequate fluid resuscitation. Vasopressin has been shown to be useful in refractory shock and diminishing responses to first-line vasopressors. Marked depression of myocardial contractility can occur, requiring inotropic support. Dobutamine has been shown to be effective in maintaining a high normal range of cardiac output and subsequently increasing SVO_2. In general, acceptable endpoints of resuscitation include establishing a mean arterial blood pressure to at least 65 mm Hg, CVP between 8 and 12 mm Hg, and SVO_2 equal to or greater than 65%.[18]

Right Ventricular Failure

Acute RV failure had been a fairly neglected entity in the ICU until recent times. The incidence has been reported to be similar to that of LV failure and can occur in a variety of clinical settings, including heart or lung transplant, acute respiratory distress syndrome (ARDS), presence of an LV assist device (LVAD), RV infarction, positive pressure mechanical ventilation, or significant pulmonary embolism.[5] Any impairment of RV preload, afterload, or LV function can result in damage to the RV. The RV is very sensitive to increased afterload. If pulmonary vascular resistance is persistently elevated, it may allow progression to RV dilation, tricuspid regurgitation, increased myocardial consumption, and worsening RV output, and initiate a degenerating cycle of RV failure. Additionally, right coronary artery perfusion of the RV, which normally continues throughout systole and diastole, degenerates into only diastolic perfusion in the presence of significant pulmonary hypertension. Increased RV end diastolic volume can also have ill effects on LV function if it is significant enough to cause interventricular septal deviation impairing LV filling. RV insufficiency during the initial few days following LVAD insertion occurs because of this leftward septal shift as the LV is unloaded.[5]

Maintaining higher filling pressures can restore normal hemodynamics if RV contractility, PVR, and interventricular septal function are normal.[7] In fact, volume loading may be counterproductive if mean pulmonary artery pressures are already greater than 30 mm Hg. Dobutamine and PDE inhibitors such as milrinone increase RV contractility while allowing pulmonary (and systemic) vasodilation and help establish improved filling of the left ventricle by increasing right-to-left blood flow. Epinephrine and isoproterenol are also effective agents in improving RV contractility. Vasopressors are indicated to increase arterial blood pressure and improve coronary perfusion. Norepinephrine has been recommended over other α adrenergic agents to enhance right coronary artery perfusion in hypotensive patients. Inhaled NO has been shown to be effective in reducing PVR, improving oxygenation, and subsequently improving RV function due to its selective pulmonary vasodilation and improved ventilation-to-perfusion (V/Q) matching.[2] Its inhaled route avoids significant effects on systemic blood pressure. However, outcome studies are lacking, and effects on mortality have not been well studied. Other provocative selective pulmonary vasodilators, such as inhaled prostacyclin with or without inhaled PDEs, have been used with anecdotal success. They boast similar pulmonary selectivity and avoidance of systemic hypotension, and are much cheaper than inhaled NO but are very labor intensive to use. Regardless of our pharmacologic treatment, the diagnosis must be determined and underlying etiology must be corrected to re-establish intrinsic RV function. Pulmonary artery monitoring and/or echocardiography can be very helpful in establishing the correct diagnosis and may aid in augmenting treatment.

Blunt Cardiac Injury

Blunt cardiac injury (BCI) infrequently requires the use of inotropic support, except in the patient with pre-existing heart disease. When it does occur, BCI results either from energy transfer from the direct blow to the chest, a deceleration-type injury, and/or a compression injury between the spine and sternum. There are no standard treatment guidelines, and care must be supportive based on injury pattern and the clinical picture. One must then familiarize oneself with all the potential causes of cardiac failure and treat accordingly. Blunt cardiac injury is a general term and encompasses all types of injury. The term "myocardial commotion" is used in the literature and occurs when no identifiable lesion exists on histology or imaging study. This is most commonly a low-impact event, such as in contact sports. Nevertheless, cardiac arrest may occur from timed impact 15–30 milliseconds before the peak of the T wave initiating ventricular fibrillation or impact during the QRS complex, causing complete heart block.[19] Contusion implies a myocardial lesion and most commonly will involve the right ventricle and septum due to its proximity anteriorly. RV dysfunction can also occur, as it is sensitive to increases in RV afterload that can result from ARDS, high levels of positive-end expiratory pressure (PEEP), or severe chest trauma and pulmonary contusions. Invasive monitoring and echocardiography can help guide treatment in the hypotensive patient, the elderly, or patients with pre-existing heart disease. There are also reports of perioperative concerns including increased risk of systemic hypotension, arrhythmias, and cardiac arrest, which have been shown to persist at least up to 1 month following injury. Treatment is largely supportive, ensuring adequate preload and inotropic support. RV contusion again is common, and dysfunction must first be suspected. Treatment of increased RV afterload must be addressed, including correction of acidosis, hypoxia, and pulmonary hypertension, and avoidance of conventional mechanical ventilation and high PEEP.

SUMMARY

Acute decompensated heart failure is a common occurrence in the surgical ICU, with urgent surgical problems becoming progressively more complicated by pre-existing heart failure or cardiac compromise. These patients bring additional challenges to the surgical intensivist. Although the pathophysiology of ADHF remains the same, treatment of the surgical patient becomes increasingly complex due to the additional, simultaneously occurring perioperative pathophysiology. Recognition and optimal pharmacologic support can improve patient outcome in ADHF and allow opportunity for recovery from the initial insult.

REFERENCES

1. American Heart Association: *Heart and Stroke Statistical Update.* Dallas, TX, American Heart Association, 2004.
2. Griffin MJ, Hines RL: Management of perioperative ventricular dysfunction. *J Cardiothorac Vasc Anesth* 15(1):90–106, 2001.
3. Southworth M: Treatment options for acute decompensated heart failure. *Am J Health Syst Pharm* 60(Suppl 4):S7–S15, 2003.
4. Ramsay JG: Cardiac management in the ICU. *Chest* 115(5):S138–S144, 1999.
5. Mebazza A, Karpait P, Renaud E, Algotsson L: Acute right ventricular failure—from pathophysiology to new treatments. *Intern Care Med* 30: 185–196, 2004.
6. Doyle AR, Dhir AK, Moors AH, Latimer RD: Treatment of perioperative low cardiac output syndrome. *Ann Thorac Surg* 59:S3–S11, 1995.
7. Via G, Veronies R, Giuseppe M, Braschi A: The need for inotropic drugs in anesthesiology and intensive care. *Ital Heart J* 4(Suppl 2):S50–S60, 2003.
8. Sutter MD: New insights into decompensated heart failure. *Emerg Med* 37:18–25, 2005.
9. Sharma M, Teerlink JR: A rational approach to the treatment of acute heart failure: current strategies and future options. *Curr Opin Cardiol* 19: 254–263, 2004.
10. Sackner-Bernstein JD, Kowalski M, Fox M, Aaronson K: Short-term risk of death after treatment with nesiritide for decompensated heart failure: a pooled analysis of randomized controlled trials. *JAMA* 293(15): 1900–1905, 2005.
11. Barnard MJ, Linter SPK: Fortnightly review: acute circulatory support. *BMJ* 307(6895):35–41, 1993.
12. Yamani MH, Haji SA, Starling RC, Kelly L, Albert N, Knack DL, Young JB: Congestive heart failure. *Am Heart J* 142(6):998–1002, 2001.
13. Holmes CL, Walley KR: Vasopressin in the ICU. *Curr Opin Crit Care* 10:442–448, 2004.
14. Klemperer JD, Klein I, Gomez M, et al: Thyroid hormone treatment after coronary-artery bypass surgery. *N Engl J Med* 333(23):1522–1527, 1995.
15. Bennett-Guerrero E, Jimenez JL, White WD, et al: Cardiovascular effects of intravenous triiodothyronine in patients undergoing coronary artery bypass graft surgery: a randomized, double-blind, placebo-controlled trial. *JAMA* 275(9):687–692, 1996.
16. Kirov MY, Evgenov OV, Evgenov NV, et al: Infusion of methylene blue in human septic shock: a pilot, randomized, controlled study. *Crit Care Med* 29:1860–1867, 2001.
17. Dellinger R: Cardiovascular management of septic shock. *Crit Care Med* 31(3):946–955, 2003.
18. Rivers E: Early goal-directed therapy in the treatment of severe sepsis and septic shock. *N Engl J Med* 345:1368–1377, 2001.
19. Gilles O, Mustapha F, Bruno R: The heart in blunt trauma. *Anesthesiology* 95:544–548, 2001.

THE DIAGNOSIS AND MANAGEMENT OF CARDIAC DYSRHYTHMIAS

Jason L. Sperry   and   **Joseph P. Minei**

With increasing frequency, patients undergoing surgery have multiple medical comorbidities, not necessarily associated with their surgical disease. Cardiac dysrhythmia in this setting can be a primary event, a secondary event related to ischemia or myocardial infarction, or may be due to toxic or metabolic abnormalities associated with perioperative care. The type of dysrhythmia can usually be diagnosed with a focused physical exam, a standard 12-lead electrocardiogram (ECG), and from the response to specific maneuvers or drug therapy. The acute management depends on the hemodynamic stability of the patient, the accurate classification of dysrhythmia, and an understanding of the underlying mechanism so that appropriate treatment can be given in an expeditious fashion. Management may include a combination of cardioversion for the acutely unstable, pharmacological intervention, percutaneous or transvenous pacing, or modalities such as aberrant pathway ablation and implantation of pacemakers or defibrillators.

INCIDENCE

The incidence of dysrhythmia following cardiac surgery can be high as 40% in some studies, with a large proportion caused by atrial fibrillation. It is well known that up to 15% of patients with inferior wall myocardial infarction present with atrioventricular (AV) nodal conduction disturbances or complete heart block. Patients with pre-existing cardiac or pulmonary disease have an increased risk of dysrhythmia, which is compounded in the face of noncardiac surgery, trauma, or other critical illness. Vasopressor requirement is associated with an increased risk of dysrhythmia due to the proarrhythmic effect of catecholamines on the heart. It has been shown that dysrhythmias, in a standard intensive care unit (ICU) that admits cardiac, noncardiac, and medical critical care patients, occur in up to 20% of patients. The vast majority are tachyarrhythmias, while 10% are bradyarrhythmias. Dysrhythmias are distributed equally between atrial and ventricular origin. Atrial fibrillation and ventricular tachycardia are by far the most common. Patients that have dysrhythmias have longer ICU stays and had worse survival overall, likely signifying that dysrhythmias in patients are an indicator of more severe critical illness.

BRADYARRYTHMIAS

Bradyarrhythmias are frequently encountered in the ICU setting, and can present as incidental findings on electrocardiogram (ECG) or as potentially life-threatening events. They can be classified according to whether they originate from the sinoatrial (SA) node or the AV node. The etiology of bradyarrhythmias is due to either extrinsic factors or intrinsic disease in the cardiac conduction system. Extrinsic causes include medications, myocardial ischemia, metabolic abnormalities, enhanced vagal tone secondary to tracheal manipulation, vomiting, or acute respiratory failure. Further classification depends on the reversibility of the rhythm, whether the patient is symptomatic due to the rhythm, and the likelihood that the rhythm will progress or recur. Management options include watchful waiting, with removal of the offending agent, pharmacological treatment for the acutely symptomatic, temporary pacing and permanent pacing, depending on the hemodynamic status and the reversibility of the rhythm.

Sinus Node

The normal heartbeat arises from the SA node that serves as the pacemaker of the heart under normal conditions. Bradycardia resulting form SA node dysfunction originates from either failure of impulse generation or failure of impulse conduction. In the past, the term "sick sinus syndrome" has been used to describe a variety of sinus bradyarrhythmias with many etiologies. More appropriate classification of SA node dysfunction includes inappropriate sinus bradycardia, sinus pause or arrest, sinus exit block, and bradycardia-tachycardia syndrome.

Sinus bradycardia (heart rate <60) does not necessarily imply SA node dysfunction, and even a heart rate less than 40 at rest can be asymptomatic in well-trained athletes. Sinus bradycardia is considered pathologic when patients are symptomatic or when there is failure to appropriately increase heart rate during activity or exercise. Sinus pause or arrest occurs when the SA node transiently fails to exhibit automaticity and does not fire. Sinus exit block similarly results in a pause but the SA node does fire. The impulse is either delayed or fails to propagate beyond the SA node, resulting in failure of atrial depolarization. Bradycardia-tachycardia syndrome refers to sinus node dysfunction with both bradycardia and tachycardia. Typically bradycardia episodes follow the termination of tachycardia events and can be associated with clinical symptoms of presyncope or syncope. Management can be challenging, as pharmacotherapy to treat fast rhythms predisposes to slow ones and vice versa. Commonly, insertion of a pacemaker for the symptomatic bradycardia, in conjunction with pharmacological treatment for the tachycardia, is required.

Treatment for SA node dysfunction depends on the clinical status of the patient and presumed etiology. If the bradycardia is transient and not associated with hemodynamic compromise, no therapy is necessary. Correction of any metabolic abnormalities, minimizing vagal-inducing maneuvers, and removal or dose reduction of medications such as beta-blockers, calcium channel antagonists, and lithium may be necessary. If the bradycardia is sustained or severe enough to cause hemodynamic instability, therapy with anti-muscarinic agents (atropine) or beta-agonist (isoproterenol) may be initiated. Percutaneous or transvenous pacing may be necessary in some patients in the acute setting and can be a bridge to permanent pacemaker placement. Patients that are relatively stable but are symptomatic from sinus node dysfunction virtually always require permanent pacing.

Atrioventricular Node

Disturbances in conduction through the AV node or His-Purkinje system are classified as atrioventricular blocks. These may be temporary or permanent, depending on the etiology of the delayed conduction. In adults, the most common causes are drug toxicity, coronary artery disease, and degenerative disease of the conduction system. Many other conditions, such as electrolyte disturbances, myocarditis, sarcoidosis, scleroderma, and hypervagal responses, can cause AV block. The P-R interval is a measure of the conduction time through the AV node and bundle of His. When the P-R interval is prolonged (>210 milliseconds), a patient has first-degree AV block. Second-degree AV block is when intermittent failure of the conduction of the impulse to the ventricles occurs. In Mobitz type I, second-degree AV block (Wenckebach block), there is progressive prolongation of the P-R interval until failure of conduction to the ventricle occurs (Figure 1). The P-R interval then shortens following the dropped beat. This failure in conduction originates from the AV node itself and the QRS complex remains narrow. In Mobitz type II, second-degree AV block, there is intermittent failure of conduction reaching the ventricles that is not associated with progressive prolongation of the P-R interval. There is not a shortened P-R interval following the dropped beat. This failure in conduction is considered "infranodal" and originates from the His-Purkinje system. The QRS complex may be prolonged, and this type of AV block is more concerning. There is a significant likelihood of progression to complete heart block associated with inadequate ventricular response with this rhythm. Third-degree or complete heart block results from failure of all impulses through the AV node and His-Purkinje system, resulting in atrioventricular disassociation. The ventricles rely on their innate automaticity which produces a typical wide QRS escape rhythm between 40 and 50 beats per minute. The atrial rate is commonly faster, producing multiple P waves with no relationship to the ventricular QRS complexes (Figure 2).

Management of AV block depends on the hemodynamic stability of the patient, the transient nature of the dysrhythmia, and where the focus originates from within the conduction system. Acute pharmacotherapy relies upon atropine and isoproterenol. Isoproterenol use

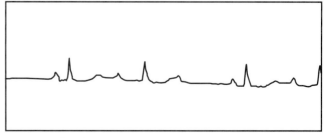

Figure I Rhythm strip shows progressive P-R prolongation and a subsequent "dropped" QRS complex, followed by shortening of the P-R interval which is diagnostic of Mobitz type I, second-degree AV block.

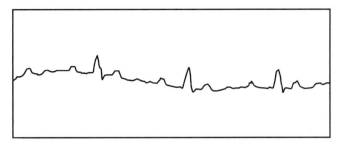

Figure 2 Rhythm strip shows atrial P waves and ventricular QRS complexes occurring at different rates and with no relationship between them, which is characteristic of third-degree AV block.

should be avoided in patients with ischemia heart disease because of the associated increase in myocardial oxygen demand. There is no long-term pharmacotherapy for AV block, and removal of any of the common offending agents, such as digitalis or beta-blockers, should first be attempted. Temporary pacing is used for those with ongoing instability, and permanent pacing is typically required for Mobitz type II second-degree AV block and third-degree AV block.

TACHYARRHYTHMIAS

Tachyarrhythmias are classified according to their anatomical origin in relation to the AV node. Those that originate at or above the AV node are considered supraventricular tachyarrhythmias; the most relevant include sinus tachycardia, paroxysmal supraventricular tachycardia, multifocal atrial tachycardia, atrial flutter, and atrial fibrillation. Ventricular tachyarrhythmias originate from below the AV

node and include ventricular tachycardia and ventricular fibrillation. Important determinants of the malignant potential of these tachyarrhythmias are the duration, the hemodynamic consequences, and the presence of significant structural heart disease. The acute management depends on a basic understanding of the mechanism, the choices for pharmacological intervention (Table 1), and the indications for urgent cardioversion for each situation. Interventional techniques, such as aberrant pathway ablation and implantation of pacemakers and defibrillators, have drastically improved long-term outcome once patients have left the ICU setting, and have added significantly to our armamentarium in treating these dysrhythmias.

The mechanism by which tachyarrhythmias arise are categorized into (1) abnormal automaticity, (2) triggered activity, or (3) re-entry. Abnormal automaticity occurs when cells outside the normal conduction system generate spontaneous impulse formation. Triggered activity occurs during "after depolarizations," which cause the membrane potential to reach threshold early and generate abnormal impulse formation. Re-entry, the most common mechanism, occurs when an impulse can travel down two pathways separated by an area of unexcitable tissue. One of the pathways contains a unidirectional block, with slowed conduction, so that recovery and further excitation can subsequently occur. This defines an area of cardiac tissue that can self-propagate and thus becomes the focus for the generation of the tachyarrhythmia (Figure 3).

Sinus Tachycardia

Sinus tachycardia should be considered a physiological reflex rather than a true dysrhythmia, but it is an important sign for which the etiology must be sought. Fever, hypovolemia, and anemia all appropriately increase heart rate to at least maintain or increase cardiac

Table 1: Classification of Common Tachyarrhythmic Drug Therapies

	Examples	Mechanism of Action	Prolong QT
Class I IA IB IC	Quinidine, procainamide, disopyramide Lidocaine, mexiletine Flecainide, propafenone	-Sodium channel blockade -Varying effects on prolongation of action potential, and dissociation from the sodium channel	Yes
Class II	Metoprolol, esmolol	-Blocks beta-adrenergic receptor -Sympatholytic	No
Class III	Amiodarone, bretylium, sotalol, ibutilide	-Blocks the delayed rectifier potassium current -Significant prolongation of action potential	Yes
Class IV	Verapamil, diltiazem	-Calcium channel blockade -Slows primarily AV node conduction	No
Other	Adenosine Digoxin	-Activation of an inward rectifier K^+ current and inhibition of calcium current -Extremely short acting, primarily on AV node -Blocks sodium-potassium ATPase and increases intracellular calcium -Slow onset of action and toxicity can be common	No

Adapted from Brunton L, editor: *Goodman & Gilman's The Pharmacological Basis of Therapeutics*, 11th ed. New York, McGraw-Hill, 2005.

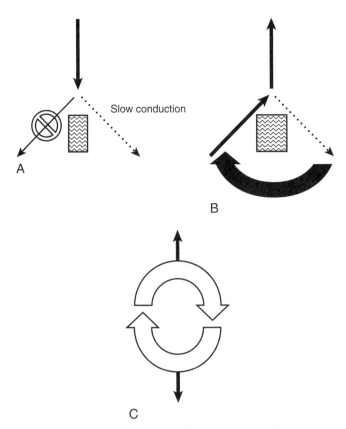

Figure 3 **(A)** Conditions required for reentry; two pathways separated by inexcitable tissue, unidirectional block, and slowed conduction. **(B)** Initiating factors allow retrograde conduction up the prior blocked pathway. **(C)** A re-entrant circuit is formed.

output. Blunting this reflex with pharmacotherapy without knowledge of the etiology can be dangerous. Thyrotoxicosis, pheochromocytomas, or side effects of sympathomimetic drugs also cause sinus tachycardia without regard for reflex mechanisms. The primary goal for management of sinus tachycardia is to find and appropriately treat the confounding condition. Sinus tachycardia will resolve with resolution of this inciting process.

Paroxysmal Supraventricular Tachycardia

The term "paroxysmal supraventricular tachycardia" actually describes a diverse group of tachyarrhythmias, the two most common being atrioventricular nodal re-entry tachycardia (AVNRT) and atrioventricular re-entry tachycardia (AVRT). They both have in common dual conduction pathways, each with different rates of conduction. As described previously, this allows for the possibility of re-entry and the potential for a self-propagating tachyarrhythmia focus. In AVNRT, the two pathways reside in or around the AV node itself. Antegrade conduction typically occurs through the slower pathway, while the retrograde conduction occurs through the faster pathway. Rates of 140–220 beats/min are typical, and P waves are not seen on ECG since retrograde atrial activation and antegrade ventricular activation occur simultaneously. The QRS complex is typically narrow because the antegrade conduction to the ventricles uses the normal AV node and His-Purkinje system. In comparison, AVRT also has two conduction pathways, but the additional pathway is remote from the AV node and resides in the atrioventricular groove, where it is commonly referred to as an "accessory pathway." Similar to AVNRT, antegrade conduction occurs through the AV node and His-Purkinje system, while retrograde conduction occurs via the

accessory pathway. The QRS complex for AVRT is also narrow, and since the accessory pathway only conducts retrograde, it is not seen on ECG and is considered "concealed."

Acute management depends on the stability of the patients with paroxysmal supraventricular tachycardia. Urgent direct-current cardioversion is indicated when myocardial ischemia, acute heart failure, or hypotension result. In hemodynamically stable patients, pharmacological intervention with the intent to slow or break AV nodal conduction is the mainstay of treatment. Intravenous adenosine is the first-line drug of choice due to its potent yet short-lived depressant effects on AV nodal conduction. Adenosine will successfully terminate greater than 90% of tachyarrhythmias due to AVNRT and AVRT. Calcium channel blockers or beta-blockers (verapamil/diltiazem or metoprolol) are also useful, particularly when adenosine is not successful, although they should be used with caution due to possible hypotensive and bradycardic effects.

When the accessory pathway has the potential for antegrade conduction, the QRS complex will be wide, since conduction occurs between the ventricular myocytes themselves rather than the His-Purkinje system. Wolfe-Parkinson-White syndrome occurs when the accessory pathway allows both antegrade and retrograde conduction, and commonly a delta wave or pre-excitation can be seen in the early QRS complex (Figure 4). This syndrome can present in early adulthood, and the initial presentation can be ventricular fibrillation. Management in these patients where conduction occurs antegrade through the accessory pathway varies from narrow complex AVRT as described previously. Adenosine will only be effective if the antegrade conduction occurs through the AV node. Otherwise it can precipitate atrial fibrillation, which can result in degeneration to ventricular fibrillation when an antegrade accessory pathway exists in these patients. Calcium channel blockers and digoxin are contraindicated, because they will slow conduction in the AV node and enhance conduction through the accessory pathway. Class I and class III antiarrhythmics, which include flecainide, procainamide, and ibutilide, are able to depress the conduction across the accessory pathway, decrease the ventricular rate, and likely terminate the wide QRS tachyarrythmia. Direct-current cardioversion is used with hemodynamic instability or if failure of antiarrhythmic therapy occurs.

Multifocal Atrial Tachycardia

Multifocal atrial tachycardia is thought to be due to abnormal automaticity and is commonly associated with chronic respiratory disease, congestive heart failure, and pulmonary embolus. It has an irregular rate and rhythm that is characterized by the presence of three or more morphological different P waves on ECG, and rates of 110–140 beat/min (Figure 5). It can easily be confused with atrial fibrillation if P waves are not prominent on a rhythm strip. First-line therapy consists of treating the underlying condition, correction of hypercarbia or hypoxia, and electrolyte repletion. Calcium channel blockers typically can provide rate control but beta-blockers should be used with caution in those with

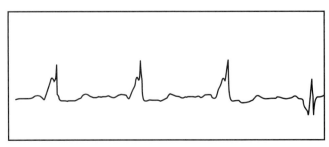

Figure 4 Lead II in this ECG shows a prominent delta wave consistent with the diagnosis of Wolfe-Parkinson-White syndrome.

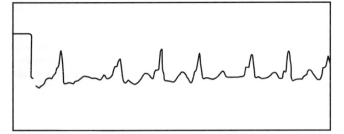

Figure 5 Rhythm strip shows an irregular tachycardia with greater than three morphologically different P waves, characteristic of multifocal atrial tachycardia (MAT).

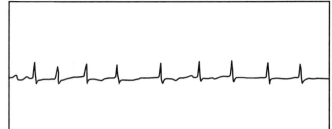

Figure 7 Rhythm strip shows an irregular, normal complex tachycardia without P waves, consistent with atrial fibrillation.

obstructive pulmonary disease. Amiodarone can be helpful in patients refractory to first-line therapies.

Atrial Flutter

Atrial flutter is due to a re-entrant circuit from within atrial tissue and is associated with atrial enlargement. It is commonly grouped with atrial fibrillation due to similar associated causes and similar treatment regimens. Atrial rates of 250–350 beats/min are typical. The AV node refractory period allows only a proportion of these atrial beats to pass to the ventricle, typically in a 2:1 ratio. When a ventricular pulse rate is measured to be 150 beats per minute, atrial flutter should be considered. By increasing AV nodal delay with adenosine or beta-blockade, the atrial "flutter waves," characterized by a saw-tooth appearance, can usually be seen on a rhythm strip (Figure 6). Adenosine may be useful for diagnosis, but as with atrial fibrillation, it rarely converts the rhythm back to sinus. Beta-blockers and calcium channel blockers allow ventricular rate control, but more commonly the use of antiarrythmic drug therapy and or electrical cardioversion is required if the rhythm remains persistent.

Atrial Fibrillation

Atrial fibrillation (AF) is the most common supraventricular tachyarrhythmia with a concerning amount of possible detrimental consequences. Atrial fibrillation and flutter account for greater than 60% of the supraventricular tachyarrhythmias in noncardiac surgical patients and affect up to 40% of patients following cardiac surgery. It is commonly associated with left atrial distension, whether from acute fluid shifts or chronic dilatation secondary to structural heart disease. Other associations that must be ruled out include electrolyte imbalances, myocardial ischemia, hyperthyroidism, hypoxia/hypercarbia, pulmonary embolus, and pneumonia. It is an "irregularly irregular" rhythm with an absence of P waves on ECG (Figure 7). It is thought to arise from multiple shifting re-entrant circuits that bombard the AV node with a mul-

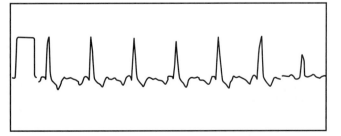

Figure 6 Lead II in this ECG shows the characteristic "saw-tooth" flutter wave of atrial flutter with 2:1 conduction. The rate is approximately 150 beats per minute.

titude of impulses, from which only a proportion initiate ventricular contraction, 110–190 beats/min. Patients without structural heart disease tolerate the loss of the atrial component of ventricular filling quite well, but in those with this history, hypotension, acute congestive failure, and myocardial ischemia can be precipitated. Another concerning consequence is the possibility of mural thrombus formation, and the associated embolic risk, from within the noncontracting left atrium. Thrombus can occur in up to 10% of patients, with new-onset AF lasting longer than 3 days.

The overall goals of treatment include ventricular rate control, resumption and maintenance of sinus rhythm, and prevention of embolic events. Acutely, if the patient is hemodynamically unstable, in acute heart failure, or the rhythm is precipitating myocardial ischemia, direct-current cardioversion should be performed. This is successful in restoring sinus rhythm in up to 90% of patients with recent-onset AF. In the hemodynamically stable patients, ventricular rate control should be the main priority. Calcium channel blockers, beta-blockers, amiodarone, and digoxin are all shown to be of benefit due to enhancement of the AV nodal refractory period. Secondary hypotension can be a common side effect, which may require concomitant fluid administration and calcium infusion. Digoxin is not associated with hypotension, but the slow mechanism of action of digoxin limits it usefulness in the semiurgent setting.

A variety of treatment methods may be used to terminate AF and restore sinus rhythm. Common options include the use of antiarrythmic drugs, alone or in conjunction with electrical cardioversion, but these must be tailored to each individual case. Therapy with class III antiarrhythmic drugs such as amiodarone, ibutilide, dofetilide, and propafenone have been shown to terminate AF, alone or in conjunction with electrical cardioversion, in 30%–80% of cases if initiated within 7 days of onset. The use of antiarrhythmic therapy must keep in mind the side-effect profile of this class of drugs, including the risk of drug-induced torsades de pointes ventricular tachycardia and other serious dysrhythmias. Controversy exists concerning what emphasis should be placed on pharmacological or electrical cardioversion of AF back into sinus rhythm. The recent results from the AFFIRM study have shown no difference in the long-term outcome in those patients treated with ventricular rate control versus rhythm control. Despite these controversies, up to one-third of patients with new-onset AF spontaneously convert to sinus rhythm without antiarrhythmic therapy in the perioperative period. In those where AF continues unabated, options include pharmacological and/or electrical cardioversion, versus ventricular rate control alone.

The risk of atrial thrombus and emboli become more concerning over time in AF, and anticoagulation therapy should be considered if return to sinus rhythm has not occurred after 48–72 hours. The potential benefits of anticoagulation must be weighed against the risk of postoperative bleeding. The embolic risk is increased when transition occurs from AF to sinus rhythm and vice versa. Typically, anticoagulation is recommended for 3–4 weeks prior to elective electrical cardioversion. If earlier cardioversion is required, it can be performed safely with only 48 hours of anticoagulation if atrial thrombus is ruled out via transesophageal echocardiogram. If this test is positive for atrial thrombus, anticoagulation should be continued for 4–6 weeks, and resolution of thrombus should be proven prior to elective cardioversion.

Ventricular Tachyarrhythmias

Appropriate management of newly diagnosed ventricular tachyarrhythmias depends on accurate rhythm classification and patient risk factor stratification so that appropriate therapy can be provided in a timely fashion. Serious ventricular tachyarrhythmias occur in less than 2% of patients following cardiac surgery, and in noncardiac surgery they are most commonly associated with postoperative myocardial ischemia and significant structural heart disease. The position of intravascular hardware should always be evaluated because dislodgement can be associated with mechanically induced dysrhythmias. Metabolic, acid-base, and oxygenation disturbances in the context of myocardial ischemia and exogenous or endogenous catecholamine excess have all been implicated in promoting triggered activity, abnormal automaticity, and re-entry phenomenon in ventricular tissue. The presence of significant structural heart disease is the most important predictor of future malignant ventricular tachyarrhythmias and sudden cardiac death. A typical ECG will show a wide QRS complex tachycardia, which can originate from a supraventricular source, or more commonly, is due to ventricular tachycardia (VT). If differentiation is not feasible, a wide complex tachycardia should be treated as probable VT. Attention to the QT interval is imperative because treatment without regard for QT prolongation can have drastic consequences. The majority, if not all, antiarrhythmic drugs are "proarrhythmic" themselves. Torsades de pointes accounts for the majority of these drug-induced ventricular tachyarrhythmias. Because of this, it is most advantageous to use single antiarrhythmic drug therapy and avoid the proarrhythmia effects of combination therapy. Ventricular fibrillation (VF) is an inherently unstable rhythm, and a detailed discussion on advanced cardiovascular life support (ACLS) is not the focus of this chapter. More pertinent is an understanding of the rhythms with the propensity to degenerate into VF, and the ability to intervene in an appropriate fashion to prevent this from happening.

Ventricular tachycardia (VT) is classified into monomorphic and polymorphic subtypes. Monomorphic VT is thought to originate from a single ventricular focus and has a wide QRS pattern, each with similar morphology (Figure 8). Polymorphic VT, in contrast, is characterized by an irregular, undulating appearance, with significant variation in QRS morphology. Differentiation is important because polymorphic VT commonly degenerates to VF. Further classification is determined by the persistence of the rhythm. Compared with sustained VT, nonsustained VT typically lasts less than 30 seconds and spontaneously terminates.

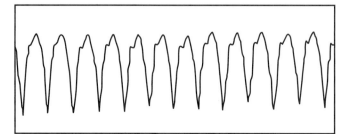

Figure 8 Rhythm strip shows a classic wide QRS tachycardia with similar QRS morphology characteristic of sustained monomorphic ventricular tachycardia.

Premature Ventricular Contractions

Premature ventricular contractions (PVCs) are common in postoperative critical care patients. They can be unifocal, present as couplets, or as bigeminy. They are associated with many electrolyte imbalances and metabolic abnormalities, such as hypokalemia, hypomagnesemia, alkalosis, hypoxia, and catecholamine excess. Correction of these abnormalities, along with the use of beta-blockers, commonly eliminates the majority of PVCs. In asymptomatic patients without structural heart disease, further treatment or suppression of PVCs is rarely required, and there are no associated short- or long-term consequences. In patients with coronary artery disease, history of myocardial infarction, or impaired left ventricular function (ejection fraction [EF] < 40%), PVCs may be a sign of more malignant dysrhythmias to come. Correction of any reversible precipitating factors, including myocardial ischemia, should first be performed, followed with attempts to reduce vasopressor or inotropic support. In symptomatic patients that do not generate sufficient stroke volumes in the face of multiple PVCs, temporary suppression with antiarrythmic drug therapy may be of benefit in critically ill patients.

Monomorphic Ventricular Tachycardia

Nonsustained monomorphic VT can be considered as a prolonged version of PVCs. The rhythm is associated with similar electrolyte and metabolic abnormalities that promote or initiate triggered activity, abnormal automaticity, or re-entry mechanisms. Beta-blockade, and reversal of any of the above precipitating factors, will reduce the frequency and duration of this rhythm. The use of antiarrythmic drug therapy or electric cardioversion is only required for those patients who manifest symptoms or hemodynamic compromise. The long-term prognosis associated with nonsustained monomorphic VT again depends on the presence of structural heart disease. There is an overall increased risk of sudden cardiac death in those with coronary artery disease and left ventricular dysfunction (EF < 40%). Due to this association, patients with structural heart disease should be referred for electrophysiologic (EP) testing. Patients found to have an inducible rhythm at the time of EP testing benefit from placement of an implantable cardioverter-defibrillator (ICD). In patients without structural heart disease, nonsustained monomorphic VT carries no added long-term risk.

The most common mechanism causing sustained monomorphic VT is re-entry. This rhythm is most commonly due to a healed scar from a prior myocardial infarction, which allows a re-entry circuit to occur. Because of this, sustained monomorphic VT is commonly recurrent and portends a poor prognosis. In-hospital mortality rates exceed 40% following surgery, with recurrence in more than 30% of patients who initially survive. As many as 20% discharged from the hospital will succumb to cardiac death within 24 months. Because the substrate for sustained monomorphic VT persists, in those that survive their acute illness, EP testing and subsequent ICD placement is similarly recommended.

The acute management for monomorphic VT is dependent on the hemodynamic status of the patient. Direct-current cardioversion is the mainstay of treatment for those symptomatic or unstable. Electric cardioversion is highly effective and is also recommended for hemodynamically stable VT in conjunction with adequate short-term anesthesia. In those patients who are stable, or where electric cardioversion is not appropriate or available, either intravenous procainamide, sotalol, or amiodarone are the current antiarrhythmic drug recommendations. Amiodarone is the drug of choice for those patients with impaired cardiac function. An important change from the most recent ACLS guidelines is that lidocaine is no longer recommended as a first-line treatment. Antitachycardia pacing is also an option in those with transvenous or an internal pacemaker already in place, although the potential for tachycardia acceleration exists and a defibrillator should be at the bedside if attempted.

Polymorphic Ventricular Tachycardia

Polymorphic ventricular tachycardia has a significant predisposition to degenerate into ventricular fibrillation. The distinction between nonsustained and sustained is less pertinent, because short bursts of this rhythm commonly evolve into sustained polymorphic VT. This rhythm is invariably symptomatic and requires prompt direct-current cardioversion. The most important step once the patient's condition is more stable is the determination of the QT interval by ECG analysis. In patients without QT prolongation, the most likely cause is acute cardiac ischemia and associated severe left ventricular dysfunction. Correction of any associated electrolyte and metabolic abnormalities must occur. Minimization of exogenous catecholamine support and beta-blockade should be initiated, and in those with severe coronary vascular disease, revascularization or intraaortic balloon counterpulsation may be required. Antiarrhythmic drug therapy with intravenous amiodarone, procainamide, or sotalol can promote maintenance of sinus rhythm, but emphasis should be placed on treating the underlying cardiac ischemia. Prognosis depends on the hemodynamic status of the patient rather than the presence of ongoing VT. In those that acutely recover, ICD placement has been shown to improve long-term outcome.

Polymorphic VT in the setting of a prolonged QT interval (QT 460 milliseconds) is commonly referred to as the syndrome of *torsades de pointes* or "twisting of the points." The ECG shows a wide QRS tachycardia that appears to twist around the ECG baseline. This syndrome requires a different management algorithm because the mechanism is attributed to triggered activity secondary to early afterdepolarizations rather than re-entry. Acquired QT prolongation can result from many electrolyte abnormalities and a myriad of medications. Common causes seen in an ICU setting include hypokalemia, hypomagnesemia, specific antibiotics and psychoactive drugs, and, most importantly, class I and III antiarrhythmics (Table 2). The first priority in the management of torsades is identification and removal of the offending agent concurrent with correction of any electrolyte abnormalities. Direct-current cardioversion is used for the hemodynamically unstable, and it is important that any medication that could further prolong the QT interval not be given. Intravenous magnesium should be given to all patients with suspected torsades. Because the length of the QT interval is proportional to the R-R interval (time between each beat), patients benefit from overdrive pacing with isoproterenol or transvenous pacing. Isoproterenol should be used with caution in patients with coronary vascular disease. Antiarrhythmic drugs that do not prolong the QT internal can be used and include lidocaine and phenytoin. Long-term management

depends on avoiding the use of drugs that prolong the QT interval. The overall prognosis is good, and no long-term therapy is typically recommended.

CONCLUSION

The diagnosis and management of cardiac dysrhythmias depends on accurate rhythm classification, knowledge of the underlying mechanisms, and a thorough understanding of appropriate treatment regimens. Measures aimed at prevention of electrolyte and metabolic disturbances that promote these dysrhythmias must not be understated. The use of antiarrhythmic drugs must be limited to those who are symptomatic or hemodynamically unstable so as to limit their potential for inducing a proarrhythmic state. Direct-current cardioversion should be used without hesitation in appropriate patients with instability and in those with a propensity to degenerate into ventricular fibrillation. Particular emphasis should be placed on diagnosis of the more uncommon dysrhythmias, including Wolfe-Parkinson-White and torsades de pointes, since following standard treatment algorithms can lead to disastrous consequences. Consultation with cardiology is essential in regard to long-term management, patient risk stratification, and the plethora of interventional procedures which can improve both acute and long-term outcomes in patients with dysrhythmias. Physical exam, ECG interpretation, and experience are the required tools necessary to manage dysrhythmias appropriately. In just about every ICU setting, these tools can be sharpened and fine-tuned so that ultimately, patients receive the maximum benefit.

Suggested Readings

Bernard EO, et al: Ibutilide versus amiodarone in atrial fibrillation: a double-blinded, randomized study. *Crit Care Med* 31(4):1031–1034, 2003.

Blomstrom-Lundqvist C, et al: ACC/AHA/ESC guidelines for the management of patients with supraventricular arrhythmias—executive summary: a report of the American College of Cardiology/American Heart Association Task Force on Practice Guidelines and the European Society of Cardiology Committee for Practice Guidelines (Writing Committee to Develop Guidelines for the Management of Patients with Supraventricular Arrhythmias). *Circulation* 108(15):1871–1909, 2003.

Chung MK: Cardiac surgery: postoperative arrhythmias. *Crit Care Med* 28(Suppl 10):N136–N144, 2000.

Curtis AB, et al: Clinical factors that influence response to treatment strategies in atrial fibrillation: the Atrial Fibrillation Follow-up Investigation of Rhythm Management (AFFIRM) study. *Am Heart J* 149(4):645–649, 2005.

Delle Karth G, et al: Amiodarone versus diltiazem for rate control in critically ill patients with atrial tachyarrhythmias. *Crit Care Med* 29(6):1149–1153, 2001.

European Resuscitation Council: Part 6: advanced cardiovascular life support. Section 5: pharmacology I: agents for arrhythmias. *Resuscitation* 46(1–3):135–153, 2000.

European Resuscitation Council: Part 6: advance cardiovascular life support. Section 7: algorithm approach to ACLS emergencies. 7A: principles and practice of ACLS. *Resuscitation* 46(1–3):163–166, 2000.

European Resuscitation Council: Part 6: advanced cardiovascular life support. Section 7: algorithm approach to ACLS. 7C: a guide to the international ACLS algorithms. *Resuscitation* 46(1–3):169–184, 2000.

European Resuscitation Council: Part 6: advanced cardiovascular life support. Section 7: algorithm approach to ACLS emergencies. 7D: the tachycardia algorithms. *Resuscitation* 46(1–3):185–193, 2000.

Fuster V, et al: ACC/AHA/ESC guidelines for the management of patients with atrial fibrillation: executive summary. A Report of the American College of Cardiology/American Heart Association Task Force on Practice Guidelines and the European Society of Cardiology Committee for Practice Guidelines and Policy Conferences (Committee to Develop Guidelines for the Management of Patients with Atrial Fibrillation): developed in collaboration with the North American Society of Pacing and Electrophysiology. *J Am Coll Cardiol* 38(4):1231–1266, 2001.

Hersi A, Wyse DG: Management of atrial fibrillation. *Curr Probl Cardiol* 30(4):175–233, 2005.

Hollenberg SM, Dellinger RP: Noncardiac surgery: postoperative arrhythmias. *Crit Care Med* 28(Suppl 10):N145–N150, 2000.

Table 2: Common ICU Drugs That Can Promote Torsades de Pointes

Drug Class	Examples
Antiarrhythmics	Procainamide, quinidine, amiodarone, sotalol, ibutilide
Antimicrobial	Erythromycin, trimethoprim-sulfamethoxazole
Psychoactive	Haloperidol, lithium, chloral hydrate, tricyclic antidepressants
Miscellaneous	Tacrolimus, vasopressin

Adapted from Parrillo J, Dellinger R, editors: *Critical Care Medicine: Principles of Diagnosis and Management in the Adult*, 2nd ed. St. Louis, Mosby, 2001.

Kaushik V, et al: Bradyarrhythmias, temporary and permanent pacing. *Crit Care Med* 28(Suppl 10):N121–N128, 2000.

Mason PK, et al: Influence of the randomized trials, AFFIRM and RACE, on the management of atrial fibrillation in two university medical centers. *Am J Cardiol* 95(10):1248–1250, 2005.

McNamara RL, et al: Management of atrial fibrillation: review of the evidence for the role of pharmacologic therapy, electrical cardioversion, and echocardiography. *Ann Intern Med* 139(12):1018–1033, 2003.

Ramaswamy K, Hamdan MH: Ischemia, metabolic disturbances, and arrhythmogenesis: mechanisms and management. *Crit Care Med* 28(Suppl 10): N151–N157, 2000.

Reinelt P, et al: Incidence and type of cardiac arrhythmias in critically ill patients: a single center experience in a medical-cardiological ICU. *Intensive Care Med* 27(9):1466–1473, 2001.

Singh BN: Atrial fibrillation following investigation of rhythm management: AFFIRM trial outcomes. What might be their implications for arrhythmia control? *J Cardiovasc Pharmacol Ther* 7(3):131–133, 2002.

Trappe HJ, Brandts B, Weismueller P: Arrhythmias in the intensive care patient. *Curr Opin Crit Care* 9(5):345–355, 2003.

Trohman RG: Supraventricular tachycardia: implications for the intensivist. *Crit Care Med* 28(Suppl 10):N129–N135, 2000.

FUNDAMENTALS OF MECHANICAL VENTILATION

Soumitra R. Eachempati, Marc J. Shapiro, and Philip S. Barie

Mechanical ventilation is often required to manage trauma or critical illness, whether for airway protection, administration of general anesthesia, or management of acute respiratory failure (ARF) (Table 1). New technology now provides several modes by which a patient may be ventilated, with the goals of improved gas exchange, better patient comfort, and rapid liberation from the ventilator. Moreover, noninvasive positive-pressure ventilation permits some cases of ARF to be managed without insertion of an artificial endotracheal airway, and some patients who are extubated with marginal reserves to avoid reintubation. Nearly all ventilators can be set to allow full support of the patient on the one hand, and periods of exercise on the other. Thus, the choice of ventilator settings is a matter of physician preference for the majority of patients (Table 2). Controlled ventilation with suppression of spontaneous breathing leads rapidly to respiratory muscle atrophy; therefore modes of assisted ventilation are preferred wherein machine-delivered breaths are triggered by the patient's own inspiratory efforts. Basic modes of assisted ventilation include assist-control ventilation (ACV), synchronized intermittent mandatory ventilation (SIMV), and pressure support ventilation (PSV).

Most patients are started on mechanical ventilation for management of ARF, during which the work necessary to initiate a breath increases by a factor of four to six. The most common reason to initiate mechanical ventilation is to decrease the work of breathing by the patient. Additional potential benefits of mechanical ventilation include improved gas exchange, enhanced coordination between support and the patient's own efforts, resting of respiratory muscles, prevention of deconditioning, and prevention of iatrogenic lung injury while promoting healing. However, unless settings are chosen carefully to synchronize with the patient's own central respiratory drive, mechanical ventilation can cause an increase in work. Regardless of the mode chosen, all mechanical ventilation is a modification of the manner in which positive pressure is applied to the airway, and the interplay of the mechanical support and the patient's own efforts.

NONINVASIVE VENTILATION

Ventilatory support delivered without establishing an endotracheal airway is "noninvasive ventilation" (NIV). Noninvasive ventilation was administered previously with intermittent negative pressure, but the current technique utilizes positive-pressure ventilation delivered through a nasal or face mask, and usage is expanding in the management of acute and chronic respiratory failure and possibly for some patients with heart failure.

Putative benefits of NIV are numerous, owing to avoidance of the complications of endotracheal intubation. Noninvasive ventilation preserves swallowing, feeding, speech, cough, and physiologic air warming and humidification by the nasooropharynx. Nonintubated patients communicate more effectively, require less sedation, and are more comfortable. In addition, patients are often able to continue with standard oral nutrition. Noninvasive ventilation eliminates complications such as trauma with tube insertion, mucosal ulceration, aspiration, infection (e.g., pneumonia, sinusitis), and dysphagia after extubation.

In a randomized, prospective trial following pulmonary resection of 48 patients with acute hypoxemic respiratory insufficiency, Auriant et al. compared standard invasive mechanical ventilation with nasal mask NIV. The need for postoperative reintubation and mortality were clearly reduced in patients receiving NIV as a part of respiratory support. Similarly, Squadrone et al. randomized 209 patients with respiratory failure in the postanesthesia care unit after major abdominal surgery to oxygen alone, or with continuous positive airway pressure (CPAP) via a mask. Patients who received oxygen plus CPAP had a significantly lower intubation rate, and also lower rates of pneumonia, infection, and sepsis.

Contraindications to Noninvasive Ventilation

Crucial to successful NIV is an awake, cooperative, spontaneously breathing patient. Airway, electrocardiographic, or hemodynamic instability argues against the use of NIV. An additional requirement is an intact cough reflex and ability to clear secretions, the absence of which is a common reason for failure of NIV. Relative contraindications include the inability to fit and seal the mask adequately, inability to cough with prompting, or inability to remove the mask in the event of emesis. A hypothetical contraindication is recent gastrointestinal surgery with aerophagia and gut distention. If pressures used to ventilate the patient are kept below 30 mm Hg, the closing pressure of the lower esophageal sphincter should not be exceeded, and aerophagia should be avoided. Morbid obesity is also a relative contraindication secondary to increased ventilatory pressure requirements arising from body habitus and the weight of the chest wall and abdominal viscera while the patient is supine.

Table 1: General Indications for Mechanical Ventilation

Airway maintenance or protection
Airway obstruction
General inhalational anesthesia
Hemodynamic instability
Hypoxemia
Metabolic acidosis
Pulmonary toilet (excessive secretions)

Complications of Noninvasive Ventilation

The most common complication of NIV is focal skin necrosis, which is most common over the bridge of the nose but may also occur over the zygoma. The incidence is 7%–10% among patients receiving full-face-mask NIV. Other complications (incidence, 1%–2% each) include gastric distention, aspiration, and pneumothorax. Conceptual concerns with gastric distention are subsequent vomiting, aspiration, and pneumonia. Conjunctivitis may develop secondary to air leaks near the eyes in around 2% of patients.

The most serious complication is failure to recognize when noninvasive ventilation is not providing a patient with adequate ventilation, oxygenation, or airway patency. Delayed placement of an artificial airway, or failure of placement thereof, may cause continued deterioration or the death of a patient.

PRESSURE SUPPORT VENTILATION

Pressure support is a method of assisting spontaneous breathing in a ventilated patient, either partially or fully. The patient controls all parts of the breath except the pressure limit. The patient triggers the ventilator, which delivers a flow of gas in response up to a preset pressure limit (for example, 10 cm H_2O) depending on the desired minute ventilation (V_E). Gas flow cycles off when a certain percentage of peak inspiratory flow (usually 25%) has been reached. Tidal volumes (V_T) may vary, just as they do spontaneously.

Positive end-expiratory pressure (PEEP, also called continuous positive airway pressure [CPAP]) is added to restore functional residual capacity (FRC) to normal for the patient. When lung volumes are low, the work of breathing during early inhalation is reduced. Noncompliant lungs require higher intrapleural pressures to inflate to a normal V_T, even with CPAP. The addition of pressure support (PS) assists the patient to move up the pressure–volume curve (larger changes in volume for a given applied pressure, i.e., increased lung compliance). The term "pressure support ventilation" describes the combination of pressure support and PEEP (or CPAP). Although useful in the patient breathing spontaneously, PS

Table 2: Glossary of Basic Terminology of Mechanical Ventilation

Control: regulation of gas flow

Volume-controlled—volume limited, volume targeted; airway pressure is variable
Pressure-controlled—pressure limited, pressure targeted; volume delivered is variable
Dual-controlled—volume targeted (guaranteed), pressure limited; seldom used in practice

Cycling: ventilator switching from inhalation to exhalation after volume or pressure target (or limit) has been reached

Time-cycled—example: pressure control ventilation
Flow-cycled—example: pressure support ventilation
Volume-cycled—example: volume-controlled ventilation

Triggering: causes the ventilator to cycle to inhalation

Time-triggered—ventilator cycles at a set frequency as determined by the controlled rate
Pressure-triggered—ventilator senses the patient's inspiratory effort from a decrease of airway pressure
Flow-triggered—constant flow of gas is delivered throughout the respiratory cycle (flow-by). Altered flow caused by patient inhalation is detected by the ventilator, which delivers a breath. Less work is done by the patient than with pressure-triggering

Breaths: cause the ventilator to cycle from inhalation to exhalation

Mandatory—controlled; determined by the respiratory rate
Assisted—examples: assist control, synchronized intermittent mandatory ventilation, pressure support
Spontaneous—no additional assistance, as in continuous positive airway pressure (CPAP)

Flow pattern: constant, decelerating, or sinusoidal

Sinusoidal—examples: spontaneous breathing and CPAP
Constant—flow continues at a constant rate until the set tidal volume is delivered, seldom used in practice
Decelerating—inhalation slows from a high initial flow rate as alveolar pressure increases; example: pressure-targeted ventilation, often used in volume-targeted ventilation, as it causes lower peak airway pressures than constant flow

Mode (breath pattern)

Controlled mechanical ventilation—controlled ventilation, without allowances for spontaneous breathing, typical of anesthesia ventilators
Assist-control—assisted breaths simulate controlled breaths
Intermittent mandatory ventilation—admixes controlled and spontaneous breaths, which may also be synchronized to prevent "stacking"
Pressure support—patient controls all aspects of breath except pressure limit

may be used to assist spontaneous breaths in SIMV. Weaning may be facilitated using this combination, as the backup (SIMV) rate is weaned initially, and then the PS.

HELIOX

Helium has significantly lower density than air or nitrogen. Substituting helium for nitrogen reduces the density of the gas in direct proportion to the amount of helium admixed. Breathing heliox (the concentration in clinical use ranges from 80:20 to 60:40) results in more laminar flow, reduced airway resistance, and reduced work of breathing. Heliox may be useful in clinical situations where resistance to airflow is high, including asthma, acute exacerbations of chronic bronchitis or chronic obstructive pulmonary disease, other causes of bronchospasm, and upper airway obstruction with stridor. Breathing heliox is well tolerated, without significant adverse effects. Disadvantages include high cost and limited utility when a high F_IO_2 is required. Ventilators must also be recalibrated when heliox is delivered by ventilator rather than nebulizer (the usual route), to ensure that the flow of gas is measured correctly.

MODES OF MECHANICAL VENTILATION

Assist Control Ventilation

The ACV mode is the most commonly used mode in medical/surgical critical care units. Set parameters in ACV mode are inspiratory flow rate, frequency (*f*), and V_T. The ventilator delivers a set number of equal breaths per minute, each of a given V_T. Tidal volume and flow determine inspiratory (I) and expiratory (E) time and the I:E ratio. Plateau or alveolar pressure is related to V_T and respiratory system compliance. The patient has the ability to trigger extra breaths by exerting an inspiratory effort exceeding a preset trigger level. Typically, each patient will display a preferred rate for a given V_T and will trigger all breaths when *f* is set a few breaths per minute below the patient's rate. In this mode, the control rate serves as adequate support should the patient stop initiating breaths. When high inspiratory effort continues during a ventilator-delivered breath, the patient may trigger a second superimposed breath. Patient effort can be increased, if desired, by increasing the triggering threshold or lowering V_T.

Synchronized Intermittent Mandatory Ventilation

In a passive patient, SIMV cannot be distinguished from ACV. Ventilation is determined by *f* and V_T. However, if the patient is not truly passive, respiratory work may be performed during mandatory breaths. In addition, the patient may trigger additional breaths by spontaneous effort. If the triggering effort comes in a brief, defined interval before the next mandatory breath, the ventilator will deliver the mandatory breath ahead of schedule to synchronize with patient inspiratory effort. If a breath is initiated outside the synchronization window, V_T, flow, and I:E are determined by patient effort and respiratory system mechanics, not by ventilator settings. These spontaneous breaths tend to be of low V_T and are variable from breath to breath. The SIMV mode is often used to augment patient work of breathing gradually by lowering the mandatory breath frequency or V_T, compelling the patient to breathe more rapidly in order to maintain adequate V_E. Some ventilators allow combinations of modes. A useful combination is SIMV plus PSV as a means to add "sigh" breaths and decrease atelectasis. Because SIMV plus PSV guarantees some backup V_E that PSV alone does not, this combination may be particularly useful for patients at high risk for deteriorating central

respiratory drive, and it is also popular as an adjunct to weaning the ventilator.

Positive End-Expiratory Pressure

Although it is a ubiquitous form of ventilatory support, positive end-expiratory pressure (PEEP) can be confusing because the positive pressure is actually applied throughout the respiratory cycle and is more correctly termed CPAP. Using PEEP accomplishes three goals: prevention of alveolar derecruitment by restoring FRC, which is decreased in acute lung injury (ALI) and atelectasis, to the physiologic range; protection against injury during phasic opening and closing of atelectatic units; and assisting cardiac performance during heart failure, by increasing mean intrathoracic pressure.

The FRC is the lung's physiologic reserve; loss of chest wall or lung compliance (the rate of change of volume in response to pressure) causes reduced FRC. The FRC is the volume of gas that remains in the lungs at the end of a normal tidal breath (~2.5 liters); gas exchange does occur. At FRC, the tendency for the lungs to collapse is balanced by the tendency for the chest wall to move outward. A small vacuum in the pleural space assists in maintaining equilibrium, which is lost when pneumothorax is present.

The FRC is determined by the compliance of the lung and chest wall. Anything that constrains chest wall expansion reduces its compliance; likewise, anything that reduces lung volume reduces lung compliance. The FRC is composed of two volumes, the expiratory reserve volume (ERV) and the residual volume (RV). Below FRC, exhalation is active; lung tissue must be compressed to express gas. The RV (~1 liter in adults) is the point where no more gas can be expressed from the lungs regardless of the pressure applied, because alveolar pressure exceeds atmospheric pressure and the gradient along the airway is reversed. Being filled with gas and coated with surfactant, alveoli are difficult to compress, but airways are compressible. When intrathoracic pressure exceeds pressure in the small airways, "dynamic airway collapse" occurs and gas is trapped in alveoli. Airway collapse increases the work of breathing and leads to ventilation-perfusion (V/Q) mismatch. Collapsed airways are difficult to reinflate, leading to a huge increase in the work of breathing and oxygen consumption.

The concept behind PEEP is to increase FRC; in essence, to allow alveoli to deflate only to the point just above where inflation remains easy (called the lower inflection point of the pressure–volume curve). The patient requires sufficient PEEP to prevent alveolar derecruitment, but not so much PEEP that alveolar overdistension, dead space ventilation from collapse of the alveolar microcirculation, or hypotension due to reduced right ventricular preload, right ventricular output, and ultimately cardiac output occur.

Auto-PEEP is caused by gas trapped in alveoli at end-expiration. This gas is not in equilibrium with the atmosphere and is at positive pressure, increasing the work of breathing. In patients with obstructive airways disease, increased bronchial tone leads to resistance to both inhalation and exhalation. Shortening of E (e.g., small airways disease, mucus plugging, pressure-controlled ventilation with inverted I:E) results in gas trapping at end-expiration, hyperinflation, and increased intrathoracic pressure, which abolishes the alveolar pressure gradient. Auto-PEEP can be ameliorated by lengthening E, shortening I, or decreasing the respiratory rate.

The ideal level of PEEP is controversial (Table 3). It may be that which prevents derecruitment of the majority of alveoli, while causing minimal overdistension; alternatively, application of PEEP is a recruitment maneuver, arguing for higher pressures to be applied to overcome alveolar collapse. Applying PEEP to put the majority of lung units on the favorable part of the pressure–volume curve will maximize gas exchange and minimize overdistension, but is easier said than done because the lower inflection point is sometimes indistinct. Undoubtedly, the combination of PEEP and low V_T prevents volutrauma, but the exact amount of PEEP to apply is controversial. The reason for

Table 3: Protocol Summary for Institution of Mechanical Ventilation for Acute Lung Injury/Acute Respiratory Distress Syndrome

Initial ventilator settings

Use a volume-controlled mode initially to ensure that V_T is delivered.

Initial V_T 8 ml/kg; reduce by 1 ml/kg/2 hours until 6 ml/kg is reached. Minimum V_T is 4 ml/kg.

Set ventilator rate at 12–20 breaths/minute. Maximum ventilator rate 35 breaths/minute.

Adjust ventilator subsequently based on goals of arterial pH (7.25–7.45; ventilator rate) and end-inspiratory plateau pressure (P_{plat}) (<30 cm H_2O; V_T).

Measure arterial pH upon admission to the ICU, every morning, and 15 minutes after each change in respiratory rate or V_T.

Alkalemia is managed by decreasing ventilator rate by at least two breaths/minute.

Mild acidemia (pH 7.15–7.25) is managed by increasing ventilator rate until pH >7.25 or $PaCO_2$ <25 mm Hg up to 35 breaths/minute. If ventilator rate = 35 or $PaCO_2$ < 25 mm Hg, give sodium bicarbonate.

Severe acidemia (pH < 7.15) is managed by increasing the ventilator rate up to 35 breaths/minute. If ventilator rate = 35 and pH < 7.15, and sodium bicarbonate has been given, increase V_T in increments of 1 ml/kg until pH > 7.15. It may be necessary to exceed the target P_{plat} under these conditions.

Keep P_{plat} < 30 cm H_2O. Measure P_{plat} at least every 8 hours, and 5 minutes after each change in PEEP or V_T, and more frequently when changes in lung compliance are likely. Accurate measurement of P_{plat} requires a patient who is not moving or coughing.

If P_{plat} cannot be measured because of an air leak, peak inspiratory pressure may be substituted.

Target ranges for PaO_2 are 55–80 mm Hg, or SaO_2 > 88%. The combination of PEEP and F_IO_2 is discretionary, but F_IO_2:PEEP should generally be <5 if F_IO_2 > 0.45.

When increasing PEEP above 10 cm H_2O, increase by 2–5 cm increments up to a maximum of 35 cm H_2O, until target ranges for PaO_2 are reached. Reduce PEEP to the previous level of PEEP if the change does not increase PaO_2 > 5 mm Hg or if decreased oxygen delivery results from a decrease of cardiac output.

Assess arterial oxygenation by blood gas determination or oximetry at least every 4 hours.

If arterial oxygenation is below the target range, increase F_IO_2 incrementally (up to 1.0), then PEEP (up to 35 cm H_2O within 30 min). Reassess every 15 min after each adjustment until target ranges for PaO_2 are regained. Brief periods of SaO_2 < 88% (<5 min) may be tolerated. F_IO_2 = 1.0 may be used transiently (<10 min) for arterial desaturation or during suctioning or bronchoscopy.

PEEP, Positive end-expiratory pressure.

Adapted from Nathens AB, Johnson JL, Mine JP, et al. Inflammation and the Host Response to Injury Investigators: Inflammation and the host response to injury, a large-scale collaborative project: patient-oriented research core—standard operating procedures for clinical care. I. Guidelines for mechanical ventilation of the trauma patient. *J Trauma* 59:764–769, 2005.

this is hysteresis—the tendency of the lungs, due to surfactant, to exist at higher volumes in exhalation than in inhalation.

Ventilator "Bundle"

Care of the patient who requires mechanical ventilation is more than just a matter of providing ventilation and oxygenation. Such patients are often critically ill and at risk of numerous complications, not all of which are related directly to acute respiratory failure or mechanical ventilation. Therefore, it is important for the clinician to bear in mind the total patient. The patient may be at prolonged bed rest, and at risk for deconditioning, venous thromboembolic complications, and the development of pressure ulcers. Neurologic compromise from disease or sedative/analgesic drugs may impair the sensorium sufficiently that the patient cannot protect his or her airway, increasing the risk of pulmonary aspiration of gastric contents. Oversedation may be one component aspect of prolonged mechanical ventilation, which is a definite risk factor for development of ventilator-associated pneumonia (VAP). Prolonged mechanical ventilation (>48 hours) is itself a marker of critical illness, specifically the development of stress-related gastric mucosal hemorrhage, a rare but serious (~50% mortality) harbinger of adverse outcomes of critical illness.

Using the principles of evidence-based medicine, several "best practices" have been combined into a "ventilator bundle" to optimize the outcomes of mechanical ventilation. The bundle consists of four maneuvers: Keeping the head of the patient's bed up at least 30 degrees from level *at all times* unless contraindicated medically; prophylaxis against venous thromboembolic disease; prophylaxis against stress-

related gastric mucosal hemorrhage; and a daily "sedation holiday" to assess for readiness to liberate from mechanical ventilation through assessment of a trial of spontaneous breathing. Careful adoption and adherence to all facets of the bundle can decrease the substantial risk of VAP, along with other maneuvers such as adherence to the principles of infection control.

Routine Settings

Ventilator settings are based on the patient's ideal body mass and medical condition. The risk of oxygen toxicity from prolonged exposure to a fraction of inspired oxygen (F_IO_2) greater than 60% is minimized by using the lowest F_IO_2 that can oxygenate arterial blood satisfactorily (e.g., arterial oxygen tension [PaO_2] of 60 mm Hg or an oxygen saturation [SaO_2] of 88%) (see Table 3).

The normal lung (e.g., during general anesthesia) may be ventilated safely with V_T 8–10 ml/kg for prolonged periods. Historically, critically ill patients with acute lung injury (ALI)/acute respiratory distress syndrome (ARDS) have been ventilated with V_T 10–15 ml/kg of ideal body mass, which is now considered inappropriate due to convincing data from experiments indicating that alveolar overdistention can produce endothelial, epithelial, and basement membrane injuries associated with increased microvascular permeability and iatrogenic lung injury (VILI). Direct monitoring of alveolar volume is not feasible. A reasonable substitute is to estimate peak alveolar pressure as obtained from the plateau pressure (P_{plat}) measured in a relaxed patient by occluding the ventilator circuit briefly at end-inspiration. In patients with pulmonary dysfunction, there is a growing tendency to reduce the V_T delivered to 4–6 ml/kg or less in order to achieve a P_{plat} no higher than 35 cm H_2O.

The incidence of VILI increases markedly when P_{plat} is high. Low V_T ventilation may lead to an increase in $PaCO_2$. Acceptance of elevated CO_2 tension in exchange for controlled alveolar pressure is termed "permissive hypercapnia." It is important to focus on pH rather than $PaCO_2$ if this approach is employed. If the pH falls below 7.25, increase V_E or administer $NaHCO_3$.

The f that is set depends on the mode. With ACV, the backup rate should be about four breaths per minute less than the patient's spontaneous rate to ensure that the ventilator will continue to supply adequate V_E should the patient have a sudden decrease in spontaneous breathing. With SIMV, the rate is typically high at first and then decreased gradually in accordance with patient tolerance.

An inspiratory flow rate of 60 l/min is used with most patients during ACV and SIMV. In patients with chronic obstructive pulmonary disease, better gas exchange may be achieved at a flow rate of 100 l/min, probably because the resulting increase in E allows for more complete emptying of trapped gas. If the flow rate is insufficient to meet the patient's requirements, the patient will strain against his or her own pulmonary impedance and that of the ventilator, with a consequent increase in the work of breathing.

In the ACV, SIMV, and pressure control modes (discussed in the next chapter), the patient must lower airway pressure below a preset threshold (usually minus 1–2 cm H_2O) in order to trigger the ventilator to deliver a tidal breath. In most situations, this is straightforward; the more negative the sensitivity the greater the effort demanded of the patient. When auto-PEEP is present, the patient must lower alveolar pressure by the amount of auto-PEEP in order to have any impact on airway opening pressure, and then further by the trigger amount to initiate a breath, increasing dramatically the work of breathing. Flow triggering systems have been used to reduce the work of triggering the ventilator. In contrast to the usual approach in which the patient must open a demand valve in order to receive assistance, continuous flow systems maintain a high continuous flow, and then further augment flow when the patient initiates a breath. These systems reduce the work of breathing slightly below that present using conventional demand valves, but do not solve the triggering problem when breath stacking occurs.

Sedation

Most patients who require mechanical ventilation will require sedation, but only a minority (~10%) will also require neuromuscular blockade. A panoply of agents are available for both (Table 4), so the choice of agent can be individualized for the patient, but caution must be exercised so that patients receive only what they need and are not oversedated. Titration of sedation such that patients are comfortable is facilitated by ordering sedation to be titrated to a sedation score of 3–4 points on the Ramsay or Riker scale (Table 5). Intermittent doses of sedatives are preferred to continuous infusions, also to attempt to minimize the amount of sedation. Neuromuscular blockade should be avoided whenever possible.

Prolonged or excessive sedation increases the duration of mechanical ventilation and increases the likelihood of tracheostomy. Protocolized weaning of sedative medications and daily sedation "holidays" to permit spontaneous breathing trials (see following) shorten the duration of mechanical ventilation and decrease the risk of VAP and other complications.

MONITORING

Blood Gases

Blood gas analyzers report a wide range of results, but the only parameters measured directly are the partial pressures of oxygen (pO_2) and carbon dioxide (pCO_2), and blood pH. The arterial blood hemoglobin saturation (SaO_2) is calculated from the pO_2 using the oxyhemoglobin dissociation curve, assuming a normal P_{50} (the pO_2 at which SaO_2 is 50%, normally 26.6 mm Hg), and that hemoglobin is normal structurally. Some blood gas analyzers incorporate a co-oximeter that measures the various forms of hemoglobin directly, including oxyhemoglobin, total hemoglobin, carboxyhemoglobin, and methemoglobin. The actual HCO_3^-, standard HCO_3^-, and base excess are calculated from the pH and pCO_2.

A freshly drawn, heparinized, bubble-free arterial blood sample is required. Heparin is acidic; if present to excess, the measured pCO_2 and calculated HCO_3^- are reduced spuriously. Delayed analysis allows continued metabolism by erythrocytes, reducing pH and pO_2 and increasing pCO_2; keeping the specimen iced preserves accuracy for up to 1 hour. Air bubbles cause a decrease in pCO_2 and an increase in pO_2.

The solubility of all gases in blood, including CO_2 and O_2, increases with a decrease in temperature. Thus, hypothermia causes the pO_2 and pCO_2 to decrease and pH to increase. As analysis of a sample taken from a hypothermic patient occurs at 37° C, the pO_2 and pCO_2 results are artificially high, but the error is usually too small to be meaningful clinically.

Pulse Oximetry

Pulse oximetry calculates SaO_2 by estimating the difference in intensity of signal between oxygenated and deoxygenated blood from the red (660 nm) and near-infrared (940 nm) regions of the light spectrum. To function accurately, pulse oximetry must detect pulsatile blood flow, but all things being equal, pulse oximetry data can be obtained from a detector on the finger, the earlobe, or even the forehead. Pulse oximetry is generally accurate (+2%) over the range of SaO_2 70%–100%, but less accurate below 70%.

Several aspects of the technology and patient physiology limit the accuracy of pulse oximetry. If the device cannot detect pulsatile flow, the waveform will be damped and unable to provide an accurate estimation. Consequently, patients with hypothermia, hypotension, hypovolemia, or peripheral vascular disease, or who are treated with vasoconstrictor medications (e.g., norepinephrine), may have inaccurate pulse oximetry readings. Additionally, an elevated carboxyhemoglobin concentration will lead to falsely elevated SaO_2 because reflected light is absorbed at the same wavelength as oxygenated hemoglobin. Other situations contributing to inaccurate pulse oximetry include the presence of ambient light and motion artifact.

Capnography

Capnography measures changes in the concentration of CO_2 in expired gas during the ventilatory cycle. This technique is most reliable in ventilated patients and employs either mass spectroscopy or infrared light absorption to detect the presence of CO_2. The gas may be collected by sidestream or mainstream sampling; the former is most common and has the advantage of a lightweight analyzer. However, sidestream sampling is susceptible to accumulation of water vapor in the sampling line. In the ICU, where respiratory gases are humidified, mainstream sampling may be preferable.

The peak CO_2 concentration occurs at end-exhalation and is regarded as the patient's "end-tidal CO_2" ($ETCO_2$), at which time $ETCO_2$ is in close approximation to the alveolar gas concentration. Capnography is useful in the assessment of successful tracheostomy or endotracheal tube placement, to monitor weaning from mechanical ventilation, and as a monitor of resuscitation. The ability to detect hypercarbia during ventilator weaning can diminish the need for serial blood gas measurements. In conjunction with pulse oximetry, many patients can be weaned successfully from mechanical ventilation, without reliance upon arterial blood gases or invasive hemodynamic monitoring.

Table 4: Selected Formulary for Analgesia, Anesthesia, and Sedation in the Intensive Care Unit

Agent	Initial IV Adult Dose	Comments
		Induction Agents
Etomidate	≥6 mg	Maintains CO and BP. Reduces ICP but maintains CPP. Short $T_{1/2}$; use infusion for maintenance. Possible adrenal suppression.
Ketamine	1–2 mg/kg	Rapid-onset, short-duration agent for induction of anesthesia. Can be given by maintaining continuous infusion, and at lower dose for sedation without anesthesia. Transiently increases BP and HR, raises ICP and intraocular pressure. Usually does not depress breathing. Generally safe in pregnancy and for neonates and children. Concurrent narcotics or barbiturates may prolong recovery. Can cause anxiety, disorientation, dysphoria, and hallucinations, which may be reduced by a short-acting benzodiazepine during emergence. Atropine pretreatment is recommended to decrease secretions, but may increase incidence of dysphoria. Hepatic metabolism.
Propofol	1.5–2.5 mg/kg	Provides no analgesia. Potent amnestic effect. Causes apnea and loss of gag reflex. Can cause marked low BP. Infuse at 0.05–0.3 mg/kg/min for prolonged sedation. Minimal accumulation (hepatic insufficiency) facilitates rapid elimination. Account for 1 kCal/ml (lipid infusion) in nutrition prescription. Use of same vial >12 hours associated with bacteremia. Safety for children still debated.
		Intravenous Sedatives/Analgesics
Midazolam	0.5–4 mg	Short $T_{1/2}$, but accumulates during infusion owing to active metabolites. Only benzodiazepine with potent amnestic effect. Can cause low BP and loss of airway. Primary use is short-term sedation for ICU procedures. Renal elimination.
Lorazepam	1–4 mg	Effective anxiolytic. Preferred agent for continuous infusion of benzodiazepine (starting dose 1 mg/hr). Can cause low BP, especially with hypovolemia, and paradoxical agitation. Hepatic elimination.
Morphine	2–10 mg	Analgesic and sedative effects. Can cause low BP, CO, and apnea. Tolerance and withdrawal possible after long-term use. Can be given as IV infusion or by PCA for analgesia or to facilitate prolonged mechanical ventilation or withdrawal of care. Hepatic elimination.
Hydromorphone	0.5–2.0 mg	Hydrated ketone of morphine with similar use and risk profiles. Approximately eight-fold more potent than morphine. Hepatic elimination.
Fentanyl	50–100 mcg	Approximately 50-fold potency compared with morphine, but less likely to cause low BP in appropriate dosage (less histamine release). Versatile for ICU use given IV or by epidural infusion or PCA. Less potent than local anesthetics for epidural analgesia or abrogation of surgical stress response. Can cause truncal rigidity and apnea with inability to ventilate by hand (use neuromuscular blockade to facilitate intubation in that setting). Hepatic elimination.
		Neuromuscular Blocking Agents
Succinylcholine	0.75–1.5 mg/kg	Only depolarizing NBMA (occupies ACh receptor). Rapid onset, effect dissipates within 10 minutes of single dose. Causes hyperkalemia. Can precipitate malignant hyperthermia. Increases ICP and intraocular pressure. Contraindicated in TBI, spinal cord injury, neuromuscular disease, and burns. Metabolized by plasma cholinesterase; absence of enzyme (relatively common) causes prolonged paralysis.
Atracurium	0.2–0.5 mg/kg	Short-acting nondepolarizing NMBAs (competitive inhibitor of ACh).
Cisatracurium	0.2–0.5 mg/kg	Relatively slow in onset (also competitive inhibitor of ACh). Atracurium and cisatracurium are similar, except that the former causes histamine release and can cause high HR and low BP. Cisatracurium now used preferentially. Short acting, requires IV infusion for prolonged effect. Effect potentiated by hypokalemia. Many drug interactions. Metabolized by Hoffman elimination/ester hydrolysis, and is thus used for patients with renal/hepatic insufficiency.
Pancuronium	0.05–0.1 mg	Rapid onset, prolonged effect. Causes increased BP and HR. Used for induction of neuromuscular blockade, but should be converted to a drug such as continuous-infusion cisatracurium for maintenance. Renal/hepatic elimination, accumulates in organ dysfunction.
Vecuronium	0.08–0.10 mg/kg	Nondepolarizing NMBA with rapid onset and short duration of action. Less potential for histamine release. Can cause malignant hyperthermia. Metabolized by liver.

Miscellaneous Agents		
Dexmedetomidine	1 mcg/kg load, then 0.2–0.7 mcg/kg/hr	Central selective α_2 agonist used for short-term (<24 hours) sedation. Sympatholysis lowers HR and BP. Can achieve light sedation, does not depress respirations. No anamnestic effect. Useful for drug/alcohol withdrawal and sedation when liberation from mechanical ventilation is imminent. Expensive.
Haloperidol	2–5 mg	Used commonly for anxiolysis (often over lorazepam), especially when respiratory depression is undesirable. IV administration, not FDA-approved, is commonplace. Antidopaminergic properties contraindicate use in Parkinson disease. Causes extrapyramidal effects. Hepatic elimination.
Ketorolac	0.5–1.0 mg/kg	Parenteral NSAID used in lieu of opioids or for opioid-sparing effect in combination. Irreversible platelet dysfunction; can cause incisional or GI hemorrhage and acute renal failure. Use strictly limited to less than 5 days in postoperative period.
Reversal Agents		
Flumazenil	0.1–0.2 mg	Benzodiazepine antagonist. Rapid onset and short duration. Adverse effect of benzodiazepine can persist after drug wears off. Repeated doses of up to 0.8 mg can be used. Abrupt antagonism of chronic benzodiazepine use can precipitate seizures.
Naloxone	0.4 mg	Opioid antagonist. Rapid onset and short duration. Often diluted 0.4 mg/10 ml and titrated 0.04–0.08 mg at a time to reverse undesirable side effects while preserving analgesia. Repeated doses of up to 0.4 mg or continuous IV infusion can be used. Abrupt opioid antagonism can precipitate hypertension, increased HR, pulmonary edema, or myocardial infarction.
Edrophonium with atropine	0.5–1.0 mg/kg 0.007–0.014 mg/kg	Anticholinesterase inhibitor with antidysrhythmic properties. Rapid onset, short duration; therefore used usually in concert with atropine, which counteracts the increased secretions, decreased HR, and bronchospasm. Not effective for reversal of neuromuscular blockade caused by depolarizing agents. Renal and hepatic elimination (edrophonium). Atropine may cause fever.
Neostigmine with glycopyrrolate	0.5-2.0 mg 0.1-0.2 mg	Neostigmine causes salivation and severe low HR. May cause laryngospasm or bronchospasm. Renal metabolism. Not effective for reversal of neuromuscular blockade caused by depolarizing agents. Because of profound low HR, given in same syringe with glycopyrrolate (or sometimes atropine). Glycopyrrolate counteracts low HR, and unopposed causes increased HR. May cause fever. Glycopyrrolate is contraindicated in GI ileus/obstruction and in neonates.

ACh, Acetylcholine; *BP*, blood pressure; *CO*, cardiac output; *CPP*, cerebral perfusion pressure; *ICP*, intracranial pressure; *FDA*, U.S. Food and Drug Administration; *GI*, gastrointestinal; *HR*, heart rate; *IV*, intravenous; *NBMA*, neuromuscular blocking agent; *NSAID*, nonsteroidal anti-inflammatory drug; *PCA*, patient-controlled analgesia; *T½*, elimination half-life; *TBI*, traumatic brain injury; *VO₂*, oxygen consumption.

Other information is acquired from capnography as well. Prognostically, an $ETCO_2$-$PaCO_2$ gradient of 13 mm Hg or more after resuscitation has been associated with increased mortality in trauma patients. A sudden decrease or even disappearance of $ETCO_2$ can be correlated with potentially serious pathology or events, such as a low cardiac output state, disconnection from the ventilator, or pulmonary thromboembolism. A gradual increase of $ETCO_2$ can be seen with hypoventilation; the converse is also true. Another cause of gradually decreasing $ETCO_2$ is hypovolemia.

INVASIVE HEMODYNAMIC MONITORING

Arterial Catheterization

Measurement of arterial blood pressure is one of the simplest, most reproducible methods of evaluating hemodynamics. Automated noninvasive blood pressure cuff devices are accurate (error, ±2%), but take measurements only periodically. If fluctuations require more frequent monitoring, continuous monitoring is available via an indwelling arterial catheter. Indications for invasive arterial monitoring include prolonged operations or prolonged mechanical ventilation (>24 hours), unstable hemodynamics, substantial blood loss, a need for frequent blood sampling, or a need for precise blood pressure control, (e.g., neurosurgical patients, patients on cardiopulmonary bypass). Although there is morbidity from insertion and from indwelling catheters, there is also morbidity from repetitive arterial punctures; the risk:benefit analysis is a matter of clinical judgment for "less-unstable" patients.

Arterial catheters may be placed in any of several locations. The catheter should be a special-purpose thin-walled catheter to maintain fidelity of the waveform and to avoid obstructing the vessel lumen; a standard intravenous cannula should not be used. The radial artery at the wrist is the most commonly used site; although the ulnar artery is usually of larger diameter, it is relatively inaccessible percutaneously. Careful confirmation of a patent collateral circulation to the hand is mandatory before cannulation of an artery at the wrist, to minimize potential tissue loss from arterial occlusion or embolization. In neonates, the umbilical artery may

Table 5: Sedation Scales in Common Usage

	Value	Clinical Correlate
Ramsay Sedation Score		
Awake scores 1–3	1	Anxious, agitated, or restless
	2	Cooperative, oriented, tranquil
	3	Responsive to commands
Asleep scores 4–6	4	Brisk response to stimulus[a]
	5	Sluggish response to stimulus
	6	No response to stimulus
Riker Sedation-Agitation Scale		
Dangerous agitation	7	Pulling at catheters, striking staff
Very agitated	6	Does not calm to voice, requires restraint
Agitated	5	Anxious, responds to verbal cues
Calm and cooperative	4	Calm, awakens easily, follows commands
Sedated	3	Awakens to stimulus
Very sedated	2	Arouses to stimulus, does not follow commands
Unarousable	1	Minimal or no response to noxious stimulus

[a]Stimulus is light glabellar tap or loud auditory stimulus.
Adapted from Ramsay M, Savege T, Simpson B, et al: Controlled sedation with alphaxalon-alphadolone. *BMJ* 2:656–659, 1974; and Riker RR, Picard JT, Fraser GL: Prospective evaluation of the Sedation-Agitation Scale for adult critically ill patients. *Crit Care Med* 27:1325–1329, 1999.

be catheterized; intestinal ischemia is a rare complication. The axillary artery is relatively spared by atheromata, supported by good collaterals at the shoulder, and easy to cannulate percutaneously, making it a suitable choice. The superficial femoral artery may also be used, but is not a location of choice because the burden of plaque (and therefore the risk of distal embolization) is higher, as is the infection rate. The superficial temporal artery is difficult to cannulate because of small caliber and tortuosity. The dorsalis pedis artery is accessible, but should be avoided in patients with peripheral vascular disease. The brachial artery should be strictly avoided, because the collateral circulation around the elbow is poor and the risk of ischemia of the hand or forearm is high. Severe peripheral vasoconstriction due to vasopressor therapy may necessitate a longer catheter at a more central location (e.g., axillary, femoral) in order to place the catheter tip into an artery in the torso that would be less affected. Nosocomial infection of arterial catheters is unusual, provided that basic tenets of infection control are honored and femoral artery catheterization is avoided. Other complications from arterial catheterization include bleeding, hematoma, and pseudoaneurysm.

Central Venous Pressure Monitoring

The central venous pressure (CVP) is an interplay of the circulating blood volume, venous tone, and right ventricular function. The CVP measures the filling pressure of the right ventricle, providing an estimate of intravascular volume status. Central venous access can be obtained via the basilic, femoral, external jugular, internal jugular, or subclavian vein. In the ICU, the internal jugular, subclavian, and femoral veins are used in decreasing frequency. The inter-

nal jugular site is the most popular because of ease of accessibility, a high technical success rate of cannulation, and a low rate of complications. However, it is difficult to keep an adherent dressing in place, and the infection rate is higher than for subclavian catheters. Subclavian insertion is technically demanding, and has the highest rate of pneumothorax (1.5%–3%), but the lowest rates of infection. The femoral vein site is least preferred, despite the relative ease of catheter placement. It is accessible during cardiopulmonary resuscitation or emergency intubation, so procedures can occur concurrently. However, the site is particularly prone to infection, and the risks of arterial puncture (9%–15%) and venous thromboembolic complications are higher than for jugular or subclavian venipuncture. Overall complications are comparable for internal jugular and subclavian vein cannulation (6%–12%), and higher for femoral vein cannulation (13%–19%). The incidence of carotid puncture during internal jugular cannulation (6%–9%) is higher than the incidence of puncture of the subclavian artery during subclavian vein catheterization (3%–5%).

PULMONARY ARTERY CATHETERIZATION

A pulmonary artery catheter (PAC) is a balloon-tipped, flow-directed catheter that is usually inserted percutaneously via a central vein and transits the right heart into the PA. Data from PACs are used mainly to determine cardiac output (Q) and preload, which is most commonly estimated in the clinical setting by the PA occlusion pressure (PAOP). Pulmonary artery diastolic pressure corresponds well to the PAOP. Diastolic pressure can exceed the PAOP when pulmonary vascular resistance is high (e.g., pulmonary fibrosis, pulmonary hypertension).

Normally, PAOP approximates left atrial pressure, which in turn approximates left ventricular end-diastolic pressure (LVEDP), itself a reflection of left ventricular end-diastolic volume (LVEDV). The LVEDV represents preload, which is the actual target parameter. Factors that may cause PAOP to reflect LVEDV inaccurately include mitral stenosis, high levels of PEEP (>10 cm H_2O), and changes in left ventricular compliance (e.g., due to myocardial infarction, pericardial effusion, or increased afterload). Inaccurate readings may result from balloon overinflation, improper catheter position, alveolar pressure exceeding pulmonary venous pressure (as with ventilation with PEEP), or severe pulmonary hypertension (which may make PAOP measurement hazardous). Elevated PAOP occurs in left-sided heart failure. Decreased PAOP occurs with hypovolemia or decreased preload.

A desirable feature of PA catheterization is the ability to measure mixed venous oxygen saturation ($S_{mv}O_2$), although controversially, sampling from the superior vena cava via a central venous catheter may provide data of comparable utility. True mixed venous blood is blood from both the superior and inferior vena cava admixed in the right atrium, which may be sampled for blood gas analysis from the distal port of the PAC. Some catheters have embedded fiberoptic sensors that measure $S_{mv}O_2$ directly. Causes of low $S_{mv}O_2$ include anemia, pulmonary disease, carboxyhemoglobinemia, low Q, and increased tissue oxygen demand. The S_aO_2:($S_aO_2 - S_{mv}O_2$) ratio determines the adequacy of O_2 delivery (DO_2). Ideally the $P_{mv}O_2$ should be 35–40 mm Hg, with a $S_{mv}O_2$ of about 70%. Values of $P_{mv}O_2$ < 30 mm Hg are critically low.

CLINICAL USE OF THE PULMONARY ARTERY CATHETER

Many indications have been championed for the PAC, but no studies have demonstrated unequivocally that PAC use decreases morbidity or mortality. Pulmonary artery catheters may still be useful in cardiomyopathy, shock of various etiologies, suspected pulmonary hypertension, or an unpredicted or poor response to conventional fluid therapy. Transesophageal echocardiography is an alternative, but it is not widely available outside cardiac surgery operating rooms. Critically ill patients receiving inotropic agents despite resuscitation with large volumes of fluid may also benefit from monitoring by PAC. However, a recent ARDSnet trial demonstrated no differences in outcome when ALI/ARDS was managed by PAC versus CVP monitoring.

LIBERATION FROM MECHANICAL VENTILATION

Objective measures and proactive strategies are available to hasten the moment when mechanically ventilated patients can be liberated from the ventilator. The stakes are high, because each day of mechanical ventilation via artificial airway (e.g., endotracheal or tracheostomy tube) increases the need for sedation, which may postpone "liberation day." Moreover, each day of mechanical ventilation increases the risk of VAP, which may prolong further the need for mechanical ventilation.

Some patients do not separate readily from the ventilator, which may be due to disease- or therapy-related reasons. Most clinical cases of failed liberation from the ventilator are multifactorial, but respiratory muscle fatigue is a common factor, in that the load on the respiratory system exceeds the capacity to breathe (Table 6). The increased load may take the form of a demand for increased V_E, or increased work of breathing. Increased V_E may result from increased CO_2 production, increased dead space (V_D) ventilation, or increased ventilatory drive. Increased CO_2 production may be caused by a catabolic state, or excess carbohydrate administered during nutritional support. Increased V_D (ventilation of unperfused or under-perfused lung) may be caused by decreased Q, pulmonary embolism, pulmonary hypertension, severe ALI, or iatrogenically from positive-pressure ventilation. Increased ventilatory drive may occur from muscle fatigue or failure, stimulation of pulmonary J receptors (usually by lung inflammation or parenchymal hemorrhage), or lesions of the central nervous system. Psychological stress is also an important factor that may manifest itself as tachypnea, hypoxemia, or agitation or delirium. Stress may be caused by inadequate analgesia or sedation, or untreated delirium. Acute alcohol or drug withdrawal is a major factor in some patients.

Increased work of breathing results from either increased airflow resistance or decreased thoracic compliance. Airway obstruction can result from reversible small airways disease (e.g., bronchospasm), tracheal stenosis, tracheomalacia, glottic edema or dysfunction, mucus plugging, or muscle weakness or fatigue. Muscle dysfunction may be caused by nutritional or metabolic causes (including hypocalcemia, hypokalemia, or hypophos-

phatemia). The *critical illness polyneuropathy* syndrome has poorly understood pathophysiology, but is associated with sepsis and multiple organ dysfunction syndrome, and is often diagnosed when sought specifically by electromyography. Other potential causes of muscular failure or weakness include hypoxemia, hypercarbia, and possible anemia.

Patients who "fight" the ventilator technically have the syndrome of *patient–ventilator dyssynchrony*. The cause can usually be found and must be sought; to sedate the patient more deeply (or administer neuromuscular blockade) before correctable causes are identified and remedied is incorrect and may be catastrophic if an unstable airway is the cause. A systematic approach to evaluation is advocated; recognizing that the patient and the ventilator are supposed to be working in concert facilitates an understanding that the problem may be the patient or the ventilator. The cause may be found anywhere on the continuum from the alveolus to the power outlet or the source of respiratory gases, and must be sought systematically (Table 7). The first step is always to ensure that the patient has a patent airway that is positioned properly.

Liberation from mechanical ventilation can be easy in patients requiring short-term support. However, as many as 25% of

Table 6: Load on Respiratory System

Demand for increased minute ventilation
Increased carbon dioxide production
Increased dead space ventilation
Increased ventilatory drive
Increased work of breathing
Airway obstruction
Decreased respiratory system compliance
Decreased respiratory system capacity
Impaired central drive to breathe
Integrity of phrenic nerve transmission
Impaired respiratory muscle force generation

Table 7: Therapies to Reverse Ventilatory Failure

Improve muscular function	
Treat sepsis—avoid aminoglycosides	
Nutritional support without overfeeding (follow indirect calorimetry)	
Replete electrolytes to normal	
Assure periods of rest—do not exhaust the patient	
Limit neuromuscular blockade	
Avoid oversedation	
Identify/correct hypothyroidism	
Reduce respiratory load	
Airway resistance	Ensure airway patency/adequate caliber
Compliance (elastance)	Treat pneumonia
	Treat pulmonary edema
	Identify/reduce intrinsic PEEP (auto-PEEP)
	Drain large pleural effusions
	Evacuate pneumothorax
	Treat ileus (promotility agents)
	Decompress abdominal distention/ treat abdominal compartment syndrome
	Position patient 30 degrees head up
Minute ventilation	Treat sepsis
	Antipyresis (temperature >40° C)
	Avoid overfeeding
	Correct metabolic acidosis
	Identify/reduce intrinsic PEEP (auto-PEEP)
	Bronchodilators
	Maintain least possible PEEP
	Resuscitate shock/correct hypovolemia
	Identify and treat pulmonary embolism

PEEP, Positive end-expiratory pressure.

patients will experience respiratory distress such that ventilation has to be reinstituted; patients recovering from acute respiratory failure, necrotizing pneumonia, or major torso trauma can be especially challenging. Patients who cannot be weaned have a characteristic response to trials of spontaneous breathing: there is an almost immediate increase in respiratory rate and decrease in V_T. As the trial of spontaneous breathing continues over 30–60 minutes, work of breathing increases substantially by four- to seven-fold. Increased oxygen demand is met by increased oxygen extraction, which eventually causes decreased DO_2 and arterial hypoxemia. Pulmonary compliance decreases, and gas trapping from lengthened I:E doubles measured auto-PEEP. The rapid, shallow breathing pattern causes CO_2 retention because of increased dead space ventilation despite increased V_E. There is considerable cardiovascular stress also, with pulmonary and systemic hypertension and increased afterload on both ventricles, likely from the extreme changes in intrathoracic pressure generated by the struggling patient.

Timing is important; if weaning is delayed unnecessarily, the patient remains at risk for a host of ventilator-associated complications. If weaning is performed prematurely, failure may lead to cardiopulmonary decompensation and further prolonged mechanical ventilation. In general, discontinuation of mechanical ventilation is not attempted in the setting of cardiopulmonary instability or $PaO_2 < 60$ mm Hg with an F_IO_2 of 0.60 or higher. However, satisfactory oxygenation does not predict successful weaning reliably; rather, a more important determinant is the ability of respiratory muscles to perform increased respiratory work. Decisions based solely on clinical judgment are frequently erroneous. Parameters gathered traditionally, including maximal negative inspiratory pressure, vital capacity, and V_E, have limited predictive accuracy. Respiratory frequency $(f)/V_T$ during 1 minute of spontaneous breathing (the Rapid Shallow Breathing Index) is a more accurate predictor (95% probability of success) if f/V_T is less than 80 after a 30-minute trial of spontaneous breathing. Calculation of f/V_T during PSV is considerably less accurate.

The process of weaning begins by determining patient readiness (Figure 1). Patients should be screened carefully for hemodynamic stability, cooperative mental status, respiratory muscle strength, consistent and adequate wakefulness, ability to manage secretions, nutritional repletion and normalization of acid–base and electrolyte status, and an artificial airway of adequate size. Particular attention should be given to acceptance of hypercapnia if chronically present and avoidance of new metabolic alkalosis. Finally, ensure normality of electrolytes affecting muscle function (e.g., calcium, phosphate, and potassium). If the aforementioned conditions are addressed, weaning may be attempted.

There are four methods of weaning. Simplest is to perform spontaneous breathing trials each day with a T-piece circuit providing oxygen-enriched gas. Initially brief (5–10 minutes), the trials can be increased in frequency and duration until the patient can breathe spontaneously for several hours. An alternative is to perform a single daily T-piece trial of up to 2 hours in duration; if successful, the patient is extubated; if not, the next attempt is the following day. Much more common (and popular) are SIMV and PSV, which in fact are often combined. Ventilatory assistance is decreased gradually by decreasing f or the amount of pressure. When combined, f is set to zero before the level of pressure is decreased. Pressure support of 5–8 cm H_2O is used widely to compensate for the resistance inherent in the ventilator circuit, and patients who can breathe comfortably at that level should be able to be extubated, although the minimal level of assistance in these modes has never been well defined. Randomized, controlled trials indicate that the process of weaning takes up to three times as long when IMV is used rather than trials of spontaneous breathing. Approximately 10%–20% of patients require reintubation, defining a subgroup of patients with mortality that is six-fold higher, which

may be a marker of more severe underlying illness. Use of NIV following extubation may improve the likelihood of successful extubation.

SPECIAL AIRWAY CONSIDERATIONS

Unplanned Extubation

Unplanned extubation (usually by the patient) is a morbid event that occurs in approximately 10% of patients receiving mechanical ventilation. Risk factors include chronic respiratory failure, poor fixation of the airway device, orotracheal intubation (which is decidedly uncomfortable), and inadequate sedation. The associated complications include reintubation (required in one-half of cases), pneumonia, vocal cord trauma, and rarely, loss of the airway with attendant cardiovascular and neurologic complications. Reintubation is more likely in the setting of accidental extubation, decreased mentation, occurrence outside a process of active weaning, and PaO_2: $F_IO_2 < 200$. The risk of unplanned extubation can be reduced by adequate, appropriate sedation, vigilance during positioning of the patient and bedside procedures, durable fixation of the airway device, and daily screening and assessment of patient readiness for liberation from the ventilator.

Reintubation

Approximately 20% of patients will require reintubation, which can occur even if protocols are followed and the patient meets all criteria for extubation. The rate varies widely among units; a rate that is "too low" may imply that patients are not being weaned aggressively enough, whereas a rate that is "too high" may reflect a high proportion of patients with neurologic impairment, who are at highest risk. Interestingly, weaning protocols, which are designed to liberate patients from mechanical ventilation sooner, are associated paradoxically with lower rates of reintubation. Reintubation may be a marker of severity of illness, but it is associated with substantially increased risks of pneumonia and death. The cause may either be airway compromise or failure of lung/chest wall mechanics (weaning failure).

Tracheostomy

Identifying patients who will not be able to be removed from the ventilator is challenging. Possible reasons include airway obstruction, anxiety or agitation (requiring heavy doses of sedatives), aspiration syndromes, alkalosis, bronchospasm/wheezing, chronic obstructive pulmonary disease, critical illness polyneuropathy or other forms of neuromuscular disease, electrolyte abnormalities heart disease, hypothyroidism, morbid obesity, nutrition (over- or under-feeding), opioids, oversedation, pleural effusion (if large), pulmonary edema, and sepsis.

The timing of tracheostomy remains controversial. There is no consensus definition of when a tracheostomy is "early" (<10 days?) or "late" (>21 days?), although trends are toward earlier performance, with decreased sedation requirements and risk of pneumonia, greater patient comfort, and facilitated weaning subsequently. The shorter tube decreases airway resistance and work of breathing, and facilitates pulmonary toilet by suctioning. Percutaneous tracheostomy has decreased the morbidity of tracheostomy substantially. However, modern high-volume, low-pressure cuffs on endotracheal tubes permit translaryngeal intubation for several weeks with relative safety. Patients who are unstable hemodynamically, coagulopathic, or on high levels of PEEP may benefit from having tracheostomy postponed until they are more stable.

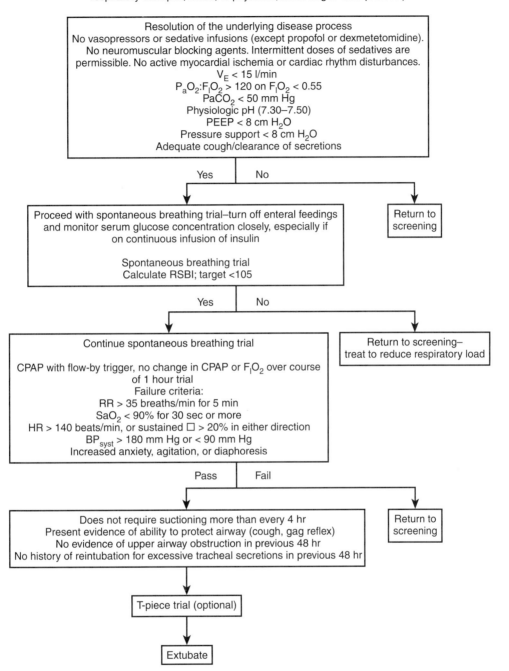

Screening (performed at least once daily, usually in early AM, by respiratory therapist, nurse, or physician, according to local protocol)

Resolution of the underlying disease process
No vasopressors or sedative infusions (except propofol or dexmetetomidine).
No neuromuscular blocking agents. Intermittent doses of sedatives are
permissible. No active myocardial ischemia or cardiac rhythm disturbances.
$V_E < 15$ l/min
$P_aO_2:F_IO_2 > 120$ on $F_IO_2 < 0.55$
$PaCO_2 < 50$ mm Hg
Physiologic pH (7.30–7.50)
PEEP < 8 cm H_2O
Pressure support < 8 cm H_2O
Adequate cough/clearance of secretions

Yes · No

Proceed with spontaneous breathing trial–turn off enteral feedings
and monitor serum glucose concentration closely, especially if
on continuous infusion of insulin

Spontaneous breathing trial
Calculate RSBI; target <105

Return to screening

Yes · No

Continue spontaneous breathing trial

CPAP with flow-by trigger, no change in CPAP or F_IO_2 over course
of 1 hour trial
Failure criteria:
RR > 35 breaths/min for 5 min
$SaO_2 < 90\%$ for 30 sec or more
HR > 140 beats/min, or sustained □ > 20% in either direction
$BP_{syst} > 180$ mm Hg or < 90 mm Hg
Increased anxiety, agitation, or diaphoresis

Return to screening–
treat to reduce respiratory load

Pass · Fail

Does not require suctioning more than every 4 hr
Present evidence of ability to protect airway (cough, gag reflex)
No evidence of upper airway obstruction in previous 48 hr
No history of reintubation for excessive tracheal secretions in previous 48 hr

Return to screening

T-piece trial (optional)

Extubate

Figure 1 Cornell protocol for liberation from mechanical ventilation.

Suggested Readings

Acton RD, Hotchkiss JR, Dries DJ: Noninvasive ventilation. *J Trauma* 53:593–601, 2002.

Antonelli M, Conti G, Rocco M, et al: A comparison of noninvasive positive-pressure ventilation and conventional mechanical ventilation in patients with acute respiratory failure. *N Engl J Med* 339:429–435, 1998.

ARDS Network: Ventilation with lower tidal volumes as compared with traditional tidal volumes for acute lung injury and the acute respiratory distress syndrome. *N Engl J Med* 342:1301–1308, 2000.

Arroliga A, Frutos-Vivar F, Hall J, et al: International Mechanical Ventilation Study Group. Use of sedatives and neuromuscular blockers in a cohort of patients receiving mechanical ventilation. *Chest* 128:496–506, 2005.

Auriant I, Jallot A, Hervé P, et al: Noninvasive ventilation reduces mortality in acute respiratory failure following lung resection. *Am J Respir Crit Care Med* 164:1231–1235, 2001.

Banner MJ, Kirby RR, MacIntyre NR: Patient and ventilator work of breathing and ventilatory muscle loads at different levels of pressure support ventilation. *Chest* 100:531–533, 1991.

Bouderka MA, Fakhir B, Bouaggad A, et al: Early tracheostomy versus prolonged endotracheal intubation in severe head injury. *J Trauma* 57:251–254, 2004.

Brochard L, Pluskwa F, Lemaire F: Improved efficacy of spontaneous breathing with inspiratory pressure support. *Am Rev Respir Dis* 136:411–415, 1987.

Brochard L: Inspiratory pressure support. *Eur J Anaesthesiol* 11:29–36, 1994.

Brochard L, Rauss A, Benito S, et al: Comparison of three methods of gradual withdrawal from ventilatory support during weaning from mechanical ventilation. *Am J Respir Crit Care Med* 150:896–903, 1994.

Consales G, Chelazzi C, Rinaldi S, De Gaudio AR: Bispectral Index compared to Ramsay score for sedation monitoring in intensive care units. *Minerva Anestesiol* 72:329–336, 2006.

Cook DJ, Meade MO, Hand LE, McMullin JP: Toward understanding evidence uptake: semirecumbency for pneumonia prevention. *Crit Care Med* 30:1472–1477, 2002.

Dodek P, Keenen S, Cook D, et al: Evidence-based clinical guideline for the prevention of ventilator-associated pneumonia. *Ann Intern Med* 141:305–313, 2004.

Eachempati SR, Barie PS: Monitoring respiratory function and weaning from the ventilator. In Bland K, editor: *The Practice of General Surgery*. Philadelphia, WB Saunders, 2001, pp. 144–150.

Ely EW, Baker AM, Dunagan DP, et al: Effect on the duration of mechanical ventilation of identifying patients capable of breathing spontaneously. *N Engl J Med* 335:1864–1869, 1996.

Ely EW: Weaning from mechanical ventilatory support. In Murray MJ, Coursin DB, Pearl RG, Prough DS, editors: *Critical Care Medicine: Perioperative Management*. Baltimore, Lippincott, Williams & Wilkins, 2002, pp. 460–474.

Epstein SK, Ciubotaru RL, Wong JB: Effect of failed extubation on the outcome of mechanical ventilation. *Chest* 112:186–192, 1997.

Esteban A, Frutos F, Tobin MJ, et al: A comparison of four methods of weaning patients from mechanical ventilation. *N Engl J Med* 332:345–350, 1995.

Freeman BD, Isabella K, Lin N, Buchman TG: A meta-analysis of prospective trials comparing percutaneous and surgical tracheostomy in critically ill patients. *Chest* 118:1412–1418, 2000.

Guidelines for the management of adults with hospital-acquired, ventilator-associated, and healthcare-associated pneumonia. *Am J Respir Crit Care Med* 171:388–416, 2005.

Habashi N, Andrews P: Ventilator strategies for posttraumatic acute respiratory distress syndrome: airway pressure release ventilation and the role of spontaneous breathing in critically ill patients. *Curr Opin Crit Care* 10:549–557, 2004.

Hillberg RE, Johnson DC: Noninvasive ventilation. *N Engl J Med* 337:1746–1752, 1997.

Jaeschke RZ, Meade MO, Guyatt GH, et al: How to use diagnostic test articles in the intensive care unit: diagnosing weanability using f/VT. *Crit Care Med* 25:1514–1521, 1997.

Keenan SP, Sinuff T, Cook DJ, Hill NS: Does noninvasive positive pressure ventilation improve outcome in acute hypoxemic respiratory failure? A systematic review. *Crit Care Med* 32:2516–2523, 2004.

Keroack MA, Cerese J, Cuny J, et al: The relationship between evidence-based practices and survival in patients requiring prolonged mechanical ventilation in academic medical centers. *Am J Med Qual* 21:91–100, 2006.

Kollef MH, Shapiro SD, Silver P, et al: A randomized, controlled trial of protocol-directed versus physician-directed weaning from mechanical ventilation. *Crit Care Med* 25:567–574, 1997.

Kress JP, Pohlman AS, O'Connor MF, Hall JB: Daily interruption of sedative infusions in critically ill patients undergoing mechanical ventilation. *N Engl J Med* 342:1471–1477, 2000.

Liesching T, Kwok H, Hill NS: Acute applications of noninvasive positive pressure ventilation. *Chest* 124:699–713, 2003.

MacIntyre NR: Respiratory function during pressure support ventilation. *Chest* 89:677–683, 1986.

MacIntyre NR, Cook DJ, Ely EW Jr, et al: Evidence-based guidelines for weaning and discontinuing ventilatory support: a collective task force facilitated by the American College of Chest Physicians, the American Association for Respiratory Care, and the American College of Critical Care Medicine. *Chest* 120:375S–395S, 2001.

Marelich GP, Murin S, Batistella F, et al: Protocol weaning of mechanical ventilation in medical and surgical patients by respiratory care practitioners and nurses: effect on weaning time and incidence of ventilator-associated pneumonia. *Chest* 118:459–467, 2000.

Mascia ME, Koch M, Medicis JJ: Pharmacoeconomic impact of rational use guidelines on the provision of analgesia, sedation, and neuromuscular blockade in critical care. *Crit Care Med* 28:2300–2306, 2000.

McCulloch TM, Bishop MJ: Complications of translaryngeal intubation. *Clin Chest Med* 12:507–521, 1991.

McGee DC, Gould MK: Preventing complications of central venous catheterization. *N Engl J Med* 348:1123–1133, 2003.

Meduri GU: Noninvasive positive-pressure ventilation in patients with acute respiratory failure. *Clin Chest Med* 17:513–553, 1996.

Nathens AB, Johnson JL, Mine JP, et al. Inflammation and the Host Response to Injury Investigators: Inflammation and the host response to injury, a large-scale collaborative project: patient-oriented research core—standard operating procedures for clinical care. I. Guidelines for mechanical ventilation of the trauma patient. *J Trauma* 59:764–769, 2005.

Nieszkowska A, Combes A, Luyt CE, et al: Impact of tracheotomy on sedative administration, sedation level, and comfort of mechanically ventilated intensive care unit patients. *Crit Care Med* 33:2527–2533, 2005.

Pieracci FM, Barie PS, Pomp A: Critical care of the bariatric patient. *Crit Care Med* 34:1796–1804, 2006.

Ramsay M, Savege T, Simpson B, et al: Controlled sedation with alphaxalone-alphadolone. *BMJ* 2:656–659, 1974.

Riker RR, Picard JT, Fraser GL: Prospective evaluation of the Sedation–Agitation scale for adult critically ill patients. *Crit Care Med* 27:1325–1329, 1999.

Schuerer DJ, Whinney RR, Freeman BD, et al: Evaluation of the applicability, efficacy, and safety of a thromboembolic event prophylaxis guideline designed for quality improvement of the traumatically injured patient. *J Trauma* 58:731–739, 2005.

Squadrone V, Coha M, Cerutti E, et al: Continuous positive airway pressure for treatment of postoperative hypoxemia: a randomized controlled trial. *JAMA* 293:589–595, 2005.

Straus C, Louis B, Isabey D, et al: Contribution of the endotracheal tube and the upper airway to breathing workload. *Am J Respir Crit Care Med* 157:23–30, 1998.

Tobin MJ: Advances in mechanical ventilation. *N Engl J Med* 344:1986–1996, 2001.

Tobin MJ, Van de Graaff WB: Monitoring of lung mechanics and work of breathing. In Tobin MJ, editors: *Principles and Practice of Mechanical Ventilation*. New York, McGraw-Hill, 1994, pp. 967–1003.

Wheeler AP, Bernard GP, Thompson BT, et al: Pulmonary-artery versus central venous catheter to guide treatment of acute lung injury. National Heart, Lung, and Blood Institute Acute Respiratory Distress Syndrome (ARDS) Clinical Trials Network. *N Engl J Med* 354:2213–2224, 2006.

Yang KL, Tobin MJ: A prospective study of indexes predicting the outcome of trials of weaning from mechanical ventilation. *N Engl J Med* 324:1445–1450, 1991.

Young CC, Prielipp RC: Sedative, analgesic, and neuromuscular blocking drugs. In Murray MJ, Coursin DB, Pearl RG, Prough DS, editors: *Critical Care Medicine: Perioperative Management*. Baltimore, Lippincott, Williams & Wilkins, 2002, pp. 147–167.

ADVANCED TECHNIQUES
IN MECHANICAL VENTILATION

Mark M. Melendez, Marc J. Shapiro,
Soumitra R. Eachempati, and Philip S. Barie

Since the introduction of mechanical ventilation using a bicycle tire and bellows about 50 years ago, the science and art of respiratory therapy has advanced dramatically—allowing the clinician to ventilate and oxygenate patients who would have died in the past due to limitations of man and machine. This chapter focuses on recent advances and future considerations in ventilatory support to allow further improvements in respiratory care and survival from acute lung injury (ALI), acute respiratory distress syndrome (ARDS), and chronic respiratory failure.

IMPROVING OXYGENATION AND PREVENTING ACUTE LUNG INJURY

Providing adequate oxygen delivery (DO_2) with minimal barotrauma is the primary goal of mechanical ventilation for patients with all types of pulmonary pathology, as well as for those with normal lungs. Noninvasive ventilation (NIV) using such modalities as bi-level positive airway pressure (BiPAP) with various degrees of inspiratory and expiratory pressure applied via a face, nasal, or combined face mask has become a more common modality to avoid endotracheal intubation or to perhaps shorten the need or period of ventilation by artificial airway. Marginal candidates for liberation from ventilation may stave off reintubation once extubated.

Peak and plateau airway pressures are crucial parameters for the clinician in managing patients on the ventilator. The ARDSnet trial examined conventional mechanical ventilation with a tidal volume (V_T) of 10 ml/kg and with V_T at a lower tidal volume of 6 ml/kg in patients with ALI/ARDS and found a significant improvement in oxygenation, a decrease in ventilator-associated lung injury (VILI), and decreased mortality related to ALI/ARDS. Tidal volumes as low as 4 ml/kg may be used to maintain the plateau pressure at less than 30 cm H_2O to minimize barotrauma (or "volutrauma," as it is called by some). In some circumstances, conventional mechanical ventilator modalities may be inadequate to the task. Modern microprocessor-controlled ventilators allow modification of flow rate and flow patterns in providing adequate and safe mechanical ventilation.

Ventilator-Associated Lung Injury

Acute lung injury and ARDS are recognized as affecting the lungs heterogeneously. The distribution of edema fluid, ventilated versus flooded alveoli, and consequently the matching of ventilation and perfusion vary among gas exchange units. Moreover, it is recognized that the lung is capable of a brisk inflammatory response when injured or when ventilated mechanically, which may have local or systemic manifestations. The ARDSnet trial demonstrated improved outcomes from ALI/ARDS after ventilation with lower V_T and minute ventilation (V_E), resulting in lower airway pressures, less overdistension of recruitable alveoli, less shear stress on lung tissue, and lower mortality despite the paradox that most patients with ALI/

ARDS do not die from an inability to oxygenate or ventilate. Rather, most such patients die in association with the multiple organ dysfunction syndrome—which has been linked closely with a rampant systemic inflammatory response. If less ventilation is better, it was hypothesized that more ventilation may be injurious or indeed provocative to the lung—leading to the concept of VILI.

Ventilator-induced lung injury occurs from excessive mechanical stress to the lung, either from excessive V_T or excessive airway pressure. Mechanical ventilation induces a pulmonary and systemic cytokine response, which can be minimized by limiting overdistension and phasic recruitment/derecruitment of lung. A substantial body of experimental and clinical data demonstrates that the mechanism of VILI is the proinflammatory response in the lung and the periphery, and that the response and injury are attenuated by lung-protective ventilation strategies. New modes of ventilation and protective ventilation are designed to minimize the deleterious effects of mechanical ventilation, which is a fundamental aspect of critical care management.

ALTERNATIVES TO CONVENTIONAL MECHANICAL VENTILATION

Proportional Assist Ventilation

Proportional assist ventilation (PAV) is a form of synchronized partial ventilatory assistance that augments the flow of gas to the patient in response to patient-generated effort. The ventilator augments the patient's inspiratory effort without using preselected target volume or pressure. The purpose of PAV is to allow the patient to achieve a pattern of ventilation and breathing that is adequate and comfortable. The patient initiates and determines the depth and frequency of the breaths independently of the ventilator. Advantages to this type of ventilator support include greater comfort; reduction of peak airway pressure required to deliver the V_T; less likelihood of overventilation and overdistension of alveoli; preservation and enhancement of the patient's own reflex, behavioral, and homeostatic control mechanisms; and improved efficiency of negative-pressure ventilation.

Effective use of PAV requires an understanding of the individual patient's ventilatory mechanics. This entails measuring the patient's airway resistance, compliance, and intrinsic positive end-expiratory pressure (auto-PEEP) to determine the ventilatory load and assistance the patient requires. Younes et al. proposed an innovative method for the noninvasive determination of passive elasticity during PAV. Once the patient's elastance and resistance are determined, the PAV parameters are set followed by PEEP, adjusting the peak pressure limit to 30 cm H_2O, adjusting volume assist to 8% of elastance measured on PAV, and finally observing the patient's ventilation, breathing pattern, and peak airway pressure. As a new ventilatory method, PAV can conceivably improve patient-ventilator interaction. Its true usefulness remains to be measured, and clinical usage is uncommon.

Pressure-Controlled Ventilation

Pressure-controlled ventilation (PCV) is pressure-limited time-cycled breathing that is completely controlled by the ventilator, with no participation by the patient. Inspiratory airway pressure increases early in the respiratory cycle, and is maintained at that specified pressure throughout the remainder of the delivery phase. The major benefit of PCV relates to the inspiratory flow pattern and its benefit in gas delivery for patients with suppressed respiratory efforts. In pressure-cycled breathing, the inspiratory flow decreases exponentially during lung inflation in order to keep the airway pressure at the preselected value. Thus, this type of flow pattern can improve gas exchange. The primary disadvantage of PCV is the tendency for inflation volumes to vary with changes in the mechanical properties of the lungs. There is a proportional relationship between the lung inflation and the peak inflation pressure. When a constant peak inflation pressure is reached, the inflation volume decreases as the airway resistance increases or lung compliance decreases. The result is fluctuation in inflation volumes due to reliance on a specific pressure target.

Inverse-Ratio Ventilation

Inverse-ratio ventilation (IRV) is a combination of PCV (hence, PC-IRV) with a prolonged inspiratory time (I). One way to increase I is to decrease the inspiratory flow rate, such as increasing the I:expiratory time (E) ratio from the usual 1:4 to 2:1 (up to 4:1). Benefits of IRV include improved oxygenation and the prevention of alveolar collapse as confirmed in cases of ARDS and neonatal respiratory distress syndrome. On occasion, the early use of PC-IRV can facilitate tapering of high fractions of inspired oxygen (F_IO_2) and decrease high PEEP and peak inspiratory pressures (PIPs). The downside to PC-IRV is that is can lead to stacking of breaths (auto-PEEP), with high airway pressures, hyperinflation and barotrauma, CO_2 retention, and metabolic acidosis. Another adverse effect observed with IRV is the potential to cause decreased cardiac output due to auto-PEEP because increased transthoracic pressure decreases venous return.

Mandatory Minute Ventilation

Mandatory minute ventilation (MMV) is a mode of mechanical ventilation in which the minimum level of V_E needed by the patient is provided. If the patient's spontaneous ventilation is insufficient to meet the predetermined V_E, the ventilator provides the difference. Conversely, if the patient's spontaneous breathing exceeds the target V_E no ventilator support is provided. This mode is one of the so-called "closed-loop" ventilation modes (Table 1) because the ventilator varies its parameters in response to the patient's own intrinsic ventilatory requirements. The major advantage of MMV is the capability to vary ventilatory support according to the response of the patient. This mode of mechanical ventilation is best suited for patients with severe neuromuscular disease or drug overdose, or patients heavily sedated. One of the main disadvantages with MMV is that alveolar ventilation may not be matched equally with exhaled V_E, thus diminishing closing volumes and leading to atelectasis. None of the closed-loop modes, MMV included, has been tested sufficiently on critically ill patients to recommend widespread incorporation into practice.

Airway Pressure Release Ventilation

Airway pressure release ventilation (APRV) (Table 2) has been used as an alternative mode of mechanical ventilation in patients with acute respiratory failure. APRV, which has been available in some ventilator models since the mid-1990s, allows for the unloading during exhalation of any positive pressure provided during inhalation in order to facilitate the egress of the tidal breath. Release of airway

Table 1: Closed-Loop Modes of Mechanical Ventilation

Mode	Principle	Theoretical Advantage	Caveat
Mandatory minute ventilation	SIMV mode in which mandatory breath rate increases or decreases in response to V_E	Guaranteed minimum V_E in patients with fluctuating or unreliable ventilatory drive	Desired V_E must be set carefully, or the patient may be over- or underventilated.
Pressure-regulated volume control	Pressure-targeted time-cycled breaths with automatic pressure adjustment to guarantee V_T	Decelerating variable pattern of gas flow combined desirable characteristics of pressure-controlled (synchrony, gas mixing) and volume-controlled (guaranteed V_T) breaths during full ventilator support	No pressure limit is set.
Volume support	Pressure-targeted flow-cycled breaths with automatic pressure adjustment to guarantee V_T	Decelerating variable pattern of gas flow combined desirable characteristics of pressure-controlled (synchrony, gas mixing) and volume-controlled (guaranteed V_T) breaths during weaning	Because V_T is the main controller, inappropriate setting of V_T may lead to inappropriate changes in pressure as patients recover.
Volume-assured pressure support	Pressure-targeted flow-cycled breaths with backup set flow to guarantee V_T	Decelerating variable pattern of gas flow combined desirable characteristics of pressure-controlled (synchrony, gas mixing) and volume-controlled (guaranteed V_T) breaths	No pressure limit is set. Inappropriate high setting of V_T may lead to inappropriately high pressure as patients recover.
Adaptive support ventilation	V_T-frequency combination set automatically based on proportion of V_E to be provided by ventilator	Automatic settings have ability to adjust to patient mechanics and effort	Untested in sick patients.

Adapted from Macintyre NR: Basic principles and new modes of mechanical ventilation. In Murray MJ, Coursin DB, Pearl RG, Prough DS, editors: *Critical care medicine: perioperative management.* Baltimore, Lippincott Williams & Wilkins, 2002, pp. 445–459.

Table 2: Comparison of Common Modes of Ventilation

Mode	Trigger	Limit	Cycle-Off	Spontaneous Breathing	Gas Flow
AC (volume)	T or P	V	T	N	C
AC (pressure)	T or P	Pr	T	N	D
SIMV	T or P	V	T	Y	C
PSV	P	Pr	Gas flow	N[a]	D
APRV	T	P	T	Y	D

[a]Can be used as a standalone modality for patients breathing spontaneously, but not in patients with alveolar hypoventilation or periods of apnea because there is no backup rate of mechanical ventilation.

AC, Assist-control ventilation; *APRV*, airway pressure release ventilation; *C*, constant; *D*, decelerating; *N*, no; *P*, patient; *Pr*, pressure; *PSV*, pressure support ventilation; *SIMV*, synchronized intermittent mandatory ventilation; *T*, time; *V*, volume; *Y*, yes.

pressure from an elevated baseline simulates exhalation. Technically, APRV is time-triggered, pressure-limited, time-cycled mechanical ventilation. Conceptualizing APRV as continuous positive airway pressure (CPAP) with regular, brief, intermittent releases of airway pressure may facilitate understanding. It can augment alveolar ventilation in the patient breathing spontaneously, or provide full support to the apneic patient.

Advantages of APRV include lower peak airway pressure, lower intrathoracic pressure, lower V_E, minimal effect on cardiac output, and improved matching of ventilation and perfusion. The mode may facilitate spontaneous breathing by the patient. Sedation requirements may be decreased, and neuromuscular blockade should be avoided altogether. Patient-ventilator dyssynchrony is believed not to develop. Disadvantages of APRV include pressure control of ventilation, increased effects of airway and circuit resistance on ventilation, decreased transpulmonary pressure, and potential interference with spontaneous ventilation. Facilitated exhalation may make APRV beneficial in patients with bronchospasm or small-airways disease. This mode of ventilation can be used as a weaning mode. Although increasingly popular, the advantage of APRV over other modes of ventilation is unproved.

The terminology of APRV differs somewhat from other modes of mechanical ventilation, and has yet to be standardized. Four important terms include pressure high (P_{high}), pressure low (P_{low}), time high (T_{high}), and time low (T_{low}). The P_{high} term describes the baseline airway pressure (the higher of the two pressures), alternatively called CPAP, inflating pressure, or the P1 pressure. The P_{low} term describes the airway pressure resulting from the release of pressure (alternatively called PEEP, release pressure, or the P2 pressure). The T_{high} time refers to the time during which P_{high} is maintained (T1), whereas T_{low} refers to the duration of time when airway pressure is released (T2). Mean airway pressure can be calculated from the following equation:

$$[(P1 \times T1) + (P2 \times T2)] / (T2 + T1)$$

Application of APRV to the patient must be individualized, as standard approaches have yet to emerge. Initial settings are deduced partly from the result of conventional mechanical ventilation, which should be attempted initially for most patients. The plateau airway pressure (P_{plat}) from conventional ventilation (if not higher than 35 cm H_2O) is converted to P_{high}, aiming for a V_E of 2–3 l/min (lower than with conventional ventilation). The P_{low} pressure is set initially at 0 cm H_2O. The setting for T_{high} is a minimum of 4 seconds, and T_{low} is set at approximately 0.8 seconds (0.5–1.0 second). Spontaneous breating is permitted. At these settings, mean airway pressure is 29 cm H_2O. Rarely, a higher P_{high} (40–45 cm H_2O) is needed for patients with low compliance (e.g., morbid obesity, abdominal distention). For all patients, T_{high} is lengthened progressively to 12–15 seconds (usually in 1- to 2-second increments as lung

mechanics improve). Longer T_{high} prevents the cyclical opening and closing of small airways that is believed to be a cause of VILI. The T_{low} parameter is optimized when expiratory flow decreases to 25%–50% of peak expiratory flow.

Clinical improvement may not be immediate after transition to APRV (as is the case with IRV). Clinical studies have shown that maximum clinical improvement may not occur until 8–16 hours after the transition. After improvement, weaning from APRV is guided by general principles of weaning. Weaning from APRV is accomplished primarily by manipulation of P_{high} and T_{high}. High pressure is decreased in increments of 2–3 cm H_2O down to about 15 cm H_2O, and T_{high} is lengthened progressively to 12–15 seconds (usually in 1- to 2-second increments). Minute ventilation must be monitored carefully for signs of hypoventilation during the transition. The goal is to switch the patient to pure CPAP of 6–12 cm H_2O, at which point the patient may be extubated—all conditions permitting.

Some confusion arises with similar modes of ventilation. BiPAP differs from APRV only in the timing of T_{high} and T_{low}. The latter is longer in BiPAP. Intermittent mandatory pressure release ventilation (IMPRV)—similar to APRV and rarely used—synchronizes the release of pressure with the patient's spontaneous effort. In IMPRV, all spontaneous breaths are pressure-supported ventilation (PSV) to reduce the work of breathing. However, the rationale for IMPRV is considered dubious by some because dyssynchrony appears not to occur with APRV.

High-Frequency Ventilation

High-frequency ventilation (HFV) is a ventilatory strategy that has been used with success for respiratory failure in neonates and children. This modality utilizes limited high mean airway pressures at low V_T (often smaller than anatomic dead space) and a high-frequency respiratory rate (2.5–30 Hz) to achieve adequate ventilation while at the same time preventing alveolar overdistension. This mode is conceptually attractive because it achieves many of the goals of lung-protective ventilation. Used most often to support complex thoracic surgical procedures (e.g., one-lung or split-lung ventilation) or to facilitate fiberoptic bronchoscopy or healing of bronchopleural fistula, HFV has been shown to be safe and effective for ventilation of small numbers of adult patients with severe ARDS who have failed conventional ventilation. However, large-scale trials are needed.

Permissive Hypercapnia

Permissive hypercapnia is an adjunctive protective ventilatory strategy. Permissive hypercapnia defines a ventilatory strategy for acute respiratory failure in which the lungs are ventilated with a low V_T, permitting $PaCO_2$ levels to increase. Permissive hypercapnia aims to avoid hyperinflation-induced lung trauma, as described initially by limiting the plateau airway pressure (as a surrogate of static alveolar pressure) to approximately 30–35 cm H_2O while allowing $PaCO_2$ to increase absent any contraindications (such as increased intracranial pressure).

Hickling et al. introduced the concept of permissive hypercapnia, reporting that reducing the peak inspiratory airway pressure to a maximum of 20–30 cm H_2O while allowing $PaCO_2$ to increase resulted in a decreased mortality rate of 16% for 50 consecutive patients with ARDS. Amato et al. reported similar results in the first controlled study on the use of permissive hypercapnia in patients with ARDS. If the ARDSnet low V_T protocol is adhered to as a ventilatory strategy, permissive hypercapnia may provide further improvement in outcomes in patients with ALI. In addition, experimental evidence suggests that VILI may cause release of inflammatory mediators—increasing the likelihood of multiple-organ dysfunction syndrome.

Permissive hypercapnia has not been widely implemented to near its physiologic limits (e.g., $PaCO_2$ up to 80 mm Hg, arterial pH down to 7.20) because of a relative paucity of controlled studies showing clear benefit from the application of this strategy in ARDS, and because of concerns over physiologic consequences of the associated hypercapnia on the central nervous, cardiovascular, and renal systems. The absolute level of $PaCO_2$ and the permissible degree of acidosis is debated, as is the concern of alveolar derecruitment and possible worsening of ventilation-perfusion mismatching. The $PaCO_2$ is directly proportional to the rate of CO_2 production by oxidative metabolism (VCO_2) and inversely proportional to the rate of CO_2 elimination by alveolar ventilation (V_A). An equation that illustrates the relationship between each source is $PaCO_2 = k\,(VCO_2/V_A)$. The three major sources of hypercapnia include increased CO_2 production, hypoventilation, and increased dead space ventilation. Metabolic CO_2 production is an essential factor in promoting hypercapnia only in patients with underlying lung disease.

Contraindications and adverse effects of permissive hypercapnia include cerebral edema or high intracranial pressure, convulsions, depressed cardiac function, arrhythmias, increased pulmonary vascular resistance, tachypnea, increased work of breathing, dyspnea, respiratory distress, headache, sweating, and biochemical disturbances related to acidosis.

PHARMACOTHERAPY

Liquid Ventilation

Use of fluids to facilitate gas exchange has been under scrutiny for many years. Due to the fact that mechanical ventilation with gas may cause barotrauma, exacerbate ALI (causing structural damage to the lungs), and induce the release of inflammatory mediators, alternative means of supporting pulmonary gas exchange while preserving lung structure and function are desirable. Much research has focused on the use of perfluorocarbon (PFC) liquids to deliver biologic agents to diseased lungs, generally by one of two modalities. The first is total liquid ventilation, in which the lungs are filled with PFC to a volume equivalent to functional residual capacity (FRC), then ventilating the PFC-filled lung with oxygen. Total liquid ventilation has been largely abandoned owing to its logistical complexity.

The second technique of liquid ventilation (partial liquid ventilation, PLV) involves intratracheal administration of PFC in a volume equivalent to FRC, followed by standard gas mechanical ventilation of the PFC-filled lung. In infants with biochemically immature lungs, liquid ventilation may minimize the effect of barotrauma. There is evidence that liquid ventilation may eliminate surface-active forces, providing effective gas exchange with minimal risk for barotrauma. Airway toilet may be improved as debris floats upward to the menis-

cus, where it can be removed. Notably, the debris can be so voluminous as to cause airway obstruction. Thus, pulmonary toilet must be diligent. However, PFC is volatile and requires frequent "topping off" to maintain sufficient volume. Moreover, PFC is radioopaque and creates a bilateral "white-out" on chest x-ray that makes radiographic interpretation impossible.

Perfluorocarbon liquids may have anti-inflammatory properties in the alveolar space. The anti-inflammatory effects of liquid ventilation in ALI are from inhibition of neutrophil and macrophage function, and the dilution of inflammatory debris in the airways. PFC liquids are currently used clinically in a number of ways, such as intravascular PFC emulsions for volume expansion, improving oxygen-carrying capacity, angiography, and intracavitary PFC liquid for image contrast enhancement and vitreous fluid replacement. However, no agent for liquid ventilation in the United States has been approved for clinical use. Several factors complicated the phase 2 and 3 clinical studies of PLV. In a prospective, randomized, controlled pilot study of 90 adults with ALI/ARDS, with $PaO_2:F_IO_2$ greater than 60 but less than 300, PLV did not affect ventilator-free days (the primary endpoint), mortality, or any other clinical factors. Criticisms of this study included slow recruitment (entry criteria were relaxed after 45 patients), lack of a weaning protocol, and a disproportionate number of patients over age 55 in the PLV group. However, a post hoc analysis found significantly more rapid discontinuation of mechanical ventilation and a trend toward more ventilator-free days in the PLV group among younger patients. The authors suggested further evaluation, particularly in certain well-defined (especially younger) patients.

In a second trial, the hypothesis was tested that PLV would increase the number of ventilator-free days compared to conventional mechanical ventilation—and would decrease 28-day all-cause mortality compared to conventional ventilation. Adult patients with ALI who had been on mechanical ventilation for less than 120 hours (with a $PaO_2:F_IO_2$ below 200, F_IO_2 above 0.5, and PEEP above 5 cm H_2O) were enrolled. There was no improvement in 28-day all-cause mortality. The mean number of ventilator-free days was reduced significantly. The aggregate results have caused a substantial loss of enthusiasm for the clinical use of PLV.

Surfactant Administration

Acute lung injury is characterized by pulmonary and endothelial inflammation, which causes pulmonary edema, destruction and impaired synthesis of surfactant with atelectasis and reduced pulmonary compliance, hypoxemia from ventilation/perfusion mismatching, and subsequent pulmonary hypertension and fibrosis. Studies have examined the intratracheal administration of surfactant as a means of improving both oxygenation and ventilation. Although surfactant is indisputably effective for neonatal respiratory distress syndrome, clinical trials of adult patients have failed to demonstrate a benefit for any of several variations of natural or synthetic surfactant or components thereof.

Inhaled Nitric Oxide

Inhaled nitric oxide (NO) is a selective pulmonary vasodilator that acts on the alveolar endothelium to produce regional vasodilation in well-ventilated lung units where it is distributed. NO at a dose of 40 parts per million (PPM) has been demonstrated to improve ventilation-perfusion mismatching, hypoxemia, and pulmonary hypertension in patients who have ALI/ARDS. In contrast, systemic vasodilators may actually cause pulmonary vasodilation in nonventilated lung, thereby abrogating hypoxic vasoconstriction and leading to hypoxemia and exacerbated ventilation-perfusion inequality. NO is also a bronchodilator and has anti-inflammatory properties that have been helpful in lung transplant patients. When inhaled, it diffuses into the blood stream—where it is metabolized rapidly and excreted via the urine, minimizing systemic effects. Three randomized controlled trials suggest that NO may improve oxygenation for up to 72 hours, but neither survival nor a shorter duration of mechanical ventilation was observed. In addition, rebound pulmonary hypertension has been reported with cessation of therapy. Therefore, inhaled NO is not recommended for therapy of ALI/ARDS even as rescue therapy.

UNCONVENTIONAL METHODS OF PULMONARY SUPPORT

Independent Lung Ventilation

Acute lung injury is recognized to be heterogeneous with the lung, but also may be heterogeneous between lungs (e.g., massive aspiration of gastric content confined to one lung). The left lung is smaller than the right in human beings. Moreover, when lung injury is asymmetric, differences in compliance exist between the lungs. Consequently, conventional mechanical ventilation delivers a larger V_T to the more compliant lung—which may cause overdistension and VILI. In addition, overdistension disrupts blood flow through alveolar vessels—diverting flow to the underventilated lung and worsening ventilation-perfusion mismatch. Independent lung ventilation (ILV) has been described to ventilate the more diseased lung while avoiding overdistension of the more normal lung.

Using a dual-lumen endotracheal tube with a bifurcated tip such that each main-stem bronchus can be intubated separately, gas can be delivered using two ventilators dedicated one to each lung. Typically, the V_T is set equal for both lungs. However, this may be an irrational approach both anatomically and physiologically because higher airway pressure may be anticipated in the more injured lung. Alternatively, ventilator settings may be adjusted to produce equal P_{plat} in both lungs. The ventilators may be managed independently, and the lungs may be monitored independently by pressure measurements, compliance calculations, and capnography.

Independent lung ventilation is seldom used anymore. Modern mechanical ventilators and lung-protective ventilation strategies have obviated many of the difficulties that made ILV attractive when described initially in the 1970s and early 1980s. The dual-lumen endotracheal tube is challenging to position and keep positioned. Patients require heavy sedation and often neuromuscular blockade. Combinations of ILV with newer modes of ventilation have not been described.

Extracorporeal Membrane Oxygenation

Extracorporeal membrane oxygenation (ECMO) provides oxygenation of blood and removal of CO_2 via an extracorporeal circuit. ECMO consists of the application of intermediate-term cardiopulmonary bypass for the treatment of potentially reversible cardiac or pulmonary failure for patients of any age. If successful, sufficient gas exchange permits reduced support of positive-pressure ventilation—thereby lowering the incidence of barotrauma-induced lung injury associated with mechanical ventilation. ECMO thus provides relative "lung rest" to the acutely injured lungs and facilitates recovery.

Conventional mechanical ventilation is the mainstay of treatment for severe respiratory failure associated with trauma. However, when extensive lung injury is present, conventional ventilation may not be sufficient to prevent hypoxia and may exacerbate pulmonary damage by barotrauma. The logic of ECMO for severe pulmonary failure is that borderline patients may be saved if their lungs are allowed to rest and heal rather than endure the morbidity of the high-level ventilator support necessary to achieve adequate gas exchange. ECMO has

been used successfully to manage critically ill adult trauma patients and offers an additional treatment modality. However, ECMO is not available in all centers.

The first adult managed successfully with prolonged ECMO was a trauma patient cared for by Hill et al., reported in 1972. Subsequently, a National Institutes of Health (NIH)-sponsored randomized multi-institutional trial (reported in 1979) failed to demonstrate improved survival in adults managed with ECMO. In contrast, Cordell-Smith et al. found that a high proportion of trauma patients treated with ECMO for severe lung injury survived. This outcome appears to compare favorably with conventional ventilation techniques and may have a role in patients who develop acute severe respiratory failure associated with trauma. ECMO may be considered for support of severe ARDS affecting adult patients when all other treatment options have failed. Injury of the thoracic aorta, even if contained, is considered a contraindication to ECMO use. The paradox is that ECMO appears to achieve the best outcomes when utilized relatively early. The mortality from respiratory failure increases the longer a patient is mechanically ventilated before initiation of ECMO.

Over the years, ECMO therapy has undergone substantial changes in indications, technique, and materials. Technical progress has been made in the pumps, oxygenators, and coating of artificial surfaces, leading to greater biocompatibility and a lower rate of procedure-related complications. The potential of new inline pumps in combination with a decreasing incidence of procedure-related complications may lead to a reevaluation of the role of ECMO in the therapy of ARDS. New techniques for insertion of intravascular oxygenators (IVOX) and extracorporeal CO_2 removal (ECCO$_2$R) devices highlight some of the technical advances being made. Unfortunately, the technical advancements have yet to translate to improved survival in clinical trials.

In a prospective controlled trial using ECMO in patients with ARDS and severe ALI, Zapol et al. showed that refractory hypoxia tempered enthusiasm for ECMO use by demonstrating no survival benefit. However, the control group and treatment group both had very high mortality rates (control 91% vs. ECMO 90%, vs. ~30% in the ARDSnet trial), and the study did not use a lung protection ventilation strategy. The only randomized, prospective, controlled study utilizing ECCO$_2$R similarly did not demonstrate any survival benefit from ECCO$_2$R use. The IVOX device attempts to accomplish the same objectives as ECMO through placement of a membrane within a major vein such as the vena cava. Its intended patient population is intensive care unit (ICU) patients with severe potentially reversible acute respiratory failure. Initially examined in its current form in 1982, the main function of IVOX is to provide transport for oxygen and CO_2 across its microporous hollow capillaries. Phase I and phase II IVOX clinical trial observations note that IVOX managed limited but statistically significant amounts of oxygen and CO_2. Further trials are pending.

Prone Positioning

Prone positioning (PP)—in which the patient is positioned prone, most commonly using a specialty bed—improves oxygenation by decreasing ventilation-perfusion mismatching. Ventilated lung segments tend to be in nondependent portions of lung, whereas perfused lung segments (and higher pulmonary vascular pressures and hence lung edema) tend to be in dependent portions of lung. Positive-pressure ventilation exacerbates the mismatching. PP reverses the dependency of the lung, and newly dependent well-ventilated lung segments are well perfused for several hours until the effects of gravity and positive airway pressures restore the previous conditions over a period of several hours. Drainage of secretions may also be facilitated in the prone position. The large multicenter randomized controlled trial by Gattinoni et al. showed significant improvement in PaO$_2$:F$_I$O$_2$ and in 10-day mortality, but this modest advantage did not persist beyond ICU discharge. Complications with PP include pressure sores, need for increased sedation, facial edema, and difficulty maintaining airway patency or restoring it when the patient is inverted. Recently, facilitated PP using a specialized bed has shown promise. Thus, this intervention may yet prove useful for management of severely hypoxic patients with ARDS.

THE FUTURE

Mechanical ventilation is crucial for oxygenation and ventilation of the critically ill patient. The use of low V_T ventilation and a mode that minimizes barotrauma is already being incorporated into practice. Microprocessor technology has increased the sophistication of mechanical ventilators, thus leading to new modes of ventilation. New modes often refine old techniques by adding devices or combining different modes. The role of these new modes in relation to conventional mechanical ventilation, and the optimal combination of the various modes and adjuncts, remains to be tested for benefit in these complex patients.

SUGGESTED READINGS

Betensley AD, Kakkar R: Noninvasive positive pressure ventilation. *Hosp Physician* 8:3–12, 2005.

Branson RD, Johannigman JA, Campbell RS: Closed-loop mechanical ventilation. *Respir Care* 47:427–451, 2002.

Burns KE, Sinuff T, Adhikari NK. et al: Bilevel non-invasive positive pressure ventilation for acute respiratory failure: survey of Ontario practice. *Crit Care Med* 33:1477–1483, 2005.

Carlucci A, Richard J, Wysocki M, et al: Noninvasive versus conventional mechanical ventilation. An epidemiological survey. *Am J Respir Crit Care Med* 163:874–880, 2001.

Cheung TM, Yam LY, So LK, et al: Effectiveness of noninvasive positive pressure ventilation in the treatment of acute respiratory failure in severe acute respiratory syndrome. *Chest* 126:845–850, 2004.

Cinnella G, Dambrosio M, Brienza N, et al: Compliance and capnography monitoring during independent lung ventilation: report of two cases. *Anesthesiology* 93:275–278, 2000.

Dellinger RP: Inhaled nitric oxide in acute lung injury and acute respiratory distress syndrome. *Intensive Care Med* 25:881–883, 1999.

Fan E, Mehta S: High-frequency oscillatory ventilation and adjunctive therapies: inhaled nitric oxide and prone positioning. *Crit Care Med* 33(Suppl 3): S182–S187, 2005.

Frawley PM, Habashi NM: Airway pressure release ventilation: theory and practice. *AACN Clin Issues* 12:234–246, 2001.

Gattinoni L, Tognoni G, Presenti A, et al: Effect of prone positioning on the survival of patients with acute respiratory failure. *N Engl J Med* 345:568–573, 2001.

Grasso S, Ranieri MV: Proportional assist ventilation. *Semin Respir Crit Care Med* 21:161–166, 2000.

Hemmila MR, Rowe SA, Boules TN: Extracorporeal life support for severe acute respiratory distress syndrome in adults. *Ann Surg* 240:595–607, 2004.

Imai Y, Parodo J, Kajakawa O, et al: Injurious mechanical ventilation and end-organ epithelial cell apoptosis and organ dysfunction in an experimental model of acute respiratory distress syndrome. *JAMA* 289:2104–2112, 2003.

Kacmarek RM, Slutsky AS, editors: *Mechanical Ventilation: Current Trends and Future Directions.* Des Plaines, IL, Society of Critical Care Medicine, 2005.

MacIntyre NR: Basic principles and new modes of mechanical ventilation. In Murray MJ, Coursin DB, Pearl RG, Prough DS, editors: *Critical Care Medicine. Perioperative Management.* Baltimore, Lippincott Williams & Wilkins, 2002, pp. 445–459.

MacIntyre NR, Ho L: Effects of initial flow rate and breath termination criteria on pressure support ventilation. *Chest* 99:134–138, 1991.

Matthay MA, editor: *Acute Respiratory Distress Syndrome.* New York, Marcel Dekker, 2003.

Needham DM, Bronskill SE, Calinawan JR, et al: Projected incidence of mechanical ventilation in Ontario to 2026: preparing for the aging baby boomers. *Crit Care Med* 33:574–579, 2005.

Sevransky JE, Levy MM, Marini JJ: Mechanical ventilation in sepsis-induced acute lung injury/acute respiratory distress syndrome: an evidence-based review. *Crit Care Med* 32(Suppl):S548–S553, 2004.

Siegel JH, Stoklosa JC, Borg U, et al: Quantification of asymmetric lung pathophysiology as a guide to the use of simultaneous independent lung ventilation in post-traumatic and septic ARDS. *Ann Surg* 202:425–439, 1985.

Sydow M, Burchardi H, Ephraim E, et al: Long-term effects of two different ventilatory modes on oxygenation in acute lung injury: comparison of airway pressure release ventilation and volume-controlled inverse ratio ventilation. *Am J Respir Crit Care Med* 149:1550–1556, 1994.

The Acute Respiratory Distress Network Investigators: Ventilation with lower tidal volumes as compared with traditional tidal volumes for acute lung injury and the acute respiratory distress syndrome. *N Engl J Med* 342: 1301–1308, 2000.

Tobin MJ, editors: *Principles and Practice of Mechanical Ventilation.* New York, McGraw-Hill, 1994.

Uhlig S, Ranieri M, Slutsky AS: Biotrauma hypothesis of ventilator-associated lung injury. *Am J Respir Crit Care Med* 169:314–315, 2004.

Varelmann D, Wrigge H, Zinserling J, et al: Proportional assist versus pressure support ventilation in patients with acute respiratory failure: cardiorespiratory responses to artificially increased ventilatory demand. *Crit Care Med* 33:1968–1975, 2005.

THE MANAGEMENT OF RENAL FAILURE: RENAL REPLACEMENT THERAPY AND DIALYSIS

Joseph M. Gutmann,   Christopher McFarren,
Lewis M. Flint,   and   Rodney Durham

Acute renal failure (ARF) is a common and devastating problem that contributes to morbidity and mortality in critically ill patients. ARF prolongs hospital stays and increases mortality. Although effective renal replacement therapy (RRT) is available, it is not ideal and the best therapy is prevention.

The kidneys are the primary regulators of volume and composition of the internal fluid environment and their excretion. Renal failure leads to regulatory function impairment, causing retention of nitrogenous waste products and disturbance in fluid, electrolyte, and acid-base balance. Renal injury in intensive care unit (ICU) patients is a progressive process, usually starting with a prerenal insult—which progresses to severe renal injury. Other systemic issues can worsen the renal injury.

Acute renal failure in critically ill patients is a growing clinical problem. Options for RRT in these patients use convective and diffusive clearance, which may be intermittent (as in classic hemodialysis) or continuous. RRT needs to be tailored to the needs of each patient. Current and future research studies are essential in improving outcomes.

INCIDENCE

Acute renal failure is defined as an abrupt and sustained decline in the glomerular filtration rate (GFR),[1] which leads to accumulation of nitrogenous waste products and uremic toxins. In critically ill patients, more than 90% of the episodes of ARF are due to acute tubular necrosis (ATN) and are the result of ischemic or nephrotoxic etiology (or a combination of both). ARF affects nearly 5% of all hospitalized patients and as many as 15% of critically ill patients.[2] Like many other medical conditions, there is no gold standard of diagnosis, no specific histopathologic confirmation, and no uniform clinical picture.

The mortality rate of an isolated episode of ARF is approximately 10% to 15%. When it occurs in association with multiple-organ dysfunction, as in the ICU setting, mortality rates are much greater and vary in published series between 40% and 90%.[3]

In some cases, preexisting conditions may worsen. New major complications, such as sepsis and respiratory failure, may also develop after the onset of renal failure. Although ARF that requires RRT carries a high mortality,[4] there is emerging evidence to suggest that milder forms of ARF that do not require supportive therapy with RRT have better patient outcomes.[5]

Many aspects of surgical diseases and their care have the potential to impair renal function, either by toxic effects on the renal parenchyma or by reducing renal perfusion (or a combination of the two). The prevention of ARF in critical patients consists of minimizing toxicity and ensuring adequate blood flow. Avoidance of renal failure is preferred to any treatment. Therefore, renal function should be monitored closely so that adverse circumstances can be limited.

Given the impact of ARF on mortality, it is important to prevent or hasten the resolution of even the mildest forms of ARF. The goals of a preventive strategy for the syndrome of ARF are to preserve renal function, to prevent death, to prevent complications of ARF (volume overload, acid–base disturbances, and electrolyte abnormalities), and to prevent the need for chronic dialysis (with minimum adverse effects).

This chapter explores preventive strategies, the major challenges ARF presents, and key issues to be considered. Can the patient be managed conservatively or will RRT be needed? If RRT is required, which form of RRT is most appropriate?

MECHANISM OF INJURY/ETIOLOGY

Diagnosis

Renal failure is measured routinely and easily in the ICU: the excretion of water-soluble waste products of nitrogen metabolism, urea and creatinine, and the production of urine. To understand renal failure, we need to reflect on some important aspects of renal physiology.

Water and Fluid Homeostasis

Because body water is the primary determinant of the osmolality of the extracellular fluid (ECF), disorders of body water homeostasis can be divided into hypo- and hyperosmolar disorders depending on whether there is an excess or deficiency of body water relative to body solute. The end result of any change in circulating blood volume is a change in sodium excretion by the kidneys. This is brought about by the activation of the sympathetic nervous system, the renin-angiotensin-aldosterone axis, and release/suppression of natriuretic peptides.

Assessment of Renal Function

Serum concentrations of blood urea nitrogen (BUN) and creatinine are the most commonly used markers of renal function. Urea is the end product of protein and amino acid catabolism. Under normal conditions, 80%–90% of total nitrogen excretion is by the kidneys. Creatinine is formed in muscle by the nonenzymatic degradation of creatine and phosphocreatine, and is excreted primarily by glomerular filtration. A small percentage of creatinine is actively secreted into the glomerular filtrate and tubular reabsorption of creatinine is negligible.[5]

Circulating concentrations of BUN and creatinine are determined not only by how efficiently they are excreted by the kidneys but by their rate of production. Urea formation depends on the amount of protein and amino acids catabolized. It is increased with high-protein diets, reabsorption of hematomas, and digestion of blood in the gastrointestinal (GI) tract. It is reduced in starvation. These factors may change the value of the BUN, even though renal function is adequate. Creatinine production reflects muscle mass. It is constant over the short term, and steadily diminishes if muscle mass is lost. Muscle mass diminishes with age, together with intrinsic renal function. Therefore, serum creatinine stays relatively constant over time.

Creatinine Clearance

Determination of the creatinine clearance (Ccr) provides a measure of renal function. Creatinine secretion and reabsorption in the kidneys is negligible. Clearance is defined as the volume of plasma or serum cleared by the kidneys over a period of time. It is calculated as

$$Ccr \ (ml/min) = (Ucr \times V) \ / \ Pcr$$

where Ucr is urine creatinine, Pcr is serum creatine, and V is volume.

The clearance reflects the net effect of GFR, which is the amount of fluid filtered from the plasma in a given time by the kidneys. The most commonly used method for estimating Ccr is the Cockcroft-Gault formula:

$$Ccr_{men} = GFR \ (ml/min) = (140 - age) \times [ideal \ body \ weight \ (kg) \ / \ 72 \times serum \ creatinine \ (mg/dl)].$$

$$Ccr_{women} = Ccr_{men} \times 0.85.$$

Normal GFR is 125 ± 15 ml/min/1.73 m^2 body surface area (BSA).

Sodium has the highest serum concentration of all cations in the ECF. Any transport of sodium necessarily involves the transport of water. Renal sodium clearance is an important mechanism for the regulation of ECF volume and tonicity. Aldosterone promotes tubular reabsorption of sodium, and it is elaborated in response to changes in hydrostatic pressure within the glomerular arterioles. If renal blood flow or pressure is reduced, tubular sodium reabsorption is increased—thus preserving ECF volume. The ratio of sodium clearance to Ccr is known as the fractional excretion of sodium (FENa):

$$FENa = [(Una \times Pcr) \ / \ (Ucr \times Pna)] \times 100.$$

Here, Una and Ucr are the urinary concentrations of sodium and creatinine, and Pna and Pcr are the serum levels of sodium and creatinine, respectively. If the FENa is very low ($<1\%$), it may indicate inadequate renal arteriolar pressure—suggesting that factors other than intrinsic renal dysfunction are responsible for clinically inadequate renal function.[6]

Urine Production and Output

The end result of renal function is the production of urine. Quantitative measurements of urine are important for assessing renal function. Urine output is highly sensitive to renal blood flow, making it a key indicator of renal function and total body vascular perfusion[7] (Table 1).

MANAGEMENT OF PATIENTS

Conservative Management

Despite many advances in medical technology, the mortality and morbidity attributed to ARF in the ICU remains high. Primary strategies to prevent ARF still include adequate hydration, maintenance of mean arterial pressure (preferably MAP >60), and minimization

Table 1: Adequate Urine Output

Age	Urine Output (ml/kg/min)
Infant (<10 kg)	2.0
Toddler (10–20 kg)	1.5
Child (20–50 kg)	1.0
Adult (>50 kg)	0.5

of exposure to potentially nephrotoxic agents. Although hydration was shown to be beneficial, the type of fluid to be used in a hydration regime remains controversial.

Considering its low cost, low toxicity, and consistent benefit, NAC (N-acetylcysteine) administration with IV hydration should be considered to decrease the prevalence of nephropathy in high-risk patients. Note that the routine use of NAC is controversial and is not well studied.

Nonpharmacologic Strategies for Acute Renal Failure Prevention

Nonpharmacologic strategies to prevent ARF include ensuring adequate hydration (limiting dehydration), maintenance of adequate mean arterial pressures, and minimizing exposure to nephrotoxic agents. Four particular strategies are worth reviewing: fluids, aminoglycoside dosing, lipid-soluble preparations of amphotericin, and nonionic contrast agents.

Fluids

Adequate hydration is the cornerstone of renal failure prevention. One randomized controlled trial ($n = 1620$) compared hydration using 0.9% saline infusion with 0.45% saline in dextrose for prevention of radiocontrast-induced nephropathy in patients who underwent coronary angiography.[8] Hydration with 0.9% saline infusion significantly reduced contrast nephropathy compared with 0.45% saline in dextrose hydration (0.7% vs. 2%, respectively; $p = 0.04$). This effect was greater in women, diabetics, and patients who received a large volume (>250 ml) of a contrast agent. A recent single-center randomized controlled trial compared the efficacy of sodium bicarbonate with 0.9% saline hydration in preventing contrast nephropathy.[9] In this study, 119 patients who had stable serum creatinine of at least 1.1 mg/dl were randomized to 154 mEq/l infusion of sodium chloride ($n = 59$) or sodium bicarbonate ($n = 60$) before and after contrast (iopamidol) administration. One of 59 patients (1.7%) in the group that received bicarbonate developed contrast nephropathy (defined as an increase of ≥25% in serum creatinine from baseline within 48 hours) compared with 8 of 60 patients (13.3%) in the group that received saline ($p = 0.02$).

Nephrotoxin Exposure

Minimizing exposure to potentially nephrotoxic agents is an important strategy to prevent ARF in the ICU setting. Aminoglycosides, other antibiotics, amphotericin, and radiocontrast are the nephrotoxins encountered most commonly in the ICU. A systematic review in patients who had neutropenic fever and received aminoglycosides, however, found no significant differences in efficacy or nephrotoxicity between once daily and three times daily dosing.[10]

The use of lipid formulations of amphotericin B seems to cause less nephrotoxicity compared with standard formulations, but direct comparisons of long-term safety are lacking. With regard to contrast media, one systematic review (31 randomized controlled trials, 5146 patients) compared low osmolality contrast media with standard contrast media.[11] The study showed that low osmolality contrast media did not influence the development of ARF or the need for dialysis.

Pharmacologic Strategies for Acute Renal Failure Prevention

Loop Diuretics

Multiple small clinical trials studied the efficacy of loop diuretics in preventing ARF and have provided conflicting results. They have been underpowered, nonrandomized, or methodologically flawed.

One systematic review that compared fluids with diuretics in people who were at risk for ARF from various causes did not show any benefit from diuretics with regard to prevalence of ARF, need for dialysis, or mortality.[12]

N-Acetylcysteine

Systematic reviews found that NAC plus hydration reduced the incidence of contrast nephropathy more than hydration alone in people who had baseline renal impairment and underwent radiocontrast studies.[13] A recent study, however, suggested that NAC could decrease serum creatinine independently without any effect on GFR (as evaluated by other surrogate outcomes, such as serum cystatin C levels).[14] Hence, the current implications of reduction in serum creatinine after contrast administration with the use of NAC remain unclear and need to be explored further.

INDICATIONS FOR RENAL REPLACEMENT THERAPY IN ACUTE RENAL FAILURE

As in chronic kidney disease, overt disturbances of ECF volume and body fluid composition remain the objective indications for initiation of RRT in patients with ARF (Table 2). These include volume overload, hyperkalemia, severe metabolic acidosis, uremia, and azotemia.

Volume Overload

Volume overload is generally recognized as an indication for RRT in ARF. All modalities of RRT are effective at diminishing intravascular volume. Subjective criteria for initiation of therapy include impairment of cardiopulmonary function by pulmonary vascular congestion or compromise of cutaneous integrity and wound healing by peripheral edema.

Mehta and colleagues[15] performed a retrospective analysis of data from 522 critically ill patients who had ARF. Fifty-nine percent of these patients had been treated with diuretics. After adjustment for relevant covariates and the propensity for diuretic use, they observed a significant increase in the risk of death or nonrecovery of renal function (odds ratio 1.77, 95% confidence interval 1.14–2.76). On the basis of this, they concluded that diuretic therapy was potentially deleterious in patients who had ARF. They noted, however, that the increased risk was borne largely by patients who were unresponsive to diuretics. This suggested that this increased risk might reflect selection for a more severe degree of renal injury.

Hyperkalemia

The treatment of hyperkalemia with evidence of myocardial toxicity was one of the early indications for hemodialysis in ARF. Hyperkalemia is a well-recognized complication of ARF, which, if not treated, may be rapidly fatal. Most medical therapies for hyperkalemia (e.g., intravenous calcium to directly antagonize the effects of hyperkalemia on the myocardial cell membrane, and intravenous insulin/

Table 2: Indications for Renal Replacement Therapy

Volume overload
Hyperkalemia
Metabolic acidosis
Uremia
Azotemia

dextrose and intravenous or inhaled β-adrenergic agonists to shift potassium into the intracellular compartment) are primarily temporizing measures. Three modalities are available to decrease the total body potassium burden: diuretic therapy, enteric potassium-binding resins, and dialysis.

In patients who have severe renal failure, diuretic therapy is generally ineffective in promoting kaliuresis due to lack of diuretic response. Although sodium polystyrene sulfonate can enhance fecal potassium losses, its use is limited in patients with recent intraabdominal or GI surgery, ileus, or bowel ischemia. Dialysis provides the most rapid means of decreasing the serum potassium concentration. However, because of variability in study design and evolution of dialysis techniques it is difficult to determine the expected potassium removal during a single dialysis treatment.[16]

Even greater clearances of potassium may be achieved by using more permeable synthetic hemodialysis membranes and greater blood flow rates. However, the rate of potassium removal is ultimately limited by the rapid decrease in the concentration gradient between plasma and dialysate.[17] As with volume status, a specific threshold level of serum potassium cannot be established as an indication for initiation of RRT. Myocardial toxicity from hyperkalemia is uncommon when the serum potassium concentration is less than 6.5 mmol/l.[16] Therefore, decisions regarding the initiation of treatment for control of hyperkalemia must take into consideration the absolute level and rate of increase of serum potassium, the patient's overall condition, and the likely efficacy of medical therapy.

Metabolic Acidosis

The role of alkali therapy in the treatment of metabolic acidosis, particularly lactic acidosis, is controversial.[18] The use of RRT as an alternative to alkali replacement in metabolic acidosis can avoid some of the deleterious effects ascribed to aggressive alkali replacement, specifically volume overload and hypernatremia. Although progressive metabolic acidosis is a generally accepted indication for RRT, clinical trials to establish a threshold blood pH or serum bicarbonate concentration or to demonstrate improved patient outcomes have not been performed.

Other Electrolyte Disturbances

RRT may be used for the treatment of a variety of other electrolyte disturbances that can occur in the setting of ARF. These include severe hypo- and hypernatremia, hyperphosphatemia, hypo- and hypercalcemia, and hypermagnesemia. In the treatment of hyponatremia, caution must be used to ensure that rapid correction does not predispose to the development of the osmotic demyelination syndrome. A rapid decrease of serum phosphate and uric acid levels and control of acidemia using RRT are necessary in patients who have the tumor lysis syndrome to support recovery of renal function.

Uremia

The development of overt uremic signs or symptoms represents an obvious indication for initiation of RRT in ARF. Early manifestations of uremia, such as anorexia, nausea and vomiting, and pruritus, are nonspecific and may be difficult to differentiate from other comorbid conditions in patients who have critical illness. Mental status changes, which may represent uremic encephalopathy, also may be difficult to differentiate from other etiologies of delirium in the critically ill patient. Uremic pericarditis is usually a late complication, but requires urgent initiation of renal support given the high risk of intrapericardial hemorrhage and tamponade. As was emphasized more than four decades ago by Teschan et al.,[19] optimally RRT should be initiated before the onset of overt uremic manifestations.

Azotemia

In many patients, the sole indication for initiation of RRT in ARF is the presence of progressive azotemia in the absence of uremia or other indications for renal support. There is no consensus, however, on the degree of azotemia that warrants initiation of therapy. In a multicenter trial that evaluated the dosing strategies for RRT in critically ill patients who had ARF, we observed substantial variation in practice regarding the degree of azotemia deemed appropriate for initiation of treatment between practitioners within individual institutions and between institutions (unpublished data). There are many experts in nephrology who feel that RRT should be initiated in critically ill patients with a BUN >60.

TIMING OF INITIATION OF RENAL REPLACEMENT THERAPY

Beginning with the studies by Paul Teschan and colleagues,[19] in the years following the Korean War numerous studies have attempted to define the criteria for timing of initiation of RRT in ARF. These studies attempted to determine the balance between three major competing risks: the inherent risk that results from delay in therapy; the potential risk of harm as a result of RRT, including complications of therapy and the potential that dialysis may prolong the course of ARF; and the risk that early initiation of therapy will result in patients undergoing treatment who, if managed conservatively, might recover renal function without requiring RRT.

In their landmark report, Teschan et al.[19] described a prospective uncontrolled series of 15 patients who had oliguric ARF who were treated with "prophylactic" hemodialysis defined as the initiation of dialysis before the serum urea nitrogen reached 100 mg/dl.[18] Patients received daily dialysis (average duration 6 hours) using twin-coil cellulosic dialyzers at a blood flow of 75–250 ml/min to maintain a predialysis serum urea nitrogen of less than 75 mg/dl. Caloric and protein intake were unrestricted. All-cause mortality was 33%. Mortality due to hemorrhage or sepsis was 20%. Although no control group was studied, the investigators reported that the results contrasted dramatically with their own past experience in patients in whom dialysis was not initiated until "conventional" indications were present.

Acute Renal Failure

ARF is a common complication in critically ill patients and is associated with a mortality rate greater than 50%.[20] As many as 70% of these patients require RRT, making it an important component of the management of ARF in the ICU. Ideally, RRT controls volume, corrects acid-base abnormalities, improves uremia through toxin clearance, promotes renal recovery, and improves survival without causing complications (such as bleeding from anticoagulation and hypotension). The available RRT options include intermittent hemodialysis (IHD), continuous RRT (CRRT), and sustained low-efficiency dialysis (SLED). Currently, there is insufficient evidence to establish which modality of RRT is best for ARF in the critically ill patient. There is a general consensus that patients receiving CRRT using lower blood flow rates and lower fluid removal rates have less cardiovascular instability/morbidity. Clearly, there is no significant difference in mortality rates with any of the available modalities. Understanding the advantages and limitations of the various dialysis modalities is essential for appropriate RRT selection in the ICU setting.

Principles of Renal Replacement Therapy

All forms of RRT rely on the principle of allowing water and solute transport through a semipermeable membrane and then discarding the waste products. Ultrafiltration is the process by which water is transported across a semipermeable membrane. Diffusion and convection are the two processes by which solutes are transported across the membrane. The available RRT modalities use ultrafiltration for fluid removal and diffusion, convection, or a combination of diffusion and convection to achieve solute clearance.

Ultrafiltration achieves volume removal by using a pressure gradient to drive water through a semipermeable membrane. This pressure gradient is known as the transmembrane pressure gradient and is the difference between plasma oncotic pressure and hydrostatic pressure. Determinants of the ultrafiltration rate include the membrane surface area, water permeability of the membrane, and transmembrane pressure gradient.[21]

Diffusion occurs by movement of solutes from an area of higher solute concentration to an area of lower solute concentration across a semipermeable membrane. The concentration gradient is maximized and maintained throughout the length of the membrane by running the dialysate (an electrolyte solution usually containing sodium, bicarbonate, chloride, magnesium, and calcium) countercurrent to the blood flow. Solutes with a higher concentration in the blood, such as potassium and urea, move down their concentration gradient across the membrane to the dialysate compartment. Conversely, solutes with a higher concentration in the dialysate (such as bicarbonate) diffuse into the blood. Solute concentrations that are nearly equivalent in the blood and dialysate, such as sodium and chloride, move very little across the membrane. Because smaller solutes (such as urea and creatinine) diffuse more rapidly than larger solutes, lower-molecular-weight molecules (<500 daltons) are cleared more efficiently than heavier molecules. The rate of solute diffusion depends on blood flow rate, dialysate flow rate, duration of dialysis, concentration gradient across the membrane, and membrane surface area and pore size.[21]

Convection occurs when the transmembrane pressure gradient drives water across a semipermeable membrane (as in ultrafiltration) but then "drags" with the water both small-molecular-weight (BUN, creatinine, potassium) and large-molecular-weight (inulin, β_2-microglobulin, tumor necrosis factor, vitamin B_{12}) solutes. Membrane pore diameter limits the size of the large solutes that can pass through. Increasing the transmembrane pressure difference allows more fluid and solutes to be "pulled" through the membrane. Because the efficiency of solute removal depends mainly on the ultrafiltration rate, typically at least 1 l of water needs to be pulled through the membrane each hour. The process of increasing the ultrafiltration rate to provide convective clearance of solutes is known as hemofiltration. Ultrafiltration rate is determined by the transmembrane pressure, water permeability of the membrane, and membrane surface area and pore size.[21]

CLASSIFICATION OF RENAL REPLACEMENT THERAPIES

RRT for ARF can be classified as intermittent or continuous, based on the duration of the treatment. The duration of each intermittent therapy is less than 24 hours, whereas the duration of continuous therapy is at least 24 hours. The intermittent therapies include IHD and SLED. The continuous therapies include peritoneal dialysis and CRRT.[22] Peritoneal dialysis is rarely used in the acute setting because it provides inefficient solute clearance in critically ill catabolic patients, increases the risk of peritonitis, compromises respiratory function by impeding diaphragmatic excursion, and is contraindicated in patients with recent abdominal surgery or abdominal sepsis.[23]

Intermittent Hemodialysis

Traditionally, nephrologists have managed ARF with IHD—empirically delivered three to six times a week, 3–4 hours per session, with a blood flow rate of 200–350 ml/min and a dialysate flow rate of

500–800 ml/min. In IHD, solute clearance occurs mainly by diffusion—whereas volume is removed by ultrafiltration. The degree of solute clearance, also known as the "dialysis dose," is largely dependent on the rate of blood flow. Increasing the blood flow increases solute clearance. Decisions regarding dialysis duration and frequency are based on patient metabolic control, volume status, and presence of any hemodynamic instability.

Advantages of IHD include rapid solute and volume removal. This results in rapid correction of electrolyte disturbances, such as hyperkalemia, and rapid removal of drugs or other substances in fatal intoxications within a matter of hours. IHD also has a decreased need for anticoagulation compared with other types of RRT because of the higher blood flow rates and shorter duration of therapy.

The main disadvantage of IHD is the risk of systemic hypotension caused by rapid electrolyte shifts and fluid removal. Hypotension occurs in approximately 20%–30% of hemodialysis treatments. Sodium modeling, cooling the dialysate, increasing the dialysate calcium concentration, IV albumin, and intermittent ultrafiltration may be used to improve hemodynamic stability during IHD. Despite this, approximately 10% of ARF patients cannot be treated with IHD because of hemodynamic instability. Systemic hypotension can limit the efficacy of IHD and result in poor solute clearance, insufficient acid-base correction, and persistent volume overload, because the rate of ultrafiltration necessary to maintain fluid balance is seldom achieved within the 4-hour dialysis session.

Rapid solute removal from the intravascular space can cause cerebral edema and increased intracranial pressure. ARF patients with head trauma or hepatic encephalopathy are at a significant risk of brain edema and even herniation.[24] Finally, there is a lack of consensus as to how to assess solute clearance (dialysis dose) and what constitutes an adequate dose in ARF because the kinetics of urea in the end-stage renal disease patient cannot be extrapolated to patients with ARF.

Although the results of some studies suggested an advantage of daily HD over conventional IHD, it is unclear whether the increased dialysis dose improved outcome by improving uremic control or by reducing the volume of fluid removed during each dialysis session and resulting in less hemodynamic instability.

Continuous Renal Replacement Therapy

Although the worldwide standard for RRT is IHD, CRRT has emerged over the past decade as a viable modality for management of hemodynamically unstable patients with ARF. Continuous therapies have evolved from systems that relied on arterial access and blood pressure to maintain blood flow through the extracorporeal circuit to pump-driven systems that use double-lumen venous catheters. The arteriovenous (CAVH) circuit is now rarely used in CRRT because of poor solute removal and complications from arterial cannulation. Unlike IHD, CRRT is a continuous treatment occurring 24 hours a day—with a blood flow of 100–200 ml/min and a dialysate flow of 17–40 ml/min if a diffusive CRRT modality is used. The different CRRT modalities can use diffusion, convection, or a combination of both for solute clearance.

All types of CRRT use membranes that are highly permeable to water and low-molecular-weight solutes. CRRT modalities are classified by access type and method of solute clearance. Venovenous circuits are now the standard, and the various venovenous modalities of CRRT differ by their mechanism of solute removal. The four main types of CRRT in order of increasing complexity are slow continuous ultrafiltration, continuous venovenous hemofiltration (CVVH), continuous venovenous hemodialysis (CVVHD), and continuous venovenous hemodiafiltration (CVVHDF).[25]

In slow continuous ultrafiltration, low-volume ultrafiltration at a rate of 100–300 ml/hr is performed to maintain fluid balance only and does not result in significant convective clearance of solutes. No fluids are administered either as dialysate or replacement fluids, and

the purpose of treatment is for volume overload with or without renal failure. Indications include volume overload in patients with congestive heart failure refractory to diuretics.

In CVVH, solute clearance occurs by convection. Solutes are carried along with the bulk flow of fluid in a hydraulic-induced ultrafiltrate of blood. No dialysate is used. Clearances are similar for all solutes that have a molecular weight in the range at which the membrane is readily permeable. The rate at which ultrafiltration occurs is the major determinant of convective clearance. The ultrafiltration rate is determined by the transmembrane pressure, water permeability, pore size, surface area, and membrane thickness. Typically, hourly ultrafiltration rates of 1–2 l/hr are used to provide adequate solute removal. These high ultrafiltration rates rapidly cause volume contraction, hypotension, and loss of electrolytes. Intravenous "replacement fluid" is provided to replace the excess volume being removed and to replenish desired solutes. Replacement fluid can be administered prefilter or postfilter.

In CVVHD, a dialysate solution runs countercurrent to the flow of blood at a rate of 1–2.5 l/hr. Solute removal occurs by diffusion. Unlike IHD, the dialysate flow rate is slower than the blood flow rate, allowing small solutes to equilibrate completely between the blood and dialysate. As a result, the dialysate flow rate approximates urea and Ccr. Ultrafiltration is used for volume control but can allow for some convective clearance at high rates. CVVHDF combines the convective solute removal of CVVH and the diffusive solute removal of CVVHD. As in CVVH, the high ultrafiltration rates used to provide convective clearance require the administration of intravenous replacement fluids.

Replacement fluids can be administered prefilter or postfilter. Postfilter replacement fluid results in hemoconcentration of the filter and increased risk of clotting, especially when the filtration fraction is greater than 30%. The filtration fraction is the ratio of ultrafiltration rate to plasma water flow rate and is dependent on the blood flow rate and hematocrit.[25] Prefilter replacement fluid dilutes the blood before the filter, resulting in reduced filter clotting. Dilution of solutes before the filter reduces solute clearance by up to 15% by lowering the diffusion driving force and convective concentration.

Advantages and Disadvantages

The advantages of CRRT include hemodynamic tolerance caused by slower ultrafiltration rates.[27] The gradual continuous volume removal makes control of volume status easier and allows administration of medications and nutrition with less concern for volume overload. Because it is a continuous modality, there is less fluctuation of solute concentrations over time and better control of azotemia, electrolytes, and acid-base status. The improved hemodynamic stability may be associated with fewer episodes of reduced renal blood flow, less renal ischemia, and more rapid renal recovery. Mehta et al.[28] examined this issue in a prospective study in which 166 ICU patients with ARF were randomized to IHD or to CRRT. CRRT patients who survived were significantly more likely to show renal recovery than those treated with IHD. Because CRRT does not cause rapid solute shifts, it does not raise intracranial pressure like IHD.

The cumulative solute removal with CRRT is greater than that achievable with IHD. Ronco et al.[29] provided convincing evidence that increasing solute clearance with CRRT can improve outcome in critically ill patients with ARF. In a prospective randomized controlled trial, 425 critically ill patients with ARF were assigned to CVVH using ultrafiltration rates of 20 ml/kg/hr (group 1), 35 ml/kg/hr (group 2), or 45 ml/kg/hr (group 3). The ultrafiltration rate of 20 ml/kg/hr was based on the average rate used in clinical practice as reported in the literature at the time of the study. The blood flow rates ranged from 120 to 240 ml/min and the replacement fluid was administered postfilter. The primary study outcome was survival at

15 days after discontinuation of CVVH. Secondary outcomes were recovery of renal function and CRRT-related complications. Patient survival after discontinuing CVVH was 41, 57, and 58% in groups 1, 2, and 3, respectively. Survival in group 1 was significantly lower than group 2 ($p = 0.0007$) and group 3 ($p = 0.001$), demonstrating a survival advantage for patients treated with CVVH at an ultrafiltration rate of at least 35 ml/kg/hr. It is unclear, however, whether the reduction in mortality was solely caused by small-molecule (urea) clearance or by both small-molecule clearance and increased middle-molecule clearance.

Intermittent Hemodialysis versus Continuous Renal Replacement Therapy: Outcomes

There are few prospective studies comparing IHD with CRRT with respect to outcomes, such as mortality or recovery of renal function. Mehta et al.[28] randomized 166 patients to CRRT (CVVH or CVVHDF) or IHD. Univariate intention-to-treat analysis revealed a higher mortality among patients receiving CRRT. Patients randomized to CRRT had higher APACHE III scores and had a higher prevalence of liver failure, confounding the results. Multivariate analysis revealed no impact of RRT modality on all-cause mortality or recovery of renal function. Instead, severity of illness scores (such as APACHE III scores and number of failed organs) were more important prognostic factors. The authors concluded that insufficient data existed to draw strong conclusions, mainly because of the lack of randomized controlled trials and the influence of biases and confounding variables.

Sustained Low-Efficiency Dialysis or Extended Daily Dialysis

SLED and extended daily dialysis are slower dialytic modalities run for prolonged periods using conventional hemodialysis machines with modification of blood and dialysate flow rates. Typically, sustained low-efficiency dialysis and extended daily dialysis use low blood-pump speeds of 200 ml/min and low dialysate flow rates of 300 ml/min for 6–12 hours daily. Sustained low-efficiency dialysis and extended daily dialysis combine the advantages of CRRT and IHD. They allow for improved hemodynamic stability through gradual solute and fluid removal, as in CRRT. At the same time, they are able to provide high solute clearances (as seen in IHD) and eliminate the need for expensive CRRT machines, costly customized solutions, and trained staff.

Because sustained low-efficiency dialysis and extended daily dialysis can be done intermittently based on the needs of the patient, they also avoid the interruption of therapy for various diagnostic and therapeutic procedures that may be required in such patients. Kumar et al.[30] described their prospective experience of 25 patients treated with extended daily dialysis and 17 patients treated with CVVH at University of California Davis Medical Center. No significant differences in mean arterial pressure or inotrope requirements were observed between the two groups. Mortality was higher in the extended daily dialysis group (84% vs. 65%). The APACHE II scores were higher, however, in the extended daily dialysis group at the onset of treatment. The authors argued that extended daily dialysis was more cost effective by removing the need for constant monitoring of dialysis equipment and reducing nursing workload.

SUMMARY

ARF in critically ill patients is a significant clinical problem. Options for RRT in these patients use convective and diffusive clearance. The renal replacement modality may be intermittent, as in classic hemodialysis, or continuous. RRT needs to be tailored to the needs of each patient. Future research studies are needed to determine criteria for RRT.

Given the impact of ARF on mortality, it is important to prevent or hasten the resolution of even the mildest forms of ARF. The main goal is a preventive strategy for the syndrome of ARF to preserve renal function, prevent death, prevent complications of ARF (volume overload, acid-base disturbances, and electrolyte abnormalities), and to prevent the need for chronic dialysis, with minimum adverse effects.

In this chapter, we discussed preventive strategies, and offered several options for treatment of ARF. Advances in RRT in the last few years have resulted in multiple RRT modalities available for treating ARF in the ICU. CRRT is gaining greater acceptance with the use of venovenous access and its advantages in hemodynamically unstable patients. There is little scientific data as to the best modality of RRT. There are few randomized controlled trials. Most existing studies are retrospective and poorly controlled. Many confounders exist, such as severity of illness and etiology of renal failure, which are probably the most important factors affecting outcome in ICU patients with ARF. Some recent studies also suggest that higher doses of dialysis confer a survival advantage.

The choice of dialytic modality to be used should be tailored to the needs of the individual patient. IHD is best for patients requiring rapid metabolic control (e.g., in hyperkalemia), whereas volume overload is best managed with CRRT. Patients who are hemodynamically unstable or who have increased intracranial pressure are best treated with CRRT. Patients in whom anticoagulation is contraindicated might be better managed with IHD unless CRRT with citrate is used. CRRT is limited by its greater cost, demands on nursing time, and the constraint it places on a patient's mobility. Theoretically, the choice of RRT might also depend on the underlying disease and etiology of ARF. The choice of modality should be based on the clinical status of the patient and the resources available in a given institution.

REFERENCES

1. Nissenson AR: Acute renal failure: definition and pathogenesis. *Kidney Int Suppl* 66:7–10, 1998.
2. Hou SH, Bushinsky DA, Wish JB: Hospital-acquired renal insufficiency: a prospective study. *Am J Med* 74:243–248, 1983.
3. Bellomo R, Ronco C: The changing pattern of severe acute renal failure. *Nephrology* 2:602–610, 1991.
4. Metnitz PG, Krenn CG, Steltzer H: Effect of acute renal failure requiring renal replacement therapy on outcome in critically ill patients. *Crit Care Med* 30:2051–2058, 2002.
5. Gehr TWB, Schoolwerth AC: Adult acute and chronic renal failure. In Ayers SM, et al, editors: *Textbook of Critical Care*, 3rd ed. Philadelphia, WB Saunders, 1995, pp. 1029–1041.
6. Mullins RJ: Acute renal failure. In Cameron JL, editor: *Current Surgical Therapy*, 6th ed. St. Louis, Mosby, 1998, pp. 1109–1114.
7. Thadhani R, Paucual M, Bonventre JV: Acute renal failure, *N Engl J Med* 334:1448–1460, 1996.
8. Mueller C, Buerkle G, Buettner HJ: Prevention of contrast media-associated nephropathy: randomized comparison of 2 hydration regimens in 1620 patients undergoing coronary angioplasty. *Arch Intern Med* 162:329–336, 2002.
9. Merten GJ, Burgess WP, Gray LV: Prevention of contrast-induced nephropathy with sodium bicarbonate: a randomized controlled trial. *JAMA* 291:2328–2334, 2004.
10. Hatala R, Dinh TT, Cook DJ: Single daily dosing of aminoglycosides in immunocompromised adults: a systematic review. *Clin Infect Dis* 24:810–815, 1997.
11. Barrett BJ, Carlisle EJ: Metaanalysis of the relative nephrotoxicity of high- and low-osmolality iodinated contrast media. *Radiology* 188:171–178, 1993.
12. Kellum JA: The use of diuretics and dopamine in acute renal failure: a systematic review of the evidence. *Crit Care* 1:53–59, 1997.
13. Alonso A, Lau J, Jaber BL: Prevention of radiocontrast nephropathy with N-acetylcysteine in patients with chronic kidney disease: a meta-analysis of randomized, controlled trials. *Am J Kidney Dis* 43:1–9, 2004.

14. Hoffmann U, Fischereder M, Kruger B: The value of N-acetylcysteine in the prevention of radiocontrast agent-induced nephropathy seems questionable. *J Am Soc Nephrol* 15:407–410, 2004.
15. Mehta RL, Pascual MT, Soroko S: Diuretics, mortality, and nonrecovery of renal function in acute renal failure. *JAMA* 288:2547–2553, 2002.
16. Greenberg A: Hyperkalemia: treatment options. *Semin Nephrol* 18:46–57, 1998.
17. Hou S, McElroy PA, Nootens J: Safety and efficacy of low-potassium dialysate. *Am J Kidney Dis* 13:137–143, 1989.
18. Forsythe SM, Schmidt GA: Sodium bicarbonate for the treatment of lactic acidosis. *Chest* 117:260–267, 2000.
19. Teschan PE, Baxter CR, O'Brien TF: Prophylactic hemodialysis in the treatment of acute renal failure. *Ann Intern Med* 53:992–1016, 1960.
20. Liano F, Junico E: The spectrum of acute renal failure in the intensive care unit compared with that seen in other settings. *Kidney IntKidney Int Suppl* 66:S16–S24, 1998.
21. Yeun J, Depner T: Principles of dialysis. In Owen WF, Pereira BJ, Sayegh MH, editors: *Dialysis and Transplantation: A Companion to Brenner & Rectors' The Kidney.* Philadelphia, WB Sanders, 2000, pp. 1–32.
22. Mehta RL, Chertow GM: Selection of dialysis modality. In Owen WF, Pereira BJ, Sayegh MH, editors: *Dialysis and Transplantation: A Companion to Brenner & Rectors' The Kidney.* Philadelphia, WB Sanders, 2000, pp. 403–417.
23. Goel S, Saran R, Nolph KD: Indications, contraindications and complications of peritoneal dialysis in the critically ill. In Ronco C, Bellomo R, editors: *Critical Care Nephrology.* Dordrecht, Kluwer Academic Publishers, 1998, pp. 1373–1381.
24. Davenport A, Will EJ, Davidson AM: Effect of renal replacement therapy on patients with combined acute renal failure and fulminant hepatic failure. *Kidney Int* 43:S245–S251, 1993.
25. Bellomo R, Ronco C, Mehta R: Nomenclature for continuous renal replacement therapies. *Am J Kidney Dis* 28:S2–S7, 1996.
26. Clark WR, Turk JE, Kraus MA: Dose determinants in continuous renal replacement therapy. *Artif Organs* 27:815–820, 2003.
27. Lameire N, Van Biesen W, Vanholder R: The place of intermittent hemodialysis in the treatment of acute renal failure in the ICU patient. *Kidney Int Suppl* 66:S110–S119, 1998.
28. Mehta R, McDonald B, Gabbai F: A randomized, clinical trial of continuous versus intermittent dialysis for acute renal failure. *Kidney Int* 60:1154–1163, 2001.
29. Ronco C, Bellomo R, Homel P: Effects of different doses in continuous veno-venous hemofiltration on outcomes of acute renal failure: a prospective, randomized trial. *Lancet* 356:26–30, 2000.
30. Kumar VCM, Depner T, Yeun J: Extended daily dialysis: a new approach to renal replacement for acute renal failure in the intensive care unit. *Am J Kidney Dis* 36:294–300, 2000.

MANAGEMENT OF COAGULATION DISORDERS IN THE SURGICAL INTENSIVE CARE UNIT

Christopher P. Michetti and Samir M. Fakhry

Surgeons commonly encounter coagulation disorders in the course of caring for patients, especially those with serious injury and those undergoing or recovering from surgery. Whereas bleeding is a condition well known to man since the beginnings of time, understanding the pathophysiology of bleeding and coagulation and developing effective therapies for them have come relatively recently and continue to undergo change as more is learned about the complex mechanism of blood coagulation and fibrinolysis. The ability to treat hemorrhage effectively had to await the discovery of blood types A, B, and O by Karl Landsteiner in 1900 and the AB blood type by Alfred Decastello and Adriano Sturli in 1902.

It would be nearly 40 years before the first blood bank was established in the United States in 1937. The development of reliable techniques of cross-matching, anticoagulation, and storage of blood was followed by the introduction of plastic bags for storage and devices for plasmapheresis making component therapy possible. The discovery of blood coagulation pathways and the development of reliable tests of coagulation made it possible to provide treatment for a variety of coagulation disorders, including those encountered as a result of the newfound ability to keep humans alive by the infusion of blood and the surgical control of bleeding.

The ability to replace blood loss is critically important in modern surgical practice and in trauma care. Equally important is the ability to provide therapy to patients who need individual blood components. Effective use of the precious resource that blood and its prod-

ucts represents is increasingly important as problems of supply continue to exist even while demand increases. The purpose of this chapter is to familiarize the practicing surgeon with the types of coagulation disorders encountered in critically ill or injured patients, reliable ways of diagnosing these disorders, and effective therapeutic strategies for treating them.

INCIDENCE

Congenital Bleeding Disorders

Von Willebrand Disease

Von Willebrand disease (vWD) is the most common inherited bleeding disorder, occurring in 1/100 to 1/1000 live births via autosomal inheritance. The disease consists of deficiency or dysfunction of von Willebrand factor (vWf), which promotes platelet adhesion to damaged endothelium and stabilizes factor VIII. There are three types of vWD. Knowing the specific type is important to direct therapy. In type 1, a deficiency of vWf exists. In type 3, vWf is absent. The main subtypes of type 2, 2a, and 2b, both consist of a qualitative functional defect in vWf.

Diagnosis of vWD is supported by prolonged partial thromboplastin time (PTT), and in types 1 and 3 reduced levels of vWf antigen. Factor VIII activity may be reduced, and bleeding time or other platelet functional assays may be abnormal. The ristocetin cofactor assay is a test that measures the ability of vWf to induce platelet aggregation.

1-deamino-8-D-arginine vasopressin (DDAVP) may be used to stimulate production of vWf and increase factor VIII levels in type 1 and type 2a disease. It is ineffective in type 3, however, and contraindicated in type 2b due to risk of thrombocytopenia and increased bleeding. Concentrates of factor VIII vWf are virus inactivated and are used commonly in types 2 and 3, but also in type 1 that is unresponsive to DDAVP. Cryoprecipitate contains vWf and factor VIII, and may be used in all types of vWD. However, it is pooled and not virus inactivated. It is only recommended as a third-line therapy. Antifibrinolytic amino acids, such as aminocaproic acid and tranexamic acid, are used as adjuvant therapy in all types of vWD along with the previously cited treatments.

Hemophilia A

Hemophilia A is a congenital bleeding disorder that results from factor VIII deficiency. It is phenotypically expressed in males due to its X-linked inheritance pattern, whereas females maintain a carrier state. Bleeding tendency is inversely related to factor VIII levels. As with most factor deficiencies, clinical coagulopathy is usually not evident until factor levels fall below 30% of normal (mild hemophilia). Spontaneous bleeding may occur at levels less than 5% (moderate hemophilia), and those with levels less than 1% (severe hemophilia) are especially at risk. Coagulation studies will show a prolonged PTT, normal prothrombin time (PT), and low factor VIII levels.

Patients with clinically significant bleeding or those undergoing surgery should receive factor VIII concentrates, preferably recombinant products. DDAVP increases endogenous factor VIII levels and may be used in mild cases. Up to 20% of individuals may develop IgG antibodies ("inhibitors") to factor VIII after factor infusion, rendering future treatments ineffective. In such cases, recombinant factor VIIa (rFVIIa) may be used to induce hemostasis. rFVIIa is discussed in more detail later in this chapter. Cryoprecipitate contains factor VIII in lower concentrations than in factor VIII concentrates, but its use is tempered by risks of viral transmission. Viral transmission from pooled factor concentrates is now extremely rare, and virtually eliminated with use of recombinant factors.

Hemophilia B

Hemophilia B (Christmas disease) is an X-linked disorder of factor IX deficiency. It is clinically similar to hemophilia A, and coagulation tests also show prolonged PTT with normal PT and low factor IX levels. Recombinant factor IX concentrates are available, as well as pooled donated concentrates. Development of inhibitors is less common (1%) than in hemophilia A, and treatment of severe bleeding may also include rFVIIa. Therapy in such cases should be given in conjunction with a hematologist.

Acquired Bleeding Disorders

Coagulopathy of Hemorrhagic Shock

Hemorrhagic shock causes a complex coagulopathy whose etiology is multifactorial, and widely misunderstood. Misinterpretation of clinical and laboratory data may lead clinicians to incorrectly label this coagulopathy as disseminated intravascular coagulation (DIC) or dilutional coagulopathy, which may misdirect treatment. In hemorrhagic shock, blood loss and tissue hypoperfusion result in acidosis from anaerobic metabolism—leading to the generation of lactate. Decreased ATP production from tissue ischemia contributes to hypothermia and inability to maintain core temperature. Coagulopathy is the result, which exacerbates bleeding and perpetuates the "bloody vicious cycle." Resuscitation with room-temperature fluids worsens hypothermia. In massive resuscitation from hemorrhagic shock, variable degrees of dilution of coagulation factors occur.

Hypothermia and acidosis are the two major contributors to the coagulopathy of hemorrhagic shock, and are discussed in more detail in material following. In the operating room and postoperatively in the intensive care unit (ICU), multiple treatments are obviously conducted simultaneously. However, the priorities in general are to stop the bleeding, resuscitate with crystalloid and blood to reverse ischemia and acidosis, and prevent and treat hypothermia. Because of the overwhelming influence of hypothermia and acidosis, coagulopathy is primarily that of ineffective clotting. This is in contrast to DIC, which implies an overactivated coagulation system with unregulated microvascular thrombosis. Attributing the bleeding to DIC may lead one to focus therapy on providing clotting factors with fresh frozen plasma (FFP), or the rarely needed cryoprecipitate, when time is much better spent on adequate resuscitation and rewarming.

Dilutional coagulopathy (the idea that microvascular bleeding can result from dilution of clotting factors) has limited scientific support. Clotting factor concentrations as low as 30% of normal are sufficient for hemostasis, as are fibrinogen levels greater than 75 mg/dL. Even replacement of an entire blood volume leaves one with about a third of the normal coagulation factor concentration. This is probably the minimum volume of transfusion that can lead to a true dilutional coagulopathy. Although dilution of factors may result in abnormalities in laboratory measures of coagulation such as PT and PTT, these alterations do not necessarily affect hemostasis in vivo. Furthermore, platelet count cannot reliably be predicted based on volume of blood loss. Formula-based replacement (X units of FFP and platelets for every Y units of blood transfused) has little rationale, and should be discouraged. In the perioperative hemorrhagic shock patient, factor replacement with FFP should be based primarily on clinical evidence of microvascular (nonsurgical) bleeding to target clinical hemostasis while efforts to correct hypothermia and acidosis are optimized.

Hypothermia

Hypothermia is often seen in the critical care setting in association with the systemic inflammatory response syndrome (SIRS), sepsis, and shock, in which decreased oxygen consumption prevents maintenance of core body temperature. It routinely accompanies major surgery for hemorrhagic shock, in which it exacerbates the coagulopathy and should prompt a "damage control" strategy. In addition, heat loss from hemorrhage is compounded by the administration of room-temperature fluids and blood products. In trauma patients, temperatures less than 32° C are associated with 100% mortality.

Hypothermia slows the rate of reaction of the proteolytic enzymes of coagulation, resulting in impaired hemostasis. Both coagulation enzyme activity and platelet function are impaired at temperatures below 34° C in trauma patients. Platelet dysfunction is multifactorial, and is caused by defective adhesion and aggregation and decreased thromboxane production.

Prompt and efficient rewarming is essential in the hypothermic coagulopathic surgical patient. Although controlled hypothermia has proven beneficial in other conditions, such as cardiac arrest, no clear benefit has been proven in trauma or general surgery. The priority of therapy is to treat the underlying cause, whether by stopping any ongoing surgical bleeding, evacuating an undrained abscess, treating infection, or debriding necrotic tissue. External rewarming methods, although slow and inefficient, help to prevent further heat loss. Ambient room temperature should be raised, and warm air blankets and fluid pads applied to the patient (including the head). Core rewarming is far more efficacious than external techniques. At the very least, all infused fluids and blood products should be run through a fluid warmer, and warm humidified air given via the mechanical ventilator. When available, the more aggressive rapid technique of continuous arteriovenous rewarming may be used. A randomized prospective study suggests improved early survival and reduced fluid resuscitation requirements with this method when compared with slower methods.

Acidosis

Metabolic acidosis has long been recognized as a consequence of, and contributor to, coagulopathy. However, the specific pathways whereby acidosis impairs coagulation have yet to be clearly defined. Animal data suggest that hypothermia induces a delayed onset of thrombin formation, whereas acidosis decreases the overall thrombin generation rate. The association of severe acidosis (pH < 7.1) with hypotension and hypothermia in severely injured patients virtually guarantees life-threatening coagulopathy. Therapy is again directed at the cause of acidosis and not merely the correction of the pH.

While simultaneously addressing the inciting events, lactic acidosis is treated with fluid resuscitation to optimize tissue perfusion. It can be guided by following the trend in base deficit or lactate level. Sodium bicarbonate administration is ineffective and potentially harmful in lactic acidosis, and is not recommended.

Thrombocytopenia

Thrombocytopenia is generally defined as a platelet count lower than 100,000/mm^3. Counts of 50,000/mm^3 to 100,000/mm^3 increase risk of bleeding with surgery or major trauma, and spontaneous bleeding is a risk below 10,000/mm^3 to 20,000/mm^3. Thrombocytopenia in the ICU setting has a lengthy differential diagnosis, but its etiology can be broadly divided into three categories: decreased production of platelets, consumption or sequestration of platelets, and dilution. Malignancies or chemotherapy may affect platelet production, and massive transfusion and fluid resuscitation can lead to dilution of the total platelet count. In critically ill surgical patients, sepsis can cause a consumptive coagulopathy that in its most severe form manifests as DIC. Platelet consumption also occurs through immune mechanisms (antibodies to platelet glycoproteins), most notably in response to certain drugs. The list of such drugs includes heparin, H$_2$ antagonists, sulfa, rifampin, quinidine, hypoglycemics, and gold salts.

Heparin-induced thrombocytopenia is a rare but highly morbid condition associated with a greatly increased risk of thrombosis. Dilutional thrombocytopenia may occur with massive transfusion because stored blood contains negligible levels of platelets. However, the decrease in platelet count is not proportional to the volume of blood transfusion. Thus, simple dilution is unlikely to be the sole determinant of the low platelet count. Release of platelets from the spleen and bone marrow may partly account for this variability. As with coagulation factors, dilutional thrombocytopenia alone does not account for microvascular bleeding. Treatment and transfusion guidelines are discussed later in this chapter.

Disseminated Intravascular Coagulation

DIC is a syndrome involving diffuse systemic hypercoagulation and fibrinolysis that occurs in response to specific clinical conditions. Disorders associated with DIC in the surgical ICU include sepsis, trauma, severe pancreatitis, malignancies, fulminant liver failure, and transfusion reactions—among others. The syndrome involves excessive fibrin deposition in the microvasculature, with platelet aggregation and microvascular thrombosis. The pathophysiology of DIC is linked to the inflammatory cascade and TF pathway, and is reviewed in more detail elsewhere. The condition ranges in severity from a subclinical low-grade acceleration of thrombosis and fibrinolysis to overt pathologic bleeding. Fulminant DIC is associated with multiple-organ dysfunction and death.

Diagnosis of DIC is made with a few laboratory tests in the proper clinical setting, after other causes of coagulopathy have been excluded. Scoring systems and algorithms have been proposed to aid the diagnosis. However, treatment is mainly supportive and targets the underlying cause, clinical endpoints, and associated laboratory abnormalities. Given the nonspecific nature of DIC, setting a defined threshold for making the diagnosis in the clinical setting is unnecessary—whereas set criteria are still needed for therapeutic trials and research. In addition, the label of DIC is often applied to patients receiving massive transfusion and resuscitation when their coagulopathy stems from other more common and reversible causes. It has also been observed that trauma patients with DIC have a thrombotic and fibrinolytic profile distinct from the usual hemostatic response to trauma.

DIC may be suspected in the setting of a generalized coagulopathy and clinical microvascular bleeding associated with an underlying process such as those described previously. The laboratory profile includes a low platelet count, prolonged PT and PTT, and elevated fibrin split products. D-dimer levels are increased in up to 94% of patients diagnosed with DIC, and the D-dimer assay is the most sensitive test for this condition. Fibrinogen levels may be maintained except in severe forms of DIC.

Therapy for DIC centers on treatment of the underlying disease process to remove the proinflammatory stimulus of the syndrome. Clinical hemostasis is the goal. Platelet counts and the PT/PTT are used to guide response to therapy, but are not endpoints themselves. FFP and platelet transfusion are indicated in patients with active bleeding and those with significant laboratory derangements undergoing surgery or procedures. Cryoprecipitate may be considered to replace fibrinogen if fibrinogen levels fall below 100 mg/dl and are not corrected with FFP infusion.

Many other therapeutic agents have been investigated, but to date no specific treatment has proven successful in improving outcome in patients with DIC. Anticoagulation has been used to attempt to control the hypercoagulation in DIC, and although improvement in certain lab parameters has been reported no survival benefit has been demonstrated with low-molecular-weight heparin, thrombin inhibitors, or antifibrinolytics.

Severe Sepsis

Research in recent years continues to elucidate the complex interrelationship of the inflammatory process and the coagulation mechanism. The initial manifestation of this relationship leads to a hypercoagulable state. Inflammation in sepsis induces tissue factor (TF) expression on circulating monocytes, tissue macrophages, and the endothelial surface—and fibrinolysis is inhibited. As fibrinolysis is impaired, fibrin deposition in the microvasculature proceeds unchecked. In addition, most patients with severe sepsis have low levels of the natural anticoagulants protein C and antithrombin III. Diffuse thrombosis leads to tissue ischemia and the multiple-organ dysfunction syndrome (MODS).

Coagulopathy in sepsis is multifactorial. Sepsis-induced thrombocytopenia occurs through immune mechanisms, platelet sequestration on activated endothelium, and consumption in DIC. Extensive thrombin generation consumes clotting factors, and fibrinogen is often reduced (although levels may be normal due to its generation as an acute-phase reactant). Pathologic bleeding may occur due to lack of circulating clotting factors and platelets that have been consumed, but this is relatively uncommon. Although DIC is estimated to occur in 15%–30% of patients with severe sepsis, the incidence of serious bleeding episodes in a recent study of septic patients was only 5%.

Transfusion of FFP or platelets in septic patients is indicated for active bleeding, or those at high risk for bleeding. As mentioned previously, transfused factors and platelets usually have only a transient impact because they are depleted by the ongoing consumption in the microvasculature. However, in the face of active bleeding aggressive therapy is warranted while every effort is made to treat or remove the source of the sepsis.

Traumatic Brain Injury

Traumatic brain injury (TBI) is associated with changes in the coagulation system, thought to result from release of the brain's abundant concentration of TF (thromboplastin). Exposed TF incites hypercoagulation, followed by fibrinolysis—similar to the changes seen in trauma patients without TBI. Although laboratory tests may confirm coagulation and fibrinolysis in many patients, the manifestations of this process have a spectrum of severity ranging from clinically undetectable to occasional pathologic bleeding from consumptive coagulopathy. Coagulopathy is associated with increased mortality in blunt and penetrating TBI, but the mechanism for this is not clear.

The importance of the hemostatic changes may lie in promotion of secondary brain injury through cerebral microvascular thrombosis, which may exacerbate cerebral ischemia. Currently, it is not known whether therapy should target hemostasis to prevent further bleeding in the injured brain or block part of the coagulation pathway to prevent microthrombosis and ischemia. Until the pathophysiology is better understood, treatment should be directed only toward clinical endpoints and maintenance of platelets and clotting factors as necessary for hemostasis (as outlined elsewhere in this chapter).

Vitamin K Deficiency

Vitamin K is a necessary cofactor in the enzymatic reactions of coagulation factors II, VII, IX, X, protein C, and protein S—known as the vitamin-K–dependent factors. When vitamin K is deficient, calcium binding is impaired—resulting in inactive factors. These factors comprise the extrinsic portion of the traditional coagulation cascade, and their function can be measured with the international normalized ratio (INR) or PT assays. Vitamin K deficiency may be due to inadequate dietary intake, malabsorption of adequate intake, destruction of vitamin-K–producing enteric bacteria by antibiotics, insufficient supplementation during parenteral nutrition, renal insufficiency, and hepatic dysfunction. Vitamin K may be given orally or parenterally to correct coagulopathy from deficiency or to reverse the effects of warfarin, and is discussed in more detail in material following.

Anticoagulant Drugs

The list of drugs that affect hemostasis is extensive and expanding rapidly. Drugs that affect platelet function and fibrinolysis have no specific antidote, but some of the thrombin inhibitors and GPIIb/IIIa blockers have short half-lives and are able to be removed by hemodialysis. Serious bleeding associated with aspirin and other antiplatelet agents may be partially ameliorated with platelet transfusion, but a functional platelet count or platelet function test may be warranted to assess the level of thrombocytopathy prior to transfusion. Heparin and warfarin are undoubtedly the most common drugs associated with bleeding complications in the surgical ICU. Reversal of these agents is discussed later in this chapter.

Cirrhosis and End-Stage Liver Disease

Severe liver disease is associated with abnormal coagulation from multiple hemostatic defects. The diseased liver's ability to synthesize coagulation factors is impaired, and fibrinogen levels are low in end-stage liver disease (ESLD) and decompensated cirrhosis but may be normalized by its acute-phase reaction to inflammation. Thrombocytopenia may be present due to decreased production of thrombopoietin in the liver, and platelets may be destroyed or sequestered. Platelet function may be altered as well, by an excess of circulating inhibitors of platelet aggregation such as nitrous oxide. Systemic fibrinolysis occurs, in part by reduced clearance in the liver of profibrinolytic enzymes. Patients with ESLD may appear to have a baseline low-grade DIC (e.g., elevated fibrin split products) and are at higher risk of declining into overt DIC. The frequency and severity of DIC generally advance with the disease stage of the liver.

Cirrhotic patients who require surgery pose a significant challenge to the surgeon. Morbidity and mortality are increased in such patients, especially for emergent operations (for which mortality may reach 50%). In one study, patients undergoing trauma laparotomy with intraoperatively diagnosed cirrhosis had 45% mortality compared to 24% in injury severity-matched controls. Postoperative ICU stay was significantly longer as well. Patients with ESLD undergoing surgery may have an enhanced fibrinolytic response due to release of tissue plasminogen activator (tPA) and other factors, hindering stable clot formation. Compounding the risk of bleeding from coagulopathy in ESLD is the presence of large intraabdominal and abdominal wall varices, which can make even the laparotomy incision itself a daunting task. Given all of these obstacles, the decision to undertake any invasive procedure on a patient with cirrhosis or ESLD must be made with the utmost discretion.

The goal of treatment of coagulopathy in ESLD should be clinical hemostasis, and not complete normalization of laboratory values (which is often not possible). Mild aberrations in lab assays are frequent and may not result in a bleeding diathesis. FFP is used for factor and fibrinogen replacement, but cryoprecipitate may be necessary if fibrinogen levels are lower than 100 mg/dl. Due to the short half-life of some clotting factors, large volumes of FFP may be needed to maintain the hemostatic state. Continuous FFP infusion is sometimes warranted, and can be titrated to clinical endpoints. In cases of life-threatening bleeding or the need for emergency surgery, recombinant human factor VIIa (rFVIIa) may be used to correct the INR acutely. However, its short half-life may necessitate repeated dosing after a few hours to maintain hemostasis. Transfusion guidelines for thrombocytopenia are the same as described elsewhere in this chapter. However, patients with splenomegaly may sequester transfused platelets and the rise in platelet count may be less than expected. The presence of microvascular bleeding with a normal platelet count may indicate platelet dysfunction, and a platelet function test may be considered. However, transfusion in these cases may result in brief or no improvement in hemostasis unless the underlying cause of the thrombocytopathy has been corrected. Administration of DDAVP may be considered, but its efficacy is unproven in this setting.

Despite an underlying coagulopathy, risk for thrombosis remains. Cirrhotic patients should not be presumed protected by an "auto-anticoagulation." In fact, hepatic and portal vein thromboses are common in these patients, especially in advanced disease. The INR may be misleading, in that an elevated INR in ESLD does not necessarily correlate with the same level of anticoagulation as if that value were achieved with warfarin therapy. Deficient factor VII synthesis may produce a measurable abnormality in laboratory tests due to its short half-life, but clinical clotting abnormalities may not be apparent. Maintenance of normal fibrinogen levels is usually sufficient to aid in coagulation, except in late stages.

Renal Failure

Renal failure and uremia impair primary hemostasis through platelet dysfunction, specifically decreased platelet adhesion to the subendothelium and platelet aggregation. However, the exact mechanisms are not known. Uremic toxins such as urea, creatinine, phenolic acids, and guanidinosuccinic acid contribute to the platelet dysfunction. Hemodialysis may be the most effective therapy for the platelet dysfunction due to uremia. However, hemodialysis is typically not used solely to correct coagulopathy. DDAVP may be used if active bleeding is present, given intravenously in a dose of 0.3 micrograms/kg. DDAVP can reduce bleeding associated with procedures in renal failure patients. Cryoprecipitate and conjugated estrogens are additional second-line treatment options. Despite their platelet dysfunction, chronic renal failure patients on dialysis may also be prone to thrombotic complications due to defective fibrinolysis.

Liver Injury

Liver injury may be indirectly associated with coagulopathy. Severe hepatic trauma may lead to hemorrhagic shock and all of its attendant causes of coagulopathy, as described previously. The liver has considerable compensatory function even with extensive direct damage, and thus a small percentage of normal parenchyma is sufficient to produce adequate amounts of coagulation factors and to clear profibrinolytic substances from the circulation. Given that normal hepatic function is maintained with resection of up to 75% of a normal liver, it is unlikely that parenchymal damage alone will result in a clotting abnormality.

■ DIAGNOSIS

Clinical Evaluation

Bleeding in a critically ill patient should be evaluated in a systematic fashion to detect the cause and direct the treatment of the bleeding (Figure 1). In the surgical ICU, the first critical decision in a bleeding patient is to differentiate surgical bleeding from nonsurgical

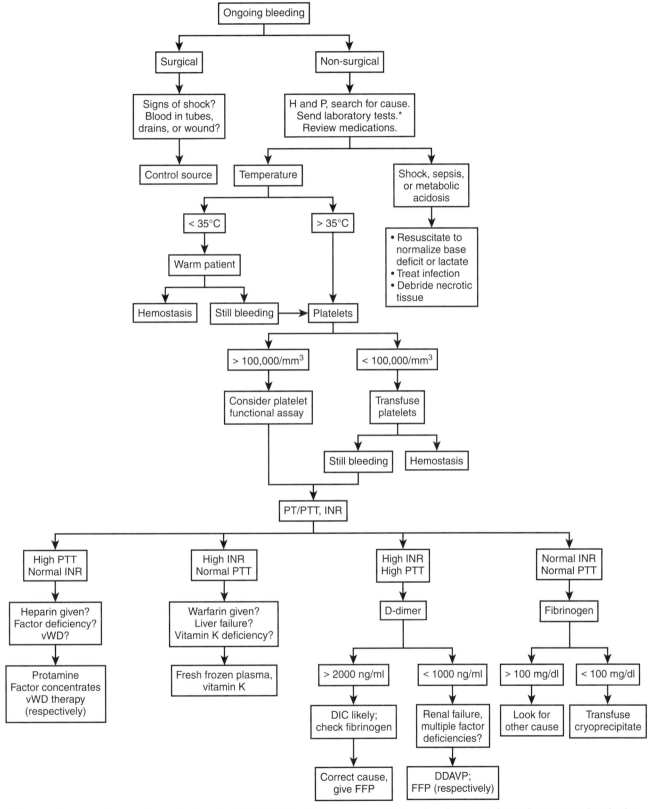

Figure 1   Approach to patients with bleeding. *INR, PT/PTT, platelet count, arterial blood gas for base deficit or lactate; consider platelet function assay and thromboelastogram. *DDAVP,* 1-deamino-8-D-arginine vasopressin; *PT,* prothrombin time; *PTT,* partial thromboplastin time; *vWD,* von Willebrand disease.

coagulopathic microvascular bleeding. This may be one of the most difficult decisions a surgeon can face. A nontherapeutic operation on a coagulopathic patient may exacerbate the vicious cycle, but leaving a surgically correctable source of bleeding untouched can prove fatal.

The evaluation begins with a detailed history, especially review of operative notes if the patient has had surgery or invasive procedures. Physical examination may reveal blood in operative wounds, tubes, or drains that indicate a source of bleeding requiring reoperation. Conversely, oozing of blood from multiple sites or seemingly minor wounds (e.g., intravenous catheter sites) may indicate coagulopathy. All recently administered medications should be reviewed for drugs that may affect hemostasis, in addition to reviewing the patient's medical history.

Postoperative bleeding may be considered in the broad categories of loss of surgical hemostasis versus coagulation disorders. Loss of surgical hemostasis is bleeding at the operative site, which may be due to technical problems such as slipped ligature or inadequate hemostasis from the procedure. During an operation, vasoconstriction may prevent visible bleeding—but with warming and resuscitation bleeding resumes. Loss of surgical hemostasis usually requires definitive control through reoperation. Postoperative surgical bleeding may be associated with signs and symptoms ranging from hypovolemia to hemorrhagic shock. The physician should intervene based on early signs of shock (tachycardia, restlessness, anxiety, pallor, oliguria), and not wait until shock is glaringly obvious. Anxiety or agitation in a postoperative surgical patient should prompt first an assessment of perfusion and oxygenation, before analgesics or sedatives are given. Hypotension is a late sign of hemorrhage, indicating severe volume deficit.

Coagulation disorders may be grouped into those affecting primary hemostasis (formation of initial platelet plug) or secondary hemostasis (clotting factors and the coagulation cascade). These groups may be subdivided into qualitative defects (e.g., dysfunctional platelets, factor inhibition by heparin) or quantitative defects (e.g., thrombocytopenia, factor deficiencies). Furthermore, these conditions may be congenital or acquired. The algorithm presented in Figure 1 represents one example of a systematic approach that can help guide therapy in most surgical patients, even if the exact cause of the coagulopathy is not evident. It is intended to aid rapid assessment and initiation of treatment in the ICU, rather than as a definitive guide to diagnosis of specific bleeding disorders.

A few basic laboratory tests are helpful in guiding diagnosis and treatment of coagulopathy. It is worthwhile first to reiterate that the primary goal of therapy is clinical hemostasis, and not complete normalization of every clotting parameter. Platelet count, PT, INR, and PTT are the minimum basic lab tests needed to help differentiate problems with primary or secondary hemostasis. A baseline hematocrit level should be checked, keeping in mind that acute hemorrhage will not be reflected by a change in hematocrit until dilution of the intravascular space occurs from fluid shifts and intravenous fluid administration. Thromboelastography (TEG) is a global test of coagulation that may help define the etiology of a coagulopathy. Fibrin split products, D-dimer, and fibrinogen levels are rarely necessary in the setting of hemorrhagic shock-induced coagulopathy but may help confirm a clinical diagnosis of DIC. Each test is discussed in more detail in the following section.

Laboratory Tests of Coagulation

PT: This test is done by adding a thromboplastin containing TF, phospholipid, and calcium to citrated plasma and measuring the time in seconds until a fibrin clot is formed compared to a control. The PT measures the activity of the extrinsic pathway (factor VII) and the common pathway (fibrinogen, factors II, IX, and X). It is used to monitor warfarin therapy, and is affected by depletion of the vitamin-K–dependent factors (factors II, VII, IX, and X, and proteins C and S).

INR: The INR is used to adjust for individual lab variation in the PT, using the formula INR = (log patient PT/log control PT) to the power of "c," where c is the international sensitivity index (ISI). The thromboplastin used in individual laboratories is thus calibrated against a reference thromboplastin. The INR was developed to monitor the degree of warfarin anticoagulation.

PTT: The PTT is done by adding a partial thromboplastin (mixture of phospholipids), an activating substance, and calcium chloride to citrated plasma. It measures the activity of the intrinsic pathway (HMW kininogen, prekallikrein, and factors VIII, IX, XI, and XII) and the common pathway (fibrinogen, factors II, IX, and X). Only factor VII activity is not measured by the PTT.

Bleeding time: The bleeding time is a test of platelet function and primary hemostasis. However, due to variation in the performance of the test it is relatively insensitive and nonspecific in identifying platelet function abnormalities and may not predict surgical bleeding.

Platelet function tests: Several tests of platelet function are available through the lab or as point-of-care tests. Our hospital has abandoned the bleeding time in favor of the PFA-100 (Platelet Function Analyzer, Dade-Behring). The PFA-100 measures platelet function by the time it takes whole blood to occlude an aperture in a filter as it flows under high shear conditions. It is a global test of primary hemostasis that may detect platelet dysfunction due to certain disorders or medications, and congenital diseases such as vWD, but its role has not yet been completely defined. Other tests measure the percentage of platelets working normally to determine the functional platelet count, and are used often during cardiac surgery. Several point-of-care tests are available to assess platelet inhibition by drugs such as aspirin or GPIIb/IIIa inhibitors. Platelet aggregation tests use several agonists in different concentrations to induce aggregation in platelet-rich plasma, and will reveal quantitative or qualitative defects. It is a gold standard test but takes hours to perform, making it less useful in acute coagulopathy management.

TEG: TEG is reported as a graph of clot formation in a sample of whole blood (Figure 2). The TEG tracing is drawn based on several factors, including rate of clot formation, fibrin cross-linking, and platelet-fibrin interaction. By measuring various parameters of the

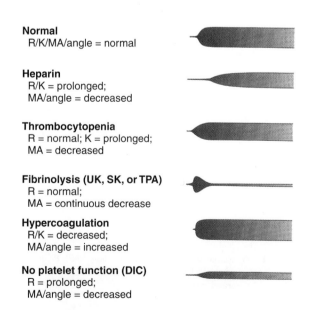

Normal
R/K/MA/angle = normal

Heparin
R/K = prolonged;
MA/angle = decreased

Thrombocytopenia
R = normal; K = prolonged;
MA = decreased

Fibrinolysis (UK, SK, or TPA)
R = normal;
MA = continuous decrease

Hypercoagulation
R/K = decreased;
MA/angle = increased

No platelet function (DIC)
R = prolonged;
MA/angle = decreased

Figure 2 Thromboelastogram (TEG). *(Adapted from Kaufmann CR, et al: Usefulness of thromboelastography in assessment of trauma patient coagulation. J Trauma 42:716, 1997.)*

tracing, TEG provides an assessment of platelet function, coagulation enzyme activity, and the overall degree of coagulability. It can identify conditions such as primary fibrinolysis, consumptive coagulopathy, anticoagulant therapy, and the effect of hypothermia. TEG is used frequently during cardiopulmonary bypass, liver transplantation, and in intensive care settings due to its rapid availability and ability to assess the components of coagulation in an integrated fashion.

TT: The TT is done by adding thrombin to citrated plasma +/− calcium. The TT measures the time for conversion of fibrinogen to fibrin, which is induced by thrombin. It is prolonged when fibrinogen is deficient (<100 mg/dl) or abnormal, in the presence of circulating anticoagulants (including fibrin split products [FSPs] and heparin), and during excessive fibrinolysis. Its high sensitivity to exogenous anticoagulants such as heparin limit its usefulness in hospitalized patients, but it can be used to detect low levels of circulating heparin that do not cause changes in the PTT.

Fibrinogen: Fibrinogen is a large protein that is cleaved by thrombin to produce fibrin monomers, which cross-link to form a fibrin clot in the presence of factor XIII. Fibrinogen levels may fall with the excess clotting seen in consumptive coagulopathy or with overanticoagulation by thrombolytic agents. It is also an acute-phase reactant, increasing in response to physiologic stress.

FSPs: FSP's are fragments of the fibrin molecule that result from breakdown of fibrin by plasmin. The test is nonspecific, but elevated levels may indicate fibrinolysis and support a clinical picture of consumptive coagulopathy. The D-dimer is a specific form of FSP that is most closely associated with DIC.

Factor assays: Specific coagulation factor levels can be used to help diagnose certain diseases or deficiencies (for example, factor VIII for hemophilia A and factor IX for hemophilia B). Other assays may detect deficiencies in factors V, VII, X, XI, and XII (Hagemann factor), prekallikrein, and HMWK, all of which are very rare. Factor assays are used infrequently in the ICU setting.

MANAGEMENT

Blood Product Transfusion

Fresh Frozen Plasma

FFP is prepared by extracting the noncellular portion of blood and freezing it within hours of donation. One 250- to 300-ml unit of FFP contains all clotting factors and about 400 mg of fibrinogen, and will increase clotting factor levels by about 3%. The PT and PTT should be used during FFP therapy to gauge the efficacy of transfusion.

Indications for FFP administration in the surgical ICU are relatively few. These include coagulopathy with clinical bleeding, accompanied by measured or suspected factor deficiency as indicated by a PT or PTT more than 1.5 times normal, and emergent correction of a prolonged PT due to acquired coagulopathy from warfarin, liver disease, or DIC. FFP should not be used for volume replacement, nutrition, to promote wound healing, hypoalbuminemia, empirically during massive transfusion, or as part of a preset formula based on number of red blood cell transfusions. Avoiding unnecessary transfusion is important to reduce risks of transfusion reaction and transfusion-related acute lung injury (TRALI), as well as for cost control. The dose of FFP should be aimed at a minimum of 30% of normal plasma factor concentration and clinical hemostasis. Practically, 10–15 ml/kg of FFP are sufficient for this purpose, although lower volumes are usually adequate (5–8 ml/kg) to reverse warfarin.

Platelets

Treatment of thrombocytopenia or platelet dysfunction centers on the underlying cause and the patient's clinical condition. In the absence of active bleeding or imminent surgery, platelet counts above

10,000/mm^3 do not require treatment—whereas counts below 10,000/mm^3 warrant platelet transfusion to prevent spontaneous bleeding. Patients with microvascular bleeding and thrombocytopenia may benefit from platelet transfusion after excluding hypothermia because the transfused platelets will not function properly at low temperatures. Evidence-based guidelines are lacking for surgical patients with platelet counts between 50,000/mm^3 and 100,000/mm^3, and therapy should take into account the patient's condition, risk of significant bleeding, and plans for surgery or high-risk invasive procedures (e.g., ventriculostomy).

In general, platelet transfusion is not indicated at these levels in the absence of microvascular bleeding. Patients with consumptive coagulopathy rarely benefit from platelet transfusion because the same process consumes newly transfused platelets. However, microvascular bleeding in the presence of sepsis or DIC usually warrants treatment. If surgery or invasive procedures are necessary in the presence of a consumptive process and low platelet count, platelet transfusion should be given just before or during the procedure to maximize the number of circulating platelets available for hemostasis.

Different platelet concentrates are available. The traditional "six-pack" from random donor concentrates contains platelets from multiple individuals and equals six units of platelet concentrates. One unit of single-donor platelets, also called apheresis platelets, contains roughly the same volume of platelets as 6 random donor units but has the advantage of originating from one person and thereby exposing the recipient to only one set of antigens. One can expect a rise in platelet count by about 30,000/mm^3 for each unit of single-donor platelets and for each 6 units of random donor. Repeated platelet transfusion may lead to alloantibody formation in some patients, making them refractory to further platelet transfusions. HLA-matched or cross-matched platelets may be required in such cases. The use of single-donor platelet transfusions has been adopted by many institutions to minimize antibody formation and preserve the response to a platelet transfusion for as long as possible.

Cryoprecipitate

Cryoprecipitate is prepared by thawing FFP to 1° C to 6° C and then removing and refreezing the insoluble precipitate that forms. Each bag of cryoprecipitate has a volume of approximately 15 ml and contains 150–250 mg fibrinogen per bag, along with 80–100 factor VIII units and other components such as vWf and fibronectin. It is usually given as a pooled product containing 8–10 bags, resulting in transfusion of 1200–2500 mg of fibrinogen. Although it is not virus inactivated, it is thoroughly screened for virus—resulting in extremely low risk of transmission. Cryoprecipitate is used for treatment of hemophilia A, vWD, hypofibrinogenemia, in DIC when serum fibrinogen levels fall below 100 mg/dl, and when the previously cited factors need to be replaced in a low volume of fluid. Cryoprecipitate has little role in treating the coagulopathy of hemorrhagic shock, where factor replacement (when needed) is accomplished with FFP because volume is not an issue and fibrinogen replacement is rarely necessary.

Reversal of Warfarin

The prevalence of preinjury warfarin use among trauma patients increases with age. The effect of this drug on morbidity and mortality in trauma is variable, but potentially significant. Emergent reversal of warfarin anticoagulation is occasionally required in patients with TBI or serious injury associated with hemorrhage, and slower reversal is often used for patients with increased risk of bleeding due to trauma or perioperative status. Before initiating therapy, several factors should be considered—including urgency of warfarin reversal, expected length of time until re-anticoagulation, and cardiac function of the patient (i.e., tolerance of volume loading).

Reversal of warfarin is guided by the INR and is best managed by standardized evidence-based guidelines. Vitamin K takes 8–12 hours to take effect, and is the first-line choice for nonemergent treatment of a high INR. However, it has a long half-life and high or repeated doses should be avoided if re-anticoagulation with warfarin is anticipated in the next several days. Oral vitamin K is preferred for nonemergent reversal of warfarin, whereas the subcutaneous route is not recommended because of inefficient absorption. Patients receiving intravenous vitamin K should have continuous cardiac monitoring due to the risk of anaphylaxis. FFP is the standard therapy for patients with a high INR and significant bleeding or need for invasive procedures.

Many elderly patients on warfarin have concomitant heart disease, and caution must be used to avoid precipitating congestive heart failure with overly aggressive fluid loading. In our experience, an INR greater than 2 is rarely normalized with only one or two units of FFP. In addition, patient factors vary considerably—resulting in an unpredictable and nonlinear dose-response relationship. Recombinant activated factor VII (rFVIIa) may be used when immediate reversal of anticoagulation is required in emergent situations such as severe TBI or life-threatening bleeding. However, data on its proper use in these conditions is limited. rFVIIa's half-life is only a fraction of that of warfarin, and thus it must be used in conjunction with FFP and vitamin K to maintain normal coagulation. Table 1 is an example of a management scheme for patients on warfarin with an elevated INR and risk of bleeding.

Reversal of Heparin

Unfractionated heparin (UFH) and low-molecular-weight heparin (LMWH) are used commonly in the surgical ICU for venous thromboembolism prophylaxis or treatment of other conditions. Although risk of major bleeding events with prophylactic doses is low, full anticoagulation is associated with higher risk. When nonsurgical bleeding occurs in patients anticoagulated with heparin, reversal of the drug's effects may be necessary. The half-life of UFH is about an hour, and thus most treatment doses are reversed by holding the infusion for 6 hours. When immediate reversal is desired, protamine may be used. Protamine binds heparin and neutralizes its effects. The dose is 1 mg of protamine for each 100 units of heparin given. The half-life of heparin must be taken into account when calculating the protamine dose, such that the dose of heparin must be halved for each hour since its injection. If a continuous infusion has been used, the cumulative dose must be estimated. Protamine administration carries risks of hypotension, which may be avoided by slow injection

over 10 minutes, and a 1% risk of anaphylaxis in patients who have had previous exposure to protamine or NPH insulin.

The half-life of LMWH varies with the particular agent used, but in general ranges from 2 to 5 hours. LMWH is only partially neutralized by protamine, which reverses most of the anti-IIa (thrombin) activity but only some of the anti-Xa activity. The reversal is based on the level of anti-Xa activity, in a dose of 1 mg protamine per 100 anti-Xa units.

Recombinant Activated Factor VIIa

rFVIIa is a synthetic form of coagulation factor VII, intended to promote hemostasis. It is an FDA-approved drug for bleeding in hemophilia patients with inhibitors, but has also been used in a variety of other conditions. The primary mechanism of action has been debated. When bound to exposed TF in the subendothelium, rFVIIa can activate factors X and IX—which then promote thrombin formation. This mechanism would explain its localized activity at sites of injury. Other data suggest that high-dose rFVIIa acts independently of TF by activating factor Xa on the platelet surface.

rFVIIa has proven efficacious in reducing blood loss and improving survival in multiple animal studies of its use for the coagulopathy of hemorrhagic shock, and in reducing blood loss and operative time in humans undergoing radical prostate surgery. In blunt trauma patients, rFVIIa reduces the need for blood transfusion and for massive transfusion. A similar significant benefit was not seen in patients with penetrating trauma, however. Initial concerns about an increased risk of thrombosis with rFVIIa have not been borne out. Studies have revealed no evidence of systemic thrombi or increased risk of thrombotic complications in animals or humans.

The optimal dose of rFVIIa for surgical patients has not yet been determined. Doses ranging from 20 to 200 micrograms/kg have been used successfully in clinical trials. Due to the drug's short half-life, certain conditions such as severe coagulopathy may require a second or third dose within a few hours of the first to maintain hemostasis while other contributing factors are aggressively treated. Until specific guidelines are developed through future large multicenter trials, use of rFVIIa should be directed in accordance with local hospital policies, economic considerations, and specific patient variables.

The current expense of the drug precludes its routine use in most bleeding conditions. We have employed a multidisciplinary approach to develop guidelines for use of rFVIIa on our Trauma Service, and have limited prescribing authority to certain specialists. Our guidelines promote use of rFVIIa in two specific conditions: severe hepatic trauma requiring surgery and coagulopathy from hemorrhagic shock (as diagnosed by operating surgeon in the presence of microvascular bleeding) that is unresponsive to standard therapy. Its use in other conditions, such as TBI, remains unspecified.

CONCLUSIONS

Coagulopathy is commonly encountered in critically ill or injured patients. When bleeding is encountered, the first priorities should be control of bleeding and resuscitation with crystalloids and blood. Congenital disorders should be considered. The patient should also be evaluated for acquired coagulopathies, including those resulting from medications. Coagulopathy frequently accompanies massive bleeding and resuscitation, and its etiology in this setting is multifactorial. Although dilution is frequently invoked as the primary pathophysiologic process, hypothermia, acidosis, and shock generally play more important roles.

The use of blood components should be guided by objective evidence of coagulation abnormalities (including clinical findings and laboratory data) rather than resorting to formula-based replacement. Selective use of components (especially platelet transfusion) will yield safer and more effective therapy. Such an approach should lead

Table 1: Management Options for Patients with Warfarin Anticoagulation and Bleeding Risk

Clinical Context	Treatment Options
INR < 5, no significant bleeding	Hold warfarin
INR > 5, no significant bleeding	Vitamin K 1–5 mg orally
INR > 1.5, bleeding or high risk of bleeding, nonemergent	FFP in 2- to 4-unit doses, recheck INR after each dose, until bleeding stopped or INR < 1.5 Consider vitamin K 5 mg orally
INR > 1.5, life-threatening bleeding or emergent surgery or invasive procedure required	FFP in 4-unit doses, recheck INR after each dose, *and* vitamin K 10 mg slow IV infusion Consider factor 7a (repeat in 2–3 hours if still bleeding)

to more effective management of coagulopathy and more judicious use of blood component therapy. Continued advances in the field present novel opportunities to affect coagulation, but the fundamental principles still apply in the patient with hemorrhage: control bleeding rapidly, expeditiously resuscitate from shock, manage temperature carefully, and monitor the patient for clinical and laboratory evidence of coagulation abnormalities.

SUGGESTED READINGS

Aird WC: Sepsis and coagulation. *Crit Care Clin* 21:417, 2005.

Ansell J, et al: The pharmacology and management of the vitamin K antagonists: the seventh ACCP conference on antithrombotic and thrombolytic therapy. *Chest* 126(Suppl 3):204S, 2004.

Bernard GR, et al: Safety and dose relationship of recombinant human activated protein C for coagulopathy in severe sepsis. *Crit Care Med* 29:2051, 2001.

Boffard KD, et al: Recombinant factor VIIa as adjunctive therapy for bleeding control in severely injured trauma patients: two parallel randomized, placebo-controlled, double-blind clinical trials. *J Trauma* 59:8, 2005.

Boccardo P, et al: Platelet dysfunction in renal failure. *Semin Thromb Hemost* 30(5):579, 2004.

Cable R, et al: Practice guidelines for blood transfusion: a compilation from recent peer-reviewed literature. American National Red Cross, 2002. http://www.redcross.org/services/biomed/profess/pgbtscreen.pdf.

Committee on Trauma of the American College of Surgeons: *Advanced Trauma Life Support Course for Doctors*, 7th ed. Chicago, American College of Surgeons, 2004, p. 69.

Cosgriff N, et al: Predicting life-threatening coagulopathy in the massively transfused trauma patient: hypothermia and acidoses revisited. *J Trauma* 42:857, 1997.

Demetriades D, et al: Liver cirrhosis in patients undergoing laparotomy for trauma: effect on outcomes. *J Am Coll Surg* 199:539, 2004.

Fakhry SM, et al: Hematologic principles in surgery. In Townsend CM, Beauchamp RD, Evers BM, Mattox KL, editors: *Sabiston Textbook of Surgery: The Biological Basis of Modern Surgical Practice*, 16th ed. Philadelphia, WB Saunders, 2001, p. 68.

Forsythe SM, Schmidt GA: Sodium bicarbonate for the treatment of lactic acidosis. *Chest* 117:260, 2000.

Gando S: Disseminated intravascular coagulation in trauma patients. *Semin Thromb Hemost* 27(6):585, 2001.

Gando S, et al: Coagulofibrinolytic changes after isolated head injury are not different from those in trauma patients without head injury. *J Trauma* 46:1070, 1999.

Gentilello LM et al: Is hypothermia in the victim of major trauma protective or harmful? A randomized, prospective study. *Ann Surg* 226(4):439, 1997.

Holcomb JB: Use of recombinant activated factor VII to treat the acquired coagulopathy of trauma. *J Trauma* 58:1298, 2005.

Jurkovich GJ, et al: Hypothermia in trauma victims: an ominous predictor of survival. *J Trauma* 27:1019, 1987.

Kashuk JL, et al: Major abdominal vascular trauma—a unified approach. *J Trauma* 22:672, 1982.

Kujovich JL: Hemostatic defects in end stage liver disease. *Crit Care Clin* 21:563, 2005.

Levi M: Disseminated intravascular coagulation: what's new? *Crit Care Clin* 21:449, 2005.

Mannucci PM: Treatment of von Willebrand's disease. *N Engl J Med* 351:683, 2004.

Mina AA, et al: Complications of preinjury warfarin use in the trauma patient. *J Trauma* 54:842, 2003.

Oung CM et al: In vivo study of bleeding time and arterial hemorrhage in hypothermic versus normothermic animals. *J Trauma* 35:251, 1993.

Owings JT, Gosselin RC: Bleeding and transfusion. In Fink MP, Jurkovich GJ, Kaiser LR, Pearce WH, Pemberton J, Soper NJ, editors: *ACS Surgery: Principles & Practice*. New York, Web MD Corp, 2003. www.acssurgery.com.

Rodgers RPC, Levin J: A critical reappraisal of the bleeding time. *Semin Thromb Hemost* 16:1, 1990.

Stein SC, Smith DH: Coagulopathy in traumatic brain injury. *Neurocrit Care* 1:479, 2004.

The American Society of Anesthesiologists Task Force on Blood Component Therapy: practice guidelines for blood component therapy. *Anesthesiology* 84(3):732, 1996.

Valeri CR, et al: Hypothermia induced reversible platelet dysfunction. *Ann Surg* 205:175, 1987.

Watts DD, et al: Hypothermic coagulopathy in trauma: effect of varying levels of hypothermia on enzyme speed, platelet function, and fibrinolytic activity. *J Trauma* 44:846, 1998.

Wolberg AS, et al: A systematic evaluation of the effect of temperature on coagulation enzyme activity and platelet function. *J Trauma* 56:1221, 2004.

Wojcik R, et al: Preinjury warfarin does not impact outcome in trauma patients. *J Trauma* 51:1147, 2001.

MANAGEMENT OF ENDOCRINE DISORDERS IN THE SURGICAL INTENSIVE CARE UNIT

Anthony J. Falvo and Mathilda Horst

The endocrine system as a part of the neuroendocrine axis (hypothalamic-pituitary axis) influences the response to stress and critical illness. Endocrine abnormalities within this axis change and modify the physiologic response to trauma and stress. Critically ill patients with a known diagnosis of an endocrine problem are treated with replacement therapy. However, an unrecognized endocrine abnormality often creates management difficulties and increases morbidity. Endocrine problems occur at all levels of the neuroendocrine axis from primary or secondary disease, medications, or end-organ failure.

The neuroendocrine axis is responsible for the stress response and is controlled by the hypothalamus, pituitary, and the autonomic nervous system (Figure 1). This axis is activated by baroreceptor response to intravascular volume, sympathetic response from tissue injury, and inflammatory mediators released from tissue trauma. The hormones released in response to injury act through binding to cell surface receptors or intracellular receptors and produce a complex series of responses and feedback loops that maintain cellular processes.[1] This chapter addresses abnormalities in the endocrine system that affect the course of critically ill patients.

BRAIN PROBLEMS: ABNORMALITIES IN HYPOTHALAMIC/PITUITARY RESPONSE

Injuries that affect the brain can interrupt the hypothalamus or pituitary production of hormone. Head injury, brain surgery, mass lesions or infiltrative diseases, vascular or hypoxic injuries, and cerebral infections cause failure of the releasing and pituitary

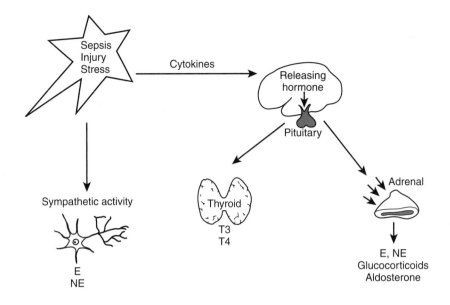

Hypothalamus: releasing hormones

- Corticotropin releasing hormone (CRH): stimulates the release of adrenocorticotropic hormone (ACTH)
- Thyrotropin releasing hormone (TRH): stimulates the release of thyroid stimulating hormone (TSH)
- Antidiuretic hormone (ADH)/vasopressin: increased production in the hypothalamus and release from the posterior pituitary

Pituitary: stimulating hormones

- Adrenocorticotropic hormone (ACTH): stimulates the adrenal gland
- Thyroid stimulating hormone (TSH): stimulates the thyroid gland
- Antidiuretic hormone (ADH)/vasopressin: multiple organs affected including the vascular system and the kidney

Figure I   Neuroendocrine axis. *E,* Epinephrine; *NE,* norepinephrine.

hormones—resulting in single or combined abnormalities. Cerebral edema or increased intracranial pressure is thought to restrict the blood flow to the hypothalamic pituitary area. Frequently encountered abnormalities are diabetes insipidus (DI), syndrome of inappropriate antidiuretic hormone (SIADH), and cerebral salt wasting. These syndromes cause abnormalities of sodium and water balance. Evaluation of volume status, urine and serum sodium, and osmolality are required to determine which syndrome is present. This evaluation is important because the treatment depends on which abnormality is present (Table 1).

Diabetes Insipidus

DI is caused by lack of vasopressin (antidiuretic hormone [ADH]), which causes water diuresis of more than 3 l/day, dehydration, and hypernatremia. The urine is dilute with urine osmolality of less than 300 mOsm/kg and urine specific gravity of less than 1.005. Urine osmolality greater than 800 mOsm/kg excludes DI. The diagnosis is usually made when dilute urine output exceeds 200 ml for 2 consecutive hours.[2] A dramatic rise in serum sodium occurs in the ICU patient population unless fluids are aggressively replaced. In the neurosurgery

Table 1: Comparison of Central Causes of Sodium and Water Abnormalities

	Diabetes Insipidus	Cerebral Salt Wasting	SIADH
Serum sodium	↑	↓	↓
Serum osmolality (mOsmo/kg)	>290	<280	<280
Urine osmolality (mOsmo/kg)	<300	>100	>100
Urinary sodium (mEq/l)	Variable	>20	>20
Volume depletion	Yes	Yes	No
Treatment	dDAVP, water replacement	Normal saline	Fluid restriction

dDAVP, 1-Desamino-8d-arginine vasopressin; *SIADH,* Syndrome of inappropriate antidiuretic hormone.

patient population, the incidence of DI is 3.7% with a mortality of 70%.[2] DI commonly occurs in association with severe brain injury and herniation. The treatment is fluid rehydration and vasopressin replacement via IV dDAVP 2 to 4 mcg/day or intranasally 10 to 60 mcg/day. Frequent monitoring of electrolytes and central venous pressure monitoring are necessary. The water deficit is calculated and slowly replaced. Caution should be used when severe hypernatremia is present, with half the water deficit replaced in 24 hours to avoid demyelination (Table 2).

SIADH and Cerebral Salt Wasting

The syndrome of inappropriate antidiuretic hormone and cerebral salt wasting are linked through a common cause—traumatic brain injury—and common result—hypotonic hyponatremia. Cerebral salt wasting is most often associated with subarachnoid hemorrhage, whereas SIADH is also associated with brain injury, tumors, and medications (Table 3).[3] The cause of SIADH is excessive release of ADH that leads to water retention and an increase in extracellular fluid volume. Volume expansion increases renal sodium excretion, producing hyponatremia. Cerebral salt wasting is thought to involve

Table 2: Formulas for Water Deficit and Sodium Deficit

Water deficit = 0.6 × (wt kg) × (Na −140/140) (0.5 for females)
Sodium deficit = 0.6 × (wt kg) × (140 − Na) (0.5 for females)

Table 3: Medications That Interfere with Thyroid Hormone and ADH

Drugs Causing Syndrome of Inappropriate Antidiuretic Hormone (SIADH):

ADH analogs: vasopressin, oxytocin, desmopressin

Stimulating ADH release: opiates, opioids, barbiturates, nicotine, thiazides, isoproterenol, cyclic antidepressants, MAO inhibitors, haloperidol, risperidone, acetylcholine

Enhancing renal sensitivity: NSAIDs, acetaminophen

Stimulating ADH release and enhancing renal sensitivity: chlorpropamide, tolbutamide, cyclophosphamide, chlorambucil

Phosphodiesterase inhibition: theophylline

Other: amiodarone, ACE inhibitors, loop diuretics, thiazide diuretics, general anesthesia

Drugs That Influence Thyroid Function:

Influence conversion: glucocorticoids, beta blockers, contrast agents, amiodarone, propylthiouracil

Increase TSH: cimetidine, dopamine antagonists, haloperidol, iodide, lithium, contrast agents, metoclopramide

Decrease TSH: adrenergic agonists, dopamine, steroids, opiates, phenytoin, phentolamine

Increase binding: estrogens, methadone, 5-FU, heroin, tamoxifen

Decrease binding: steroids, androgens, heparin, salicylates, seizure medications, furosemide

NSAID, Nonsteroidal anti-inflammation drug.

disruption of the neural input to the kidney or central secretion of a natriuretic factor. Sodium is wasted by the kidney, causing extracellular volume depletion and stimulation of ADH secretion. Hyponatremia develops with extracellular volume depletion.

In both syndromes, the diagnosis begins with serum sodium less than 135 mmol/l. Measurement of serum osmolality is less than 280 mOsm/kg, and the urine osmolality is greater than 100 mOsm/kg in both diseases. The differentiating factor is the effective blood volume, which is normal in SIADH and low in cerebral salt wasting. Low effective blood volume causes orthostatic blood pressure, tachycardia, low central venous pressure (CVP), low urine sodium, chloride, and fractional excretion of sodium with high BUN. Both disease states have low uric acid level. With correction of the salt deficit, uric acid levels normalize in SIADH and not in cerebral salt wasting.[3] The treatment of SIADH is fluid restriction (800–1000 ml/day) and occasional hypertonic saline. Demelocycline, phenytoin, and lithium are used for chronic SIADH. The treatment for cerebral salt wasting is normal saline fluid replacement to expand the extracellular fluid compartment (see Table 1).

ABNORMALITIES IN THYROID RESPONSE

Untreated or unrecognized thyroid problems (excess or deficit) create life-threatening illness in critically ill patients. Thyroid hormones are responsible for the metabolic rate in all tissues. Critical illness may alter the production of thyroid hormone through thyroid-stimulating hormone (TSH) regulation, peripheral metabolism, or alteration in binding proteins. Cytokines as well as commonly used intensive care unit (ICU) medications (see Table 3) affect thyroid hormone function.

Nonthyroidal illness has been described in critically ill patients. Symptoms from thyroid function abnormalities are a continuum from hyperthyroidism to thyroid storm and hypothyroidism to myxedema coma.

Thyroid Excess

Hyperthyroidism with a 3% incidence in out-patients is caused by Grave's disease, goiter, and adenoma. Treatment with amiodarone increases the incidence to 9%.[4] Thyroid storm (severe hyperthyroidism) was first recognized after thyroidectomy in unprepared patients and now encompasses 1%–2% of all admissions for thyrotoxicosis (with a mortality of 20%–30%).[5] It is precipitated by physiologic stress related to specific events such as surgery, trauma, childbirth, severe illness, overdose of thyroid medication, iodine in medications, and contrast. The classic symptomatology includes fever, cardiovascular abnormalities, and mental status changes. The tachycardia is out of proportion to the fever. Fever is the hallmark of this disease, with temperatures to 106° F. A state of high-output cardiac failure can develop with bounding pulses, rales and hepatomegaly, and thyroidal bruit. Atrial fibrillation and congestive heart failure are common in elderly patients with hyperthyroidism and can occur without fever (thyrocardiac crisis). The mental status changes include a broad spectrum, from anxiety to coma. There can be nonspecific gastrointestinal (GI) complaints and clinical findings of Grave's disease.

This syndrome is recognized by clinical signs and symptoms. Laboratory test turnaround time is long, and treatment should be started based on clinical suspicion. The TSH is not detectable, and both T3 and T4 are elevated (with T3 > T4).[6] There is an associated elevation of white blood counts (WBCs), calcium, blood glucose, and liver function tests. The treatment is directed toward decreasing the production of thyroid hormone and preventing its release, blocking the peripheral action, supportive care, and treating the cause (Table 4).[7]

Table 4: Treatment of Thyroid Storm

Inhibit hormone synthesis: propylthiouracil 1000 mg loading dose, and then 300 mg orally every 6 hours

Blunt end-organ effects: propranolol 1–10 mg IV push, then 20–120 mg orally every 6 hours *or* esmolol 250 mcg/kg loading dose IV over 1 minute, and then 50 mcg/kg/minute infusion

Stop hormone release: sodium iodide 500 mg orally or IV every 8 hours

Block peripheral conversion: propranolol or hydrocortisone 50–100 mg IV every 8 hours

Supportive treatment:

    Intensive care unit monitoring

    Treat congestive heart failure

    Treat hyperthermia with cooling blanket or acetaminophen

Thyroid Deficit

Hypothyroidism occurs in patients over age 50 years, 8% females and 2% males.[8] Previous surgery, radiation, and autoimmune disease are the most common causes. Myxedema coma is severe hypothyroidism. Myxedema coma is rare, but has a mortality rate of more than 60%.[5] It is precipitated by physiologic stress of trauma, surgery, burns, infections, cardiovascular events or cold temperatures, or failing to take thyroid medication. Medications can decrease hormone production and function (see Table 3). The cardinal findings relate to reduced metabolic rate and oxygen consumption and include hypothermia, bradycardia, hypotension, hypoventilation, and mental status changes.[8] The mental status changes range from lethargy to coma and are associated with decreased deep tendon reflexes. Low cardiac output with both right- and left-sided failure and decreased myocardial contractility occur. There is slowing of the GI system, with constipation or ileus. Skin, nail, and hair changes associated with hypothyroidism are present. The name myxedema comes from the infiltration of mucopolysaccharide infiltration of the skin. This is a clinical diagnosis with elevated TSH, very low T4 and hyponatremia, low blood glucose, elevated CPK, low PaO_2, and elevated PCO_2. There are characteristic EKG changes (Table 5).

The treatment of myxedema coma includes supportive care in an ICU setting and replacement of thyroid hormone. ICU care includes EKG monitoring and possibly cardiac pacing, arterial blood gas monitoring with possible intubation and ventilation, warming with blankets and external warmers and IV fluid with glucose, temperature monitoring, and neurologic checks. Thyroxine is given

Table 5: EKG Findings in Hypothyroidism

Sinus bradycardia

Low-voltage QRS complex

Flat or inverted T waves

Prolonged intervals of PR, QRS, QT

Heart block

300 to 500 mcg IV on day 1 and then 50 to 100 mcg IV every day until oral replacement is started.[7,8] Adrenal insufficiency should be tested for with the rapid cosyntropin test and treated with 100 mg of hydrocortisone IV every 8 hours.[5]

Sick Euthyroid Syndrome

Sick euthyroid or nonthyroidal illness is a common finding in the ICU patient population. It is not completely clear if this syndrome represents a pathologic process or a means of adapting to critical illness. There are three patterns of abnormal thyroid function, which represent a progression of disease severity: decreased T3, decreased T3 and T4, and decreased T3, T4, and TSH (Table 6).[7] Patients with decreased T3 alone usually have mild to moderate illness. This pattern is the most common pattern of the sick euthyroid syndrome. The peripheral conversion of T4 to T3 is decreased. Mainly this pattern is the effect of medications (see Table 3). Serum T4 levels are increased early in acute illness related to decreased conversion or increased binding levels. This pattern is seen with elderly patients and patients with psychiatric problems. The most severe pattern has decreased T3, T4, and TSH. The free T4 may be low, normal, or elevated. In addition to conversion problems, the binding proteins are low (as is TSH). The decline in T4 correlates with prognosis. Mortality increases as the T4 level drops below 4 mcg/dl and is 80% at T4 levels of 2 mcg/dl.[1,7]

The diagnosis requires trending thyroid function tests. These tests may serve as markers of the severity of disease rather than treatable thyroid disease. The treatment of sick euthyroid syndrome is unclear. Both thyroid replacement and no treatment are advocated.[9] Animal studies show improvement with thyroid replacement, but human studies have not shown similar results. Therefore, currently treatment is not advised.

ABNORMALITIES OF ADRENAL FUNCTION

The adrenal glands are an important part of the neuroendocrine axis. The adrenals produce glucocorticoids, catecholamines, mineralcorticoids, and sex hormones. Clinical problems arise with either excess production or insufficient production. Cortisol is required for normal function of all cells, and deficiency states in critical illness are associated with increased morbidity and mortality. Catecholamines are produced in the adrenal medulla and require cortisol for synthesis. Sex hormones are not required for recovery from critical illness and there is some compensation for loss of mineral-corticoid activity. The two abnormalities discussed here are pheochrocytoma and adrenal insufficiency.

Pheochromocytoma

Pheochromocytomas produce excess catecholamines and follow the rule of 10s: 10% are malignant, 10% are extraadrenal, 10% are incidental findings on radiographic studies, and 10% are multiple. Less than 0.2% of patients with hypertension have pheochromocytoma as their diagnosis.[10] The diagnosis is usually not made in the ICU, but patients

Table 6: Abnormalities in Thyroid Response

	Myxedema Coma	Thyroid Storm	Sick Euthyroid		
			Mild	**Moderate**	**Severe**
TSH	↑	↓	↔	↔	↓
T3	↓	↑	↓	↓	↓
T4	↓	↑	↔	↓	↓

require ICU management for hypertensive crisis or perioperative care. The patients usually have the classic triad of headache, sweating, and tachycardia or palpitations. Weekly paroxysms of hypertension occur in at least 75% of patients.[11] This is due to rapid release of catecholamines from an inciting event. Other symptoms include blurred vision, orthostatic hypotension, weight loss, polyuria, and polydipsia.

Clinical suspicion leads to urinary and plasma evaluation for catecholamines and metabolites. These tests confirm the diagnosis 95% of the time.[12] If these tests are inconclusive, a clonidine suppression test is performed with 0.3 mg of clonidine given orally 12 hours after antihypertensives have been stopped. No beta blockers, diuretics, or tricyclic antidepressants can be used. Alpha blockers will not affect the test. The patients without a pheochromocytoma have a fall of the plasma catecholamines to less than 500 pg/ml.[13] The tumor is localized with a computed tomography (CT) scan or magnetic resonance imaging (MRI). The CT has a risk of exacerbating the hypertension with its contrast. Failure to detect the tumor with these studies leads to an MIBG, octreoscan, total body MRI, or selected venous sampling.

Acute hypertensive crisis requires treatment with sodium nitroprusside or phentolamine. Phentolamine is given as an IV bolus of 2.5–5 mg, repeated every 5 minutes until the blood pressure is controlled. Nitroprusside is dosed at 0.5–10 mcg/kg/minute.[11]

Preparation for surgery requires alpha blockade, which is initiated with phenoxybenzamine 10 mg orally daily and increased every few days until symptoms and blood pressure are under control. B-blockade can then be initiated to control the tachycardia, but only after alpha blockade has been performed. Surgery will generally proceed in 10–14 days. Postoperatively, patients require monitoring and fluid resuscitation. The alpha blockade is continued.

Adrenal Insufficiency

Controversy exists over the incidence, diagnosis, and treatment of adrenal insufficiency in ICU patients.[14] The incidence is less than 0.01% in the general population but up to 28% in seriously ill patients.[15] Reported mortality is as high as 25%, but this mortality rate may be reduced with early recognition to 6%–11%.[16] Cortisol is needed in the critically ill patient for appropriate response to acute inflammation and vasomotor stability. Cortisol has metabolic, catabolic, anti-inflammatory, and vasoactive properties. The most common cause of adrenal insufficiency remains adrenal suppression from the administration of steroids. This effect lasts up to a year after the discontinuation of steroids. In the ICU, adrenal gland destruction can occur from infection, bleeding, or system inflammation. However, decreased cortisol concentration during critical illness without anatomic disruption is the more common cause. This secondary adrenal insufficiency is usually related to sepsis.[7,17]

In critically ill patients, the usual signs and symptoms of adrenal insufficiency are not usually apparent. These critically ill patients often have hemodynamic instability despite fluid resuscitation and vasopressor use. This is a tip-off to adrenal insufficiency and should lead to evaluation of cortisol level and treatment. The most common abnormalities in ICU patients with adrenal insufficiency are listed in Table 7.[18] Several signs and symptoms exist if the patient had preexisting adrenal insufficiency. These include fatigue, weight loss, nausea, abdominal pain, arthralgias, syncope, hyperpigmentation of the skin, vitiligo, anorexia, and decreased libido.

In ICU patients, clinical suspicion leads to a random cortisol test. If the cortisol level is low with a random level less than 15 mcg/dl, adrenal insufficiency is present and treatment begins. With a random level greater than 35 mcg/dl, adrenal insufficiency is unlikely. If the level is between these two values, a stimulation test is performed with 250-mcg IV synthetic ACTH. Cortisol levels are drawn at 0, 30, and 60 minutes after the ACTH. If the cortisol level changes 9 mcg/dl or more, adrenal insufficiency is unlikely. If the cortisol changes less than 9 mcg/dl, adrenal insufficiency is likely and treatment occurs.[17]

Table 7: ICU Patient Suspicious for Adrenal Insufficiency

Hypotension unresponsive to vasopressors and fluids
Abdominal pain
Nausea/vomiting
Recent steroid use
Tachycardia
Fever
Hypoglycemia
Hyponatremia
Hyperkalemia
Eosinophilia

The patient is treated immediately after a stimulation test is performed. Dexamethasone is used. It will not interfere with the stimulation test as hydrocortisone does. Do not wait for the results. If the stimulation test comes back as normal, the steroids can be discontinued. Hydrocortisone 50 mg IV every 6 hours with 50 mcg fluorocortisone daily orally is used for those patients with adrenal insufficiency in shock on vasopressors. This therapy is continued for 7 days (Figure 2).[19] For patients with proven adrenal insufficiency but not in shock, hydrocortisone 50 mg IV every 6 hours is given. This dose can then be tapered over several days as the illness subsides. Retesting after the illness can determine if this was a primary adrenal problem and transient or if it is a secondary adrenal insufficiency and requires further workup and treatment.

PROBLEMS WITH HYPERGLYCEMIA

Hyperglycemia occurs in most critically ill patients. Diabetes and undiagnosed diabetes may contribute to hyperglycemia. However, in critically ill patients increased sympathetic activity and the activation of the cytokine cascade are the major causes of elevated blood glucose. Medications (total parenteral nutrition, beta blockers, cyclosporine, catecholamines, and glucocorticoids) promote hyperglycemia. Electrolyte imbalance (hypokalemia) decreases insulin release and contributes. The stress-induced increased sympathetic activity leads to increased glycogenolysis, increased hepatic gluconeogenesis, and peripheral insulin resistance—which cause an increase in the serum glucose. Cytokines produced by the inflammatory process promote insulin resistance and/or activate the hypothalamic-pituitary-adrenal axis.[14] All or many of these factors come into play in the critically ill patient and produce an imbalance between glucose production and uptake, resulting in hyperglycemia.

Regardless of the mechanism of hyperglycemia, organ system dysfunction occurs in the cardiovascular, cerebrovascular, neuromuscular, and immunologic systems. Hyperglycemia in the cardiovascular population has been widely studied.[20,21] An increased risk of in-hospital mortality has been found in patients with myocardial infarction and hyperglycemia. Insulin deficiency/resistance is associated with increased free fatty acids, which the heart uses as a fuel source. These free fatty acids are toxic to the ischemic myocardial cells and lead to arrhythmias. Hyperglycemia also causes an osmotic diuresis, leading to volume depletion and increased oxygen consumption from increased contractility.[7]

Hyperglycemic patients with ischemic stroke and head injury have worse outcomes than patients who are euglycemic. With elevated blood glucose levels, there is an increased risk of in-hospital mortality after ischemic stroke in nondiabetic patients. Persistent hyperglycemia is an independent predictor of infarct expansion and is associated with worse functional outcome in patients with ischemic stroke.[22] There may be an association with tissue plasminogen activator and hemorrhagic transformation in hyperglycemic patients with ischemic

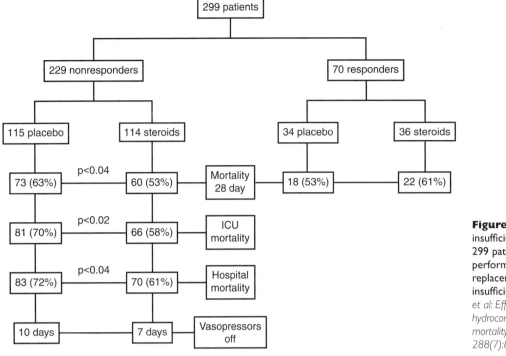

Figure 2 Outcome of proven adrenal insufficient patients. Study including 299 patients with ACTH stimulation test performed showing the results of steroid replacement to those with adrenal insufficiency. *(Data from Annane D, et al: Effect of treatment with low doses of hydrocortisone and fludrocortisone on mortality in patients with septic shock.* JAMA *288(7):862–869, 2002.)*

stroke. In patients with head injury, both the Glasgow coma scale and mortality appear related to blood glucose levels—with an inverse relationship to the Glasgow coma scale and survival.[23]

Increased brain glucose levels contribute to the acidosis from the glycolysis induced by anaerobic metabolism of the ischemic brain tissue. The lactic acidosis promotes the formation and accumulation of free radicals, which impede mitochondrial activity. This effect is most important at the edge of the infarct, where neurons that may survive are recruited into the infarct. Many animal models have shown infarct size increasing with hyperglycemia. Both disruption of the blood/brain barrier and hemorrhagic infarct conversion are suggested mechanisms for deterioration of brain function.[24]

Polyneuropathy of critical illness appears to be related to blood glucose levels. Van den Berghe et al. screened for polyneuropathy in critically ill patients and found that patients with control of hyperglycemia were less likely to have critical-illness neuropathy.[25] They also found that in those patients who developed neuropathy there was more rapid resolution. There was a positive linear correlation between blood glucose levels and risk of polyneuropathy. The mechanism of polyneuropathy and its association with hyperglycemia has yet to be defined.

Postoperative wound infections, pneumonias, urinary tract infections, and bacteremias are increased in patients with hyperglycemia. The immunologic system is impaired by hyperglycemia through action on the white blood cells. Polymorphonuclear cells have impaired chemotaxis, phagocytosis, and oxidative burst pathways. Macrophages have impaired phagocytosis and deceased complement fixation. Collagen deposition is impaired, granulocyte adherence is irregular, and there is decreased bactericidal activity.[7]

Evidence is accumulating that control of blood glucose in the normal range improves outcome from critical illness (Figure 3). Van den Berghe et al. showed that tight glycemic control of blood glucose 80 to 110 mg/dl reduced morbidity and mortality in the surgical ICU, with reduction of episodes of septicemia and length of stay in the ICU.[25] Two large patient population studies showed that control of blood glucose to less than 200 mg/dl in cardiothoracic surgery patients reduced the incidence of deep wound infections.[26,27] Improved survival after myocardial infarction occurs with glycemic control. Evidence is lacking for improved neurologic outcomes with glycemic control.

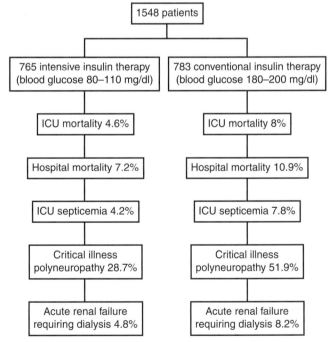

Figure 3 Outcome of tight glycemic control. *(Data from Van Den Berghe, et al: Intensive insulin therapy in critically ill patients.* N Engl J Med *345(19):1359–1367, 2001.)*

The hyperglycemia should be rapidly controlled with IV insulin to a normal glucose range (Table 8). Rapid control can easily be achieved with continuous insulin infusion.[28] Patients with renal failure, liver failure/resection, and transplantation are susceptible to hypoglycemia.

Although the neuroendocrine axis is important for maintaining homeostasis, abnormalities in hormone production occur frequently in the critically ill. Clinical suspicion is required to diagnosis the abnormalities. Early aggressive treatment appears to improve morbidity and mortality related to these disorders.

Table 8: Tight Glycemic Control Protocol for the Surgical ICU of Henry Ford Hospital, Detroit, MI

A. Starting Insulin Infusion		
Glucose	151–219 mg/dl	>220 mg/dl
Starting insulin dose	Give 2 units regular insulin IVP and start 2 units/hr. If renal failure (creatinine >2), liver failure, liver transplant or kidney transplant, start at 1 unit/hr.	Give 4 units regular insulin IVP and start 4 units/hr. If renal failure (creatinine >2), liver failure, liver transplant, or kidney transplant, start at 2 units/hr.

B. Maintenance Insulin Drip for Glucose ≤110 mg/dl		
Glucose Level	**Insulin Rate 1–3 Units/Hr**	**Insulin Rate >3 Units/Hr**
<41 mg/dl	D/C infusion. Give 1 amp dextrose 50% IVP. Notify physician. Check glucose hourly until glucose greater than 80, then every 2 hours. When >100, restart drip at 1 unit/hr. Notify physician when glucose greater than 80.	D/C infusion. Give 1 amp dextrose 50% IVP. Notify physician. Check glucose hourly until glucose greater than 80, then every 2 hours. When >100, restart drip but reduce rate by 50%. Notify physician when glucose greater than 80.
41–60 mg/dl	D/C infusion. Give ½ amp dextrose 50% IVP. Notify physician. Check glucose hourly until glucose greater than 80, then every 2 hours. When >100, restart drip at 1 unit/hr. Notify physician when glucose greater than 80.	D/C infusion. Give ½ amp dextrose 50% IVP. Notify physician. Check glucose hourly until glucose greater than 80, then every 2 hours. When >100, restart drip but reduce rate by 50%. Notify Physician when glucose greater than 80.
61–80 mg/dl	D/C infusion: Recheck glucose *every hour*. When glucose greater than 100, restart drip at 1 unit/hr.	D/C infusion: Recheck glucose *every hour*. When glucose greater than 100, restart insulin infusion but decrease dose rate 50%.

If insulin drip turned off for glucose less than 80 and three checks in a row are less than 100 (every 2 hours × 3), restart protocol from beginning. Change glucose check to every 4 hours, and cover with regular insulin IV push 2 units for glucose 110–150 mg/dl and start insulin drip for first glucose greater than 150 mg/dl.

| 81–110 mg/dl | No change unless: If previous glucoses higher, reduce drip by 1 unit/hr. (If current dose 1 unit/hr, do not change.) | No change unless: If previous glucose higher, reduce per below: |

Infusion Rate	Decrease Dose by
4–7 units/hr	1 unit/hr
8–12 units/hr	2 units/hr
13–17 units/hr	3 units/hr
18–22 units/hr	4 units/hr
>22 units/hr	5 units/hr

C. Maintenance Insulin Drip for Glucose ≥111 mg/dl		
Glucose	**Insulin Dosage All Others**	**Insulin Dosage for: Renal Failure (Creatinine >2), Liver Failure, or Liver or Kidney Transplant**
111–150 mg/dl	Increase drip rate by 0.5 unit/hr (no bolus). Continue same rate if last glucose was higher value.	No change.
151–200 mg/dl	Give 2 units regular insulin IVP and increase drip rate by 1 unit/hr.	Give 2 units regular insulin IVP and increase drip rate by 0.5 unit/hr.
201–250 mg/dl	Give 4 units regular insulin IVP and increase drip rate by 1 unit/hr.	Give 4 units regular insulin IVP and increase drip rate by 0.5 unit/hr.
251–300 mg/dl	Give 6 units regular insulin IVP and increase drip rate by 1 unit/hr.	Give 6 units regular insulin IVP and increase drip rate by 0.5 unit/hr.
301–400 mg/dl	Give 8 units regular insulin IVP and increase drip rate by 1 unit/hr.	Give 8 units regular insulin IVP and increase drip rate by 0.5 unit/hr.
>400 mg/dl	Call MD for new order.	Call MD for new order.

REFERENCES

1. Nylen ES, Muller B: Endocrine changes in critical illness. *J Intensive Care Med* 19(2):67–82, 2004.
2. Boughey JC, Yost MJ, Bynoe RP: Diabetes insipidus in the head-injured patient. *Am Surg* 70(6):500–503, 2004.
3. Palmer BF: Hyponatremia in a neurosurgical patient: syndrome of inappropriate antidiuretic hormone secretion versus cerebral salt wasting. *Nephrol Dial Transplant* 15:262–268, 2000.
4. Braithwaite SS: Thyroid Disorders. In Parrillo JE, Dellinger RP, editors: *Critical Care Medicine: Priniciples of Diagnosis and Management in the Adult*, 2nd ed. St. Louis, Mosby, 1235–1256, 2002.
5. Sarlis NJ: Loukas gourgiotis: thyroid emergencies. *Rev Endocr Metabol Disord* 4:129–136, 2003.
6. Franklyn J: Thyrotoxicosis. *Clin Med* 3(1):11–14, 2003.
7. Goldberg PA, Inzucchi SE: Clinical issues in endocrinology. *Clin Chest Med* 24:583–606, 2003.
8. Ringel MD: Management of hypothyroidism and hyperthyroidism in the intensive care unit. *Crit Care Clin* 17(1):59–75, 2001.
9. Stathotos N, Levetan C, Burman KD, et al: The controversy of the treatment of critically ill patients with thyroid hormone. *Best Pract Res Clin Endocrinol Metab* 15(4):465–478, 2001.
10. Rusnak RA: Adrenal and Pituitary Emergencies. *The Emeregency Medicine Clinic of North America* 7(4):903–925, 1989.
11. Brouwers FM, Lenders JW, Eisenhofer G, et al: Pheochromocytoma as an endocrine emergency. *Rev Endocr Metabol Disord* 4:121–128, 2003.
12. Vaughn ED: Diseases of the adrenal gland. *Med Clin North Am* 88:443–466, 2004.
13. Grossman E, Goldstein DS, Hoffman A, Keiser A: Glucagon and clonidine testing in the diagnosis of pheochromocytoma. *Hypertension* 17:733, 1991.
14. Gropper MA: Evidence-based management of critically ill patients: analysis and implementation. *Anesth Analg* 99(2):566–572, 2004.
15. Rivers EP, Gaspari M, Saad GA, et al: Adrenal insufficiency in high-risk surgical ICU patients. *Chest* 119:889–896, 2001.
16. Barquist E, Kirton O: Adrenal insufficiency in the surgical intensive care unit. *J Trauma* 42(1):27–31, 1997.
17. Cooper MS, Stewart PM: Corticosteroid insufficiency in acutely ill patients. *N Engl J Med* 348(8):727–734, 2003.
18. Angelis M, Yu M, Takanishi D, et al: Eosinophilia as a marker of adrenal insufficiency in the surgical intensive care unit. *J Am Coll Surg* 183:589–596, 1996.
19. Annane D, Sebille V, Charpentier C, et al: Effect of treatment with low doses of hydrocortisone and fludrocortisone on mortality in patients with septic shock. *JAMA* 288(7):862–871, 2002.
20. Capes SE, Hunt D, Malmberg, et al: Stress hyperglycemia and increased risk of death after myocardial infarction in patients with and without diabetes: a systematic overview. *Lancet* 355:773–778, 2000.
21. Malmberg K: Prospective randomised study of intensive insulin treatment on long term survival after acute myocardial infarction in patients with diabetes mellitus. *BMJ* 314(7093):1512–1515, 1997.
22. Baird TA, Parsons MW, Phanh T, et al: Persistent poststroke hyperglycemia is independently associated with infarct expansion and worse clinical outcome. *Stroke* 2208–2214, 2003.
23. Laird AM, Miller PR, Kilgo PD, et al: Relationship of early hyperglycemia to mortality in trauma patients. *J Trauma* 56(5):1058–1062, 2004.
24. De Courten-Myers GM, Kleinholz M, Holm P, et al: Hemorrhagic infarct conversion in experimental stroke. *Annals of Emergency Medicine* 21(2):120–126, 1992.
25. Van den Berghe G, Wouters P, Weekers F, et al: Intensive insulin therapy in critically ill patients. *N Engl J Med* 345(19):1359–1367, 2001.
26. Furnary AP, Zerr KJ, Grunkemeier GL, et al: Continuous intravenous insulin infusion reduces the incidence of deep sternal wound infection in diabetic patients after cardiac surgical procedures. *Ann Thorac Surg* 67:352–362, 1999.
27. Zerr KJ, Furnary AP, Grunkemeier GL, et al: Glucose control lowers the risk of wound infection in diabetics after open heart operations. *Ann Thorac Surg* 63:356–361, 1997.
28. Zimmerman CR, Mlynarek ME, Jordan JA, et al: An insulin infusion protocol in critically ill cardiothoracic surgery patients. *Ann Pharmacother* 38:1123–1129, 2004.

TRANSFUSION: MANAGEMENT OF BLOOD AND BLOOD PRODUCTS IN TRAUMA

Lena M. Napolitano

Approximately 15% of all blood transfusions in the United States are used in the care of patients that have sustained traumatic injury. Blood transfusion in trauma is life-saving for those patients in hemorrhagic shock who are unresponsive to crystalloid fluid resuscitation. Importantly, concomitant attempts at prompt cessation of hemorrhage are also necessary. Blood transfusion in trauma has also been identified as an independent predictor of multiple-organ failure (MOF), systemic inflammatory response syndrome (SIRS), increased postinjury infection, and increased mortality in multiple studies. The cumulative risks of blood transfusion have been related to the number of units of packed red blood cells (PRBCs) transfused, increased storage time of transfused blood, and possibly donor leukocytes. Lack of efficacy of red blood cell transfusion in critically ill patients has also been documented.[1] Therefore, once hemorrhage control has been established in acute trauma we should attempt to minimize the use of blood transfusion for the treatment of asymptomatic anemia in trauma patients.

A number of potential mechanisms that may mediate adverse affects associated with blood transfusion in trauma have been proposed, including increased systemic inflammatory response, immunomodulation, microcirculatory dysfunction due to altered RBC deformability, increased nitric oxide binding by free hemoglobin and vasoconstriction, and others. These data have led some to conclude that blood transfusion in the injured patient should be minimized whenever possible.[2]

INCIDENCE: WHO NEEDS BLOOD TRANSFUSION IN TRAUMA?

Trauma patients in hemorrhagic shock have an absolute indication for PRBC transfusion if they are unresponsive to isotonic crystalloid fluid resuscitation, have ongoing significant hemorrhage, and manifest physiologic signs of persistent shock (hypotension, tachycardia, oliguria, lactic acidosis, abnormal base deficit)—indicating that oxygen consumption is dependent on hemoglobin concentration (critical oxygen delivery).[3] In these patients, the prompt transfusion of PRBCs in conjunction with prompt hemorrhage control can be life-saving.

Patients with hemorrhagic shock, identified by a metabolic acidosis and increasing base deficit, have been documented to require increased blood and plasma transfusion (Table 1). A single-institution study in calendar year 2000 documented that 8% (479 of 5645) of acute trauma

Table 1: Blood Transfusion Requirements in Trauma Patients and Admission Base Deficit

Admission Base Excess	Interpretation	Units PRBCs in First 24 Hours	Total Units PRBCs	Total Units FFP
≥–2	Normal	0–1	1–2	0–1
–3 to –5	Mild base deficit	1–2	2–3	0–1
–6 to –9	Moderate base deficit	3–4	5–6	1–2
≤–10	Severe base deficit	8–9	9–10	3–4

FFP, Fresh frozen plasma; *PRBC,* packed red blood cells.
Modified from Davis JW, Parks SN, et al: Admission base deficit predicts transfusion requirements and risk of complications. *J Trauma* 41:769–774, 1996.

patients received PRBCs, using 5219 units. The majority (62%) of transfusions were administered in the first 24 hours of care. Only 3% of patients (*n* = 147) received more than 10 units of PRBCs, and these patients also received plasma and platelet transfusions to treat actual or anticipated dilutional coagulopathy. Mortality rates in trauma patients who require blood transfusion is high, ranging from 27% to 39%.[4]

A recent study identified independent risk factors for blood transfusion in trauma (*n* = 1103), including increased age, admission from scene, trauma mechanisms of motor vehicle crash or fall from height, admission systolic blood pressure <120 mm Hg, free fluid on abdominal ultrasound, and unstable pelvis on clinical examination (Table 2). The probability of RBC transfusion in the emergency

Table 2: Risk Factors Associated with Blood Transfusion in Emergency Room After Severe Trauma

Variable	Score	Odds Ratio (95% CI)
Age (Years)		
0–20	0	2.0 (0.9–4.3)
20–60	0.5	5.6 (2.3–13.4)
>60	1.5	
Admission		
From scene	1.0	2.4 (1.3–4.5)
From other hospital	0	
Trauma Mechanism		
Traffic	1	3.2 (1.7–6.0)
Fall from height >3 m	1	2.4 (1.1–5.2)
Blood Pressure (mm Hg)		
0–90	2.5	12.2 (6.4–23.4)
90–120	1.5	4.1 (2.3–13.4)
>120	0	
Abdominal Ultrasound		
Free fluid	2	8.4 (4.3–16.2)
No fluid	0	
Pelvis on Clinical Examination		
Unstable	1.5	
Stable	0	4.7 (2.1–10.3)
Total risk factor points	9.5	

Adapted from Como JJ, Dutton RP, Scalea TM, Edelman BB, Hess JR: Blood transfusion rates in the care of acute trauma. *Transfusion* 44(6):809–813, 2004.

department was significantly increased if these risk factors were present, and increased substantially with multiple risk factors. An Emergency Room Transfusion Score (ETS) was calculated from these rapidly assessable parameters, ranging from 1 point to 9.5 points maximum. The probability of blood transfusion exponentially increased with the sum of points in the ETS (i.e., from 0.7% at 1 point to 5% at 3 points and 97% at the maximum of 9.5 points).[5]

For severe hemorrhagic shock, type O blood should be transfused.[6] Rh-negative blood should be used in women of childbearing age if possible. A prompt transition to the use of type-specific (ABO, Rh-matched) blood should be accomplished as quickly as possible, and use is continued until fully cross-matched units of blood are available. Once a trauma patient has been administered more than one blood volume and the initial antibody screen is negative, there is no point attempting compatibility testing except for ABO matching.

Once hemorrhage control has been established and the patient has completed resuscitation from hemorrhagic shock, all efforts to restrict RBC transfusion in trauma are advisable. Anemia is common in critically injured trauma patients and persists throughout the duration of critical illness, as documented in a post hoc analysis of a subset of trauma patients (*n* = 576) from a prospective multicenter observational cohort study in the United States.[7] While in the intensive care unit (ICU), 319 (55.4%) trauma patients received a total of 1858 units of blood (or 5.8 ± 5.5 units of blood each) on average. The majority (87.1%, *n* = 278) of all ICU trauma patients requiring transfusions received them within the first 4 days, accounting for almost half of all ICU transfusions. However, 5%–10% of patients continued to receive blood transfusions. Importantly, this study documented that a large number of blood transfusions were administered when the hemoglobin concentration was greater than 10 g/dl.

National guidelines regarding blood transfusion differ, such that the American Society of Anesthesiology[8] recommends maintaining hemoglobin (Hb) greater than 6 gm/dl—whereas the National Institutes of Health[9] (NIH) recommends maintaining Hb greater than 7 g/dl for patients who are critically ill. A Cochrane Database Systematic Review titled *Transfusion Thresholds and Other Strategies for Guiding Allogeneic Red Blood Cell Transfusion* concluded that the limited published evidence (10 trials, *n* = 1780 patients) supports the use of restrictive transfusion triggers (blood transfusion only if Hb <7 g/dl) in patients who are free of cardiac disease.[10]

An analysis from the prospective multicenter randomized controlled trial (Transfusion Requirements in Critical Care, TRICC) compared the use of restrictive (transfuse if Hb <7 g/dl) and liberal (transfuse if Hb <10 g/dl) transfusion strategies in resuscitated critically ill trauma patients (*n* = 203). The average hemoglobin concentrations (8.3 ± 0.62 g/dl vs. 10.4 ± 1.2 g/dl; *p* < 0.0001) and the RBC units transfused per patient (2.3 ± 4.4 vs. 5.4 ± 4.3; *p* < 0.0001) were significantly lower in the restrictive group than in the liberal group. No differences in mortality, multiple-organ dysfunction, or ICU or hospital length of stay were identified—suggesting that a restrictive RBC transfusion strategy appears to be safe for critically ill multiple trauma patients.[11]

RISKS OF BLOOD TRANSFUSION

The blood supply in the United States has never been as safe as it is now. During the past several decades, there have been dramatic progressive reductions in the risk of transfusion-transmitted clinically significant blood-borne infections.[12] Figure 1 summarizes the significant decline in human immunodeficiency virus (HIV), hepatitis B (HBV), and hepatitis C (HCV) risks of transmission through blood transfusion.

Although there has been a 10,000-fold reduction in the risk to patients from transfusion-transmitted infectious diseases in recent decades, there has been little progress in reducing the risk of noninfectious hazards of transfusion. A recent analysis of 366 spontaneously reported deaths and major complications of transfusion in the United Kingdom and Ireland identified that the majority (53%) of these adverse events were related to the incorrect blood component being transfused (i.e., a clerical or human-related error).[13] As a result, patients today are harmed from noninfectious serious hazards of transfusion at a rate that exceeds infectious hazards by 100-fold to 1000-fold (Table 3).

Emerging risks of blood transfusion include West Nile virus (WNV) transmission via blood transfusion. Between August of 2002 and January of 2003, there were 23 confirmed cases of transfusion-associated WNV from 14 donors. Experimental WNV nucleic acid amplification test assays were implemented for blood donor testing in July of 2003. Reports through September 2003 indicated that more than 600 infected units of blood were identified from 2.5 million donations during a period of 4137 known WNV infections reported to the Centers for Disease Control and Prevention (CDC).[14] Although nucleic acid amplification testing of blood donations prevented hundreds of cases of WNV infection, it failed to detect units with a low level of viremia—some of which were antibody negative and infectious. These data sup-

port the use of targeted nucleic acid amplification testing of individual donations in high-prevalence WNV regions, a strategy that was implemented successfully in 2004.[15]

Transfusion-Related Acute Lung Injury

Transfusion-related acute lung injury (TRALI) is a life-threatening complication of blood transfusion. TRALI is now the leading cause of transfusion-related mortality, even though it is probably still underdiagnosed and underreported. The National Heart, Lung and Blood Institute of the NIH convened a working group on TRALI, and a common definition has been established—defined as new acute lung injury occurring during or within 6 hours after a blood transfusion.[16] TRALI, like the acute respiratory distress syndrome (ARDS), may be a two-event phenomenon—with both recipient predisposition and factors in the stored blood units playing major roles.[17] The overall prevalence has been reported as 1 in 1120 cellular components transfused.

A recent prospective cohort study documented a significant independent association between the amount of transfused blood and the development of ARDS and hospital mortality. The association between the amount of transfused blood and the development of ARDS remained significant in a multivariable logistic regression model accounting for differences in severity of illness, type of trauma, race/ethnicity, gender, and base deficit.[18] A larger study in 5260 blunt trauma patients documented that delayed blood transfusion (defined as no blood transfusion received within the initial 48 hours after admission) was independently associated with ventilator-associated pneumonia, ARDS, and death in trauma regardless of injury severity.[19] Similarly, an additional study that examined clinical predictors of ARDS identified that PRBC transfusion was an independent risk factor for increased development of and increased mortality in ARDS.[20] All of these studies mandate a judicious transfusion policy after trauma resuscitation, and emphasize the need for safe and effective blood substitutes and transfusion alternatives.

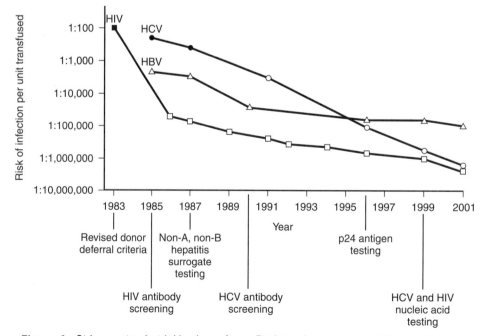

Figure 1 Risks associated with blood transfusion. Decline in human immunodeficiency virus (HIV), hepatitis B (HBV) and hepatitis C (HCV) risks of transmission through transfusion. Data were derived from studies sponsored by the National Heart, Lung and Blood Institute. Estimated risk of infection per unit transfused in 2000–2001 was 1:220,000 for HBV; 1:1,600,000 for HCV; and 1:1,800,000 for HIV. *(From Busch MP, Kleinman SH, Nemo GJ: Current and emerging infectious risks of blood transfusions. JAMA 26;289(8):959–962, 2003.)*

Table 3: Risks Associated with Transfusion

Type of Risk	Incidence
Noninfectious Risks	
Depressed erythropoiesis	Universal
Volume overload, pulmonary edema	10%–40%
Febrile reaction	1/10–1/100
Urticarial reaction	1/33–1/100
Transfusion-related acute lung injury (TRALI)	1/1120–1/5000
Delayed hemolytic transfusion reaction	1/2500
Hemolytic transfusion reactions	1/38,000–1/70,000
Fatal hemolytic transfusion reactions	1/600,000
Anaphylactic shock	1/500,000
Immunosuppression	Unknown
Graft-versus-host disease	1/400–1/10,000
Alloimmunization (RBCs)	1/100
Alloimmunization (platelets)	1/10
ABO-Rh mismatch	
Occurrence	1/6,000–1/20,000
Mortality	1/100,000–1/600,000
Infectious Risks	
Cytomegalovirus conversion	7%
Epstein-Barr virus	0.5%
Bacterial contamination (PRBCs + platelets)	1/2000
Hepatitis B transmission	1/220,000
PRBC-related bacterial sepsis	1/500,000–1/786,000
Hepatitis A transmission	1/1,000,000
West Nile Virus transmission	1/1,400,000
Hepatitis C transmission	1/1,600,000
HIV transmission	1/1,800,000

Adapted from Klein HG: Allogenic transfusion risks in the surgical patient. *Am J Surg* 170;6A:21S–26S, 1995; Silliman CC, Moore EE, Johnson JL, et al: Transfusion in the injured patient: proceed with caution. *Shock* 21(4):291–299, 2004; Busch MP, Kleinman SH, Nemo GJ: Current and emerging infectious risks of blood transfusions. *JAMA* 289(8):959–962, 2003; and Spiess BD: Risk of transfusion: outcome focus. *Transfusion* 44:4S–14S, 2004.

MASSIVE TRANSFUSION

Massive blood transfusion is most commonly defined as complete replacement of a patient's blood volume within a 24-hour period or more than 10 units of PRBCs in 24 hours. Newer definitions include an ongoing blood loss of more than 150 ml/min, or the replacement of 50% of the circulating blood volume in 3 hours or less.[21] These newer definitions have the benefit of allowing early recognition of major blood loss and of the need for effective intervention to prevent hemorrhagic shock and other complications of massive hemorrhage and transfusion.

Massive transfusion therapy for the treatment of hemorrhagic shock requires a coordinated and detailed approach with the fundamental components listed in Table 4. In the absence of a predefined massive transfusion protocol, access to the appropriate blood products (and adequate volume of these products) may be significantly delayed. Without prompt replacement of these blood products, the resultant coagulopathy may worsen and bleeding will continue. In fact, the implementation of an organized "Massive Transfusion Policy" to address exsanguinating hemorrhage in

Table 4: Management of Massive Transfusion for Hemorrhagic Shock

- Provide adequate ventilation and oxygenation.
- Control the source of hemorrhage.
- Restore the circulating volume.
- Start blood component therapy:
  Early transfusion of red blood cells (RBCs) will be required.
  Anticipate coagulopathy, thrombocytopenia.
- Maintain or restore normothermia.
- Evaluate the therapeutic response.
  Test for coagulopathy, thrombocytopenia, and disseminated intravascular coagulation (DIC).
- Know and implement specific local procedures for dealing with the logistic demands of massive transfusion.

the trauma population has proven of benefit in patient outcomes and in reducing blood product utilization. Studies have demonstrated an increase in survival (16%–45%) in patients with exsanguinating hemorrhage following the implementation of such a protocol.[22,23] Guidelines for the treatment of acute massive blood loss are listed in Table 5.

Blood Component Therapy: Fresh Frozen Plasma, Platelets, and Cryoprecipitate

Coagulopathy and thrombocytopenia are a common occurrence during major trauma resuscitation, and hemorrhage remains a major cause of traumatic deaths. Current coagulation factor replacement practices vary, and may be inadequate. A recent pharmacokinetic model was used to simulate the dilutional component of coagulopathy during hemorrhage and compared various fresh frozen plasma (FFP) transfusion strategies for the prevention or correction, or both, of dilutional coagulopathy. This study documented that once excessive deficiency of factors has developed and bleeding is unabated 1–1.5 units of FFP must be given for every unit of PRBC transfused. If FFP transfusion should start before plasma factor concentration drops below 50% of normal, an FFP:PRBC transfusion ratio of 1:1 would prevent further dilution. They concluded that during resuscitation of a patient who has undergone major trauma the equivalent of whole-blood transfusion is required to correct or prevent dilutional coagulopathy.[24]

Ultimately, additional blood product administration for the treatment of dilutional and consumptive coagulopathy and thrombocytopenia in trauma must be guided by blood coagulation testing, with regular monitoring of hemoglobin, platelet count, prothrombin time (PT), partial thromboplastin time (PTT), and fibrinogen levels (see Table 5). Component replacement therapy recommendations differ in many institutions. Some advocate 1:1:1 unit replacements of PRBCs, FFP, and platelets. Others recommend platelet concentrates (1 pack/10 kg) if platelet count falls below 50,000, recognizing that each platelet concentrate also provides about 50 ml of fresh plasma. FFP (12 ml/kg) is administered if the INR, PT, or PTT are greater than 1.5 times control levels. Cryoprecipitate (1–1.5 packs/10 kg) is administered if fibrinogen concentrations are lower than 0.8 g/l. Some suggested massive transfusion protocols include:

- Initial massive transfusion response: 10 units PRBCs, 2 units platelets, 4 units plasma
- Subsequent massive transfusion response: 6–8 units PRBCs, 2 units platelets, 4 units plasma
- Cryoprecipitate requested in patients with reduced fibrinogen concentration

Table 5: Acute Massive Blood Loss: Template for Guidelines

Goal	Procedure	Comments
■ Arrest bleeding.	■ Prompt cessation of hemorrhage ■ Surgical intervention ■ Interventional radiology ■ Angiographic embolization	■ All attempts at early hemorrhage cessation should be initiated, and may include multiple modalities.
■ Restore circulating volume. ■ Resuscitate to a level that restores or maintains vital organ perfusion, but restoration of normal blood pressure should not be attempted until definitive measures have been taken to control hemorrhage	■ Insert large-bore peripheral venous lines. ■ Give adequate volumes of warmed crystalloid, colloid, blood. ■ Aim to maintain adequate mean arterial pressure and urine output (0.5 ml/kg/hour).	■ 14 gauge or larger. ■ Blood loss often underestimated. ■ Refer to Advanced Trauma Life Support guidelines. ■ Keep patients warm.
■ Request laboratory testing.	■ PT, PTT, INR, CBC, blood bank sample for type and cross-match, DIC screen. ■ Ensure correct sample identity. ■ Repeat testing after each one-third blood volume replacement, every 4 hours. ■ Repeat testing after component infusion.	■ Take initial samples on admission. ■ Misidentification is the most common transfusion risk. ■ May need to give FFP and platelets before coagulation tests available if clinical evidence of coagulopathy.
■ Request red blood cells.	■ Severity of hemorrhage determines choice. ■ Immediate need: use group O Rh D neg. ■ Need in 15–60 min: uncross-matched ABO group-specific will be provided when blood group known. ■ Need in 60 min or longer: fully cross-matched blood. ■ When time permits, use blood warmer and/or rapid infusion device. ■ Employ blood salvage if available and appropriate (i.e., minimal contamination).	■ Emergency use of Rh D-positive blood is acceptable if patient is male or postmenopausal female. ■ Laboratory will complete cross-match after issue. ■ Further cross-match not required after replacement of one blood volume (8–10 units PRBCs). ■ Blood warmer indicated if large volumes are transfused rapidly to prevent hypothermia. ■ Salvage contraindicated if wound heavily contaminated.
■ Request platelets. ■ 10 ml/kg body weight for neonate/child). ■ One adult therapeutic dose.	■ May have delayed delivery time. ■ Anticipate platelet count <50 × 10⁹/l after 2 × blood volume replacement. ■ Repeat platelet count 10 minutes and 1 hour after platelet transfusion to assess efficacy.	■ Target platelet count: >100 × 10⁹/l for multiple/CNS trauma or if platelet function abnormal. ■ >50 × 10⁹/l for other situations. ■ May need to use platelets before lab results available (take sample before platelets transfused).
■ Request FFP. ■ 15 ml/kg body weight or 4 units (1 liter) for an adult.	■ Anticipate coagulation factor deficiency after blood loss of 1.5 × blood volume. ■ Aim for PT and PTT <1.5 × control. ■ Allow for 30 minutes thaw time (if pre-thawed FFP not available in hospital).	■ PT and PTT >1.5 × control correlates with increased surgical bleeding. ■ May need to use FFP before lab results available (take sample before FFP transfused).
■ Request cryoprecipitate.	■ To replace fibrinogen and factor VIII. ■ Aim for fibrinogen >1 g/l. Allow for delivery and 30 min thaw time.	■ Fibrinogen <0.8 g/l strongly associated with microvascular bleeding. ■ Fibrinogen deficiency develops early when plasma-poor PRBCs transfused for hemorrhage.
■ Suspect disseminated intravascular coagulation (DIC).	Treat underlying cause if possible.	■ Shock, hypothermia, acidosis leading to risk of DIC. ■ Mortality from DIC is high.

Adapted from Stainsby D, Maclennan S, Hamilton PJ: Management of massive blood loss: a template guideline. *Br J Anaesth* 85:487–491, 2000; and McClelland DBL: Clinical use of blood products. In McClelland DBL, editor: *The Handbook of Transfusion Medicine*, 3rd ed. London, The Stationery Office, 2001, p. 79.

MANAGEMENT OF COMPLICATIONS RELATED TO BLOOD TRANSFUSION

The aim of massive blood transfusion treatment is to restore adequate blood volume, to support hemostasis, maintain oxygen-carrying capacity, and restore or maintain oncotic pressure. Although survival with massive transfusion in trauma has improved, a number of complications related to blood transfusion may occur. Physicians caring for patients that require massive transfusion must anticipate, identify, and rapidly treat these complications to ensure optimal patient outcome.

Thrombocytopenia

Dilutional thrombocytopenia is inevitable following massive transfusion because platelet function declines to zero after only a few days of storage. It has been shown that at least 1.5 times blood volume must be replaced for this to become a clinical problem. However, thrombocytopenia can occur following smaller transfusions if disseminated intravascular coagulation (DIC) occurs or there is pre-existing thrombocytopenia.

Coagulation Factor Depletion

Stored blood contains all coagulation factors except V and VIII. Production of these factors is increased by the stress response to trauma. Therefore, only mild changes in coagulation are due to the transfusion per se, and supervening DIC is more likely to be responsible for disordered hemostasis. DIC is a consequence of delayed or inadequate resuscitation, and the usual explanation for abnormal coagulation indices out of proportion to the volume of blood transfused.

Hypocalcemia

Each unit of blood contains approximately 3 g citrate, which binds ionized calcium. The healthy adult liver will metabolize 3 g citrate every 5 minutes. Transfusion at rates higher than 1 unit every 5 minutes or impaired liver function may thus lead to citrate toxicity and hypocalcemia. Hypocalcemia does not have a clinically apparent effect on coagulation, but patients may exhibit transient tetany and hypotension. Calcium should only be given if there is biochemical, clinical, or electrocardiographic evidence of hypocalcemia.

Hypokalemia and Hyperkalemia

The plasma potassium concentration of stored blood increases during storage and may be greater than 30 mmol/l. Hyperkalemia is generally not a problem unless very large amounts of blood are given quickly. On the contrary, hypokalemia is more common as red cells begin active metabolism and intracellular uptake of potassium restarts.

Acid/Base Disturbances

Lactic acid levels in the blood pack give stored blood an acid load of up to 30–40 mmol/l. This, along with citric acid, is usually metabolized rapidly. Indeed, citrate is metabolized to bicarbonate, and a profound metabolic alkalosis may ensue. The acid-base status of the recipient is usually of more importance, final acid/base status being dependent on tissue perfusion, rate of administration, and citrate metabolism.

Hypothermia

Hypothermia leads to reduction in citrate and lactate metabolism (leading to hypocalcemia and metabolic acidosis), increase in affinity of hemoglobin for oxygen, impairment of red cell deformability, platelet dysfunction, and an increased tendency to cardiac dysrhythmias.

Blood Transfusion and Postinjury Multiple-Organ Failure

Blood transfusion was first identified as an independent risk factor for MOF in a 3-year single-institution prospective cohort study (n = 394) aimed at finding a predictive model for postinjury MOF.[25]

Trauma patients (n = 394) with Injury Severity Score (ISS) of greater than 15 and survival over 24 hours were examined. The following variables were identified as early independent predictors of MOF: age greater than 55 years, ISS 25 or higher, and more than six units of RBCs in the first 12 hours after admission. In addition, base deficit greater than 8 mEq/l (0–12 hours) and lactate greater than 2.5 mmol/l (12–24 hours) were independent predictors of MOF in the subgroup of patients that had these measurements obtained. Whether blood transfusion was simply a surrogate measure of severity of hemorrhagic shock in this study was not fully explored.

A subsequent prospective study by this group confirmed that blood transfusion was an independent risk factor of postinjury MOF, controlling for other indices of shock—including base deficit and lactate.[26] This study had a similar experimental design, with 513 trauma patients with ISS greater than 15 admitted to the ICU who survived >48 hours. A dose–response relationship between early blood transfusion and postinjury MOF was identified and blood transfusion was confirmed as an independent risk factor in 13 of the 15 multiple logistic regression models tested. The odds ratios were high, especially in the early MOF models.

Most recently, this group identified that the incidence, severity, and attendant mortality of postinjury MOF has decreased over the last 12 years despite an increased MOF risk. This is related to improvements in trauma and critical care and to the decreased use of blood transfusion during resuscitation.[27]

Blood Transfusion and SIRS/Mortality

Blood transfusion (in the first 24 hours) in trauma was associated with an increased incidence of systemic inflammatory response syndrome (SIRS, defined as SIRS score ≥2) in 7602 trauma patients studied at a single institution.[28] Blood transfusion within the first 24 hours was administered to 954 patients, comprising 10% of the study cohort. Blood transfusion and increased total volume of blood transfusion was a significant independent predictor of SIRS, ICU admission, and mortality in trauma patients by multinomial logistic regression analysis after stratification for ISS, Glasgow Coma Scale (GCS), and age. Trauma patients who received blood transfusion had a two- to nearly six-fold increase in SIRS ($p < 0.0001$) and more than a four-fold increase in ICU admission (odds ratio [OR] 4.62) and mortality (OR 4.23, $p < 0.0001$), as well as significantly longer ICU and hospital length of stay compared to nontransfused trauma patients.

A recent prospective study confirmed that trauma patients are heavily transfused with allogeneic blood throughout the course of their hospital stay and transfusions are administered at relatively high pretransfusion hemoglobin levels (mean of 9 g/dl). One hundred and four patients (87%) received a total of 324 transfusions, 20 (6%) of which were given in the emergency room, 186 (57%) in the SICU, 22 (7%) post-SICU, and 96 (30%) in the operating room. The mean volume of blood per patient transfused was 3144 (± 2622 ml). Transfusion of more than four units of blood was an independent risk factor for SIRS. Strategies for limiting blood transfusions should be investigated in this population.[29]

BLOOD TRANSFUSION AND MORTALITY

A follow-up study assessed the effect of blood transfusion within the first 24 hours postinjury on outcome in trauma in a larger sample size (n = 15,534, 3-year study, 1998–2000). The study controlled for all potential confounding shock variables (including base deficit, serum lactate, and shock index [heart rate/systolic blood pressure]) on admission, as well as stratification by age, gender, race/ethnicity, GCS, and ISS.[30] Blood transfusion was a strong independent predictor of mortality (OR 2.83, 95% confidence interval [CI] 1.82–4.40, $p < 0.001$), ICU admission (OR 3.27, 95% CI 2.69–3.99, $p < 0.001$), ICU length of stay (LOS) ($p < 0.001$), and hospital LOS (coefficient 4.37, 95% CI 2.79–5.94, $p < 0.001$) when stratified by indices of shock (base deficit, serum lactate, shock index, and anemia). Patients who underwent blood transfusion were almost three times more likely to die. Blood transfusion early after injury (within the first 24 hours) was therefore confirmed as an independent predictor of mortality, ICU admission, ICU LOS, and hospital LOS in trauma after controlling for severity of shock by admission base deficit, lactate, shock index, and anemia.

We also examined blood transfusion and outcome in trauma, dependent on whether patients were transfused less than or more than 24 hours postinjury (Table 6).[31] This retrospective study confirmed our trauma registry data with blood bank data, and delineated the association of blood transfusion and mortality—which was higher (OR 4.13 vs. OR 3.10) when patients were transfused early (<24 hours) after injury.

A retrospective 4-year single-institution review of all adults with blunt hepatic and/or splenic injuries admitted to a Level I trauma recently examined blood transfusion as an independent risk factor for outcome.[32] Of 316 patients presenting with blunt hepatic and/or splenic injuries, 143 (45%) received blood transfusion within the first 24 hours. Of the total, 230 patients (72.8%) were selected for nonoperative management, of whom 75 (33%) required transfusion in the first 24 hours. Transfusion was an independent predictor of mortality in all patients (OR 4.75, 95% CI 1.37–16.4, $p = 0.014$) and in those managed nonoperatively (OR 8.45, 95% CI 1.95–36.53, $p = 0.0043$) after controlling for indices of shock and injury severity. The risk of death increased with each unit of PRBCs transfused (OR per unit 1.16, 95% CI 1.10–1.24, $p < 0.0001$). Blood transfusion was also an independent predictor of increased hospital length of stay (coefficient 5.45, 95% CI 1.64–9.25, $p = 0.005$). Transfusion-associated mortality risk was highest in the subset of patients managed nonoperatively. The authors suggested that prospective examination of transfusion practices in treatment algorithms of blunt hepatic and splenic injuries is warranted.

Another single-institution study examined whether elderly patients are disproportionately affected by blood transfusion in trauma.[33] To determine the possible interaction among age, PRBC transfusion volume, and mortality after injury, a 6-year retrospective review (January 1995 through December 2000) of adult patients who received blood transfusion within the first 24 hours after injury was completed. Of the 1312 patients who received PRBCs in the first 24 hours postinjury, 1028 (78%) were aged 55 years and younger and 284 (22%) were over 55—and overall mortality was 21.2%. Age, ISS, GCS, and PRBC transfusion volume emerged as independent predictors of mortality. Mean PRBC transfusion volume for elderly survivors (4.6 units) was significantly less than that of younger survivors (6.7 units). No patient aged over 75 years with a PRBC transfusion volume greater than 12 units survived. The authors concluded that age and PRBC transfusion volume act independently, yet synergistically, to increase mortality following injury.

Most recently, a 5-year single-institution study confirmed that low hemoglobin, abnormal prothrombin and partial thromboplastin time, and physiologic signs of shock (low systolic blood pressure and elevated base deficit) were independent predictors of mortality in trauma.[34] Currently, the only treatment available for low hemoglobin and signs of hemorrhagic shock in a trauma patient is the transfusion of stored RBCs. Blood transfusions are also associated with increased mortality in two large prospective multicenter studies quantifying the incidence of anemia and the use of RBC transfusions in critically ill patients.[35,36]

BLOOD TRANSFUSION AND INFECTION

Immunosuppression is a consequence of allogeneic blood transfusion in humans and is associated with an increased risk in cancer recurrence rates after potentially curative surgery, as well as with an increase in the frequency of postoperative bacterial infections. A recent metaanalysis has been reported demonstrating the relationship of allogeneic blood transfusion to postoperative bacterial infection.[37] Twenty peer-reviewed articles published from 1986 to 2000 were included in a metaanalysis. Criteria for inclusion included a clearly defined control group (nontransfused) compared with a treated (transfused) group and statistical analysis of accumulated data that included stepwise multivariate logistic regression analysis. In addition, a subgroup of publications that included only the traumatically injured patient was included in a separate metaanalysis.

The total number of subjects included in this metaanalysis was 13,152 (5215 in the transfused group and 7937 in the nontransfused group). The common odds ratio for all articles included in this metaanalysis evaluating the association of allogeneic blood transfusion to the incidence of postoperative bacterial infection was 3.45 (range 1.43–15.15), with 17 of the 20 studies demonstrating a value of $p = 0.05$. These results provide overwhelming evidence that allogeneic blood transfusion is associated with a significantly increased risk of postoperative bacterial infection in the surgical patient.

The common odds ratio of the subgroup of trauma patients was 5.263 (range 5.03–5.43), with all studies showing a value of $p < 0.05$ (range 0.005–0.0001). These results demonstrate that allogeneic blood transfusion is associated with a greater risk of postoperative bacterial infection in the trauma patient when compared with those patients receiving allogeneic blood transfusions (ABTs) during or after elective surgery.

A recent single-institution study documented that blood transfusions (within the first 28 hours after admission) correlate with infections in trauma patients in a dose-dependent manner.[38] All adult patients ($n = 1593$) admitted to the trauma service of a Level I trauma center from November 1996 to December 1999 were studied. Of these, 12.6% developed at least one infection. The overall transfusion rate

Table 6: Blood Transfusion and Outcome After Trauma ($n = 16,824$, 1998–2000)

	Mortality (OR, p)	ICU Admission (OR, p)	ICU LOS (Coef, p)	Hospital LOS (Coef, p)
Blood Tx <24 hours $n = 1618$ Mean 6.64 ± 8.58 U	4.13, <0.001	3.50, <0.001	3.33, <0.001	6.81, <0.001
Blood Tx >24 hours $n = 2427$ Mean 8.37 ± 12.04 U	3.10, <0.001	6.54, <0.001	7.29, <0.001	8.91, <0.001

Notes: Stratified for age, Injury Severity Score, Glasgow Coma Scale, gender, race/ethnicity, base deficit, lactate, and shock index. Statistical analysis by multiple logistic and linear regression. Data excludes patients who died within 24 hours.
ICU, Intensive care unit; *LOS,* length of stay; *OR,* odds ratio; *Tx,* transfusion.

was 19.4%. The infection rate in patients who received at least one transfusion was significantly higher ($p < 0.0001$), at 33.0 versus 7.6% in patients receiving no blood transfusion. Transfusions per patient ranged from 0 to 46 units. There was a clear exponential correlation in patients receiving between 0 and 15 transfusions ($R^2 = 0.757$). Multivariate logistic regression, which was used to identify risk factors for the development of infection, confirmed that transfusion of PRBCs was an independent risk factor for infection (OR 1.084, 95% CI 1.028–1.142, $p = 0.0028$). This study documented a clear dose-dependent correlation between PRBC transfusion and the development of infection in trauma patients. Similarly, studies in critically ill patients have documented increased rates of nosocomial infection in transfused patients compared to nontransfused patients after stratification of severity of illness and age.[39,40]

POTENTIAL MECHANISMS FOR TRANSFUSION-ASSOCIATED ADVERSE OUTCOME

A number of potential mechanisms have been delineated regarding adverse effects of blood transfusion, including increased storage time of blood, decreased RBC deformability resulting in reduced microcirculatory perfusion, increased inflammatory response, immunosuppression and microchimerism (related to donor leukocytes in nonleuko reduced blood), and increased free hemoglobin with nitric oxide binding. Discussion of each of these potential mechanisms is beyond the scope of this chapter.

A recent review of blood transfusion in the critically ill concluded the following: (1) RBC transfusion does not improve tissue oxygen consumption consistently in critically ill patients, either globally or at the level of the microcirculation; (2) RBC transfusion is not associated with improvements in clinical outcome in the critically ill and may result in worse outcomes in some patients; (3) specific factors that identify patients who will improve from RBC transfusion are difficult to identify; and (4) lack of efficacy of RBC transfusion is likely related to storage time, increased endothelial adherence of stored RBCs, nitric oxide binding by free hemoglobin in stored blood, donor leukocytes, host inflammatory response, and reduced RBC deformability.[1]

Decreased Red Blood Cell Deformability

Erythrocyte aggregation parameters and deformability and shape descriptors were analyzed in blood stored for 35 days.[41] RBC deformability was reduced up to 5% compared with that of fresh samples.

Hovav et al.[42] reported that blood storage induced changes in RBCs associated with a continuous increase in their aggregability (Figure 2). Another recent study demonstrated that human RBC deformability decreased by 34% after 4 weeks of storage.[43] During storage, erythrocytes underwent a time-dependent echinocytic shape transformation in another investigation.[44] This transformation increased the suspension viscosity at high and low shear rates. These investigators also confirmed that prestorage leukocyte depletion decreased these effects.

Traumatic injury is also accompanied by a decrease in RBC deformability. RBC shape was examined by scanning electron microscopy in 43 patients with multisystem trauma.[45] Blood samples were taken at admission and every 24 hours afterward for 4–10 days. A significant decrease in the percentage of discoid erythrocytes, compared with the volunteers, was observed in both groups of patients at admission ($p < 0.01$). The percentage of irreversibly changed RBC (spherostomatocytes, spherocytes) was lower in survivors (12.9 ± 2.0% vs. 20.3 ± 9.4%, $p < 0.01$). This study confirmed that RBC shape alterations appear within the first hours after trauma and persist for at least 7–10 days (Figure 3), and these changes are more severe in patients with secondary septic complications.

Hemoglobin-Based Oxygen Carriers

The potential role for hemoglobin-based oxygen carriers (HBOCs) in trauma care is significant. Most authorities believe that the greatest need for HBOCs is in patients with unanticipated acute blood loss, and trauma is the most likely scenario.[46] The advantage of HBOCs is that they do not require blood typing, testing, or crossmatching; can be readily available; do not require refrigeration; and have long shelf lives. Some disadvantages to the HBOCs include their short half-life in the circulation; the possibility of hemoglobin binding to nitric oxide, resulting in vasoconstriction (less likely with the current products due to polymerization); inaccuracy of oxygen saturation monitoring because of methemoglobin; and potential interference with laboratory tests that are based on colorimetric changes from the dissolved plasma hemoglobin. The newer HBOCs currently in clinical investigation and their characteristics compared to stored PRBCs are listed in Table 7.

Clinical trials and preclinical animal studies have documented that HBOCs attenuate the systemic inflammatory response associated with transfusion of stored RBCs, and decrease neutrophil priming, endothelial activation, and systemic release of interleukin 6 (Figure 4).[47] A multicenter prehospital trial is currently ongoing in

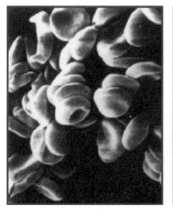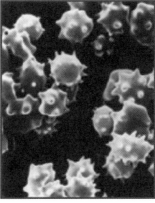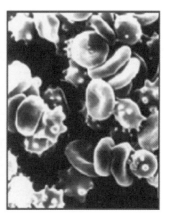

| Day 1 | Day 21 | Day 35 |

Figure 2 Changes in red blood cell shape after traumatic injury. *(From Hovav T, Yedgar S, Manny N, Barshstein G: Alteration of red cell aggregability and shape during blood storage. Transfusion 39(3):277–281, 1999.)*

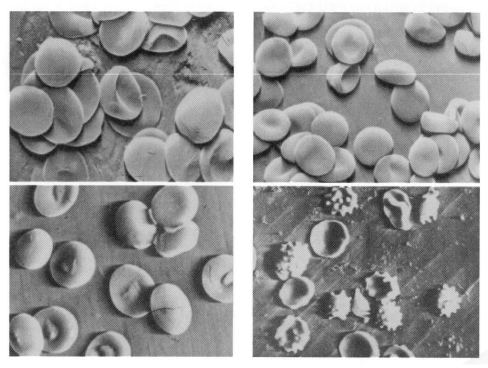

Figure 3 Changes in endogenous red blood cell shape and deformability in trauma patients. *(From Berezina TL, Zaets SB, Machiedo GW: Alterations of red blood cell shape in patients with severe trauma. J Trauma 57(1):82–87, 2004.)*

Table 7: Characteristics of Hemoglobin-Based Oxygen Carriers Used in Phase III Clinical Trials Versus Stored Red Blood Cells

Characteristic	Hemopure	Hemolink	PolyHeme	PRBCs
Source	Bovine	Human outdated PRBCs	Human outdated PRBCs	Human
Manufacturer	Biopure, Inc.	Hemosol, Inc.	Northfield Laboratories, Inc.	—
Polymerization	Yes, glutaraldehyde	Yes, cross-linked with oxidized raffinose	Yes, glutaraldehyde	—
Hemoglobin (g/dl)	13	10	10	13
Unit volume (ml)	250	250	500	250
Unit equivalent (g)	30	25	50	50
P50 (mm Hg)	38	34	29	27
Methemoglobin (%)	<10	<7	<8	<1
Half-life	19 hours	18 hours	24 hours	31 days
Shelf life at 4° C	≥3 years	≥1 year	≥1.5 years	42 days
Shelf life at 21° C	≥2 years	—	≥6 weeks	<6 hours

P50, Oxygen tension when hemoglobin-binding sites are 50% saturated; *PRBC*, packed red blood cells.

which severely injured patients with major blood loss (systolic blood pressure <90 mm Hg) are randomized to initial field resuscitation with crystalloid versus a human polymerized HBOC (PolyHeme). During the hospital phase, the control group is further resuscitated with stored PRBCs—whereas the study group receives HBOC (up to 6 units) in the first 12 hours. The primary study endpoint is 30-day mortality, with secondary endpoints including reduction in allogeneic RBC transfusion, hemoglobin concentrations <5 g/dl, uncrossmatched RBC use, and MOF. A bovine HBOC (Hemopure) is also undergoing additional clinical investigation.

CONCLUSIONS

Despite evolving evidence that transfusion risks outweigh benefits in some patients, the critically injured continue to receive large quantities of blood. Transfusion of the injured patient with stored PRBCs requires careful vigilance during the acute resuscitative and recovery phases postinjury. At present, blood transfusion is the only option for treatment of severe hemorrhagic shock. A more conservative approach to blood transfusion should be utilized in the trauma patient with stable asymptomatic anemia. Development of institutional protocols for transfusion of blood (Figure 5) can assist in appropriate

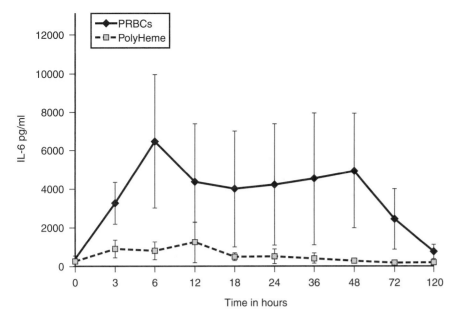

Figure 4 Plasma IL-6 concentrations in critically injured patients randomized to receive packed red blood cell transfusion (PRBCs) versus the human hemoglobin-based oxygen carrier PolyHeme. *(From Johnson J, et al: Alteration of the postinjury hyperinflammatory response by means of resuscitation with a red cell substitute. J Trauma 54:133–140, 2003.)*

A   **Transfusion Guideline for Trauma Patient***

Inflammation and the Host Response to Injury

1. Identify critically ill patient with hemoglobin < 7 gm/dL (or Hct < 21%).
2. If hemoglobin < 7 gm/dL transfusion of PRBCs is appropriate.
   a. For patients with severe cardiovascular disease, a higher transfusion trigger may be appropriate.
3. If hemoglobin > 7gm/dL assess the patient for hypovolemia.
   a. If the patient is hypovolemic, administer IV fluids to achieve normovolemia.
   b. If the patient is not hypovolemic, determine whether there is evidence of impaired oxygen delivery (low S_vO_2, persistent/worsening base deficit, presence/worsening of lactic acidosis).
4. If impaired O_2 delivery present, consider pulmonary artery catheter placement, measure cardiac output, and optimize O_2 delivery.
5. If impaired O_2 delivery not present, monitor hemoglobin as clinically indicated.

* This protocol assumes that acute hemorrhage has been controlled, the initial resuscitation has been completed, and the patient is stable in the ICU without ongoing hemorrhage.

B   **Transfusion Guidelines for Trauma Patient** (excludes immediate resuscitation)

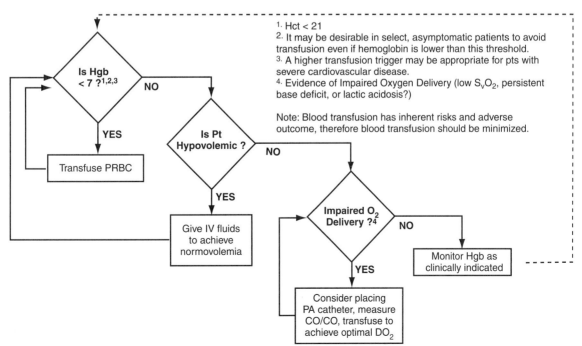

1. Hct < 21
2. It may be desirable in select, asymptomatic patients to avoid transfusion even if hemoglobin is lower than this threshold.
3. A higher transfusion trigger may be appropriate for pts with severe cardiovascular disease.
4. Evidence of Impaired Oxygen Delivery (low S_vO_2, persistent base deficit, or lactic acidosis?)

Note: Blood transfusion has inherent risks and adverse outcome, therefore blood transfusion should be minimized.

Figure 5 Trauma transfusion guideline. Summary of Protocol for Bedside Use. *(From West MA, et al: Inflammation and the host response to injury, a large-scale collaborative project: Patient-oriented research core-standard operating procedures for clinical care. IV. Guidelines for transfusion in the trauma patient. J Trauma 61(2):436–439, 2006.*

utilization of this scarce resource. In an effort to minimize adverse events, immunosuppression, and hyperinflammation, all attempts to minimize the use of blood transfusion in trauma patients is warranted. The future of HBOCs in the treatment of hemorrhagic shock holds great promise and may ultimately lead to better outcomes for injured patients.

REFERENCES

1. Napolitano LM, Corwin HL: Efficacy of red blood cell transfusion in the critically ill. *Crit Care Clin* 20(2):255–268, 2004.
2. Silliman CC, Moore EE, Johnson JL, Gonzalez RJ, Biffl WL: Transfusion of the injured patient: proceed with caution. *Shock* 21(4):291–299, 2004.
3. Napolitano LM: Resuscitation endpoints in trauma. *Transfus Alternatives Transfus Med* 6(4):6–14, 2005.
4. Como JJ, Dutton RP, Scalea TM, Edelman BB, Hess JR: Blood transfusion rates in the care of acute trauma. *Transfusion* 44(6):809–813, 2004.
5. Ruchholtz S, Pehle B, Lewan U, et al: The emergency room transfusion score (ETS): prediction of blood transfusion requirements in initial resuscitation after severe trauma. *Transfus Med* 16(1):49–56, 2006.
6. Dutton RP, Shih D, Edelman BB, et al: Safety of uncrossmatched type-O red cells for resuscitation from hemorrhagic shock. *J Trauma* 59(6):1445–1449, 2005.
7. Shapiro MJ, Gettinger A, Corwin HL, Napolitano LM, et al: Anemia and blood transfusion in trauma patients admitted to the intensive care unit. *J Trauma* 55:269–274, 2003.
8. Practice guidelines for blood component therapy: a report by the American Society of Anaesthesiologists Task Force on Blood Component Therapy. *Anesthesiology* 84:732–747, 1996.
9. National Institutes of Health Consensus Conference. Perioperative red blood cell transfusion. *JAMA* 2700–2703, 1988.
10. Hill SR, Carless PA, Henry DA, Carson JL, Hebert PC, McClelland DBL, Henderson KM: Transfusion thresholds and other strategies for guiding allogeneic red blood cell transfusion. *Cochrane Database Syst Rev* 1:CD002042, 2000.
11. McIntyre L, Hebert PC, Wells G, Canadian Critical Care Trials Group: is a restrictive transfusion strategy safe for resuscitated and critically ill trauma patients? *J Trauma* 57:563–568, 2004.
12. Busch MP, Kleinman SH, Nemo GJ: Current and emerging infectious risks of blood transfusion. *JAMA* 289(8):959–962, 2003.
13. Williamson LM, Lowe S, Love EM, et al: Serious hazards of transfusion (SHOT) initiative: analysis of the first two annual reports. *BMJ* 319(7201):16–19, 1999.
14. Goodnough LT: Risks of blood transfusion. *Crit Care Med* 31(Suppl):S678–S686, 2003.
15. Busch MP, Caglioti S, Robertson EF, et al: Screening the blood supply for West Nile virus RNA by nucleic acid amplification testing. *N Engl J Med* 4;353(5):460–467, 2005.
16. Toy P, Popovsky MA, Abraham E, National Heart, Lung and Blood Institute Working Group on TRALI: Transfusion-related acute lung injury: definition and review. *Crit Care Med* 33(4):721–726, 2005.
17. Silliman CC, Boshkov LK, Mehdizadehkashi Z, et al: Transfusion-related acute lung injury: epidemiology and a prospective analysis of etiologic factors. *Blood* 101(2):454–462, 2003.
18. Silverboard H, Aisiku I, Martin GS, Adams M, Rozycki G, Moss M: The role of acute blood transfusion in the development of acute respiratory distress syndrome in patients with severe trauma. *J Trauma* 59(3):717–723, 2005.
19. Croce MA, Tolley EA, Claridge JA, Fabian TC: Transfusions result in pulmonary morbidity and death after a moderate degree of injury. *J Trauma* 59(1):19–23, discussion 23–24, 2005.
20. Gong MN, Thompson BT, Williams P, Pothier L, Boyce PD, Christiani DC: Clinical predictors of and mortality in acute respiratory distress syndrome: potential role of red cell transfusion. *Crit Care Med* 33(6):1191–1198, 2005.
21. National Blood Users Group: A guideline for the use of blood and blood components in the management of massive haemorrhage. November 2002. http://www.ibts.ie/docs/120-MassiveHaemorrhageGuideline.pdf.
22. Cinat ME, Wallace WC, Nastanski F, et al: Improved survival following massive transfusion in patients who have undergone trauma. *Arch Surg* 134:964–970, 1999.
23. Vaslef SN, Knudson NW, Neligan PJ, et al: Massive transfusion exceeding 50 units of blood products in trauma patients. *J Trauma* 53:291–296, 2002.
24. Ho AM, Dion PW, Cheng CA, et al: A mathematical model for fresh frozen plasma transfusion strategies during major trauma resuscitation with ongoing hemorrhage. *Can J Surg* 48(6):470–478, 2005.
25. Sauaia A, Moore FA, Moore EE, Haenel JB, Read RA, Lezotte DC: Early predictors of postinjury multiple organ failure. *Arch Surg* 129(1):39–45, 1994.
26. Moore FA, Moore EE, Sauaia A: Blood transfusion. An independent risk factor for postinjury multiple organ failure. *Arch Surg* 132(6):620–624, discussion 624–625, 1997.
27. Ciesla DJ, Moore EE, Johnson JL, Burch JM, Cothren CC, Sauaia A: A 12-year prospective study of postinjury multiple organ failure: has anything changed? *Arch Surg* 140(5):432–438, discussion 438–440, 2005.
28. Dunne JR, Malone DL, Tracy JK, Napolitano LM: Allogenic blood transfusion in the first 24 hours after trauma is associated with increased systemic inflammatory response syndrome (SIRS) and death. *Surg Infect (Larchmt)* 5(4):395–404, 2004.
29. Beale E, Zhu J, Chan L,, et al: Blood transfusion in critically injured patients: a prospective study. *Injury* 37:455–465, 2006.
30. Malone DL, Dunne J, Tracy JK, Putnam AT, Scalea TM, Napolitano LM: Blood transfusion, independent of shock severity, is associated with worse outcome in trauma. *J Trauma* 54(5):898–905, discussion 905–907, 2003.
31. Malone D, Edelman B, Hess J, Tracy JK, Scalea T, Napolitano L: Age of blood transfusion in trauma: does it alter outcome? *Crit Care Med* 30(Suppl)72:A21, 2003.
32. Robinson WP 3rd, Ahn J, Stiffler A, Rutherford EJ, Hurd H, Zarzaur BL, Baker CC, Meyer AA, Rich PB: Blood transfusion is an independent predictor of increased mortality in nonoperatively managed blunt hepatic and splenic injuries. *J Trauma* 58(3):437–444, discussion 444–445, 2005.
33. Mostafa G, Gunter OL, Norton HJ, McElhiney BM, Bailey DF, Jacobs DG: Age, blood transfusion, and survival after trauma. *Am Surg.* 70(4):357–363, 2004.
34. MacLeod J, Lynn M, McKenney MG, Jeroukhimov I, Cohn SM: Predictors of mortality in trauma patients. *Am Surg* 70(9):805–810, 2004.
35. Vincent JL, Baron JF, Reinhart K, Gattinoni L, Thijs L, Webb A: Anemia and blood transfusion in critically ill patients. *JAMA* 288:1499–1507, 2002.
36. Corwin HL, Gettinger A, Pearl RG, Fink MP, Levy MM, Abraham E, et al: Anemia and blood transfusion in the critically ill: current clinical practice in the United States. The CRIT study. *Crit Care Med* 32:39–52, 2004.
37. Hill GE, Frawley WH, Griffith KE, Forestner JE, Minei JP: Allogeneic blood transfusion increases the risk of postoperative bacterial infection: a meta-analysis. *J Trauma* 54(5):908–914, 2003.
38. Claridge JA, Sawyer RG, Schulman AM, McLemore EC, Young JS: Blood transfusions correlate with infections in trauma patients in a dose-dependent manner. *Am Surg* 68(7):566–572, 2002.
39. Taylor RW, Manganaro LA, O'Brien J, Trottier SJ, Parkar N, Veremakis C: Impact of allogeneic packed red blood cell transfusion on nosocomial infection rates in the critically ill patient. *Crit Care Med* 30:2249–2254, 2002.
40. Shorr AF, Duh MS, Kelly KM, Kollef MH, CRIT Study Group: Red blood cell transfusion and ventilator-associated pneumonia: a potential link? *Crit Care Med* 32(3):666–674, 2004.
41. Nagaprasad V, Singh M: Sequential analysis of the influence of blood storage on aggregation, deformability and shape parameters of erythrocyte. *Clin Hemorheol Microcirc* 18(4):273–284, 1998.
42. Hovav T, Yedgar S, Manny N, Barshstein G: Alteration of red cell aggregability and shape during blood storage. *Transfusion* 39(3):277–281, 1999.
43. d'Almeida MS, Jagger J, Duggan M, White M, Ellis C, Chin-Yee IH: A comparison of biochemical and functional alterations of rat and human erythrocytes stored in CPDA-1 for 29 days: implications for animal models of transfusion. *Transfus Med* 10(4):291–303, 2000.
44. Solberger T, Walter R, Brand B: Influence of prestorage leucocyte depletion and storage time on rheologic properties of erythrocyte concentrates. *Vox Sang* 82(4):191–197, 2002.
45. Berezina TL, Zaets SB, Machiedo GW: Alterations of red blood cell shape in patients with severe trauma. *J Trauma* 57(1):82–87, 2004.
46. Moore EE, Johnson JL, Cheng AM, Masuno T, Banerjee A: Insights from studies of blood substitutes in trauma. *Shock* 24(3):197–205, 2005.
47. Moore EE: Blood substitutes: the future is now. *J Am Coll Surg* 196(1):1–17, 2003.

CRITICAL CARE II, SPECIAL ISSUES AND TREATMENTS

ACUTE RESPIRATORY DISTRESS SYNDROME

Booker T. King,   Alexander Becker,   George D. Garcia, and   Juan A. Asensio

There have not been many topics in critical care medicine that have received as much as attention as the acute respiratory distress syndrome (ARDS). Recently, there has been significant medical progress in this area—due in part to a better understanding of the pathophysiology of ARDS as well as earlier diagnosis and initiation of therapy. The "open lung" concept of mechanical ventilation has revolutionized the management of these patients. Newer modes of ventilation and novel strategies to improve oxygenation and reduce lung compliance have also contributed substantially.[1] Despite these advances, a 30%–40% mortality can be attributed to ARDS.[2] ARDS can occur directly from traumatic chest trauma or as a sequela of a host of disease processes (sepsis, fat emboli syndrome, pneumonia, severe blunt chest trauma, and so on). Therefore, a thorough understanding of the clinical presentation and treatment options for ARDS is essential for every practitioner who manages critically ill patients.

EPIDEMIOLOGY

The first estimate of the incidence of ARDS, 75 cases per 100,000 person per year population correlating with 150,000 cases per year in this country, was published in an expert panel report by the National Institute of Health in 1972.[3] The American European Consensus Conference (AECC) redefined ARDS in 1992. Recent studies based on the AECC criteria found incidence rates that varied from 4.9 to 22 per person years. More recent studies reported high incidence rate of ARDS among ventilated patients. In a large multicenter study including 5183 mechanically ventilated patients, 9% of patients met ARDS criteria at the beginning or over the course of the ventilatory support.[4] In a more recent prospective study, Estenssoro et al.[5] found that 8% of patients admitted to an intensive care unit (ICU) and 20% of mechanically ventilated patients fulfilled criteria for ARDS.

The reported rate of mortality from ARDS ranges from 31% to 74%. Several investigators have observed a reduction in mortality rates over time, from more than 60% in the 1980s to less than 40% in the 1990s.[2,6] Most studies have indicated that nonsurvivors of ARDS usually die of nonrespiratory causes. In 1985, Montgomery et al.[7] highlighted that only 16% of deaths were caused by respiratory failure. In most cases, early death was caused by underlying disease, whereas late death was caused by sepsis. Recently, Bersten et al.[8] showed that

respiratory failure was the cause of death in only 9% of ARDS cases. Thus, ARDS is a systemic disease and the main cause of death is related to multiorgan failure. It is interesting that degree of hypoxemia is unimportant in terms of predicting mortality. Valta et al.[9] showed that age, right ventricular dysfunction, and the presence of acute renal failure were found to have important prognostic value.

DEFINITION AND CLINICAL DIAGNOSIS

The definition of ARDS has been simplified over the past few years, allowing clinicians to identify patients earlier. Ashbaugh's 1967 original description consisted of respiratory distress, cyanosis, decreased lung compliance, and bilateral infiltrates on chest radiograph.[10] In 1988, Murray and Mathay devised a four-point scoring system that included the level of positive end expiratory pressure (PEEP), the ratio of partial pressure of arterial oxygen to the fraction of inspired oxygen (PaO_2/FiO_2), lung compliance, and chest x-ray findings.[11] In 1994, the AECC modified the 1988 definition and their new definition included the following major components[12]:

- Hypoxia defined specifically as PaO_2/F_1O_2 of less than 200
- Bilateral diffuse alveolar infiltrates on chest x-ray
- Pulmonary artery occlusion pressure (PAOP) of less than 18

The new definition also introduced a classification for a lesser form of ARDS: acute lung injury (ALI). The diagnosis of ALI is identical except in one respect: PaO_2/FiO_2 of less than 300. This distinction is important because a greater portion of ARDS patients will require mechanical ventilation.

Acute respiratory distress syndrome presents with dyspnea, usually developing within 72 hours of the initial insult. Some patients may progress to moderate or severe respiratory failure necessitating intubation. Stable patients with mild to moderate ALI can be cautiously managed with a trial of noninvasive ventilation.[13] Arterial blood gas will often reveal hypoxia with respiratory alkalosis. The diagnosis is confirmed by chest x-ray, which shows bilateral infiltrates resembling pulmonary congestion. Infrequently, the chest x-ray will have an atypical pattern that will be asymmetric or unilateral. Computer tomography of the chest, if obtained, shows consolidation with atelectasis in the dependent zones.[14]

Acute respiratory distress syndrome is associated with several clinical disorders, sepsis being the most common among them (40%).[5] Two clinical disorders often found in trauma patients are pulmonary contusion and multiple blood transfusions, which can lead to ARDS. Pulmonary contusion is a direct insult to the lung parenchyma, leading to the accumulation of blood and proteinaceous fluid at the alveolar-capillary interface.[15] This will lead to ALI in many patients, with some patients progressing to ARDS. Trauma patients requiring multiple transfusions of packed red cells are at risk for ARDS. Transfusion-related ALI (TRALI) accounts for a small percentage of cases of ARDS. The exact mechanism of TRALI is still unclear.

PATHOPHYSIOLOGY

Acute respiratory distress syndrome is a devastating form of acute respiratory failure that frequently develops in patients with pulmonary and nonpulmonary organ failure. Experimental and clinical data regarding the pathogenesis of disease have evolved significantly over the past decade. ARDS is an extremely severe form of ALI that occurs as a result of systemic inflammation caused by either direct or indirect lung injury. Direct lung injury is associated with high mortality rate. Some causes of direct lung injury include pneumonia, aspiration, and pulmonary contusion. Common causes of indirect lung injury are sepsis, multiple blood transfusion, shock, and acute pancreatitis.[16] Regardless of the initial etiology, ARDS is characterized histologically by diffuse alveolar damage with interstitial and alveolar infiltration with neutrophils and macrophages. On the other hand, it is a progressive disease and has indistinct stages with different histologic features.

The acute exudative phase is manifested by the rapid onset of respiratory failure. Arterial hypoxemia that is refractory to oxygen is a characteristic feature. Pathologically, this picture is characterized by injury of the alveolar-capillary membrane and accumulation of protein-rich fluid with neutrophils, macrophages, and disruption of the endothelial-epithelial barrier—ending with the development of the pulmonary interstitial edema secondary to microcapillary circulatory injury.[17] The resulting interstitial accumulation of fluid and protein impairs diffusion capacity and thus oxygenation. These changes are responsible for the decreasing pulmonary compliance and hypoxemia. Disruption of the alveolar epithelium and loss of types 1 and 2 pneumocytes lead to loss of the mechanical barrier integrity, leading to bacterial translocation and sepsis.

The key role of the activated neutrophils and macrophages has been established based on analyses of bronchoalveolar (BAL) fluid in the acute phase of ARDS.[18] Several recent studies stressed that activated neutrophils and macrophages produce cytokines, including TNF-α, interleukins IL-1βm IL-6, IL-8, and IL-10 (all of these playing essential roles in pathophysiology of ARDS).[19] Recovery from ARDS is characterized by the resolution of the alveolar edema and recuperation of the alveolar epithelial barrier. During the acute phase of inflammation, alveolar epithelial cells undergo apoptosis. Once recovery begins, type 2 cells proliferate—producing surfactant. The type 2 cells then differentiate to type 1 cells. After the acute phase, some patients make uncomplicated and rapid recovery—whereas others progress to the fibrotic stage, which has been observed early in the course of disease.[20] The alveolar space filled with mesenchymal cells (producing procollagen 3 peptide, collagen, and fibronectin, along with new blood vessels) gives a histologic picture of fibrosing alveolitis associated with poor outcome and an increased risk of death.[21]

TREATMENT

The initial steps in the treatment of ARDS include early recognition of the disorder, followed by the initiation of therapies designed to treat the underlying insult or condition that caused the ARDS to develop. In the case of pneumonia, this may entail early aggressive initiation of broad-spectrum antibiotics. In sepsis, early resuscitation and optimization as well as treatment of the septic focus are essential. All cases of ALI and ARDS will require the trauma surgeon or surgical critical care specialist to continually assess the need for mechanical ventilatory support. In addition to the therapies previously cited, other areas must be addressed—including the nutritional status of the patient, comorbid conditions, and extrapulmonary sites of end-organ failure.

The first major decision for the trauma surgeon or surgical critical care specialist caring for a patient developing ARDS is whether or not mechanical ventilation is necessary. This will depend of course on the severity of the patient's symptoms. Patients who cannot be supported by noninvasive therapies (supplemental oxygen and continuous positive airway pressure mask) will definitely require intubation and mechanical ventilation.

The use of PEEP in the treatment of ARDS patients dates back to the original description of the disease.[10] The effectiveness of PEEP is due to its ability to recruit lung units, thereby increasing functional residual capacity (FRC) and hence increasing lung compliance. PEEP also increases the proportion of alveoli actively engaged in gas exchange, leading to a decrease in shunt fraction.[22] PEEP has a third advantage of protecting against ventilator-associated lung injury (VALI) by preventing the derecruitment-recruitment cycle that ultimately leads to alveolar damage. There has been much interest in the past few years in determining the optimum level of PEEP (a PEEP level that yields maximum oxygenation without overdistending the lung).

The use of upper and lower inflection points on the pressure-volume curve has been advocated by some as a more accurate way of determining this PEEP level.[23,24] This method is highly sophisticated, often requiring computer software designed to graphically display pressure-volume curves. Therefore, this method has not gained widespread appeal. The current recommendation is to adjust PEEP to a level at which the F_IO_2 can be decreased to less than 60% and oxygen saturation can be maintained at 88% or greater.[25] The ARDS network recently conducted a trial comparing lower to higher PEEP levels and there was no difference in mortality between the two groups.[26] The use of high PEEP in ARDS remains controversial.

A landmark study conducted by the ARDS Network compared ventilating ARDS patients with tradition tidal volume (12 ml/kg) with lower tidal volume (6 ml/kg). A 22% reduction in risk was seen in patients ventilated with lower tidal volume.[27] No other single ventilator strategy has been shown to impact survival dramatically in ARDS. Additional recommendations derived from the ARDS Network study included keeping plateau pressure less than 30 mm Hg and adjusting the PEEP to keep to oxygen saturation between 88% and 95%. Together, these recommendations comprise the "open lung" strategy of management of patients with ARDS.

Permissive hypercapnia has emerged as another important tool in the treatment of ARDS patients. With permissive hypercapnia, the partial pressure of carbon dioxide (PCO_2) is allowed to rise as high as 70 mm Hg—and in some cases higher. Several studies have shown that this level of PCO_2 is well tolerated and that attempts to normalize the PCO_2 by increasing the respiratory rate or using bicarbonate replacement are unnecessary and perhaps detrimental. Permissive hypercapnia is thought to be lung protective.[28]

Pressure-controlled ventilation (PCV) was once thought to provide an advantage over volume-controlled ventilation in ARDS patients. It has been suggested that the rapid inspiratory flow characteristic of PCV leads to better oxygenation. A prospective randomized trial failed to show that PCV was superior.[29] Inverse ratio ventilation (IRV) is used to improve oxygenation by allowing a greater time for inspiration to occur, this allowing more time for oxygen exchange. A longer inspiratory time can lead to hypercapnia and auto-PEEP. Some studies have found a small benefit to IRV, but others have failed to show a survival advantage.[30] Other newer modes of ventilation are being used for ARDS. One mode that has recently attracted attention is airway pressure release ventilation (APRV). In this mode, continuous positive airway pressure is delivered for prolonged periods with exhalation allowed to occur over a fraction of a second.[31] APRV has been successful in improving oxygenation in ARDS in anecdotal reports, but it can result in profound hypercapnia and auto-PEEP. No data exists to show this newer modality increasing survival.

It is important for the critical care team caring for ARDS patients on mechanical ventilation to be mindful of the potential to create

VALI. VALI is an insult that arises in the lung as a result of the ventilator pressures causing alveoli to overdistend. This leads to not only physical stress-related injury to the alveolus but to activation of the proinflammatory response.[32] The main components of VALI are oxygen toxicity and "volutrauma." VALI is often seen after attempts to ventilate ARDS patients with high tidal volumes and when higher levels of oxygen (>60%) are used unnecessarily. The ARDS patient must be managed with a strategy that minimizes VALI.

Alternative Therapies

Inhaled nitric oxide improves oxygenation in respiratory failure by several mechanisms. First, it selectively vasodilates the pulmonary capillaries of well-ventilated alveoli—leading to a reduction in shunt and decreasing pulmonary vascular resistance. Second, inhaled nitric oxide may have some anti-inflammatory properties.[33] It is usually delivered at concentrations of 1 to 10 parts per million, although concentrations as high as 40 parts per million can be delivered without toxicity. Several randomized clinical trials failed to show an outcome benefit.[34] To date, the use of inhaled nitric oxide in ARDS is confined mostly to patients who are severely hypoxemic despite maximal efforts with conservative therapy.

Prone positioning has the theoretical benefit of improving oxygenation by redistributing lung ventilation and perfusion. Other important mechanisms include improving ventilation mechanics and alleviating the medial compression of the lung by the heart and mediastinum. A recent multicenter randomized trial conducted by Gattinoni et al.[35,36] showed improved oxygenation in ARDS patients who were ventilated in the prone position. No improvement in mortality was shown in this study. Prone positioning is associated with several complications, including risk of pressure necrosis of facial structures, difficulty assessing sedated patients, and the possibility of dislodging the airway. Currently, there is no recommendation advising the routine use of prone positioning.

High-frequency ventilation (HFV) is achieved with a special ventilator or oscillator designed to deliver tidal volume of 1 to 5 ml/kg at rates of 60 to 300 breaths per minute. Ventilating the lung at such high frequency and with small tidal volumes is believed to have a lung-protective effect that reduces VALI.[37] Multiple clinical trials of HFV in ARDS patients have failed to show a survival benefit. Its use is highly individualized and is often applied to patients who do not respond to conservative therapies.[38]

Partial liquid ventilation is a process in which the lungs are filled with perflouro-carbon (PFC) liquid and ventilated with conventional mechanical ventilator. PFC is an inert liquid with high affinity for oxygen. Partial liquid ventilation improves oxygenation by distributing PFC throughout the lung, allowing gas exchange in areas where gaseous oxygen will not.[39] Previous studies have shown some promise for this modality in children with severe respiratory failure.[40] A recent randomized study performed by Kacmerak et al.,[41] which compared conventional mechanical ventilation with partial liquid ventilation, failed to show outcome benefit. With no large randomized studies to show efficacy partial liquid, ventilation remains investigational but it has been used as a salvage therapy at some institutions.

Extra corporeal membrane oxygenation (ECMO) utilizes a mechanical membrane oxygenator to directly oxygenate blood while blood is circulated through the machine by roller pumps. This is an appealing strategy potentially allowing the lung to "rest" while continuing to maintain maximal oxygenation. This procedure is fraught with logistical difficulties and is not available at many medical centers. The procedure also carries the risk of injury to vasculature from insertion of venous and/or arterial cannulas and the risk of bleeding because full anticoagulation is necessary. Clinical studies have not shown a benefit to using ECMO.[42] ECMO is reserved almost exclusively for patients who fail conservative therapy and cannot be oxygenated by any other method.

Enthusiasm for the use of surfactant arose as a result of its beneficial effects on neonatal respiratory distress syndrome.[43] Attempts to apply this therapy to adults have not proven fruitful. A recent randomized study comparing aerosolized surfactant to placebo in ARDS patients failed to show improvement in survival or an increase in ventilator-free days.[44] To date, surfactant has no role in the management of adult patients with ARDS.

A significant proportion of patients with ARDS will begin to develop fibrosis early as a result of a deranged healing process. These patients may exhibit poor lung compliance, elevated peak airway pressures, and pulmonary hypertension—and have a "honeycomb" appearance on chest x-ray indicating fibrotic lung. It has been postulated that corticosteroids may arrest this process and possibly reverse it. Clinical studies looking at high-dose steroid (methylprednisolone 30 mg/kg every 6 hours) failed to show improvement.[45] A recent study conducted by the ARDS Network used low-dose methylprednisolone (2 mg/kg) tapered over 25 days.[46] The steroid group had higher 60-day mortality but was shown to have improved oxygenation, increased ventilator-free days, and increased shock-free days. However, despite these benefits the ARDS Network did not advocate the use of corticosteroids for fibroproliferative ARDS.

CONCLUSIONS

ARDS is a common life-threatening disorder with a significant influence on the morbidity and mortality of ICU patients. It has been clinically recognized for nearly 30 years. During that time, the understanding of the risk, pathophysiology, and outcomes has changed and improved. In the last years, important randomized controlled trials in patients with ARDS have been conducted and have shown that mechanical ventilation with low tidal volume is better than mechanical ventilation with high tidal volume. High PEEP pressure has not been shown to offer any survival benefit. Different modes of ventilation (such as APRV and HFPV) have some disadvantages, but their benefits have to be proven. No drug therapy has been shown to improve survival in patients with ARDS. Despite the success of a low tidal volume strategy in reducing mortality, ARDS patients still have increased risk of death as well as significant functional disability and decrements in quality of life. Therefore, new therapies are still needed.

REFERENCES

1. Amato MRP, Barbas CSV, Medeiros DM, et al: Beneficial effects of the "open lung approach" with low distending pressures in acute respiratory distress syndrome. *Am J Respir Crit Care Med* 152:1835, 1995.
2. Milberg JA, Davis DR, Steinberg KR, et al: Improved survival of patients with acute respiratory distress syndrome (ARDS): 1983–1993. *JAMA* 273:306–309, 1995.
3. Conference report: mechanism of acute respiratory failure. *Am Rev Respir Dis* 115:1071–1078, 1977.
4. Esteban A, Anzueto A, Frutos F, et al: Characteristics and outcomes in adult patients receiving mechanical ventilation: a 28-day international study. *JAMA* 287:345–555, 2002.
5. Estenssoro E, Dubin A, Laffaire E, et al: Incidence, clinical course, and outcome in 217 patients with acute respiratory distress syndrome. *Crit Care Med* 30:2450–2456, 2002.
6. Abel SJ, Finney SJ, Steinberg KR, et al: Reduced mortality in association with the acute respiratory distress syndrome (ARDS). *Thorax* 53:292–294, 1998.
7. Montgomery BA, Stager MA, Carrico J, et al: Causes of mortality in patients with the adult respiratory distress syndrome. *Am Rev Respir Dis* 132:485–491, 1985.
8. Bersten AD, Edibam C, Hunt T, et al: Incidence and mortality of acute lung injury and the acute respiratory distress syndrome in three Australian states. *Am J Respir Crit Care Med* 165:443–448, 2002.
9. Valta P, Uusaro A, Nunes S, et al: Acute respiratory distress syndrome: frequency, clinical course, and costs of care. *Crit Care Med* 27:2367–2374, 1999.

10. Ashbaugh DG, Bigelow DB, Petty TL, et al: Acute respiratory distress in adults. *Lancet* 2:319–323, 1967.
11. Murray JF, Mathay MA, Luce JM, et al: An expanded definition of the adult respiratory distress syndrome. *Am Rev Respir Dis* 138:720–723, 1988.
12. Bernard GR, Artigas A, Brigham KL, et al: The American-European consensus conference of ARDS: definitions, mechanisms, relevant outcomes, and clinical trial coordination. *Am J Respir Crit Care Med* 149:818, 1994.
13. Patrick W, Webster K, Ludwig L, et al: Noninvasive positive pressure ventilation in acute respiratory distress without prior chronic respiratory failure. *Am J Respir Crit Care Med* 153:1005, 1996.
14. Gattinoni L, Pesenti A, Bombino M: Relationships between lung computed tomographic density, gas exchange and PEEP in acute respiratory failure. *Anesthesiology* 69:824, 1988.
15. Wanek S, Mayberry JC: Blunt thoracic trauma: flail chest, pulmonary contusion, and blast injury. *Crit Care Clin* 20(1):71–81, 2004.
16. Ware LB, Mathay MA: The acute respiratory distress syndrome. *N Engl J Med* 134(18):1334–1349.
17. Goodman LR: Congestive heart failure and adult respiratory distress syndrome: new insight using computed tomography. *Radiol Clin North Am* 34:33–46, 1996.
18. Bachofen M, Weibel ER: Structural alterations of lung parenchyma in the adult respiratory distress syndrome. *Clin Chest Med* 2:35–56, 1982.
19. Martin TR: Lung cytokines and ARDS: Roger S. Mitchell Lecture. *Chest* 116:2S–8S, 1999.
20. Fukuda Y, Ishizaki M, Masuda Y, et al: The role of intraalveolar fibrosis in the process of pulmonary structural remodeling in patients with diffuse alveolar damage. *Am J Pathol* 126:171–182, 1987.
21. Zapol WM, Trelstad RL, Coffey JW, et al: Pulmonary fibrosis in severe acute respiratory failure. *Am Rev Respir Dis* 119:547–554, 1979.
22. Marini JJ: Mean airway pressure: physiologic determinants and clinical importance. Part 1: physiologic determinants and measurements. *Crit Care Med* 20:1461–1472, 1992.
23. Benito S, Lemaire F: Pulmonary pressure-volume relationship in acute respiratory distress syndrome in adults: role of positive end expiratory pressure. *Crit Care* 5:27, 1990.
24. Gattinoni L, Pelosi A, Crotti S, et al: Effects of positive end expiratory pressure on regional distribution of tidal volume and recruitment in adult respiratory distress syndrome. *Am J Respir Crit Care Med* 151:1807, 1995.
25. Pepe PE, Hudson LD, Carrico CJ: Early application of positive of end-expiratory pressure in patients at risk for the adult respiratory distress syndrome. *N Engl J Med* 311:281–286, 1982.
26. Acute Respiratory Distress Syndrome Network: Higher versus lower positive end-expiratory pressures in patients with acute respiratory distress syndrome. *N Engl J Med* 351(4):327–336, 2004.
27. Acute Respiratory Distress Syndrome Network: Ventilation with low tidal volumes as compared with traditional tidal volumes for acute lung injury and the acute respiratory distress syndrome. *N Engl J Med* 342:1301–1308, 2000.
28. Kregenow DA, Rubenfeld GD, et al: Hypercapnic acidosis and mortality in acute lung injury. *Crit Care Med* 34(1):1–7, 2006.
29. Stewart TE, Mead MO, Cook DJ, et al: Evaluation of a ventilation strategy to prevent barotraumas in patients at high risk for acute respiratory distress syndrome. Pressure- and Volume-Limited Ventilation Strategy Group. *N Engl J Med* 338(6):355–361, 1998.
30. Morris AH, Wallace CJ, et al: Randomized clinical trial of pressure controlled inverse ratio ventilation and extracorporeal CO_2 removal for acute respiratory distress syndrome. *Am J Respir Crit Care Med* 149:295, 1994.
31. Frawley PM, Habashi NM: Airway pressure release ventilation: theory and practice. *AACN Clin Issues* 12(2):234–246, 2001.
32. van Soeren MH, et al: Pathophysiology and implications for treatment of acute respiratory distress syndrome. *AACN Clin Issues* 11(2):179–197, 2000.
33. Griffiths MJ, Evans TW: Inhaled nitric oxide therapy in adults. *N Engl J Med* 353(25):2683–2695, 2005.
34. Gerlach J, Semmerow A, Busch T, et al: Dose–response characteristics of during long-term inhalation of nitric oxide in patients with severe acute respiratory distress syndrome: a prospective, randomized, controlled study. *Am J Respir Crit Care Med* 167:1008–1015, 2003.
35. Gattinoni L, Pesenti A, Taccone P, et al: Effect of prone positioning on the survival of patients with acute respiratory failure. *N Engl J Med* 345:568–573, 2001.
36. Mancebo J, Fernandez R, Gordo F, et al: Prone vs supine position in ARDS patients: results of a randomized multicenter trial. *Am J Respir Crit Care Med* 167:A180, 2003.
37. Derdak S, Mehta S, Stewart TE, et al: High frequency oscillatory ventilation for acute respiratory distress syndrome in adults: a randomized, controlled trial. *Am J Respir Crit Care Med* 166:801, 2002.
38. Velmahos GC, Chan LS, Tatevossian R, et al: High-frequency percussive ventilation improves oxygenation in patients with ARDS. *Chest* 116(2):440–446, 1999.
39. Hirschl RB, Panikoff T, Wise C, et al: Initial experience with partial liquid ventilation in adult patients with acute respiratory distress syndrome. *JAMA* 275:383, 1996.
40. Greenspan JS, Wolfson MR, Shaffer TH: Liquid ventilation. *Semin Perinatol* 24(6):396–405, 2000.
41. Kacmerak RM, Wiederman HP, Lavin PT et al: Partial liquid ventilation in adult patients with acute respiratory distress syndrome. *Am J Respir Crit Care Med* 173(8):882–829, 2006.
42. Mols G, et al: Extracorporeal membrane oxygenation: a ten year experience. *Am J Surg* 180:144–154, 2000.
43. Perspectives for use of surfactant in children and adults. *J Matern Fetal Neonatal Med* 16(Suppl 2):29–31, 2004..
44. Kesecioglu J, Schultz MJ, Lundberg D: Treatment of acute lung injury (ALI/ARDS) with surfactant. *Am J Respir Crit Care Med* 163:A819, 2001.
45. Meduri GU, et al: Corticosteroid rescue treatment of progressive fibroproliferative in late ARDS. Patterns of response and predictors of outcome. *Chest* 105(5):1516–1527, 1994.
46. Acute Respiratory Distress Syndrome Network: Efficacy and safety of corticosteroids for persistent acute respiratory distress syndrome. *N Engl J Med* 354(16):1671–1684, 2006.

SYSTEMIC INFLAMMATORY RESPONSE SYNDROME AND MULTIPLE-ORGAN DYSFUNCTION SYNDROME: DEFINITION, DIAGNOSIS, AND MANAGEMENT

Anthony Watkins   and   Edwin A. Deitch

In 1973, Tilney et al.[1] described 18 patients who developed "sequential system failure" following surgery for ruptured abdominal aneurysms. It was at this time that the idea that severe physiologic insults could lead to multiple-organ failure (MOF) was first established. Several decades later, MOF (or multiple organ dysfunction syndrome [MODS]) remains a major source of postinjury morbidity and a leading cause of death in surgical intensive care units (SICUs). Although the pathogenesis of this syndrome remains to be fully defined, it is evident that sepsis, systemic inflammatory response syndrome (SIRS), acute respiratory distress syndrome (ARDS), and MODS are closely related phenomena. Consequently, the goal of this chapter is to review SIRS and MODS, focusing on current strategies for diagnosing, managing, and (most importantly) preventing these syndromes.

INCIDENCE

The concept that death from trauma has a trimodal distribution (with these deaths being caused by hemorrhage, head injury, and sepsis/organ failure) is well established. Because MODS is the most common cause of late trauma deaths, it has been the subject of intense investigation. It is now clear that certain clinical risk factors can be used to predict the likelihood of a patient developing MODS. These include age, injury severity score (ISS), number of blood transfusions, and lactate/base deficit levels.[2] However, it is only over the last decade that the incidence of MODS in high-risk trauma patients appears to have decreased. This decrease appears to be due to a better knowledge of the factors predisposing patients to its development, as well as to the immunoinflammatory response to shock and trauma. For example, a 12-year prospective study examining 1344 trauma patients noted that the actual incidence of MODS (25%) was lower than its predicted rate.[3]

The authors concluded that this decrease was likely due to the concomitant drop in the liberal use of blood transfusions, which have been shown to be an independent predictor of MODS, SIRS, and mortality.[4,5] Not only does the incidence of MODS appear to be decreasing but there is emerging data to suggest that the mortality rate of patients with MODS is also declining—as reflected in a retrospective study of MODS-related death after blunt multiple trauma during a 25-year period. This study revealed an approximately 50% reduction in MODS-related mortality, from 29% to 14% over this time period.[6] As will be discussed later in this chapter, several therapeutic interventions have been developed that have been shown to reduce mortality or to attenuate organ dysfunction, which would help explain this decline in mortality. In spite of these improvements, once MODS has become established the risk of death is significant—with the patient's prognosis being more closely related to the number of organs that have failed than to any other variable, including the underlying processes that initiated the MODS.[7]

MECHANISMS OF MODS

The clinical picture of MOF is indicative of a generalized systemic inflammatory response, which typically occurs as a result of infection or uncontrolled inflammation in the patient with severe trauma. Several distinct and often conflicting hypotheses have been proposed to explain the mechanisms underlying MODS.[7] Nonetheless, MOF can be viewed as a systemic process involving the excessive stimulation of certain inflammatory responses mediated by circulating factors whose effects contribute to injury or dysfunction in organs not involved in the initial insult. To a large extent, the cascade of events culminating in MOF is likely to be mediated by the same factors irrespective of the exact nature of the triggering insult. In fact, it is the host's inflammatory response to injury or infection that is probably more important in the genesis of SIRS, ARDS, and MODS than the microbial agent or the initiating insult. Thus, an appreciation of the role of the inflammatory response of the host in the pathogenesis of MOF is vital in order to develop new and effective modalities for the prevention and treatment of this syndrome.

The earliest reports of postinjury MODS identified occult intra-abdominal infection as the etiology in approximately half of the cases. However, the recognition that more than 50%–70% of patients with MOF do not have an identifiable focus of infection meant that uncontrolled infection could not be the universal cause of MODS. From this early work came the recognition that only a fraction of septic-appearing patients were infected and that the host's own response to tissue injury or shock could result in a noninfectious septic state. In turn, this recognition that the host's immunoinflammatory response to microbial infection, tissue injury, necrotic tissue, or shock was similar led to the hypotheses that immune cell products, such as cytokines, contributed to the development of MODS.

This hypothesis was based on the concept that an excessive immuno-inflammatory response due to activated macrophages and other immune cells led to cytokine-mediated tissue injury and thereby the development of SIRS and MODS. This hypothesis was supported by several experimental and clinical observations. For example, cytokine levels were increased in trauma patients and the administration of tumor necrosis factor alpha (TNF-α) to humans elicited a clinical response similar to SIRS, whereas preclinical animal studies documented that TNF-neutralization improved survival in animals receiving a lethal dose of endotoxin. However, things were not this simple—as soon became apparent from multiple failed clinical trials of anti-inflammatory agents and the results of more complex preclinical animal studies. In fact, it is now recognized that cytokines have many beneficial functions, such as the control of infection. It is also recognized that elevated cytokine levels appear to be more markers or predictors of the host response than inducers of MODS.

Another mechanism by which hemorrhagic shock and trauma could predispose to the developments of MODS is through an ischemia-reperfusion injury and/or damage to the microcirculation. Because shock is essentially a total-body ischemia-reperfusion insult and the microcirculation of various tissues and organs are highly susceptible to ischemia-reperfusion–mediated insults, this process has been termed the microcirculatory hypothesis of MODS.[7]

Physiologically, circulatory shock could contribute to MOF through inadequate global oxygen delivery, the ischemia-reperfusion phenomenon, and/or the promotion of deleterious endothelial-leukocyte interactions.

Although prolonged tissue hypoxia leads to inadequate ATP generation and potentially irreversible cell damage, under most clinical conditions the shock period is not long enough for this process to occur. Thus, in clinical situations it appears that most of the tissue damage occurs after ischemia is relieved by reperfusion and that this damage is due to the production of reperfusion-induced oxygen radicals and proinflammatory factors (such as oxidants, nitric oxide, chemokines, and cytokines). In fact, recent studies show that the combination of reperfusion-induced increased levels of nitric oxide and superoxide anion synergistically increase cell injury via the production of peroxynitrite, which is a long-lasting and potent oxidant that causes direct cell injury through lipid peroxidation. This notion that increased nitric oxide production is important in the pathogenesis of MODS is supported by clinical studies showing that serum nitrate levels (an index for the systemic production of nitric oxide) correlated well with MOF scores in critically ill patients.[8]

Endothelial-leukocyte interactions leading to tissue injury also seem to be a key step in the pathogenesis of SIRS, ARDS, and MODS. Many factors related to shock and tissue injury, including cytokines, necrotic tissue, endotoxins, and oxidants, can convert endothelial cells from a quiescent state to a proinflammatory procoagulant one and can activate neutrophils. The combination of these changes in endothelial cell phenotype and neutrophil activation has been documented to lead to increased neutrophil adherence to the microcirculatory endothelium, thereby promoting neutrophil-mediated microvascular injury.[7] Experimentally, inhibition of neutrophil-endothelial interactions has been shown to limit shock- and sepsis-induced injury to a number of organs, including the lung. Furthermore, neutrophil activation in trauma patients has been identified as a predictor of the development of SIRS, ARDS, and MODS. Therefore, endothelial cell–neutrophil interactions, whether induced by shock, sepsis, or an augmented inflammatory response, appear to be an important effector mechanism in the development of ARDS and MODS.

The gut hypothesis of MOF has been used to explain why no identifiable focus of infection can be found in as many as 30% of bacteremic patients who die from MOF.[9] An extensive body of experimental as well as clinical studies supports this hypothesis. For example, clinical studies indicate that intestinal permeability is increased in patients with sepsis after major thermal injury or trauma and that loss of intestinal barrier function correlates with the development of systemic infection, ARDS, and MODS.[10] Likewise, studies in intensive care unit (ICU) and trauma patients indicated that gut ischemia, as measured by gastric tonometry, is a better predictor of the development of ARDS and MODS than global indices of oxygen delivery.[11] Although both clinical and experimental studies implicated intestinal injury and bacterial translocation in the development of SIRS and MODS, a study by Moore et al.[12] began to cast doubt on the clinical relevance of bacterial translocation.

These investigators failed to find bacteria or endotoxin in the portal blood of severely injured patients, including a subgroup of patients developing MODS. One potential explanation for this failure to find endotoxin or bacteria in the portal blood was that the gut-derived factors contributing to SIRS, ARDS, and MODS were exiting the gut via the lymphatics. Studies testing this possibility have documented that nonbacterial factors exiting the ischemic gut contribute to acute ARDS, MODS, neutrophil activation, and endothelial cell injury/activation in both rodent and primate models of trauma-hemorrhagic shock and have led to the gut-lymph hypothesis of MODS.[10] This gut lymph hypothesis of MODS proposes that nonbacterial noncytokine factors released from the stressed gut via the lymphatic system activate neutrophils and endothelial cells, thereby leading to organ dysfunction. Thus, over the last several years the gut hypothesis has expanded beyond bacterial translocation and now also implicates gut-derived nonbacterial proinflammatory

and tissue-injurious factors in the pathogenesis of SIRS, ARDS, and MODS.

Although each of the various MODS hypotheses was presented individually, in patients many of these pathways overlap and the induction of one pathway can lead to activation of others. For example, severe bacterial infection activates the immuno-inflammatory response, which in turn leads to microcirculatory dysfunction and gut ischemia. Likewise, nonbacterial gut-derived factors have been shown to activate neutrophils, lead to an augmented inflammatory response, and promote microcirculatory dysfunction. Furthermore, shock states are associated with microcirculatory failure, gut injury, induction of an inflammatory response, and augmented neutrophil-endothelial cell interactions. In addition, in many patients who develop MOF no one major insult seems to have occurred. Instead, it appears that the development of MODS is related to the summation of several minor insults rather than one major event.

This clinical observation has led to the "two-hit" hypothesis of MODS, where potentially clinically modest events prime the host so that the host's response to subsequent secondary events becomes exaggerated, culminating in SIRS, ARDS, and MOF. Although this two-hit theory needs to be further understood, it is a feasible explanation of how trauma or burn injury can convert a nonlethal infectious or hypoxic challenge into a lethal insult. In fact, as illustrated in Figure 1 it is clear that the difficulty in finding an effective therapy to prevent or treat MODS relates to the overlapping nature of the multiple systems activated by shock and trauma as well as the ability of one system to prime other systems for an exaggerated physiologic response to secondary insults. Nonetheless, the knowledge gained from these basic studies of the physiology of inflammation and MODS have provided important therapeutic insights. For example, they highlight the importance of prompt and adequate volume resuscitation and microcirculatory blood flow to prevent organ ischemia, the need for early excision of nonviable tissue to limit systemic inflammation, and the need for therapies to better preserve gut barrier dysfunction and limit uncontrolled inflammation.

DIAGNOSIS

A key step in the treatment of a disease process is the establishment of an accurate diagnosis. To that end, a number of consensus conferences have been held in an attempt to provide classification schemes that allow SIRS, ARDS, and MODS to be accurately diagnosed.

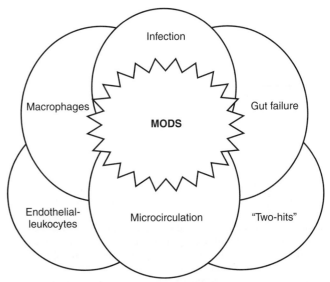

Figure 1 Overlapping nature of multiple hypotheses believed to be responsible for causing MODS.

Based on these conferences, SIRS is defined as the response to a variety of severe clinical insults, which is manifested by two or more of the four conditions listed in Table 1.[13] Furthermore, SIRS should be viewed as an evolved dynamic process that has adaptive survival value for the host under most circumstances because it signals the body to respond to injury or to an external threat such as a bacterial infection. However, if this protective inflammatory response becomes uncontrolled or excessive it has maladaptive consequences due to its potential to injure the host's own tissues.

The term "MODS" was introduced by a consensus conference of the American College of Chest Physicians (ACCP) and the Society of Critical Care Medicine (SCCM) in 1991.[14] Prior to that time, this syndrome had many different names, including *sequential organ dysfunction syndrome* and *multiple-organ failure syndrome*. Several MODS scoring systems have been established that grade the severity of MODS and emphasize the concept that there exists a continuous spectrum from mild to full-blown dysfunction that correlates, on a patient population level, with mortality and morbidity (Table 2).[15–18]

These systems, much like the sequential organ failure assessment (SOFA) score developed by Vincent et al.,[18] score organ failure by assigning a numerical scale in which more points are given to the higher degree of organ dysfunction in several organ systems (Table 3).[16,19] Although not developed to predict mortality in individual patients, there are several areas where the use of such scoring systems can be beneficial in critically ill patients. This includes their use in the daily clinical evaluation of a patient's response, in research involving epidemiologic studies, and in the assessment of new therapies in clinical trials. Although these scoring systems use slightly different parameters to grade organ failure, most studies have found that the clinical utility of these scoring systems is comparable.[20,21]

MANAGEMENT

At the current time, the treatment of patients with established MODS is largely symptomatic and dedicated to supporting organs and systems that have failed. Because there is no "cure" for MODS,

once it is present—and because the mortality rate of patients with established MODS is high—prevention becomes a key strategy in the care of the high-risk trauma patient. Therefore, it is important to understand and utilize certain strategies and approaches that have been shown to reduce the risk for developing MODS. In trauma patients, prevention begins in the field, with rapid transport to a medical facility, and extends throughout the resuscitative, operative, and ICU phases of care (Table 4). Because the approaches and strategies used at different phases of patient care may vary to some extent, each of these phases is discussed individually—although in actual clinical practice these phases often overlap.

Resuscitative Phase

The resuscitative phase has as its central goal the restoration of an effective blood volume, optimization of microcirculatory blood flow (and hence tissue perfusion), and the prevention/limitation of ischemia-reperfusion injury. Recognition that shock causes a global ischemia-reperfusion injury, which directly and indirectly leads to cellular and hence organ injury, has led to an increasing emphasis on the adequacy of volume resuscitation as well as a search for more effective resuscitation fluids. The primary endpoint of resuscitation, however, remains controversial. Parameters such as base deficit and lactate levels, oxygen delivery, gastric intramucosal pH (pHi), and invasive monitoring using pulmonary artery catheters have all been used in an attempt to optimize volume resuscitation.

This is because blood pressure and urine output may not reflect the adequacy of volume resuscitation in the severely injured trauma patient. In this setting, arterial blood base deficit and serum lactate levels have been shown to be useful markers with which to monitor the response to resuscitation. A worsening base deficit or serum lactate has been shown to correlate with ongoing blood loss or inadequate volume resuscitation, whereas improvements in these parameters are indicative of adequate volume resuscitation. Because in severely injured patients the period of volume resuscitation may last up to 48 hours, serial measurements are important. Based on prospective studies demonstrating that patients who cleared their base deficient or lactate levels within 48 hours had a reduced incidence of ARDS and MODS plus a higher survival rate than those who did not,[22,23] the resuscitative goal should be to reduce and keep the base deficit below −2 mmol/l and/or the serum lactate less than 1.5 mEq/l.

The choice of resuscitative fluid has become a more controversial subject with the recognition that Ringers lactate is proinflammatory and thus may exacerbate the inflammatory response and contribute to the development of organ injury in shock states.[24–27] Given these

Table 1: Definition of Systemic Inflammatory Response Syndrome

Temperature >38°C or <36°C
Heart rate >90 bpm
$PaCO_2$ <32 torr (<4.3 kPa)
WBC of >12,000 or <4,000 cells/mm³; >10% immature forms

Table 2: Comparison of Scores Evaluating Multiple-Organ Dysfunction

System	Brussels Score	MODS Score	LOD Score	SOFA Score
Respiratory	P_aO_2/F_IO_2 ratio	P_aO_2/F_IO_2 ratio	P_aO_2/F_IO_2 ratio	P_aO_2/F_IO_2 ratio
Cardiovascular	■ Arterial pressure ■ Response to fluids ■ Acidosis	Pressure-adjusted heart rate	■ Arterial pressure ■ Heart rate	■ Arterial pressure ■ Vasoactive drugs
Renal	Creatinine	Creatinine	Creatinine, urea, UO	Creatinine, UO
Hematologic	Platelets	Platelets	Platelets, leukocytes	Platelets
Hepatic	Bilirubin	Bilirubin	Bilirubin, PT	Bilirubin
Neurologic	GCS	GCS	GCS	GCS

Brussels score,[15]; *GCS*, Glasgow Coma Scale; *LOD*, logistic organ dysfunction[16]; *MODS*, multiple organ dysfunction score[20]; *PT*, prothrombin; *SOFA*, sequential organ failure assessment[18]; *UO*, urine output.

Table 3: The Sequential Organ Failure Assessment (SOFA) Score

Organ System	Indicator of Dysfunction	Degree of Dysfunction				
		0	1	2	3	4
Respiratory	PaO$_2$/FIO$_2$ ratio (torr)	>400	≤400	≤300	≤200 With respiratory support	100 With respiratory support
Renal	Creatinine (mg/dl) or urine output	<1.2	1.2–1.9	2.0–3.4	3.5–4.9 <500 ml/day	>5.0 <200 ml/day
Hepatic	Bilirubin (mg/dl)	<1.2	1.2–1.9	2.0–5.9	6.0–11.9	>12.0
Cardiovascular	Hypotension	No hypotension	MAP <70 mm Hg	Dopamine 5 or dobutamine (any dose)[a]	Dopamine >5 or epi 0.1 or norepi 0.1[a]	Dopamine >15 or epi >0.1 or norepi >0.1[a]
Hematologic	Platelet count (mm^3)	>150,000	≤150,000	≤100,000	≤50,000	20,000
Neurologic	Glasgow Coma Score	15	13–14	10–12	6–9	<6

Note: To convert torr to kPa, multiply the value by 0.1333.

[a]Adrenergic agents administered for at least 1 hour (doses given are in micrograms per kilogram per minute).

epi, Epinephrine; *norepi,* norepinephrine.

Adapted from Vincent JL, de Mendonca A, Cantraine F, et al.: Use of the SOFA score to assess the incidence of organ dysfunction/failure in intensive care units: Results of a multicenter, prospective study. Working group on "sepsis-related problems" of the European Society of Intensive Care Medicine. *Crit Care Med* 26:1793–1800, 1998.

concerns, plus the recent recognition that large-volume resuscitation with crystalloid solutions contributes to the development of the abdominal compartment syndrome (ACS),[28] attention has refocused on the early resuscitation of trauma patients with hypertonic (7.5%) saline. The largest clinical trial comparing hypertonic saline versus Ringer's lactate when administered in the field demonstrated similar survival between the two groups.[29] However, there were decreased complications (such as renal failure and ARDS) in the hypertonic saline group.[29]

Nonetheless, at the current time due to the paucity of clinical trials there is not enough data to determine whether or not initial hypertonic saline resuscitation is superior to standard crystalloid resuscitation of the trauma patient. Another encouraging approach is the use of resuscitation fluids containing antioxidants, with three clinical trials, including a recent prospective randomized trial, showing that splanchnic-directed antioxidant therapy helps prevents MODS in trauma patients.[30] As investigations into novel resuscitation fluids with pharmacologic actions (i.e., gut-protective, immune modulatory) continues, it is likely that the initial resuscitative approach of the trauma patient will evolve from Ringer's lactate to include new fluid formulas.

The role of blood transfusions in trauma patients has also undergone an intense reevaluation based on clinical studies showing that blood is immune-suppressive and that blood transfusions are an independent predictor of MODS, especially when blood older than 2 weeks is administered.[31] These observations, plus the fact that ICU patients as well as trauma patients can be safely managed with hemoglobin levels in the range of 7 g/dl, has led to the emergence of a selective transfusion policy in which prophylactic transfusions for anemia are no longer routinely administered. In fact, the TRICC trial demonstrated a significant reduction in the severity of new organ dysfunction in a critical care setting when transfusion was withheld unless the hemoglobin concentration was less than 7 g/dl.[32,33]

Thus, based on the existing literature regarding the clinical efficacy of prophylactic red blood cell (RBC) transfusions for anemia in the critically ill two general conclusions can be made:prophylactic RBC transfusions to raise the hemoglobin above 7 g/dl does not improve tissue oxygen consumption consistently in critically ill patients, either globally or at the level of the microcirculation, and prophylactic RBC transfusion is not associated with improvements in clinical outcome in the critically ill and may result in worse outcomes in several patient subgroups.

A large amount of the research that was carried out on the physiology of volume resuscitation involved attempts to identify optimal central hemodynamic values, especially cardiac index, oxygen delivery, and oxygen consumption values. This research also attempted to identify tissue-specific regional resuscitation endpoints, such as the gastric pH using gastric tonometry. Although the early studies suggested that resuscitating patients to supranormal levels of cardiac output and oxygen delivery to meet increased tissue oxygen demands will improve survival, these early results have been refuted by numerous prospective randomized trials. In fact, it is now clear that the use of prophylactic blood transfusions, inotropes, and large volumes of crystalloids to reach supranormal levels of oxygen delivery may be deleterious rather than beneficial. Likewise, although there is data suggesting that patients with low gastric mucosal pHs have a worse outcome measuring gastric mucosal pH has not been shown to be as effective as measuring base deficit or lactate as markers of the adequacy of volume resuscitation. Thus, at the current time there is no compelling reason to use gastric tonometry to guide resuscitation effects.

Operative Intervention

In an early article on multiple organ failure, Eiseman et al. described a series of 42 surgical patients with MODS, 24 of whom developed MODS as a result of intraoperative error or postoperative mismanagement.[34] This study emphasizes one of the key elements in the perioperative care of trauma patients: missed injuries are not uncommon in trauma patients and they can have dire consequences, including the development of ARDS, MODS, and death.[35–37] Although the specifics of the operative care of the trauma patient are covered elsewhere, certain aspects are important in the context of MODS. An example is the judicious use of damage-control laparotomy to limit both acute and delayed

MODS. The rationale behind a damage-control laparotomy is the clinical observation that prolonged attempts at definitive control of intra-abdominal injuries can result in hemodynamic instability, acidosis, and coagulopathy.

If the patient survives the operation, the incidence of postoperative MODS is high. In contrast, a planned reoperation is safer and easier in patients who have been warmed and fully resuscitated and have had their acidosis and coagulopathy corrected. Although the morbidity and mortality rate of patients undergoing damage-control laparotomies is significant, the incidence of MODS appears to be reduced and survival increased.[36] A second example of operative intervention to reduce the incidence of ARDS and MODS is early fixation of long-bone fractures.[38] In fact, beginning as early as 1985, numerous prospective and retrospective clinical trials have documented that early fixation of long-bone fractures compared with delayed fracture fixation is associated with lower rates of renal, respiratory, and liver failure and lower rates of death.

Early fracture fixation in the presence of major thoracic or head injury is controversial. Proponents of early fixation have shown no added morbidity in the presence of either chest or head injury, whereas opponents have cited increases in the risk for secondary brain injury and ARDS associated with early orthopedic intervention in these specific patient subpopulations. Despite these subgroups, most evidence supports early fracture fixation as an effective method of reducing organ failure in patients with long-bone fractures, although in the individual patient caution must be exercised in the timing of secondary operations.

Intensive Care Unit Management Phase

The incidence of postoperative and postinjury MOF can be prevented through strategies such as continued resuscitation, management of infectious complications, and early nutritional and specific organ support. Although some organs (such as the pulmonary system) have randomized prospective data supporting certain therapies that improve outcome, other systems (such as the hepatic system) rarely require specific treatment. In this section we focus on preventive and therapeutic strategies that appear to have reduced the incidence of MODS and/or improved outcome in patients with MODS (Tables 4 and 5).

Because infections can contribute to the development of MODS and can increase mortality, several key concepts must be kept in

Table 4: Prevention of Multiple Organ Failure

Resuscitative Phase

Shock resuscitation

Base deficit and lactate monitoring

Restrictive strategy for blood transfusion

Operative Phase

Vigilance in preventing missed injuries

Damage-control laparotomy

Early fracture fixation

ICU Phase

Infection-related issues

Early nutritional support and glucose control

Specific organ support

Recognition of abdominal compartment syndrome

Pharmacologic therapy

ICU, Intensive care unit.

Table 5: ICU Interventions That Reduce Mortality or Attenuate Organ Dysfunction

Objective	Intervention
Resuscitation	Early goal-directed resuscitation
Prophylaxis	SDD
ICU support	Restrictive transfusion strategy
	Low tidal volume ventilation
	Daily awakening
	Tight glucose control
	Enteral feeding
Mediator-targeted therapy	Activated protein C
	Low-dose corticosteroids

ICU, Intensive care unit; *SDD*, selective decontamination of digestive tract.

mind to limit infection-related MODS. The use of early empiric antibiotics in patients suspected of having pneumonia is important because the use of early adequate empiric antibiotic has been shown to reduce pneumonia-related mortality.[39] Interestingly, although not used much in the United States it appears that selective decontamination of the digestive tract (SDD) reduces infectious complications as well as mortality in critically ill trauma and other surgical patients.[40]

The concept behind SDD is that the gut is a major reservoir for organisms causing pneumonias and bacteremias. By controlling the intestinal bacterial flora, including the upper gastrointestinal tract flora, the incidence of infections and hence mortality will be reduced. The reason for the failure to employ SDD appears to relate to the fact that this therapy is very labor intensive and has only recently been shown by meta-analyses to improve survival. In addition, when MODS develops in the postoperative or post-trauma period a meticulous search for a source of infection should be made, with particular attention to wounds, incisions, sites of previous injury or surgery, and intravenous catheter sites because the development of ARDS or MODS is not an uncommon manifestation of an occult infection. Despite extensive research involving various pharmacologic therapies of severe sepsis, with the exception of activated protein C, the results of clinical trials of immunomodulatory agents have been distressing.

In contrast, a prospective randomized trial documented that the recombinant form of activated protein C improved 28-day survival and led to a more rapid resolution of cardiovascular, respiratory, and hematologic dysfunction in patients with severe sepsis.[41] The reason activated protein C was effective where other agents were not may relate to the fact that it has both anticoagulant and anti-inflammatory activity, thereby protecting the microcirculation as well as limiting the inflammatory response. Last, the use of low-dose steroids has emerged as an effective therapy in patients with pressor-refractory septic shock and an impaired response to ACTH stimulation because controlled trials have documented that in this patient group the administration of 50 mg of hydrocortisone every 6 hours and 50 mcg of fludrocortisone improves survival.[42]

In addition to infectious issues, other non organ-specific therapies that appear to be beneficial include early enteral alimentation, glucose control, elevation of the head of the bed, and daily cessation of sedative infusions in ventilated patients. The notion of early enteral feeding is based on the concept of limiting gut-origin sepsis because the fed gut is more resistant to stress-induced injury and parenteral alimentation is associated with gut atrophy, increased permeability, and loss of barrier function.[7] Based on the results of multiple prospective randomized trials, early enteral nutrition has been found to effectively reduce infectious complications, ICU, and total hospital length of stay, although it does not appear to improve survival.[43] Thus, in an attempt to further improve the beneficial effects of enteral feedings a number of immune-enhancing enteral formulas were produced and tested in trauma and ICU patients.

Although some studies comparing standard to immune-enhancing enteral formulas suggested that immune-enhancing diets are associated with a further decrease in infectious complications, others did not.[44] Thus, at the current time the institution of early enteral feeding seems to be the key factor in reducing infectious complications—with the composition of the enteral formula being of secondary importance. A second metabolic approach has been the institution of tight glucose control in which insulin is liberally used to keep the serum glucose less than 120 mg/dl.

Since the original prospective randomized controlled study showing that tight glucose control (<120 mg/dl) was associated with a survival advantage compared to a more liberal glucose control regimen (<215 mg/dl),[45] numerous other studies (including several in trauma patients) have validated the concept that elevated serum glucose levels are associated with an increased incidence of infectious complications and poorer clinical outcomes.[46] Other easily instituted ICU therapies have been shown to reduce complications. For example, daily interruption of sedative infusions in critically ill patients undergoing mechanical ventilation reduces ICU length of stay and morbidity,[47] whereas elevation of the head of the bed of ventilated patients reduces the incidence of pneumonia and helps to preserve pulmonary function.[48]

In addition to elevating the head of the bed and daily sedative cessation, other advances in the care of the patient with respiratory failure have been made over the last several years. The most important of these was the recognition that high tidal volumes and increased airway pressures cause, rather than prevent, lung injury by inducing lung inflammation. This process has been termed *ventilator-induced lung injury* (VILI). Consistent with this physiologic concept, multicenter randomized controlled trials confirmed that mechanical ventilation of patients with acute lung injury and ARDS with a lower tidal volume (i.e., 6 ml/kg) than traditionally used results in decreased mortality and attenuates the local and systemic release of proinflammatory mediators.[49,50] In addition, further clinical trials documented that outcomes in patients with acute lung injury or ARDS are similar whether lower or higher PEEP levels are used when an end-inspiratory plateau-pressure limit of 30 cm of water is maintained.[51]

While oxygenation is maintained with low tidal volumes, permissive hypercapnia and increased CO_2 levels may develop as a result of decreased ventilation, but this does not appear to be harmful.[52,53] Thus, the use of low-tidal volume ventilation that maintains the inspiratory plateau pressure below 30 cm of water is effective both in the prevention and treatment of acute lung injury and ARDS. A number of other ventilatory strategies have either failed to show consistent benefit (such as inhaled nitric oxide) or remain to be proven beneficial (such as prone ventilation or high-frequency ventilation).

Renal replacement therapy has been effective in critically ill patients with MODS by allowing regulation of fluid and electrolytes. Renal replacement therapy also has the potential to remove toxins and circulating mediators of inflammation. Methods of supporting renal function, such as the prophylactic use of low-dose dopamine, have not been found to be effective.[54] Thus, currently the best way to limit renal failure is to avoid underresuscitation and to promptly diagnose and treat infectious complications. Once renal failure has occurred, continuous venovenous hemodialysis appears to be superior to hemodialysis because it avoids the need for systemic anticoagulation and is less likely to cause hypotensive episodes in the fragile patient.[55]

A recently recognized and important treatable cause of MODS is the abdominal compartment syndrome (ACS). The ACS can be viewed as a reversible mechanical cause of MODS that is related to increased intra-abdominal pressure.[56,57] As the intra-abdominal pressure rises, abdominal visceral perfusion decreases, ventilation is impaired, and cardiac output declines. Clinically, the ACS is manifested

as a decreasing urine output, inadequate ventilation associated with elevated peak airway pressures, and hypotension. Patients at highest risk of developing ACS are those suffering from multiple trauma, massive hemorrhage, and prolonged operations with massive volume resuscitation, as well as those requiring intra-abdominal packing to control bleeding.

ACS can also develop in patients after severe hemorrhagic shock without an abdominal or retroperitoneal injury, and this phenomenon is known as secondary ACS. Secondary ACS is due to progressive visceral and retroperitoneal edema in shocked patients with the capillary leak syndrome who receive massive crystalloid fluid resuscitation. The diagnosis of ACS is made or confirmed by measuring the abdominal pressure through a Foley catheter placed in the bladder, with ACS being defined as the combination of a urinary bladder pressure >25 mm Hg, progressive organ dysfunction (urinary output <0.5 ml/kg/hr or PaO_2/F_1O_2 <150 or peak airway pressure >45 cm H_2O or cardiac index <3 L/min/m² despite resuscitation), and improved organ function after surgical abdominal decompression. Surgical treatment, consisting of opening the abdomen, leads to rapid and profound correction of the physiologic abnormalities in most cases, whereas untreated the ACS is highly lethal, with a mortality rate approaching 100%.

CONCLUSIONS AND ALGORITHM

The development of SIRS and MODS in trauma patients remains relatively common. However, due to advances in understanding the biology of the host's immunoinflammatory system as well as the mechanisms involved in the pathogenesis of SIRS, ARDS, and MODS progress in the treatment and prevention of these syndromes has occurred. This progress is reflected both as a decrease in the incidence of MODS and an improvement in the survival of patients with MODS. The strategies used to accomplish these goals involve both preventive and therapeutic approaches that begin in the resuscitative phase of the operative care of these patients and continue through the operative and ICU phase (Figure 2).

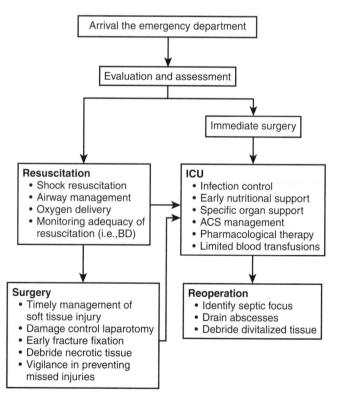

Figure 2 Algorithm for preventing and managing MODS.

REFERENCES

1. Tilney NL, Bailey GL, Morgan AP: Sequential system failure after rupture of abdominal aortic aneurysms: an unsolved problem in postoperative care. *Ann Surg* 178:117–122, 1973.
2. Sauaia A, Moore FA, Moore EE, et al: Early predictors of postinjury multiple organ failure. *Arch Surg* 129:39–45, 1994.
3. Ciesla DJ, Moore EE, Johnson JL, et al: A 12-year prospective study of postinjury multiple organ failure: has anything changed? *Arch Surg* 140:432–439, 2005.
4. Dunne JR, Malone DL, Tracy JK, Napolitano LM: Allogenic blood transfusion in the first 24 hours after trauma is associated with increased systemic inflammatory response syndrome (SIRS) and death. *Surg Infect* 5:395–404, 2004.
5. Moore FA, Moore EE, Sauaia A: Blood transfusion. An independent risk factor for postinjury multiple organ failure. *Arch Surg* 132:620–625, 1997.
6. Nast-Kolb D, Aufmkolk M, Rucholtz S, et al: Multiple organ failure still a major cause of morbidity but not mortality in blunt multiple trauma. *J Trauma* 51:835–842, 2001.
7. Deitch EA: Multiple organ failure. Pathophysiology and potential future therapy. *Ann Surg* 216:117–134, 1992.
8. Groeneveld PH, Kwappenberg KM, Langermans JA, et al: Nitric oxide (NO) production correlates with renal insufficiency and multiple organ dysfunction syndrome in severe sepsis. *Intensive Care Med* 22:1197–1202, 1996.
9. Goris RJ, te Boekhorst TP, Nuytinck JK, Gimbrere JS: Multiple-organ failure. Generalized autodestructive inflammation? *Arch Surg* 120:1109–1115, 1985.
10. Deitch EA: Role of the gut lymphatic system in multiple organ failure. *Curr Opin Crit Care* 7:92–98, 2001.
11. Ivatury RR, Simon RJ, Islam S, et al: A prospective randomized study of end points of resuscitation after major trauma: global oxygen transport indices versus organ-specific gastric mucosal pH. *J Am Coll Surg* 183:145–154, 1996.
12. Moore FA, Moore EE, Poggetti R, et al: Gut bacterial translocation via the portal vein: a clinical perspective with major torso trauma. *J Trauma* 31:629–638, 1991.
13. Bone RC, Sibbald WJ, Sprung CL: The ACCP-SCCM consensus conference on sepsis and organ failure. *Chest* 101:1481–1483, 1992.
14. Bone RC, Cerra FB, Dellinger RP, Fein AM, Knaus WA, Schein RM, Sibbald WJ: Definitions for sepsis and organ failure and guidelines for the use of innovative therapies in sepsis. The ACCP/SCCM Consensus Conference Committee. *Chest* 101:1644–1655, 1992.
15. Bernard G: The Brussels Score. *Sepsis* 1:43–44, 1997.
16. Le Gall JR, Klar J, Lemeshow S, et al: The Logistic Organ Dysfunction system. A new way to assess organ dysfunction in the intensive care unit. ICU Scoring Group. *JAMA* 276:802–810, 1996.
17. Marshall JC: Multiple organ dysfunction syndrome. *ACS Surgery: Principles and Practice*, November 3, 2003.
18. Vincent JL, de Mendonca A, Cantraine F, et al: Use of the SOFA score to assess the incidence of organ dysfunction/failure in intensive care units: results of a multicenter, prospective study. Working group on "sepsis-related problems" of the European Society of Intensive Care Medicine. *Crit Care Med* 26:1793–1800, 1998.
19. Marshall JC, Cook DJ, Christou NV, et al: Multiple organ dysfunction score: a reliable descriptor of a complex clinical outcome. *Crit Care Med* 23:1638–1652, 1995.
20. Peres Bota D, Melot C, Lopes Ferreira F, et al: The Multiple Organ Dysfunction Score (MODS) versus the Sequential Organ Failure Assessment (SOFA) score in outcome prediction. *Intensive Care Med* 28:1619–1624, 2002.
21. Pettila V, Pettila M, Sarna S, et al: Comparison of multiple organ dysfunction scores in the prediction of hospital mortality in the critically ill. *Crit Care Med* 30:1705–1711, 2002.
22. Davis JW, Kaups KL, Parks SN: Base deficit is superior to pH in evaluating clearance of acidosis after traumatic shock. *J Trauma* 44:114–118, 1998.
23. Davis JW, Shackford SR, Mackersie RC, Hoyt DB: Base deficit as a guide to volume resuscitation. *J Trauma* 28:1464–1467, 1988.
24. Rhee P, Wang D, Ruff P, et al: Human neutrophil activation and increased adhesion by various resuscitation fluids. *Crit Care Med* 28:74–78, 2000.
25. Rhee P, Burris D, Kaufmann C, et al: Lactated Ringer's solution resuscitation causes neutrophil activation after hemorrhagic shock. *J Trauma* 44:313–319, 1998.
26. Koustova E, Stanton K, Gushchin V, et al: Effects of lactated Ringer's solutions on human leukocytes. *J Trauma* 52:872–878, 2002.
27. Alam HB, Sun L, Ruff P, et al: E- and P-selectin expression depends on the resuscitation fluid used in hemorrhaged rats. *J Surg Res* 94:145–152, 2002.
28. Balogh Z, McKinley BA, Cocanour CS, et al: Supranormal trauma resuscitation causes more cases of abdominal compartment syndrome. *Arch Surg* 138:637–643, 2003.
29. Mattox KL, Maningas PA, Moore EE, et al: Prehospital hypertonic saline/dextran infusion for post-traumatic hypotension. The U.S.A. Multicenter Trial. *Ann Surg* 213:482–491, 1991.
30. Nathens AB, Neff MJ, Jurkovich GJ, et al: Randomized, prospective trial of antioxidant supplementation in critically ill surgical patients. *Ann Surg* 236:814–822, 2002.
31. Moore EE. Blood substitutes: the future is now. *J Am Coll Surg* 196:1–17, 2003.
32. Hebert P, Wells G, Blajchman M, et al: A multicenter, randomized, controlled clinical trial of transfusion requirements in critical care. Transfusion Requirements in Critical Care Investigators, Canadian Critical Care Trials Group. *N Engl J Med* 340:409–413, 1999.
33. Hebert PC, McDonald BJ, Tinmouth A: Clinical consequences of anemia and red cell transfusion in the critically ill. *Crit Care Clin* 20:225–235, 2004.
34. Eiseman B, Beart R, Norton L: Multiple organ failure. *Surg Gynecol Obstet* 144:323–326, 1977.
35. Brooks A, Holroyd B, Riley B: Missed injury in major trauma patients. *Injury* 35:407–410, 2004.
36. Hirshberg A, Wall MJ Jr, Mattox KL: Planned reoperation for trauma: a two year experience with 124 consecutive patients. *J Trauma* 37:365–369, 1994.
37. Houshian S, Larsen MS, Holm C: Missed injuries in a level I trauma center. *J Trauma* 52:715–719, 2002.
38. Carlson DW, Rodman GH Jr, Kaehr D, et al: Femur fractures in chest-injured patients: is reaming contraindicated? *J Orthop Trauma* 12:164–168, 1998.
39. Garnacho-Montero J, Garcia-Garmendia JL, Barrero-Almodovar A, et al: Impact of adequate empirical antibiotic therapy on the outcome of patients admitted to the intensive care unit with sepsis. *Crit Care Med* 31:2742–2751, 2003.
40. De Jonge E: Effects of selective decontamination of digestive tract on mortality and antibiotic resistance in the intensive-care unit. *Curr Opin Crit Care* 11:144–149, 2005.
41. Vincent JL, Angus DC, Artigas A, et al: Effects of drotrecogin alfa (activated) on organ dysfunction in the PROWESS trial. *Crit Care Med* 31:834–840, 2003.
42. Annane D, Sebille V, Charpentier C, et al: Effect of treatment with low doses of hydrocortisone and fludrocortisone on mortality in patients with septic shock. *JAMA* 288:862–871, 2002.
43. Marik PE, Zaloga GP: Early enteral nutrition in acutely ill patients: a systematic review. *Crit Care Med* 29:2264, 2003.
44. Kieft H, Roos AN, van Drunen JD, et al: Clinical outcome of immunonutrition in a heterogeneous intensive care population. *Intensive Care Med* 31:524–532, 2005.
45. Van den Berghe G, Wouters P, Weekers F, et al: Intensive insulin therapy in the critically ill patients. *N Engl J Med* 345:1359–1367, 2001.
46. Laird AM, Miller PR, Kilgo PD, et al: Relationship of early hyperglycemia to mortality in trauma patients. *J Trauma* 56:1058–1062, 2004.
47. Schweickert WD, Gehlbach BK, Pohlman AS, et al: Daily interruption of sedative infusions and complications of critical illness in mechanically ventilated patients. *Crit Care Med* 32:1272–1276, 2004.
48. Drakulovic MB, Torres A, Bauer TT, et al: Supine body position as a risk factor for nosocomial pneumonia in mechanically ventilated patients: a randomised trial. *Lancet* 354:1851–1858, 1999.
49. Ranieri VM, Suter PM, Tortorella C, et al: Effect of mechanical ventilation on inflammatory mediators in patients with acute respiratory distress syndrome: a randomized controlled trial. *JAMA* 282:54–61, 1999.
50. The Acute Respiratory Distress Syndrome N: Ventilation with lower tidal volumes as compared with traditional tidal volumes for acute lung injury and the acute respiratory distress syndrome. *N Engl J Med* 342:1301–1308, 2000.
51. Brower RG, Lanken PN, MacIntyre N, et al: Higher versus lower positive end-expiratory pressures in patients with the acute respiratory distress syndrome. *N Engl J Med* 351:327, 2004.
52. Hickling KG, Walsh J, Henderson S, Jackson R: Low mortality rate in adult respiratory distress syndrome using low-volume, pressure-limited

ventilation with permissive hypercapnia: a prospective study. *Crit Care Med* 22:1568–1578, 1994.

53. Laffey JG, Tanaka M, Engelberts D, et al: Therapeutic hypercapnia reduces pulmonary and systemic injury following in vivo lung reperfusion. *Am J Respir Crit Care Med* 162:2287–2294, 2000.

54. Friedrich JO, Adhikari N, Herridge MS, Beyene J: Meta-analysis: low-dose dopamine increases urine output but does not prevent renal dysfunction or death. *Ann Intern Med* 142:510–524, 2005.

55. Swartz RD, Bustami RT, Daley JM, et al: Estimating the impact of renal replacement therapy choice on outcome in severe acute renal failure. *Clin Nephrol* 63:335–345, 2005.

56. Balogh Z, McKinley BA, Holcomb JB, et al: Both primary and secondary abdominal compartment syndrome can be predicted early and are harbingers of multiple organ failure. *J Trauma* 54:848–861, 2003.

57. Burch JM, Moore EE, Moore FA, Franciose R: The abdominal compartment syndrome. *Surg Clin North Am* 76:833–842, 1996.

SEPSIS, SEPTIC SHOCK, AND ITS TREATMENT

Preya Ananthakrishnan and **Edwin A. Deitch**

Sepsis and septic shock, especially when associated with single or multiple organ dysfunction, are important causes of morbidity and mortality in trauma patients. Thus, an organized approach directed at preventing infectious complications as well as a strategy ensuring early diagnosis and treatment of infections, when they occur, are important components of trauma care. Over the last decade, progress has been made in developing such strategies, not just in trauma patients, but in all intensive care unit (ICU) patient populations. In fact, because sepsis and septic shock are such a major cause of mortality, an international group of experts from nine different societies met, and, through a Delphi-type process, developed a series of guidelines for the optimal treatment of sepsis and septic shock. These evidence-based recommendations were published in 2004 and are called the Surviving Sepsis Campaign guidelines.[1]

INCIDENCE

In trauma patients, injury not only predisposes to infection by promoting bacterial contamination of normally sterile tissues and spaces, but also induces the development of an immunocompromised state with infection and infection-related multiple organ failure being common causes of late death after trauma. Although the exact incidence of sepsis and septic shock in trauma patients is not fully known, the incidence of sepsis and septic shock is increasing nationally and affects an estimated 751,000 patients per year in the United States with an overall mortality in excess of 30%.[2] This mortality rate is even higher in the presence of multiple organ failure, where mortality rates up to 85% have been reported. This increase in the incidence of sepsis and septic shock appears to involve trauma patients as well and can be attributed to several factors, including the aging of the population, which results in more elderly patients with significant comorbidities sustaining trauma. Additionally, advances in medical and surgical care have resulted in more severely injured patients surviving their initial injuries and thus being at risk for the subsequent development of infectious complications. Lastly, certain trauma-related variables appear to increase the risk of developing an infectious complication and these include the presence of preoperative shock, colon injuries, central nervous system (CNS) injuries, and injury to multiple organs as well as the administration of blood transfusions, due to their immunosuppressive effects.[3]

MECHANISM OF INFECTION

Infections in trauma patients may occur for many reasons. These include the global immunosuppressive effects of a major injury, patient-related factors, consequences of injuries to specific organs such as the intestine, as well as infections occurring after operations or due to the need for invasive monitoring or mechanical ventilation. For example, risk factors for sepsis include extremes of age and chronic underlying medical conditions, such as malnutrition, alcoholism, malignancy, and diabetes mellitus, all of which compromise the immune system.[2] There is also evidence to suggest that some patients may have a genetic predisposition for the development of sepsis, as well as increased mortality when an infection is acquired.[4] For example, genetic polymorphisms have been identified in the genes for TNF, IL-6, IL-10, IL-1 receptor antagonist, heat shock protein, CD14, and lipopolysaccharide binding proteins.[2] There is even evidence that gender influences the risk of post-trauma sepsis with males being more susceptible than premenopausal females.[5] Thus, genetic factors and to a lesser extent sex hormonal status may help explain the heterogeneity observed among patients developing infections after trauma as well as in the evaluation of new therapeutic molecules in patients with sepsis.

Another reason why infectious complications are relatively common in trauma patients is that traumatic injury itself leads to bacterial contamination of spaces that are normally sterile, while the presence of hematomas and devitalized or necrotic tissue causes an anoxic microenvironment that impairs the ability of the host's antibacterial factors to effectively clear bacteria if these hematomas or devitalized tissue sites become infected. Clinical examples of this phenomenon are secondary infections of major liver injuries or splenic injuries treated with splenic artery embolization. Likewise, pulmonary contusions, which occur in 10%–25% of patients after blunt chest injury, are associated with impaired immune function and an increased susceptibility to infectious complications. Additionally, many of our therapeutic maneuvers potentially predispose patients to an increased risk of infection. For example, invasive monitoring lines allow bacteria colonizing the skin surface direct access to the bloodstream, while endotracheal tubes and Foley catheters also promote the development of pneumonia and urinary tract infection (UTI). In fact, the incidence of nosocomial infections in mechanically-ventilated trauma patients is relatively high and increases as the ICU length of stay increases, reaching over 50% in patients in the ICU more than 7–10 days. This increased infection rate appears to be associated with up to a three-fold increase in mortality, especially in patients with moderately severe injuries who might otherwise be expected to survive.[6]

DIAGNOSIS

The making of an early and accurate diagnosis of infection or septic shock is an important, but potentially difficult, aspect of the care of the trauma patient. One reason for this difficulty is that the common signs of infection, such as fever, leukocytosis, and tachycardia are relatively common in noninfected trauma patients and represent the host's inflammatory response to injury. The fact that noninfectious septic responses are common after major trauma and can be indistinguishable from an infectious-mediated septic response therefore confounds diagnostic decision making. Furthermore, the need for ventilatory support and sedation in many of these patients further impairs the ability of the clinician to accurately question and examine the patient. Additionally, the presence of postoperative pain after procedures, such as a laparotomy, further limits the accuracy of abdominal symptoms or physical examination in the patient at risk for developing abdominal sepsis. For all of these reasons, vigilance, a high level of suspicion and knowledge of the likely sites of infection in each specific patient are required to facilitate the early diagnosis of an infection. Likewise, it is important to recognize that certain physiologic changes in the otherwise stable patient may be an early sign of a serious infection. Examples of these physiologic derangements, in addition to the standard signs of fever and tachycardia, include new onset ileus, a change in sensorium, fluid sequestration manifesting as an increasing need for fluids to maintain urine output, the development of a metabolic acidosis, or worsening of the patient's respiratory status.

Since pneumonia, line sepsis, and infections at the sites of injury or previous operations are especially common in severely injured trauma patients, special attention should be focused on these areas in the at risk patient in whom infection is suspected. In fact, ventilator-associated pneumonia is one of the most common causes of infection-related death in the ICU and can be difficult to diagnose, as are episodes of life-threatening line sepsis. Whenever an infection is suspected, diagnostic studies to determine the causative organisms should be performed before the start of antibiotic therapy, although commencement of antibiotic therapy should not wait for diagnostic studies to be completed since the early treatment of an infection appears to reduce morbidity and mortality (Figure 1). Specifically, when infection is suspected, two sets of blood cultures should be drawn—one percutaneously, and one through any intravascular

catheter more than 48 hours old. The rationale for drawing cultures from existing vascular lines is to screen for line sepsis and if the blood culture from the vascular line comes back positive earlier than the percutaneously drawn blood culture (i.e., >2 hours), this suggests that the vascular access device is a likely source of the infection.[7] Additionally, as appropriate, cultures of urine, cerebrospinal fluid, and body fluids should be obtained. Bronchoscopy and bronchoalveolar lavage with quantitative cultures should be used for the diagnosis of ventilator-associated pneumonia. Radiologic imaging studies with sampling of potential sources of infection can also be helpful, especially in patients at risk of having intra-abdominal septic sites.

Since the response to empiric antibiotics is also important in validating that a patient's septic response is infectious and not related to an excessive inflammatory response or a nonbacterial etiology, such as pancreatitis, the initial antibiotic therapy should be broad enough to be effective against the most likely causative organisms and have good penetration into the presumed infectious source. When used appropriately, antibiotics are effective in the treatment of certain infections, yet they can also predispose to superinfections or antibiotic-resistant strains by disrupting the host's normal microflora. The key strategy to minimize the development of antibiotic resistant strains is to use the narrowest spectrum of agents for the shortest time possible. Consequently, the empiric antibiotic regimen should be reassessed after culture data is available (usually after 48 to 72 hours), and broad-spectrum antibiotics should be tapered to a more narrow spectrum as soon as possible if an infection is documented or stopped completely if there is no evidence of an infection.

STAGING

An international sepsis definitions consensus conference of the American College of Chest Physicians and the Society of Critical Care Medicine attempted to define a staging system for sepsis. This was called PIRO (predisposition, insult or infection, response, and organ dysfunction). Predisposition includes premorbid conditions that influence the likelihood of infection, sepsis, morbidity, and survival. Insult or infection refers to the specific organism causing the septic response, the sensitivity pattern, and whether the infection is community acquired or nosocomial. Response attempts to quantify the clinical manifestations of the systemic inflammatory response syndrome (SIRS), by using markers such as procalcitonin, IL-6, HLA-DR, TNF, PAF, and C-reactive protein. Organ dysfunction refers to the type and number of dysfunctional organs, and whether it is reversible or irreversible.[8] Organ dysfunction is judged by other scoring systems discussed elsewhere in this text, including multiple organ dysfunction syndrome (MODS) score, logistic organ dysfunction system (LODS), and sequential organ failure assessment (SOFA). Although the PIRO classification is not in wide use, it provides a conceptual framework for staging sepsis (Table 1).

MEDICAL AND SURGICAL MANAGEMENT

Management of sepsis due to an infectious process begins with prompt recognition that an infection is likely, determination of the probable site of infection and assessment of the severity of the physiologic derangements. Based on the source and cause of the infection, specific therapy may be limited to antibiotics or require a combination of antibiotics plus operative or interventional source control. The choice of antibiotics depends on the suspected site of infection and the organisms that commonly inhabit that location (Table 2). Antibiotic choice may have to be modified for patients likely to have an abnormal flora, such as patients who have had a previous course of antibiotics or those who have been colonized by hospital-acquired pathogens. In these circumstances, treatment is

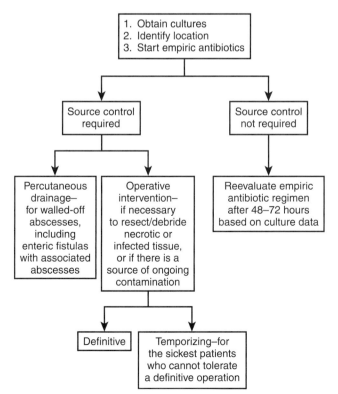

Figure 1 Diagnosis and treatment of sepsis.

Table 1: *PIRO* Staging of Sepsis

Predisposition	Premorbid conditions influencing the likelihood of infection, sepsis, morbidity, or survival (age, sex, hormonal state, genetic polymorphisms)
Insult/infection	Insult or organism associated with the sepsis response (type of organism, sensitivity pattern, community or nosocomial acquisition)
Response	Clinical manifestation of the SIRS response (procalcitonin, IL-6, TNF, C-reactive protein)
Organ dysfunction	Type and number of dysfunctional organs (reversible vs. irreversible dysfunction), severity of dysfunction (judged by scoring systems such as MODS, LODS, and SOFA)

IL, Interleukin; *LODS,* logistic organ dysfunction score; *MODS,* multiple organ dysfunction score; *SIRS,* systemic inflammatory response syndrome; *SOFA,* sequential organ failure assessment; *TNF,* tumor necrosis factor.
Adapted from Magnotti LJ, Croce MA, Fabian TC: Is ventilator-associated pneumonia in trauma patients an epiphenomenon or a cause of death? *Surg Infect (Larchmt)* 5:237–242, 2004.

Table 2: Common Organisms and Antibiotic Choice Based on Location of Suspected Infection

Site	Common Community-Acquired Organisms and Treatment	Common Nosocomial Organisms and Treatment
Lung	*Streptococcus pneumoniae, Haemophilus influenzae, Legionella, Chlamydia, Pneumocystic carinii*	Aerobic Gram-negative bacilli
	Macrolide and third-generation cephalosporin or levofloxacin	Cefepime or imipenem-cilastatin with aminoglycoside
Abdomen	*Escherichia coli, Bacteroides fragilis*	Aerobic Gram-negative rods, anaerobes, *Candida*
	Imipenem-cilastatin or piperacillin-tazobactam with or without aminoglycoside	Imipenem-cilastatin with or without aminoglycoside, or piperacillin-tazobactam with or without amphotericin B
Skin/soft tissue	Group A *Streptococcus, Staphylococcus aureus, Clostridium,* polymicrobial, enteric Gram-negative rods, *Pseudomonas Aeruginosa,* anaerobes, *Staphylococci*	*Staphylococcus aureus,* aerobic Gram-negative rods
	Vancomycin with or without imipenem-cilastatin or piperacillin-tazobactam	Vancomycin with cefepime
Urinary tract	*Escherichia coli, Klebsiella* sp., *Enterobacter* sp., *Proteus* sp.	Aerobic Gram-negative rods, *Enterococci*
	Ciprofloxacin with or without aminoglycoside	Vancomycin with cefepime
CNS	*S. pneumoniae, Neisseria meningitidis, Listeria monocytogenes, E. coli, H. influenzae*	*P. aeruginosa, E. coli, Klebsiella, Staphylococcus*
	Vancomycin, third-generation cephalosporin, or meropenem	Cefepime or meropenem with vancomycin

Adapted from Balk RA: Optimum treatment of severe sepsis and septic shock: evidence in support of the recommendations. *Dis Month* 50:163–213, 2004.

initiated with a single agent or combination of agents with the lowest possible toxicities, whose spectrum of activity is broad enough to cover all suspected pathogens. Since victims of major trauma are at increased risk of developing multiple infections, it is crucial that antibiotics are stopped as soon as possible to limit the emergence of antibiotic-resistant bacteria. There is no good evidence to suggest that antibiotic treatment should exceed 7–10 days, except in unusual circumstances. Likewise, in determining the length of antibiotic use, it is also important to differentiate between prophylaxis and therapy, especially in the trauma patient in whom injury-induced bacterial contamination may have occurred. For example, in a trauma patient undergoing laparotomy for blunt or penetrating trauma, the patient receives preoperative antibiotics (usually a second-generation cephalosporin), which are usually stopped within 24 hours postoperatively. However, if a major degree of contamination is present, as in a colon injury where the incidence of abdominal abscess formation reaches over 25%,[9] the antibiotics should be continued for 3–5 days, since they serve both prophylactic (for the wound) and therapeutic roles (for the peritoneum).

In addition, antibiotics play only a secondary role in certain infections, and their effectiveness can be influenced by local factors. For example, certain antibiotics, such as the aminoglycosides, are inactivated by purulent material and thus are not fully effective in treating abscesses. Furthermore, since many antibiotics as well as host phagocytic cells require oxygen for optimal activity, antibiotics play only a supportive role to operative drainage in the treatment of infections associated with a low oxygen tension such as abscesses. Antibiotics are also secondary to surgical intervention in infections complicated by the presence of necrotic tissue or hematomas, in which case debridement of necrotic tissue and removal of hematomas in combination with source control is of the utmost importance. Source control is also critical in cases of leaking anastomoses or injured intestinal viscera.

However, even in spite of appropriate initial surgical management, postoperative intra-abdominal infections remain a major cause of morbidity and mortality in the trauma victim. Although the peritoneal cavity is relatively resistant to a bacterial challenge, the presence of adjuvant substances such as fibrin or hemoglobin allows bacteria to evade the normal host defenses and can result in intra-abdominal infection. Thus, if there is suspicion of a postoperative intra-abdominal infection, the primary goal is to determine whether the patient has intra-abdominal sepsis, and if so, to determine the necessity and timing of reoperation versus percutaneous therapy. In this situation, the most useful diagnostic modality in a stable patient is a helical abdominal computed tomography (CT) scan. Abdominal CT scan has a sensitivity of 97% and a specificity of 65% in diagnosing an intra-abdominal source of sepsis.[10] If there are no signs of overwhelming sepsis and the CT scan shows evidence of a localized abscess, whether in the peritoneal cavity or at the site of an injured organ, such as the liver, the intra-abdominal infection usually can be managed nonoperatively with fluid resuscitation, CT-guided drainage of the abscess and broad-spectrum antibiotics. This is especially useful in the patient who has undergone multiple abdominal operations, where relaparotomy can be difficult. Even though anastomotic leaks and breakdowns may result in severe sepsis or the formation of an enterocutaneous fistula, these patients still may be candidates for percutaneous drainage if there is no evidence of continuing contamination, if the catheter drainage route does not traverse bowel or uncontaminated organs and the infectious source is controlled by catheter drainage.[11] In contrast, when these conditions can not be met, or in the patient with diffuse peritonitis, prompt reoperation to control the source of infection and provide drainage is mandatory and can be life-saving.

MORBIDITY AND COMPLICATIONS MANAGEMENT

Two of the major complications of infection are the development of septic shock and/or MODS. In fact, the development of shock and/or organ dysfunction can even be the first sign that a patient has a serious infection. Consequently, this section will focus on the treatment of septic shock as well as on MODS.

Septic Shock

The therapeutic approach to a patient with septic shock has several components and begins with fluid administration (Figure 2). Fluids are the initial component of therapy since septic shock is characterized by excessive vasodilation and a decrease in systemic vascular resistance, although the cardiac output may be greatly increased. Septic shock is also associated with an increase in capillary permeability resulting in a decrease in intravascular volume secondary to third-spacing of fluid. In spite of the ongoing debate as to the relative value of crystalloids versus colloids, they both have similar effects on preload, stroke volume, and oxygen delivery, thereby restoring tissue perfusion to the same degree, although approximately three times more volume of crystalloid is required than colloid, because of the propensity of crystalloid to leak into the extravascular space. Despite this debate, no difference has been shown in length of stay, mortality, or pulmonary edema when comparing colloid to crystalloid.[12] Consequently, it is the adequate and rapid administration of volume that appears more important than the fluid administered. To that end, it is important to try to reach certain specific physiologic goals to ensure that the amount of volume administered is adequate (Table 3). The importance of the early institution of goal-directed volume resuscitation in patients with septic shock was recently shown in a prospective, randomized, controlled trial where patients resuscitated to a central venous pressure of 8–12 (or 12–15 in mechanically ventilated patients due to the increased intrathoracic pressure), a mean arterial pressure above 65 mm Hg, a urine output above 0.5 ml/kg/hr, and a mixed venous oxygen saturation of over 70% had a significant reduction in hospital mortality (30% vs. 46%) as compared to patients treated with standard therapy.[13] The major difference between the two groups was that the patients in the early goal-directed group received more volume in the first 6 hours than the standard therapy group, reinforcing the importance of early and adequate volume resuscitation.

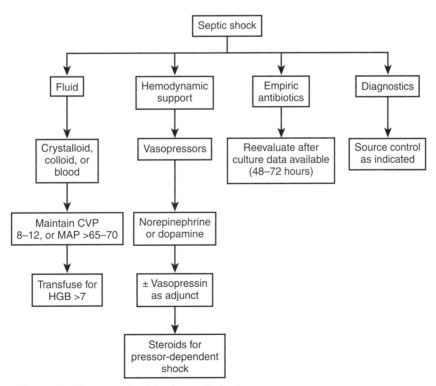

Figure 2 Treatment algorithm for septic shock.

Table 3: Goals of Resuscitation

Mixed venous O_2 saturation $> 70\%$
CVP 8–12 or CVP 12–15 on ventilator
MAP $> 65–70$ mm Hg
UOP > 0.5 ml/kg/hr
Hemoglobin > 7 g/dl
Lactate <2 mMol/l
Base deficit <-2.0 mMol/l

Adapted from Dellinger RP, Carlet JM, Masur H, et al: Surviving sepsis campaign guidelines for management of severe sepsis and septic shock. *Crit Care Med* 32:858–873, 2004 and Rivers E, Nguyen B, Havstad S, Ressler J, Muzzin A, Knoblich B, et al: Early goal-directed therapy in the treatment of severe sepsis and septic shock. *N Engl J Med* 345:1368–1377, 2001.

The role of blood products in the resuscitation of patients with septic shock should be limited to patients with significant anemia or evidence of cardiac ischemia. There is no physiologic benefit to routine RBC transfusion in the critically ill patient to maintain a hemoglobin level above 9–10 g/dl and banked blood may actually be harmful in light of its documented immunesuppressive effects,[3] and the fact that blood transfusions have been shown to be an independent predictor of MODS. In fact, the Transfusion Requirements in Critical Care Investigators (TRICC) trial demonstrated that the patients who only received blood transfusions to maintain a hemoglobin level of 7 gm/dl had a decrease in the incidence and severity of new organ dysfunction as compared to the liberal transfusion group.[14]

The role of vasopressors in septic shock continues to be an area of active investigation and they are the second line of therapy. Currently vasopressors are indicated when appropriate fluid resuscitation fails to restore adequate arterial pressure or organ perfusion (see Figure 2). They also should be used when life-threatening hypotension is present, even if fluid resuscitation is not complete.[15] In this latter situation, vasopressors are used as a bridge to temporarily maintain blood pressure while fluid resuscitation is completed. The choice of agents includes dopamine, norepinephrine, epinephrine, phenylephrine, vasopressin, and dobutamine. Dopamine and norepinephrine are the first-line pressors in septic shock, since they have limited directed cardiac effects and there are no consistent, hard data supporting the use of one over the other.[1,16] Dopamine is a precursor of epinephrine and norepinephrine with dose-dependent pharmacologic effects. At moderate doses, it stimulates beta-adrenergic receptors, and thereby increases heart rate and contractility with minimal effects on systemic vascular resistance. At high doses, the alpha-adrenergic effects predominate causing vasoconstriction with increased mean arterial pressure. Norepinephrine is an alpha-adrenergic agonist with some beta effects. Overall it causes vasoconstriction, so it was traditionally thought to have negative effects on splanchnic and renal perfusion. Recent studies, however, show that this is not true, and there are data to suggest that norepinephrine actually improves renal perfusion. A drawback with norepinephrine use is that there can be an adrenergic receptor down-regulation in sepsis, which may require large doses of the drug to be administered in order to achieve the desired physiologic effects. Norepinephrine increases mean arterial pressure without changing heart rate and cardiac output is either unchanged or increased, while systemic vascular resistance is increased. However, the increase in afterload observed with norepinephrine use may be problematic in those patients with underlying cardiac dysfunction.

Although epinephrine increases cardiac index, heart rate, and stroke volume, it is not a first-line treatment for septic shock because it decreases splanchnic blood flow and oxygen delivery. It has also been shown to be associated with transiently elevated lactate levels and can cause tachyarrhythmias. Phenylephrine is a potent alpha-adrenergic agonist, but is not a first-line agent because it can decrease cardiac output and heart rate as well as decrease splanchnic blood flow. Thus, in the patient who is refractory to dopamine or norepinephrine, the next option is to add vasopressin. The rationale for vasopressin use is based on small patient series where it was effective in patients with otherwise pressor-refractory septic shock.[17] Physiologically, endogenous vasopressin is rapidly depleted in patients with septic shock, and it has been shown to have a permissive effect on adrenergic agents increasing their vasoconstrictive effects. Specifically, low-dose vasopressin (0.01 and 0.04 units/min) has been shown to improve mean arterial pressure, cardiac index, and left ventricular stroke work when added to norepinephrine. Currently, clinical trials are investigating the clinical efficacy of vasopressin use in conjunction with dopamine or norepinephrine to augment their vasopressor effects.

Another approach to the patient with pressor-refractory septic shock is the use of low-dose steroids. This option is based on the recent recognition that patients with vasopressor-dependent septic shock often have an inappropriately low cortisol response to the shock state and are in a state of relative adrenal insufficiency. While absolute adrenal insufficiency in the septic state is rare (0%–3%), relative adrenal insufficiency is present in 50%–75% of patients in septic shock, and several recent studies have shown that low-dose corticosteroids improve survival in septic shock.[18–20] There is some controversy in defining adrenal insufficiency in patients with shock, with most series using the corticotropin stimulation test to establish the diagnosis of relative adrenal insufficiency. In this test, a baseline cortisol level is drawn, and the patient is then stimulated with 250 micrograms of corticotropin. Cortisol levels are drawn 30 and 60 minutes after administration of the corticotropin. An absolute incremental increase of less than 9 micrograms/dl 30–60 minutes after stimulation indicates relative adrenal insufficiency. Random cortisol levels of less than 25 microgram/dl have also been used as a marker for relative adrenal insufficiency in septic patients. Furthermore, since a subgroup of patients who were not found to have adrenal insufficiency responded to low-dose steroid therapy, it is unclear at this time whether the use of low-dose corticosteroids should be limited to patients with relative adrenal insufficiency or given to all patients with vasopressor-dependent septic shock, in light of the beneficial hemodynamic effects. On the other hand, there are no data to support the use of corticosteroids in septic patients without shock.

Practically speaking, empiric steroid therapy is generally begun as soon as the diagnostic tests are complete and blood has been obtained for cortisol measurements. Since the results of these tests may not return for more than 24 hours, it is also possible to use the patient's response in deciding whether the steroid therapy should be continued. The preferred glucocorticoid in patients with septic shock is hydrocortisone because it is the most closely related to the active cortisol molecule, and consequently does not rely on metabolic transformation in order to directly replace cortisol. In addition, it is the only steroid with intrinsic mineralocorticoid activity for those with absolute primary adrenal insufficiency. Several studies recommend daily dosages of 200–300 mg of hydrocortisone given in divided doses (q6–q8 hours) administered for 5–7 days or longer. There is no established protocol for cessation of steroid therapy, and since a rebound effect has been noted with abrupt cessation of steroid treatment, the dose is generally tapered over a few days. The European Corticus trial recommends halving the steroid dosage over a 3-day period with complete cessation after 6 days. Restarting of therapy is recommended if shock reoccurs during weaning of the steroid.[20]

The use of recombinant human activated protein C (rhAPC) in the treatment of septic shock is another potential option based on a large clinical trial showing that it improved survival in patients with severe sepsis, some of whom had septic shock.[21] In this phase III trial, termed the PROWESS study, rhAPC reduced the absolute 28-day mortality by 6% in patients with severe sepsis and evidence of organ failure in two or more organs (19% relative risk reduction). However, due to its ability to cause severe bleeding complications, it is contraindicated in patients with head injury, an increased risk of life-threatening bleeding, and with epidural catheters or recent active bleeding. Thus, although rhAPC is the only immunomodulatory treatment shown to date to improve survival in patients with a high risk of death (Apache II score above 25 or multiple organ failure), little information is available on its effectiveness in trauma patients. Furthermore, in contrast to the PROWESS study, no 28-day mortality benefit was shown in septic patients with a low risk of death (Apache II scores <25 or single organ failure); however, it doubled the risk of the development of a bleeding complication.[22] Thus, it appears that the use of rhAPC may not be appropriate for many trauma patients, but it should be considered in selected patients.

Multiple Organ Dysfunction Syndrome

Since infections can contribute to the development of MODS as well as increase mortality, several key concepts must be kept in mind to limit as well as to treat infection-related organ dysfunction. For example, sepsis is one of the most common clinical precursors to ARDS. Tachypnea and hyperventilation are frequent manifestations of severe sepsis, and increased work of breathing and abnormalities of oxygenation often make oxygen delivery difficult. Thus, one of the primary goals in severe sepsis is to ensure adequate oxygen delivery and oxygenation; however, the timing of mechanical ventilation is controversial. Clearly, patients with clinically evident acute lung injury or ARDS should be intubated early; however, the benefits of early ventilatory support should be weighed against the risks of ventilator-associated complications. In mechanically ventilated patients, the goal is to keep the oxygen saturation above 88%–95% while keeping the FiO_2 less than 0.6. Lung-protective strategies for improved outcome include volume-cycled ventilation in the assist control mode, with a low tidal volume (6 ml/kg of body weight). In the ARDSNET trial, low tidal volume strategies produced significantly decreased in-hospital mortality with an increase in ventilator-free and organ failure–free days.[23] In this trial, plateau pressures were kept below 30 cm of water, and tidal volumes were approximately 6 ml/kg; however, if necessary, tidal volumes were dropped to 4 ml/kg and permissive hypercapnia was allowed to achieve this goal. Permissive hypercapnia has not been shown to be detrimental, except in patients with elevated intracranial pressures. Once intubated, the only preventive strategy for decreasing the incidence of ventilator-associated pneumonia is semirecumbent positioning.[24] Patients may be laid flat for procedures, hemodynamic measurements, or episodes of hypotension, but the remainder of the time they should be semirecumbent. In addition, sedation and neuromuscular blockade should be frequently evaluated. Neuromuscular blockade should be avoided due to prolonged paralysis and skeletal muscle weakness. If necessary, depth of blockade with train-of-four monitoring should be used. Sedation should also be monitored with sedation scales and daily periods of lightening or interrupting continuous sedation, which has been shown to decrease the length of mechanical ventilation and ICU stays.[25]

Sepsis can also lead to cardiac dysfunction and associated myocardial depression, manifested as both diastolic dysfunction and a decreased cardiac response to catecholamines. This causes a decreased ejection fraction despite an increased cardiac index. This reversible biventricular myocardial dysfunction has been attributed to TNF-alpha, IL-1, or nitric oxide. Hypovolemia also exacerbates cardiac dysfunction and thus must be avoided. During this period of myocardial depression, the ventricles dilate and the ejection fraction is decreased. Even in the presence of normal or increased cardiac output, cardiac function is not always adequate to provide sufficient oxygen to the tissues to meet metabolic needs. Thus, a goal of therapy is to maintain oxygen delivery at sufficient levels to allow optimization of oxygen consumption at the tissue level. Consequently, if there

is evidence of inadequate systemic oxygen delivery associated with a low cardiac output despite adequate fluid therapy, then the use of inotropes is indicated with dobutamine being the agent of choice.[1] On the other hand, attempts to drive oxygen delivery to supranormal levels should not be done, since this strategy has been shown to increase rather than decrease mortality.[26]

While renal dysfunction is common in the setting of severe sepsis or septic shock, renal failure requiring renal replacement therapy occurs in less than 5% of patients with severe sepsis. The development of acute renal failure requiring replacement therapy, either hemodialysis or continuous venovenous hemofiltration, in severe sepsis is associated with an increased risk of death. Although it has been hypothesized that plasma exchange may be beneficial in removing molecules in the bloodstream that initiate or propagate the sepsis cascade, there are no compelling data to support the efficacy of this approach. When acute renal failure occurs in the septic patient, it is generally a consequence of inadequate volume resuscitation, the use of nephrotoxic drugs or a prolonged period of shock. Thus, prevention of renal failure is primarily aimed at maintenance of effective renal perfusion, including volume administration and cardiovascular support. In contrast, multiple studies have shown that there is no role for "renal-dose" dopamine in the prevention or treatment of acute renal failure.[27] Since the mortality rate of nonoliguric renal failure is about half that of oliguric renal failure, once renal failure becomes manifest it is important to attempt to convert oliguric to nonoliguric renal failure. Therapeutic strategies that can be used include volume administration to maintain pulmonary arterial wedge pressure of 15–18 and the administration of mannitol or high-dose continuous loop diuretics to convert nonoliguric to oliguric renal failure.[28] In addition, in patients with renal failure, drug dosing is modified and levels of drugs such as aminoglycosides are monitored. Lastly, endogenously produced nephrotoxic substances such as myoglobin must be cleared, and continued attempts are made to control the infectious process.

Since the early studies performed by Moore et al. in 1989 documenting that early enteral nutrition is associated with a reduction in infectious complications and length of stay in trauma patients,[29] many other studies have validated the concept that early enteral feeding reduces infection rates in trauma as well as other ICU patient populations. Not only is there evidence that enteral nutrition is beneficial, but there is also evidence from several clinical trials that total parenteral nutrition (TPN) may be harmful as illustrated in the VA cooperative perioperative trial of 395 malnourished surgical patients.[30] In this study, the TPN-treated patients had an infection rate that was almost 2.5-fold higher than the saline controls (14% vs. 6%), thereby highlighting the potential risk of parenteral nutrition. The mechanisms by which enteral nutrition appears to exert its beneficial effects appears to be multifactorial, and is related to the ability of enteral nutrition, in contrast to TPN, to directly feed the gut as well as the rest of the body.[31] More recent studies using newer enteral diets containing higher levels of various nutrients, such as glutamine, arginine, fiber, or omega-fatty acids, have documented that early enteral nutrition is associated not just with less infectious complications but also with a reduction in organ dysfunction.[31] When choosing an enteral formula, the following nutritional guidelines for patients with sepsis should be considered: (1) caloric intake 25–30 kcal/kg of lean (not total) body weight, (2) protein 1.3–2.0 g/kg/day, (3) glucose 30%–70% of total nonprotein calories, and (4) lipids 15%–30% of total nonprotein calories.

The reason why TPN was associated with an increased incidence of infectious complications was initially unclear when these clinical TPN studies were performed; however, it has now become clear that hyperglycemia is a major risk factor in critically ill patients and TPN was commonly associated with hyperglycemia. Since then, another component of metabolic management that has been shown to improve survival in ICU patients is tight glucose control, where the blood glucose is maintained at 90–110 mg/dl.[32] Consequently, the nutritional support of the septic as well as the nonseptic trauma patient includes enteral alimentation as well as the liberal use of insulin to avoid hyperglycemia.

CONCLUSIONS

The mortality associated with sepsis and septic shock remains high, ranging from 13% to 50% and as high as 85% when complicated by multiple organ failure. After recovery from severe sepsis, mortality is higher during the first year of follow-up.[13] The challenge remains to prevent infections and limit the development of SIRS and MODS. Although our understanding of the pathophysiologic changes that occur in septic shock continues to increase, we are just beginning to employ novel therapeutic strategies with a significant survival benefit.

The therapeutic goals for management of sepsis and septic shock include early recognition, prompt initiation of antibiotic therapy, and source control. Restoration of volume status and hemodynamic function is accomplished with volume administration and the addition of vasoactive medications when volume fails to restore adequate hemodynamic function, remembering that vasopressor-dependent patients with septic shock are candidates for steroid replacement therapy. Early support of oxygenation with lung-protective ventilatory strategies, as well as metabolic support, with early enteral feeding and tight glucose control, also appears to impart a survival benefit. Lastly, selected patients with sepsis and no contraindications might benefit from the use of activated protein C as an antithrombotic agent that restores normal fibrinolytic pathways and reduces inflammation.

REFERENCES

1. Dellinger RP, Carlet JM, Masur H, et al: Surviving sepsis campaign guidelines for management of severe sepsis and septic shock. *Crit Care Med* 32:858–873, 2004.
2. Angus DC, Linde-Zwirble WT, Lidicker J, Clermont G, Carcillo J, Pinsky MR: Epidemiology of severe sepsis in the United States: analysis of incidence, outcome, and associated costs of care. *Crit Care Med* 29:1303–1310, 2001.
3. Hebert PC, McDonald BJ, Tinmouth A: Clinical consequences of anemia and red cell transfusion in the critically ill. *Crit Care Clin* 20:225–235, 2004.
4. Holmes CL, Russell JA, Walley KR: Genetic polymorphisms in sepsis and septic shock. *Chest* 124:1103–1115, 2003.
5. Ananthakrishnan P, Deitch EA: Gut origin sepsis and MODS: the role of sex hormones in modulating intestinal and distant organ injury. *XX vs XY* 1:108–117, 2003.
6. Magnotti LJ, Croce MA, Fabian TC: Is ventilator-associated pneumonia in trauma patients an epiphenomenon or a cause of death? *Surg Infect (Larchmt)* 5:237–242, 2004.
7. Blot F, Schmidt E, Nitenberg G, et al: Earlier positivity of central venous versus peripheral blood cultures is highly predictive of catheter-related sepsis. *J Clin Microbiol* 36:105–109, 1998.
8. Levy MM, Fink MP, Marshall JC, Abraham E, Angus D, Cook D, et al: International Sepsis Definitions Conference 2001. *Crit Care Med* 31:1250–1256, 2003.
9. Miller PR, Fabian TC, Croce MA, Magnotti LF, Pritchard E, Minard G, Stewart RM: Improving outcomes following penetrating colon wounds: application of a clinical pathway. *Ann Surg* 23:775–781, 2002.
10. Velmahos GC, Kamel E, Berne TV, Yassa N, Ramicone E, Song Z, Demetriades D: Abdominal computed tomography for the diagnosis of intraabdominal sepsis in critically injured patients: fishing in murky waters. *Arch Surg* 134:831–836, 1999.
11. Men S, Akhan O, Koroglu M: Percutaneous drainage of abdominal abscess. *Eur J Radiol* 43:204–218, 2002.
12. Schierhout G, Roberts I: Fluid resuscitation with colloid or crystalloid solutions in critically ill patients: a systematic review of randomized trials. *BMJ* 961–964, 1998.
13. Rivers E, Nguyen B, Havstad S, Ressler J, Muzzin A, Knoblich B, et al: Early goal-directed therapy in the treatment of severe sepsis and septic shock. *N Engl J Med* 345:1368–1377, 2001.
14. Hebert PC, Wells G, Blajchman MA, Marshall J, Martin C, et al: A multicenter, randomized, controlled clinical trial of transfusion requirements in critical care. *N Engl J Med* 340:409–417, 1999.
15. Vincent JL: Hemodynamic support in septic shock. *Intensive Care Med* 27:S80–S92, 2001.
16. Steel A, Bihari D: Choice of catecholamine: does it matter? *Curr Opin Crit Care* 6:347–353, 2000.
17. Beale RJ, Hollenberg SM, Vincent JL, Parrillo JE: Vasopressor and inotropic support in septic shock: an evidence-based review. *Crit Care Med* 32:S455–S465, 2004.
18. Annane D, Sebille V, Charpienter C, et al: Effect of treatment with low doses of hydrocortisone and fludrocortisone on mortality in patients with septic shock. *JAMA* 288:862–871, 2002.
19. Keh D, Boehnke T, Weber-Carstens S, et al: Immunologic and hemodynamic effects of "low-dose" hydrocortisone in septic shock: a double-blinded, randomized, placebo-controlled crossover study. *Am J Respir Crit Care Med* 167:512–520, 2003.
20. Keh D, Sprung CL: Use of corticosteroid therapy in patients with sepsis and septic shock: an evidence-based review. *Crit Care Med* 32:S527–S533, 2004.
21. Bernard GR, Vincent JL, Laterre PF, LaRosa SP, Dhainaut JF, Lopez-Rodriguez A, et al: Recombinant human protein C worldwide evaluation in severe sepsis (PROWESS) study group: efficacy and safety of recombinant human activated protein C for severe sepsis. *N Engl J Med* 344:699–709, 2001.
22. Abraham E, Laterre PF, Garg R, et al: Drotrecogin alfa (activated) for adults with severe sepsis and a low risk of death. *N Engl J Med* 353:1332–1341, 2005.
23. The Acute Respiratory Distress Syndrome Network: Ventilation with lower tidal volumes as compared with traditional tidal volumes for acute lung injury and the acute respiratory distress syndrome. *N Engl J Med* 342:1301–1308, 2000.
24. Drakulovic MB, Torres A, Bauer TT, et al: Supine body position as a risk factor for nosocomial pneumonia in mechanically ventilated patients: a randomized trial. *Lancet* 354:1851–1858, 1999.
25. Schweickert WD, Gehlbach BK, Pohlman AS, et al: Daily interruption of sedative infusions and complications of critical illness in mechanically ventilated patients. *Crit Care Med* 32:1272–1276, 2004.
26. Gattinoni L, Brazzi L, Pelosi P, et al: A trial of goal-oriented hemodynamic therapy in critically ill patients. *N Engl J Med* 333:1025–1032, 1995.
27. Bellomo R, Chapman M, Finfer S, et al: Low-dose dopamine in patients with early renal dysfunction: a placebo-controlled randomized trial. *Lancet* 356:2139–2143, 2000.
28. Shilliday IR, Quinn KJ, Allison ME: Loop diuretics in the management of acute renal failure: a prospective, double-blind, placebo-controlled, randomized study. *Nephrol Dial Transplant* 12:2592–2596, 1997.
29. Moore FA, Moore EE, Jones TN, et al: TEN versus TPN following major torso trauma reduced septic morbidity. *J Trauma* 29:916–923, 1989.
30. VA Cooperative Study Group: Perioperative total parenteral nutrition in surgical patients. *N Engl J Med* 325:525–532, 1991.
31. Deitch EA, Sambol JT: The gut-origin hypothesis of MODS. In Deitch EA, Vincent JL, Windsor A, editors: *Sepsis and Multiple Organ Dysfunction: A Multidisciplinary Approach.* Philadelphia, WB Saunders, 2002, pp. 105–116.
32. Van der Berghe G, Wouters P, Weekers F, et al: Intensive insulin therapy in the critically ill patient. *N Engl J Med* 345:1359–1367, 2001.
33. Balk RA: Optimum treatment of severe sepsis and septic shock: evidence in support of the recommendations. *Dis Month* 50:163–213, 2004.

THE IMMUNOLOGY OF TRAUMA

S. Rob Todd   and   Christine S. Cocanour

Following trauma, the immune system is called into action by signals from injured tissues. Injuries, hypoxia, and hypotension, as well as secondary insults such as ischemia/reperfusion injuries, compartment syndromes, operative interventions, and infections induce a host response that is characterized by local and systemic release of proinflammatory cytokines, arachidonic acid metabolites, and activation of complement factors, kinins, and coagulation as well as hormonal mediators. Clinically, this is the systemic inflammatory response syndrome (SIRS). Paralleling SIRS is an anti-inflammatory response referred to as the compensatory anti-inflammatory response syndrome (CARS). An imbalance between these responses appears to be responsible for increased susceptibility to infection and organ dysfunction. The aim of this chapter is to provide an overview of the immune response following trauma.

In this chapter we will discuss the two-hit model, SIRS, CARS, cytokine response, cell-mediated response, leukocyte recruitment, proteases and reactive oxygen species, and acute phase reaction.

TWO-HIT MODEL

In the two-hit model, the inciting injury induces a systemic inflammatory response (Figure 1). This "first hit" primes the immune system for an exaggerated and potentially lethal inflammatory reaction to a secondary, otherwise nonlethal, stimulus ("second hit"). This secondary stimulus may be either endogenous or exogenous. Endogenous second hits include cardiovascular instability, respiratory distress, metabolic derangements, and ischemia/reperfusion injuries. In contrast, exogenous second hits include surgical interventions, blood product transfusions, and missed injuries. The two-hit model proposes that this second hit results in destructive inflammation leading to multiple organ failure (MOF) and potentially death. This model has been supported by the work of Moore and colleagues who linked postinjury opportunistic infections to SIRS and MOF.

SYSTEMIC INFLAMMATORY RESPONSE SYNDROME

In 1991, a consensus conference of the American College of Chest Physicians and the American Society of Critical Care Medicine (ACCP/SCCM) defined SIRS as a generalized inflammatory response triggered by a variety of infectious and noninfectious events. They arbitrarily established clinical parameters through a process of consensus. Table 1 summarizes the diagnostic criteria for SIRS. At least two of the four criteria must be present to fulfill the diagnosis of SIRS. Note that this definition emphasizes the inflammatory process regardless of the presence of infection. The term sepsis is reserved for SIRS when infection is suspected or proven. Subsequent studies have validated these criteria as predictive of increased intensive care unit (ICU) mortality, and that this risk increases concurrent with the number of criteria present.

Systemic inflammatory response syndrome is characterized by the local and systemic production and release of multiple mediators, including proinflammatory cytokines, complement factors, proteins of the contact phase and coagulation system, acute-phase proteins, neuroendocrine mediators and an accumulation of immunocompetent cells at the local site of tissue damage. The severity of trauma, duration of the insult, genetic factors, and general condition of the individual determine the local and systemic release of proinflammatory cytokines and phospholipids.

COMPENSATORY ANTI-INFLAMMATORY RESPONSE SYNDROME

Trauma not only stimulates the release of proinflammatory mediators, but also the parallel release of anti-inflammatory mediators. This compensatory anti-inflammatory response is present concurrently with SIRS (Figure 2). When these two opposing responses are appropriately balanced, the traumatized individual is able to effectively heal the injury without incurring secondary injury from the autoimmune inflammatory response. However, overwhelming CARS appears responsible for post-traumatic immunosuppression, which leads to increased susceptibility to infections and sepsis. With time, SIRS ceases to exist and CARS is the predominant force.

CYTOKINE RESPONSE

Cytokines exert their effects in both a para- and auto-crine manner. Proinflammatory cytokines, tumor necrosis factor-α (TNF-α), and interleukin-1β (IL-1β) are released within 1–2 hours. Secondary proinflammatory cytokines are released in a subacute fashion and include IL-6, IL-8, macrophage migratory factor (MMF), IL-12, and IL-18. Clinically, IL-6 levels correlate with injury severity score (ISS) and the development of MOF, acute respiratory distress syndrome (ARDS), and sepsis.

Interleukin-6 also acts as an immunoregulatory cytokine by stimulating the release of anti-inflammatory mediators such as IL-1 receptor antagonists and TNF receptors which bind circulating proinflammatory cytokines. IL-6 also triggers the release of prostaglandin E2 (PGE2) from macrophages. Prostaglandin E2 is potentially the most potent endogenous immunosuppressant. Not only does it suppress T-cell and macrophage responsiveness, it also induces the release of IL-10, a potent anti-inflammatory cytokine that deactivates monocytes. Serum IL-10 levels correlate with ISS as well as the development of post-traumatic complications.

Following trauma, IL-12 production is decreased, stimulating a shift in favor of T_H2 cells and the subsequent production of anti-inflammatory mediators IL-4, IL-10, IL-13, and transforming growth factor beta (TGF-β). This decrease in IL-12 and resultant increase in T_H2 cells correlates with adverse outcomes. A listing of pro and anti-inflammatory mediators appears in Tables 2 and 3.

CELL-MEDIATED RESPONSE

Trauma alters the ability of splenic, peritoneal, and alveolar macrophages to release IL-1, IL-6, and TNF-α leading to decreased levels of these proinflammatory cytokines. Kupffer cells however, have an enhanced capacity for production of proinflammatory cytokines. Cell-mediated immunity not only requires functional macrophage

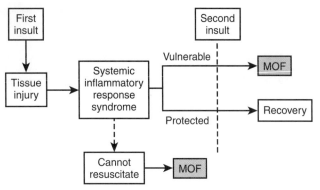

Figure 1   Pathogenesis of postinjury multiple organ failure.

Table 1: Clinical Parameters of Systemic Inflammatory Response Syndrome

Heart rate > 90 beats/min

Respiratory rate > 20 breaths/min, or $PaCO_2$ < 32 mm Hg

Temperature > 38° C or <36° C

Leukocytes > 12,000/mm³ or < 4000/mm³ or ≥10% juvenile neutrophil granulocytes

$PaCO_2$, Arterial CO_2 partial pressure.

and T cells but also intact macrophage–T-cell interaction. Following injury, human leukocyte antigen (HLA-DR) receptor expression is decreased leading to a loss of antigen-presenting capacity and decreased TNF-α production. Prostaglandin E2, IL-10, and TGF-β all contribute to this "immunoparalysis."

T-helper cells differentiate into either T_H1 or T_H2 lymphocytes. T_H1 cells promote the proinflammatory cascade through the release of IL-2, interferon-γ (IFN-γ), and TNF-β, while T_H2 cells produce anti-inflammatory mediators. Monocytes/macrophages, through the release of IL-12, stimulate the differentiation of T-helper cells into T_H1 cells. Because IL-12 production is depressed following trauma, there is a shift toward T_H2, which has been associated with an adverse clinical outcome.

Adherence of the leukocyte to endothelial cells is mediated through the upregulation of adhesion molecules. Selectins such as leukocyte adhesion molecule-1 (LAM-1), endothelial leukocyte adhesion molecule-1 (ELAM-1), and P-selectin are responsible for polymorphonuclear leukocytes (PMNL) "rolling." Upregulation of integrins such as the CD11/18 complexes or intercellular adhesion molecule-1 (ICAM-1) is responsible for PMNL attachment to the endothelium. Migration, accumulation, and activation of the PMNL are mediated by chemoattractants such as chemokines and complement anaphylotoxins. Colony-stimulating factors (CSFs) likewise stimulate monocyte- or granulocyto-poiesis and reduce apoptosis of PMNL during SIRS. Neutrophil apoptosis is further reduced by other proinflammatory mediators, thus resulting in PMNL accumulation at the site of local tissue destruction.

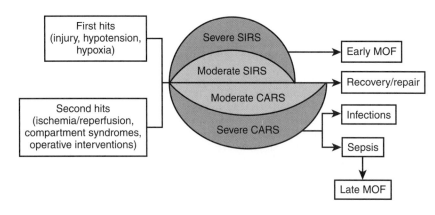

Figure 2   Postinjury multiple organ failure occurs as a result of a dysfunctional inflammatory response. *CARS*, Compensatory anti-inflammatory response syndrome; *MOF*, multiple organ failure; *SIRS*, systemic inflammatory response syndrome.

Table 2: Proinflammatory Mediators

Mediator	Action
IL-1	IL-1 is pleiotropic. Locally, it stimulates cytokine and cytokine receptor production by T cells as well as stimulating B-cell proliferation. Systemically, IL-1 modulates endocrine responses and induces the acute phase response.
IL-6	Il-6 induces acute-phase reactants in hepatocytes and plays an essential role in the final differentiation of B cells into Ig-secreting cells. Additionally, IL-6 has anti-inflammatory properties.
IL-8	IL-8 is a major mediator of the inflammatory response. It functions as a chemoattractant and is also a potent angiogenic factor.
IL-12	IL-12 regulates the differentiation of naive T cells into TH1 cells. It stimulates the growth and function of T cells and alters the normal cycle of apoptotic cell death.
TNF-α	TNF-α is pleiotropic. TNF-α and IL-1 act alone or together to induce systemic inflammation as above. TNF-α is also chemotactic for neutrophils and monocytes, as well as increasing neutrophil activity.
MIF	MIF forms a crucial link between the immune and neuroendocrine systems. It acts systemically to enhance the secretion of IL-1 and TNF-α.

Ig, Immunoglobulin; *IL*, interleukin; *MIF*, migration inhibitory factor; *TNF*, tumor necrosis factor.

Table 3: Anti-Inflammatory Mediators

Mediator	Action
IL-4	IL-4, IL-3, IL-5, IL-13, and CSF2 form a cytokine gene cluster on chromosome 5q, with this gene particularly close to IL-13.
IL-10	IL-10 has pleiotropic effects in immunoregulation and inflammation. It downregulates the expression of T_H1 cytokines, MHC class II antigens, and costimulatory molecules on macrophages. It also enhances B-cell survival, proliferation, and antibody production. In addition, it can block NF-kappa B activity, and is involved in the regulation of the JAK-STAT signaling pathway.
IL-11	IL-11 stimulates the T-cell–dependent development of immunoglobulin-producing B cells. It is also found to support the proliferation of hematopoietic stem cells and megakaryocyte progenitor cells.
IL-13	IL-13 is involved in several stages of B-cell maturation and differentiation. It upregulates CD23 and MHC class II expression, and promotes IgE isotype switching of B cells. It downregulates macrophage activity, thereby inhibiting the production of proinflammatory cytokines and chemokines.
IFN-α	IFN-α enhances and modifies the immune response.
TGF-β	TGF-β regulates the proliferation and differentiation of cells, wound healing, and angiogenesis.
α-MSH	α-MSH modulates inflammation by way of three mechanisms: direct action on peripheral inflammatory cells, actions on brain inflammatory cells to modulate local reactions, and indirect activation of descending neural anti-inflammatory pathways that control peripheral tissue inflammation.

CSF, Colony-stimulating factor; *IFN,* interferon; *Ig,* immunoglobulin; *IL,* interleukin; *MHC,* major histocompatibility complex; *MSH,* melanocyte stimulating hormone; *TGF,* transforming growth factor; *T_H,* T helper.

LEUKOCYTE RECRUITMENT

Proinflammatory cytokines enhance PMNL recruitment, phagocytic activity, and the release of proteases and oxygen-free radicals by PMNL. This recruitment of leukocytes represents a key element for host defense following trauma, although it allows for the development of secondary tissue damage. It involves a complex cascade of events culminating in transmigration of the leukocyte, whereby the cell exerts its effects. The first step is capture and tethering, mediated via constitutively expressed leukocyte selectin denoted L-selectin. L-selectin functions by identifying glycoprotein ligands on leukocytes and those upregulated on cytokine-activated endothelium.

Following capture and tethering, endothelial E-selectin and P-selectin assist in leukocyte rolling or slowing. P-selectin is found in the membranes of endothelial storage granules (Weibel-Palade bodies). Following granule secretion, P-selectin binds to carbohydrates presented by P-selectin glycoprotein ligand (PSGL-1) on the leukocytes. In contrast, E-selectin is not stored, yet it is synthesized de novo in the presence of inflammatory cytokines. These selectins cause the leukocytes to roll along the activated endothelium, whereby secondary capturing of leukocytes occurs via homotypic interactions.

The third step in leukocyte recruitment is firm adhesion, which is mediated by membrane expressed β_1- and β_2-integrins. The integrins bind to ICAM resulting in cell-cell interactions and ultimately signal transduction. This step is critical to the formation of stable shear-resistant adhesion, which stabilizes the leukocyte for transmigration.

Transmigration is the final step in leukocyte recruitment following the formation of bonds between the aforementioned integrins and Ig-superfamily members. The arrested leukocytes cross the endothelial layer via bicellular and tricellular endothelial junctions in a process coined diapedysis. This is mediated by platelet–endothelial cell adhesion molecules (PECAM), proteins expressed on both the leukocytes and intercellular junctions of endothelial cells.

PROTEASES AND REACTIVE OXYGEN SPECIES

Polymorphonuclear lymphocytes and macrophages are not only responsible for phagocytosis of microorganisms and cellular debris, but can also cause secondary tissue and organ damage through degranulation and release of extracellular proteases and formation of reactive oxygen species or respiratory burst. Elastases and metalloproteinases which degrade both structural and extracellular matrix proteins are present in increased concentrations following trauma. Neutrophil elastases also induce the release of proinflammatory cytokines.

Reactive oxygen species are generated by membrane associated nicotinamide adenine dinucleotide phosphate (NADPH) oxidase, which is activated by proinflammatory cytokines, arachidonic acid metabolites, complement factors, and bacterial products. Superoxide anions are reduced in the Haber-Weiss reaction to hydrogen peroxide by superoxide dismutase located in the cytosol, mitochondria, and cell membrane. Hydrochloric acid is formed from H_2O_2 by myeloperoxidase, while the Fenton reaction transforms H_2O_2 into hydroxyl ions. These free reactive oxygen species cause lipid peroxidation, cell membrane disintegration, and DNA damage of endothelial and parenchymal cells. Oxygen radicals also induce PMNL to release proteases and collagenase as well as inactivating protease inhibitors.

Reactive nitrogen species cause additional tissue damage following trauma. Nitric oxide (NO) is generated from L-arginine by inducible nitric oxide synthase (iNOS) in PMNL or vascular muscle cells and by endothelial nitric oxide synthase in endothelial cells. Nitric oxide induces vasodilatation. Inducible nitric oxide synthase is stimulated by cytokines and toxins, whereas endothelial nitric oxide synthase (eNOS) is stimulated by mechanical shearing forces. Damage by reactive oxygen and nitrogen species leads to generalized edema and the capillary leak syndrome.

COMPLEMENT, KININS, AND COAGULATION

The complement cascade, kallikrein-kinin system, and coagulation cascade are intimately involved in the immune response to trauma. They are activated through proinflammatory mediators, endogenous endotoxins, and tissue damage. The classical pathway of complement is normally activated by antigen-antibody complexes (immunoglobulins [Ig] M or G) or activated coagulation factor XII (FXII), while the alternative pathway is activated by bacterial products such as lipopolysaccharide. Complement activation following trauma is most likely from the release of proteolytic enzymes, disruption of the endothelial lining, and tissue ischemia. The degree of complement activation correlates with the severity of injury. The cleavage of C3 and C5 by their respective convertases results in the formation of opsonins, anaphylotoxins, and the membrane attack complex (MAC). The opsonins C3b and C4b enhance phagocytosis of cell debris and bacteria by means of opsonization. The anaphylotoxins C3a and C5a support inflammation via the recruitment and activation of phagocytic cells (i.e., monocytes, polymorphonuclear cells, and macrophages), enhancement of the hepatic acute-phase reaction, and release of vasoactive mediators (i.e., histamine). They also enhance the adhesion of leukocytes to endothelial cells, which results in increased vascular permeability and edema. C5a induces apoptosis and cell lysis through the interaction of its receptor and the membrane attach complex (MAC). Additionally, C3a and C5a activate reparative mechanisms. C1-inhibitor inactivates C1s and C1r, thereby regulating the classical complement pathway. However, during inflammation, serum levels of C1-inhibitor are decreased via its degradation by PMNL elastases.

The plasma kallikrein-kinin system is a contact system of plasma proteases related to the complement and coagulation cascades. It consists of the plasma proteins FXII, prekallikrein, kininogen, and factor XI (FXI). The activation of FXII and prekallikrein occurs via contact activation when endothelial damage occurs exposing the basement membrane. Factor XII activation forms factor XIIa (FXIIa), which initiates the complement cascade through the classical pathway, whereas prekallikrein activation forms kallikrein, which stimulates fibrinolysis through the conversion of plasminogen to plasmin or the activation of urokinase-like plasminogen activator (u-PA). Tissue plasminogen activator (t-PA) functions as a cofactor. Additionally, kallikrein supports the conversion of kininogen to bradykinin. The formation of bradykinin also occurs through the activation of the tissue kallikrein-kinin system, most likely through organ damage as the tissue kallikrein-kinin system is found in many organs and tissues including the pancreas, kidney, intestine, and salivary glands. The kinins are potent vasodilators. They also increase vascular permeability and inhibit the function of platelets.

The intrinsic coagulation cascade is linked to the contact activation system via the formation of factor IXa (FIXa) from factor XIa (FXIa). Its activation leads to the consumption of FXII, prekallikrein, and FXI while plasma levels of enzyme-inhibitor complexes are increased. These include FXIIa-C1 inhibitor and kallikrein-C1 inhibitor. C1-inhibitor and α1-protease inhibitor are both inhibitors of the intrinsic coagulation pathway.

Although the intrinsic pathway provides a stimulus for activation of the coagulation cascade, the major activation following trauma is via the extrinsic pathway. Increased expression of tissue factor (TF) on endothelial cells and monocytes is induced by the proinflammatory cytokines TNF-α and IL-1β. The factor VII (FVII)–TF complex stimulates the formation of factor Xa (FXa) and ultimately thrombin (FIIa). Thrombin-activated factor V (FV), factor VIII (FVIII), and FXI result in enhanced thrombin formation. Following cleavage of fibrinogen by thrombin, the fibrin monomers polymerize to from stable fibrin clots. The consumption of coagulation factors is controlled by the hepatocytic formation of antithrombin (AT) III. The thrombin–antithrombin complex inhibits thrombin, FIXa, FXa, FXIa, and FXIIa. Other inhibitors include TF pathway inhibitor (TFPI) and activated protein C in combination with free protein S. Free protein S is decreased during inflammation due to its binding with the C4b binding protein.

Disseminated intravascular coagulation (DIC) may occur following trauma. After the initial phase, intra- and extra-vascular fibrin clots are observed. Hypoxia-induced cellular damage is the ultimate result of intravascular fibrin clots. Likewise, there is an increase in the interactions between endothelial cells and leukocytes. Clinically, coagulation factor consumption and platelet dysfunction are responsible for the diffuse hemorrhage. Consumption of coagulation factors is further enhanced via the proteolysis of fibrin clots to fibrin fragments. The consumption of coagulation factors is further enhanced through the proteolysis of fibrin clots to fibrin fragments by the protease plasmin.

ACUTE-PHASE REACTION

The acute-phase reaction describes the early systemic response following trauma and other insult states. During this phase, the biosynthetic profile of the liver is significantly altered. Under normal circumstances, the liver synthesizes a range of plasma proteins at steady state concentrations. However, during the acute phase reaction, hepatocytes increase the synthesis of positive acute-phase proteins (i.e., C-reactive protein [CRP], serum amyloid A [SAA], complement proteins, coagulation proteins, proteinase inhibitors, metal-binding proteins, and other proteins) essential to the inflammatory process at the expense of the negative acute-phase proteins. The list of acute-phase proteins is in Table 4.

The acute-phase response is initiated by hepatic Kupffer cells and the systemic release of proinflammatory cytokines. Interleukin-1, IL-6, IL-8, and TNF-α act as inciting cytokines. The acute phase reaction typically lasts for 24–48 hours prior to its downregulation. Interleukin-4, IL-10, glucocorticoids, and various other hormonal stimuli function to downregulate the proinflammatory mediators of the acute-phase response. This modulation is critical. In instances of chronic or recurring inflammation, an aberrant acute-phase response may result in exacerbated tissue damage.

The major acute-phase proteins include CRP and SAA, the activities of which are poorly understood. C-reactive protein was so named secondary to its ability to bind the C-polysaccharide of *Pneumococcus*. During inflammation, CRP levels may increase by up to 1000-fold over several hours depending on the insult and its severity. It acts as an opsonin for bacteria, parasites, and immune complexes, activates complement via the classical pathway, and binds chromatin. Binding chromatin may minimize autoimmune responses by disposing of nuclear antigens from sites of tissue debris. Clinically, CRP levels are relatively non-specific and not predictive of post-traumatic complications. Despite this fact, serial measurements are helpful in trending a patient's clinical course.

Serum amyloid A interacts with the third fraction of high-density lipoprotein (HDL3), thus becoming the dominant apolipoprotein during acute inflammation. This association enhances the binding of HDL3 to macrophages, which may engulf cholesterol and lipid debris. Excess cholesterol is then utilized in tissue repair or excreted. Additionally, SAA inhibits thrombin-induced platelet activation and the oxidative burst of neutrophils, potentially preventing oxidative tissue destruction.

SUMMARY

Injury triggers a tremendously complex response involving a multitude of systems. The individual's immune system must balance the proinflammatory response, which is necessary to clear injured tissue, yet not cause overwhelming endogenous injury with a necessary downregulation of the inflammatory process in order to provide an environment of minimal inflammation that can nurture the cell proliferation and tissue remodeling needed for healing. A loss of this

Table 4: Acute-Phase Proteins

Group	Individual Proteins
Positive Acute-Phase Proteins	
Major acute phase proteins	C-reactive protein, serum amyloid A
Complement proteins	C2, C3, C4, C5, C9, B, C1 inhibitor, C4 binding protein
Coagulation proteins	Fibrinogen, prothrombin, von Willebrand factor
Proteinase proteins	α_1-Pntitrypsin, α_1-antichymotrypsin, α_2-antiplasmin, heparin cofactor II, plasminogen activator inhibitor I
Metal-binding proteins	Haptoglobin, hemopexin, ceruloplasmin, manganese superoxide dismutase
Other proteins	α_1-acid glycoprotein, heme oxygenase, mannose-binding protein, leukocyte protein I, lipoprotein (a), lipopolysaccharide-binding protein
Negative Acute-Phase Proteins	Albumin, prealbumin, transferrin, apolipoprotein AI, apolipoprotein AII, α_2-Heremans-Schmid glycoprotein, inter–α-trypsin inhibitor, histidine-rich glycoprotein, protein c, protein s, antithrombin III, high-density lipoprotein

Note: Positive acute-phase proteins increase production during an acute-phase response. Negative acute-phase proteins have decreased production during an acute-phase response.

balance can cause additional tissue injury from the immune response itself, or leave the individual susceptible to infection and sepsis. As our understanding of the immune response following injury grows, the more likely that we will be able to monitor and effectively manage the traumatized, critically ill patient.

SUGGESTED READINGS

Angele MK, Chaundry IH: Surgical trauma and immunosuppression: pathophysiology and potential immunomodulatory approaches. *Arch Surg* 390:333–341, 2005.

Ayala A, Chung C-S, Grutkoski PS, Song GY: Mechanisms of immune resolution. *Crit Care Med* 31:S558–S571, 2003.

Cook MC: Immunology of trauma. *J Trauma* 3:79–88, 2001.

DeLong WG, Born CT: Cytokines in patients with polytrauma. *Clin Orthop Relat Res* 422:57–65, 2004.

Faist E, Angele MK, Wichmann M: *The Immune Response.* In *Trauma,* 5th ed. McGraw Hill, New York, 2004, pp. 1383–1396.

Faist E, Schinkel C, Zimmer S: Update on the mechanisms of immune suppression of injury and immune modulation. *World J Surg* 20:454–459, 1996.

Fosse E, Pillgram-Larsen J, Svennevig JL, Nordby C, Skulberg A, Mollnes TE, Abdelnoor M: Complement activation in injured patients occurs immediately and is dependent on the severity of the trauma. *Injury* 29:509–514, 1998.

Goris RJA: MODS/SIRS: result of an overwhelming inflammatory response? *World J Surg* 20:418–421, 1996.

Gruys E, Toussaint MJM, Niewold TA, Koopmans SJ: Acute phase reaction and acute phase proteins. *J Zhejiang Univ Sci* 6B 11:1045–1056, 2005.

Harris BH, Gelfand JA: The immune response to trauma. *Semin Pediatr Surg* 4:77–82, 1995.

Keel M, Trentz O: Pathophysiology of trauma. *Injury* 36:691–709, 2005.

Kubes P, Ward PA: Leukocyte recruitment and the acute inflammatory response. *Brain Pathol* 10:127–135, 2000.

Matzinger P: The danger model: a renewed sense of self. *Science* 296:301–305, 2002.

Menger MD, Vollmar B: Surgical trauma: hyperinflammation versus immunosuppression? *Arch Surg* 389:475–484, 2004.

Moore FA, Moore EE: Evolving concepts in the pathogenesis of postinjury multiple organ failure. *Surg Clin North Am* 75:257–277, 1995.

Murphy TJ, Paterson HM, Kriynovich S, et al: Linking the "two-hit" response following injury to enhanced TLR4 reactivity. *J Leukocyte Biol* 77:16–23, 2005.

Nathens AB, Marshall JC: Sepsis, SIRS, and MODS: what's in a name? *World J Surg* 20:386–391, 1996.

Sauaia A, Moore FA, Moore EE, Lezotte DC: Early risk factors for postinjury multiple organ failure. *World J Surg* 20:392–400, 1996.

Schinkel C, Wick M, Muhr G, Köller: Analysis of systemic interleukin-11 after major trauma. *Shock* 23:30–34, 2005.

Schlag G, Redl H: Mediators of injury and inflammation. *World J Surg* 20:406–410, 1996.

Simon SI, Green CE: Molecular mechanics and dynamics of leukocyte recruitment during inflammation. *Annu Rev Biomed Eng* 7:151–185, 2005.

Sugimoto K, Hirata M, Majima M, Katori M, Ohwada T: Evidence for a role of kallikrein-kinin system in patients with shock after blunt trauma. *Am J Physiol Regul Integr Comp Physiol* 274:R1556–R1560, 1998.

NOSOCOMIAL PNEUMONIA

D. Brandon Williams, Amritha Raghunathan, David A. Spain, and Susan I. Brundage

The two broad classes of pneumonia are nosocomial and community-acquired pneumonia. Nosocomial pneumonia is often referred to as hospital-acquired pneumonia (HAP), defined as pneumonia occurring 48 hours or more after admission that was not incubating at the time of admission. Postoperative pneumonia is essentially HAP, except in a patient who has undergone a surgical procedure. Finally, ventilator-associated pneumonia (VAP) refers to pneumonia occurring 48 hours or more after initiating mechanical ventilation via endotracheal intubation or tracheostomy.

Our goals in this chapter are to review the incidence of nosocomial pneumonia in the trauma patient, risk factors contributing to pneumonia, proven prevention strategies, the specifics of diagnosis, appropriate management of pneumonia once diagnosed, and associated morbidity and mortality relevant to the trauma population such as the relationship between prophylactic antibiotics, tube thoracostomy, and pneumonia.

INCIDENCE/MORBIDITY AND MORTALITY

Nosocomial infections cause significant mortality and morbidity in the critical care setting. HAP is the most common infection in the intensive care unit (ICU), causing between 25% and 48% of all nosocomial infections. Pneumonia is the leading cause of death due to hospital-acquired infections, with an estimated associated mortality ranging from 20% to 50%. The majority of nosocomial pneumonia episodes, 80%–90%, are associated with mechanical ventilation. While VAP makes up 90% of all infections in intubated patients, the overall reported incidence of VAP varies, with rates between 6% and 52%. The incidence varies due to differences in the definition of VAP in studies as well as differences in patient populations. There is, for example, a lower incidence in respiratory and medical ICUs (4.2 and 7.4 cases per 1000 ventilator days, respectively) as compared to trauma, neurosurgical, and burn units (15–16.3 cases per 1000 ventilator days). Although there is approximately a 1% cumulative risk per day of mechanical ventilation, the risk is highest in the first 5 days (approximately 3% per day), and steadily decreases after that. A number of studies place nosocomial pneumonia's risk ratio for death around 2.0. Developing pneumonia increases the overall hospital stay by approximately 9–11.5 days, and for critically ill patients, increases the ICU stay by 4–6 days. In addition to prolonging hospital and ICU stays, pneumonia increases hospital cost by requiring more antibiotics, chest radiographs, and days of mechanical ventilation, with all its associated care. The attributable cost of a single episode of HAP is estimated to be between $12,000 and $16,000.

RISK FACTORS AND PREVENTIVE MEASURES

Nonmodifiable versus Modifiable Risk Factors

While the greatest risk factor for VAP is the duration of mechanical ventilation, there are many other independent predictors, including modifiable and nonmodifiable risk factors (Table 1).

These risk factors are directly related to the pathogenesis of VAP. As the lower respiratory tract is sterile under basal conditions, the introduction of pathogens into the lungs and the impairment of traditional host defenses are necessary to cause infection. There is growing evidence that aspiration of pathogens colonizing or contaminating the oropharynx or gastrointestinal tract results in lower respiratory tract infection. Colonization of the endotracheal tube itself also may lead to alveolar infection during suctioning or bronchoscopy. Other less frequent sources include bacteremia and hematogenous spread or inhalation of infected aerosols.

Mechanical Ventilation

Mechanical ventilation is the greatest risk factor for HAP and is associated with a 6- to 20-fold increase in the risk of lung infection. Intubation itself increases the risk of pneumonia due to the potential for direct inoculation of pathogens into the lungs during the procedure. Therefore, intubation should be avoided, with noninvasive positive-pressure ventilation being the preferred alternative to mechanical ventilation, when clinically feasible. A prospective survey of those who underwent mechanical ventilation versus noninvasive ventilation showed that even after adjusting for the severity of illness using the Simplified Acute Physiology Score (SAPS II), both the risk of VAP as well as the risk of nosocomial infections in general were reduced. Other invasive procedures such as tracheostomy, bronchoscopy, placement of a nasogastric (NG) tube, and chest tube thoracostomy also increase the risk. Thoracic trauma and chest operations lead to a disproportionately higher incidence of VAP, likely due to direct inoculation of pathogens, as well as infection due to chest tube placement.

In a trauma or surgical unit, the majority of patients are mechanically ventilated secondary to the need for surgery. However, all efforts to decrease sedation and wean the patient to extubation postoperatively should be made. The risk of reintubation and emergency intubation should be minimized, as these events are also associated with increased risk of VAP.

Subglottic secretions are also potential sources of infection. A recent meta-analysis showed that continuous aspiration of subglottic secretions resulted in a 50% decrease in incidence of VAP. This was particularly beneficial in those who were mechanically ventilated for longer than 72 hours. If mechanical ventilation is necessary, this technique should be utilized. Besides this, the ventilator circuit can also become contaminated due to patient secretions. Many prospective randomized trials have shown that the incidence of VAP is not associated with the frequency of ventilator circuit changes. However, care should be taken to frequently clean the circuit and prevent aspiration of accumulated secretions. The endotracheal tube cuff pressure should also be greater than 20 mm H_2O to prevent tracking of bacterial pathogens around the cuff and into the lower respiratory tract.

Impaired Host Defenses

Markers of impaired host defenses, such as increased age, the presence of lung disease and other comorbidities including sepsis, steroid use, and a history of multiple blood transfusions have been shown to be risk factors. Patients with these risk factors should be carefully monitored with all precautionary measures implemented to prevent pneumonia.

Table 1: Risk Factors for Ventilator-Associated Pneumonia

Nonmodifiable Factors	Modifiable Factors Affording Prevention Strategies
Age > 60	Duration of mechanical ventilation (>3 days)
Male gender	Self-extubation
History of COPD	Re-intubation
Presence of significant comorbidity	Tracheostomy
Steroid use	Bronchoscopy
Admitting diagnosis of burns	Nasogastric tube
Admitting diagnosis of trauma	Thoracoabdominal surgery
Head trauma and other central nervous system disease	Endotracheal intracuff pressure of <20 cm H_2O
Emergency or field intubation	Supine positioning
Need for emergency surgery	Antacids or histamine type-2 antagonists
	Elevated gastric pH
	Aspiration
	Use of paralytic agents
	Glasgow Coma Scale < 9
	Septic shock
	Hypoalbuminemia
	No prophylactic antibiotics in first 48 hours of ICU stay
	Patient transport out of ICU
	Hemodialysis
	Blood transfusions
	Acute Physiology and Chronic Health Evaluation (APACHE) II score

ICU, Intensive care unit.

Oropharyngeal Colonization

While the oropharynx is not colonized by enteric Gram-negative bacteria under normal conditions, such colonization is present in 75% of the ICU population within the first 48 hours of admission. Studies monitoring oropharyngeal colonization in the ICU have further shown that colonization with specific pathogens like *Acinetobacter baumannii* results in increased risk for subsequent development of VAP.

Oropharyngeal colonization can be reduced by aggressive oral hygiene and the use of the oral antiseptic chlorhexidine. Oral inspections, tooth brushing and mouth swabs should all be utilized on a regular basis. Multiple randomized trials have shown a 60% decrease in VAP in postoperative patients with the use of chlorhexidine.

Aspiration

Due to the association between VAP and aspiration, factors involved in increased risk of aspiration such as continuous sedation, a low Glasgow Coma Scale, use of paralytic agents, and a supine position have all been shown to increase the risk of VAP. All efforts should be made to reduce the aspiration of gastric and oropharyngeal contents. One randomized trial was stopped ahead of schedule when it was apparent that the supine position results in increased aspiration and increased incidence of VAP compared to the semirecumbent position. Therefore, patients should be semirecumbent with the head of the bed raised to an angle of 30–45 degrees whenever possible. Continuous lateral rotation of ICU patients has also shown a protective effect and is another possibility. Transporting patients out of the ICU for procedures also leads to increased risk of VAP. This is potentially due to the fact that they are supine during transport. Thus, patients should be kept semirecumbent during transport whenever possible.

While it has been postulated that enteral nutrition would result in increased risk of VAP compared to parenteral nutrition due to aspiration, the evidence goes against that hypothesis, with VAP odds ratios of 2.65 and 3.27, respectively. As parenteral feeding is associated with many other risks like bacteremia as a complication of intravascular lines, and bacterial overgrowth and translocation, enteral feeding is preferred. As enteral feeding in the supine position maximizes risk, with a 50% incidence of VAP, feeding in the semirecumbent position is preferable. Other hypotheses include a benefit to smaller nasogastric tubes as well as a benefit to postpyloric or small intestine feeding. However, neither of those techniques has been proven to decrease the risk of VAP.

Gastrointestinal Tract Bacterial Overgrowth

Given their associated predisposition to bacterial overgrowth in the gastrointestinal tract, antacids and histamine type-2 antagonists are also associated with increased risk of VAP. There have been multiple trials comparing various stress ulcer prophylaxis agents. While there have been controversial results on the effect of sucralfate on VAP, the latest large randomized trial showed that while sucralfate resulted in a significantly lower rate of VAP compared to ranitidine and antacids, it is associated with a higher incidence of gastrointestinal bleeding. Therefore, sucralfate is recommended in all patients except those with risk factors for gastrointestinal bleeding.

Selective decontamination of the digestive tract (SDD) may be effective in reducing incidence of VAP. It attempts to reduce oropharyngeal and gastric colonization with aerobic Gram-negative bacilli and *Candida* species, without affecting anaerobic flora. Most regimens include a combination of an aminoglycoside, amphotericin B, or nystatin, and a nonabsorbable antibiotic like polymyxin. Systemic cefuroxime was also added in a few trials. Multiple randomized controlled trials have shown that SDD results in reduced incidence of VAP, decreased hospital mortality, and a decrease in antibiotic-resistant microorganism infections as well. However, these preventive effects were inversely related to study quality, and were much less pronounced in hospitals with high levels of antibiotic resistance. Therefore, SDD is not recommended for routine use, particularly for patients with risk factors for resistant pathogens.

It has been postulated that the intravenous antibiotic component of SDD is the main cause of improved survival, and current randomized trials are evaluating the effect of prophylactic IV antibiotics around the time of intubation. Intravenous cefuroxime reduced the incidence of early-onset hospital-acquired pneumonia in one recent trial. Intravenous antibiotics are currently not recommended for routine use, pending results from further trials.

Resistant Organisms

There has recently been an increase in the incidence of VAP caused by resistant organisms. Risk factors for infection with one of these pathogens include a recent history of antibiotic use, hospitalization of 5 days or more, admission from an allied health facility, immunosuppressive disease or therapy, presence of a severe, chronic comorbidity, and a high frequency of antibiotic resistance in that particular hospital or community. Another recent study also showed that aspiration, emergency intubation, and a Glasgow Coma Score of 9 or less are specific risk factors for early-onset VAP that is caused by resistant organisms.

Putting All Risk Factors Together

Croce et al. recently reported a post-trauma VAP probability calculation formula incorporating many of these risk factors. The probability of VAP (P_{VAP}) equals $e^{f(x)} / (1 + e^{f(x)})$, where $f(x) = -3.08 - 1.56$

(mechanism of injury, penetrating = 1, blunt = 0) − 0.12 (Glasgow Coma Scale score) + 1.37 (spinal cord injury where yes = 1, no = 0) + 0.30 (chest abbreviated injury score) + 1.87 (emergency laparotomy where yes = 1, no = 0) + 0.67 (units of blood transfused in the resuscitation room) + 0.05 (Injury Severity Score) + 0.66 (intubation in either the field or the resuscitation room, where yes = 1, no = 0). Over 2 months, this formula was 95% accurate in predicting subsequent development of VAP.

General Prophylaxis

Maximizing hand hygiene protocols and barrier precautions is crucial in preventing the spread of nosocomial infections. Compliance with hand hygiene protocols has improved with the introduction of alcohol

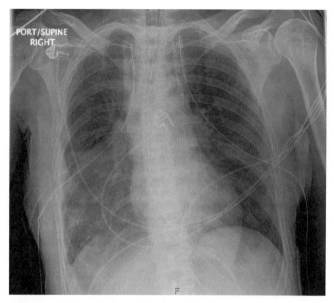

Figure 1 Chest x-ray with right lower lobe consolidation.

foams and gels. These products have improved efficacy and take substantially less time to use compared to thorough hand washing. Health care personnel should use these products before and after any contact with patients who are being mechanically ventilated. Gowns and gloves should also be used appropriately in any situation where contamination with respiratory secretions or other bodily fluids is possible.

Effectiveness of Preventive Measures

Preventive measures are very effective in preventing VAP. One institution showed that the incidence of VAP decreased by 58% after an educational session emphasizing positioning (head of bed elevated >30 degrees), appropriate use of sedation, routine oral hygiene, and management of respiratory devices. As VAP routinely results in increased hospital stays and therefore cost, this program was very cost-effective and the estimated savings were over $400,000.

DIAGNOSIS

Pneumonia is suspected when a patient develops new or progressive radiographic lung infiltrates (Figure 1), along with a clinical scenario of pulmonary infection (i.e., fever, leukocytosis, purulent sputum, respiratory distress, and a worsening of oxygenation) (Table 2). Of note, in patients diagnosed with acute respiratory distress syndrome (ARDS), the suspicion of pneumonia should be especially high. Several studies have noted a higher incidence of pneumonia in patients with ARDS. For example, one study showed a pneumonia rate of 55% in patients with ARDS, versus 28% in those without. Another study noted a 60% incidence of pneumonia in patients with severe ARDS (Pa_{O2}/FI_{O2} ratio < 150 mm Hg).

Diagnostic Strategies

However, ventilated ICU patients often have radiographic infiltrates, fever, and thick respiratory secretions in the absence of pneumonia. To assess the diagnostic efficacy of clinical criteria alone for VAP, one study reviewed 25 patients who died while on mechanical ventilation

Table 2: Centers for Disease Control and Prevention Criteria for Defining Hospital-Acquired Pneumonia

Radiology	Signs/Symptoms	Laboratory
Two or more serial chest radiographs with at least one of the following: New or progressive and persistent infiltrate Consolidation Cavitation Pneumatoceles, in infants <1 year old Note: In patients without underlying pulmonary or cardiac disease (e.g., respiratory distress syndrome, bronchopulmonary dysplasia, pulmonary edema, or chronic obstructive pulmonary disease), one definitive chest radiograph is acceptable.	At least one of the following: Fever (>38° C or >100.4° F) with no other recognized cause Leukopenia (<4000 WBC/mm³) or leukocytosis (>12,000 WBC/mm³) For adults >70 years old, altered mental status with no other recognized cause *and* At least one of the following: New onset of purulent sputum, or change in character of sputum or increased respiratory secretions, or increased suctioning requirements New onset or worsening cough, or dyspnea, or tachypnea Rales or bronchial breath sounds Worsening gas exchange (e.g., O₂ desaturations [e.g., PaO2/FiO2 < 240], increased oxygen requirements, or increased ventilation demand)	At least one of the following: Positive growth in blood culture not related to another source of infection Positive growth in culture of pleural fluid Positive quantitative culture from minimally contaminated specimen (e.g., BAL or PSB) ≥5% BAL-obtained cells contain intracellular bacteria on direct microscopic exam (e.g., Gram stain) Histopathologic exam shows at least one of the following evidences of pneumonia: Abscess formation or foci of consolidation with intense PMN accumulation in bronchioles and alveoli Positive quantitative culture of lung parenchyma Evidence of lung parenchyma invasion by fungal hyphae or pseudohyphae

BAL, Bronchoalveolar lavage; *PMN,* polymorphonuclear leukocytes; *PSB,* protected specimen brush; *WBC,* white blood cells.

and used lung histology plus quantitative lung culture as the standard for pneumonia. The presence of radiographic chest infiltrates plus two of three clinical criteria (leukocytosis, purulent secretions, fever) had a sensitivity of 69% and a specificity of 75%. Thus, it is important to obtain sputum cultures to confirm the diagnosis of VAP; additionally, identifying the causative organism(s) aids in selecting appropriate antibiotics.

Looking at trauma patients in particular, the utility of obtaining a sputum culture was illustrated in a study of 43 patients undergoing mechanical ventilation and demonstrating symptoms of pneumonia, namely fever, leukocytosis, purulent sputum, and changing radiographic infiltrates. Of this group, 20 had positive cultures with greater than or equal to 10^5 colony-forming units (CFU) per milliliter. Antibiotics were discontinued in the other 23 patients, and 65% showed improvement after stopping the antibiotics. Overall, there was no difference in mortality between the two groups.

Methods of Obtaining Sputum Cultures

Samples for sputum culture may be obtained noninvasively, via tracheal aspiration, or invasively with bronchoscopy and either bronchoalveolar lavage (BAL) or a protected specimen brush (PSB). Positive tracheal cultures may reflect simple tracheal colonization, and overestimate the rate of pneumonia. Invasive cultures are more accurate in diagnosing pneumonia. In one multicenter, randomized trial of 413 patients, those receiving invasive, bronchoscopic management had a lower mortality at day 14, but not at 28, and lower mean sepsis-related organ failure assessment scores on days 3 and 7. At 28 days, the invasive management group had significantly more antibiotic-free days (11 ± 6 vs. 7 ± 7). A multivariate analysis showed a significant difference in mortality (hazard ratio 1.54, 95% confidence interval 1.10–2.16). Both BAL and PSB have sensitivities and specificities greater than 80%. Studies have shown these two techniques yield similar results (Table 3).

Most studies involving BAL have used 10^4 or 10^5 CFU/ml as the threshold for a positive culture. The presence of numerous squamous epithelial cells suggests upper pharyngeal contamination, and calls into question the utility of the specimen. The presence of intracellular organisms can be detected by Gram stain, and is particularly useful as it provides a rapid result with high predictive value (see Table 3).

However, if bronchoscopic sampling is not immediately available, nonbronchoscopic techniques can reliably obtain lower respiratory tract quantitative cultures. Blinded bronchial sampling, mini-BAL, and blinded protected-specimen brush involve blindly wedging a catheter into a distal bronchus and obtaining a sample. A review of several studies suggests that the sensitivities and specificities of these techniques are similar to those involving fiberoptic bronchoscopy.

Bronchial sampling techniques aside, when there is a high suspicion of pneumonia, or the patient is clinically unstable or septic, antibiotic therapy should be initiated promptly regardless of whether bacteria is detected from the distal respiratory tract.

Impact of Prior Antibiotic Use on Diagnosis

As one might expect, prior antibiotic therapy can impair the ability to obtain accurate culture results. The key factor appears to be the duration of antibiotics. Initiation of antibiotic therapy within the preceding 24 hours decreases the chances of obtaining a positive sputum culture, although this impact is less pronounced for BAL than with other methods. However, in patients receiving antibiotics for more than 72 hours, the sensitivity and specificity of BAL and PSB are essentially unaffected. Thus, these modalities are still just as useful for diagnosing pneumonias in those patients in the midst of a course of antibiotics for some other site of infection.

Value of Clinical Pulmonary Infection Score in Trauma Patients

Lastly, the clinical pulmonary infection score (CPIS) is an attempt to optimize a noninvasive diagnostic approach by pooling several clinical indicators of pneumonia (Table 4). A CPIS greater than 6 has been shown to be highly suggestive of pneumonia and correlates with a high concentration of bacteria from invasive cultures. The main criticisms of the CPIS are that all elements are weighted equally even though some are stronger predictors of pneumonia, and that some elements are necessarily subjective, such as the interpretation of chest x-rays. Furthermore, most of the components of the CPIS may be altered by the systemic effects of trauma, and therefore simply reflect the systemic inflammatory response syndrome (SIRS). A recent study of 113 trauma patients with suspected pneumonia found the average CPIS score to be 7.0 in those with VAP confirmed by BAL versus 6.9 in those with a negative BAL. In this study the sensitivity and specificity of using a CPIS greater than 6 to diagnose VAP were only 65% and 41%, respectively.

MANAGEMENT

Adequate Initial Antibiotics

Effective treatment for HAP depends on rapid institution of an appropriate initial antibiotic. At least three separate studies have shown mortality to almost double when the initial choice of antibiotics was

Table 3: Quantitative Cultures and Microscopic Examination of Lower Respiratory Tract Secretions in Diagnosis of Ventilator-Associated Pneumonia

Diagnostic Techniques	Sensitivity (%)	Specificity (%)	Positive Predictive Value (%)	Negative Predictive Value (%)
PSB cultures ($>10^3$ CFU/ml)	82	89	90	89
BAL cultures ($>10^4$ CFU/ml)	91	78	83	87
Microscopic examination of BAL fluid ($>5\%$ intracellular organisms)	91	89	91	89

BAL, Bronchoalveolar lavage; *CFU,* colony-forming units; *PSB,* protected specimen brush.

Table 4: Calculation of Clinical Pulmonary Infection Score

Variable	Finding	Points
Temperature (° C)	≥365 and ≤384	0
	≥385 and ≤389	1
	≥39 or ≤36	2
Blood leukocytes (n/mm^3)	≥4,000 and ≤11,000	0
	<4,000 or >11,000	1
	Plus band forms ≥50%	Add 1
Tracheal secretions	Absent	0
	Nonpurulent secretions present	1
	Purulent secretions present	2
Oxygenation (P_aO_2/F_1O_2)	>240 or ARDS[a]	0
	≤240 and no ARDS	2
Pulmonary radiography	No infiltrate	0
	Diffuse (or patchy) infiltrate	1
	Localized infiltrate	2
Progression of pulmonary in-filtrates	No radiographic progression	0
	Radiographic progression (after CHF and ARDS excluded)	2
Culture of tracheal aspirate	Pathogenic bacteria cultured in very low to low quantity or not at all	0
	Pathogenic bacteria cultured in moderate or high quantity	1
	Same pathogenic bacteria seen on Gram stain	Add 1

[a]Defined as P_aO_2/F_1O_2 ≥200 and PAWP ≥18 mm Hg, with acute bilateral infiltrates.
ARDS, Acute respiratory distress syndrome; *CHF,* congestive heart failure; F_1O_2, fraction of inspired oxygen; P_aO_2, arterial oxygen tension; *PAWP,* pulmonary arterial wedge pressure.

inadequate. Another study looked at patients receiving appropriate initial antibiotics, but with a delay of more than 24 hours from the time of meeting diagnostic criteria for VAP. In this group, VAP-attributable mortality was 39.4%, compared to 10.8% in those receiving antibiotics in a timely manner.

The first step in treating pneumonia is to determine whether the responsible organism is likely to demonstrate antibiotic resistance. Hospitalization for 5 days or more and recent antibiotic or health care exposure are common risk factors for developing multidrug-resistant (MDR) pneumonia (Table 5).

After determining the likelihood of antibiotic resistance, an appropriate initial therapy is selected. If the likelihood of antibiotic resistance is low, suitable initial choices include a third- or fourth-generation cephalosporin, a fluoroquinolone, an antipseudomonal penicillin with

a beta-lactamase inhibitor, or a carbapenem (Table 6). Also, knowing hospital-specific or even ICU-specific patterns of antibiotic resistance can be particularly useful in guiding antibiotic choices.

If the patient has risk factors for MDR pneumonia, initial antibiotics should include double coverage for Gram-negatives and an agent for MRSA. The necessity of double antipseudomonal coverage is controversial. Evidence of in vitro synergy with combination therapy has been inconsistently demonstrated, and proof of clinical relevance is lacking. Also, prevention of emergent drug resistance during therapy has not been well demonstrated. However, one good reason to initiate double coverage is simply to increase the odds that at least one of the drugs will have activity against the suspected MDR organism. For

Table 5: Risk Factors for Multidrug-Resistant Pathogens Causing Hospital-Acquired Pneumonia and Ventilator-Associated Pneumonia

Antimicrobial therapy in preceding 90 days
Current hospitalization of 5 days or more
High frequency of antibiotic resistance in community or the specific hospital unit
Recent health care exposure
Hospitalization for 2 days or more in the preceding 90 days
Residence in a nursing home or extended care facility
Home infusion therapy (including antibiotics)
Chronic dialysis within 30 days
Home wound care
Family member with multidrug-resistant pathogen
Immunosuppressive disease and/or therapy

Table 6: Initial Empiric Antibiotic Therapy for Hospital-Acquired Pneumonia or Ventilator-Associated Pneumonia in Patients with No Known Risk Factors for Multidrug-Resistant Pathogens

Potential Pathogens	Recommended Initial Antibiotics
Streptococcus pneumonia, *Haemophilus influenzae,* Methicillin-sensitive *Staphylococcus aureus* (MSSA) Enteric Gram-negative bacilli	Ceftriaxone *or* Levofloxin or moxifloxin *or* Ampicillin/sulbactam *or* Ertapenem
Escherichia coli	
Klebsiella pneumoniae	
Enterobacter sp.	
Proteus sp.	
Serratia marcescens	

MRSA coverage, it is important to remember that vancomycin has relatively poor lung penetration, and serum drug levels should be measured to ensure adequate dosage. Linezolid is another option, and two retrospective analyses comparing vancomycin to linezolid in treating MRSA nosocomial pneumonia showed improved survival and clinical cure rates with linezolid therapy (Table 7).

De-Escalation of Antibiotics

While starting therapy with broad-spectrum antibiotics is necessary to ensure adequate coverage, it is inappropriate to routinely continue these agents for the duration of therapy. Sputum culture results should be closely monitored to allow tailoring antibiotic therapy based upon the sensitivities as soon as they become available. The question remains, however, regarding how to tailor antibiotics when the culture results are negative. These patients are often categorized into two broad groups, those with clinical improvement on broad-spectrum therapy, and those with deterioration or lack of improvement. In those of the first group with good evidence of pneumonia, antibiotics may be de-escalated to simply Gram-negative coverage. MRSA is relatively easy to culture, so its absence justifies discontinuation of vancomycin or linezolid. In the second group, repeat cultures should be sent, and a nonpulmonary source of infection should be sought.

Duration of Therapy

To help determine the optimal duration of therapy, a prospective, randomized trial assessed 401 patients with VAP in 51 ICUs. Antibiotics were discontinued at either 8 or 15 days of therapy, regardless of the patient's condition, except in the situation of a documented pneumonia recurrence. The two groups had similar results regarding ventilator-free days, length of stay, and 60-day mortality. The only apparent disadvantage to the shorter course of therapy was a higher recurrence rate in those with nonfermenting Gram-negative bacilli (e.g., *Pseudomonas aeruginosa*). Otherwise, pneumonia recurrence rates were similar between the two groups. However, in those receiving 15 days of treatment, if there was a recurrence, it was much more likely to be associated with multidrug resistant organisms.

From a hospital systems standpoint, the use of protocols for initial empiric therapy and scheduled rotation of antibiotics have shown promise for improving effective treatment and reducing resistance. Protocols can help by incorporating local antibiotic resistance patterns and ensuring appropriate de-escalation of therapy. A study involving antibiotic rotation on a quarterly basis reduced infection-related mortality from 9.6 to 2.9 deaths per 100 admissions, and reduced rates of resistant Gram-positive coccus infection (14.6–7.8 per 100 admissions) and Gram-negative bacillus infection (7.7–2.5 per 100 admissions).

ANTIBIOTIC PROPHYLAXIS AND TUBE THORACOSTOMY

As previously mentioned, thoracic trauma is an important risk factor for ventilator-associated pneumonia. The risk of empyema and pneumonia is increased after thoracic trauma due to multiple etiologies. Direct infection may occur due to penetrating thoracic wounds. Secondary infection from an intra-abdominal source is also a possibility both due to direct spread after diaphragmatic rupture or hematogenous or lymphatic spread of disease. Finally, infection of undrained hemothoraces can occur.

Tube thoracostomy secondary to hemothorax or pneumothorax is necessary in up to 15% of thoracic trauma patients. While chest tube placement reduces the chance of infection due to undrained hemothoraces, it presents a risk of direct iatrogenic infection and bacterial inoculation of the pleural space and lung. The overall complication rate of thoracostomy has been reported to be approximately 20%, and the incidence of empyema up to 18%.

Prophylactic Antibiotics for Chest Tube Placement

Multiple studies have investigated the efficacy of prophylactic antibiotics in reducing the incidence of pneumonia and empyema related to chest tube placement. An evidentiary review performed by the Eastern Association for the Surgery of Trauma (EAST) Practice Management

Table 7: Initial Empiric Therapy for Hospital-Acquired Pneumonia and Ventilator-Associated Pneumonia in Patients with Late-Onset Disease or Risk Factors for Multidrug-Resistant Pathogens

Potential Pathogens	Combination Antibiotic Therapy
Pathogens listed in Table 6 and MDR pathogens	Antipseudomonal cephalosporin (cefepime, ceftazidime)
Pseudomonas aeruginosa	*or*
Klebsiella pneumoniae (ESBL+)[a]	Antipseudomonal carbepenem (imipenem or meropenem)
	or
Acinetobacter species[a]	β-Lactam/β-lactamase inhibitor (piperacillin–tazobactam)
	plus
	Antipseudomonal fluoroquinolone (ciprofloxacin or levofloxacin)
	or
	Aminoglycoside (amikacin, gentamicin, or tobramycin)
	plus
Methicillin-resistant	Linezolid or vancomycin
Staphylococcus aureus (MRSA)	
Legionella pneumophila[b]	

[a]If an ESBL+ strain, such as *K. pneumoniae*, or an *Acinetobacter* species is suspected, a carbepenem is a reliable choice.
[b]If *L. pneumophila* is suspected, the combination antibiotic regimen should include a macrolide (e.g., azithromycin) or a fluoroquinolone (e.g., ciprofloxacin or levofloxacin) should be used rather than an aminoglycoside.

group included nine prospective series and two meta-analyses. Their analysis showed that overall, the incidence of pneumonia was significantly reduced from 14% in the placebo group to 4.1% in the group receiving prophylactic antibiotic therapy, and the incidence of empyema was also significantly reduced from 8.7% in the placebo group to 0.6% in the antibiotic group.

The studies included in the meta-analysis varied considerably with regards to the antibiotic of choice, duration of therapy, definition of empyema and pneumonia, the location in which the procedure was performed and the experience of the medical personnel involved in the procedure. Those factors, particularly the location of tube placement, whether in the field, emergency room, operating room, or ICU, as well as the training of the medical personnel involved have been shown to impact the risk of infection. Further well-designed trials taking these factors into account should be done to provide a better understanding of this issue.

However, based on the data available, the EAST Practice group has recommended 24 hours of therapy with a first-generation cephalosporin after tube thoracostomy. The calculated number needed to treat to prevent a pulmonary infection is six. As chest tube placement is a known risk factor for ventilator-associated pneumonia, such treatment may well decrease the incidence of VAP as well as empyema, and should be practiced on a regular basis.

SUGGESTED READINGS

American Thoracic Society: Guidelines for the management of adults with hospital-acquired, ventilator associated, and healthcare-associated pneumonia. *Am J Respir Crit Care Med* 171(4):388–416, 2005.

Chastre J, Wolff M, Fagon JY, et al: Comparison of 8 vs 15 days of antibiotic therapy for ventilator-associated pneumonia in adults: a randomized trial. *JAMA* 290(19):2588–2598, 2003.

Croce MA, Fabian TC, Schurr MJ, et al: Using bronchoalveolar lavage to distinguish nosocomial pneumonia from systemic inflammatory response syndrome: a prospective analysis. *J Trauma* 39(6):1134–1139, discussion 1139–1140, 1995.

Croce MA, Fabian TC, Waddle-Smith L, Maxwell RA: Identification of early predictors for post-traumatic pneumonia. *Am Surg* 67(2):105–110, 2001.

Croce MA, Tolley EA, Fabian TC: A formula for prediction of posttraumatic pneumonia based on early anatomic and physiologic parameters. *J Trauma* 54(4):724–729, discussion 729–730, 2003.

Croce MA, Fabian TC, Mueller EW, et al: The appropriate diagnostic threshold for ventilator-associated pneumonia using quantitative cultures. *J Trauma* 56(5):931–934, discussion 934–936, 2004.

Dezfulian C, Shojania K, Collard HR, Kim HM, Matthay MA, Saint S: Subglottic secretion drainage for preventing ventilator-associated pneumonia: a meta-analysis. *Am J Med* 118(1):11–18, 2005.

Etoch SW, Bar-Natan MF, Miller FB, Richardson JD: Tube thoracostomy. Factors related to complications. *Arch Surg* 130(5):521–525;discussion 525–526, 1995.

Fagon JY, Chastre J, Vuagnat A, Trouillet JL, Novara A, Gibert C: Nosocomial pneumonia and mortality among patients in intensive care units. *JAMA* 275(11):866–869, 1996.

Kearns PJ, Chin D, Mueller L, Wallace K, Jensen WA, Kirsch CM: The incidence of ventilator-associated pneumonia and success in nutrient delivery with gastric versus small intestinal feeding: a randomized clinical trial. *Crit Care Med* 28(6):1742–1746, 2000.

Kollef MH, Von Harz B, Prentice D, et al: Patient transport from intensive care increases the risk of developing ventilator-associated pneumonia. *Chest* 112(3):765–773, 1997.

Kollef MH: Prevention of hospital-associated pneumonia and ventilator-associated pneumonia. *Crit Care Med* 32(6):1396–1405, 2004.

Luchette FA, Barrie PS, Oswanski MF, et al: Practice management guidelines for prophylactic antibiotic use in tube thoracostomy for traumatic hemopneumothorax: the EAST Practice Management Guidelines Work Group. Eastern Association for Trauma. *J Trauma* 48(4):753–757, 2000.

Marik PE, Zaloga GP: Gastric versus post-pyloric feeding: a systematic review. *Crit Care* 7(3):R46–R51, 2003.

Safdar N, Dezfulian C, Collard HR, Saint S: Clinical and economic consequences of ventilator-associated pneumonia: a systematic review. *Crit Care Med* 33(10):2184–2193, 2005.

Shaw MJ: Ventilator-associated pneumonia. *Curr Opin Pulm Med* 11(3):236–241, 2005.

Spain DA: Pneumonia in the surgical patient: duration of therapy and does the organism matter? *Am J Surg* 179(Suppl 1):36–39, 2000.

Spain DA: Ventilator-associated pneumonia and surgical patients. *Chest* 121(5):1390–1391, 2002.

Torres A, Aznar R, Gatell JM, et al: Incidence, risk, and prognosis factors of nosocomial pneumonia in mechanically ventilated patients. *Am Rev Respir Dis* 142(3):523–528, 1990.

Torres A, Gatell JM, Aznar E, et al: Re-intubation increases the risk of nosocomial pneumonia in patients needing mechanical ventilation. *Am J Respir Crit Care Med* 152(1):137–141, 1995.

ANTIBACTERIAL THERAPY: THE OLD, THE NEW, AND THE FUTURE

Philip S. Barie, Soumitra R. Eachempati, and Marc J. Shapiro

Infections remain the leading cause of death in hospitalized patients, and antimicrobial therapy is a mainstay of treatment. However, widespread overuse and misuse of antibiotics have led to an alarming increase in multiple-drug-resistant (MDR) pathogens. New agents may allow shorter courses of therapy and prophylaxis, which are desirable for cost control and control of microbial flora. Moreover, antibiotics are second only to analgesic agents in the number of adverse drug reactions.

PRINCIPLES OF PHARMACOKINETICS

The goal of pharmacotherapy is an effective response with no toxicity. The prescriber must have knowledge of the principles of drug absorption, distribution, and elimination. The dose-response relationship is influenced by dose, dosing interval, and route of administration. The plasma drug concentration is influenced by absorption, distribution, and elimination—which in turn depend on drug metabolism and excretion. The plasma concentration may not reflect tissue concentrations, as penetration into individual tissues is variable. Finally, the relationship between local drug concentration and effect is defined by several pharmacodynamic (PD) principles (see following discussion).

A few basic concepts of pharmacokinetics (PK) are useful to the practitioner. *Bioavailability* is defined as the percentage of an administered dose of a drug that reaches the systemic circulation. By definition, bioavailability is 100% after intravenous administration. However, this varies among drugs after oral administration, being affected by absorption (a function of product formulation and gastric emptying time), intestinal transit time, and the degree of hepatic first-pass metabolism.

Half-life refers to the amount of time required for the drug concentration to reduce by half, and thus is a hybrid of considerations of both clearance and volume of distribution. Half-life is useful to estimate when a steady-state drug concentration will be achieved. If a "loading dose" is not administered intravenously, thereby creating instantaneously a desired drug concentration to be maintained throughout therapy, four to five half-lives must elapse to achieve a steady state. Changes in dosage and changes in half-life owing to disease state (e.g., renal failure) must be accounted for. Interpretation of drug concentration data is difficult if the patient is not at a steady state, especially so in critical illness characterized by fluctuating organ function and *volume of distribution*.

Volume of distribution (V_D) is a proportionality constant that relates to plasma concentration and the amount of drug in the body. V_D is useful for estimating achievable plasma drug concentrations that result from a given dose. It is a derived parameter that is independent of a drug's clearance or half-life. It does not have particular physiologic significance, but pathophysiologic conditions can alter V_D substantially. A reduction of V_D will result in a higher plasma drug concentration for a given dose. However, the "third space" extravascular volume redistribution, fluid overload, and hypoalbuminemia (with decreased drug binding) of surgical illness act to increase V_D, all of which makes dosing a complex matter.

Clearance refers to the volume of liquid from which drug is eliminated completely per unit of time (whether by distribution to tissues, metabolism, or elimination) and is important for determining the amount of drug necessary to maintain a steady-state concentration. Drug elimination may be by metabolism, excretion, or dialysis. Most drugs are metabolized by the liver to polar compounds that can then be excreted by the kidney, but metabolism does not imply inactivation. For example, metronidazole is metabolized to a bactericidal metabolite with a prolonged half-life that has dosing implications. The kidneys are most important for excretion of metabolized drugs, although some drugs are metabolized or conjugated by the kidneys. Renal excretion may occur by filtration or by active or passive transport. The degree of filtration is determined by molecular size and charge and by the number of functional nephrons. In general, if greater than 40% of administered drug or its active metabolites is eliminated unchanged in the urine, decreased renal function will require a dosage adjustment. Active reabsorption and concentration of aminoglycosides by proximal tubular cells is a likely component of its well-recognized nephrotoxicity.

PRINCIPLES OF PHARMACODYNAMICS

The variable responses to drugs administered to a heterogeneous patient population can be described and perhaps reduced by an understanding of PD, the relationship of a drug to its intended effect. The PD of antibiotic therapy is especially complex because drug-patient, drug-microbe, and microbe-patient interactions must be accounted for. Knowledge of how patient characteristics influence absorption, distribution, and elimination of a drug—and how an antibiotic interacts with the targeted microbe—can increase the likelihood of a salutary clinical response. In turn, antimicrobial effects on bacteria are highly variable. Microbial physiology, inoculum size, microbial growth phase, intrinsic and extrinsic mechanisms of resistance, microenvironmental factors such as the pH at a local site of infection, and the patient's immune response are important factors. In the case of antimicrobial therapy, the key drug interaction is not with the host but with the microbe.

Because of microbial ability to alter the nature of the interaction with antimicrobial agents (principally via the development of resistance), mere delivery of drug may not be microbicidal. Factors that may contribute to the development of resistance are the production of drug-inactivating enzymes, alteration of cell surface receptor target molecules, and altered bacterial permeability to antimicrobial penetration. Critical to the microbe-patient interaction is the patient's immune system. Also inseparable are drug-patient factors that may influence PK, such as hepatic and renal function, serum albumin concentration, and extracellular volume status.

Antibiotic PD is determined by laboratory analysis, and thus the extrapolation of in vitro results to the patient may be challenging because the interaction with the host immune system is isolated from the analysis of the drug-microbe interaction. Analyses from in vitro study include the minimal inhibitory concentration (MIC). The MIC is the minimal serum drug concentration necessary for inhibition of bacterial growth, expressed as the proportion of the inoculum inhibited (MIC_{90} refers to 90% inhibition). However, some antibiotics may have important effects on bacteria at subinhibitory concentrations. Moreover, MIC testing may not detect the presence of resistant bacterial subpopulations (a particular problem with "heteroresistance" of Gram-positive bacteria, particularly *Staphylococcus aureus*).

Sophisticated analytic strategies draw upon the principles of both PK and PD; for example, by determination of the peak serum concentration:MIC ratio, the duration of time plasma concentration remains above the MIC, and the area of the plasma concentration-time curve above the MIC (the "area under the curve," or AUC). With some agents, antibacterial effects may persist for prolonged periods after the plasma drug concentration has become "subtherapeutic." The persistent inhibition of bacterial growth (but not killing) that persists after the serum drug concentration has fallen below the MIC for the organism is known as the postantibiotic effect (PAE). Appreciable PAE can be observed with aminoglycosides and fluoroquinolones for Gram-negative bacteria, and with some β-lactam drugs (notably carbapenems) against *S. aureus*. Through analyses of this type, certain drugs (e.g., aminoglycosides) have been characterized as having concentration-dependent killing whereby a higher peak concentration increases the efficacy of bacterial killing (up to a point). Other agents (most β-lactam agents) exhibit bactericidal properties that are independent of concentration. Rather, efficacy is determined by the duration of time the plasma concentration remains above the MIC. Other agents (e.g., fluoroquinolones) exhibit both properties such that bacterial killing may increase as drug concentration increases up to a point of saturation, after which the effect becomes independent of concentration.

EMPIRIC ANTIBIOTIC THERAPY

The decision to administer empiric antibiotic therapy must be considered carefully. An injudicious approach could result in nontreatment of established infection or therapy when the patient has only sterile inflammation or colonization with bacteria. Inappropriate therapy (e.g., delay, therapy misdirected against usual pathogens, failure to treat MDR pathogens) leads unequivocally to increased mortality. Several questions should be asked in each circumstance where empiric therapy is being considered.

Are antibiotics indicated at all? The answer is ultimately often no, but the decision to start treatment of the unstable patient must often be made before definitive information becomes available. The decision to start antibiotics empirically is based on the likelihood of infection, its likely source, and whether the patient's condition is sufficiently precarious that a delay will be detrimental. Outcome from serious infections is improved if antibiotics are started promptly, but on the other hand only about 50% of fever episodes in hospitalized patients are caused by infection. Many causes of the systemic inflammatory response syndrome are not due to infection (e.g., aspiration pneumonitis, burns, trauma, pancreatitis), although they may be complicated later by infection. Multiple organ dysfunction syndrome may progress even after an infectious precipitant has been controlled, due to a dysregulated host response.

Must antibiotics be started immediately? If the presumed infection is not destabilizing, this decision also depends on the overall status of the patient and should take into consideration such host factors as age, debility, renal and hepatic function, and immunosuppression. Culture yields are highest before antibiotics are administered, which for certain types of specimens (e.g., blood, cerebrospinal fluid) can be crucial. However, for many infections (e.g., bacteremia, intraabdominal infection, pneumonia) early appropriate therapy improves outcome.

Which organisms are the likely pathogens, and are they likely to be MDR? The clinical setting must be considered (e.g., nosocomial versus community-acquired infection, recent antimicrobial therapy), as must the patient's environment (e.g., recent hospitalization, proximity to another infected patient, the presence of MDR pathogens in the unit) and any recent microbial cultures obtained from the patient.

Will a single antibiotic suffice? The likely diagnosis and the nature of the probable pathogens are crucial determinants. If a nosocomial Gram-positive pathogen is suspected (e.g., wound or surgical site infection, catheter-related infection, prosthetic device infection, pneumonia) and methicillin-resistant *S. aureus* (MRSA) is endemic, empiric vancomycin (or linezolid) is appropriate. Some authorities recommend dual-agent therapy for serious *Pseudomonas* infections (i.e., an antipseudomonal β-lactam drug plus an aminoglycoside). It is important to use at least two antibiotics for empiric therapy of any infection that may be caused by a Gram-positive or Gram-negative infection (e.g., nosocomial pneumonia).

Duration of Therapy

Perhaps the most difficult issue is identifying the endpoint. If bona fide evidence of infection is evident, treatment is continued as indicated clinically. Often, however, the cultures will return negative and the decision must be arbitrary. The decision is complicated further when the patient has had a clinical response to antibiotic therapy in the absence of corroborating evidence, which may be coincident with or a result of false-negative cultures. Moreover, the bias to do *something* to treat the patient (i.e., continue antibiotic therapy) can be compelling in a patient who is deteriorating.

It must be recognized that careful culture techniques and specimen handling, combined with current sophisticated microbiology laboratory support, make it unlikely that substantive pathogens will be missed. Therefore, continuing empiric antibiotic therapy beyond 48 hours becomes difficult to justify. There are two possible exceptions. One occurs when fungal infection is suspected because the organisms can be difficult to culture, and the other occurs when deep cultures are needed from areas that are inaccessible without radiologic-guided aspiration and some time is necessary to make appropriate arrangements (but is not an excuse for procrastination).

How long should a course of therapy be continued? Effective broad-spectrum antibiotics are widely available, and many infections can be treated with therapy lasting 5 days or fewer. It is important that every decision to start antibiotics must be accompanied by a decision regarding the duration of therapy. A reason to continue therapy beyond the predetermined endpoint must be compelling. Bacterial killing is rapid in response to effective agents, but the host response may not subside immediately. Therefore, the clinical response of the patient should not be the sole determinant for continuation of therapy. If a patient still has sepsis syndrome at the end of a defined course of therapy, it is more useful to stop therapy and obtain a new set of cultures to look for new sites of infection, resistant pathogens, and noninfectious causes of inflammation.

There is a clear trend toward shorter courses of antibiotics for established infections. Broad-spectrum antibiotics that achieve excellent tissue penetration have been an important clinical development, but they also carry morbidity. The worldwide emergence of MDR Gram-positive and Gram-negative bacteria, superinfections in immunosuppressed patients, and the increased mortality associated with nosocomial infections in general make it important that adequate therapy be provided rapidly and for the shortest possible duration. Unfortunately, duration of therapy is not well established in the literature—and new studies are seldom designed with duration of therapy as a primary endpoint. Much depends on expertise and clinical judgment, which is accumulating in favor of shorter courses

of therapy. Nowhere is this clearer than for peritonitis and intra-abdominal abscess, for which the previous standard 7- to 10-day courses of therapy have been reduced to 5 days.

Infections that require 24 hours of therapy or less (sometimes just a single dose) include uncomplicated acute appendicitis or cholecystitis, uncomplicated bacterial cystitis (with some agents), and intestinal infarction without perforation. There is seldom justification to continue antibacterial therapy for more than 10 days. Examples of bacterial infections that require more than 14 days of therapy include tuberculosis of any site, endocarditis, osteomyelitis, and selected cases of brain abscess, liver abscess, lung abscess, some cases of postoperative meningitis, and some cases of endophthalmitis. Among the many reasons to limit therapy to only that which is needed is that antibiotic therapy has adverse consequences, despite a widespread perception that therapy is safe if not entirely benign. Adverse consequences of antibiotics include allergic reactions; development of nosocomial superinfections, including fungal infections, enterococcal infections, and *Clostridium difficile*–related disease; organ toxicity; promotion of antibiotic resistance; reduced yield from subsequent cultures; and induced vitamin K deficiency with coagulopathy or accentuation of warfarin effect.

CHOICE OF ANTIBIOTIC

The choice of which antibiotic to prescribe is made based on several interrelated factors. Paramount is activity against identified pathogens, presuming that a distinction between infecting and colonizing organisms can be made and that narrow-spectrum coverage is always most desirable. Knowledge of antimicrobial resistance patterns, nationally and especially in one's own institution and unit, is essential. Also important is an assumption regarding likely pathogens, which is paramount in cases where empiric therapy is necessary. Estimation of likely pathogens depends on the disease process believed responsible, whether the infection is community- or hospital-acquired, whether MDR organisms are present, and proximity to other infected patients. Also important are patient-specific factors, including age, debility, immunosuppression, intrinsic organ function, prior allergy or another adverse reaction, and recent antibiotic therapy. Institutional factors that may play a role include the existence of guidelines or practice parameters that may specify a particular therapy, or the availability of specific agents as defined by inclusion on the formulary or restriction by antibiotic control programs (Figure 1).

Development of Bacterial Resistance

In general, bacteria use four different mechanisms to develop resistance to antibiotics. Cell wall permeability to antibiotics is decreased by changes in porin channels (especially important for Gram-negative bacteria with complex cell walls, affecting aminoglycosides, β-lactam drugs, chloramphenicol, sulfonamides, tetracyclines, and possibly quinolones). Production of specific antibiotic-inactivating enzymes by plasmid-mediated or chromosomally mediated mechanisms affects aminoglycosides, β-lactam drugs, chloramphenicol, and macrolides. Alteration of the target for antibiotic binding in the cell wall affects β-lactam drugs and vancomycin, whereas alteration of target enzymes can inhibit β-lactam drugs, sulfonamides, quinolones, and rifampin. Drugs that bind to the bacterial ribosome (aminoglycosides, chloramphenicol, macrolides, lincosamides, streptogramins, and tetracyclines) are also susceptible to alteration of the receptor on the ribosome. Antibiotics may be extruded actively once entry to the cell is achieved in the case of macrolides, lincosamides, streptogramins, quinolones, oxazolidinones, and tetracyclines.

Cephalosporin resistance among Gram-negative bacilli can be the result of induction of chromosomal β-lactamases after exposure to the antibiotic. The extended-spectrum cephalosporins are rendered ineffective when bacteria such as enteric Gram-negative bacilli mutate to constitutively produce a β-lactamase that is normally an inducible enzyme. Although resistance to cephalosporins can occur by several

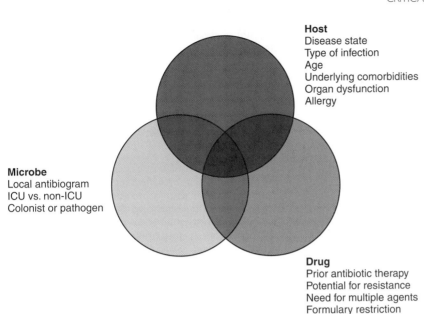

Host
Disease state
Type of infection
Age
Underlying comorbidities
Organ dysfunction
Allergy

Microbe
Local antibiogram
ICU vs. non-ICU
Colonist or pathogen

Drug
Prior antibiotic therapy
Potential for resistance
Need for multiple agents
Formulary restriction
Cost

Figure I   Host factors, microbe-specific factors, and drug-related factors all influence the selection of antibacterial agents. *ICU,* Intensive care unit.

mechanisms, the appearance of chromosomally mediated β-lactamases has been identified as a consequence of the use of third-generation cephalosporins. Resistance rates decline when use is restricted. The induction of an extended-spectrum β-lactamase (ESBL) in *Klebsiella* by ceftazidime was first reported approximately 20 years ago, but more than 200 mutations have now been described in several species of Gram-negative bacteria. The mutant bacteria develop resistance rapidly not only to all cephalosporins but to entire other classes of β-lactam antibiotics. It is therefore justifiable to restrict the use of ceftazidime, especially in institutions grappling with an ESBL-producing bacterium. The carbapenems generally retain useful microbicidal activity against ESBL-producing strains. Increasingly, *Pseudomonas aeruginosa* produces beta-lactamases of the ampC type.

Quinolone resistance, which is increasing rapidly, is for the most part chromosomally mediated, primarily by changes in the target sites for the antibiotic (DNA gyrase or topoisomerase IV). Changes in permeability or efflux may sometimes cause resistance to quinolones as well. Quinolone resistance is relatively easy to induce if a less-than-maximally effective drug is chosen for initial therapy. Resistance to one quinolone may also increase the MIC for the other quinolones against the organism, and thus if a quinolone is used, a highly active agent given in adequate dosage is essential.

ANTIBIOTIC SPECTRUM OF ACTIVITY

Susceptibility testing of specific organisms is necessary for management of serious infections (including all nosocomial infections). Recommended agents for specific organisms are guidelines only because in vitro susceptibilities may not correlate with clinical efficacy. The necessary concentration of antibiotics may not be achieved in tissue because of underdosing or poor tissue penetration. Moreover, bacterial killing correlates well with peak serum antibiotic concentrations for some drugs (e.g., aminoglycosides) and disorders (e.g., bacterial endocarditis) but correlates better with the duration of bactericidal drug concentrations for other antibiotics (e.g., β-lactam agents).

Cell-Wall–Active Agents: β-lactam Antibiotics

The β-lactam antibiotic group consists of penicillins, cephalosporins, monobactams, and carbapenems. Within this group, several agents have been combined with β-lactamase inhibitors to broaden the spectrum and increase the efficacy of the drugs. Several subgroups of anti-

biotics are recognized within the group, notably several "generations" of cephalosporins and penicillinase-resistant penicillins.

Penicillins

With the exception of carboxy- and ureidopenicillins, penicillins do not retain important activity against most strains of Gram-negative bacilli. Penicillin G (parenteral) and V (oral) are useful against most strains of aerobic and anaerobic streptococci (except for the increasingly important problem of penicillin-resistant pneumococci [PRSP, up to 40% of isolates] in bacteremia, recurrent otitis, and upper respiratory tract infections). Penicillins also have activity against *Enterococcus faecalis* (but not *E. faecium*), *Corynebacterium diphtheriae*, and *Listeria monocytogenes*. Gram-negative bacteria that are susceptible to penicillins include *Neisseria meningitidis* (highly resistant strains exist), some strains of *Proteus mirabilis*, and *Pasturella multocida*. In addition to anaerobic streptococci, penicillins are effective against other anaerobes, such as *Bacteroides melaninogenicus* (but not *B. fragilis*) and all clostridial species other than *C. difficile*.

The penicillinase-resistant semisynthetic penicillins include methicillin, nafcillin, oxacillin, cloxacillin, and dicloxacillin. Although these agents have useful activity against streptococci, *C. diphtheriae*, and anaerobic streptococci, the primary use of these agents is as therapy for sensitive strains of staphylococci. Hospitalized patients who need empiric therapy should not be treated with these agents because 60% of strains of *S. aureus* (MRSA), 90% of strains of *S. epidermidis* (MRSE), and virtually all enterococcal strains are resistant. However, these drugs are the treatment of choice for infections caused by susceptible isolates of *S. aureus*.

Activity against Gram-negative organisms was achieved initially by the addition of an amino group to the penicillin nucleus, thereby creating such drugs as ampicillin and amoxicillin. These drugs retain their antistreptococcal activity and a similar spectrum against most other Gram-positive pathogens, including anaerobic streptococci, but do not have appreciable activity against staphylococci. Ampicillin is highly effective against *E. faecalis*, including some vancomycin-resistant strains (VRE), but only rarely effective against *E. faecium*. Useful activity remains against *N. meningitidis*, *Moraxella catarrhalis*, community-acquired strains of *E. coli* and *Klebsiella* spp., *Salmonella* and *Shigella* spp., and *Proteus* spp. Ampicillin remains reasonably effective against community-acquired strains of *Hemophilus influenzae*, but *H. influenzae* is increasingly important as a nosocomial pathogen and resistant strains are recognized.

The carboxypenicillins (ticarcillin and carbenicillin) and ureidopenicillins (azlocillin, mezlocillin, and piperacillin; sometimes referred to as acylampicillins) have enhanced activity against Gram-negative bacteria and some activity against *P. aeruginosa*. Ureidopenicillins have greater intrinsic activity against *Pseudomonas*, but with the advent of β-lactamase inhibitor combination drugs none of these agents is used widely anymore. Beta-lactamase inhibitors (sulbactam, tazobactam, and clavulanic acid) result in enzymatic inactivation and enhanced effectiveness of the antibacterial agent. The effectiveness of these drugs as antibacterial agents is primarily a function of the inherent antibacterial properties of the parent compound (ampicillin < ticarcillin < piperacillin), and to a lesser extent of the effectiveness of the inhibitor (sulbactam ~ clavulanic acid < tazobactam). The spectrum of activity varies as a result, and the treating clinician needs to be familiar with each of the drugs in this class.

All of these drugs are effective against streptococci, methicillin-sensitive strains of *S. aureus*, *Listeria monocytogenes*, *Salmonella*, *Proteus*, and *Providentia* spp., *P. multocida*, and widely effective against anaerobes—including anaerobic cocci, *B. fragilis*, *Bacteroides and Prevotella* spp., and *Clostridium* spp. (except for *C. difficile*). Piperacillin/tazobactam has the widest spectrum of activity against Gram-negative bacteria, and the most potency against *P. aeruginosa*. Although ampicillin/sulbactam has excellent activity against community-acquired Gram-negative bacilli, it has major shortcomings against hospital-acquired strains of *E. coli* and *Klebsiella* (as many as 50% of strains may be resistant). However, sulbactam has useful activity against *Acinetobacter* spp., making ampicillin/sulbactam an option for therapy of infections caused by susceptible strains.

Cephalosporins

More than 20 antibiotics comprise this class of agents. The characteristics of the drugs thus vary widely when considered individually. It is useful to consider these drugs within four broad "generations" whose general characteristics are similar. For example, the first-generation agents retain useful activity against Gram-positive organisms—whereas the second-generation agents generally lose that activity in favor of antianaerobic activity. In contrast, the third-generation agents generally have enhanced activity against Gram-negative bacilli—and some have specific antipseudomonal activity. However, most lack efficacy against Gram-positive organisms and none is effective against anaerobic bacteria.

Cefepime, the fourth-generation cephalosporin available in the United States, has enhanced antipseudomonal activity and has regained activity against most Gram-positive cocci but not MRSA. None of the cephalosporins, regardless of class, has clinically useful activity against any of the enterococci. Regardless, there is sufficient heterogeneity of spectrum (especially among the third-generation agents) such that the clinician should be familiar with all of these drugs. Collectively, they account for a majority of prescriptions for parenteral antibiotics. Ceftriaxone, a third-generation agent unique in its class for excellent activity against Gram-positive organisms and once-daily dosing, was at one time the most-prescribed injectable antibiotic worldwide.

First-Generation Cephalosporins

First-generation cephalosporins include cefadroxil, cefazolin, cephalexin, cephalothin, cephapirin, and cephradine. Parenteral agents may be used against selected community-acquired Gram-negative infections, but they are of limited use against nosocomial pathogens. Parenteral first-generation cephalosporins still have a major role in surgical prophylaxis. Oral first-generation cephalosporins are used mostly for outpatient therapy of skin and soft-tissue and urinary tract infections. First-generation cephalosporins are the most active of the cephalosporin classes against

staphylococci (not methicillin-resistant strains) and streptococci, but they are not active against anaerobes other than anaerobic streptococci. Against Gram-negative bacilli, first-generation cephalosporins are active against some strains of *E. coli*, *Klebsiella*, *H. influenzae*, and *P. mirabilis*.

Second-Generation Cephalosporins

Second-generation cephalosporins have activity that makes them useful to the abdominal surgeon, but they are in increasingly short supply. These agents include cefaclor, cefamandole, cefmetazole, cefonicid, cefotetan (manufactured intermittently in the United States), cefoxitin (technically a cephamycin), and cefuroxime. These drugs retain activity against aerobic and anaerobic streptococci, but lose some activity against methicillin-sensitive staphylococci. Activity against *Neisseria gonorrheae* is reliable, although resistant strains do exist. However, only cefuroxime has appreciable activity against *Neisseria meningitidis*. Activity against Gram-negative bacilli is intermediate between that of the first- and third-generation agents, and thus the clinician must be familiar with the activity of specific agents. In general, there is activity against the *Enterobacteriaceae* except for *Enterobacter* but no activity against *Acinetobacter*, *Pseudomonas*, or *Stenotrophomonas*. As a class, there is good activity against *E. coli* and *K. pneumoniae* for all agents. Cefmetazole, cefotetan, and cefoxitin have appreciable activity against anaerobic Gram-negative bacilli—including *Bacteroides fragilis*. The spectrum of antianaerobic activity is a bit broader for cefoxitin compared to cefotetan. Both are more effective than clindamycin against anaerobes, but neither is as effective as β-lactamase–combination drugs, carbapenems, or metronidazole.

Third-Generation Cephalosporins

Rightly or wrongly, third-generation cephalosporins dominate prescribing practices for parenteral antibiotics. These agents include cefoperazone, cefotaxime, cefpodoxime, cefprozil, ceftazidime, ceftibuten, ceftizoxime, ceftriaxone, and lorcarbacef. They are relatively resistant to β-lactamases, and therefore have an extended spectrum of activity against Gram-negative bacilli. Despite this, these agents lack efficacy against Gram-positive bacteria (except for ceftriaxone) and anaerobic bacteria. Activity is reliable against non-ESBL–producing species of *Enterbacteriaceae*, including *Enterobacter*, *Citrobacter*, *Providencia*, and *Morganella*. Activity is variable against *Acinetobacter* and the pseudomonads, with broad activity against *Aeromonas*, reasonable albeit variable activity against *P. aeruginosa* (cefoperazone and ceftazidime), but no activity against *S. maltophilia*. Ceftriaxone and ceftazidime have activity against *Borrelia burgdorferi*, the agent of Lyme disease.

Paradoxically, third-generation cephalosporins (particularly ceftazidime) have been associated with the induction of ESBLs among many of the *Enterobacteriaceae*. Production of ESBLs was first reported in strains of *Klebsiella pneumoniae*, but now is so well recognized that susceptible pathogens are now referred to commonly as "inducible enteric" bacteria. The resistance induced by ESBL production is not just against other third-generation cephalosporins but affects entire other classes of β-lactam antibiotics. Third-generation cephalosporins, especially ceftazidime, have also been implicated (in concert with the widespread overuse of vancomycin; see material following) in the emergence of VRE. Because resistance can be transferred between enterococci and staphylococci, staphylococci of intermediate susceptibility to glycopeptides (GISA) or resistant to vancomycin (VRSA) have now been reported. Because of the potential to induce resistance of hospital flora, many centers no longer use third-generation cephalosporins as empiric therapy but rather reserve them for directed narrow-spectrum monotherapy of known susceptible organisms.

Fourth-Generation Cephalosporins

Cefepime is considered a fourth-generation agent because it has the broadest in vitro activity of any cephalosporin. The Gram-negative spectrum is more broad than that of the third-generation cephalosporins, the antipseudomonal activity exceeds that of ceftazidime, and the Gram-positive activity is comparable to that of a first-generation cephalosporin. The excellent safety profile of the cephalosporins is retained, and the potential for induction of ESBL production appears to be less. In common with all other cephalosporins, there is no meaningful activity against either enterococci or enteric anaerobic pathogens. Similar to the carbapenems, cefepime appears to be intrinsically more resistant to hydrolysis by β-lactamases. However, cefepime has variable activity against ESBL-producing bacteria. As a zwitterion, tissue penetration of cefepime is rapid.

Monobactams

Monobactams possess only the β-lactam nucleus. The single clinically available agent of this class, aztreonam, has a spectrum of activity against Gram-negative bacilli (including *Pseudomonas aeruginosa* and *Aeromonas* but not *P. cepacia* or *Stenotrophomonas*) that is similar to the third-generation cephalosporins—with no activity against either Gram-positive organisms or anaerobes. Aztreonam is not a potent inducer of β-lactamases. Resistance to aztreonam is widespread, but the drug may be useful for directed therapy against known susceptible strains and may be used safely for penicillin-allergic patients because the incidence of cross-reactivity is low.

Carbapenems

Carbapenems have a five-carbon ring attached to the β-lactam nucleus. The alkyl groups are oriented in a trans-configuration rather than the cis-configuration characteristic of other β-lactam agents, making these drugs resistant to β-lactamases. Four drugs (imipenem/cilastatin, meropenem, doripenem, and ertapenem) are available for clinical use in the United States and other agents are in clinical trials. Imipenem/cilastatin does induce β-lactamase production, but because it is resistant itself to ESBLs the activity of the drug is undiminished and little cross-resistance develops. Cilastatin is irrelevant to the antibacterial activity of imipenem/cilastatin, but it inhibits renal dihydropeptidase I, thereby abrogating the profound nephrotoxicity of the parent compound.

Imipenem-cilastatin, meropenem, and doripenem have the widest antibacterial spectrum of any antibiotics, with excellent activity against aerobic and anaerobic streptococci, methicillin-sensitive staphylococci, and virtually all Gram-negative bacilli except *Legionella*, *P. cepacia*, and *S. maltophilia*. Activity against the *Enterobacteriaceae* exceeds that of all antibiotics, with the possible exceptions of piperacillin/tazobactam and cefepime—and activity of meropenem against *P. aeruginosa* is approached only by that of amikacin. All of the carbapenems are superlative antianaerobic agents, and thus there is no reason to combine a carbapenem with metronidazole except for example to treat concurrent *C. difficile* colitis in a patient with a life-threatening infection that mandates continuance of the carbapenem. Other differences in spectra between imipenem-cilastatin and meropenem are trivial except that imipenem is an effective drug against *E. faecalis* (but not *E. faecium*). Meropenem is ineffective against enterococci.

Meropenem and doripenem appear not to have the same potential for neurotoxicity that is recognized with imipenem-cilastatin, which is contraindicated in patients with active central nervous system disease or injury (excepting the spinal cord) because of the rare (~0.5%) appearance of myoclonus or generalized seizures in patients who have received doses of more than 3 g/day (with normal renal function) or who have not had dosage reductions in the setting of renal insufficiency. With both drugs, the widespread disruption of the host microbial flora

inherent in such broad-spectrum therapy may lead to superinfections (e.g., fungi, *C. difficile*, *Stenotrophomonas*, or resistant enterococci).

Ertapenem is not active against *Pseudomonas* spp., *Acinetobacter* spp., *Enterobacter* spp., or MRSA, but is a useful drug nonetheless by virtue of its long half-life and substantial PAE—permitting once-daily dosing. In addition, ertapenem is highly active against ESBL-producing *Enterobacteriaceae* and has less potential for neurotoxicity than imipenem-cilastatin.

Cell-Wall–Active Agents

Lipoglycopeptides

Vancomycin is a soluble lipoglycopeptide with a complex bactericidal mechanism of action. The drug inhibits synthesis and assembly of the second phase of cell wall peptidoglycan synthesis, and it may also injure protoplasts by altering the permeability of their cytoplasmic membrane. There is some evidence that RNA synthesis may be impaired as well. These multiple mechanisms, along with a lack of cross-resistance with other antibiotics, may explain the historic low resistance rate for Gram-positive bacteria. Vancomycin is rapidly bactericidal, but only on dividing organisms. A PAE persists for about 2 hours. Unfortunately, tissue penetration of vancomycin is poor for almost all tissues—which can limit its effectiveness.

Both *S. aureus* and *S. epidermidis* are susceptible to vancomycin, although MICs for *S. aureus* are increasing and may require higher doses for therapeutic effect. *Streptococcus pyogenes*, group B streptococci, *S. pneumoniae* (including penicillin-resistant strains), and *C. difficile* are also susceptible. *Listeria monocytogenes*, anaerobic cocci, other clostridial species, and *Actinomyces* are usually susceptible. Most strains of *E. faecalis* are inhibited (but not killed) by concentrations attainable in serum, but *E. faecalis* is increasingly resistant to vancomycin. Resistant enterococci have emerged because of prolonged or indiscriminate use of vancomycin (Table 1), occasioned by the ubiquity of MRSA/MRSE. Both GISA and strains of *S. aureus* fully resistant to vancomycin are recognized, but so far only in association with prolonged (i.e., weeks to months) exposure to vancomycin.

Vancomycin usage is often inappropriate, and it is important for the public health that inappropriate usage should be curtailed. Bona fide indications include serious infections caused by MRSA/MRSE, Gram-positive infections in patients with serious penicillin allergy, and oral therapy (or by enema in patients with ileus) for *C. difficile*-related colitis in patients who have failed or are intolerant to

Table 1: Situations in Which Use of Vancomycin Is Discouraged

- Routine surgical prophylaxis in the absence of life-threatening allergy to β-lactam antibiotics
- Empiric therapy of febrile neutropenia in the absence of evidence for a Gram-positive infection
- Continued empiric use when microbiologic data suggest a reasonable alternative
- Systemic or local (i.e., catheter flush) prophylaxis of indwelling vascular catheters
- Selective decontamination of the digestive tract
- Eradication of colonization of methicillin-resistant staphylococci
- Primary treatment of antibiotic-associated colitis due to *Clostridium difficile*
- Routine prophylaxis for patients on hemodialysis or continuous ambulatory peritoneal dialysis
- Use for topical irrigation or application

metronidazole. Parenteral vancomycin is now usually administered in a dose of 15 mg/kg actual body weight q12h. The infusion must be performed over the course of at least 1 hour. The dose must be reduced in renal failure, and monitoring of serum concentrations may be helpful in that circumstance. New high-flux hemodialysis membranes dialyze vancomycin partially, and a 500-mg dose should be given after each dialysis.

Dalbavancin is a second-generation lipoglycopeptide agent that has a mechanism of action similar to vancomycin, resulting in disruption of the bacterial cell wall. Advantages of dalbavancin over vancomycin include a long elimination half-life in human beings, which makes once-weekly dosing feasible. For example, a phase III randomized trial demonstrated that two doses of dalbavancin (1 g initially, followed by 500 mg 7 days later) in complicated skin infections can take the place of other antibiotics requiring up to 28 doses. An additional possible advantage is that dalbavancin is bactericidal, whereas vancomycin is bacteriostatic, against most Gram-positive cocci.

Cyclic Lipopeptides

Daptomycin is a cyclic lipopeptide antibiotic with potent bactericidal activity against most gram-positive organisms, including MDR strains. The unique structure of daptomycin consists of a 13-member amino acid cyclic lipopeptide with a decanoyl side chain. This distinctive structure confers a novel mechanism of action, believed to involve insertion of the lipophilic daptomycin tail into the bacterial cell membrane—causing rapid membrane depolarization and a potassium ion efflux. This is followed by arrest of DNA, RNA, and protein synthesis, resulting in bacterial cell death. The bactericidal effect of daptomycin is rapid, with greater than 99.9% of both MRSA and MSSA bacteria dead in less than 1 hour without appreciable bacterial cell lysis.

Daptomycin is effective in a concentration-dependent manner, has a long half-life (8 hours), and demonstrates a prolonged PAE (up to 6.8 hours). Once-daily dosing of daptomycin results in linear PK with minimal drug accumulation. A dosing regimen of 4 mg/kg once daily is recommended for complicated skin/skin structure infections (cSSSI). Daptomycin is excreted renally. Therefore, the dosing interval should be increased to every 48 hours in patients with a creatinine clearance of less than 30 ml/min. Because of daptomycin's unique mechanism of action and because it is not metabolized by cytochrome p450 or other hepatic enzymes, no antagonistic drug interactions have been observed.

In vitro potency of daptomycin has been demonstrated against many aerobic and anaerobic Gram-positive bacteria, including MDR strains. Daptomycin's spectrum of activity encompasses difficult-to-treat antibiotic-resistant Gram-positive cocci, including MRSA and VRE. Daptomycin demonstrates activity against vancomycin-resistant *S. aureus*, as well as against linezolid- and quinupristin/dalfopristin-resistant *S. aureus* and *E. faecium*. Furthermore, daptomycin is also effective against a variety of streptococci—including *S. pyogenes* (group A) and *S. agalactiae* (group B) as well as other *Streptococcus* spp.—and against a variety of anaerobic species, including *Peptostreptococcus* spp., *C. perfringens*, and *C. difficile*. Daptomycin's efficacy is enhanced by the near absence thus far of antibiotic resistance, as verified by both in vitro and clinical studies. No transferable elements conferring daptomycin resistance have been isolated to date.

Daptomycin has been approved in the United States for the treatment of cSSSI associated with *S. aureus* (both MSSA and MRSA), *S. pyogenes*, *S. agalactiae*, *S. dysgalactiae* subsp. *equisimilis*, and *E. faecalis* (vancomycin-susceptible only) and for bacteremia caused by susceptible pathogens. Importantly, daptomycin must not be used for the treatment of pneumonia or empiric therapy when pneumonia is in the differential diagnosis (even when caused by a susceptible organism) because daptomycin penetrates lung tissue poorly and is inactivated by pulmonary surfactant.

▌ PROTEIN SYNTHESIS INHIBITORS

Several classes of antibiotics, although dissimilar structurally and having widely divergent spectra of activity, exert their antibacterial effects via the similar mechanism of binding to bacterial ribosomes to inhibit protein synthesis. This classification is valuable mechanistically and serves to link several classes of antibiotics conceptually that have few clinically useful members.

Aminoglycosides

With a reputation as toxic agents that have been superceded by newer antibiotics, it is ironic that the resurgence of aminoglycoside use has occurred as resistance to these newer antibiotics (especially third-generation cephalosporins and quinolones) has developed. Aminoglycosides exert their microbicidal activity by binding to the bacterial 30S ribosomal subunit, thereby inhibiting protein synthesis. With the exception of slightly better activity against Gram-positive cocci possessed by gentamicin, the spectrum of activity for the various agents is nearly identical. Differences among the agents are based on differences in toxicity, and efficacy is based on local resistance patterns. Gentamicin, tobramycin, and amikacin are still used frequently. Netilmycin is comparable in toxicity, but seldom used. Neomycin and kanamycin are quite toxic, and are now used only topically. Streptomycin is also quite toxic, but is still used in regimens for antimycobacterial therapy.

Nevertheless, the potential toxicity is real and aminoglycosides are seldom first-line therapy anymore except in a synergistic combination to treat a serious *Pseudomonas* infection, enterococcal endocarditis, or an infection caused by a MDR Gram-negative bacillus. As second-line therapy, these drugs are efficacious against the *Enterobacteriaceae*, *M. catarrhalis*, *H. influenzae*, *Salmonella* spp., and *Shigella* spp. Notably, there is somewhat less activity against *Acinetobacter*, and limited activity against *P. cepacia*, *Aeromonas* spp., *S. maltophilia*, and anaerobic organisms.

Aminoglycosides kill bacteria most effectively when the peak concentration of antibiotic is high. Therefore, a loading dose is necessary and serum drug concentration monitoring is often performed. Synergistic therapy with a β-lactam agent is theoretically effective because damage to the bacterial cell wall caused by the β-lactam drug enhances intracellular penetration of the aminoglycoside. However, evidence of improved clinical outcomes is scant. Serious infections require 5 mg/kg/day of gentamicin or tobramycin after a 2-mg/kg loading dose, or 15 mg/kg day of amikacin after a loading dose of 7.5 mg/kg. Clearance and volume of distribution are variable and unpredictable in critically ill patients, and doses that are higher still are sometimes necessary (e.g., burn patients). High doses (e.g., gentamicin 7 mg/kg/day) administered as part of a single-daily-dose protocol can obviate these problems in selected patients. Marked dosage reductions are necessary in renal failure, but the drugs are dialyzed and a maintenance dose should be given after each hemodialysis treatment.

Tetracyclines

Tetracyclines bind irreversibly to the 30S ribosomal subunit, but unlike aminoglycosides are bacteriostatic agents. Widespread resistance limits their utility in the hospital setting (with two exceptions), but they are still prescribed as oral agents. Short-acting oral tetracyclines include oxytetracycline and tetracycline HCl. Intermediate-acting oral agents of this class include demeclocycline, whereas those with a long half-life include the semisynthetic lipophilic congeners doxycycline and minocycline. Most pneumococci and *H. influenzae* are inhibited by achievable concentrations in serum. Thus, the tetracyclines may be used for management of sinusitis and acute exacerbations of chronic bronchitis. Gonococci and meningococci are quite susceptible. Unfortunately, penicillin-resistant gonococci tend also to be resistant to tetracycline. Outpatient urinary isolates of *E. coli* can be treated with tetracyclines, as can most infections caused by *Vibrio* spp. Most recently, doxycycline has been used with some success against VRE.

Tetracyclines are active against anaerobic pathogens. *Actinomyces* can be treated successfully. Doxycycline has activity against *B. fragilis*, but is it seldom used for the purpose. Many spirochetes are susceptible, including the Lyme disease pathogen *Borrelia burgdorferi*. The drugs can be used against rickkettsiae, *Chlamydophila* spp., mycoplasmas, and to some extent protozoa (*Entamoeba histolytica*).

Tigecycline is a novel glycycline antibiotic derived from minocycline. The drug shares with other tetracyclines its bacteriostatic mechanism of action and toxicities, including the contraindicated administration to children under the age of 8 years owing to dental toxicity. With the major exception of *Pseudomonas* spp., the spectrum of activity is broad—including many MDR Gram-positive and Gram-negative bacteria. Tigecycline is able to overcome typical bacterial resistance to tetracyclines because of modification at position 9 of its core structure. This enables it to bind to the bacterial 30S ribosomal unit with greater affinity than earlier-generation tetracyclines. The modification at position 9 provides additional steric hindrance, giving tigecycline a broader spectrum of activity than traditional tetracyclines. In vitro Gram-positive activity is directed against streptococci (including anaerobic species), staphylococci (including methicillin- and fully vancomycin-resistant strains), and enterococci (including VRE, *E. avium*, *E. casseliflavus*, and *E. gallinarum*). Activity against Gram-negative bacilli is directed against *Enterobacteriaceae* (including ESBL-producing strains), *P. multocida*, *A. hydrophila*, *S. maltophila*, *E. aerogenes*, and *Acinetobacter* spp. Activity against anaerobic bacteria is excellent.

Tigecycline has been approved in the United States for treatment of cSSSI and complicated intraabdominal infection caused by susceptible organisms. As clinical experience accrues, the utility of tigecycline for therapy of MDR organisms will become clear.

Oxazolidinones

Oxazolidinones bind to the 50S subunit of the prokaryotic ribosome, preventing it from complexing with the 30S subunit, mRNA initiation factors, and formylmethionyl-tRNA. The net result is to block assembly of a functional initiation complex for protein synthesis, thereby preventing translation of mRNA. This mode of action differs from that of existing protein synthesis inhibitors such as chloramphenicol, macrolides, lincosamides, and tetracyclines—which allow mRNA translation to begin but then inhibit peptide elongation. This difference may seem trivial, but is important in two respects. First, linezolid (the first oxazolidinone to be marketed) appears to be particularly effective in preventing the synthesis of staphylococcal and streptococcal virulence factors (e.g., coagulase, hemolysins, and protein A). Second, linezolid has a target that does not overlap with those of existing protein synthesis inhibitors. Consequently, its activity is unaffected by the rRNA methylases that modify the 23S rRNA so as to block the binding of macrolides, clindamycin, and group B streptogramins. Preventing the initiation of protein synthesis is no more inherently lethal than prevention of peptide elongation. Consequently, linezolid (similar to chloramphenicol, clindamycin, macrolides, and tetracyclines) is essentially bacteriostatic. The only protein synthesis inhibitors to achieve strong bactericidal activity are the aminoglycosides, which cause misreading of mRNA—leading to the manufacture of defective proteins that, among other effects, destabilize the membrane structure and cause leakage of cell content. The ribosomes of *E. coli* are as susceptible to linezolid as those of Gram-positive cocci. However, with minor exceptions Gram-negative bacteria are oxazolidinone-resistant—apparently because oxazolidinones are excreted by endogenous efflux pumps.

Linezolid is equally active against methicillin-susceptible and -resistant staphylococci; against vancomycin-susceptible enterococci and those with VanA, VanB, or VanC resistance determinants (VRE); and against pneumococci with susceptibility or resistance to penicillins or macrolides. Most Gram-negative organisms are resistant to linezolid, but susceptibility is observed for many *Bacteroides* spp., *M. catarrhalis*, and *Pasteurella* spp.

Linezolid exhibits excellent tissue penetration, and does not require a dosage reduction in renal insufficiency. Some class II and class III evidence suggests that linezolid may produce better outcomes compared with vancomycin for hospital-acquired pneumonia and cSSSI. Confirmation of these observations is required for linezolid to supplant vancomycin definitively as first-line therapy for serious infections caused by Gram-positive cocci.

Chloramphenicol

Chloramphenicol is a bacteriostatic agent that binds to the 50S ribosomal subunit. The drug has limited activity against the *Enterobacteriaceae* but remains effective against *Salmonella/Shigella* spp., including *S. typhimurium*. Chloramphenicol retains useful activity against most anaerobic organisms except for *C. difficile*. A resurgence in the use of chloramphenicol was occasioned by the emergence of VRE, but newer agents have supplanted that usage. Chloramphenical penetrates well into cerebrospinal fluid, and receives occasional usage for meningitis—especially when caused by *H. influenzae*. The bone marrow toxicity of chloramphenicol is feared, but rare in actuality. Reversible dose-related bone marrow toxicity is more common than aplastic anemia, which occurs in only about 1/25,000 courses of therapy. It is one of only a few antibiotics that require a dosage reduction in liver disease (Table 2) but not in renal insufficiency.

The Macrolide-Lincosamide-Streptogramin Family

Clindamycin

The lincosamide antibiotics in clinical use include lincomycin and clindamycin, but lincomycin is no longer widely available. Clindamycin also binds to the 50S ribosome and has good antianaerobic activity (although *B. fragilis* resistance is increasing), but in contrast to chloramphenicol it is devoid of activity against Gram-negative organisms while possessing reasonably good activity against Gram-positive cocci. Clindamycin is used occasionally for anaerobic infections, and it is a preferred choice to vancomycin for prophylaxis of clean surgical cases in penicillin-allergic patients (where the primary concern is the prevention of Gram-positive surgical site infections). Because clindamycin inhibits production of exotoxins in vitro, it has been advocated in preference to penicillin as first-line therapy of

Table 2: Antimicrobials Requiring Dosage Reduction in Hepatic Disease

Aztreonam
Cefoperazone
Chloramphenicol
Clindamycin
Erythromycin
Isoniazid
Metronidazole
Nafcillin
Quinupristin/dalfopristin
Rifampin
Tigecycline

invasive infections caused by *S. pyogenes*. The toxicity of clindamycin is far less than that of chloramphenicol, but its use has been associated with the development of antibiotic-associated colitis due to overgrowth of *C. difficile*.

Macrolides and Ketolides

Azithromycin, clarithromycin, dirithromycin, and erythromycin (the available macrolide antibiotics) and telithromycin (the first ketolide) are characterized by a macrocyclic lactone ring. Clarithromycin was developed against atypical mycobacteria in immunosuppressed patients, for which it is indeed effective. However, the macrolides are now used broadly in the outpatient setting—largely for upper respiratory tract infections and sometimes for uncomplicated skin infections. Clarithromycin and telithromycin are only available orally. Erythromycin has been available for more than 40 years, but its toxicities (e.g., nausea, vomiting, diarrhea for the oral form and gastrointestinal upset, cholestasis, and phlebitis for the parenteral form) and an unfavorable drug interaction profile make low cost the only advantage erythromycin possesses over the other agents in the class. Azithromycin is also available orally and parenterally.

All of these agents have excellent activity against aerobic streptococci, but azithromycin and clarithromycin are better against methicillin-sensitive *Staphylococcus aureus*. There is no appreciable activity against coagulase-negative staphylococci or methicillin-resistant strains of either organism. For Gram-positive organisms, susceptibility to erythromycin reflects activity of the newer drugs. Azithromycin is approved in the United States for treatment of sexually transmitted diseases caused by *C. pneumoniae*. The usefulness of these drugs for community-acquired upper respiratory tract infections is reflected by activity against *M. catarrhalis* and *L. pneumophilia*, but only azithromycin, clarithromycin, and telithromycin (especially) have useful activity against *H. influenzae*. Clarithromycin is extremely active against *Helicobacter pylori*. The penicillin-resistant pneumococci are almost always resistant to macrolides.

Macrolides inhibit the function of the cytochromes P$_{450}$. Patients on theophylline should be monitored carefully when clarithromycin and erythromycin are used concurrently, but neither azithromycin nor dirithromycin alters the PK profile. Interactions between erythromycin or clarithromycin and other drugs that prolong the Qtc interval, such as quinolones, may precipitate ventricular dysrhythmias such as torsades de pointes. Serum concentration of the anticonvulsant carbamazepine must be monitored carefully during clarithromycin therapy.

Streptogramins

The streptogramin group is a separate family of antimicrobials within the macrolide-lincosamide-streptogramin (MLS) framework. Thus, they rarely exhibit cross-resistance with other anti-infective agents. Several compounds are known, but antimicrobial activity depends on a tertiary complex of two agents with the ribosome. Pristinamycin, one such combination, has been available in Europe for many years as an oral antistaphylococcal agent. Quinupristin/dalfopristin has been approved for clinical use in the United States. Quinupristin (a derivative of pristinamycin IA) and dalfopristin (a derivative of pristinamycin IIA) are admixed in a fixed 30:70 ratio for administration. Each component binds to a different site on the 50S ribosomal subunit to form the stable tertiary complex. The drug exhibits rapid bactericidal activity against Gram-positive cocci, and a prolonged PAE.

The in vitro activity of quinupristin/dalfopristin includes most Gram-positive pathogens, including methicillin-resistant *S. aureus* and *S. epidermidis*, penicillin- and macrolide-resistant pneumococci, and most strains of VRE (including the *vanA* and *vanB* phenotypes of *E. faecium*). Some Gram-negative respiratory tract pathogens are covered, including *M. catarrhalis*, *N. meningitides*, and *H. influenzae* and the intracellular respiratory pathogens *Legionella* spp., *Mycoplasma pneumoniae*, and *Chlamydophila* spp.

Both components are converted rapidly in the liver to active metabolites. Although the elimination half-lives for quinupristin and dalfopristin are ~0.9 and 0.75 hours, respectively, the prolonged PAE is ~10 hours for *S. aureus* and ~9 hours for pneumococci. The clearance for both drugs is similar (0.7 l/kg), as is the volume of distribution (1 l/kg). Less than 20% is excreted by the kidneys. The usual adult dose is 7.5 mg/kg q8 hours. Dosage reductions for renal dysfunction are not needed, but are necessary in hepatic insufficiency. Musculoskeletal toxicity or phlebitis may require cessation of therapy.

DRUGS THAT DISRUPT NUCLEIC ACIDS

Quinolones

The quinolones inhibit bacterial DNA synthesis rapidly by inhibiting DNA gyrase, which serves to fold DNA into a superhelix in preparation for the initiation of replication. These are potent antimicrobial agents with an unfortunate propensity to develop resistance rapidly. The fluoroquinolones enjoy a broad spectrum of activity, demonstrate excellent oral absorption and bioavailability, and are generally well tolerated.

Numerous quinolones are available, and more are in development. Oral agents include ciprofloxacin, gatifloxacin, gemifloxacin, levofloxacin, and moxifloxacin, whereas parenteral formulations are available for ciprofloxacin, levofloxacin, and moxifloxacin.

Currently available quinolones are most active against enteric Gram-negative bacteria, particularly the *Enterobacteriaceae* and *Hemophilus* spp. There is activity against *P. aeruginosa*, *S. maltophilia*, and Gram-negative cocci. Activity against Gram-positive cocci is variable, being least for ciprofloxacin and best for the so-called "respiratory quinolones" (gatifloxacin, gemifloxacin, and moxifloxacin). Among commonly prescribed fluoroquinolones, ciprofloxacin is most active against Gram-negative isolates, particularly *P. aeruginosa*. The in vitro susceptibility to moxifloxacin is comparable to metronidazole for *B. fragilis*, and acceptable for bacteria of the *B. fragilis* group. However, rampant overuse (particularly in the outpatient setting) is leading to rapidly increasing resistance that may limit severely the future usefulness of these agents.

Rifampin

The rifamycins, of which rifampin is widely used clinically, inhibit DNA-dependent RNA polymerase at the β-subunit—which prevents chain initiation. Rifampin, a zwitterion that is soluble in acidic aqueous solution, is highly diffusable through lipid membranes. It penetrates well almost all body tissues. Rifampin has a unique ability to penetrate living neutrophils and to kill phagocytosed intracellular bacteria. Rifampin is available both orally and parenterally, and is active against a wide range of pathogens. Oral bioavailability approaches 100% with the usual dose of 600 mg once daily. Unfortunately, the rapid development of resistance relegates this agent to combination therapy in virtually all circumstances.

Rifampin is active against staphylococci (including some activity against MRSA) and against other Gram-positive and Gram-negative cocci, including the gonococcus and the meningococcus. Among the Gram-negative bacilli, it is most active against *Hemophilus influenzae*, with little activity against the *Enterobacteriaceae*. It is the most active known agent against *Legionella* spp., more so than the macrolides (which are the drugs of choice). It is as active as vancomycin in vitro against *C. difficile*, and is useful against *M. tuberculosis* and *C. pneumoniae*.

In addition to antituberculosis chemotherapy, rifampin is used for meningococcal meningitis prophylaxis of close contacts, synergistic therapy of MSSA endocarditis (this is controversial because of questions about antagonism and a propensity to develop resistance), the staphylococcal carrier state (including MRSA), chronic staphylococcal arthritis or osteomyelitis, synergistic therapy of Legionnaire's disease, brucellosis, and staphylococcal prosthetic device infections. Synergistic therapy with rifampin and vancomycin is controversial for MRSA endocarditis, and there are no data to support synergistic therapy for other MRSA infections.

Rifampin is a potent inducer of the hepatic microsomal enzyme system. Reduced oral bioavailability and decreased serum half-life occurs for a number of drugs, including barbiturates, benzodiazepines, calcium channel blockers, chloramphenicol, cyclosporine, digitalis, estrogens, fluconazole, haloperidol, histamine H2-antagonists, metoprolol, phenytoin, prednisone, propranolol, quinidine, theophylline, and warfarin (Table 3).

CYTOTOXIC ANTIBIOTICS

Metronidazole

Metronidazole is active against nearly all anaerobic infections, and against many protozoa that are human parasites. Against anaerobes, metronidazole has the best bactericidal activity of all—including activity against *B. fragilis*, *Prevotella* spp., *Clostridium* spp. (including *C. difficile*), and anaerobic cocci. The most notable exception to the antianaerobic efficacy of metronidazole is a lack of activity in actinomycosis. Potent bactericidal activity is characterized by killing often at the same concentration required for inhibition. Resistance has been reported, but it remains rare and of negligible clinical significance. Also sensitive are *Campylobacter fetus*, *Gardnerella vaginalis*, *H. pylori*, *Giardia lamblia*, *Trichomonas vaginalis*, and *E. histolytica*.

Metronidazole causes DNA damage after intracellular reduction of the nitro group of the drug. Acting as a preferential electron acceptor, it is reduced by low-redox potential electron transport proteins—decreasing the intracellular concentration of the unchanged drug and maintaining a transmembrane gradient that favors uptake of additional drug. Toxicity is mediated directly by short-lived intermediate compounds or free radicals.

The drug diffuses well into nearly all tissues, including the central nervous system—thus making it an effective agent for deep-seated infections, even against bacteria that are not multiplying rapidly. Absorption after oral or rectal administration is rapid and nearly complete. Historically, a loading dose of 15 mg/kg followed by 7.5 mg/kg every 6 hours by intravenous administration was recommended. However, the loading dose was seldom administered in practice. This short dosing interval is also difficult to reconcile considering that the half-life of the drug is 8 hours owing to the production of an active hydroxy metabolite. Increasingly, intravenous metronidazole is administered every 8–12 hours in recognition of the active metabolite.

No dosage reduction is required for patients with renal insufficiency, but the drug is dialyzed effectively and administration should be timed to follow dialysis if twice-daily dosing is used. PK studies of patients with hepatic impairment performed at higher doses indicated that dosage reduction of 50% was necessary, but this is probably not the case when twice-daily dosing is used.

Trimethoprim-Sulfamethoxazole

Sulfonamides exert bacteriostatic activity by interfering with bacterial folic acid synthesis, a necessary preliminary step in purine synthesis and ultimately in DNA synthesis. Resistance is widespread, and the agents are seldom used for infections other than of the urinary tract. The addition of sulfamethoxazole to trimethoprim, which prevents the conversion of dihydrofolic acid to tetrahydrofolic acid by the action of dihydrofolate reductase (downstream from the action of sulfonamides), accentuates the inherent bactericidal effects of trimethoprim.

Trimethoprim-sulfamethoxazole (TMP-SMX) is active in vitro against *S. aureus*, *S. pyogenes*, *S. pneumoniae*, *E. coli*, *P. mirabilis*, *Salmonella*, *Shigella* spp., *Pseudomonas* spp. (but not *P. aeruginosa*), *Yersinia enterocolitica*, *S. maltophilia*, *L. monocytogenes*, and *Pneumocystis carinii*. The combination is useful in urinary tract infections, acute exacerbations of chronic bronchitis, and *Pneumocystis* infections in immunocompromised patients, and is the treatment of choice for infections caused by *S. maltophilia*. The drug may be used as a second-line therapy for many other infections caused by susceptible organisms because tissue penetration is generally excellent.

A fixed-dose combination of TMP-SMX of 1:5 is available for parenteral administration. The standard oral formulation is 80:400 mg, but lesser- and greater-strength tablets are available. Oral absorption is rapid and bioavailability is nearly 100%. Ten ml of the parenteral formulation contains 160:800 mg drug. Full doses (15–30 mg/kg TMP in three to four divided doses) may be given as long as the creatinine clearance is greater than 30 ml/minute, but the drug is not recommended when the creatinine clearance is less than 15 ml/min.

ANTIBIOTIC TOXICITIES

Beta-Lactam Allergy

Allergic reaction, although less common than generally believed, is the most common toxicity of β-lactam antibiotics. The incidence is approximately 7–40/1000 treatment courses of penicillin. Reactions of four distinct types are recognized, but certain reactions are not easily classified. Immediate hypersensitivity reactions occur because of an interaction with preformed β-lactam-specific IgE antibodies bound to mast cells or circulating basophils via high-affinity receptors. Cytotoxic antibody reactions occur when β-lactam-specific IgG (usually) or IgM antibodies bind to red blood cells or renal interstitial cells that have bound to antigen, resulting in complement-dependent cell lysis.

Complement-independent toxicity may result from binding to neutrophil or macrophage cell membranes. Examples include leukopenia, thrombocytopenia, hemolytic anemia, and interstitial nephritis. Immune complex (Arthus) reactions occur when circulating antigen-antibody (IgG, IgM) complexes fix complement and lodge in various tissue sites, causing serum-sickness–like reactions and possibly drug fever. The onset of these reactions is usually 7–14 days after therapy has begun, even if drug has already been stopped. In cell-mediated hypersensitivity, β-lactam antigen-specific T-cell receptors bind the antigen—causing cytokine release and lymphocyte proliferation. Contact dermatitis is the usual manifestation. Certain reactions do not fall under these classifications, including pruritis, maculopapular reactions,

Table 3: Antimicrobial Interactions with Oral Anticoagulants

Potentiated Effect of Oral Anticoagulants

Cephalosporins
Chloramphenicol
Erythromycin
Fluoroquinolones
Metronidazole
Sulfonamides
Tetracyclines
Trimethoprim/sulfamethoxazole

Attenuated Effect of Oral Anticoagulants

Nafcillin
Rifampin

erythema multiforme, erythema nodosum, photosensitivity, and exfoliative dermatitis.

The immunochemistry of penicillin reactions has been well defined. Penicillin binds with tissue proteins to produce multivalent hapten-protein complexes, which are required for induction of immunity. The most common hapten form of penicillin in vivo is the penicilloyl derivative, which is called the *major determinant*. Accelerated (1–72 hours) and late reactions are usually in response to the major determinant. Small quantities of other *minor determinants* may be formed by metabolic activity, and these induce a variable response. Anaphylactic reactions are usually in response to a minor determinant.

Parenteral therapy causes more clinical allergic reactions, but this is a function of the dose administered. Most serious reactions occur in patients with no history of an allergic reaction, simply because a history of penicillin allergy is often sought specifically. Patients with a prior reaction have a four- to sixfold increased risk of another reaction compared to the general population. However, this risk decreases with time—from 80%–90% skin test reactivity at 2 months to 20% reactivity at 10 years. An estimated 5%–20% of patients give a history of penicillin allergy. The risk of cross-reactivity between penicillins and cephalosporins is 5%–10%, being higher for first-generation agents. There is a low incidence of cross-reactivity between carbapenems and penicillins, but negligible cross-reactivity to monobactams.

"Red Man" Syndrome

Tingling and flushing of the face, neck, or thorax may occur with parenteral vancomycin therapy. However, these symptoms are less common than fever, rigors, or local phlebitis. Although it is a hypersensitivity reaction, it is not an allergic phenomenon owing to the clear association with too-rapid infusion of the drug (which can also cause hypotension)—particularly of the now-common 1-g dose. Parenteral vancomycin should be administered over a 1-hour period. The cause is believed to be histamine release due to local hyperosmolality rather than an allergic reaction. A maculopapular rash due to hypersensitivity does occur in about 5% of patients. It may persist for weeks after the drug is discontinued in patients with renal failure.

Nephrotoxicity

Aminoglycosides

The inherent potential of aminoglycosides for nephrotoxicity is related to the degree of positive electrical charge at physiologic pH. There is little if any clinical difference among commonly used agents in terms of potential nephrotoxicity. Aminoglycosides do not provoke inflammation, and thus there are no allergic components to this or any other manifestation of aminoglycoside toxicity.

The mechanisms of clinical toxicity relate to ischemia and to toxicity to of renal proximal tubular cell (PTC). Aminoglycosides cause afferent arteriolar vasoconstriction. Thus, ischemia is a prominent component of the response. Aminoglycosides bind to the brush border membrane of PTC after glomerular filtration, leading to enzymuria, excretion of calcium and magnesium, and internalization by pinocytosis. The consequence is perturbation of the phosphatidyl inositol "middle messenger" system, with membrane damage and increased excretion of membrane phospholipids. Subsequently, there is rapid perinuclear localization of drug—with disturbed protein synthesis and mitochondrial respiration. Ultimately, the injury is manifested by necrosis of the PTC, reduction of the glomerular filtration rate (GFR), and decreased creatinine clearance. Postulated mechanisms of reduced GFR include release of vasoconstrictive hormones, transepithelial back-leak of toxins, obstruction by necrotic cellular debris, or a change in glomerular fenestrae and the ultrafiltration coefficient.

The PTC is actually relatively resistant to injury, which is usually reversible. It generally takes several days of therapy to induce a clinically important injury.

Most patients develop a non-oliguric decrease in creatinine clearance. Progression to dialysis dependence is rare. Aminoglycoside nephrotoxicity is accentuated by frequent dosing, older age, sodium and volume depletion, acidemia, hypokalemia, hypomagnesemia, coexistent liver disease, and other nephrotoxic drugs. The risk of injury is ameliorated by single-daily-dose therapy. If renal function deteriorates, it is advisable to discontinue therapy. If necessary (i.e., life-threatening *Pseudomonas* infection), therapy may be continued.

Vancomycin

Vancomycin nephrotoxicity is less common than previously. Multiple courses of therapy, administration of very high doses (substantial dosage reductions are necessary in renal insufficiency), and concurrent administration of aminoglycosides are known risk factors for toxicity.

Ototoxicity

Aminoglycosides

Aminoglycosides can cause cochlear and vestibular toxicity. Ototoxicity is usually irreversible, and may develop after the cessation of therapy. Repeated exposures create cumulative risk. Most patients develop cochlear toxicity or a vestibular lesion. Rarely are both organs injured. Cochlear toxicity can be a subtle diagnosis to make because baseline audiograms are virtually never available and formal screening programs are undertaken seldom. Few patients complain of hearing loss, yet when sought the incidence of cochlear toxicity may be more than 60%. Clinical hearing loss may occur in 5%–15% of patients.

The outer hair cells of the basal turn of the cochlea, where high-frequency detection is located, are most susceptible to aminoglycosides. Amikacin and netilmicin are less ototoxic than gentamicin and streptomycin, and tobramycin is intermediate in toxicity. Neomycin is extremely ototoxic, and caution must be used when the drug is administered topically or orally to patients with renal insufficiency. Risk factors include treatment duration, high serum drug concentrations, a large cumulative dose, concomitant ototoxic drug therapy (especially vancomycin or furosemide), hypovolemia, and renal or liver disease. Cochlear injury may be unilateral or bilateral, and may occur days to weeks after termination of therapy. There is no apparent correlation with the development of nephrotoxicity.

The target of vestibular toxicity is the type I hair cell of the summit of the ampullar cristae. The true incidence of vestibular toxicity has been impossible to determine, but the best estimate is about 5%. Whether different agents have different potential for injury is unknown. Patients can suffer considerable injury before the onset of symptoms, owing to the compensatory contribution of visual and proprioceptive cues (symptoms may therefore be worse at night). Complaints of nausea, vomiting, and vertigo are most common—and patients may exhibit nystagmus.

Vancomycin

Ototoxicity caused directly by vancomycin is accepted as fact, but poorly documented in the literature. Hearing loss attributed to vancomycin is better described as neurotoxicity, manifesting as auditory nerve damage, tinnitus, and loss of acuity for high-frequency tones. Particular caution must be exercised with concurrent administration of other ototoxic drugs, especially aminoglycosides and furosemide, because synergistic injury is possible.

Metronidazole Toxicity

Metronidazole is generally well tolerated. Minor adverse reactions include gastrointestinal upset and metallic taste, which sometimes necessitate stopping the drug. Discolored urine, rash, urticaria, urethral or vaginal burning, gynecomastia, and reversible neutropenia have also been noted. Rare but serious adverse neurologic reactions include seizures, encephalopathy, ataxia, and peripheral neuropathy. Other rare but potentially serious reactions include disulfiram-like reactions in the presence of alcohol, potentiation of warfarin effect (see Table 2), *C. difficile*-associated disease (despite its therapeutic efficacy), and acute pancreatitis. Suggestions of mutagenicity from in vitro studies have not been borne out clinically, but the drug crosses the placenta readily and should be used in pregnancy only when necessary.

Quinolone Toxicity

Quinolones are generally well tolerated. For the most part, adverse effects increase with higher doses and prolonged therapy. Gastrointestinal side effects are common (up to 13%), and *C. difficile*-related disease has been reported.

Adverse central nervous system effects are also common (up to 7%). Headache and dizziness predominate, followed by insomnia and mood alteration. Hallucinations, delirium, and seizures are rare. Allergic and skin reactions occur in up to 2% of patients. Phototoxicity after exposure to ultraviolet A light (sunlight is sufficient exposure) occurs in some patients. Anaphylactoid reactions are rare. Arthopathy and tendinitis, reversible bone marrow depression, leukopenia, and hemolytic anemia have been reported. Rare but important is prolongation of the electrocardiogram Qtc interval, which may precipitate the dangerous ventricular dysrhythmia torsades de pointes.

Tetracycline Toxicity

Hypersensitivity reactions to tetracyclines can manifest as anaphylaxis, fixed drug eruptions, or morbilliform reactions. Allergy to one agent in the class indicates allergy to all. Photosensitivity is most common with demeclocycline, but can occur with any of the drugs. It appears to be a toxic reaction rather than an allergic one.

Permanent gray-brown discoloration of the teeth of children represents toxicity to the tooth enamel. Therefore, it is important not to administer any tetracycline to pregnant women or children up to the age of eight unless alternative therapies for a serious illness are more toxic (i.e., Rocky Mountain spotted fever). Depression of skeletal growth has been reported in premature infants exposed to tetracycline.

Gastrointestinal toxicities are common. Nausea, vomiting, and epigastric pain are dose related. Administration with food can reduce the symptoms but seriously reduces the bioavailability of the drug. *Clostridium difficile* superinfection has been reported.

Symptoms of renal failure can be aggravated by azotemia related to disrupted amino acid metabolism. Nephrogenic diabetes insipidus is caused by demeclocycline, which fact has been taken advantage of clinically in the management of chronic inappropriate antidiuretic hormone secretion.

Trimethoprim-Sulfamethoxazole Toxicity

The toxicity symptoms of TMP-SMX include all of those characteristic of sulfonamides, including nausea, vomiting, diarrhea, anorexia, and hypersensitivity reactions. Skin eruptions are common in patients with the acquired immunodeficiency syndrome, and transient diffuse pulmonary infiltrates and hypotension have been described upon rechallenge in such patients. Prolonged administration may disrupt folic acid metabolism in patients (megaloblastic anemia, hypersegmented neutrophils, leukopenia, thrombocytopenia). Administration

of folinic acid is protective. *Clostridium difficile*-related disease has been reported. Dose-related reversible increases in serum creatinine concentration have been reported, especially with concomitant cyclosporine administration—as have drug-induced hepatitis and cholestasis. Phenytoin concentrations increase markedly during therapy. Elderly patients are more susceptible to toxicity, especially in the presence of hepatic or renal dysfunction. The parenteral formulation contains metabisulfites, to which some people are allergic. Allergy to sulfites has a higher incidence in asthmatic patients.

AVOIDING TOXICITY

Adjustment of Antibiotic Therapy in Hepatic Insufficiency

The liver is crucial for metabolism and elimination of drugs that are too lipophilic for renal excretion. This metabolism is carried out by several different sets of enzymes. For example, the cytochromes P_{450} (a gene superfamily consisting of more than 300 different enzymes) carry out oxidative reactions that convert lipophilic compounds to water-soluble products. Other enzymes convert drugs or metabolites by conjugating them with sugars, amino acids, sulfates, or acetate to facilitate biliary or renal excretion—whereas enzymes such as esterases and hydrolases act by other distinct mechanisms. Many of these functions are disrupted when liver function is impaired.

The clinical problem of drug dosing is complicated by several factors. The wide variability of severity of injury, the insensitivity for clinical assessments of liver function to quantify the degree of impairment, the fact that few if any hepatic clearance functions are performed at 100% capacity, and changing metabolism as the degree of impairment fluctuates (e.g., resolving cholestasis) must all be considered. Changes in renal function that develop as the liver becomes progressively impaired must also be taken into account. Renal blood flow is decreased in cirrhosis, and glomerular filtration is decreased in cirrhosis with ascites. Clinical studies indicate that adverse drug reactions are more frequent in patients with cirrhosis than in patients with other forms of liver disease or with renal disease.

Liver disease has the greatest effect on those drugs that undergo extensive oxidative metabolism. With such a multiplicity of factors involved, it is difficult to predict the effect of disease on drug disposition in individual patients. There is no useful clinically available test of liver function that can be used as a guide to dosage, such as glomerular filtration rate in the case of renal failure. A general rule is that dosage reduction should be up to 25% of the usual dose if hepatic metabolism is 40% or less and renal function is normal, the drug is given acutely, and has a large therapeutic index (see Table 2). Greater dosage reductions (up to 50%) are advisable if the drug is administered chronically, there is a narrow therapeutic index, protein binding is significantly reduced, or the drug is excreted renally and renal function is severely impaired. In circumstances where renally excreted therapeutic substitutes exist for patients with liver disease, such drugs should be used.

Adjustment of Antibiotic Therapy in Renal Insufficiency

Drug elimination by the kidneys depends on the GFR, tubular secretion, and reabsorption. Renal dysfunction may alter any or all of these parameters, which in turn may be influenced by nonrenal organ dysfunction. Different types of renal disease, or acute versus chronic renal failure, may result in different drug clearance rates among patients with the same GFR. The management of antibiotics in renal failure must be individualized because most antibiotics are excreted via the kidneys. Relatively precise estimates of renal function are especially important in patients with impaired renal function who have not yet come to dialysis

Table 4: Dosing of Selected Parenteral Antibiotics Applied After Dialysis

Antibiotic	Dose
Amikacin	2.5–3.75 mg/kg
Ampicillin	1 g
Azlocillin	3 g
Aztreonam	0.125 g
Cefamandole	0.5–1 g
Cefepime	0.5 g
Cefoxitin	1 g
Ceftazidime	1 g
Ceftizoxime	1–3 g
Cefuroxime	0.75 g
Chloramphenicol	1 g
Gentamicin	1.0–1.7 mg/kg
Imipenem/cilastatin	0.25–0.5 g
Meropenem	0.5 g
Mezlocillin	2–3 g
Netilmicin	2 mg/kg
Piperacillin	2 g
Piperacillin/tazobactam	2.25 g
Ticarcillin	3 g
Ticarcillin/clavulanic acid	3.1 g
Tobramycin	1.0–1.7 mg/kg
Trimethoprim/sulfamethoxazole	5 mg/kg trimethoprim
Vancomycin	0.5 g if using polysulfone dialysis membrane; otherwise no supplement

because the clearance of many drugs by dialysis actually makes management easier.

Volume of distribution can change in renal failure due to fluid overload or hypoproteinemia. Antimicrobials known to have an increased volume of distribution in renal failure are aminoglycosides, azlocillin, cefazolin, cefoxitin, cefuroxime, cloxacillin and dicloxacillin, erythromycin, trimethoprim, and vancomycin. Few antimicrobials have a decreased volume of distribution in renal failure, but chloramphenicol and methicillin are notable examples.

Renal failure may affect hepatic as well as renal drug metabolic pathways. Drugs whose hepatic metabolism is likely to be disrupted in renal failure include aztreonam, cefmetazole, cefonicid, cefotaxime, ceftizoxime, erythromycin, and imipenem/cilastatin. Some potential for disruption exists for cefamandole and cefoperazone.

Factors influencing drug clearance by hemofiltration include molecular size, aqueous solubility, plasma protein binding, equilibration kinetics between plasma and tissue, and the apparent volume of distribution. Generally, drugs that have a molecular weight greater than 500 daltons are less efficiently dialyzed by standard dialysis membranes. However, the new high-flux polysulfone membranes can clear efficiently molecules up to 5 kD (the molecular weight of vancomycin is 1.486 kD) (Table 4).

Cefaclor, cefoperazone, ceftriaxone, chloramphenicol, clindamycin, cloxacillin and dicloxacillin, doxycycline, erythromycin, linezolid, methicillin/nafcillin/oxacillin, metronidazole, rifampin, and tigecycline do not require dosage reductions in renal failure. Many penicillins and cephalosporins require a dosage reduction only when severe renal insufficiency (variously defined as a creatinine clearance <30–50 ml/min) exists (Table 5). Tetracyclines other than doxycycline and tigecycline are contraindicated in renal failure.

When adjusting therapy in renal failure, the dose can be reduced or the interval between doses can be prolonged. The initial dose should be the same regardless, in order to obtain adequate peak serum concentrations. It is preferred to maintain the dose and prolong the interval with aminoglycosides because of the importance of maintaining a high peak concentration. However, it makes sense to reduce dose but maintain the

Table 5: Dosage Reductions for Selected Antimicrobials in Renal Insufficiency

Drug (Usual Dose)	Dose for CCr 10–50 ml/min	Dose for CCr <10 ml/min	Dialyzed?
Aminoglycosides	Individualize	Individualize	Yes
Ampicillin (1–2 g g4hr)	0.5–1 g q6hr	0.5–1 g q12hr	Yes
Aztreonam (1 g q8hr)	0.5 g q8hr	0.5 g q12hr	HD only
Cefamandole (1–2 g q6hr)	1–2 g q8–12hr	1–2 g q8–24hr	HD/CAVHD
Cefazolin (1 g q8hr)	1 g q12–24hr	1 g q48hr	HD only
Cefepime (2 g q12hr)	1 g q12hr	1 g q24hr	Yes
Cefotaxime (1 g q 6hr)	1 g q8–12hr	1 g q24hr	HD only
Cefotetan (1 g q12hr)	1 g q24hr	0.5–1g q24hr	No
Cefoxitin (1–2 g q6hr)	1–2 g q8–12hr	1–2 g q24hr	HD/CAVHD
Ceftazidime (1 g q8hr)	1 g q24hr	1 g q48hr	Yes
Ceftizoxime (1 g q8hr)	1 g q12–24hr	1 g q48hr	HD only
Ciprofloxacin (0.4 g q8–12hr)	0.4 g q8hr	0.4 g q16hr	No

Drug (Usual Dose)	Dose for CCr 10–50 ml/min	Dose for CCr <10 ml/min	Dialyzed?
Imipenem/ cilastatin (0.5 g q6hr)	0.25–0.5 g q6–8hr	0.25–0.5 g q12hr	HD only
Levofloxacin (0.5–0.75 g q12hr)	0.5g q24hr	0.5 g q248hr	CAVHD only
Piperacillin (2–4 g q4hr)	2–4 g q6hr	2–3 g q8hr	HD/CAVHD
Vancomycin (1 g q12hr)	Individualize	Individualize	High–flux HD only

Notes: Formula for estimation of creatinine clearance [C_{Cr}]: [140 – age $\times$ (1.00 [male] or 0.85 [female]) $\times$ weight (kg). C_{Cr} (ml/min) = serum Cr concentration (mg/dl) $\times$ 72,
CAVHD, Continuous arteriovenous or venovenous hemodialysis; *HD,* hemodialysis; *PD,* peritoneal dialysis.

interval when administering β-lactam drugs (especially those with no PAE) in order to maintain a constant drug concentration. The need to dose patients during or after a renal replacement therapy treatment must be borne in mind. During continuous renal replacement therapy, the estimated creatinine clearance is 15 ml/minute in addition to the patient's intrinsic clearance.

SUGGESTED READINGS

American Thoracic Society: Guidelines for the management of adults with hospital-acquired, ventilator-associated, and healthcare-associated pneumonia. *Am J Respir Crit Care Med* 171:388–416, 2005.

Anstead GM, Owens AD: Recent advances in the treatment of infections due to resistant *Staphylococcus aureus. Curr Opin Infect Dis* 17:549–555.

Bartlett JG, Perl TM: The new *Clostridium difficile*—what does it mean? *N Engl J Med* 343:2503–2505, 2005.

Benko AS, Cappelletty DM, Kruse JA, et al: Continuous infusion versus intermittent administration of ceftazidime in critically ill patients with suspected Gram-negative infections. *Antimicrob Agents Chemother* 40:691–695, 1996.

Bosso JA: The antimicrobial armamentarium: evaluating current and future treatment options. *Pharmacotherapy* 25:55S–62S, 2005.

Carlet J, Ben Ali A, Chalfine A: Epidemiology and control of antibiotic resistance in the intensive care unit. *Curr Opin Infect Dis* 17:309–316, 2004.

Chastre J, Wolff M, Fagon JY, et al: Comparison of 15 vs. 8 days of antibiotic therapy for ventilator-associated pneumonia in adults: a randomized trial. *JAMA* 290:2588–2598, 2003.

Clark NM, Hershberger E, Zervosc MJ, et al: Antimicrobial resistance among Gram-positive organisms in the intensive care unit. *Curr Opin Crit Care* 9:403–412, 2003.

Dellinger EP: Duration of antibiotic treatment in surgical infections of the abdomen. Undesired effects of antibiotics and future studies. *Eur J Surg* 576(Suppl):29–31, 1996.

DiPiro JT, Edmiston CE, Bohnen JMA: Pharmacodynamics of antimicrobial therapy in surgery. *Am J Surg* 171:615–622, 1996.

Evans RS, Pestotnik SL, Classen DC, et al: A computer-assisted management program for antibiotics and other antiinfective agents. *N Engl J Med* 338:232–238, 1998.

Fry DE: The importance of antibiotic pharmacokinetics in critical illness. *Am J Surg* 172(Suppl):20S–25S, 1996.

Garnacho-Montero J, Garcia-Garmendia JL, Barrero-Almodovar A, et al: Impact of adequate empirical antibiotic therapy on the outcome of patients admitted to the intensive care unit with sepsis. *Crit Care Med* 31:2742–2751, 2003.

Gold HS, Moellering RC: Antimicrobial drug resistance. *N Engl J Med* 335:1445–1453, 1996.

Harbarth S, Ferriere K, Hugonnet S, et al: Epidemiology and prognostic determinants of bloodstream infections in surgical intensive care. *Arch Surg* 137:1353–1359, 2002.

Jones RN: Microbiological features of vancomycin in the 21st century: minimum inhibitory concentration creep, bactericidal/static activity, and applied breakpoints to predict clinical outcomes or detect resistant strains. *Clin Infect Dis* 42:S13–S24, 2005.

Kollef MH, Micek ST: Strategies to prevent antimicrobial resistance in the intensive care unit. *Crit Care Med* 33:1845–1853, 2005.

LeDell K, Muto CA, Jarvis WR, et al: SHEA guideline for preventing nosocomial transmission of multidrug-resistant strains of *Staphylococcus aureus* and *Enterococcus. Infect Control Hosp Epidemiol* 24:639–641, 2003.

Livermore DM: Bacterial resistance: origins, epidemiology, and impact. *Clin Infect Dis* 36:S11–S23, 2003.

Loo V, Poirier L, Miller MA, et al: A predominantly clonal multi-institutional outbreak of *Clostridium difficile*–associated diarrhea with high morbidity and mortality. *N Engl J Med* 353:2442–2449.

McDonald LC, Kilgore GE, Thompson A, et al: An epidemic, toxin gene-variant strain of Clostridium difficile. *N Engl J Med* 353:2433–2441, 2005.

Naiemi NA, Duim B, Savelkoul PH, et al: Widespread transfer of resistance genes between bacterial species in an intensive care unit: implications for hospital epidemiology. *J Clin Microbiol* 43:4862–4864, 2005.

Naimi TS, LeDell KH, Como-Sabetti K, et al: Comparison of community- and health care-associated methicillin-resistant *Staphylococcus aureus* infection. *JAMA* 290:2976–2984, 2004.

Neuhauser MM, Weinstein RA, Rydman R, et al: Antibiotic resistance among Gram-negative bacilli in US intensive care units: implications for fluoroquinolone use. *JAMA* 289:885–888, 2003.

Nseir S, Di Pompeo C, Soubrier S, et al: First-generation fluoroquinolone use and subsequent emergence of multiple drug-resistant bacteria in the intensive care unit. *Crit Care Med* 33(2):283–289, 2005.

Padmanabhan RA, Larosa SP, Tomecki KJ: What's new in antibiotics? *Dermatol Clin* 23:301–312, 2005.

Paul M, Benuri-Silbiger I, Soares-Weiser K, et al: Beta-lactam monotherapy versus beta-lactam-aminoglycoside combination therapy for sepsis in immunocompetent patients: systematic review and meta-analysis of randomized trials. *BMJ* 328:(7441):668, 2004.

Rello J, Ollendorf DA, Oster G, et al: Epidemiology and outcomes of ventilator-associated pneumonia in a large US database. *Chest* 122:2115–2121, 2002.

Raymond DP, Pelletier SJ, Crabtree TD, et al: Impact of a rotating empiric antibiotic schedule on infectious mortality in an intensive care unit. *Crit Care Med* 29:1101–1108, 2001.

Schentag JJ, Gilliland KK, Paladino JA: What have we learned from pharmacokinetic and pharmacodynamic theories? *Clin Infect Dis* 32:S39–S46, 2001.

Schlaes DM, Gerding DN, John JF Jr, et al: Society for Healthcare Epidemiology of America and Infectious Diseases Society of America Joint Committee on the Prevention of Antimicrobial Resistance: guidelines for the prevention of antimicrobial resistance in hospitals. *Clin Infect Dis* 25:584–599, 1997.

Sehulster L, Chinn RY, et al: Guidelines for environmental infection control in health-care facilities. Recommendations of CDC and the Healthcare Infection Control Practices Advisory Committee (HICPAC). *MMWR Recomm Rep* 6:1–42, 2003.

Shorr AF, Sherner JH, Jackson WL, et al: Invasive approaches to the diagnosis of ventilator-associated pneumonia: a meta-analysis. *Crit Care Med* 33:46–53, 2005.

Trouillet JL, Chastre J, Vuagnat A, et al: Ventilator-associated pneumonia caused by potentially drug-resistant bacteria. *Am J Respir Crit Care Med* 157:531–539, 1998.

Viviani M, Silvestri L, van Saene HK, et al: Surviving Sepsis Campaign Guidelines: selective decontamination of the digestive tract still neglected. *Crit Care Med* 33:462–463, 2005.

FUNGAL INFECTIONS AND ANTIFUNGAL THERAPY IN THE SURGICAL INTENSIVE CARE UNIT

Marc J. Shapiro, Eduardo Smith-Singares,
Soumitra R. Eachempati, and Philip S. Barie

The first clinical description of *Candida* infection can be traced to Hippocrates, with Parrot recognizing a link to severe illness. Langenbeck implicated fungus as a source of infection, and Berg established causality between this organism and thrush by inoculating healthy babies with aphthous "membrane material." The first description of a deep infection caused by *Candida albicans* was made by Zenker in 1861, even though it was not named until 1923 by Berkout. On the other hand, the genus *Aspergillus* was first described in 1729 by Michaeli, and the first human cases of aspergillosis were described in the mid-1800s.

Invasive mycoses have emerged as a major cause of morbidity and mortality in hospitalized surgical patients. It is estimated that the incidence of nosocomial candidemia in the United States is about 8 per 100,000 inhabitants. Excess attributable health care costs are approximately $1 billion per year. Average medical costs per episode of candidemia have been estimated at $34,123 for Medicare patients and $44,536 for privately insured patients. In the United States, *Candida* is the fourth most common cause of catheter-related infection. A recent prospective, observational study reported the incidence of fungemia in the surgical intensive care unit (SICU) to be nearly 10 cases per 1000 admissions with an unadjusted mortality rate of 25%–50%.

Fungemia is the fourth most common type of bloodstream infection in the United States. Outside the United States, several studies have reported a rise in candidemia and other forms of *Candida* infections. In Canada, there has been an increase in the number of *Candida* isolates since 1991, where currently it constitutes 6% of all blood isolates. In general, the rates reported from European hospitals are slightly less than those from North America. In a meta-analysis of randomized, placebo-controlled trials with fluconazole prophylaxis, the incidence of fungal infections was significantly reduced; however, there was no survival advantage, raising the issue of the value of prophylaxis.

With the introduction of antibiotics and the subsequent appearance of intensive care units (ICUs), new examples of opportunistic fungal infections have emerged. The use of immunosuppression, organ transplantation, implantable devices, and human immunodeficiency virus infection has also radically changed the spectrum of fungal pathogenicity.

Fungi are ubiquitous heterotrophic eukaryotes, quite resilient to environmental stress and able to thrive in numerous environments. They may belong to the *Chromista* or *Eumycota* kingdom.[1] For identification purposes, the separation of taxa is based on the method of spore production, assisted by molecular biology techniques (rRNA and rDNA) that further refine fungal phylogeny and establish new relationships between groups. The most important human pathogens are the yeasts and the molds (from the Norse *mowlde*, meaning fuzzy). The dual modality of fungal propagation (sexual/teleomorph and asexual/anamorph states) has meant that since the last century there has been a dual nomenclature.

PREDICTORS OF FUNGAL INFECTIONS

The National Nosocomial Infection Surveillance program (NNIS) of the U.S. Centers for Disease Control and Prevention (CDC) has reported that whereas the rate of hospital-acquired fungal infections nearly doubled in the past decade compared with the previous decade, the greatest increase occurred in critically ill surgical patients, making the surgical population in the ICU an extremely high risk group.[2] Several conditions (both patient-dependent and disease-specific) have been recognized as independent predictors for invasive fungal complications during critical illness. ICU length of stay was associated with *Candida* infection as were the degrees of morbidity, alterations of immune response, and the number of medical devices involved. Neutropenia, diabetes mellitus, new-onset hemodialysis, total parenteral nutrition, broad-spectrum antibiotic administration, bladder catheterization, azotemia, diarrhea, use of corticosteroids, and cytotoxic drug utilization are also associated with candidemia.[2–5]

Diabetes Mellitus

Diabetes mellitus is an independent predictor for mucosal candidiasis, invasive candidiasis, and aspergillosis. Diabetic ketoacidosis has a strong association with rhinocerebral mucor (produced by *Zygomycetes*) and other atypical fungal infections, with hyperglycemia being the strongest predictor of candidemia after liver transplantation and cardiac bypass. It has been postulated that hyperglycemia produces several alterations in the normal host response to infection and in the fungus itself, increasing its virulence. Glycosylation of cell surface receptors facilitates fungal binding and subsequent internalization and apoptosis of the targeted cells. Glycosylation of opsonins renders them unable to recognize fungal antigens. Diabetic serum has diminished capacity to bind iron (therefore making it available to the pathogen). There is evidence that altered Th-1 lymphocyte recognition of fungal targets impairs the production of interferon-gamma (IFN-γ), and that *Candida* spp. overexpress a C_3-receptor–like protein that facilitates fungal adhesion to endothelium and mucosal surfaces. Dendritic cells and other antigen-presenting cells have been postulated as crucial in the induction of cell-mediated responses to fungi, and diabetic patient vaccination studies have showed an impaired antigen—T-cell interaction.

Neutropenia

There is a direct correlation between the degree of neutropenia and the risk for developing invasive fungal infections. Although a recent meta-analysis concluded that there is little benefit from prophylaxis or preemptive treatment in neutropenic cancer patients, this is a regular practice in the United States. Empirical antifungal therapy is the standard of care for febrile neutropenia patients after chemotherapy or bone marrow transplantation. When profound neutropenia exists, the risk for breakthrough candidemia (during antifungal therapy) is significantly higher, and the response to voriconazole (and likely other antifungals) is decreased. Novel therapies for the treatment of invasive fungal infections in neutropenic patients include granulocyte transfusions and infusion of IFN-γ.

Organ Transplantation and Immunosuppression

The two most common opportunistic fungal infections in transplant patients are caused by *Candida* spp. and *Aspergillus* spp., generally by the inhalation route *(Aspergillus)* or from gastrointestinal sources *(Candida)*. Interestingly, the risk of fungal infection decreases six months after transplantation, unless a rejection episode requires intensification of the immunosuppression. In the solid organ transplant recipient, the graft itself is often affected. In liver transplantation, the risk of fungemia increases with the duration of the surgery and the number of transfusions. Other risk factors include the type of bile duct anastomosis (Roux-en-Y), the presence of tissue ischemia, infection with cytomegalovirus (CMV), and graft-versus-host disease. The most common place of occurrence for *Aspergillus* tracheobronchitis in lung transplant patients is at the bronchial anastomosis. Anastomotic colonization is both a risk factor for subsequent disruption or hemorrhage and a predictor for rejection and diminished graft survival. Surveillance bronchoscopies are recommended in this setting. *Aspergillus* is also the main organism responsible for fungemia after heart transplantation, and second only to CMV as the cause of pneumonia in the first month after operation.

Infectious complications are the main cause of morbidity and mortality in pancreas and kidney–pancreas transplantation. The most common organisms are gram-positive cocci, closely followed by gram-negative bacilli and *Candida*. Risk factors for fungal infections include bladder drainage (in cases of pancreas transplantation) and use of OKT-3 for rejection treatment. Kidney recipients, of all solid organ transplant recipients, have the lowest incidence of infectious complications. However, the risk is sufficiently high that all solid organ transplant recipients (kidney recipients included) receive fungal prophylaxis with fluconazole.

Solid and Hematological Malignant Tumors

Cancer patients are susceptible to opportunistic infections. Cancer and chemotherapy produce three types of immune dysfunction that render the patient vulnerable to opportunistic infections: neutropenia (see previously), deficits in lymphocyte cell-mediated immunity (e.g., Hodgkin disease and during corticosteroid treatment), and humoral immunodeficiency (e.g., multiple myeloma, Waldenström macroglobulinemia, and after splenectomy). The first two types are the most relevant in terms of fungal vulnerability. As many as one-third of the cases of febrile neutropenia after chemotherapy for malignant disease are due to invasive fungemia (see following treatment discussion). The type of lymphopenia is as important as the nadir of the lymphocyte count: Whereas Th-1 type responses (TNF-α, IFN-γ, and interleukin [IL]-12) confer protection against fungal infections, Th-2 (IL-4 and -10) responses are associated with progression of disease. Corticosteroids have anti-inflammatory properties, related to their inhibitory effects on the activation of various transcription factors, in particular NF-κB. In murine models, steroid treatment increases the production of IL-10 in response to a fungal insult, and decreased the recruitment of mononuclear cells to the site of infection. It does not, however, inhibit recruitment of neutrophils to sites of inflammation (IL-8-mediated).

Long-Term Use of Central Venous Catheters

Numerous studies have shown that many, if not most, episodes of candidemia are catheter-related; one of the largest prospective treatment studies of fungemia implicated a catheter 72% of the time. The isolation of *C. parapsilosis* from blood cultures is strongly associated with central venous catheter infection, parenteral nutrition, or prosthetic devices. The source of the fungal contaminants is different in neutropenic patients when compared with their non-neutropenic counterparts. In non-neutropenic

subjects the most common portals of entry for catheter contamination (and subsequent infection) is the skin during catheter placement, manipulation of an indwelling catheter, and cross-infection among ICU patients attributed to hand carriage of microbial flora from health care workers. Other possible sources for primary catheter colonization include contaminated parenteral nutrition solution, multiple medication administration with repetitive violation of the sterile fluid path, and the presence of other medical devices. The secondary route of contamination for intravascular catheters and other foreign bodies in direct contact with the bloodstream (e.g., pacemakers, cardiac valves, orthopedic joint prostheses) is candidemia originating via translocation from the gastrointestinal tract. Endogenous flora are also the most common source in neutropenic and other immunosuppressed patients. Once the catheter becomes contaminated, a well-studied series of events takes place: The yeast adheres to the surface of the catheter and develops hyphal forms that integrate into a matrix of polysaccharides and proteins (biofilm) that increases in size and tridimensional complexity. This biofilm is the main reservoir for candidemia secondary to contaminated medical devices, as it sequesters the fungi from antimycotic medication and against the protective immune response.

In general, the removal of all central venous catheters is indicated following the diagnosis of systemic fungal infections and fungemia. Removal may not be necessary in neutropenic patients in whom the fungi originated from the GI tract. Antifungals in general are continued after the catheter is removed, and it is recommended that *Candida* ocular dissemination be ruled out (see following discussion of endophthalmitis).

Candida Colonization

The overgrowth and recovery of *Candida* spp. from multiple sites (without clinical symptoms of disease) has been linked to a high likelihood of invasive candidiasis, and the cumulative risk of death in these two conditions is similar. Risk factors for the development of *Candida* colonization include prior use of antibiotics or a bacterial infection prior to ICU admission, a prolonged stay in the ICU, and multiple gastrointestinal operations. The source of most of the outbreaks of systemic candidiasis in the context of colonization is frequently the gastrointestinal tract.

Because colonization with *Candida* spp. is not benign in the context of critical illness, it is desirable to identify and characterize patients further in terms of risk for invasive candidiasis. Screening techniques include routine surveillance cultures in ICU patients. The method proposed by Pittet et al., the colonization index, has been validated in surgical patients. A threshold index of 0.5 has been proposed for the initiation of empiric antifungal therapy in critically ill patients (see following treatment section), although some authorities suggest that the presence of multiple *Candida* isolates is an epiphenomenon.[6]

Use of Broad-Spectrum Antibiotics

The use of broad-spectrum antibiotics is one of the best-documented risk factors for fungal overgrowth and invasive infections, but the precise mechanism is not understood completely. In evaluating the effect of antibiotic use, one must consider first the complex interrelations between bacteria and fungi in human disease. At least three experimental models have been created to investigate and characterize possible interactions between bacterial and fungal pathogens. In murine models, ticarcillin-clavulanic acid and ceftriaxone (both of which have some antianaerobic therapy) are associated with substantial increases in colony counts of yeast flora of the gut. On the other hand, antibiotics with poor anaerobic activity are less likely to produce this effect (examples are ceftazidime and aztreonam). This observation was validated in a clinical review of the quantitative colonization of stool in immunocompromised patients treated with those antibiotics. However, this interaction between fungi overgrowth and anaerobic suppression is different from the well-studied model of *Escherichia coli* and *Bacteroides fragilis* in intra-abdominal abscess formation. The work of Sawyer et al. showed that *C. albicans* induces bacterial translocation into abscesses, but the relationship is one of direct competency, rather than synergy or cooperation.[7,8] This is different than the cooperation between *C. albicans* and *Staphylococcus aureus*, *Serratia marcescens*, and *Enterococcus faecalis*, where an amplification-type interaction has been documented. A number of immunomodulatory and immunosuppressive viruses have been shown to facilitate superinfections with opportunistic fungi, the most notable examples being CMV and human herpes virus (HHV)-6, because they induce the production of immunosuppressive cytokines. It seems that *C. albicans* thrives in situations where immunocompromise is present and adds virulence and mortality to existent bacterial infections in a species-specific manner. This hypothesis has been validated from clinical observations, where antifungal treatment adds little to the therapeutic effect of antibacterial agents alone. Thus, the use of antibiotics (three or more), especially those with anti-anaerobic properties, constitute a risk factor for fungal colonization and overgrowth, which in turn is a predictor for systemic fungal infections. The precise mechanism of action for this observation is unknown but is probably related to fungi-to-microbe competence and growth suppression. *Candida* may enhance the pathogenicity of certain bacteria, but not others, and this interaction remains to be elucidated.[7]

Duration of ICU Care and Invasive Mechanical Ventilation

Epidemiological observations correlating the duration of mechanical ventilation and the amount of intensive care required correlate with the occurrence of both systemic fungal infections and fungal colonization. Other factors involved in the pathogenesis and susceptibility of systemic candidiasis are total parenteral nutrition, use of H_2 blockers, acquired immunodeficiency syndrome (AIDS), radiation therapy, previous bacteremia, abdominal surgery, hemodialysis, extremes of age, recurrent mucocutaneous candidiasis, and duration of cardiopulmonary bypass greater than 120 minutes.[2]

PATHOGENIC ORGANISMS

Candida albicans

The most common fungal pathogen both in the United States and abroad, and ranked among the most common sources of ICU sepsis, *C. albicans* is a common cause of human disease.[9] *Candida albicans* accounts for 59% of *Candida* isolates, followed by *C. glabrata* (15%–25% of all *Candida* infections). Both colonization and invasive candidiasis can be focal or disseminated. Multifocal candidiasis is the simultaneous isolation of *Candida* from two or more of the following locations: respiratory, digestive, urinary, wounds, or drainage. Disseminated candidiasis is microbiological evidence of yeast in fluids from normally sterile sites such as cerebrospinal, pleural, pericardial, or peritoneal fluid, histologic samples from deep organs, or diagnosis of endophthalmitis or candidemia with negative catheter-tip cultures. The incidence of candidemia has increased over the past 30 years, with mortality rates reported in some series to be as high as 80%. The NNIS system of the CDC found *Candida* species responsible for 8%–15% of all nosocomial bloodstream infection episodes in the United States in 1993, which ranked fourth among commonly isolated pathogens in bloodstream infections.

It is well established that a morphological transition in *C. albicans*, from yeast to hyphal forms, is the most important determinant of dissemination, because the mycelial phase is invasive.[10] Both host and pathogen play a role on this dimorphism. The fungus produces several proteins during the hyphal transition, which are currently the focus of research. The thiol-specific antioxidant, or TSA-1, has shown an increased survival capability in an antioxidant environment created by host cells. Host recognition molecules (adhesins), secreted aspartyl proteases and phospholipases, and phenotypic switching accompanied by changes in antigen expression, colony morphology, and tissue affinities are other recognized virulence factors. The inducer mechanisms and the multiple stimuli that trigger this change are unknown.

From the host side, the presence of the enzyme indoleamine 2,3-dioxygenase (IDO) has been linked to antifungal defense mechanisms, by blocking the morphological transition. The enzyme is induced in infectious sites and in dendritic cells by IFN-γ. Interferon serves in a pivotal position in immunity from *C. albicans* invasion. Other immune mechanisms blocking the transformation include salivary histidine, other gastrointestinal inhibitory peptides, and the resident population of dendritic cells. The dimorphic change produces disseminated candidiasis (also known as hepatosplenic candidiasis) and specific end-organ involvement in susceptible hosts. Of those metastatic infections, among the most devastating is fungal endophthalmitis.

Disseminated candidiasis and fungemia can lead to septic shock, similar to that seen with other microorganisms. The dimorphic transition generates shock and end-organ failure in susceptible individuals, and these events are independent of TNF-α. The diagnosis of fungemia as the cause of a patient's sepsis depends on a strong clinical suspicion. Only 50% of blood cultures for invasive candidiasis are positive and bacterial pathogens may interfere with the recovery of *Candida*. There are no reliable laboratory tests to differentiate between *Candida* colonization and invasive candidiasis, and no single site of isolation is superior to others in predicting which patients are likely to have developed systemic infection. The diagnostic criteria for fungemia are a combination of positive tissue cultures (including burn excision cultures and peritoneal cultures), endophthalmitis, osteomyelitis, and candiduria. Purpura fulminans and unexplained myalgias are suggestive of candidiasis in the appropriate clinical context. The presence of three or more colonized sites or two positive blood cultures at least 24 hours apart, with one obtained after the removal of any central venous catheters are strong indicators of fungemia.[10] Whereas asymptomatic recovery of *Candida* in urine rarely requires therapy, candiduria should be treated in symptomatic patients, neutropenic patients, renal transplant patients, and after instrumentation. The removal or at least changing of the Foley catheter is required.

Fungal endophthalmitis usually occurs as a result of hematogenous spread from systemic fungemia. *Candida* spp. are the most common offenders, although *Aspergillus*, *Cryptococcus*, *Fusarium*, *Scedosporium*, and others have been reported to lead to endophthalmitis. Retinal involvement has been diagnosed in 28%–45% of all known candidemic patients, and may actually be the first sign of clinically undetected fungemia. The early initiation of systemic treatment for deep tissue fungal infection appears to decrease dramatically the incidence of endogenous fungal endophthalmitis. It is mandatory for all individuals with systemic candidiasis and fungemia to have a formal ophthalmologic assessment to rule out eye involvement. The observation of a classic three-dimensional retina-based vitreal inflammatory process is virtually diagnostic of endogenous endophthalmitis due to *Candida* spp.

Treatment consists of aggressive intravenous antifungal therapy, and may require intraocular injections of amphotericin B, caspofungin, or voriconazole. In cases where extension to the vitreous or pars anterior are evident, surgical debridement or vitrectomy will be required. Delay in treatment leads frequently to blindness.

Non–albicans Candida

The incidence of non-*Candida* fungemia and sepsis syndrome has been increasing in recent years, accounting for up to one-half of non–*albicans Candida* adult ICU infections. The reasons for this are likely multifactorial. Undoubtedly, one explanation for the emergence of *C. glabrata* and *C. krusei* is the selection of less-susceptible species by the pressure of antifungal agents.[11] Other species of yeast are related to specific events, such as the presence of an indwelling central venous catheter and *C. parapsilosis*. The increased incidence of *C. tropicalis* in oncology patients is secondary to the increased invasiveness of the organism, especially in damaged gastrointestinal mucosa. The clinical features of this infection are indistinguishable from *C. albicans*.

Aspergillus

The noninvasive types of aspergillosis include allergic bronchopulmonary aspergillosis (a form of hypersensitivity reaction in asthmatics) and aspergilloma. These entities, without tissue invasion, usually do not require antifungal therapy. Invasive aspergillosis has experienced an increased incidence over the last decade, and has become a major cause of death among patients with liquid tumors. Although invasive *Aspergillus* infections usually occur via inhalation of conidia, the fungus is also frequently present on food (i.e., pepper, regular and herbal tea bags, fruits, corn, and rice). The thermotolerant spores of *Aspergillus* and other fungi present are difficult to eradicate, and represent a threat to the immunocompromised host. Conidia that fail to be cleared by alveolar macrophages germinate in the alveolar space, and hyphal forms invade the pulmonary parenchyma, with prominent vascular invasion and early dissemination (Figures 1 through 3).[12]

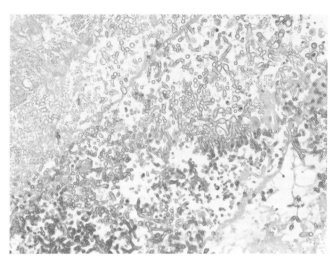

Figure 2 Microphotograph of invasive *Aspergillus* infection in the lungs of the patient in Figure 1. *(Courtesy Minick CR, Loyd E, Amin B: Department of Pathology and Laboratory Medicine, NewYork-Presbyterian Hospital-Weill Cornell Medical College.)*

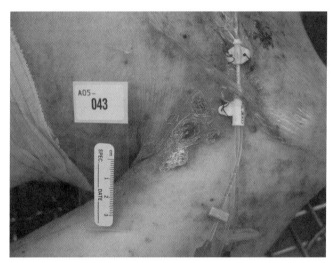

Figure 3 Purpura fulminans in a victim of hepatosplenic candidiasis. *(Courtesy Minick CR, Loyd E, Amin B: Department of Pathology and Laboratory Medicine, NewYork-Presbyterian Hospital-Weill Cornell Medical College.)*

Other Emerging Fungal Pathogens

Zygomycetes (mucor) are becoming increasingly important in ICU patients. The portal of entry in the immunocompromised host is usually inhalation of aerosolized, thermotolerant spores, although percutaneous exposure (i.e., surgical or traumatic wounds and burns) has been reported. The source of these spores is usually decaying organic matter in the soil, but they can be found in hospital food, including fruit, bread, sweet biscuits, regular and herbal tea, and pepper. The major risk factors for mucormycosis are diabetic ketoacidosis, neutropenia, iron overload, deferoxamine therapy, and protein-calorie malnutrition. Treatment includes surgical debridement, depending on the extent of the disease.

PRINCIPLES OF THERAPY

The past 10 years has seen a major expansion in the repertoire of antifungal agents with the introduction of less-toxic formulations of amphotericin B, improved triazoles, echinocandins, and other agents that

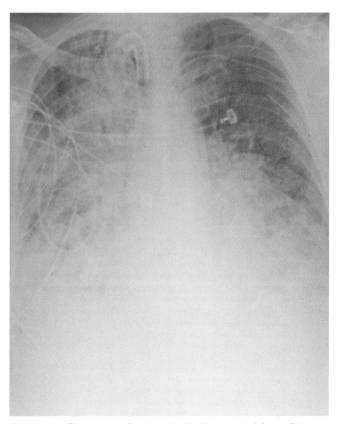

Figure 1 Chest x-ray of a patient with disseminated *Aspergillus* infection and pneumonia. The image is identical to that of acute respiratory distress syndrome. *(Courtesy of Smith-Singares E, Barie PS, Eachempati SR: The Anne and Max A. Cohen Surgical Intensive Care Unit, New York-Presbyterian Hospital-Weill Cornell Medical College.)*

target the fungal cell wall. As described by Flanagan and Barnes, therapy for fungal infections in the ICU can be directed using four different strategies: prophylactic, preemptive, empiric, and definitive. Some data suggest a decrease in invasive fungal infections with prophylactic antifungal therapy in non-neutropenic critically ill surgical patients with *Candida* isolates from sites other than blood and the presence of risk factors mentioned previously. Others have suggested that use of antifungal prophylaxis in unselected SICU patients increases mortality, length of stay, and the appearance of resistance in previously susceptible fungi, not to mention the increase in cost this approach generates.[13] Prophylactic fluconazole treatment in the SICU leads to secondary mycoses, with up to 80% of the pathogens resistant to fluconazole.[14,15] Tables 1 and 2 and Figures 4 and 5 show one schema used in the SICU at NewYork-Presbyterian Hospital-Weill Cornell Medical Center. Independent of the species, infection by fluconazole-resistant *Candida* doubles the mortality rate. The colonization index developed by Pittet et al. and Ostrosky-Zeichner suggests that high-risk patients are those who remain in the ICU for 4 days or more and who either have a central venous catheter in place or are treated with antibiotics in addition to two of the following: use of total parenteral nutrition, need for dialysis, recent major surgery, diagnosis of pancreatitis, and treatment with systemic corticosteroids or other immunosuppressive agents.[15,16] Studies have documented the lack of benefit for fluconazole prophylaxis in unselected trauma patients, and in ICU patients, for whom the contribution of mortality by candidemia is surpassed by that of age and severity of illness.[17,18]

Table 3 presents a list of available antifungal agents. Amphotericin B is a natural polyene macrolide that binds primarily to ergosterol, the principal sterol in the fungal cell membrane, leading to disruption of ion channels, production of oxygen free radicals, and apoptosis. It is active against most fungi, including in cerebrospinal fluid. Due to its high level of protein binding, tissue concentrations are not usually affected by hemodialysis. Infusion-related reactions can occur in up to 73% of patients with the first dose and often diminish during continued therapy. Amphotericin B–associated nephrotoxicity can lead to azotemia and hypokalemia, although acute potassium release with rapid infusion can occur and lead to cardiac arrest. Amphotericin B lipid formulations allow for higher dose administration with lessened nephrotoxicity, but whether outcomes are enhanced is unproved. Nystatin is a polyene similar in structure to amphotericin B, and is currently used topically for *C. albicans*. A parenteral formulation is under investigation. Flucytosine is a fluorinated pyrimidine analog that is converted to 5-fluorouracil, which causes RNA miscoding and inhibits DNA synthesis. It is available in the United States in oral form only and has been used with amphotericin B for synergism against *Candida* spp.

The azoles inhibit the cytochrome P_{450}–dependent enzyme, 14-alpha reductase, altering fungal cell membranes through accumulation of abnormal 14-alphamethyl sterols. Ketoconazole comes only in tablet form and is indicated for candidiasis and candiduria. Fluconazole and itraconazole are available in oral and parenteral formulations and are active against *Candida* spp. except *C. krusei*, and *Fusarium* spp. Itraconazole is active against *Aspergillus* spp. As mentioned previously, *C. glabrata* and *C. krusei* resistance has been seen with fluconazole. The tissue concentration of both drugs is influenced by many agents such as antacids, H_2-antagonists, isoniazid, phenytoin, and phenobarbitol.

Table 1: Usual Susceptibilities of *Candida* **Species to Selected Antifungal Agents**

Candida spp.	Fluconazole	Itraconazole	Voriconazole (not standardized)	Amphotericin B	Caspofungin (not standardized)
C. albicans	S	S	S	S	S
C. tropicalis	S	S	S	S	S
C. parapsilosis	S	S	S	S	S to I (?R)
C. glabrata	S-DD to R	S-DD to R	S to I	S to I	S
C. krusei	R	S-DD to R	S to I	S to I	S
C. lusitaniae	S	S	S	S to R	S

I, Intermediate; *R*, resistant; *S*, susceptible; *S-DD*, susceptible-dose dependent (increased MIC may be overcome by higher dosing, such as 12 mg/kg/day fluconazole).

Modified from Pappas PG, Rex JH, Sobel JD, Filler SG, Dismukes WE, Walsh TJ, Edwards JE: Guidelines for treatment of candidiasis. *Clin Infect Dis* 38(2): 161–189, 2004.

Table 2: Approximate Antifungal Daily Costs, 2005

Antifungal	Approximate Cost/Dose	Usual Adult Dose	Approximate Cost/Day
Fluconazole 400 mg IV	$30	400 mg IV daily	$30
Fluconazole 400 mg PO	$1	400 mg PO daily	$1
Itraconazole 200 mg PO solution	$17	200 mg PO twice daily	$34
Voriconazole 400 mg IV	$195	400 mg IV twice daily (load)	$390
Voriconazole 280 mg IV	$136	280 mg IV twice daily (maintenance)	$272
Caspofungin 70 mg IV	$440	70 mg IV daily (load)	$440
Caspofungin 50 mg IV	$345	50 mg IV daily (maintenance)	$345
Amphotericin B conventional 70 mg IV	$26	70 mg IV daily	$26
Amphotericin B lipid (Abelcet®)	$292	350 mg IV daily	$292

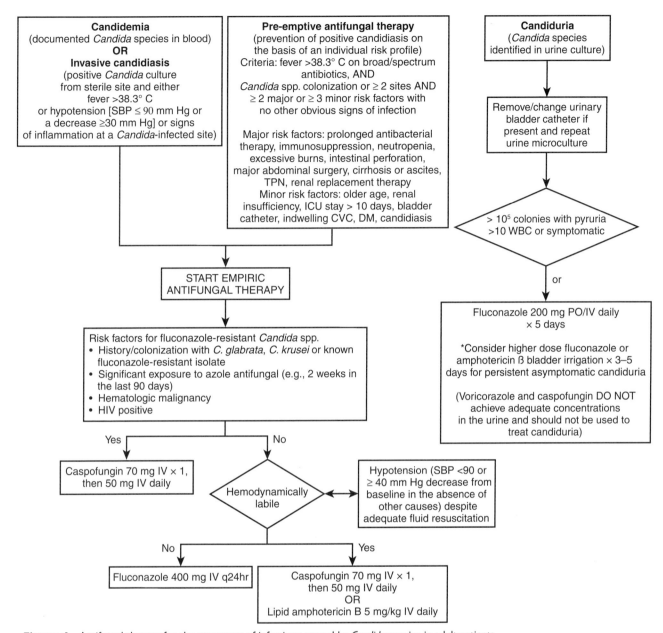

Figure 4 Antifungal therapy for the treatment of infections caused by *Candida* species in adult patients.

Second-generation antifungal triazoles include posaconazole, ravuconazole, and voriconazole. They are active against *Candida* spp., including fluconazole-resistant strains, and *Aspergillus* spp. For the latter, voriconazole is emerging as the treatment of choice.[19,20]

The echinocandins include caspofungin, micafungin, and anidulafungin, each of which is approved therapy for candidiasis and candidemia, but third-line treatment for invasive aspergillosis. Due to their distinct mechanism of action, disrupting the fungal cell wall by inhibiting β(1,3)-D-glucan synthesis, the echinocandins can theoretically be used in combination with other standard antifungal agents. The echinocandins have activity against *Candida* spp. and *Aspergillus* spp., but are not reliably active against other fungi. Echinocandin activity is excellent against most *Candida* spp., but moderate against *C. parapsilosis, C. guillermondi,* and *C. lusitaniae*. Echinocandins exhibit no cross-resistance with azoles or polyenes.[21]

Invasive fungal infections in non-neutropenic ICU patients are treated if histology or cytopathology show yeast cells or pseudohyphae from a needle aspiration or biopsy (excluding mucous membranes), a positive culture obtained aseptically from a normally sterile and clinically or radiologically abnormal site consistent with infection (excluding urine, sinuses, and mucous membranes), or positive percutaneous blood culture in patients with temporally related clinical signs and symptoms compatible with the relevant organism.

Neutropenic Patients and Preemptive Therapy

A novel approach in the use of antifungal therapy in patients who do not exhibit clinical evidence of systemic candidiasis is the concept of preemptive therapy.[16] Being more than just semantics, prophylaxis is defined as treatment triggered by risk stratification (thus directed at patients with "possible" fungal infection), whereas preemptive therapy is the early treatment of identified infection, without clinical signs, detected by the use of surrogate markers or

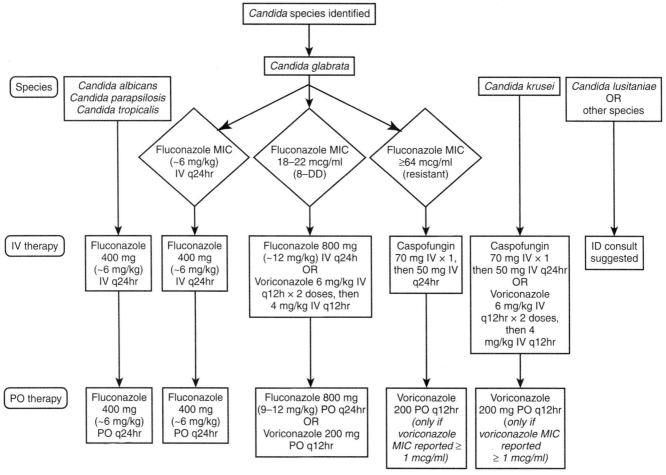

Figure 5 Treatment algorithm when *Candida* spp. are identified.

non–culture-based methods. The appeal of preemptive therapy (for patients with "probable" fungal infection) is that it theoretically combines the best of the evidence for fungal prophylaxis with the benefits of early treatment, mitigating against the increase in fungal resistance and recovery of resistant strains. Given that there is little evidence that prophylactic use of fluconazole confers benefit in the management of nonfebrile neutropenic patients, the development of new protocols using frequent surveillance and screening (instead of therapy) for patients at high risk is imperative.

Antifungal Prophylaxis in Solid Organ Transplant Recipients

Invasive fungal infections remain a frequent complication among the recipients of solid organs. The risk is greater during the early post-transplant period, decreasing after six months from the date of the operation. Liver transplantation carries the highest risk, followed by heart and lung. Other risk factors have been identified, including hepatic and renal dysfunction, retransplantation, rejection, surgical complications, and CMV infections. Fluconazole is effective for prevention of invasive fungal infections, but without any reduction in mortality. In liver transplant patients, the number necessary to treat (NNT) in order to prevent one infection is 14, given an incidence of 10%. Meta-analysis also concluded that, for lower-risk recipients (i.e., renal homograft recipients), the NNT increases to 28. Prophylaxis should be reserved for those patients with a higher stratified risk and in settings where fungal complica-

tions are highly prevalent. For those immunosuppressed patients who have developed a noncandidal systemic fungal infection, prolonged suppressive antifungal therapy may be required to prevent a relapse.

Acquired Immunodeficiency Syndrome and Empiric Antifungal Therapy

The incidence of invasive candidiasis is low in the acquired immunodeficiency syndrome (AIDS), which is surprising considering the almost ubiquitous presence of mucocutaneous candidiasis in HIV-infected patients. This underscores that the host defense mechanisms required for resistance against mucocutaneous and invasive candidiasis are different. Therefore, patients who develop AIDS and associated *Candida* infections frequently have additional risk factors, such as parenteral nutrition catheters, broad-spectrum antibiotics, or neutropenia due to HIV-related lymphoma or cytotoxic therapy. The use of empiric fluconazole for these patients is not cost effective, and should be discouraged.

Therapy Tailored to Specific Risk Factors and Likely Offending Organisms

The New York–Presbyterian Hospital, Weill Cornell Medical Center has developed algorithms and guidelines for the use of antifungal agents (see Tables 1 and 2, Figures 4 and 5) based on epidemiological considerations. Table 3 lists the antifungal agents most

Table 3: Antifungal Agents

Antifungal Agent	Indications	Routes/Dosage
Amphotericin B	*Candida albicans* (>95%) *C. glabrata* (95%), *C. parapsilosis* (>95%) *C. krusei* (>95%), *C. tropicalis* (99%) *C. guillermondi*; *C. lusitaniae* Variable activity: *Aspergillus* spp., ferrous *Trichosporon beigelii* *Fusarium* spp., *Blastomyces dermatidis*	IV: 0.5 mg/kg/day over 2–4 hours Oral: 1 ml oral suspension, swish and swallow 4× daily, times 2 weeks
Amphotericin B liposomal (less nephrotoxicity)	*C. albicans* (>95%), *C. glabrata* (>95%) *C. parapsilosis* (>95%), *C. krusei* (>95%) *C. tropicalis* (99%), *C. guillermondi*, *C. lusitaniae* Variable activity: *Aspergillus*	IV: 3–5 mg/kg/day
Amphotericin B colloidal dispersion (more infusional)	*C. albicans* (>95%), *C. glabrata* (>95%) *C. parapsilosis* (>95%), *C. krusei* (>95%) *C. tropicalis* (99%), *C. guillermondi*; *C. lusitaniae* Variable activity: *Aspergillus*	IV: 3–4 mg/kg/day
Amphotericin B Lipid Complex	*C. albicans* (>95%), *C. glabrata* (>95%) *C. parapsilosis* (>95%), *C. krusei* (>95%) *C. tropicalis* (99%), *C. guillermondi*, *C. lusitaniae* Variable activity: *Aspergillus*	IV: 5 mg/kg/day
Ketoconazole	*C. albicans*	PO: 200–400 mg/daily
Voriconazole	*Aspergillus*, *Fusarium* spp., *C. albicans* (99%) *C. glabrata* (99%), *C. parapsilosis* (99%) *C. tropicalis* (99%), *C. krusei* (99%), *C. guillermondi* (>95%) *C. lusitaniae* (95%)	IV: 6 mg/kg Q12 ×2, then 4 mg/kg IV every 12 hours PO: >40 kg, 200 mg every 12 hours <40 kg, 100 mg every 12 hours
Fluconazole	*C. albicans* (97%) *C. glabrata* (85%–90% resistant/intermediate) *C. parapsilosis* (99%) *C. tropicalis* (98%) *C. krusei* (5%) Fungistatic against *Aspergillus*	Candidiasis: Prophylaxis (IV or oral): 100–400 mg/day Invasive: 400–800 mg/day Oropharyngeal: 200 mg day 1, then 100 daily × 2 weeks
Itraconazole	Fungicidal to *Aspergillus*, *C. albicans* (93%) *C. glabrata* (50%), *C. parapsilosis* (45%), *C. tropicalis* (58%), *C. krusei* (69%), *C. guillermondi*, *C. lusitaniae* Blastomycoses, histoplasmosis, chromomycosis	IV: Load 200 mg IV 2× daily × 4 doses, then 200 mg 4× daily maximum 14 days Oral: 200 mg every daily or 2× daily Life-threatening: load 600–800/day × 3–5/days then 400–600 mg/day
Caspofungin	*C. albicans*, *C. glabrata*, *C. parapsilosis*, *C. tropicalis*, *C. krusei*, *C. guillermondi*, *C. lusitaniae*	IV: 70 mg IV, then 50 mg IV every day
Flucytosine	Not effective for *C. krusei* Effective for *C. albicans*, *C. tropicalis*, *C. parapsilosis*, *C. lusitaniae*	PO: 50–150 mg/kg/day divided QID
Nystatin	*C. albicans*	100,000 units swish and swallow QID
Clotrimazole	Thrush	Oral troches 5× daily × 14 days

commonly in use in the United States. Several studies have demonstrated that azole antifungals have immunosuppressive activity in that imidazoles interfere with neutrophil and lymphocyte function. Ketoconazole has been used to attempt to reduce the frequency of the acute respiratory distress syndrome in high-risk patients, possibly as a thromboxane synthase inhibitor. Itraconazole and miconazole are potent inhibitors of 5-lipoxygenase. Fluconazole, which has no effect on plasma thromboxane and leukotriene concentrations, has been shown in animals and in vitro to augment the bactericidal activity of neutrophils, suggesting a possible role in treating patients with sepsis.

Fungi as an Epiphenomenon

Recent advances in critical care have produced a selected population of very ill individuals that in previous years would have succumbed to their disease processes. Many of these improvements in survival have preceded (and in some cases paralleled) the explosive growth of fungal colonization and infection in ICU patients, and the availability of antifungal therapy. As antibiotic choice has become more complex and resistance has developed, so too has the complexity of fungal infections and the expanded multimodality therapy. Whereas there is little argument that invasive fungal infections are associated with increased mortality, morbidity, and length of stay (both in the ICU and hospital), the mortality attributable to these infections remains controversial. More problematic is the fact that, although antifungal prophylaxis is effective in preventing fungal colonization and invasive infections, this does not translate into a difference in mortality. Data on length of stay are also contradictory, with staunch supporters for both sides of the debate. Localized fungal infections and colonization have different natural histories depending on the severity of illness, but they remain predictors of invasive infection in very ill patients as defined by higher APACHE scores.

SUMMARY

Fungal infections are increasingly prevalent among ICU patients. The most common offending fungi are *C. albicans*, other *Candida* spp., and *Aspergillus* spp. Therapy should be directed toward patients' specific risk factors, but the use of antifungal prophylaxis is controversial. Empiric antifungal therapy is discouraged in non-neutropenic patients, as well as the treatment of isolated positive non-blood cultures.

REFERENCES

1. Guarro J, Gene J, Stchigel AM, et al: Developments in fungal taxonomy. *Clin Microbiol Rev* 12:454–500, 1999.
2. Vincent JL, Anaissie E, Bruining H et al: Epidemiology, diagnosis and treatment of systemic *Candida* infections in surgical patients under intensive care. *Intensive Care Med* 24:206–216, 1998.
3. Cornwell EE, Belzberg H, Berne TV, et al: The pattern of fungal infections in critically ill surgical patients. *Am Surg* 61:847–850, 1995.
4. Blumberg HM, Jarvis WR, Soucie JM, et al: Risk factors for candidal bloodstream infections in surgical intensive care unit patients: the NEMIS prospective multicenter study. *Clin Infect Dis* 33:177–186, 2001.
5. Paphitou NI, Ostrosky-Zeichner l, Rex JH: Rules for identifying patients at increased risk for candidal infections in the surgical intensive care unit: approach to developing practical criteria for systematic use in antifungal prophylaxis trials. *Med Mycol* 43:235–243, 2005.
6. Piarroux R, Grenouillet F, Balvay P, et al: Assessment of preemptive treatment to prevent severe candidiasis in critically ill surgical patients. *Crit Care Med* 32:2443–2449, 2004.
7. Holzheimer RG, Dralle H: Management of mycoses in surgical patients: review of the literature. *Eur J Med Res* 7:200–226, 2002.
8. Sawyer RG, Adams RB, May AK, et al: Development of candida albicans and C. albicans/escherichia coli/bacteroides fragilis intraperitoneal abscess models with demonstration of fungus-induced bacterial translocation. *J Med Vet Mycol* 33:49–52, 1995.
9. Lipsett PA: Clinical trials of antifungal prophylaxis among patients in surgical intensive care units: concepts and considerations. *Clin Infect Dis* 39:S193–S199, 2004.
10. Dean DA, Burchard KW: Surgical perspective on invasive *Candida* infections. *World J Surg* 22:127–134, 1998.
11. Eggimann P, Garbino J, Pittet D. Epidemiology of *Candida* species infections in critically ill non-immunosuppressed patients. *Lancet Infect Dis* 3:685–702.
12. Meersseman W, Vandecasteele SJ, Wilmer A, et al: Invasive aspergillosis in critically ill patients without malignancy. *Am J Respir Crit Care Med* 170:621–625, 2004.
13. Rocco TR, Reinert SE, Simms HH: Effects of fluconazole administration in critically ill patients: analysis of bacterial and fungal resistance. *Arch Surg* 135:160–165, 2000.
14. Gleason TG, May AK, Caparelli D et al: Emerging evidence of selection of fluconazole-tolerant fungi in surgical intensive care units. *Arch Surg* 132:1197–1201, 1997.
15. Shorr AF, Chung K, Jackson WL et al: Fluconazole prophylaxis in critically ill surgical patients: a meta-analysis. *Crit Care Med* 33:1928–1935, 2005.
16. Ostrosky-Zeichner L: New approaches to the risk of *Candida* in the intensive care unit. *Curr Opin Infect Dis* 16:533–537, 2003.
17. Groll AH, Gea-Banacloche JC, Glasmacher A, et al: Clinical pharmacology of antifungal compounds. *Infect Dis Clin North Am* 17:159–191, 2003.
18. Rex JH, Walsh TJ, Sobel JD, et al: Practice guidelines for the treatment of candidiasis. Infectious Diseases Society of America. *Clin Infect Dis* 30: 662–678, 2000.
19. Herbrecht R, Denning DW, Patterson TF, et al: Vooriconazole versus amphotericin B for primary therapy of invasive aspergillosis. *N Engl J Med* 347:408–415, 2002.
20. Kullberg BJ, Sobel JD, Ruhnke M, et al: Voriconazole versus a regimen of amphotericin B followed by fluconazole for candidaemia in non-neutropenic patients: a randomised non-inferiority trial. *Lancet* 366: 1435–1442, 2005.
21. Anidulafungin. *Med Lett Drugs Ther* 48:43–44, 2006.
22. Cochran A, Morris SE, Edelman LS, et al: Systemic *Candida* infection in burn patients: a case–control study of management patterns and outcomes. *Surg Infect* 4:367–374, 2002.

PREOPERATIVE AND POSTOPERATIVE NUTRITIONAL SUPPORT: STRATEGIES FOR ENTERAL AND PARENTERAL THERAPIES

Patricia M. Byers   and   S. Morad Hameed

Nutritional support is an integral part of trauma and critical care management. Its role has undergone a dramatic evolution over the past two decades as we have developed a deeper understanding of the complex inflammatory and metabolic pathways that accompany surgical stress. The manipulation of this stress response and its inherent catabolic reaction is the focus of emerging nutritional therapies.

MALNUTRITION

Malnutrition may be defined as a state of relative nutrient deprivation and metabolic perturbation that compromises host defenses and increases the risk of complications and death. For years, protein-calorie malnutrition has been characterized by weight loss, hypoalbuminemia, decreased skeletal muscle mass, reduced fat stores, and decreased total lymphocyte counts. In 1936, Hiram O. Studley first identified preoperative malnutrition as a specific operative risk factor in patients with peptic ulcer disease. He noted a ten-fold increase in mortality in patients who had lost over 20% of their body weight, and wondered if this might be reversible with a preoperative method for overcoming this deficit. Multiple studies performed since his time have confirmed that malnutrition results in poor wound healing, increased infection rates, and prolonged postoperative ileus with resultant lengthened hospital stays and increased mortality.

METABOLIC STRESS

Patients who are injured or submitted to extensive and complicated surgery manifest a pronounced acute phase reaction in response to tissue injury, reperfusion, and hemodynamic disturbances. A metabolic environment of increased catecholamines and cortisol orchestrates an increase in energy expenditure and protein turnover. The resultant insulin resistance is responsible for the decreased peripheral use of glucose and an increase in the rates of lipolysis and proteolysis for the provision of amino acids and fatty acid subunits as fuel. The conversion of peripherally mobilized amino acids (primarily alanine) to glucose by gluconeogenesis is not suppressed by hyperglycemia or the infusion of glucose solutions in this environment. The amino acid pool rapidly becomes depleted of essential amino acids as the high-branched chain amino acids are used as fuel in skeletal muscle while large amounts of the conditionally-essential amino acid glutamine are required for metabolic processes in the intestinal mucosa. Decreased protein synthesis in skeletal muscle and eventually in the intestine, is accompanied by increased breakdown, with the shuttling of amino acids to lung, cardiac, liver, and splenic tissue, where protein synthesis is maintained. As this catabolic process is perpetuated by cytokine activation, the critically ill and injured patient remains catabolic and consumes muscle and fat reserves rapidly. The previous disturbances can deplete important trace elements and vitamins, whose deficiencies may be associated with end-organ dysfunction.

In the stress state, malnutrition may be manifest as a functional deterioration in organ system function along with poor wound healing or wound breakdown. Respiratory muscle weakness can predispose to atelectasis, pneumonia and prolonged ventilator dependence. In addition, all aspects of the immune response may be impaired by malnutrition. Host barrier function may be compromised along with cell-mediated and humoral immunity as cell growth and turnover are diminished.

PREOPERATIVE NUTRITION

There are two circumstances in which preoperative nutritional support should be considered. One is for patients who will require major operative intervention, but cannot undergo immediate surgery and will have a prolonged fast for more than 5 days. The other circumstance is when operative intervention is delayed to treat patients with significant nutritional deficits that could increase postoperative morbidity (Figure 1).

In the preoperative patient, the response to starvation is associated with a redistribution of substrate flow from peripheral tissues to meet metabolic demands. The falling level of insulin promotes the release of fatty acids and amino acids from adipose tissue and skeletal muscle. Although most peripheral tissues can utilize fatty acids as fuel, proteolysis continues to fuel gluconeogenesis in order to support the fuel requirements of the glucose dependent tissues (Figure 2). Over time, there is adaptation to starvation as the brain becomes able to use ketones for 50% of its fuel needs. As fat-derived fuel sources are utilized more, the dependence on protein catabolism decreases from 85% to 35% (Figure 3).

Patients with upper gastrointestinal tract malignancies have the highest incidence of protein-calorie malnutrition, with over 30% of patients demonstrating significant nutritional deficits. Preoperative chemotherapy and radiation, combined with cancer cachexia, obstruction, increased nutrient losses, and abnormal substrate metabolism, increase nutritional risk.[1]

Prospective studies have shown a decrease in major complications such as anastomotic leak and wound disruption when surgery is delayed and preoperative parenteral nutrition is administered to severely malnourished patients. However, there is an increase in infectious complications without clinical benefit when preoperative parenteral nutrition is administered to patients who are well nourished or only

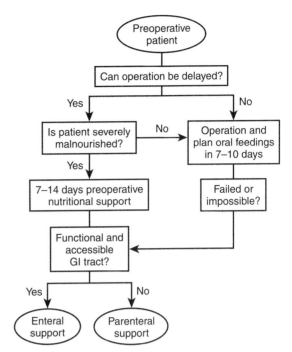

Figure 1 Algorithm for preoperative nutritional support.

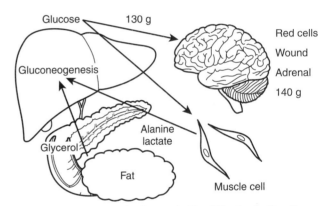

Figure 2 Fasting state: the Cori cycle. The falling level of insulin promotes the release of fatty acids and amino acids from adipose tissue and skeletal muscle. Although most peripheral tissues can utilize fatty acids as fuel, proteolysis continues to fuel gluconeogenesis in order to support the fuel requirements of the glucose-dependent tissues.

mildly malnourished. It is important, therefore, to precisely define malnutrition to appropriately select patients for this treatment modality.[2]

Severe malnutrition can be diagnosed using a clinical nutritional evaluation tool, such as the Subjective Global Assessment.[3] In 1982, Baker demonstrated the validity of a clinical assessment relative to one made on the basis of more objective laboratory values. The clinician uses historical information about recent food intake or unintentional weight loss and examines the patient for signs of nutritional depletion. Patients with multiple or severe stigmata of malnutrition or more than 15% weight loss within six months would be considered as seriously depleted. However, in patients with biopsy proven carcinoma, a weight loss of more than 10% in six months would indicate a high-risk group that would benefit from a course of preoperative nutritional support.

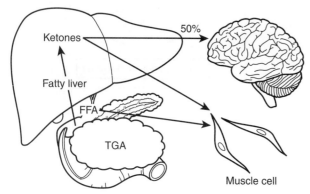

Figure 3 Fasting state: fatty acids. Over time, there is adaptation to starvation as the brain becomes able to use ketones for 50% of its fuel needs. As the use of fat-derived fuel sources increases, dependence on protein catabolism decreases from 85% to 35%. *FFA*, Free fatty acids; *TGA*, triglycerides.

After selection of a patient for preoperative nutrition, it is necessary to decide on a formulation and treatment course. Although the optimal duration of therapy has yet to be determined, preoperative therapy from 7–15 days is standard. Total nonprotein calories should be calculated at 150% of basal energy expenditure as measured using indirect calorimetry or derived from the Harris-Benedict equations (Table 1). It is prudent to start patients with severe malnutrition and starvation at a basal energy rate for several days to prevent refeeding syndrome before increasing support to goal rates. After 3 days, support may be increased to 125% of basal requirements and then increased to goal as tolerated.

Preoperative Total Parenteral Nutrition

Total parenteral nutrition (TPN) should be administered to patients who are severely malnourished with nonfunctioning gastrointestinal tracts. Dextrose and lipid formulas are used to provide nonprotein calories, usually in a 70:30 ratio. The caloric values of TPN substrates can be found in Table 2. The amount of dextrose administered should be 4–6 mg/kg/min. However, in patients with chronic obstructive pulmonary disease or diabetes, it is recommended to keep the dextrose administration at 4 mg/kg/min or less. Blood sugars must be monitored and kept tightly controlled between 85 and 120 mg/dl.

Table 1: Harris-Benedict Equations

BEE Women = 655 + (9.6 × weight in kg) + (1.7 × height in cm) − (4.7 × age in years)
BEE Men = 66 + (13.7 × weight in kg) + (5 × height in cm) − (6.8 × age in years)

Data from Van Way CW 3rd: Variability of the Harris-Benedict equation in recently published textbooks. *J Parenter Enteral Nutr* 16:566–568, 1992.

Table 2: Caloric Value of Parenteral and Enteral Nutrients

Nutrient	Parenteral (kcal/g)	Enteral (kcal/g)
Carbohydrate	3.4	4.0
Fat	9.0	9.0
Protein	3.4	4.0

Intravenous fat can be utilized to supplement nonprotein calories; however, there is data to suggest that preoperative lipid therapy should be limited to less than 30% of the total calories. Lipids are administered as a 20% emulsion and depending upon caloric needs anywhere from 100 to 250 ml may be prescribed daily.

Protein is administered as a free amino acid solution at 1.5 g/kg of body weight daily to promote protein anabolism, and should not be calculated as a source of calories. Adequate nonprotein calories must be administered to support protein synthesis in a 150/1 calorie to nitrogen ratio, along with multivitamins and trace elements as part of the nutritional regimen.

While providing preoperative parenteral nutrition for patients with gastrointestinal dysfunction, it is important to consider fluid requirements. A more dilute solution may be needed in patients with large fluid losses, while more concentrated solutions will be necessary in patients who have volume restrictions due to heart failure, renal failure, or hepatic insufficiency.

With protein-calorie malnutrition there is loss of the intracellular ions potassium, magnesium, and phosphorus, and a gain in sodium and water. During refeeding, sodium balance may become markedly positive and cause water retention. Potassium, phosphorus, and magnesium levels may drop precipitously upon initiation of nutritional support. It is important to monitor electrolytes and fluid balance to avoid the risk of refeeding syndrome. In addition, potassium and magnesium deficiencies must be corrected if anabolism is to occur (Table 3).

Trace minerals are inorganic compounds, and vitamins are complex organic compounds that regulate metabolic processes (Table 4). The majority act as coenzymes or as essential elemental constituents of enzyme complexes regulating the use of carbohydrates, proteins, and fats. Iron, zinc, copper, chromium, selenium, iodine, and cobalt are known to be necessary for health in man. However, in malnourished and seriously ill patients, requirements for zinc and selenium should be assessed and replenished as necessary.[4]

If the patient's fluid and electrolyte status stabilizes on parenteral support with blood glucose levels in good control, the patient may be discharged home on cyclic overnight feedings while awaiting surgery. The parenteral cycle is gradually decreased from 24 to 18 hours and then to 14–16 hours daily. A permanent access port will be needed for home care.

Preoperative Enteral Nutrition

Enteral nutritional support is the delivery of nutrients into the gastrointestinal tract and may require a temporary or permanent feeding tube. Enteral feeding is the preferred route of nutritional support and should be used whenever possible. Surgical patients benefit from enteral nutrition due to the maintenance of the gut-associated lymphoid tissue, enhancement of mucosal blood flow, and maintenance of the mucosal barrier.

The initial gastrointestinal barrier function is provided by mucous containing lactoferrin and lysozyme, both of which are effective, nonspecific inhibitors of microbial growth. Normal, undisturbed bacterial flora exert a similar effect. Epithelial tight junctions form the next line of nonspecific defense, with junctional integrity being energy dependent, and at least partially reliant on the presence of intraluminal energy substrates. Specific intestinal immunity is governed by the gut-associated lymphoid tissue (GALT). The inductive sites in the Peyer's patches provide an interface between antigen-presenting cells and circulating lymphocytes. Animal studies have demonstrated improved immunity in enterally fed groups.[5]

Patients may have inadequate appetite or gastrointestinal function to maintain optimal nutrition on oral intake alone. Enteral feeding has been used successfully to meet the nutritional needs of patients with a wide range of surgical diseases including cancer, inflammatory bowel disease, and pancreatic disorders. However, its use is contraindicated in cases of bowel obstruction, persistent intolerance, hemodynamic

Table 3: Electrolyte Requirements, Compartments, and Sequelae of Abnormal Levels

Electrolyte	Daily Requirement	Fluid Compartment	Effects of Excessive Levels	Effects of Diminished Levels
Sodium (Na^+)	60–120 meq	Extracellular	Dry mucous membranes, maniacal behavior	Seizures, altered mental status
Potassium (K^+)	40–120 meq	Intracellular	Cardiac arrest, peaked T waves, wide QRS on electrocardiogram	Cardiac dysrhythmias, muscle weakness
Magnesium (Mg^{2+})	10–20 mmole	Intracellular	Cardiac dysrhythmias, hypotonia	Hypokalemia, hypocalcemia, seizures
Phosphorus (PO_4^{2-})	14–20 mmole	Intracellular	Calcium phosphate salt deposits	Altered mental status, muscle weakness, hemolysis, paresthesias
Calcium (Ca^{2+})	5 mg	Intracellular	Lethargy, constipation	Tetany, hyperreflexia, seizures, cardiac dysrhythmias

Table 4: Vitamins and Minerals

Vitamin or Mineral	Function	Daily Requirement
Biotin	Coenzyme of carboxylase	60 mcg
Chromium	Insulin utilization	10–20 mcg
Copper	Enzyme systems and ceruloplasmin	0.1–0.5 mcg
Folic acid	Nucleic acid synthesis	600 mcg
Iron	Porphyrin-based compounds, enzymes, mitochondria	0–2 mg
Niacin	Component of nicotinamide adenine dinucleotide and its phosphate (NADP)	50 mg
Pantothenate	Component coenzyme A	15 mg
Pyridoxine	Coenzyme of amino acid metabolism	5 mg
Riboflavin	Coenzymes in redox enzyme system	5 mg
Selenium	Component of glutathione peroxidase	20–200 mcg
Thiamine (B1)	Cocarboxylase enzyme system	5 mg
Vitamin A	Epithelial surfaces, retinal pigments	2500 IU
Vitamin B12	Nucleic acid synthesis	12 mcg
Vitamin C	Redox reactions, collagen, immune function	1000 mg
Vitamin D	Bone metabolism	–
Vitamin E	Membrane phospholipids	50 IU
Vitamin K	Coagulation factors	1–2 mg
Zinc	Enzyme systems	1–15 mcg

instability, major gastrointestinal bleeding, and inability to access the gastrointestinal tract safely.

Once it has been decided to administer enteral nutrition, the optimal type of enteral access must be selected. Factors that determine the choice of enteral access include which components of the gastrointestinal tract are available, how long a course of enteral therapy is planned, whether the patient is at risk for aspiration, and finally, the nutritional status of the patient. When available, the gastric route is usually preferred. Postpyloric feeding into the duodenum or jejunum may be indicated when there is early satiety, gastric pathology or a risk of aspiration. Nasogastric and nasoenteral tubes are recommended for short-term feeding because of their ease of placement, low cost and low complication rate. Percutaneous endoscopic gastrostomy has become one of the most common methods for placing gastrostomy tubes. Interventional radiology can also place feeding tubes percutaneously into the stomach as well as in the jejunum. If these less-invasive techniques are not successful, feeding tubes may be placed by open or laparoscopic techniques; however, this approach is less desirable in the preoperative patient with severe malnutrition.

The appropriate selection of enteral formulation requires knowledge of the physiologic mechanisms of the digestion and absorption of each macronutrient. Sources of carbohydrate found in enteral formulas range from simple sugars to starches. The larger molecular weight of starches exert less osmotic pressure in the intestinal lumen, are less sweet and require more time for digestion prior to absorption. Different enteral formulas contain variable amounts of carbohydrates that can range anywhere from 28% to 70% of total calories. Patients with diabetes or carbon dioxide retention due to chronic obstructive pulmonary disease should be given formulas with fewer carbohydrate calories. (See "Preoperative Total Parenteral Nutrition" section.)

Many enteral formulas now contain fiber, which may be soluble or insoluble. Insoluble fiber improves colonic function and bowel transit time, but there is no nutritional benefit or requirement. In contrast, soluble fiber binds to cholesterol and bile salts, and thus lowers serum cholesterol levels. Colonic bacteria digest soluble fiber and produce short-chain fatty acids that are utilized by the colonocyte as a fuel source.

Enteral formulas contain fats derived from corn, soy, and safflower oil. Fat serves as a concentrated energy source and enhances the flavor of enteral formulas without increasing osmolality. The absorption of fat-soluble vitamins requires the intake of a minimum of 15–25 g of fat per day. Linoleic or linolenic acid must be provided to prevent essential fatty acid deficiency. Because omega-6 fatty acids have been shown to have immunosuppressive effects due to the production of inflammatory end-products, omega-3 fatty acids have been added to some enteral products. Medium-chain triglycerides may be a useful caloric source for patients with fat malabsorption, as they do not require pancreatic lipase for hydrolysis, are absorbed without micelle formation, and do not require carnitine for transport into the mitochondria.

Enteral protein may be in the form of intact protein such as casein, partially hydrolyzed oligopeptides, or crystalline L-amino acids. Intact and protein hydrolysates require further digestion by pancreatic and brush-border pancreases into short peptides and amino acids. These nutrients are then freely absorbed by the enterocyte, primarily in the proximal intestine. Patients with malabsorption may benefit from enteral protein in the form of short peptides and free amino acids. Preoperatively, patients should be given 1.5 g/kg/day to support protein synthesis.

Currently, there are over a hundred enteral products on the market. Most formulas have a caloric density of 1-2 kcal/ml, are lactose-free, and provide the recommended daily allowances of vitamins and minerals in less than 2 liters of formula per day. The majority of patients tolerate standard enteral formulas; however, elemental formulas may be necessary in patients with malabsorption. Recently, excellent results with improved immune function and surgical outcomes have been obtained with the preoperative administration of immunoenhancing formulas.[6] Other disease specific formulations have been created for patients with liver disease, renal failure, pulmonary insufficiency, and diabetes. Formulas for patients with liver disease and encephalopathy contain a higher percentage of protein in the form of branched-chain amino acids with almost no aromatic amino acids. Renal failure formulas have very low levels of potassium and phosphorus. However, hepatic and renal formulas have a very low protein content, which must be considered. Patients with advanced pulmonary disease need to receive most of their calories as fat in order to decrease carbon dioxide production. Diabetic formulas also contain additional calories as fat, but also contain soluble fiber to decrease blood sugar levels. It is important to note that all of these specialty formulas are very expensive, and should only be used when a standard formulation with an appropriate nutrient profile has failed.

It is important to monitor patients on enteral feeding for improvement in nutritional status, gastrointestinal tolerance, and fluid and electrolyte balance. When gastric feedings are administered, it is important to monitor gastric residual volumes. Increased residual volumes lead to vomiting, aspiration, pneumonia, prolonged hospital stays, and mortality. Another complication that can occur in the malnourished patient is diarrhea, which may precipitate fluid and electrolyte abnormalities. Diarrhea may be due to medications, formula composition, or infections. If infectious causes are eliminated and there are no offending medications, the formula should be changed to one that is more elemental to increase absorption. If necessary, medications can be tried in incremental dosages to slow down intestinal transit time.

Because most formulas only contain 65% water, it may be necessary to administer hypotonic enteral fluid boluses to achieve satisfactory fluid and electrolyte balance. Electrolyte levels should be monitored to avoid hyperosmolar states and to replete serum levels of potassium, phosphorus, and magnesium during refeeding. Patients may develop fluid retention and electrolyte imbalances that can result in life-threatening cardiac dysrythmias. Blood sugars must be

carefully monitored, and hyperglycemia should be treated to avoid the increased risk of infections and the development of hyperosmolar states.

Preoperative enteral feedings have been demonstrated to decrease postoperative complication rates by 10%–15% of controls, but there is debate over the length of therapy needed to achieve this. The literature supports a course of enteral feedings for 5–20 days prior to surgery. Recently, it has been shown that there may be an advantage to utilizing immune-enhancing formulas, either alone as preoperative supplements, or in combination with postoperative support.[6]

Postoperative Nutrition

When developing a plan for postoperative nutrition, it is important to anticipate the length of time that the patient may require ventilatory support or have an intestinal ileus. The condition of the patient with attention to premorbid nutrition, and the state of hypermetabolism and catabolism must be assessed to maximize the opportunity for intraoperative enteral access (Figure 4). However, this type of detailed assessment may not be possible in patients scheduled for emergency surgery or those with traumatic injury. In order to simplify these decisions, we developed a model for use in patients who have suffered from traumatic injury (Figure 5). This simple algorithm using the indication for emergency surgery and Injury Severity Score has an accuracy of 88% in selecting trauma patients that are candidates for early nutritional support. In our series, we found that 80% of all trauma patients admitted to the intensive care unit met criteria for nutritional support following traumatic injury.[7]

Although protein requirements in stable adults are only 0.6 g/kg/day, the increased catabolism that occurs during critical illness raises the basal needs for balance. Improved nitrogen equilibrium occurs with increased protein synthesis in the majority of postoperative patients when 25–30 kcal/kg of total calories is provided along with 1.5–2.0 g/kg of protein daily. Carbohydrates should be administered with a maximum of 4–6 mg of dextrose per kilogram per minute with serum blood sugars maintained between 85 and

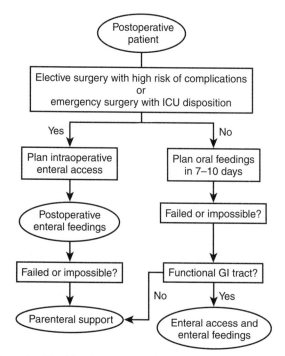

Figure 4 Algorithm for postoperative nutritional support. *GI,* Gastrointestinal; *ICU,* intensive care unit.

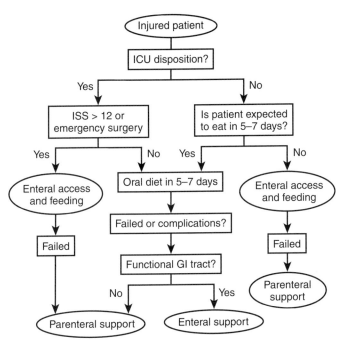

Figure 5 Trauma care nutritional support algorithm. *ICU,* Intensive care unit; *ISS,* Injury Severity Score. *(Data from Byers P, Block E, Albornoz J, et al: The need for aggressive nutritional intervention in the injured patient: the development of a predictive model. J Trauma 39:1103, 1995.)*

Table 6: Nitrogen Balance

Nitrogen (N) balance = N (in) − N (out)
N (in) = protein / 6.25 (g/day)
N (out) = total urinary N[a] (g/day) + gastrointestinal losses (2–4 g/day) + cutaneous losses (0–4 g/day)

[a]Total urinary N can either be measured directly or estimated by measuring urine urea N and dividing by 0.8

Table 7: Estimation of Creatinine Height Index

Creatinine height index (CHI) % = measured 24-hour urinary creatinine / predicted 24-hour urinary creatinine × 100
Predicted 24-hour urinary creatinine: men = 20–25 mg/kg; women = 15–20 mg/kg

Data from Heymsfield SB, Arteaga C, McManus C, Smith J, Moffitt S: Measurement of muscle mass in humans: validity of the 24-hour urinary creatinine method. *Am J Clin Nutr* 37:478–494, 1983.

120 mg/dl. Fat should be used to meet less than 30% of total calories.[8] If indirect calorimetry is available, it should be utilized to measure caloric needs to avoid overfeeding. Supplements of enteral glutamine should be given in doses of 0.5 g/kg/day, as well as multivitamins and trace minerals, including zinc and selenium.

In addition to monitoring blood sugar, electrolytes, and fluid balance, patients receiving postoperative nutrition should be monitored for efficacy of therapy. Serum protein markers with short half-lives are most effective in measuring improvement in the visceral protein compartment (Table 5). Failure to achieve improvement in these values should prompt assessment of the nutrition administered over the past several days along with a search for untreated infection or inflammation. Nitrogen balance studies may be performed where the amount of protein administered is evaluated against the amount of nitrogen lost in the urine, stool, and wound drainage (Table 6). Critically ill patients should be kept in neutral nitrogen balance while anabolic patients should be kept in a slightly positive balance. After visceral protein markers have normalized, it may become important to evaluate the somatic muscle compartment. If renal function is stable, this can be done by performing a 24-hour urine creatinine measurement and calculating the creatinine height index (Table 7). Improvement in this value will require aggressive physical therapy in addition to nutritional support.

Table 5: Visceral Protein Markers

Protein Marker	Normal Values	Half-Life (Days)
Albumin	>3.5 g/dl	20
Transferrin	>200 mg/dl	8.5
Prealbumin	20–30 mg/dl	1.3
Retinol-binding protein	4–5 mg/dl	0.4

Postoperative Parenteral Nutrition

Because most well-nourished patients tolerate inadequate nutrition postoperatively for 7–10 days, there is no justification for the use of routine postoperative parenteral nutrition (see Figure 4). Well-nourished patients with severe stress or preoperatively depleted patients should receive postoperative nutrition when a 7–10-day period of inadequate intake is anticipated. Additional candidates for postoperative parenteral feedings are patients who have been treated with preoperative parenteral nutrition, but are unable to receive postoperative enteral feedings and patients who develop complications that preclude utilization of the gastrointestinal tract. Parenteral nutrition may be life-saving in patients with high-output proximal enterocutaneous fistulae, massive intestinal resection, and end-jejunostomy syndrome.

Central venous access with a designated port for parenteral nutrition must be established. For patients that do not require fluid restriction, dextrose concentrations may be kept between 12%–18% with 5%–6% amino acid solutions. Lipids should be limited to 20% of total calories.[8]

There are new modalities that may increase the efficacy of postoperative parenteral nutrition. The addition of growth hormone has been shown to improve wound healing in burn patients, but has been harmful in critically ill surgical patients, and cannot be routinely recommended. Intravenous glutamine has also shown promise. In the future, antioxidants may be indicated as part of a nutritional regimen.[9] Although scientific studies demonstrating potential benefit are available, more clinical trials proving efficacy are needed.

Postoperative Enteral Nutrition

There is a substantial amount of data supporting the enteral route of postoperative nutrition following elective and emergency surgery as well as in patients who have sustained trauma and thermal injury. Delivery of nutrients by the enteral route attenuates the metabolic response to stress, yields better control of blood sugar, reduces clinical infections, and has been found to be associated with increased intestinal anastomotic strength.

In patients who undergo laparotomy, enteral access can be best achieved intraoperatively. Postoperative enteral support should begin 12–72 hours following surgery or injury. Hemodynamic stability should always be attained first to avoid intestinal necrosis from ischemia. Continuous tube feedings usually start at 10–20 ml/hr and may be increased by the same amount every 8–24 hours depending on the clinical scenario. Abdominal distension should prompt the immediate decrease in the tube feeding rate by half, and should prompt cessation of feedings if it persists. Gastric feedings should only be advanced if the residual volumes are 200 ml or less. Bolus feedings into the stomach of 200–300 ml every 2–6 hours may also be given and may help to maintain adequate amounts of feeding despite daily care and diagnostic tests. Enteral feedings should be continued until it has been documented that the patient has an adequate dietary intake.

When feeding directly into the jejunum, fully or partially elemental formulas should be utilized. Standard formulas are better tolerated in the stomach and duodenum. Immune-enhancing formulas are now available and have been developed by enriching enteral formulas with specific micronutrients. Newer formulas have added omega-3 fatty acids which decrease inflammation and the resultant tendency toward multisystem organ dysfunction. These formulas also contain glutamine, arginine, and nucleotides. Wound-healing formulas contain higher levels of zinc, Vitamin C, and Vitamin A. Although studies have demonstrated improved outcomes in length of stay and infectious morbidity, there has been no effect on mortality.[10]

TECHNICAL ASPECTS OF PARENTERAL AND ENTERAL ACCESS

Central Venous Access

Central venous access catheters should be performed by an experienced operator with full aseptic precautions including gown, gloves, mask, and cap after antibacterial handwashing. These antimicrobial catheters may be placed temporarily at the bedside or permanently in an operative suite. In addition, the catheters may be placed by accessing a central vein directly, or by utilizing a peripheral route. The routine use of venous Doppler devices has been demonstrated to decrease complications from venipuncture.

Peripherally inserted central venous catheters (PICC) can be placed by trained clinical specialists. These catheters may be made of silicone or polyurethane and are available in single a double lumen in gauges 16–23. A flexible stylette or guidewire is provided in the kit to help with insertion using a Seldinger technique with a peel-away sheath or by using a catheter-over-the-needle technique. Veins at or below the antecubital space are used for venipuncture. A supine position with the arm at a 90-degree angle from the body is recommended. Catheter advancement should stop if any resistance is encountered. A radiograph of the chest following the procedure is required to document catheter tip position in the central venous system.

Femoral vein cannulation is relatively safe and may not be associated with increased risk of infection. However, it is not a preferred site for long-term venous access due to the morbidity of thrombotic complications. Thoracic venous access can be obtained, and if tolerated, should be performed with the patient in Trendelenburg's position. The internal jugular vein is a preferred site of venous access, with three different approaches available: anterior to the sternocleidomastoid muscle, centrally between the bellies of the sternocleidomastoid, and posterior to the sternocleidomastoid. The external jugular vein may also be used; however, successful cannulation is only achieved 50% of the time. Due to stability of location, the subclavian route, although the most treacherous, is the preferred site for long-term venous access with tunneled catheters, such as the Hickman and Groshong.

Gastrointestinal Access

In patients with adequate gastric emptying, nasogastric feedings with small-bore, flexible, weighted tubes are adequate. These tubes are 5–8 French in diameter, made of polyurethane, and have a stylette for insertion. The tube should be lubricated and the patient should have a topical anesthetic placed in the nostril. The tube is placed through the nostril, advanced through the pharynx and esophagus for approximately 50 cm. Next, 50–100 ml of air are injected, and the tube is advanced along the greater curvature toward the pylorus. An abdominal radiograph should always be obtained prior to initiating feeds through a small-bore tube.

This technique can be modified for postpyloric placement. Intravenous metoclopramide is given prior to the procedure. As the tube is advanced along the greater curvature of the stomach, a point of resistance at the pylorus is met. Gentle pressure is maintained until the pylorus opens and the tube is advanced. Again, an abdominal radiograph is obtained.

If long-term gastrointestinal access is needed, a more invasive approach will be needed. The endoscopic placement of percutaneous gastrostomy tubes is standard and can be performed at bedside in the intensive care unit. This procedure can also be performed safely in patients with a history of previous abdominal surgery, if additional care is taken. First, it is important to know of any gastrointestinal anatomic changes that have resulted from the previous surgery. It is important to obtain abdominal films and review prior scans to be certain that the stomach is approachable through a safe window. During endoscopy, a bright light should be seen in an area accessible for tube placement. A finder needle should be used to ensure that as air is aspirated into the syringe, the needle is visualized in the lumen of the stomach. Gastrostomy tubes may be placed with a push or a pull technique and should have a bolster holding them in place. Combination tubes are made so that an inner jejunostomy portion of the gastrostomy tube can be placed transpylorically. These tubes can also be placed in the radiology suite by the interventional radiology team. It is important to remember that tubes placed by fluoroscopy alone puncture the stomach, but do not fasten it to the abdominal wall. When using the radiology approach, using a postpyloric tube and feeding distally are recommended to guard against gastric distension, until a tract has formed in approximately 3–5 days following puncture.

Patients should have enteral access placed during the primary operative abdominal procedure when it is anticipated that nutritional support will be needed postoperatively. The type of access selected depends on the procedure performed and the gastrointestinal function anticipated. A gastrostomy is easily placed in the left upper quadrant when there is sufficient gastric remnant to do so. Stamm sutures should be placed to bring the stomach up to the abdominal wall. An inner jejunostomy tube can be placed if post-pyloric feedings are desired along with gastric drainage. A jejunostomy tube can also be placed, but may be associated with torsion and potential volvulus. To avoid this risk, it is better whenever possible to access the jejunum via the stomach with long gastrojejunostomy catheters.

MORBIDITY AND COMPLICATIONS MANAGEMENT

Metabolic Complications

Some complications arise due to administration on exogenous substrates. Malnourished patients may develop electrolyte derangements and congestive heart failure when fed too aggressively. This can be avoided by limiting fluids and sodium, and carefully monitoring phosphorus, potassium, and magnesium, while hypocaloric feedings are initially administered. In addition, feeding with excessive carbohydrates can cause the development of hyperglycemia with an increase in infections, electrolyte derangements, and polyuria with dehydration. Patients with compromised respiratory function may develop hypercarbia and respiratory failure.

Complications of Enteral Nutrition

It is important to be aware of complications that can arise with enteral access. There is a 45% incidence of dislodgment of nasoenteral tubes in intensive care units. Dislodgment of percutaneous enteral access catheters into the peritoneum is more serious and may be associated with peritonitis. Radiographic confirmation of tube placement or replacement with contrast studies should be obtained to help avoid this complication. Another problem that may occur with gastrointestinal access is catheter occlusion. Care of these catheters must include frequent flushes with water. Long-standing enteral tubes may leak and cause skin breakdown. The placement of a smaller catheter will usually allow the stoma to contract and thus prevent leaking when the original catheter is replaced.

Adynamic ileus may occur in postoperative patients due to decreased splanchnic perfusion, injury, manipulation, sympathetic tone, inflammatory response, or high-dose opiates. Gastrointestinal tract dysmotility can also result in aspiration and pneumonia. Aspiration can be minimized by keeping the head of the bed elevated whenever clinically feasible.

Nonocclusive intestinal necrosis can occur when splanchnic perfusion is severely compromised. The most common signs are tachycardia, fever, leukocytosis, and distension. Tolerance of tube feeding may be optimized by minimizing opioid use, utilizing epidural anesthetics to blunt sympathetic outflow, and by using promotility agents. However, abdominal distension must be addressed with decreasing the rate or stopping the feedings. When intestinal necrosis occurs, early intervention and definitive surgical therapy have a survival rate of 56%.

Frequent interruption of tube feedings has been shown to impair adequate delivery of nutritional support and result in malnutrition. In one series, only 52% of the feeding goal was administered in a 24-hour period. Feedings are stopped due to procedures, diagnostic tests, and nursing care protocols. New feeding pumps allow nurses to record the exact amount of feedings administered each shift, so that this problem can be recognized and treated.

Complications of Parenteral Nutrition

It is important to be aware of complications that may occur while obtaining central access for total parenteral nutrition. An air embolus may occur and present with hemodynamic collapse. The patient should be immediately placed in Trendelenburg's position with the right side up. If possible, an attempt may be made to aspirate air. This complication can be avoided by hydrating the patient and creating venous hypertension with Trendelenburg's position. Adjacent anatomic structures may be injured; subclavian and internal jugular line placements may result in the development of hemothoraces or pneumothoraces due to vascular or lung injuries. Access on the left side may be associated with thoracic duct injury with clear lymph drainage from the insertion site or chylothorax formation. After catheter removal, the pleural space must be evacuated until lymphatic drainage ceases. Misplacement of the catheter into the pleural space or mediastinum is another complication that may occur. Malposition of a catheter tip into the atrium may cause dysrhythmias, injury, or infected thrombosis, and has been associated with atrial perforation and pericardial tamponade.

Line sepsis is the most common complication of indwelling central catheters and necessitates catheter removal. Primary catheter infections are usually characterized by the development of fever and positive blood cultures. In the presence of bacteremia, lines should be removed, but may be changed over a guide wire with a semiquantitative culture of the intracutaneous portion if there is doubt about the diagnosis. A semiquantitative tip culture is diagnostic when there are 15 or more colony-forming units reported. Typically, removal of the catheter results in resolution of symptoms; however, intravenous antibiotic therapy may be required for 2 weeks with bacteremia due to *Streptococcal* line sepsis or other organisms.

Another common complication of indwelling central venous catheters is venous thrombosis, which may occur with resultant thrombophlebitis and extremity edema. This can usually be treated by catheter removal and extremity elevation. Patients with subclavian vein thrombosis have a risk up to 30% for the development of pulmonary embolism and should receive anticoagulation. Catheter thrombosis is another complication and may be treated successfully with the instillation of thrombolytic agents.

SUMMARY AND ALGORITHMS

Preoperative parenteral nutrition should be given to patients who are severely malnourished and need a major operative intervention where healing complications would pose major risk, as long as enteral support is not an option and a course of 7–15 days of support is feasible (see Figure 1). Postoperative parenteral nutrition should be utilized when the postoperative or post-injury period without enteral nutrition is expected to surpass 7–10 days, when the patient has received preoperative nutrition and is not a candidate for postoperative enteral feedings, and when surgical complications develop in the postoperative period that are associated with gastrointestinal dysfunction. Tight serum glucose control is critical in order to use this therapy with minimal morbidity. Enteral feeding is the preferred method of providing nutrients to patients with a functional gastrointestinal tract and is feasible in the majority of patients. Enteral feeding preserves the structure and function of the intestine, and is associated with fewer infectious and metabolic complications (see Figure 4).

REFERENCES

1. Studley HO: Percentage of weight loss: a basic indicator of surgical risk in patients with chronic peptic ulcer. *JAMA* 106:458–460, 1936.
2. Veterans Affairs Total Parenteral Nutrition Cooperative Study Group: Perioperative total parenteral nutrition in surgical patients. *N Engl J Med* 325:525–532, 1991.
3. Baker JP, Detsky AS, Wesson DE, et al: Nutritional assessment: a comparison of clinical judgement and objective measure. *N Engl J Med* 306:969–972, 1982.
4. Byers PM, Jeejeebhoy KN: Enteral and parenteral nutrition. In Civetta JM, Taylor RW, Kirby RR, editors: *Critical Care*, 3rd ed. Philadelphia, Lippincott-Raven, 1997, pp. 457–473.
5. Alverdy J, Zaborina O, Wu L: The impact of stress and nutrition on bacterial–host interactions at the intestinal epithelial surface. *Curr Opin Clin Nutr Metab Care* 8(2):205–209, 2005.
6. Gianotti L, Braga M, Nespoli L, Radaelli G, Beneduce A, DiCarlo V: A randomized controlled trial of preoperative oral supplementation with specialized diet in patients with gastrointestinal cancer. *Gastroenterology* 122:1763–1770, 2002.
7. Byers PM, Block EJ, Albornoz JC, Pombo H, Martin LC, Kirton OC, Augenstein JS: The need for aggressive nutritional support in the injured patient—the development of a predictive model. *J Trauma* 39(6):1103–1109, 1995.
8. Hasselmann M, Reimund JM: Lipids in the nutritional support of the critically ill patients. *Curr Opin Crit Care* 10(6):449–455, 2004.
9. Heyland DK, Dhaliwal R, Suchner U, Berger MM: Antioxidant nutrients: a systematic review of trace elements and vitamins in the critically ill patient. *Intensive Care Med* 31(3):327–337, 2004.
10. Moore FA, Moore EE, Kudsk KA, Brown RO, Bower RH, Koruda MJ, Baker CC, Barbul A: Clinical benefits of an immune-enhancing diet for early postinjury enteral feeding. *J Trauma* 37:607–615, 1994.

Diagnosis and Treatment of Deep Venous Thrombosis: Drugs and Filters

Felicia A. Ivascu   and   George D. Garcia

The association between injury and venous thromboembolic events is well accepted in trauma patients. The incidence in deep venous thrombosis varies from 7% to 58% depending on the demographics of the patients, nature of the injuries, method of detection, and the type and timing of prophylaxis used in the study population.[1–4] It is thought that the high incidence of deep venous thrombosis in the trauma population can be attributed to the altered physiologic states and anatomic derangements that often coexist in these patients. Virchow's triad of stasis, vessel injury, and hypercoagulability often are present in these patients. Venous stasis is promoted by prolonged bed rest, patient immobilization, paralysis, and hypoperfusion, none of which are uncommon in trauma patients. In addition, hypercoagulability may be induced by diminished levels of antithrombin III, suppression of fibrinolysis, or other alterations in the coagulation system. Finally, the presence of endothelial damage, caused by direct vascular injury, can result in intimal damage and eventually thrombus.

Prevention of thromboembolic events in patients that are simultaneously at high risk for deep venous thrombosis (DVT) formation and bleeding poses a difficult challenge to the trauma surgeon. This challenge is compounded by the fact that more than 60% of DVTs are clinically occult.[5,6] The usual signs and symptoms of DVT, such as swelling and pain, are often obscured by injury.

Many studies have been completed in an attempt to stratify trauma patients into high-risk subgroups for the development of DVT. Traditionally, pelvic and lower extremity fractures, head injury, and prolonged immobilization are considered critical risk factors for DVT formation.[1,2,4,7,8] In addition, large volume blood transfusions raise the likelihood of DVT. Current evidence clearly implicates spinal cord injury and spinal fractures as high-risk conditions.[9] Older age also predisposes to thrombosis, although the exact transition point is unclear.[10–12] Other factors that may also place patients at a higher risk for DVT development, but are not well studied or agreed upon, include injury severity score (ISS) and large transfusion volume.

The nidus for thrombus formation occurs at the time of injury, thus trauma patients do not have the opportunity for true prophylaxis. Concomitant conditions may prohibit usual prophylaxis techniques by days to weeks. In contrast, patients undergoing elective surgery receive preemptive intervention prior to any inciting event. This differentiation likely explains the sharp difference in the incidence of DVT in the trauma population as well as why standard methods of prophylaxis are less effective in preventing posttraumatic venous thromboembolism.

CURRENT THERAPIES

Definitive randomized controlled clinical studies on prophylactic measures in trauma patients with multiple injuries do not exist. Unlike other surgical patients, injured patients are a heterogeneous group who have an isolated injury or any combination of injuries making stratification extremely complicated. Additionally many patients are excluded from one type of prophylactic measure or another by the nature of their injury. With these limitations in mind, there is literature to help guide the development of prophylactic regimens.

SEQUENTIAL COMPRESSION DEVICES

The use of sequential compression devices (SCD) is attractive because of the low complication rate associated with their use. However, with the exception of head injured patients, SCDs have been shown to offer little benefit over no specific prophylaxis.[13] Problems with mechanical compression devices in trauma patients are accessibility and compliance. Many trauma patients require casting or external fixation limiting accessibility to the lower extremity, making use of mechanical compression devices difficult or impossible. Shackford et al.[7] noted that venous compression devices could not be placed at all in 35% of trauma patients because of traction, edema, external fixators, or casts. Lack of compliance is a major contributing factor in the failure of mechanical compression devices in trauma patients. Given the short-lived antithrombotic effect of SCD, even limited periods of noncompliance may encourage clot formation.[7,14] In a prospective study of 227 patients, only 19% were fully compliant with physician orders for SCD prophylaxis.[15] Venous foot pumps, once thought of as a substitute for SCD in situations in which the calves were inaccessible, have been shown to be insufficient prophylaxis.

LOW-DOSE HEPARIN

In the general surgery population, low-dose heparin decreases the rate of DVT formation. Although the low rate of bleeding complications associated with the use of low-dose heparin would make it well suited for use in trauma, several studies reveal low-dose heparin to be relatively ineffective in preventing DVT in the subset of higher-risk trauma patients.[16–18]

LOW-MOLECULAR-WEIGHT HEPARIN

Low-molecular-weight heparin (LMWH) gained popularity in the late 1990s as an effective method of DVT prophylaxis in trauma patients. In a randomized double-blinded trial comparing LMWH to low-dose heparin in trauma patients, LMWH reduced the overall DVT rate by 30%, although both groups had a high incidence of DVT formation.[17] Subsequent clinical evaluations and recent guidelines support the safety and efficacy of enoxaparin in trauma patients who do not have substantial bleeding risk.[16,19–23] Clinical experience with other LMWH is increasing in the trauma population. A single-center evaluation of 743 high-risk trauma patients who received dalteparin 5000 IU SQ daily reported rates of proximal DVT and nonfatal PE as 3.9% and 0.8%, with a corresponding 3% rate of significant bleeding.[24] Preliminary data in spinal cord injury suggest that dalteparin 5000 IU daily and enoxaparin 30 mg twice daily have comparable bleeding risks while providing similar protection from DVT.[25] Caution is necessary in extrapolating therapeutic equivalence among LMWH agents, due to differences in dose equivalences, pharmacokinetics, administration times and DVT/PE diagnosis used in clinical trials.

INFERIOR VENA CAVA FILTERS

Trauma patients are often not candidates for adequate pharmacologic prophylaxis or therapeutic anticoagulation when a DVT is documented. These patients may, however, be candidates for the placement of an inferior vena cava filter. Currently there are no randomized and very few prospective studies on the use and long-term outcomes of inferior vena cava filters (IVC filters). IVC filters do not prevent DVT formation. They are intended to reduce the risk of pulmonary embolism (PE), and specifically, fatal pulmonary embolism. It should be noted that this has not been consistently proven, especially when used prophylactically. Some, in fact, argue that IVC filters actually promote DVT formation and may result in caval thrombosis and the long-term postphlebitic syndrome.[26–28] Other authors report a decrease in the incidence of pulmonary embolism versus historical controls. Still others cite no change in the incidence of pulmonary embolism, persistence of morbidity from DVT, or long-term outcomes. Filter complications include migration, tilt, caval perforation, and PE.[26,29–33] In 2002, the Eastern Association for the Surgery of Trauma published its practice management guidelines for the prevention of venous thromboembolism in trauma patients. Although there were no class I data to support prophylactic vena cava filter placement in high-risk trauma patients, there was a reasonable amount of retrospective and case series data to support the recommendation for consideration of prophylactic vena cava filter insertion in high-risk patients who cannot receive anticoagulation.[22] DVT formation in the trauma patient is theorized to result from local effects of the inflammatory response in combination with venous stasis. The at-risk period in these patients is relatively short and well-defined, making the use of permanent vena cava filters, with their associated risks, less appealing. Retrievable vena cava filters, on the other hand, are thought to offer the same protection as permanent filters during the period of greatest risk, while later retrieval might avoid long-term risk.[34,35] Although several filters have the indication for temporary use and, therefore, would be appropriate in trauma patients, recent literature shows a significant number of "temporary filters" are not retrieved for reasons including lack of follow-up by patients, technical difficulty, and ongoing risk that exceed the time window for filter removal.[36–39] There are also concerns about embolization and the need for anticoagulation during retrieval of temporary IVC filters, which may outweigh the benefit that these temporary filters provide.

SURVEILLANCE

The diagnosis of DVT or PE in the trauma population is plagued by the insidious onset, frequent lack of clinical signs or symptoms, and nonspecific presentation. Physical examination is unreliable and insufficient.[39] Several studies of DVT surveillance assert an overwhelming number of asymptomatic DVTs in trauma patients. Duplex scanning, which combines ultrasound imaging with Doppler measurement of flow velocity, is now the most commonly used method to detect DVT formation. It has been shown to have an 89%–100% sensitivity and specificity comparable to traditional lower extremity venography.[40] This bed-side procedure can be performed easily and repeatedly.[5,41,42] Lower extremity fixators or casts limit or prohibit visualization of the pelvic veins. Several studies have cast some doubt on the routine use of duplex surveillance, while others advocate its use in high-risk patients, particularly those with spinal cord and/or major pelvic/lower extremity orthopedic injuries.[43–49] Arguments against routine screening include the low clinical yield, minimal reduction in PE incidence, and a relatively high cost associated with serial scanning.[49–51] Perhaps strict evidence-based protocols for DVT prophylaxis, centered on risk stratification, are better at reducing the incidence and complication of DVTs than routine screening.

RECOMMENDATION

Prophylactic therapy for DVT formation in high-risk trauma patients needs to be individualized, weighing the potential risks and benefits of each intervention. It is generally accepted that low-dose heparin has no role in this patient population. SCDs, although they have not been shown to have a significant, or even any, benefit in this patient population, are essentially risk-free. The largest hurdle to the routine use of SCDs is access and compliance. Although we are limited in cases of lower extremity injuries, compliance can be improved with education for both health care providers and patients. When anticoagulation is reasonably safe, therapy with LMWH should be implemented as soon as feasible. A recent multicenter prospective cohort study of multi-injured patients, prophylaxis was initiated within 48 hours of injury in only 25% of patients and another one-quarter had no prophylaxis for at least 7 days. Furthermore, a delay in initiation of prophylaxis of more than 4 days resulted in a 300% higher risk of venous thromboembolism.[52] Thus, in high-risk patients who cannot be safely anticoagulated, the placement of an inferior vena cava filter for prophylaxis must be carefully considered early in the patient's hospital course.

As outlined previously, routine radiologic surveillance for all trauma patients is unrealistic and costly. Therefore, a high clinical suspicion for DVT formation must be maintained by the trauma surgeon. If a DVT or PE is diagnosed, the options for treatment are full anticoagulation or IVC filter placement. In patients for whom anticoagulation is prudent, an IVC filter should be considered, and if not contraindicated, immediately placed. Finally, the early placement of an IVC filter should be contemplated in patients with a tenuous pulmonary status for definitive protection from a PE.

The optimal treatment for DVT prophylaxis in patients with multiple injuries continues to be controversial and complex. It requires constant attention and flexible management on the part of the clinician, as the patient's clinical risk of treatment and DVT formation evolves.

REFERENCES

1. Knudson MM, Collins JA, Goodman SB, et al: Thromboembolism following multiple trauma. *J Trauma* 32:2–11, 1992.
2. Knudson MM, Lewis FR, Clinton A, et al: Prevention of venous thromboembolism in trauma patients. *J Trauma* 37:480–487, 1994.
3. Rogers FB: Venous thromboembolism in trauma patients: a review. *Surgery* 130:1–12, 2001.
4. Geerts WH, Code KI, Jay RM, et al: A prospective study of venous thromboembolism after major trauma. *N Engl J Med* 331:1601–1606, 1994.
5. Napolitano LM, Garlapati VS, Heard SO, et al: Asymptomatic deep venous thrombosis in the trauma patient: is an aggressive screening protocol justified? *J Trauma* 39:651–657, discussion 657–659, 1995.
6. Gearhart MM, Luchette FA, Proctor MC, et al: The risk assessment profile score identifies trauma patients at risk for deep vein thrombosis. *Surgery* 128:631–640, 2000.
7. Shackford SR, Davis JW, Hollingsworth-Fridlund P, et al: Venous thromboembolism in patients with major trauma. *Am J Surg* 159:365–369, 1990.
8. Knudson MM, Ikossi DG: Venous thromboembolism after trauma. Current opinion in critical care. 10:539–548, 2004.
9. Velmahos GC, Kern J, Chan LS, et al: Prevention of venous thromboembolism after injury: an evidence-based report—part II: analysis of risk factors and evaluation of the role of vena caval filters. *J Trauma* 49: 140–144, 2000.
10. Abelseth G, Buckley RE, Pineo GE, et al: Incidence of deep-vein thrombosis in patients with fractures of the lower extremity distal to the hip. *J Orthop Trauma* 10:230–235, 1996.
11. Spannagel U, Kujath P: Low molecular weight heparin for the prevention of thromboembolism in outpatients immobilized by plaster cast. *Semin Thromb Hemost* 19(Suppl 1):131–141, 1993.
12. Schultz DJ, Brasel KJ, Washington L, et al: Incidence of asymptomatic pulmonary embolism in moderately to severely injured trauma patients. *J Trauma* 56:727–731, discussion 731–723, 2004.
13. Fisher CG, Blachut PA, Salvian AJ, et al: Effectiveness of pneumatic leg compression devices for the prevention of thromboembolic disease in

orthopaedic trauma patients: a prospective, randomized study of compression alone versus no prophylaxis. *J Orthop Trauma* 9:1–7, 1995.

14. Jacobs DG, Piotrowski JJ, Hoppensteadt DA, et al: Hemodynamic and fibrinolytic consequences of intermittent pneumatic compression: preliminary results. *J Trauma* 40:710–716, discussion 716–717, 1996.

15. Cornwell EE, 3rd, Chang D, Velmahos G, et al: Compliance with sequential compression device prophylaxis in at-risk trauma patients: a prospective analysis. *Am Surg* 68:470–473, 2002.

16. Knudson MM, Morabito D, Paiement GD, et al: Use of low molecular weight heparin in preventing thromboembolism in trauma patients. *J Trauma* 41:446–459, 1996.

17. Geerts WH, Jay RM, Code KI, et al: A comparison of low-dose heparin with low-molecular-weight heparin as prophylaxis against venous thromboembolism after major trauma. *N Engl J Med* 335:701–707, 1996.

18. Mammen EF: Pathogenesis of venous thrombosis. *Chest* 102:640S–644S, 1992.

19. Greenfield LJ, Proctor MC, Rodriguez JL, et al: Posttrauma thromboembolism prophylaxis. *J Trauma* 42:100–103, 1997.

20. Norwood SH, McAuley CE, Berne JD, et al: Prospective evaluation of the safety of enoxaparin prophylaxis for venous thromboembolism in patients with intracranial hemorrhagic injuries. *Arch Surg* 137:696–701, discussion 701–692, 2002.

21. Norwood SH, McAuley CE, Berne JD, et al: A potentially expanded role for enoxaparin in preventing venous thromboembolism in high risk blunt trauma patients. *J Am Coll Surg* 192:161–167, 2001.

22. Rogers FB, Cipolle MD, Velmahos G, et al: Practice management guidelines for the prevention of venous thromboembolism in trauma patients: the EAST practice management guidelines work group. *J Trauma* 53:142–164, 2002.

23. Ginzburg E, Cohn SM, Lopez J, et al: Randomized clinical trial of intermittent pneumatic compression and low molecular weight heparin in trauma. *Br J Surg* 90:1338–1344, 2003.

24. Cothren CC, Smith WR, Moore EE, et al: Utility of once-daily dose of low-molecular-weight heparin to prevent venous thromboembolism in multisystem trauma patients. *World J Surg* 31:98–104, 2007.

25. Chiou-Tan FY, Garza H, Chan KT, et al: Comparison of dalteparin and enoxaparin for deep venous thrombosis prophylaxis in patients with spinal cord injury. *Am J Phys Med Rehab* 82:678–685, 2003.

26. Rodriguez JL, Lopez JM, Proctor MC, et al: Early placement of prophylactic vena caval filters in injured patients at high risk for pulmonary embolism. *J Trauma* 40:797–802, discussion 802–794, 1996.

27. Patton JH Jr, Fabian TC, Croce MA, et al: Prophylactic Greenfield filters: acute complications and long-term follow-up. *J Trauma* 41:231–236, discussion 236–237, 1996.

28. Decousus H, Leizorovicz A, Parent F, et al: A clinical trial of vena caval filters in the prevention of pulmonary embolism in patients with proximal deep-vein thrombosis. Prevention du Risque d'Embolie Pulmonaire par Interruption Cave Study Group. *N Engl J Med* 338:409–415, 1998.

29. Kinney TB: Update on inferior vena cava filters. *J Vasc Interv Radiol* 14:425–440, 2003.

30. McMurtry AL, Owings JT, Anderson JT, et al: Increased use of prophylactic vena cava filters in trauma patients failed to decrease overall incidence of pulmonary embolism. *J Am Coll Surg* 189:314–320, 1999.

31. Gosin JS, Graham AM, Ciocca RG, et al: Efficacy of prophylactic vena cava filters in high-risk trauma patients. *Ann Vasc Surg* 11:100–105, 1997.

32. Carlin AM, Tyburski JG, Wilson RF, et al: Prophylactic and therapeutic inferior vena cava filters to prevent pulmonary emboli in trauma patients. *Arch Surg* 137:521–525, discussion 525–527, 2002.

33. Bochicchio GV, Scalea TM: Acute caval perforation by an inferior vena cava filter in a multitrauma patient: hemostatic control with a new surgical hemostat. *J Trauma* 51:991–992, discussion 993, 2001.

34. Rosenthal D, Wellons ED, Lai KM, et al: Retrievable inferior vena cava filters: initial clinical results. *Ann Vasc Surg* 20:157–165, 2006.

35. Johns JS, Nguyen C, Sing RF: Vena cava filters in spinal cord injuries: evolving technology. The journal of spinal cord medicine 29:183–190, 2006.

36. Kirilcuk NN, Herget EJ, Dicker RA, et al: Are temporary inferior vena cava filters really temporary? *Am J Surg* 190:858–863, 2005.

37. Antevil JL, Sise MJ, Sack DI, et al: Retrievable vena cava filters for preventing pulmonary embolism in trauma patients: a cautionary tale. *J Trauma* 60:35–40, 2006.

38. Hoff WS, Hoey BA, Wainwright GA, et al: Early experience with retrievable inferior vena cava filters in high-risk trauma patients. *J Am Coll Surg* 199:869–874, 2004.

39. Karmy-Jones R, Jurkovich GJ, Velmahos GC, et al: Practice patterns and outcomes of retrievable vena cava filters in trauma patients: an AAST multicenter study. *J Trauma* 62:17–24, discussion 24–15, 2007.

40. Hammers LW, Cohn SM, Brown JM, et al: Doppler color flow imaging surveillance of deep vein thrombosis in high-risk trauma patients. *J Ultrasound Med* 15:19–24, 1996.

41. Wibbenmeyer LA, Hoballah JJ, Amelon MJ, et al: The prevalence of venous thromboembolism of the lower extremity among thermally injured patients determined by duplex sonography. *J Trauma* 55:1162–1167, 2003.

42. Burns GA, Cohn SM, Frumento RJ, et al: Prospective ultrasound evaluation of venous thrombosis in high-risk trauma patients. *J Trauma* 35:405–408, 1993.

43. Velmahos GC, Nigro J, Tatevossian R, et al: Inability of an aggressive policy of thromboprophylaxis to prevent deep venous thrombosis (DVT) in critically injured patients: are current methods of DVT prophylaxis insufficient? *J Am Coll Surg* 187:529–533, 1998.

44. Gathof BS, Picker SM, Rojo J: Epidemiology, etiology and diagnosis of venous thrombosis. *Eur J Med Res* 9:95–103, 2004.

45. Kadyan V, Clinchot DM, Colachis SC: Cost-effectiveness of duplex ultrasound surveillance in spinal cord injury. *Am J Phys Med Rehab* 83:191–197, 2004.

46. Liu LT, Ma BT: Prophylaxis against venous thromboembolism in orthopedic surgery. *Chin J Traumatol* 9:249–256, 2006.

47. Hums W, Blostein P: A comparative approach to deep vein thrombosis risk assessment. *J Trauma Nurs* 13:28–30, 2006.

48. Borer DS, Starr AJ, Reinert CM, et al: The effect of screening for deep vein thrombosis on the prevalence of pulmonary embolism in patients with fractures of the pelvis or acetabulum: a review of 973 patients. *J Orthop Trauma* 19:92–95, 2005.

49. Piotrowski JJ, Alexander JJ, Brandt CP, et al: Is deep vein thrombosis surveillance warranted in high-risk trauma patients? *Am J Surg* 172:210–213, 1996.

50. Spain DA, Richardson JD, Polk HC Jr, et al: Venous thromboembolism in the high-risk trauma patient: do risks justify aggressive screening and prophylaxis? *J Trauma* 42:463–467, discussion 467–469, 1997.

51. Stawicki SP, Grossman MD, Cipolla J, et al: Deep venous thrombosis and pulmonary embolism in trauma patients: an overstatement of the problem? *Am Surg* 71:387–391, 2005.

52. Nathens AB, McMurray MK, Cuschieri J, et al: The practice of venous thromboembolism prophylaxis in the major trauma patient. *J Trauma* 62:557–562, discussion 562–553, 2007.

HYPOTHERMIA AND TRAUMA

Larry M. Gentilello   and   R. Lawrence Reed

Human beings, as homeotherms, normally maintain their body temperature within a narrow range around a core temperature of 37° C. A variety of built-in mechanisms work to either preserve or lose heat. The failure of these mechanisms can result in abnormal temperatures and associated pathophysiologic consequences.

Hypothermia, defined as a core temperature of 35° C or less, is a strong predictor of mortality after injury.[1-3]

INCIDENCE

A recent analysis of the National Trauma Data Bank (NTDB) provides the most comprehensive perspective on the incidence of hypothermia among trauma patients.[4] Of 1,126,238 injured patients, the admission body temperature was recorded in 701,491 (62.3%). A total of 11,026 patients (1.57% of all patients with a recorded temperature) were hypothermic, defined as a core temperature lower than 35° C.

MECHANISM OF INJURY

Trauma patients are disrobed in the emergency department, where most heat loss occurs, and are frequently administered cold intravenous (IV) fluids. Hypothermia is more common and more profound in the more seriously injured patients. Therefore, there is uncertainty over whether the increase in mortality is primarily attributable to the hypothermia itself, or to the underlying injuries. Some have proposed that hypothermia is actually protective in trauma patients, and that mortality rates would not be higher in cold patients if comorbid factors were equal.[5] However, recent studies have documented an adverse effect of hypothermia on outcome, and a significantly improved likelihood of surviving initial resuscitation when hypothermia is aggressively treated.[1,3,4,6,7]

EFFECTS ON COAGULATION

Perhaps the most serious effect of hypothermia in the trauma victim is its effect on coagulation. Uncontrollable hemorrhage, often compounded by coagulopathy, is the most frequent cause of early death in these patients. Dilutional thrombocytopenia is usually cited as the primary cause of coagulopathic bleeding when trauma victims undergo massive transfusion.[8] However, a prospective, randomized, double-blind controlled clinical trial indicated that dilutional thrombocytopenia is relatively infrequent and that prophylactic administration of platelets was not beneficial.[9] Consumptive coagulopathy appeared to be the more common problem associated with massive transfusion.

The extent to which hypothermia causes coagulation problems is often underestimated because of the multiplicity of potential etiologies for coagulation impairment that are usually present. These patients often have conditions such as acidosis, tissue trauma, shock, and dilution of the circulating blood volume with components containing reduced concentrations of clotting factors.

Systemic hypothermia affects coagulation in a variety of ways. Normal coagulation requires adequacy of vasoconstriction, platelet counts and function, and clotting factor levels and activity. Theoretically, hypothermia could affect blood coagulation in each of these domains.

EFFECTS ON VASCULAR PHASE OF COAGULATION

Systemic hypothermia has long been known to provoke cutaneous vasoconstriction. Because of this observation, the topical application of cold has been used as a method to stop external bleeding. The assumption was that because systemic hypothermia induced vasoconstriction, that local vasoconstriction might reduce bleeding. Yet, topical exposure to cold appears to be quite different from systemic hypothermia in that local cooling elicits skin and skeletal muscle vascular dilation at 33° C.

This phenomenon makes sense from a physiologic standpoint. With total body cold exposure, the risk of developing systemic hypothermia produces generalized vasoconstriction as a means of reducing heat and protecting core temperature. Topical administration of cold produces a regional hypothermia that provokes the flow of blood into the hypothermic region through vasodilation in order to reduce the risk of local tissue damage such as frostbite.

Thus, with systemic (but not local) hypothermia, peripheral blood vessels go into vasospasm, a process that limits external heat loss. While this could help coagulation seal bleeding vessels, it can only do so if the remaining components of the coagulation system are working effectively. However, this effect is often counteracted by the adverse impacts hypothermia has on the other components of the coagulation process.

EFFECTS ON PLATELET COUNT AND FUNCTION

During development of hypothermic cardioplegia for cardiac surgery, there was a surge of research interest in the effects of hypothermia on coagulation in the late 1950s. Experimental studies in dogs at that time demonstrated a reversible thrombocytopenia associated with systemic hypothermia.[10,11] However, the thrombocytopenia observed actually occurred at very deep levels of hypothermia, well below that typically seen in a trauma setting.[11-15] Yoshihara et al.[16] reported that platelet counts dropped by only 20%-30% at an esophageal core temperature of 30° C.

In contrast, levels of hypothermia commonly encountered in clinical practice have been shown to have a significant effect on platelet function. Platelets experience a reversible inhibition of their function under conditions of local or systemic hypothermia, mediated at least in part through the temperature dependence of thromboxane B_2 by platelets.[17] Thromboxane B_2 is a potent vasoconstrictor and platelet aggregating agent. Valeri et al.[17] demonstrated this when they induced systemic hypothermia to 32° C in baboons, but kept one forearm warm using heating lamps and a warming blanket. Simultaneous bleeding time measurements in the warm and cold arm were 2.4 and 5.8 minutes, respectively. The authors concluded that warming to restore wound temperature to normal should be tried before resorting to transfusion therapy with platelets and clotting factors when treating hypothermic patients with nonsurgical bleeding.

EFFECT ON CLOTTING FACTOR LEVELS AND FUNCTION

Several studies performed on humans undergoing hypothermic open-heart surgery failed to demonstrate significant alterations in clotting test times except at extreme degrees of hypothermia (i.e., <20° C).[16,18–21] Yet, clinical experience suggests otherwise. Many patients with less severe degrees of hypothermia will have a serious coagulopathy that appears related to the presence of the hypothermia. This apparent inconsistency has been resolved by the realization that coagulation during mild hypothermia is disturbed more from enzymatic dysfunction than it is from altered clotting factor levels in blood. This explains the inability for the experimental data from the 1950s and 1960s to correlate with the clinical experience, as the clotting tests performed by the early experimenters were routinely performed at 37° C instead of at hypothermic temperatures.

In recent years, a number of studies have been performed wherein the clotting tests were performed at hypothermic temperatures. Bunker and Goldstein,[18] in a study previously mentioned of controlled hypothermia in 10 patients, measured clotting tests at the hypothermic temperature of the patients as well as at 37° C. While they found no significant changes in clotting times when performed at 37° C, they state that "prolongation of the clotting times for all coagulation tests except whole blood clotting times was consistently observed when performed at the hypothermic temperatures."

A detailed study of the kinetic effects of hypothermia on clotting factor function was undertaken by Reed et al.[22] These studies were done by performing standardized clotting tests in a modified coagulation timer (fibrometer). Because the heat block of fibrometers used clinically are set by the manufacturer at 37° C, an external digital temperature controller was connected to the heat block power source to enable measurement of clotting times at the range of hypothermic temperatures typically encountered in trauma patients. Measurement of the prothrombin time, partial thromboplastin time, and thrombin time performed on assayed reference human plasma containing normal levels of all the clotting factors at temperatures ranging from 25° C to 37° C showed a significant slowing of clotting factor function that was proportional to the degree of hypothermia (Figure 1).

These results were later confirmed by Gubler et al.,[23] in a study using a similar modified fibrometer that demonstrated an additive effect of hypothermia on dilutional coagulopathy (Figure 2).

A subsequent study demonstrated that hypothermia could produce a coagulopathy functionally equivalent to a severe clotting factor deficiency, even at intermediate levels of hypothermia and even though there was no actual deficiency of clotting factors[24] (Figure 3).

In summary, hypothermia does little to affect platelet and clotting factor levels, but it does a great deal to affect the function of these coagulation components. A recent analysis indicates that at mild temperature reductions between 33° C and 37° C, platelets are more profoundly affected than are clotting factors, although clotting factor dysfunction becomes increasingly severe as temperature cools further.[25] Because of the potent effect that severe hypothermia has on platelet and clotting factor function, it is essential that body temperature be normalized before exogenous platelets or clotting factors are administered. Even though clotting studies may demonstrate severe clotting factor deficiencies, there is no value in transfusing coagulation components to severely hypothermic patients. This is because normal levels of clotting factors fail to clot effectively in the setting of severe hypothermia. Thus, administration of platelets or clotting factors to moderately or severely hypothermic patients is essentially futile, as the coagulation components will not function in a hypothermic environment (i.e., below 34° C).

EFFECTS ON OTHER ORGANS

The organ systems that are most commonly affected by hypothermia include the circulatory, immunologic, neurologic, and coagulation systems. Cardiac function can be affected by hypothermia in the form

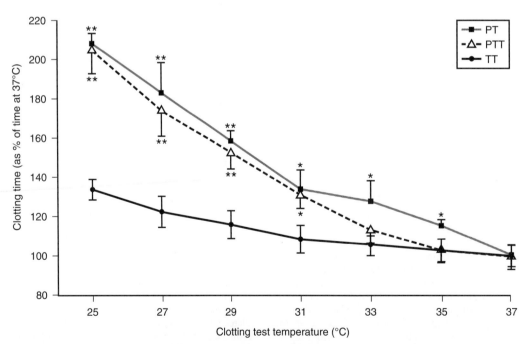

Figure 1 Comparison of effects of clotting test temperature with progressive degrees of hypothermia. Clotting times were performed on standard concentrations of assayed reference plasma using a fibrometer modified to enable control of the temperature at which the clotting test was conducted. *PT*, Prothrombin time; *PTT*, partial thromboplastin time; *TT*, thrombin time. *p, <0.001 vs. thrombin time prolongation. **p, <0.0001 vs. thrombin time prolongation. *(Adapted from Reed R, Bracey A, Hudson J, Miller T, Fischer R: Hypothermia and blood coagulation: dissociation between enzyme activity and clotting factor levels. Circ Shock 32:141–152, 1990.)*

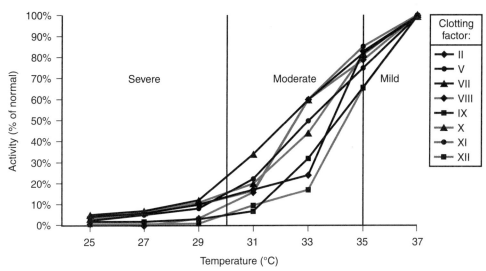

Figure 2 Prolongation of partial thromboplastin time (PTT) that results from cooling of the blood in samples with normal clotting factor levels, and in samples of blood with diluted clotting factor levels.   *(Data from Gubler K, Gentilello L, Hassantash S, Maier R: The impact of hypothermia on dilutional coagulopathy. J Trauma 36:847–851, 1994.)*

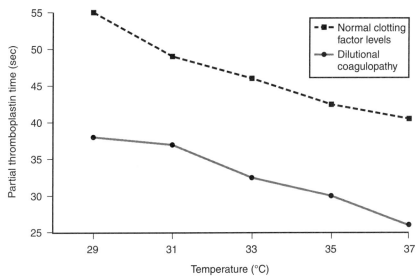

Figure 3   Relative clotting factor activities at various temperatures expressed as percentage of normal clotting factor activity.   *(Data from Johnston T, Chen Y, Reed R: Functional equivalence of hypothermia to specific clotting factor deficiencies. J Trauma 37: 413–417, 1994.)*

of bradyarrhythmias and, at a core temperature below 28° C–30° C, ventricular fibrillation. The body's attempt at restoring normothermia results in an elevation of oxygen that takes place primarily in muscles through shivering. Because of the excessive oxygen consumption required to maintain or restore normothermia in an environment with significant cold stress, organ dysfunction can occur due to a relative undersupply of oxygen, with a resultant increased risk of cardiac complications in elderly patients.[26]

The potential immunologic consequences of hypothermia have been extensively studied. Because of the enzymatic nature of most immunologic functions, it makes sense that hypothermia would inhibit many of these processes. Moreover, our immunologic system is often pitted against bacteria that are not homeotherms as humans are, and may therefore not suffer as severe a functional deterioration in the presence of a hypothermic environment. Some relatively

well-done clinical studies provide evidence that mild hypothermia is associated with increased risk for surgical site infection.[27,28] Laboratory studies of the neuroprotective effects of hypothermia appeared promising, but clinical trials have been disappointing, and the immunologic effects of hypothermia were associated with an increase in pneumonia and septic complications.[29–31]

MANAGEMENT

The relatively high specific heat of the body makes hypothermia very difficult to treat. The rapidity and aggressiveness with which treatment is provided should be based on how severely the hypothermia is affecting the patient. There are a number of clinical studies that describe the efficacy of currently available rewarming techniques. However, many were conducted on healthy, nonvaso-constricted volunteers, and most did not take into account the patient's initial body temperature and mass, the rate of endogenous heat production, and the presence or absence of anesthetics, vasodilating agents, shock, or shivering, all of which are important determinants of the rewarming rate.

Passive Rewarming

Since the specific heat of the body is 0.83 kcal/kg/° C, a 70-kg patient has to gain 58.1 kcal to raise average body temperature by one degree. Since basal heat production is approximately 1 kcal/kg/hr, endogenous heat production will produce a rewarming rate of roughly 1.2° C/hr if the patient is sufficiently insulated to prevent all heat loss. Shivering can increase heat production by three-fold, so that a spontaneous rewarming rate of 3.6° C/hr is theoretically possible.

Active External Rewarming

Heat flows from an area of higher temperature to one of lower temperature as a function of the laws of thermodynamics. Since the temperature of the skin is generally 10° C–20° C cooler than the core, the skin must first be warmed to a temperature greater than that of the core before central heat transfer can occur. Since external rewarming has little immediate effectiveness, it should not be relied upon as the principle means of rewarming patients who are suffering adverse effects of hypothermia.

Standard fluid-circulating heating blankets are a commonly used external rewarming technique. Based upon observed rewarming rates in hypothermic patients, it has been estimated that roughly 2.5 kcal/hr per degree Celsius temperature difference between blanket and skin occurs.[32] Roughly 25–35 kcal/hr of heat transfer can be expected, which is enough to rewarm body temperature by approximately 0.5° C/hr. Convective air rewarmers provide a larger surface area for heat exchange than fluid circulating heating blankets. However, the density of air is so low that it contains very little thermal energy. For example, one can tolerate a 150° F sauna for 10 minutes, but inserting a hand in 150° F water for 10 seconds results in an immediate scald injury.

The very low heat-carrying capacity of air means that little heat can be transferred to a patient by blowing warm air over the skin. However, an additional consequence of the laws of thermodynamics is that when two masses are in contact with one another, heat always flows from the area of higher temperature to the area of lower temperature, regardless of differences in heat content (law of entropy). The purpose of a convective warmer is to establish a microenvironment around the patient that is warmer than skin temperature. This prevents heat loss from the skin (except through sweating). These devices may be used to minimize heat loss from covered areas, but are ineffective means of treating hypothermia, and most of the actual warming that is observed is due to the patient's own heat generation. In a randomized treatment study hypothermic patients did not warm faster with a convective heating blanket than with a standard cotton hospital blanket.[33]

Aluminum space blankets are made of material often used as a lining in survival apparel, and are designed to minimize radiant heat loss by reflecting emitted photons back to the patient. The distance between the emitting and reflective surface is an important determinant of effectiveness. Proper use requires wrapping the blanket relatively tightly over the patient, and placement of an additional standard blanket on top of the space blanket to minimize underlying air movement. Since scalp vessels do not vasoconstrict even in hypothermic patients, a large amount of radiant heat loss occurs from the neck up.

Overhead radiant warmers can produce intense local heat in vasoconstricted patients if there is not enough circulation to carry the heat away, which can cause severe thermal injury. Patients must be fully exposed for radiant warming to occur. A blanket is often placed over the patient to diminish the risk of thermal injury, but radiant heat is then supplied only to the blanket, and the patient is warmed in a very inefficient manner by the air trapped underneath the blanket. Based on observed rewarming rates in hypothermic patients, Henneberg et al.[34] have calculated an approximate heat transfer of 17.7 kcal/hr with the use of an overhead radiant warmer.

Active Core Rewarming

Airway rewarming using humidified air at 41° C is one of the most frequently used core rewarming techniques. Fully saturated 41° C air can hold 0.05 ml H_2O per liter. At 30° C, air can only hold only 0.03 ml H_2O per liter. If a 30° C patient inspires a liter of saturated 41° C air, then 0.02 ml H_2O condenses within the airway when the air cools down to the patient's temperature. With a ventilation of 10 l/min, 12 ml of H_2O will condense each hour. When water condenses heat is liberated at a rate of 0.58 kcal/ml H_2O (latent heat of vaporization). Thus, the amount of heat contributed by airway rewarming under these conditions will be only 7 kcal/hr (0.58 kcal/ml H_2O × 12 ml H_2O/hr). An additional 1–2 kcal will be transferred by the warming effect of the inspired air, independent of condensation. Since 58 kcal is required to increase core temperature by 1° C in a 70-kg patient, as with external techniques, airway rewarming has limited effectiveness.

Pleural or peritoneal lavage should be considered for use in unstable patients with a deleterious response to hypothermia. The amount of heat transferred depends on the difference between the inlet and outlet water temperature and the water flow rate. Since the specific heat of water is 1 kcal/kg/° C, if 1 liter of 42° C water that is infused into a body cavity exits at 35° C, 7 kcal of heat will have been left in the body. However, prolonging operative time in order to irrigate the open peritoneal cavity with warm fluids is counter-productive, as most of the heat that is lost from the water will be transferred to the 21° C operating room environment rather than to the patient.

The high specific heat of water makes it important to warm cold IV fluid prior to administration. A patient will have to generate 16 kcal to warm 1 liter of crystalloid infused into the body at room temperature (21° C). When patients are under anesthesia, their metabolic rate is relatively fixed. If they cannot increase their metabolic rate sufficiently to generate this additional heat, the loss of 16 kcal will decrease body temperature by 0.28° C, which is enough to cause vigorous shivering.

Warm IV fluids also provide a simple means of transferring significant amounts of heat to cold patients requiring massive fluid resuscitation. Warm IV fluids equilibrate with body temperature, liberating heat in the process. A 1-liter infusion of 40° C crystalloid infused into a 32° C patient is, in effect, equivalent to a transfusion of 8 kcal. Since hypothermic trauma patients frequently require massive fluid resuscitation, using warm IV fluids can provide a significant quantity of heat.

Rewarming with cardiopulmonary bypass is, in effect, a means of rewarming via the provision of a continuous infusion of warmed IV fluids. The limitations imposed by the patient's fluid requirements are circumvented by recirculating the patient's own blood. Continuous arteriovenous rewarming (CAVR) is a newly described means of performing extracorporeal circulatory rewarming that does not require a mechanical pump.[6,35,36] CAVR uses percutaneously placed 8.5-Fr femoral arterial and venous lines and the patient's own blood pressure to create an extracorporeal AV fistula through the heating mechanism of a counter current fluid warmer. The tubing circuit is heparin bonded, and no additional heparinization is needed (Figure 4).

Unlike cardiopulmonary bypass, this technique requires an intact circulation, and its effectiveness is limited when arterial

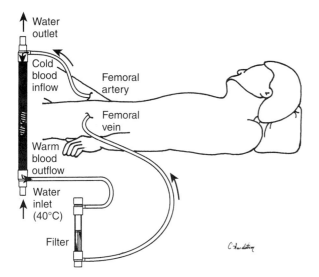

Figure 4 Diagram of continuous arteriovenous rewarming (CAVR) circuit.

pressure falls below 80 mm Hg. However, hypotensive patients generally require additional fluids, which can be "piggybacked" into the heat exchanger to supplement the fistula flow rate. The typical flow rate in normotensive individuals is between 250 and 350 ml/min. If the patient's temperature is 32° C and blood is reinfused at a temperature of 39° C approximately 6 kcal of heat will be transferred every 3–4 minutes.

Rewarming efficacy can be analyzed using standard thermodynamic and heat transfer equations to provide a more accurate assessment various rewarming techniques. A mathematical model has been developed which takes into account body mass and surface area, the specific heat of tissues, the various conductivities of body tissues as a function of temperature, endogenous heat production, and the thermophysical properties of air, water, radiation, and other heat transfer media.[37] A computer simulation provides the expected rewarming rates based on the properties of the technique used (Figure 5).

MORTALITY

Hypothermia has two well-known clinical effects: to preserve life and to kill. Which one of these properties is most active in the trauma patient has been debated for centuries. Hippocrates recommended packing injured soldiers in snow and ice. Baron de Larrey, a battlefield surgeon during Napoleon's campaigns, noted that injured soldiers who sat closest to the fire were usually the first to die. Animal studies repeatedly demonstrate that hypothermic animals are better able to survive shock than normothermic counterparts.[38,39]

Despite these observations, current recommendations for treatment of injured patients call for strict efforts to prevent hypothermia, and for aggressive treatment to reverse it once it has occurred.[40] These recommendations are based on findings of repeated clinical studies demonstrating that mortality is significantly higher in trauma patients who develop hypothermia.[1,2,4,41] One study controlled for magnitude of injury using the Injury Severity Score (ISS), the presence or absence of shock, and fluid and blood product requirements. Patients who became hypothermic had significantly higher mortality rates than similarly injured patients who remained warm. Mortality was 100% if core body temperature dropped to 32° C, even in mildly injured patients.[1] A large study analyzing the NTDB (National Trauma Data Bank) found that hypothermia was an independent predictor of mortality by using stepwise logistic regression (odds ratio 1.54, 95% CI 1.40-1.71) (Figure 6).[4]

One study compared the mortality of hypothermic patients (<35° C) admitted over a 10-month period who were treated with a combination of airway rewarming, fluid circulating or convective heating blankets, an aluminized head covering, and warm IV fluids with a consecutive sample of patients who were rapidly rewarmed with CAVR.[6] Time to rewarming (T > 35° C) was 3.23 hours with standard rewarming techniques and 39 minutes with CAVR. Rapid rewarming with CAVR resulted in a 57% decrease in blood product requirements, a 67% decrease in crystalloid requirements, and a reduction in mortality in trauma patients. In a more recent randomized, prospective clinical trial comparing slow versus rapid rewarming in critically injured patients, significantly more patients in the rapid rewarming (CAVR) group were able to be successfully resuscitated.[7] Two additional prospective, but nonrandomized studies have demonstrated improvements in outcome in trauma patients when protocols designed to minimize heat loss were utilized.[42,43]

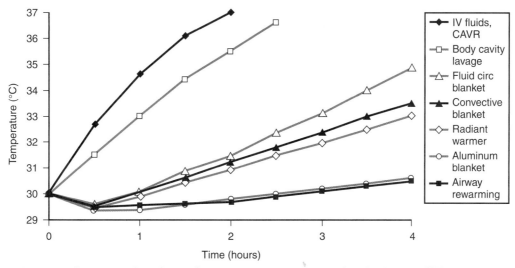

Figure 5 Computerized simulation of rewarming rates using various clinical techniques. *CAVR,* Continuous arteriovenous rewarming; *circ,* circulating. *(Adapted from Gentilello LM, Moujaes S: Treatment of hypothermia in trauma victims: thermodynamic considerations. J Intensive Care Med 10(1):5–14, 1995.)*

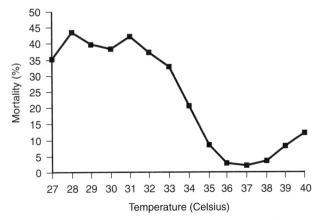

Figure 6 Mortality at each admission body temperature determined from the National Trauma Data Bank (NTDB).

CONCLUSIONS

The relatively high specific heat of the body makes hypothermia very difficult to treat. Early attention to the mechanisms of heat loss outlined previously remains the best form of therapy. Based on current data hypothermia has an adverse effect on outcome from trauma, and every attempt should be made to aggressively treat it once it has occurred.

REFERENCES

1. Jurkovich GJ, Greiser WB, Luterman A, Curreri PW: Hypothermia in trauma victims: an ominous predictor of survival. *J Trauma* 27: 1019–1024, 1987.
2. Psarras P, Ivatury RR, Rohman M, et al. Presented at the Eastern Association for the Surgery of Trauma, Longboat Key, Florida.
3. Luna GK, Maier RV, Pavlin EG, Anardi D, Copass MK, Oreskovich MR: Incidence and effect of hypothermia in seriously injured patients. *J Trauma* 27(9):1014–1018, 1987.
4. Martin RS, Kilgo PD, Miller PR, Hoth JJ, Meredith JW, Chang MC: Injury-associated hypothermia: an analysis of the 2004 National Trauma Data Bank. *Shock* 24(2):114–118, 2005.
5. Britt LD, Dascombe WH, Rodriguez A: New horizons in management of hypothermia and frostbite injury. *Surg Clin North Am* 71:345–370, 1991.
6. Gentilello LM, Cobean RA, Offner PJ, Soderberg RW, Jurkovich GJ: Continuous arteriovenous rewarming: rapid reversal of hypothermia in critically ill patients. *J Trauma* 32:316–325, discussion 325–317, 1992.
7. Gentilello LM, Jurkovich GJ, Stark MS, Hassantash SA, O'Keefe GE: Is hypothermia in the victim of major trauma protective or harmful? A randomized, prospective study. *Ann Surg* 226:439–447, discussion 447–439, 1997.
8. Counts RB, Haisch C, Simon TL, Maxwell NG, Heimbach DM, Carrico CJ: Hemostasis in massively transfused trauma patients. *Ann Surg* 190(1): 91–99, 1979.
9. Reed RL 2nd, Ciavarella D, Heimbach DM, et al: Prophylactic platelet administration during massive transfusion. A prospective, randomized, double-blind clinical study. *Ann Sur* 203:40–48, 1986.
10. Villalobos T, Adelson E, Barila T: Hematologic changes in hypothermic dogs. *Proc Soc Exp Biol Med* 89:192–196, 1955.
11. Willson J, Miller W, Eliot T: Blood studies in the hypothermic dog. *Surgery* 43:979–989, 1958.
12. Helmsworth J, Stiles W, Elstun W: Leukopenic and thrombocytopenic effect of hypothermia in dogs. *Proc Soc Exp Biol Med* 90:474–476, 1955.
13. Helmsworth J, Stiles W, Elstun W: Changes in blood cellular elements in dogs during hypothermia. *Surgery* 38(5):843–846, 1955.
14. Couves C, Overton R, Eaton W: Hematologic changes in hypothermic dogs. *Surg Forum* 6:102–106, 1955.
15. Wensel R, Bigelow W: The use of heparin to minimize thrombocytopenia and bleeding tendency during hypothermia. *Surgery* 45:223–228, 1959.
16. Yoshihara H, Yamamoto T, Mihara H: Changes in coagulation and fibrinolysis occurring in dogs during hypothermia. *Thromb Res* 37:503–512, 1985.
17. Valeri C, Feingold H, Cassidy G, Ragno G, Khuri S, Altschule M: Hypothermia-induced reversible platelet dysfunction. *Ann Surg* 205(2): 175–181, 1987.
18. Bunker J, Goldstein R: Coagulation during hypothermia in man. *Proc Soc Exp Biol Med* 97:199–202, 1958.
19. von Kaulla K, Swan H: Clotting deviations in man associated with open-heart surgery during hypothermia. *J Thorac Surg* 36(6):857–868, 1958.
20. Ahmad N, Agarwal GP, Dube RK: Comparative studies of blood coagulation in hibernating and non-hibernating frogs *(Rana tigrina)*. *Thromb Haemostas (Stuttg)* 42:959–964, 1979.
21. Bahn S, Mursch P: The effects of cold on hemostasis. *Oral Surg Oral Med Oral Pathol* 49:294–300, 1980.
22. Reed R, Bracey A, Hudson J, Miller T, Fischer R: Hypothermia and blood coagulation: dissociation between enzyme activity and clotting factor levels. *Circ Shock* 32:141–152, 1990.
23. Gubler K, Gentilello L, Hassantash S, Maier R: The impact of hypothermia on dilutional coagulopathy. *J Trauma* 36:847–851, 1994.
24. Johnston T, Chen Y, Reed R: Functional equivalence of hypothermia to specific clotting factor deficiencies. *J Trauma* 37:413–417, 1994.
25. Wolberg A, Meng Z, Monroe D, Hoffman M: A systematic evaluation of the effect of temperature on coagulation enzyme activity and platelet function. *J Trauma* 56(6):1221–1228, 2004.
26. Frank SM, Fleisher LA, Breslow MJ, et al: Perioperative maintenance of normothermia reduces the incidence of morbid cardiac events. A randomized clinical trial. *JAMA* 277(14):1127–1134, 1997.
27. Kurz A, Sessler DI, Lenhardt R: Perioperative normothermia to reduce the incidence of surgical-wound infection and shorten hospitalization. Study of Wound Infection and Temperature Group. *N Engl J Med* 334(19):1209–1215, 1996.
28. Flores-Maldonado A, Medina-Escobedo CE, Rios-Rodriguez HM, Fernandez-Dominguez R: Mild perioperative hypothermia and the risk of wound infection. *Arch Med Res* 32(3):227–231, 2001.
29. Clifton GL, Miller ER, Choi SC, et al: Lack of effect of induction of hypothermia after acute brain injury. *N Engl J Med* 344:556–563, 2001.
30. Shiozaki T, Hayakata T, Taneda M, et al: A multicenter prospective randomized controlled trial of the efficacy of mild hypothermia for severely head injured patients with low intracranial pressure. Mild Hypothermia Study Group in Japan. *J Neurosurg* 94:50–54, 2001.
31. Shiozaki T, Nakajima Y, Taneda M, et al: Efficacy of moderate hypothermia in patients with severe head injury and intracranial hypertension refractory to mild hypothermia. *J Neurosurg* 99(1):47–51, 2003.
32. Morrison RC: Hypothermia in the elderly. *Int Anesthesiol Clin* 26(2): 124–133, 1988.
33. Ereth MH, Lennon RL, Sessler DI: Limited heat transfer between thermal compartments during rewarming in vasoconstricted patients. *Aviat Space Environ Med* 63(12):1065–1069, 1992.
34. Henneberg S, Eklund A, Joachimsson PO, Stjernstrom H, Wiklund L: Effects of a thermal ceiling on postoperative hypothermia. *Acta Anaesthesiol Scand* 29(6):602–606, 1985.
35. Gentilello LM, Cortes V, Moujaes S, et al: Continuous arteriovenous rewarming: experimental results and thermodynamic model simulation of treatment for hypothermia. *J Trauma* 30(12):1436–1449, 1990.
36. Gentilello LM, Rifley WJ: Continuous arteriovenous rewarming: report of a new technique for treating hypothermia. *J Trauma* 31:1151–1154, 1991.
37. Gentilello LM, Moujaes S: Treatment of hypothermia in trauma victims: thermodynamic considerations. *J Intensive Care Med* 10(1):5–14, 1995.
38. Wu X, Kochanek PM, Cochran K, et al: Mild hypothermia improves survival after prolonged, traumatic hemorrhagic shock in pigs. *J Trauma* 59(2):291–299, discussion 299–301, 2005.
39. Tisherman SA, Safar P, Radovsky A, Peitzman A, Sterz F, Kuboyama K: Therapeutic deep hypothermic circulatory arrest in dogs: a resuscitation modality for hemorrhagic shock with 'irreparable' injury. *J Trauma* 30:836–847, 1990.
40. American College of Surgeons: *Advanced Trauma Life Support*, 7th ed. Chicago, American College of Surgeons, 2005.
41. Tyburski JG, Wilson RF, Dente C, Steffes C, Carlin AM: Factors affecting mortality rates in patients with abdominal vascular injuries. *J Trauma* 50:1020–1026, 2001.
42. Satiani B, Fried SJ, Zeeb P, Falcone RE: Normothermic rapid volume replacement in traumatic hypovolemia. A prospective analysis using a new device. *Arch Surg* 122:1044–1047, 1987.
43. Satiani B, Fried SJ, Zeeb P, Falcone RE: Normothermic rapid volume replacement in vascular catastrophes using the Infuser 37. *Ann Vasc Surg* 2:37–42, 1988.

SURGICAL PROCEDURES IN THE SURGICAL INTENSIVE CARE UNIT

Ziad C. Sifri   and   Alicia M. Mohr

Bedside procedures are an integral part of the care delivered to critically ill patients. Whether performed for diagnostic or therapeutic purposes, bedside procedures have specific indications and complications. With the pressure of more effective utilization of the operating rooms (ORs), bedside procedures in the surgical intensive care unit (SICU) have become more frequent.

This chapter is not intended to provide a comprehensive review of all the bedside procedures and monitoring that can be performed in the SICU. Rather, we will illustrate the indications, management, and complications of common surgical procedures that can be performed outside of the OR at the patient's bedside.

HISTORICAL PERSPECTIVE

The basic concept of bringing the surgeon to the site of the injured patient is not a novel one. During the Korean War, mobile army surgical hospitals (MASH) units allowed injured soldiers to receive essential surgical care close to the battlefield before they could be transported to hospitals for definite care. This concept is widely used today by the military around the world, and more recently has been adopted by humanitarian organizations to provided medical care to injured civilians. It has also been recently modified and used in response to new challenges of trauma care.

Critically injured patients are more likely to survive their injuries today due to a multitude of improvements in trauma systems and critical care.[1] As a result, "diseases of survivorship" have become more prevalent and are posing new and complex challenges to the trauma surgeon. Clearly, surgeons are most comfortable operating in the OR where conditions are optimal. However, the safe performance of bedside elective surgical procedures has already been demonstrated with tracheostomy and percutaneous feeding access. Currently, there are now circumstances where it is not safe to transport the patient to the OR, and the surgeon is forced to operate under less optimal conditions, in the patient's best interest, in the SICU. This situation arises if the patient is too critical to travel to the OR but needs urgent or emergent surgery, or if the patient needs an emergent surgery but the OR is not immediately available due to other emergencies. This chapter will provide indications and management of both elective and emergent bedside procedures.

SURGICAL PROCEDURES

Bedside Tracheostomy

Patients with persistent respiratory failure following major trauma frequently require tracheostomy since the complications related to the presence of an endotracheal tube for more than 7 days increases and can be life threatening. Patients who have a high likeli-hood of requiring prolonged mechanical ventilation undergo tracheostomy at the earliest possible time when conditions are stable and optimal. Some of the theoretic and proven benefits of tracheostomy include reduction of dead space and airway resistance, facilitation of weaning, improved pulmonary toilet and oral care, and better toleration by the patient, and establishing a secure long-term airway.[2]

Indications

The indications for tracheostomy include (1) prolonged mechanical ventilation (>7 days); (2) an inability to protect airway such as in severe traumatic brain injury, severe maxillofacial trauma, extensive neck, or vocal cord edema/trauma/injury; (3) complex tracheal repair; (4) cervical spinal cord injuries; and (5) respiratory failure and the need for multiple and frequent trips to the OR.

Procedure Options, Contraindications, and Preparation

Bedside tracheostomy can be performed via an open or percutaneous technique based on the surgeon's preference. Tracheostomy is not recommended at times when respiratory complications related to the procedure will be poorly tolerated by the patient. These include situations such as severe hypoxemia, severe hypercarbia, or respiratory acidosis. Redo tracheostomies in patients with difficult anatomy (short neck, goiter) should preferably be performed in the OR under more favorable conditions with optimal lighting. Specific relative contraindications to the percutaneous tracheostomy include a redo tracheostomy, moderate to severe coagulopathy, and unstable cervical spine injuries or an inability to extend the neck.

Adequate preparation for this procedure is critical, as errors can quickly lead to major complications. A complete surgical tracheostomy set and percutaneous tracheostomy kit are present at the bedside (Table 1). Lighting in the SICU should be optimized or surgeons may prefer using a headlight. Assisting personnel include a surgical team with an operating surgeon attending and one or two assistant surgeons, one respiratory therapist, one anesthesiologist, and a nurse. All personnel in the room have protective headwear, masks, and gloves, and the surgeons also wear sterile gowns and gloves.

Open Tracheostomy Technique

Once the patient is paralyzed and sedated, the neck is prepped and draped. Local anesthetic is injected at the surgical site, and then a 2-cm vertical midline incision is made below the cricoid. The platysma is divided and the strap muscles are retracted laterally. The second to fourth tracheal rings are exposed by retracting the isthmus of thyroid superiorly (using a vein retractor) or by dividing the isthmus of the thyroid. Stay sutures can be placed at the lateral aspect of trachea; note that the balloon of endotracheal tube should be deflated while placing stay sutures. Before the procedure begins, the surgeon should test the balloon of the tracheostomy, and ensure that the anesthesiologist suctions the endotracheal tube and mouth and that all equipment works and is within reach. A tracheotomy is performed using an 11-blade scalpel, the opening is dilated, and under direct vision the endotracheal tube is pulled back to just above the tracheotomy site. The tracheostomy is inserted, the inner cannula is placed, and the balloon is inflated. Then capnography is performed, adequate return of tidal volume is assessed, and chest wall movement is visualized. When placement is confirmed, the tracheostomy is sutured to the skin and secured with tracheal ties, and then the endotracheal tube is removed (Figure 1).

Table 1: Equipment Required for Bedside Tracheostomy

Bedside Tracheostomy	Equipment
Tracheal set	Retractors
	Hemostats
	Right-angle clamps
	Metzenbaum and suture scissors
	Tracheal hook and dilator
	Electrocautery
	#11- and #15-blade scalpels
Airways	8F tracheostomy and 6F tracheostomy
	Lubricating gel
	Capnometer
	Anesthesia kit with endotracheal tubes
Sutures	Nylon skin sutures
	Silk sutures and silk ties
Anesthesia	Paralytic and sedatives
	1% lidocaine anesthetic
Field	Sterile drapes and Betadine prep
	Sterile towels
Percutaneous Tracheostomy	
	Percutaneous tracheostomy kit
	Bronchoscope

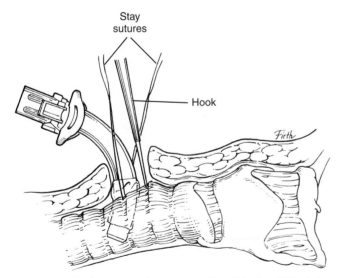

Figure 1 Tracheostomy tube insertion. *(From Velmahos GC: Bedside tracheostomy. In Shoemaker WC, Velmahos GC, Demetriades D, editors: Procedures and Monitoring in the Critically Ill. Philadelphia, WB Saunders, 2001, figure 5-4, p. 34.)*

Percutaneous Dilatation Technique

There are several kits available today with various modifications for the percutaneous tracheostomy using the Ciaglia technique. The authors recommend the following percutaneous technique, which includes making a 2-cm vertical midline incision below the cricoid, and gentle dissection and retraction of the strap muscles with the ability to identify the thyroid and palpate the tracheal rings. With or without the use

of a bronchoscope in the endotracheal tube, the endotracheal tube is pulled back superiorly so that a 10-ml saline-filled syringe is inserted into the trachea just below the endotracheal tube at about the second or third tracheal ring. Once air bubbles enter the syringe, the syringe is removed and a guidewire is advanced into the tracheal lumen. The needle is removed and the tract is dilated with the short dilator. With the use of a guiding catheter, either serial dilation (12–36 Fr) or a single tapered dilation is performed. The 28-Fr dilator within a #8 tracheostomy tube is placed over the guiding catheter and the entire unit is inserted into the trachea (Figure 2). Once in place, the guidewire, the guiding catheter, and the 28-Fr dilator are removed; the inner cannula is placed; and the balloon is inflated. Placement is confirmed and securing of the tracheostomy is performed as previously explained.

Mortality, Morbidity, and Complications

Bedside tracheostomy is considered a safe procedure when performed meticulously and using the suggestions stated above. It has a low mortality rate (0.1%–1%) and minimal morbidity (up to 3%).[3] Complications related to tracheostomy occur intraoperatively, early postoperatively, and late postoperatively. Intraoperative complications include bleeding, perforation of posterior wall of the trachea or anterior wall of esophagus, hypoxia, and loss of the airway. Early postoperative complications include bleeding, hematoma, pneumothorax, and tracheoesophageal fistula. Late postoperative complications include subglottic stenosis, laryngeal nerve injury, tracheal granulation, and tracheoinnominate fistula.

A meta-analysis comparing open surgical and percutaneous tracheostomies found that the rate of serious complication was similar in the two groups.[4] The authors also noted that perioperative complications occurred more often with the percutaneous technique, but that postoperative complications were more frequent with the open surgical tracheotomy. However, most of the differences in complication rates were attributed to minor complications. Another meta-analysis by Freeman et al.[5] found no difference in overall operative complication rates, but found lower postoperative complications and bleeding in the percutaneous technique. Currently, there are no prospective data to support the use of bronchoscopy to reduce complications related to percutaneous tracheostomy, but using it is advocated during the learning curve.

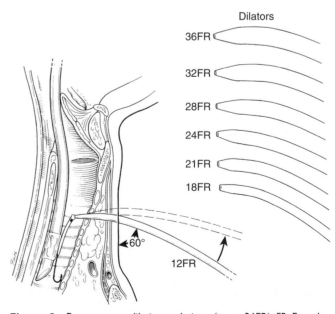

Figure 2 Percutaneous dilation technique (up to 36FR). *FR*, French. *(From Velmahos GC: Bedside tracheostomy. In Shoemaker WC, Velmahos GC, Demetriades D, editors: Procedures and Monitoring in the Critically Ill. Philadelphia, WB Saunders, 2001, figure 5-9, p. 37.)*

Percutaneous Feeding Catheters

Seriously injured patients are at risk for malnutrition and all of its complications. In addition, failure to use the gastrointestinal tract for a prolonged period leads to atrophy of the intestinal mucosa and bacterial translocation.[6] Short-term enteral nutrition is often provided via a naso- or oro-gastric tube. Due to the high incidence of patient discomfort, accidental dislodgment, and sinusitis from prolonged use of nasoenteric tubes, percutaneous cannulation of the gastrointestinal tract is preferred for long-term feeding access. Percutaneous endoscopic gastrostomy (PEG) can be performed by the surgeon at the bedside in the SICU. PEG was introduced in 1980 as an alternative to laparotomy for placement of gastrostomy.[7-9] The surgeon intensivist operator has the advantage of being familiar with the patient's condition and possible recent abdominal surgery.

Indications

Many patients undergoing major surgery for trauma will have a jejunostomy tube or gastrostomy tube inserted at the time of surgery. In the SICU setting, patients needing access to the gastrointestinal tract are those who remain ill and are unable to eat. Any organ failure may cause inability to tolerate oral feedings, especially failure resulting from prolonged ventilatory dependency, traumatic brain injury, or prolonged sepsis. If the duration of injury is expected to be 1–2 weeks, feeding can be given by naso- or oro-gastric tube. Longer periods of naso- or oro-gastric intubation are associated with sinusitis, increased reflux, aspiration, and rarely esophageal stricture. Other indications for PEG include facial trauma and dysphagia.

Procedure Options, Contraindications, and Preparation

If there is no access to the stomach via the mouth, an open procedure is indicated. If a special situation exists in which the stomach is needed for subsequent reconstruction after esophageal injury, it is better to perform an open jejunostomy tube. If there is no barrier to the upper gastrointestinal endoscopy, PEG is indicated unless the stomach is nonfunctional. An absolute contraindication to PEG is an inability to bring the anterior gastric wall in apposition to the anterior abdominal wall. In patients with prior subtotal gastrectomy, ascites or marked hepatomegaly require special consideration. Relative contraindications to PEG include proximal small bowel fistula, gastric varices, obstructive gastrointestinal lesions, and coagulation defects that are not correctable.

The stomach is the most accessible part of the gastrointestinal tract for percutaneous cannulation and the stomach should be empty prior to cannulation. The patient should also receive one dose of antibiotic prophylaxis. In the SICU, sedation is easy to administer.

Technique

The basic elements of all PEG techniques include gastric insufflation to bring the stomach into apposition with the abdominal wall, percutaneous placement of a cannula into the stomach, passage of a guidewire into the stomach, placement of the gastrostomy tube by "push" or "pull" techniques, and verification of the proper position of the gastrostomy button (see Figure 1).

In an intubated patient, the easiest way to introduce the gastroscope is to stand at the patient's head and elevate the tongue and the endotracheal tube. This may be facilitated with the use of a laryngoscope. Gently using the inflation button, the scope is passed down through the esophagus into the stomach under direct visualization. With the stomach insufflated, a place in the antrum is selected for cannulation. This location is generally two fingerbreadths below the xiphoid and two finger-breadths below the left costal margin in most patients. After placing the needle, a guidewire is thread through the needle and with the gastroscope a snare is used to secure the guidewire (Figure 3). The endoscope is removed from the mouth with snare secured to the guidewire.

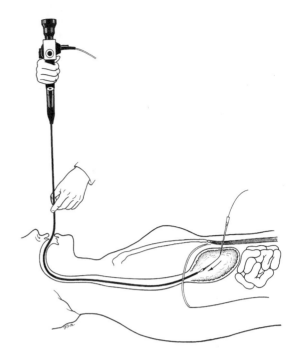

Figure 3 Basic elements of PEG technique. *(From Crookes P: Percutaneocus feeding catheters. In Shoemaker WC, Velmahos GC, Demetriades D, editors: Procedures and Monitoring in the Critically Ill. Philadelphia, WB Saunders, 2001, figure 9–7, p. 65.)*

In the "push" method, a gastrostomy tube is placed over the guidewire and the assistant pulls the wire and gastroscope out through the anterior abdominal wall after making a 1-cm incision. Typically, the gastrostomy tube can be pulled until the 3-cm mark appears at the skin. The gastroscope is replaced in the stomach and the position of the gastrostomy button is confirmed. In the "pull" method, when brought out of the mouth with the snare, a looped guidewire attaches to the end of the gastrostomy tube and pulled through the anterior abdominal wall.

Mortality, Morbidity, and Complications Management

This procedure is safe and effective with a mortality rate of 0.3%–1% and a morbidity rate of 3%–6%.[10-12] Complications are often related to the initial endoscopic procedure, the puncturing of the stomach, and the administering of feedings. There are no specific complications related to performing the procedure at bedside in the SICU, in the endoscopy suite, or in the OR. Specifically, aspiration is an important risk in all SICU patients, and gastroparesis, esophageal trauma, retention of tube feeds, and bacterial overgrowth in an acid-suppressed stomach all contribute to the risk. This risk is minimized by keeping the stomach empty, minimizing air insufflation, and carefully inserting the endoscope. Perforation with the gastroscope is rare if the gastrointestinal tract is anatomically normal. Other structures can be punctured including the colon and liver; however, if the stomach is distended enough and there is clear transillumination of the skin, this complication is rare.

Early dislodgment of feeding access can lead to gastric perforation with the infusion of feedings into the peritoneal cavity leading to peritonitis. This diagnosis may be difficult to make in obtunded SICU patients, but must be considered during a fever work-up. It is therefore important to note the level of the PEG at the time of initial placement so that it may be noted during a daily physical exam. This complication has the highest associated mortality rate.

Wound infection is the most common complication and occurs in 5% of patintents.[13] This complication may be reduced by avoidance of overtight placement of silastic cuff, and adequate skin incision surrounding PEG and possibly prophylactic antibiotics. A rare but potentially life-threatening complication is the development of necrotizing fasciitis. The area of cellulites should be assessed for crepitance as the treatment includes wide surgical debridement and broad-spectrum antibiotics.

Buried bumper syndrome refers to the clinical picture resulting from partial or complete growth of the gastric mucosa over the internal bolster and occurs in 0.3%–2.4% of patients.[14,15] The bumper may migrate through the gastric wall. The buried bumper syndrome presents with leakage or infection around the gastrostomy and is usually caused by excessive tension on the bolsters.

Inferior Vena Caval Filter Placement

Trauma patients are at increased risk for deep-vein thrombosis (DVT) and pulmonary embolism (PE). The principal methods that have reduced DVT incidence include anticoagulation, the use of sequential compression devices, and early mobilization after surgery. At least three groups of trauma patients at high risk for PE have been consistently identified: severe head injury with coma, spinal cord–injured patients with deficits, and severe pelvic and long bone fractures.[15–17] Vena caval interruption has been an effective method of PE prophylaxis, and advances in technology have allowed insertion of inferior vena caval (IVC) filters is done percutaneously. IVC filters are routinely placed under fluoroscopic guidance in the OR or in the interventional radiology suite. Bedside placement of IVC filters alleviates transportation risks and has been shown to be a safe and more cost-effective treatment.[18]

Indications

High-risk trauma patients who have IVC filter insertion are often in the SICU and require mechanical ventilation, intracranial pressure monitoring, multiple intravenous infusions, and other invasive monitoring modalities, which puts them at risk when transported from the SICU. Absolute indications for IVC filter placement include the presence of a contraindication to anticoagulation in patients with a known PE or DVT and recurrent PE despite adequate anticoagulation. The relative indications for IVC filters include a chronic PE in a patient with pulmonary hypertension and a large free-floating iliofemoral thrombus. Prophylactic indications for IVC filter placement include spinal cord injury with paralysis, spinal trauma without paralysis, severe closed head injury, severe pelvic trauma, extensive lower extremity trauma, and prolonged immobilization. The indications for IVC filter placement are no different if the IVC filter is placed in the OR or interventional radiology suite. The secondary benefits of bedside IVC filter insertion include avoiding the hazards of intrahospital transport as well as cost-effectiveness due to less resource use.[19]

Procedure Options, Contraindications, and Preparation

All patients should have an initial duplex ultrasound of both lower extremities to confirm femoral vein patency and the presence or absence of DVT. This will help to determine the proper access site. Preoperative antibiotics are not routinely indicated. Bedside IVC filter placement can be done with either ultrasound or fluoroscopic assistance. Portable fluoroscopy is very difficult at the bedside and most SICUs are not equipped for the radiation exposure. Therefore, ultrasound-assisted bedside IVC filter placement is more easily performed. An absolute contraindication is inability to visualize the renal veins as well as IVC size greater than 2.8 cm. The right groin is the preferred site for insertion due to the ease of cannulation.

Technique

The IVC and the right renal vein are imaged first. The diameter of the IVC was measured, and ensured that the maximal size limitation of 2.8 cm was not exceeded. After cannulation of the femoral vessel, a guidewire is placed with ultrasound guidance. The dilator-introducing system is then placed with the aid of ultrasound, and the guidewire and dilator are then removed. The tip of the IVC filter is deployed caudal to the confluence of the IVC and the right renal vein. After deployment, the sheath is removed and digital pressure is placed at the puncture site.

Mortality, Morbidity, and Complications Management

Failure of bedside placement is a common complication. Placement may fail if the renal vein is inadequately visualized, which may occur due to morbid obesity or intraluminal bowel gas. Inexperience recognizing landmarks can lead to delay in placement. Another common complication is bleeding at the placement site. To avoid this complication, adequate digital pressure should be applied. There is 5% incidence of filter tilting, either at the time of placement or over a follow-up period.[20] The change in position may be due to migration of the filter or fracture of a strut. Penetration of the IVC can occur during any step of insertion and its incidence is 0.1%–9%.[20]

Insertion site complications include local thrombosis of the femoral vessel, arterial-venous fistula, and pseudoaneurysm formation.[20] Long-term caval thrombosis is reported in 3%–9% of IVC filter placements. The incidence of PE with an IVC filter in position has been reported to occur in 0.1%–10% of patients.[20]

Diagnostic Peritoneal Lavage and Laparoscopy

Diagnosis of intra-abdominal injury in critically ill patients is a challenge. Diagnostic peritoneal lavage (DPL) is useful in detecting intra-abdominal injuries in trauma patients. While the use of DPL occurs primarily in the emergency room, the technique does a have a role in the ICU as well. DPL can provide cell counts and Gram stains of the fluid effluent. Similarly, laparoscopy allows for the direct intra-abdominal visualization of pathology, which is more specific in determining the etiology of the injury. Often these unstable critically ill patients cannot be transported to CT scan, and diagnostic plain radiographs are often not helpful. The importance of diagnosing intra-abdominal injuries in critically ill patients can be overstated since the mortality of missed injuries exceeds 25%.[21] The intent is to avoid a nontherapeutic laparotomy in a critically ill patient with no intra-abdominal cause for the patient's acidosis, sepsis, or clinical deterioration.

Indications

Diagnostic peritoneal lavage is used in hemodynamically unstable patients in whom clinical examination of the abdomen is unreliable due to intoxication, spinal cord injury, traumatic brain injury, or multiple associated injuries. Both DPL and bedside laparoscopy may be used in SICU patients who have clinical deterioration after an initial diagnostic evaluation with either no CT scan or an equivocal initial CT scan result as well as in patients with multiple organ failure and sepsis with no clear etiology.

Procedure Options, Contraindications, and Preparation

Both DPL and laparoscopy are diagnostic options. DPL is accurate in diagnosing the presence of bleeding and peritonitis. It can also be completed in less than 15 minutes, and results are obtained from the laboratory rather quickly. The disadvantage of DPL is its lack of specificity. Laparoscopy has the advantage of directly visualizing the peritoneal cavity and diagnosing intra-abdominal pathology. Its disadvantages include the transport of the equipment to the SICU as well as the use of pneumoperitoneum. The brevity of the procedure should result in minimal hemodynamic instability related to the pneumoperitoneum. Also, significant respiratory acidosis and hypercarbia can occur in these patients. Hypercarbia occurs due to the peritoneal absorption of CO_2. Changes in airway pressures directly correlate with intra-abdominal pressures and should encourage low-pressure insufflation for the procedure.

Relative contraindications to both DPL and laparoscopy include the presence of abdominal scars from previous surgery, advanced pregnancy, and pelvic fracture with suspicion of a large pelvic hematoma. These relative contraindications can be surpassed if the incision is moved to a supraumbilical location. Prior to performing a DPL or laparoscopy, the stomach and the bladder should be empty, and most patients in the SICU have a Foley catheter and naso- or oro-gastric tube for decompression.

Technique

After preparation of the skin, an incision is made and dissection proceeds through the anterior and posterior fascia until the peritoneum is encountered. Under direct visualization, the peritoneal cavity is entered, the catheter is placed toward the pelvis, and an initial aspiration is performed. If no fluid is encountered, 1000 ml of lactated Ringer's are instilled into the peritoneal cavity, and then the bag of fluid is placed on the floor and through passive drainage the saline instilled is recovered in the crystalloid bag.

The results of DPL are considered positive in blunt trauma if gross blood is found on aspiration; there are more than 100,000 red blood cells/ml; there are more than 500 white blood cells/ml; amylase, urea, or bilirubin levels are higher than that of blood; and/or food particles or feces are encountered. For penetrating trauma, the threshold for the red blood cell count is lowered to 1000–10,000 cells/ml. DPL is a sensitive technique for the presence of blood, and as little as 50 ml of blood will cause the red blood cell count to be more than 100,000 cells/ml.

A 10–11-mm trochar is placed in the infra- or supra-umbilical position. The abdomen is insufflated with CO_2 to 15 mm Hg. A camera is then introduced through this trochar. Additional 5-mm trochars are placed under direct visualization in the location needed to completely visualize the stomach, small intestine, colon, gallbladder, liver, spleen, and bladder. Other procedure options include the use of a 3.3- or 5-mm laparoscope if available.

Mortality, Morbidity, and Complications Management

The most worrisome complication for both DPL and laparoscopy is injury to the underlying viscera. Although the incidence of this complication is only 1%–2%, this complication is easily avoided by use of the open technique. Proponents of the closed technique cite a shorter procedure time as its greatest advantage. Another potential complication of DPL is the subcutaneous placement of the DPL catheter, which may provide a false negative result. While no deaths have been reported during these bedside procedures, this high-risk group is difficult to compare.

Intra-Abdominal Pressure Monitoring, Decompressive Laparotomy, and the Open Abdomen

Abdominal compartment syndrome following major trauma is usually due to significant intra-abdominal swelling secondary to extensive abdominal or pelvic injuries, prolonged shock, or massive resuscitation. The elevated pressure within the abdominal cavity limits regional circulation resulting in poor tissue and intra-abdominal organ perfusion, ischemia, and ultimately death. The incidence of abdominal compartment syndrome is on the rise due to increased awareness and recognition of its existence, more aggressive fluid resuscitation, the use of damage control surgery, and improved trauma systems leading to prolonged survival of severely injured patients.

Intra-abdominal pressure of less than 10 cm of water is considered normal. Pressures in the 10–20 cm of water are considered abnormal but do not require intervention. Abdominal pressures in excess of 20 cm of water require intervention. Intra-abdominal hypertension results in a series of clinical signs such as a distended abdomen, elevated peak airway pressure, decreased urine output, and hemodynamic instability. Intra-abdominal hypertension affects multiple organ systems including the cardiac, respiratory, renal, and abdominal visceral system, and its early diagnosis is important in the prevention of multiple organ failure. When the diagnosis is suspected, objective measurement of the intra-abdominal pressure is essential.

Indications

Currently indirect measurements of intra-abdominal pressure are performed. This assessment can be performed by assessing gastric or urinary bladder pressure. Less is currently known about the value of rectal pressure. Measurement of intra-abdominal pressure is critical when the diagnosis of abdominal compartment syndrome is suspected or cannot be excluded. In addition, it is recommended in postoperative patients with a tense abdomen and/or signs of organ failure.

Decompressive laparotomy is indicated in patients with elevated intra-abdominal pressures of 25–35 cm of water and signs of compromised organ function, such as oliguria, hypoxemia with elevated peak airway pressure, or hemodynamic instability. Emergent decompressive laparotomy is indicated with intra-abdominal pressures exceeding 35 cm of water due to risk of severe hemodynamic compromise. Decompressive laparotomy is an emergency procedure, and is the only current treatment for abdominal compartment syndrome. It can easily be performed in the SICU, which is often the case because the patient is too critical to be safely transported to the OR.

Procedure Options, Contraindications, and Preparation

The options for intra-abdominal pressure measurement include the direct measurement of pressure in the inferior vena cava. This method is invasive and not currently recommended because of the risk of complications. Indirect measurement of intra-abdominal pressure can be performed via the stomach or the urinary bladder.

Technique

Gastric intra-abdominal pressure can be transmitted to the stomach when it is partially filled. The patient is placed in a supine position, and then 50–100 ml of saline is infused via a nasogastric tube to fill the stomach. A pressure transducer, calibrated at the midaxillary line, is used to measure the pressure at the end of expiration. A ruler can also be used to measure the height of the column of fluid in the NG tube.

Urinary bladder pressures are the preferred and most commonly performed measurement. There are two techniques. The standard technique involves emptying the bladder and placing the patient in a supine position. The Foley is then double-clamped and 50–100 ml of saline are infused into the bladder via the aspiration port. A transducer attached to an 18-gauge needle is set to zero at the level of the symphysis pubis and then inserted into the aspiration port to measure bladder pressure. The U-tube technique involves raising the Foley catheter above the patient, allowing for a U-shaped loop to develop, and then measuring the height of the urine column from the symphysis pubis to the meniscus. The main advantage of this technique is that it does not require violation of the Foley catheter continuity, which can increase the risk of infection; however, the pressure measurement is less accurate.

Decompressive laparotomy is performed with a midline incision and opening of the peritoneal cavity. Temporary abdominal closure of the open abdomen is done with the use of the Bogota bag or prosthetic mesh. Continued urinary bladder pressure measurement should be performed with an open abdomen.

Mortality, Morbidity, and Complications Management

Although complications related to this procedure are rare, there are pitfalls worth noting. Falsely elevated intra-abdominal pressures occur in agitated or straining patients. Measurements are most accurate in sedated or chemically paralyzed patients. Abnormal values may occur in patients who are not supine, or if a transducer is not set to zero at the symphysis pubis.

Management of Extremity Trauma and Vascular Injuries

Additionally, traumatic injuries to the extremity have been rarely managed at the bedside in the SICU. These procedures include washout of open fractures, beside placement of external fixators, fasciotomies, open amputations, and placement of vascular shunts for limb salvage. The need for these procedures in unstable trauma patients, often with severe respiratory failure, may justify the risk:benefit ratio of performing these procedures at the bedside. Open-fracture washouts can be performed with pulse lavage and dressings. The performance of external fixation is done with the use of a portable C-arm.

Just as in the abdominal compartment syndrome, extremity compartment is a surgical emergency. In an unstable critically ill patient, extremity fasciotomies may be performed at the bedside with the use of a Bovie electrocautery and Metzenbaum scissors, which are not that dissimilar from bedside escharotomies in the burn patient. While the placement of extremity vascular shunts can be the most technically challenging of these procedures, it is often done as an exhaustive attempt at limb salvage.

CONCLUSIONS

The development of guidelines for performance of bedside surgery is currently in evolution. Performance of these surgical procedures by the surgeon intensivist is safe because of their awareness of need for these procedures as well as the physiologic effects on these critical patients. Complication rates of "road trips" for critically ill patients from the ICU to other parts of the hospital (i.e., radiology department or OR) can result in a mishap rate of 5%–30%.[19] These factors have made it easy to "bring the procedure to the patient," which is particularly advantageous in critically ill ICU patients.

REFERENCES

1. Sluys K, Haggmark T, Iselius L: Outcome and quality of life 5 years after major trauma. *J Trauma* 59:223–232, 2005.
2. Shoemaker WC, Velmahos GC, Demetriades D, editors: *Procedures and Monitoring in the Critically Ill.* Philadelphia, WB Saunders, 2002.
3. Dulguerov P, Gysin C, Perneger TV, et al: Percutaneous or surgical tracheostomy: a meta-analysis. *Crit Care Med* 27:1617–1625, 1999.
4. Feller-Kopman D: Acute complications of artificial airways. *Clin Chest Med* 24:445–455, 2003.
5. Freeman BD, Isabella K, Lin N, et al: A meta-analysis of prospective trials comparing percutaneous and surgical tracheostomy in critically ill patients. *Chest* 118:1412–1418, 2000.
6. Deitch EA: Bacterial translocation or lymphatic drainage of toxic products from the gut: what is important in human beings? *Surgery* 131:241–244, 2002.
7. Gauderer MWL, Ponsky JL, Izant RJ Jr: Gastrostomy without laparotomy: a percutaneous endoscopic technique. *J Pediatr Surg* 15:872, 1980.
8. Crookes P: Percutaneous feeding catheters.
9. Ponsky JL, Gauderer MWL: Percutaneous endoscopic gastrostomy: a nonoperative technique for feeding gastrostomy. *Gastrointest Endosc* 27:9, 1981.
10. Ponsky JL, Gauderer MWL, Stellato TA, et al: Percutaneous approached to enteral alimentation. *Am J Surg* 149:102, 1985.
11. Foutch PG, Haynes WC, Bellapravalu S, Sankowski RA: Percutaneous endoscopic gastrostomy (PEG). A new procedure comes of age. *J Clin Gastroenterol* 8:10, 1984.
12. Larson DE, Burton DD, Schroeder KW, Dimagno EP: Percutaneous endoscopic gastrostomy. *Gastroenterology* 93:4852, 1987.
13. Jones SK, Neimark S, Panwalker AP: Effect of antibiotic prophylaxis in percutaneous endoscopic gastrostomy. *Am J Gastroenterol* 80:438–441, 1985.
14. Venu RP, Brown RD, Pastika BJ, Erickson LW Jr: The buried bumper syndrome: a simple management approach in two patients. *Gastrointest Endosc* 56:582–584, 2002.
15. Rodrigues JL, Lopez JM, Proctor MC, et al: Early placement of prophylactic vena caval filters in injured patients at high risk for pulmonary embolism. *J Trauma* 40:797–804, 1996.
16. Khansarinia S, Dennis JW, Veldenz HC, et al: Prophylactic Greenfield filter placement in selected high-risk patients at high for pulmonary embolism. *J Trauma* 22:231–236, 1995.
17. Rogers FB, Shackford SR, Ricci MA, et al: Routine prophylactic vena cava filter insertion in severely injured trauma patients decreases the incidence of pulmonary embolism. *J Am Coll Surg* 180:641–647, 1995.
18. Ebaugh JL, Chiou AC, Morasch MD, et al: Bedside vena cava filter placement with intravascular ultrasound. *J Vasc Surg* 34:21–26, 2001.
19. Sing RF, Jacobs DG, Heniford BT: Bedside insertion of inferior vena cava filters in the intensive care unit. *J Am Coll Surg* 192:570–576, 2001.
20. Rowe VL, Hood DB: Inferior vena caval filter placement. In Shoemaker WC, Velmahos GC, Demetriades D, editors: *Procedures and Monitoring in the Critically Ill.* Philadelphia, WB Saunders, 2001.
21. Walsh RM, Popovich MJ, Hoadley J: Bedside diagnostic laparoscopy and peritoneal lavage in the intensive care unit. *Surg Endosc* 12:1405–1409, 1998.

ANESTHESIA IN THE SURGICAL INTENSIVE CARE UNIT—BEYOND THE AIRWAY: NEUROMUSCULAR PARALYSIS AND PAIN MANAGEMENT

Michael Andreae,   Jay Berger,   Ricardo Verdiner, and   Ellise Delphin

MUSCLE RELAXANTS

Historic Perspective

One of the first documented uses of a neuromuscular blocking agent (NMBA) to aid in surgical closure of the abdomen occurred in 1912 in Germany.[1] In the 1940s, the use of NMBAs during surgery started to become commonplace. Since the 1940s, the safety profile of NMBAs has significantly improved, and their use in the operating room (OR) has become routine. The introduction of mechanical ventilation in the intensive care unit (ICU) was closely followed by the use of NMBAs in the ICU. Most of our clinical experience with the use of NMBAs comes from the care of relatively healthy patients for a finite period of time in the OR. In contrast to patients in the OR, patients in the ICU are typically critically ill with multiple organ systems failing, require prolonged neuromuscular paralysis, and are receiving a large number of concomitant medications. Clinical studies have only recently started to examine indications for and complications of NMBAs in the ICU.

Current Epidemiology

Retrospective surveys reported by intensivists in 1991 and 1992 revealed that 10 patients per ICU per month required prolonged neuromuscular blockade.[2] However, a study by Murray et al.[3] in 1993 showed the probability of receiving a NMBA ranged from 0% in the neurosurgical ICU to 14% in the neonatal ICU. Several different situations have been identified that require short- or long-term neuromuscular paralysis.

Indications

Despite adequate sedation, some patients will not be able to tolerate mechanical ventilation, which can lead to unsafe peak inspiratory airway pressures. In a retrospective survey, Klessing[4] reported that 89% of the cases requiring the use of NMBAs were related to the facilitation of mechanical ventilation, making it the most common reason for the use of neuromuscular paralysis. Other indications for NMBA use are the facilitation of endotracheal intubation, control of increased intracranial pressure (ICP), decrease of high muscle tone in certain medical conditions, and facilitation of needed medical procedures or diagnostic studies[5] (Table 1). Short-acting NMBAs such as succinylcholine can be used to quickly secure an unprotected airway. However, many critically ill patients can have an airway secured by endotracheal intubation without the use of NMBAs. In patients with increased ICP, agitation or coughing caused by tracheobronchial suctioning can cause dangerous increases in ICP. Werba et al.[6] demonstrated that pretreatment with vecuronium attenuated transient increases in ICP during suctioning.

Concerns Regarding Overuse of Paralysis

Nevertheless, a retrospective study of 514 patients with severe head injuries demonstrated that the use of NMBAs resulted in longer ICU stays and increased morbidities.[7] Symptomatic muscle rigidity found in tetanus, neuroleptic malignant syndrome, and status epilepticus can be ameliorated with NMBAs; however, treating the underlying cause of the symptoms is paramount. In addition, NMBAs can be used to facilitate minor bedside surgical procedures or diagnostic studies when immobility is critical for success, in particular in situations where adequate sedation levels to prevent movement cannot be achieved with analgesics and anesthetics alone, perhaps due to hemodynamic instability.

The long-term use of NMBAs has continued to increase over the last several years.[8] New agents with improved safety profiles have been developed. A better understanding of the differences between surgical patients who are generally in good health and the critically ill patients found in the ICU is currently under active investigation. Appropriate medication selection will require a comprehensive understanding of the pharmacodynamics and pharmacokinetics of the various NMBAs as well as the physiologic status of the patient. Adequate sedation and analgesia are paramount because these patients are unable to communicate their distress. Sedation and analgesia and their monitoring are discussed further.

Mode of Action

In general, NMBAs function by competing with acetylcholine (ACh) at the nicotinic cholinergic receptor (nAChR) at the neuromuscular motor end plate (Figure 1). NMBAs are classified as either depolarizing or nondepolarizing agents. The nondepolarizing agents are further divided into short, intermediate, and long acting, and classified according to their chemical structure as aminosteroidal or benzyl-isoquinoline compounds.[9] The ideal muscle relaxant would have rapid onset, with predictable and controllable duration of action, and lack adverse effects on hemodynamics or significant toxicity. Its elimination should be independent of liver and renal function without accumulation over time. The ideal paralytic agent would have no interactions with other medications, as well as being cost effective with a long shelf life.

Depolarizing Neuromuscular Blocking Agents

The only commercially available depolarizing NMBA is succinylcholine. Succinylcholine results in a lasting depolarization of the motor end plate, leading to an initial uncoordinated contraction of the muscle fibers, observed as "fasciculations," but preventing subsequent activation. Through the continued stimulation of the nAChRs, repolarization of the receptors and subsequent muscle contractions are inhibited.[9] The rapid onset and short duration of succinylcholine make it ideal for rapid-sequence intubations (dose 1–1.5 mg/kg IV bolus)[9] (Table 2). But the concomitant potassium release as a result of the initial depolarization can be dangerous even in normal patients with borderline elevated potassium levels, but in particular in stroke, paralysis, burn, and spinal trauma patients 24 hours after the initial insult. This is because extrajunctional ACh receptors will have developed at denervated muscle

Table 1: Indications for Use of Neuromuscular Blocking Agents in Intensive Care Unit

1. Facilitation of mechanical ventilation
2. Facilitation of endotracheal intubation
3. Control of increased intra-cranial pressure
4. Decrease high muscle tone in certain medical conditions (tinnitus)
5. Facilitation of needed medical procedures
6. Facilitation of needed diagnostic procedures

fibers; they respond to succinylcholine by opening their potassium channels. Adverse effects of succinylcholine include the previously mentioned hyperkalemia, cardiac arrhythmias (in particular, bradycardia in children), myalgias, myoglobinemia, increased ICP, intraocular and gastric pressure, allergic reaction, and prolonged paralysis in patients with acquired or genetic plasma-cholinesterase deficiencies. Succinylcholine is a triggering agent for malignant hyperthermia in susceptible patients.

Nondepolarizing Neuromuscular Blocking Agents

Unlike succinylcholine, nondepolarizing NMBAs prevent muscle contraction by competitively inhibiting the binding of ACh to nAChRs. Structurally, the nondepolarizing NMBAs are classified as aminosteroidal compounds (vecuronium and pancuronium) or as benzyl-isoquinolinium compounds (atracurium and cis-atracurium). Because of similarities in their chemical structure, various commonly used medications can imitate or alter the action of NMBAs or interfere with their elimination (see Table 2). Clinically the nondepolarizing NMBAs are classified by duration of action. ACh receptors are present in both the central nervous system (CNS) and the peripheral nervous system. Because nondepolarizing NMBAs are large charged molecules, they are unable to

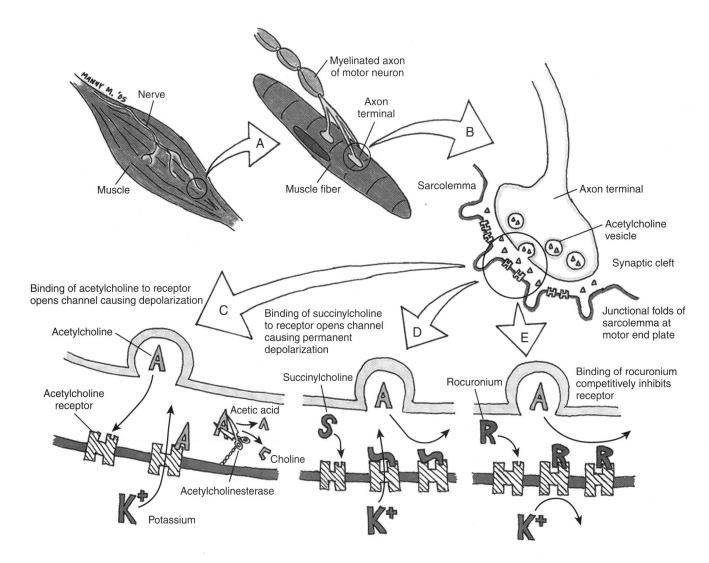

Figure 1 Neuromuscular end plate. Nerve impulse travels down the nerve (**A**) to the axon terminal (**B**), which triggers the release of ACh into the synaptic cleft (**C**). The ACh molecules traverse the synaptic cleft and bind the nicotinic ACh receptors (nAChRs), which result in a muscle contraction. When succinylcholine binds to the nAChRs (**D**) a muscle contraction results; however, succinylcholine does not readily dissociate from the receptor as ACh does. As a result, the receptors are unable to repolarize, preventing further muscle contractions. In contrast to succinylcholine, the binding of nondepolarizing muscle relaxants such as rocuronium (**E**) to the receptor does not cause a muscle contraction and blocks the binding of ACh to the receptors, preventing a muscle contraction. *ACh,* Acetylcholine.

Table 2: Drugs that Alter Neuromuscular Blocking Agent Action

Classification				Medication		
	Succinylcholine	Pancuronium	Doxacurium	Vecuronium	Atracurium	Cis-atracurium
Mechanism	Depolarizing	Nondepolarizing	Nondepolarizing	Nondepolarizing	Nondepolarizing	Nondepolarizing
Structure	Acetylcholine homolog	Aminosteroidal	Benzyl iso-quinolinium	Aminosteroidal	Benzyl isoquino-linium	Benzyl isoquino-linium
Duration		Long	Long	Intermediate	Intermediate	Intermediate
Initial intravenous dose (mg/kg)	0.6–1.5	0.04–0.1	0.1	0.08–0.1	0.4–0.5	0.15–0.2
Onset	0.5–1 minutes	3–5 minutes	4–6 minutes	3–4 minutes	3–4 minutes	3–4 minutes
Duration	6–10 minutes	90–100 minutes	60–90 minutes	34–45 minutes	25–35 minutes	20 minutes
Supplemental doses	N/A	0.01 mg/kg q 25–60 minutes	N/A	0.01–0.015 mg/kg q 12–15 minutes	0.08–0.1 mg/kg q 15–25 minutes	0.03 mg/kg
Infusion rate	0.5–10 mg/min			1 mcg/kg/min	5–9 mcg/kg/min	1–3 mcg/kg/min
Active metabolites		Yes		Yes	No	No
Toxic metabolites					Possible	Possible

N/A, Not available.

cross the brain–blood barrier into the CNS or enter across the placenta into the fetal circulation. Hence, ACh binds to receptors in the nerve ganglia and at the neuromuscular junction. NMBAs bind preferentially to the ACh receptor in the neuromuscular junction, but minimal interactions with the ACh receptors found at the autonomic ganglia help explain some side effects like the mild tachycardia observed with vecuronium and pancuronium or the bradycardia associated with the use of succinylcholine.

Pancuronium

Pancuronium (Pavulon®) is the principal long-acting aminosteroidal nondepolarizing NMBA used in the ICU. The chief advantages of pancuronium are its relatively low cost per dose and its comparatively long duration of action allowing for intermittent bolus dosing.[8] Pancuronium is partially metabolized in the liver and excreted as the parent compound or as a metabolite by the kidneys. Significant renal or hepatic dysfunction may lead to prolonged paralysis. Other complications of pancuronium result from its vagolytic effect, which can result in tachycardia and hypertension.[9]

Doxacurium

Doxacurium (Nuromax®) is a relatively new long-acting benzyl-iso-quinoline compound that causes little to no histamine release or cardiovascular side effects. In addition, duration of effect does not seem to accumulate with repeated dosing. Elimination appears to be independent of renal function.[10]

Vecuronium

Vecuronium (Norcuron®) is an intermediate-acting aminosteroid NMBA that is structurally related to pancuronium. The loss of a methyl group considerably decreases its vagolytic effect. Vecuronium is metabolized by the liver with three known metabolites retaining paralytic activity. The parent compound and its metabolites are ex-creted by the kidneys. Vecuronium can be administered either as intermittent IV boluses or as a continuous infusion.[9]

Atracurium

Atracurium (Tacrium®) and its isomer cis-atracurium (Nimbex®) are benzyl-isoquinolinium NMBAs. The advantage of these compounds is their elimination via Hoffmann degradation independent of both hepatic and renal function. Essentially, the drug spontaneously disintegrates in the warm physiochemical environment of blood (hence, unlike other NMBAs, atracurium needs to be cooled for storage). A metabolite common to both compounds is laudanosine, which in vitro has been shown to cause seizures. However, there are currently no documented occurrences of a seizure in a human receiving either of these medications. Cis-atracurium is the cis-isomer of atracurium[9] and as a result lacks the histamine release, the major side effect of atracurium. Both compounds can be administered as intermittent boluses or as a continuous infusion.

Summary

In our institution, the most frequent neuromuscular blocker used in the surgical ICU is cis-atracurium because of its independence of renal and hepatic function for elimination and the lack of hemodynamic effects, even though a more individualized selection of an appropriate alternative agent might be more cost effective in many of our patients.

Monitoring of Neuromuscular Blockade

The primary use of NMBAs in the ICU is to facilitate mechanical ventilation.[4] The degree of neuromuscular blockade required to reach this clinical goal will vary from patient to patient. The first set of guidelines detailing the use of NMBAs in the ICU was published in 1995 and later reevaluated in 2002. The current guidelines state that any patient receiving a NMBA should be assessed both clinically and by train-of-four (TOF) monitoring, with the clinical goal of NMBA titration to one or two twitches.[11] Daily clinical assessment involves the observation of skeletal muscle movement and respiratory effort by the patient. Peripheral nerve stimulation by four equal electrical charges delivered at 0.5-second intervals can be evaluated with visual, tactile, or mechanical means (Figure 2). The TOF count is the observed number of twitches out of four. A TOF count of one out of four signifies that 90%–95% of the nAChRs are occupied. A TOF count of three out of four signifies that 75%–80% of the nAChRs are occupied. At 50% occupancy of the nAChRs, the patient can be safely extubated.[12] This translates clinically to a sustained head lift for 10 seconds or to a train of four of four plus sustained tetanus to a 5-second stimulation with 100 Hz. Complete resolution of neuromuscular blockade is important not only to ensure adequate respiratory muscle power to sustain the work of breathing without ventilator support, but even more for the patient to protect the airway by unimpaired activity the bulbar muscles. Ulnar nerve innervation of the adductor pollicis muscle of the thumb is the most frequently used site to monitor TOF. The electrical stimulus should flow through the nerve, reach the neuromuscular junction, and release ACh, leading to a muscle contraction. If the electrodes are too close to the muscle tested, the current may directly cause a false-positive contraction. Hence any nerve/muscle pair that is at a certain distance apart can be used, such as the facialis/orbicularis oculi or the peroneus nerve/tibialis anterior. The monitoring of the degree of neuromuscular blockade may allow for the lowest NMBA dose and may minimize the adverse effects of prolonged NMBA use.[11]

Complications of Prolonged Neuromuscular Blockade

Complications related to the prolonged use of NMBAs include prolonged recovery from NMBAs, critical illness myopathy, and critical illness polyneuropathy.[11] Prolonged recovery from NMBAs is defined as the time to recovery requiring 50%–100% more than predicted by pharmacologic parameters, and is most likely due to the accumulation of NMBAs or their metabolites (American Society of Anesthesiologists [ASA] guidelines). As detailed previously, the steroid-based NMBAs undergo hepatic metabolism yielding active metabolites. Interaction of the NMBAs or their metabolites with other concurrent medications may also explain the prolonged blockade (see Table 1).

Critical Illness Myopathy

Critical illness myopathy (CIM), also referred to as acute myopathy of intensive care and acute quadriplegic myopathy, is believed to be an acute primary myopathy. This myopathy results in diffuse weakness or flaccid paralysis with distal and proximal muscle groups equally affected. The muscle weakness persists long after the discontinuation of the NMBA and the elimination of the NMBA and its metabolites. The respiratory muscles are commonly involved, which prevents weaning from the ventilator.[13] The majority of patients recover within 4 months; however, permanent neurologic deficits have been reported.[14] An association of concurrent administration of NMBAs and corticosteroids with CIM exists.[15–18] In addition, the prolonged use of both NMBAs and corticosteroids beyond 1–2 days increases the risk of myopathy (ASA guidelines). The ASA guidelines on the use of NMBAs in the ICU recommend that for patients receiving both NMBAs and corticosteroids, every effort should be made to discontinue the NMBAs as quickly as possible. The use of drug holidays may decrease the incidence of CIM.[11]

Critical Illness Polyneuropathy

Critical illness polyneuropathy (CIP) occurs due to diffuse axonal polyneuropathy. The mechanism is thought to involve impaired peripheral nerve perfusion, which leads to microvascular ischemia of the nerve.[11,19] The electroneurographic pattern demonstrates a decrease in the amplitude of the nerve action potential with preserved normal conduction velocities. This condition is contrasted with Guillain-Barre syndrome (GBS), demyelinating polyradiculoneuritis, in which the amplitude of the nerve action potential is preserved and the conduction velocity is decreased.[20] The occurrence of both CIP and CIM in critically ill patients is high; however, the occurrence of CIP has not been associated with the use of NMBAs (Table 3).

Functional Defects of Neuromuscular Junction

A last potential cause of motor dysfunction in ICU patients could be due to alterations in the neuromuscular junction. Conditions such as spinal cord injuries, cerebral vascular accidents, burns, crush injuries, and immobilization result in increased expression of abnormal

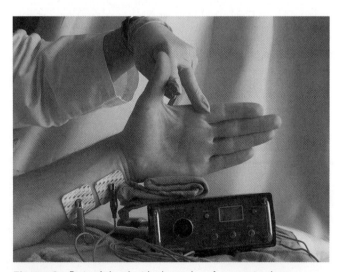

Figure 2 Patient's hand with electrodes of nerve stimulator attached on volar side of forearm over the ulnar nerve. After stimulation of the ulnar nerve, the gloved hand of the medical practitioner senses the adduction of the thumb to the index. This is the response of interest to monitor the neuromuscular junction. Caution: the flexors of the hand often contract in response to direct stimulation of the muscles, even in the presence of neuromuscular blockers.

Table 3: Risk Factors for Critical Illness Myopathy and Polyneuropathy

Sepsis
Multiorgan dysfunction syndrome
Multiorgan failure
Female gender
Corticosteroid use
Severe asthma
Electrolyte abnormalities
Malnutrition
Immobility

Adapted from Latronico N, et al: Critical illness myopathy and neuropathy. *Curr Opin Crit Care* 11(2):126–132, 2005.

nAChRs. These abnormal receptors are more sensitive to depolarizing NMBAs (succinylcholine) and more resistant to nondepolarizing NMBAs.[21] The infusion of subparalytic doses of NMBAs has been shown to increase the expression of nAChRs in the absence of immobilization.[22]

SEDATION AND ANALGESIA IN CRITICAL CARE SETTING

Analgesic Agents and Their Advantages

Morphine and fentanyl are the most widely used and appropriate opioid analgesics for use in the critical care setting (Table 4). Both are cleared by the liver. Although morphine is less costly, it has an active metabolite, morphine-6-glucoronide, that is renally excreted and can hence accumulate leading to renal failure. Fentanyl is eliminated by the liver only, and hence is safe even for long infusions in renal failure. Fentanyl, being very lipophilic, also has a more rapid onset compared to morphine, making it very suitable for the titration of acute pain at the bedside. Caution is warranted, however, as its rapid offset after a single dose is due to redistribution, not metabolism: This means that a few single small dose of fentanyl will only last for about 30 minutes, but with a continuous infusion fentanyl will behave similarly to other long acting narcotics like morphine and may take several hours to wear off. Hydromorphine may be preferable in patients with hemodynamic compromise, because of morphine's potential for histamine release or preload reduction. Meperidine and the mixed agonist/antagonist opioids should be avoided. The former because of its renally cleared proconvulsant metabolite, normeperidine. The latter because they can precipitate withdrawal in opioid habituated patients.

Indications and Patient-Controlled Analgesia

Narcotics are indicated for pain relief and their beneficial or adverse side effects include sedation, depression of respiratory drive, and euphoria. Patient-controlled analgesia (PCA) is superior in pain control and reduces both side effects and total medication administered, because the patient can administer only the pain medication needed. Two features limit the risk of patient overdose: the PCA device lockout is set to the time of peak effect of the drug chosen (at least 10 minutes for morphine, and at least 2 minutes for fentanyl), so the patient will experience the full drug effect, before being able to initiate a second dose. And obviously, an oversedated patient can no longer trigger the device. However, this limits the use of PCA to patients who can cooperate. While in chronic opioid users, converting regular (methadone) use to a baseline infusion may be a good idea, anesthesiologists normally advise against the use of a baseline background infusion in a PCA, because the pain will gradually wane (reducing the need for analgesia), while the background infusion is constant, and in the heat of action the junior staff may omit adjusting it. This would lead to gradual overdose and could result in severe respiratory depression and even death. Patients generally prefer PCA because they feel that they are in control.

Nonopioid Analgesics

Nonsteroidal anti-inflammatory drugs (NSAIDs), namely aspirin and the only intravenous NSAID ketorolac, are potent analgesics, lacking some negative side effects of narcotics such as respiratory depression, gut immobilization, and sedation. Wherever possible they are preferred over opioid analgesics. However, most of these compounds interfere with platelet function, they tilt the balance against gastric mucosal integrity, and some orthopedists fault them for interfering with bone growth. Also, prostaglandins are contraindicated in renal dysfunction, in particular in fluid under resuscitation and reduced perfusion states.

Ketamine, a phencyclidine derivative and NMDA antagonist, has many negative side effects, including delirium; increases in heart rate and in blood pressure and ICP, hypersalivation, and airway secretions, among others. Its primary use for analgesia and sedation is not recommended in national guidelines. However because of its short-acting potent analgesic properties, while lacking the respiratory depression of its opioid equivalent, it may be used in small boluses (0.5–1 mg/kg IV) in limited but painful procedures, such as dressing changes for burns, and always in conjunction with an anxiolytic or hypnotic.

Epidural and Regional Analgesia

To administer analgesics only where the pain originates makes intuitive sense. Besides, local anesthetics lack the respiratory and sedative side effects of their narcotic counterparts. By blocking the conduction of nerves reporting the nociception to the CNS, superior analgesia can be achieved (Figure 3). Limitations are the need for expertise in performing regional blocks or epidural anesthesia. Currently, duration of action of local anesthetic agents is only a matter of hours, making repeated blocks necessary. While longer-acting agents in depot formulations are on the horizon, they are not yet clinically available. Leaving catheters in place for continuous infusions may work well, but is fraught with infectious risks, particularly in septic patients. In addition, in the current

Table 4: Comparison of Typical Opioid Analgesic Agents Used in the Intensive Care Unit

	Single Dose/Patient-Controlled Analgesia Bolus	Continuous Infusion	Comments
Fentanyl (short acting)	25–100 mcg	1 mcg/kg/hr	Continuous infusion leads to a longer (morphine-like) duration of action.
Morphine (longer acting)	1–10 mg	1–5 mg/hr	Morphine-6-glucoronide is an active metabolite and can accumulate in renal failure.
Hydromorphone	0.5–1 mg	0.5–2 mg/hr	Less hemodynamic side effects compared to morphine.

Although less costly, morphine has an active metabolite, morphine-6-glucoronide, that is renally excreted, which can accumulate leading to renal failure. Caution is warranted with fentanyl's kinetics, as its rapid offset after a single dose is due to redistribution, not metabolism. This means that a few single small doses of fentanyl will only last for about 30 minutes, while a continuous infusion will behave similarly to other long-acting narcotics (e.g., morphine) and may take several hours to wear off.

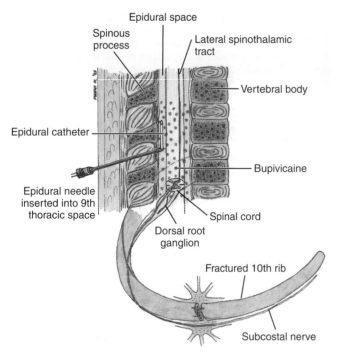

Figure 3   Placement of thoracic epidural catheter. Tip of Tuohy needle is introduced into the epidural space. Once the location of the tip is confirmed by loss of resistance of either water or air, the epidural catheter is advanced into position as shown. Through the catheter the epidural space is infused with local anesthetics that will bathe the spinal nerve roots, blocking the transmission of pain via the lateral spinothalamic tract.

litigious climate many anesthesiologists are wary about performing procedures on sedated or unconscious patients who cannot give feedback during block performance. Many critically ill patients are anticoagulated or coagulopathic. In particular, in the tight epidural space a hematoma can have devastating neurological outcomes. Hence, epidural and regional blocks and catheters can only be placed in time windows when the benefits outweigh the bleeding risk or when the anticoagulation is held for a few hours. Once the catheter is in place, prophylactic anticoagulation may be resumed, and indeed may even become superfluous. This is because epidural anesthesia has intrinsic antithrombotic effects

by its action on the autonomic system (and consequently blood flow), and because regional anesthesia may significantly enhance patient mobilization. In particular, for the pain of rib fractures and thoracotomies, the superior epidural analgesia in the absence of respiratory depression will convey a significant survival benefit in the elderly critically ill and in patients with respiratory comorbidities like chronic obstructive lung disease or pulmonary fibrosis.

Sedatives

Benzodiazepines and propofol have anxiolytic, sedative, and anticonvulsive properties, but *no* analgesic properties. Indeed, good pain control will significantly reduce, if not eliminate, the need for sedation. The sedative agent is chosen based on the clinical need for short-term reversible or prolonged sedation, taking into account comorbidities such as renal failure that might prolong the agent's duration of action (Table 5).

If there is a need for frequent neurological assessment and swift titration of sedation in intubated patients, propofol is a good choice. Typical doses range from 30 mcg/kg/hr for sedation to 120 mcg/kg/hr for general anesthesia and very invasive procedures (calculations are based on lean body weight). Propofol reduces preload and afterload and can lead to hemodynamic compromise, in particular in under-resuscitated patients or in those with septic shock. While infusions over hours and days can lead to slower recovery because of the accumulation of propofol in fat tissue, its elimination in renal or hepatic failure is not reduced. Propofol is unsafe in patients without a secured airway, except under constant observation by personnel experienced with the drug and airway management, because propofol can lead to rapid respiratory depression and airway obstruction. Propofol's lipid carrier emulsion is similar to the lipid component of total parenteral nutrition. As such, it supports bacterial growth, has similar effects on the liver and pancreas, and needs to be factored in for nutritional assessments.

Midazolam is favored for short-term sedation. But, particularly in the context of renal failure, the active metabolite 1-hydroxymidazolam can accumulate. In contrast, lorazepam has less potential for accumulation and a faster recovery profile after longer infusions, but also slower onset. Lorazepam is also the cheapest of the most frequently used sedatives. Consequently, a lorazepam drip and subsequent dose increases are best initiated with a bolus, such as 2 mg. A bolus helps prevent oversedation by an initial rate set too high due to the delayed onset of lorazepam. All benzodiazepines can be competitively antagonized at the GABA receptor by flumazenil (0.2 mg intravenously over 15 seconds). However, flumazenil does not reverse opioid overdose, and can lower the seizure threshold.

Table 5: Sedatives for Use in the Intensive Care Unit

	Bolus Dose	Continuous Infusion	Comments
Propofol (10 mg/cc)	10–50 mg ($\approx$1–5 cc)	30–120 mcg/kg/min ($\approx$10–40 cc/hr for 70-kg patient)	Ideal titration supports bacterial growth
Midazolam	1–4 mg	1–5 mg/hr initially	Active metabolite is renally cleared
Lorazepam	0.5–2mg	1–5 mg/hr, after initial bolus	Slower offset
Haloperidol	2–5 mg	2–25 mg/hr reported	QT prolongation, extrapyramidal side effects
Dexmedetomidine	Start at 0.2 mcg/kg/hr, titrate up to 0.7 mcg/kg/hr		May continue after extubation, analgesic, bradycardia

With the exception of dexmedetomidine, all sedatives are supplemented with analgesics. Propofol is ideal for frequent neurological assessments. Dexmedetomidine can be continued through and after extubation because it lacks the respiratory depression of propofol and midazolam. Haloperidol is the drug of choice for intensive care unit psychosis.

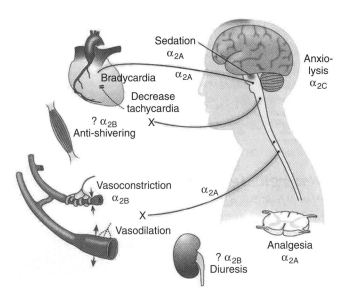

Figure 4 α_2-receptor subtypes: physiology of α_2 adrenoceptors. *(Adapted from Kamibayashi T, Maze M: Clinical uses of α_2-adrenergic agonists. Anesthesiology 93:1346, 2000.)*

mia that is triggered exclusively by succinylcholine and volatile anesthetics such as halothane.

Initial doses of haloperidol are in the order of milligrams, but because of its good safety profile and its lack of cardiovascular or respiratory depression, it can be acutely titrated on occasions to cumulative doses up to 1 mg/kg. It is also antiemetic and dissociative and may be used in conjunction with morphine for terminal sedation.

Dexmedetomidine is a new centrally active alpha-2 agonist, available for intravenous administration (Figure 4). Unlike all other sedative agents discussed previously, it has analgesic properties, yet unlike opioids it does not depress the respiratory drive. Unlike most other sedative and analgesic medications, it can be continued during trials of spontaneous ventilation and even during the actual extubation itself. Many self-extubations occur precisely when the analgesic and anxiolytic coverage is reduced to assess the patient's suitability for extubation. On the other hand, dexmedetomidine is sometimes by itself not strong enough in trauma patients to control pain, or in patients habituated to ethanol, benzodiazepine, or other recreational drugs, to achieve adequate sedation, and hence supplementation may be necessary (Figure 5). Theoretically, dexmedetomidine might be a suitable drug for analgesia and sedation by nonanesthesia personal for minor procedures in patients with an unsecured airway like dressing changes in burn patients. However, dexmedetomidine is not approved by the Food and Drug Administration (FDA) for this indication, nor can this approach be recommended as long as there is no more evidence in the literature supporting its safety profile under these circumstances. Dexmedetomidine is started as an infusion with or without initial bolus. Depending on the dose, dexmedetomidine can cause hypertension as well as hypotension, and may lead to bradycardia. The latter is often a desired effect in patients with a history of coronary artery disease, as this prolongs the time of myocardial perfusion during diastole and reduces myocardial oxygen demand, but it can reduce

Haloperidol is the drug of choice for treating ICU psychosis. It is a neuroleptic with strong antidopaminergic activity, and hence patients need to be monitored for extrapyramidal side effects, neuroleptic malignant syndrome, and QT prolongation on the electrocardiogram. Neuroleptic malignant syndrome (NMS) is a rare potentially fatal central neural disorder characterized by hyperthermia, rigidity, autonomic instability, and altered mental status, mediated by central and postganglionic dopamine agonism. NMS is different from the anesthesia-related muscular disorder malignant hyper-

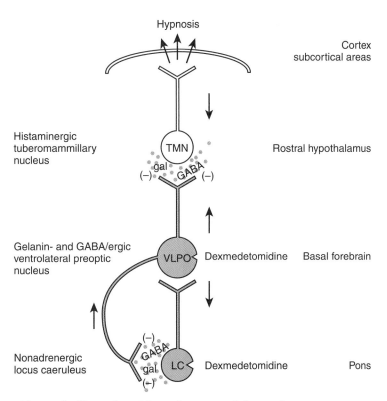

Figure 5 Dexmedetomidine activates natural sleep pathways.

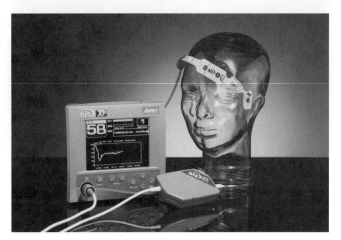

Figure 6 Bispectral index monitor.

cardiac output in patients depending on heart rate for cardiac output.

BISPECTRAL INDEX MONITORING

The bispectral index (BIS) is a neurophysiologic monitor that was designed with the intention of measuring unconsciousness under what would otherwise be an uncomfortable perioperative experience. It received FDA clearance in 1996 with studies correlating the BIS index to response to verbal command and to a lesser extent, movement upon surgical incision with various modes of anesthesia. Since then, it has become ubiquitous with prevention of perioperative awareness, and has found a niche among monitoring equipment in ORs across the country. While the popularity of this instrument has become synonymous with outpatient procedures, a new frontier has slowly developed, that is, the use of the BIS monitor in the critical care setting (Figure 6).

Although sedation monitors such as the Physiometrix PSA 4000 and Datex Entropy State are available, more studies have been focused on the Aspect Bispectral Monitor. For this reason, the subsequent discussion will primarily focus on the Aspect Bispectral Monitor.

Benefits of Bispectral Index in Critical Care Setting

Sleep disruption in critically ill patients is a well-documented phenomenon. It has been shown to increase the state of confusion, more eloquently termed ICU psychosis, in addition to contributing to respiratory dysfunction. A review by Eveloff[23] and Gabor et al.[24] concluded that sleep disruption in the ICU can cause increased respiratory muscle fatigue and decreased ventilatory responsiveness to hypercapnia, which could prolong mechanical ventilation. Another study by Rundshagen and colleagues[25] found that recall of nightmares and hallucinations in sedated and ventilated patients discharged from the ICU approached 9.3% and 6.6%, respectively. Sleep disruption with decreased slow wave patterns has also been suggested to predispose for post-traumatic stress disorder. The common element in these investigations is the value of attaining near normal sleep patterns, while preventing awareness of stressful stimuli during the ICU period, both of which could be assessed by the BIS monitor.

Minimization of drug withdrawal symptoms is another unforeseen benefit of the BIS index in the ICU. In a study by Cammarano and colleagues,[26] 9 of 28 patients mechanically ventilated for more than 7 days were found to exhibit withdrawal reactions including insomnia and sleep disturbances. This association was attributed to high-dose opioids and benzodiazepines. The implementation of sedation scores theoretically should minimize the risk of excessive doses; however, the major drawback to the traditional scoring systems is their reliance on the subjectivity of the practitioner. Several studies have shown that nurses rely on previous experiences with sedation for their population of patients, which is further complicated by a lack of scientific evidence for a particular sedative practice. In addition, most cues used by critical care nurses to judge sedation are inadequate. The importance of objective data is therefore paramount to the optimal management of sedation and convalescence in the critically ill. With the BIS monitor, an objective method for the titration of sedation transforms the realm of abstract theory to tangible and practical clinical application (Table 6).

Computing the Bispectral Index

The BIS is a single dimensionless number that incorporates information of electroencephalograph (EEG) power and frequency along with beta activation, burst suppression, and bicoherence. During sleep, a portion of the cortical EEG reflects activity in deeper structures. The bispectral analysis filters out the components of the EEG that provide information on the interaction between cortical and subcortical neural generators. The frequencies are derived from the EEG signals using a mathematical technique known as Fourier analysis. As sedation increases, more in-phase coupling occurs within signal frequencies. The degree of coupling represents bicoherence patterns. With increasing amounts of hypnotic drugs, changes in unique bicoherence patterns occur, which serve as markers for sedation level. These patterns are collected and analyzed by the monitor and compared with a database that contains a multivariate statistical model. From the comparison, the monitor assigns a number that designates a hypnotic state.

Table 6: BIS Values and EEG Patterns Correlated to Hypnotic States at Administration of Sedative Agents

Clinical State	BIS Value	EEG Pattern
Awake	100	Alpha wave predominance
Moderate hypnotic state	60	Decreased alpha / increased beta wave
Deep hypnotic state	40	Predominance of delta and theta waves
Cortical silence, coma, brain death	0	Isoelectric EEG, burst suppression

BIS, Bispectral index; *EEG,* electroencephalograph.

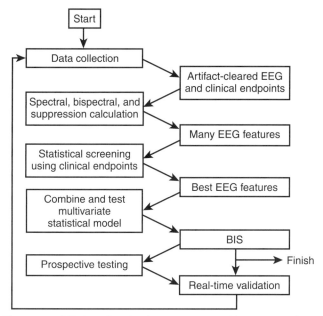

Figure 7 BIS algorithm development process. Key steps used during development phase of the BIS algorithm. The importance of statistical analysis and modeling to identify and combine key EEG parameters is noted. The circular path shows the "iterative" process by which the BIS algorithm was prospectively tuned and improved to maximize the clinical correlation of the EEG analysis. *BIS,* Bispectral index; *EEG,* electroencephalogram. *(Courtesy of Aspect Medical Systems.)*

The BIS is derived empirically based on a statistical model; it is not a physiologic parameter. It was attained by analyzing a large database of EEGs from healthy *volunteers* who had received one or more of the most commonly used hypnotic agents (Figure 7). EEG features were identified that characterized some portion of the EEG spectrum that changed as the subjects went from the awake state to anesthetized (Figure 8). Multivariate statistical models were then used to derive the optimum combination of these features, which were then transformed into a dimensionless 0–100 linear scale. Details of the algorithm and statistical model are proprietary information. However, a brief four-step model of the process is described in the following (Figure 9):

1. Data are collected and filtered.
2. EEG calculations are performed.
3. Statistical screening using clinical endpoints awake and unconscious.
4. A bispectral number is assigned using multivariate statistical modeling.

With a BIS number designation, an assessment can then be made on the hypnotic state of the patient.

Several trials were undertaken that compared the effectiveness of the BIS in measuring hypnotic drug effect. In each trial, healthy patients were given increased doses of propofol, midazolam, isoflurane, or the combinations midazolam-alfentanil, propofol-alfentanil, or propofol-nitrous oxide. The agents were increased and decreased systematically to various steady-state plasma concentrations. Clinical measurements of sedation, hypnosis, and memory were simultaneously recorded. The results supported the BIS index as a better predictor of hypnotic state compared to measured or targeted drug concentrations.

Limitations

The BIS monitor, although novel in its approach on quantifying the level of sedation, is not impervious to the setbacks of derivation and statistical models (Table 7). Namely, the instrument's ability to assess a given level of sedation is only as good as the database with which it compares the filtered EEG. Recalling the aforementioned development process, it is reasonable to presume that the differences between healthy volunteers and critically ill patients undergoing sedation may increase the margin of error, especially when considering that a portion of these patients have neurologic dysfunction or injury. Comparing these EEGs to a database of healthy patients does not seem to be an ideal scenario for assessing the hypnotic state in these patients.

Some authors have even expressed caution about using the BIS as a predictor of response. Because the BIS number is a derivation of EEG data from 15–30 seconds previously, its number reflects the state prior to the reading. Therefore, strong stimulation common during procedures in the ICU setting could lead to rapidly changing brain states. These changes can result in a response to stimulation despite a previously low BIS score.

Other authors have scrutinized the heterogeneity of the clinical endpoints and the subtleties of recall as a cause of the poor correlation between movement response and cerebrally derived parameters. The endpoints typically used include hemodynamic response to noxious stimulus, movement in response to stimulus, and response to command and recall. These endpoints are independent of one another. To add further complications, explicit (conscious) and implicit (unconscious) memory are not readily stratified on a continuum. Therefore, unconsciousness and inability to respond to commands does not equate to loss of recall.

Because BIS monitors the state of the brain and not the concentration of the drug, value ranges will vary among anesthetic regimens. This may lead, for example, to a BIS of 60 with the use of propofol having similar effects to a BIS of 40 with morphine and midazolam when assessing response to stimulation. The difference in values could lead to overestimation or underestimation in sedative dosing if the numbers were followed without taking the drug regimen into consideration.

Finally, electromyographic activity as seen in nonparalyzed sedated patients has been shown to increase BIS values. Studies have shown that BIS values in sedated patients are further decreased with the administration of muscle relaxants. One hypothesis is that the BIS inevitably interprets a portion of muscle activity as cerebral EEG activity, which causes a higher calculated number to be displayed. This is but one source of artifacts that does not include the possibility of nonphysiologic artifacts derived from lighting, pacemakers, monitors, infusion pumps, and radios. These variables contribute to what might seem an insurmountable challenge to overcoming the limitations of sedation monitoring.

Prospective Uses

The BIS monitor, an instrument designed for the quantification of sedation, has prospective uses as both an endpoint determinant of pentobarbital therapy and as a diagnostic tool. Traumatic head injury, cerebral hemorrhagic events, and neoplasms are significant causes of increased intracranial pressures. Pentobarbital-induced coma is a second-line treatment for intracranial hypertension refractory to osmotic or diuretic agents and cerebrospinal fluid drainage. Up to one-third of medical centers within the United States use barbiturates as a treatment modality for ICP. Pentobarbital-induced coma can be confirmed by an isoelectric pattern with intermittent "bursts" of activity—burst suppression—on the EEG. This pattern serves as a guide to therapy that minimizes

Awake—Low voltage–Random, fast

Drowsy–8 to 12 cps–Alpha waves

REM sleep (D sleep)–Low voltage–Random, fast

Sawtooth waves

Stage 1–3 to 7 cps–Theta waves

Theta waves

Stage 2–12 to 14 cps–Sleep spindles and K complexes

Sleep spindle

K Complex

Delta sleep (S sleep)–$\frac{1}{2}$ to 2 cps–Delta waves

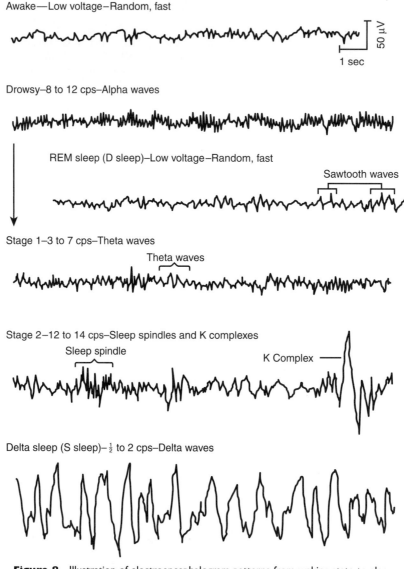

Figure 8 Illustration of electroencephalogram patterns from waking state to sleep sleep. *(Modified from Hauri P: The sleep disorders. Kalamazoo, MI, 1977.)*

barbiturate dosage and the likelihood of toxicity. The BIS monitor has the capacity to collect raw EEG data and display burst suppression ratios as a percentage of isoelectric episodes over a 63-second period. The size of the monitor and its ability to express burst suppression ratios as a numerical value make it an ideal bedside monitor in the ICU. Riker and colleagues'[27] prospective study of 12 patients comparing EEG monitoring values to BIS values found that BIS values correlated well with the standard EEG-based method used to titrate barbiturate therapy. With the BIS monitor, titration of a pentobarbital infusion could occur on a minute-to-minute basis without the use of special technicians, bulky equipment, or interpretation of the EEG by a neurologist hours later. This could significantly reduce overall cost and improve care of patients with increased ICP.

Conclusion

The BIS monitor has its limitations in terms of quantifying the hypnotic state. However, it does provide an objective method for the titration of sedation, which could lead to improved patient comfort, decreased sleep disruption, decreased withdrawal symptoms, and hopefully lower incidence of post-traumatic stress disorder. As more attention is focused on defining the endpoints to therapy, monitors that can provide insight on physiologic effect on a minute-to-minute basis will become a growing trend. Such is the case now for the BIS monitor and its potential uses as a guide to barbiturate therapy in patients with increased intracranial pressure.

SUMMARY

The care of critically ill patients in the ICU at times may require the use of NMBAs for any number of reasons. As with any medication, the risk:benefit ratio of using NMBAs must be calculated on a patient-by-patient basis. Using the lowest dose possible for the shortest time period required can minimize the complications of using NMBAs. In addition, it must be remembered that NMBAs do not provide analgesia or amnesia, and require the concurrent use of sufficient dosages of pain medication and sedation. EEG monitoring is now commercially available for assessment of adequate sedation,

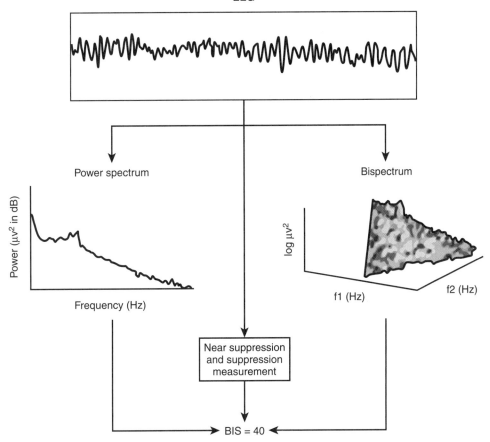

Figure 9 Schematic diagram of signal processing paths integral to generating a single BIS value. Original EEG epochs (following digitization and artifact processing) undergo three primary paths of analysis—power spectral analysis, bispectral analysis, and time-based analysis for suppression/ near-suppression—to look for key EEG features. The BIS algorithm, based on statistical modeling, combines the contribution of each of the identified features to generate the scaled BIS. *BIS,* Bispectral index; *EEG,* electroencephalogram. *(Courtesy of Aspect Medical Systems.)*

Table 7: Potential Sources of Erroneous BIS Values

Circumstance(s)	BIS Reading	Description
Electromyographic activity	Falsely increased	EMG artifact misinterpreted as cerebral activity.
Neuromuscular blockade	Falsely decreased	Removal of EMG artifact.
Electronic devices	Falsely increased	Electromagnetic fields, vibrations, and electric interference interpreted as increased cerebral activity.
Cerebral injury	Falsely decreased	Decreased cerebral perfusion, neurological damage, and abnormal mental function leads to lower EEG activity.
Alzheimer's	Falsely decreased	Decreased beta waves equate to overall decreased collection of EEG data.
Lack of stimulation	Fails to predict movement upon stimulation	BIS readings are retrospective but not predictive. They only assess adequacy of sedation at current level of stimulation.
Various combination of sedatives and opioids in critically ill patients	BIS value studied mostly for healthy volunteers, general anesthesia, and pure drug regimes	BIS values change for a given clinical endpoint depending on medication combination used.

Note: This table organizes the most common reasons for erroneous BIS-Monitor readings. Included are the potential root causes and a brief description of why they occur.

BIS, Bispectral index; *EEG,* electroencephalograph; *EMG,* electromyogram.

and also for burst suppression in pentobarbital coma, even though its use in the ICU is still being developed. Good analgesia, including regional techniques where indicated, will reduce the need for sedation and improve outcomes most if individualized and include the use of patient-controlled administration of analgesics. Adequate sedation that is adjusted with frequent patient assessment or participation and daily wake-up tests will help prevent excess morbidity from oversedation as well as recall of unpleasant experiences and post–intensive care, traumatic stress disorders.

REFERENCES

1. Lawen A: Ueber die Verbindung der Lokalanasthesie mit der Narkose, uber hohe Extraduralanasthesie and epidurale Injektionen Anasthesia render Losungen bei tabischen Magenfrisen. *Beitr Klin Chir* 80: 168–189, 1912.
2. Helliwell TR, et al: Necrotizing myopathies in critically ill patients. *J Pathol* 164:307–314, 1991.
3. Murray MJ, et al: The use of neuromuscular blocking drugs in the intensive care unit: a U.S. perspective. *Intensive Care Med*19:S40–S44, 1993.
4. Klessing HT, et al: A national survey on the practice patterns of anaesthesiologist intensivists in the use of muscle relaxants. *Crit Care Med* 20: 1341–1345, 1992.
5. Murphy GS, Vender JS: Neuromuscular-blocking drugs: use and misuse in the intensive care unit. *Crit Care Clin* 17:925–942, 2001.
6. Werba A, et al: Vecuronium prevents increases in intracranial pressure during routine tracheobronchial suctioning in neurosurgical patients. *Anaesthesist* 40:328–331, 1986.
7. Hsiang JK, et al: Early, routine paralysis for intracranial pressure control in severe head injury: is it necessary? *Crit Care Med* 22:1471–1476, 1994.
8. Ohlinger MJ, Rhoney DH: Neuromuscular blocking agents in the neurosurgical intensive care unit. *Surg Neurol* 49:217–221, 1998.
9. Stoelting RK: *Pharmacology and Physiology in Anesthetic Practice*, 3rd ed. Philadelphia, Lippincott-Raven, 1999.
10. Murray MJ, et al: Double-blind, randomized, multicenter study of doxacurium vs. pancuronium in intensive care unit patients who require neuromuscular blocking agents. *Crit Care Med* 23:450–458, 1995.
11. Murray MJ, et al: Clinical guidelines for sustained neuromuscular blockade in the adult critically ill patient. *Crit Care Med* 30:142–156, 2002.
12. Frankel H, et al: The impact of implementation of neuromuscular blockade monitoring standards in a surgical intensive care unit. *Am Surg* 62:503–506, 1996.
13. Douglass DA, et al: Myopathy in severe asthma. *Am Rev Respir Dis* 146:517–519, 1992.
14. Kordas M: The effect of procaine on neuromuscular transmission. *J Physiol* 209:689–696, 1970.
15. Road J, et al: Reversible paralysis with status asthmaticus, steroids, and pancuronium: clinical electophysiological correlates. *Muscle Nerve* 20:1587–1590, 1997.
16. David W, et al: EMG findings in acute myopathy with status asthmaticus, steroids, and patalytics: clinical and electrophysiologic correlation. *Electromyogr Clin Neurophysiol* 38:371–376, 1998.
17. Zochodne DW, et al: Acute necrotizing myopathy of intensive care: electrophysiologic studies. *Muscle Nerve* 17:285–292, 1994.
18. Marik PE: Doxacurium-corticosteroid acute myopathy: another piece to the puzzle. *Crit Care Med* 24:1266–1267, 1996.
19. Bolton CF: Sepsis and the systemic inflammatory response syndrome: neuromuscular manifestations. *Crit Care Med* 24:1408–1416, 1996.
20. Latronico N, et al: Critical illness myopathy and neuropathy. *Curr Opin Crit Care* 11:126–132, 2005.
21. Yanaz P, Martyn JAJ: Prolonged D-tubocurarine infusion and/or immobilization cause upregulation of acetylcholine receptors and hyperkalemia to succinylcholine in rats. *Anesthesiology* 84:384–391, 1996.
22. Hogue CW, et al: Tolerance and upregulation of acetylcholine receptors following chronic infusions of d-tubocurarine. *J Appl Physiol* 72: 1326–1331, 1992.
23. Eveloff SE: The disruptive ICU. An issue to lose sleep over? *Chest* 107: 809–818, 1995.
24. Gabor JY, et al: Sleep disruption in the intensive care unit. *Curr Opin Crit Care* 7:21–27, 2001.
25. Rundshagen I, et al: Incidence of recall, nightmares, and hallucinations during analgosedation in intensive care. *Intensive Care Med* 28:38–43, 2002.
26. Cammarano WB, et al: Acute withdrawal syndrome related to the administration of analgesic and sedative medications in adult intensive care unit patients. *Crit Care Med* 26:676–684, 1998.
27. Riker RR, et al: Comparing the bispectral index and suppression ratio with burst suppression of the electroencephalogram during pentobarbital infusions in adult intensive care patients. *Pharmacotherapy* 23: 1087–1093, 2003.

PALLIATIVE CARE IN THE TRAUMA INTENSIVE CARE UNIT

Anne C. Mosenthal

Despite many recent advances in trauma resuscitation and surgery, surgeons continue to care for critically injured patients who will succumb to their injuries. The mortality rate for trauma patients who require admission to the intensive care unit (ICU) remains at 10%–20%, and an additional percentage of those who survive will be significantly disabled or functionally impaired. Appropriate and compassionate care for the dying trauma patient as well as management of pain and symptoms in all critically ill patients are now part of good-quality trauma care. Aggressive pain management or comfort measures causing physiologic hemody- namic derangements or masking symptoms in the critically injured are no longer of great concern. Newer information and selection of appropriate medications now make clear that attention to pain management and comfort can be successfully provided *during* ongoing resuscitation without ill effects. The skills of the trauma surgeon encompass basic palliative care principles as they apply to the critically ill trauma patient; facility with an interdisciplinary team approach, communication of bad news, pain and symptom management, and withholding and withdrawal of life support.

▮ WHEN TO START PALLIATIVE CARE IN ICU

While mortality from injury is correlated with Injury Severity Score and increasing age, prognosis on admission to the ICU is not always clear for every patient. The majority of trauma deaths in the ICU occur in the first 48 hours secondary to traumatic brain injury or traumatic hemorrhage, while another significant proportion (20%–30%) will linger in the ICU only to die weeks later from sepsis and multiple organ failure. In the first group, catastrophic injuries have a rapid trajectory toward death, usually with prognostic certainty; here palliative care should be started early in the ICU course, shortly after admission. In this context, bereavement support and communication with the family while attending to patient care are crucial. This early support sets the stage for later decision making, minimizes conflict and has a salutary effect on family grief, bereavement, and even organ donation rates. For patients who have a protracted course and uncertain prognosis, waiting for death to be imminent before instituting palliative care means that many patients will receive end-of-life care late, have untreated suffering and symptoms, or remain on life support long after it is futile. Thus, palliative care in some form should start early in this group as well, regardless of ultimate outcome.

All trauma patients are admitted to the ICU with the hope and expectation for life-saving care, not only on the part of their families, but physicians and nurses as well. The transition in goals of care to palliative can seem daunting in the face of these hopes. This transition is best initiated on admission with a simple palliative care *assessment* for likely prognosis, even if the possible outcomes are uncertain. Assessment should include not just survival and mortality risk, but expected long-term quality of life and function. If a poor outcome is possible or expected, an interdisciplinary assessment should follow of pain and symptoms, family psychosocial needs, proxy decision makers, presence of advance directives or patient preferences regarding care, and spiritual issues (Table 1).

Table 1: Palliative Care Assessment on Admission to Trauma ICU

Pain and symptom assessment

1. Pain score_____ 2. Anxiety _____ 3. Agitation score_____
4. Dyspnea _____

Outcome and prognosis assessment

1. Is patient likely to die on this admission?
2. What is expected quality of life or functional outcome?
3. What are patient's preferences for life-sustaining therapy?
4. Is there an advance directive?

Family assessment

1. Who is patient's surrogate for medical decisions?
2. Has the health care team communicated information to family?
3. What are family support needs?

Cultural and spiritual assessment

WHAT IS PALLIATIVE CARE IN THE ICU?

Palliative care in the ICU integrates and applies the principles of shared decision making and relief of suffering to critical care practice. The family *and* the patient are the unit of care; this requires an interdisciplinary approach with team members from not only trauma surgery and critical care nursing, but pain management, social work, psychosocial support, and pastoral care. The unique nature of traumatic injury suggests four main domains of palliative care that are essential in the management of critically ill patients in the trauma ICU: communication and shared decision making, withholding and withdrawal of life support, bereavement and family support, and pain and symptom management. Depending on the injury and trajectory of illness, some domains may predominate. For example, palliative care may primarily focus on the family and their support, as in traumatic brain injury with rapid progression to brain death. Here minimal attention to patient comfort is required, and care is refocused on family crisis and grief, death rituals, and spiritual issues. Conversely, in the patient with sepsis and respiratory failure, palliative care will focus on pain and symptom management and shared decision making around goals of care and life support, often in parallel with ongoing aggressive critical care.

These four components of palliative care are essential for good quality care for trauma patients in the ICU. Evidence suggests that implementation of these components in a pathway or bundle improves many aspects of care. Integration of these four areas of assessment and management into standard critical care in a timed sequence ensures their application when appropriate. Assessment of patient, family, and prognosis is the first step, followed by appropriate family support, communication, and family meetings. From these steps, goals of care should be developed. This should be completed within 72 hours of admission (Table 2).

COMMUNICATION AND SHARED DECISION MAKING

The foundation of end-of-life care is shared decision making between physician and the patient/patient's family. In its simplest form, the patient or family report the patient's wishes and preferences, while the physician contributes information on prognosis, outcomes, and treatment options, and all parties *together* make medical decisions that are consistent with the patient's wishes and hopes. Through this process, goals of care are established that will guide specific therapies, procedures, use of life support, and comfort care.

Table 2: Integrated Care Pathway: Essential Steps in Trauma ICU

First 24 Hours	First 72 Hours	End-of-Life Care for Dying
Palliative care assessment: Likely outcomes Pain and symptoms Patient preferences	Family meeting: (physician, nurse, family) Discuss patient condition, prognosis, patient preferences	Discussion of do not resuscitate (DNR) Family support Spiritual support
Family support and communication	Goals of care discussion Plan of care to meet goals	Update goals of care Stop therapies that do not meet goals of care
Pain and symptom management	Pain and symptom management	Pain and symptom management

Skills in communication, negotiation, and consensus building are essential for this process to be effective in the trauma ICU. The vast majority of critically ill patients lack capacity for communication due to injury or sedation, and their families must function as proxy decision makers. Direct communication with the family about the patient's condition, proposed treatments, prognosis, and range of possible outcomes with each therapy should commence as soon as possible in the intensive care course. Questions on advance directives and patient preferences for or against life support should be posed. The earlier this happens, the less conflict will ensue in later discussions on end-of-life decisions, do-not-resuscitate orders, and withholding of life support. Conflict is most common between family and health care staff, usually when families want life-prolonging care that physicians deem to be futile. Good communication, education, and support in many cases will resolve conflict. Evidence is clear that a structured family meeting or communication within 72 hours of admission focused on goals of care improves quality of care, length of ICU stay, and patient and family satisfaction. Studies suggest that this meeting is most effective when it includes a proper setting and appropriate members of the team, and then assessment of family understanding, discussion of prognosis and goals of care, and provision of support, and concludes with recommendations for care (Table 3). In many instances, facilitation of the meeting is best done by social workers, bereavement counselors, or nurses who can provide emotional support for the family during difficult or conflicted decisions. The physician plays a critical role, however, in discussing prognosis and medical treatment options in a clear and direct fashion, and how each may or may not meet the patient's goals of care. It is important also for the physician to make a recommendation for a care plan based on these discussions.

Table 3: Family Meeting in ICU

Preparations

Find a private setting.

Decide who will be present (family, physician, nurse, pastoral caregiver, social worker).

Review patient's condition, prognosis, treatment options.

Review family's knowledge of patient condition.

Meeting

Find out what family understands.

Review patient's condition, likely outcomes, prognosis, and treatment options.

Acknowledge uncertainty if present.

Find out patient's preferences for treatment "what would the patient want."

Discuss goals of care in light of outcomes and preferences.

Acknowledge emotions and listen.

Allow time for questions and reflection.

Conclusion of Meeting

Come to common understanding of patient's condition and decision making.

Make a recommendation for treatment, time-limited trials if appropriate.

Have follow-up plan in place.

Adapted from Curtis JR, Patrick DL, Shannon SE, Treece PD, Engelberg RA, Rubenfeld GD: The family conference as a focus to improve communication about end-of-life care in the intensive care unit: opportunities for improvement. *Crit Care Med* 29(Suppl 2):N26–N33, 2001.

WITHHOLDING AND WITHDRAWAL OF LIFE SUPPORT

In the last decade, withdrawal and withholding of life support before death in the ICU has become common practice. Now more than 80% of patients who die in ICU do so in the setting of withdrawal or withholding of life support. Discussion and management of do-not-resuscitate orders are standard practice in critical care, and require expertise in both decision making and its clinical applications. Ethical and legal precedents in the United States clearly place patient autonomy and the right to refuse therapy as prominent principles in end-of-life care, even if withdrawal of therapy ultimately results in the patient's death. In addition, withdrawal of support is ethically equivalent to withholding it; once a therapy is initiated, it can still be withdrawn later if such decision meets the patient's goals.

The decision to withdraw or withhold any therapy is based on (1) the patient's preference, advance directives and goals of care, and (2) the benefits versus burdens of each therapy in achieving these goals. Each individual therapy is evaluated as to whether it meets the goals of care; the decision to forego cardiopulmonary resuscitation, for instance, does not necessarily imply refusal of surgery, particularly if proposed surgery would relieve burdensome symptoms. Life support can be used in time-limited trials, particularly if it is uncertain if improvement will result, and then withdrawn if it does not accomplish goals. Concerns have been raised regarding traumatic brain injuries that progress to brain death, as the issue of organ donation can complicate the palliative care plan. In reality, the option of organ donation needs to be integrated into the end-of-life discussions; if organ donation is part of the goals of care, then withdrawal of life support is not appropriate.

Once decisions have been made to withdraw life support, withdrawal should be accomplished in an appropriate setting, that is, in a manner that ensures comfort and is not unnecessarily prolonged. This is a critical care procedure that requires planning and skill. The withdrawal of the ventilator deserves special mention as it raises fears on the part of physicians and nurses that it will hasten death, and on the part of families that it will cause breathlessness and feelings of suffocation. Families need to be reassured that dyspnea can be treated, and in most cases comfort is assured for a peaceful death. Several procedures for ventilator withdrawal have been described. The terminal wean involves slowly weaning (15–20 minutes) ventilator support as well as oxygen so that opioids can be titrated to control symptoms, but the endotracheal tube is left in place to prevent airway compromise from secretions. Immediate extubation and treatment with humidified air or oxygen via face mask is preferred in many situations, since it has the advantage of removing unsightly tubes and allows the patient to communicate. The choice again is guided by the goals of the patient and family for the end of life. The patient should be premedicated with opioids for dyspnea prior to extubation and then reassessed after ventilator withdrawal for symptoms, initially every 10–15 minutes. There is no role for neuromuscular blockers, as they only mask symptoms and do not ameliorate them. Anxiety from breathlessness or hypoxia can be treated with small doses of benzodiazepines as well. There is no evidence that appropriate treatment of dyspnea in this situation hastens death. Families usually want to be present at the bedside and this should be encouraged and accommodated, although they need to be prepared for the dying process and how it looks.

PAIN AND SYMPTOM MANAGEMENT

Quality care of the trauma patient in the ICU includes good pain and symptom management. Attention to relief of suffering is not only ethical and compassionate, but also abbreviates the sympathetic response and physiologic and immunologic derangements associated with surgical stress and painful injury. Studies suggest that inadequate treatment of pain and anxiety in the ICU can lead to long-term sequelae with post-traumatic stress disorder and poor psychosocial outcomes and function. Concerns that treatment of pain in the ICU will lead to hemodynamic or neurologic compromise are for the most part unfounded, and aggressive symptom control can be delivered in parallel with resuscitation in unstable patients. Short-acting agents such as fentanyl and propofol provide pain relief and deep sedation, respectively, in such situations. Newer agents such as dexemetomidine that sedate without respiratory compromise show promise as well.

Assessment of pain and symptoms can be difficult in the critically ill, particularly trauma patients with brain injury. Unconscious, sedated, and noncommunicative patients cannot report their pain. This is a barrier to good pain management in the ICU. Little is known of the importance of other non-pain symptoms, but evidence suggests that symptoms such as thirst, anxiety, and sleeplessness are not only common, but distressing, even to patients who already are receiving pain management. Other studies have noted that even routine nursing and medical procedures such as suctioning and turning are distressing and painful.

Pain management is based on assessment and frequent reassessment of patient. Communicative patients should be assessed based on a numerical rating score (0–10) as reported by the patient. Noncommunicative patients must be assessed by observed behavioral response cues such as grimacing, splinting, restlessness, and so on. Behavioral response scales have been validated but are not in wide use. Sedation may make them less reliable. These in combination with intuitive judgment, physiologic variables, and family input may be helpful, although they are highly subjective.

Response to therapy must be gauged by consistent objective parameters and reassessed frequently. Opioids are the mainstay of therapy, and continuous infusions are first choice for administration, particularly for ventilated patients. Titration should be based on objective pain scores, and infusion increases accompanied by a bolus to produce a more immediate effect. In the end-of-life situation, if intravenous lines are to be avoided, opioids can be delivered via a patch, subcutaneous infusion, or oral suspensions with good effect, although it is difficult to achieve rapid titration with these modalities.

Treatment of anxiety, agitation, and delirium is also important for the critically ill. The presence of these symptoms is clearly associated with complications and longer ICU stay. Therapy with psychotropic drugs to reinstitute or preserve the sleep–wake cycle may be helpful, although in some patients benzodiazepines only exacerbate the situation. Tricyclic and serotonin reuptake inhibitors may be better, but data are scarce. For the terminally ill and imminently dying, sometimes terminal sedation is necessary. In these conditions, a combination of haloperidol and benzodiazepines is useful. Scopolamine is also indicated for its anticholinergic effects in the treatment of secretions.

FAMILY AND BEREAVEMENT SUPPORT

Palliative care adheres to the concept that the patient *and* the family are considered the unit of care. This is a useful construct in the trauma ICU, as families of critically injured are often in crisis, bereaved, and require lots of support and communication during the ICU stay. This is particularly important when surviving family members are called on to make end-of-life decisions for the patient. Professionals who can provide emotional support as well as consistent communication are essential. Attention to this early in the patient's course in the ICU can help support the family but also avoid or prevent conflict around decisions later. This role can be fulfilled by various members of the health care team: social workers, pastoral caregivers, bereavement counselors, but also nurses and physicians.

Communication skills in breaking bad news are important for the trauma surgeon, as the manner in which this is done and support offered in this process can have significant impact on family members' bereavement process.

It is now clear that the presence of family in the ICU is important both to the patient's recovery but also the family's well-being. The opportunity to say "goodbye" to the dying patient is important for long-term bereavement, even if the circumstances of death and dying seem traumatic or unsightly. Open family visiting hours in ICUs are fast becoming the standard of care and should be encouraged. Family presence at resuscitation is more controversial, but again appears to have a salutary effect. This can be encouraged in selected situations. Someone from the health care team should accompany the family to provide support during the resuscitation. When a patient is expected to die in the ICU, attention should be paid to spiritual care and rituals. Assistance with these matters should be part of the interdisciplinary care provided by ICU staff.

SUGGESTED READINGS

Clarke EB, Curtis JR, Luce JM, et al: Quality indicators for end-of-life care in the intensive care unit. Robert Wood Johnson Foundation Critical Care End of Life Peer Workgroup Members. *Crit Care Med* 31:2255–2262, 2003.

Curtis JR, Patrick DL, Shannon SE, et al: The family conference as a focus to improve communication about end-of-life care in the intensive care unit: opportunities for improvement. *Respir Care* 45:1385–1394, 2000.

Lilly CM, De Meo DL, Sonna LA, et al: An intensive communication intervention for the critically ill. *Am J Med* 109:469–475, 2000.

Meyers TA, Eickhard DJ, Guzzzetta C, et al: Family presence during intensive procedures and resuscitation: the experience of family members, nurses and physicians. *Am J Nurs* 100:32–42, 2000.

Mosenthal AC, Lee KF, Huffman J: Palliative care in the surgical intensive care unit. *J Am Coll Surg* 194:75–83, 2002.

Mosenthal AC, Murphy PA: Interdisciplinary Model of Palliative Care in the Trauma/Surgical ICU. Princeton, NJ, Robert Wood Johnson Foundation, 2006. www.promotingexcellence.org.

Prendergast T, Luce J: Increasing incidence of withholding and withdrawal of life support from the critically ill. *Am J Respir Crit Care Med* 155: 2130–2136, 1997.

Puntillo KA: Dimensions of procedural pain and its analgesic management in critically ill surgical patients. *Am J Crit Care* 3:116–122, 1994.

Puntillo KA, Miazkowski C, Kehrle K, et al: Relationship between behavioral and physiological indicators of pain, critical care patient's self-reports of pain and opioid administration. *Crit Care Med* 25:1159–1166, 1997.

Rubenfeld GD, Crawford SW: Principles and practice of withdrawing life-sustaining treatment in the ICU. In Curtis JR, Rubenfeld GD, editors: *Managing Death in the Intensive Care Unit.* New York, Oxford University Press, 2001, pp. 127–147.

Schneiderman LJ, Gilmer T, Teetzel HD, et al: Effect of ethics consultations on nonbeneficial life-sustaining treatments in the intensive care setting: a randomized controlled trial. *JAMA* 290:1166–1172, 2003.

Simpson T, Wilson T, Mucken N, et al: Implementation and evaluation of a liberalized visiting policy. *Am J Crit Care* 5:420–426, 1996.

The SUPPORT Investigators: A controlled trial to improve care for the seriously ill and hospitalized patients. Study to Understand Prognoses and Preferences for Outcomes and Risks of Treatments. *JAMA* 224: 1591–1598, 1995.

von Gunten CF, Weissman DE: *Fast Fact and Concept #33: Ventilator Withdrawal Protocol (Part I).* 2nd ed. Milwaukee, WI, End-of-Life Palliative Education Resource Center, Medical College of Wisconsin, July 2005. www.eperc.mcw.edu.

von Gunten CF, Weissman DE: *Fast Fact and Concept #34: Symptom Control for Ventilator Withdrawal in the Dying Patient (Part II),* 2nd ed. Milwaukee, WI, End-of-Life Palliative Education Resource Center, Medical College of Wisconsin, July 2005. www.eperc.mcw.edu.

von Gunten CF, Weissman DE: *Fast Fact and Concept #35: Information for patients and families about ventilator withdrawal (Part III),* 2nd ed. Milwaukee, WI, End-of-Life Palliative Education Resource Center, Medical College of Wisconsin, July 2005. www.eperc.mcw.edu.

DEATH FROM TRAUMA—MANAGEMENT OF GRIEF AND BEREAVEMENT AND THE ROLE OF THE SURGEON

Patricia A. Murphy   and   Anne C. Mosenthal

Death from trauma is a tragic event, often affecting young and previously healthy people. It is rarely peaceful or dignified. Traumatic sudden death leaves in its wake confused, disoriented, angry, sad, and overwhelmed survivors. Their reactions separate hem from life, from reality, and sometimes from caring about themselves. This is grief. When death occurs from sudden, unexpected events such as car crashes, suicide, or murder, grief reactions are more severe, exaggerated, and complicated. The griever's ability to use adaptive coping mechanisms is limited.

Despite all life-saving efforts, trauma surgeons must occasionally deliver news of the death or impending death of the patient. In reality, 10%–15% of trauma patients who present to the hospital will die from their injuries. The majority succumb during resuscitation or surgery within hours, but others will linger in the intensive care unit and die days to weeks after injury. Physicians often are called on to communicate with grief-stricken families and support them. The manner in which this is done can have long-term consequences for the bereaved families as well as influence end-of-life decisions. Good trauma management must include knowledge of basic grief and bereavement theory as well as skills in communication of bad news.

INCIDENCE

Violence and motor vehicle crashes continue to be a leading cause of death in young people in the United States. This leaves many survivors to cope with lifelong grief and bereavement. Increasing evidence suggests that traumatic injury and death are not necessarily isolated events, but can be part of larger social conditions (poverty, substance abuse) in some communities and families. In inner city neighborhoods, children are exposed to violence and loss at an early age. This may influence a family's ability to cope with a new loss or death. In order to care for the survivors of violent death, the trauma surgeon must be aware of the family's loss history: Is this the first (or second, third, etc.) member of the immediate family to die violently? How has the survivor coped in the past? This assessment is essential to providing competent grief support.

Even if patients die after weeks of a long illness or injury, this is still an acutely disruptive event for the family. Some trauma patients spend weeks in the surgical intensive care unit hovering near death. During this time the family is desperate for any information that gives them hope. They ride the rollercoaster of hope and despair with every conversation they have with the trauma surgeon. They are exhausted, and frequently ignore their own needs for rest and food. If their loved one dies, it is perceived as a sudden event—even if weeks have gone by since the trauma. This is because they have probably coped using the defense of denial, and the death shatters that defense.

Profound grief occurs not only after death, but after any major loss. Even if the patient survives, grief may complicate recovery and care, especially after spinal cord injury, brain injury, or traumatic amputation where lifelong loss of function means loss of hopes and dreams and expectations. This can be devastating—families and patients may experience the same sequence of grief and coping mechanisms as is apparent after the death of the patient.

GRIEF

Bereavement refers to the objective situation of having lost someone significant to death. Throughout their lives people have to face the death of parents, siblings, partners, friends, or even their own children. Bereavement is associated with intense distress for most people. This distress is grief, defined as a primarily emotional reaction to the loss of a loved one. It includes diverse psychological and physical manifestations (Table 1).

TRAUMATIC GRIEF

When the death of a loved one occurs under traumatic circumstances, the survivor's grief is predisposed to be complicated by many factors. The suddenness of the loss, violent circumstances, preventability, and/or randomness of the event and the survivor's sense of vulnerability to harm are all factors that complicate the grief. Sudden, unexpected, or violent death is a significant factor in complicated mourning. Researchers have studied the relationship of post-traumatic stress disorder (PTSD) and bereavement. PTSD was found among the bereaved and frequently correlated with the perceived inadequacy of the goodbye said to the deceased. The overlay of PTSD-type symptoms in some individuals who have lost someone to death from trauma may complicate the bereavement and capacity to grieve. Theorists have suggested that there are many issues inherent in sudden, unanticipated death that complicate mourning. Those relevant to trauma surgery in the acute care setting follow:

- The capacity to cope is diminished as the shock of the death overwhelms the self.
- The assumptive world of the mourner is violently shattered (the world as orderly, predictable, and meaningful), and causes intense reactions of fear, anxiety, and loss of control.
- The loss does not make sense and cannot be absorbed.
- There is no chance to say goodbye and finish unfinished business with the deceased.
- Symptoms of acute grief and physical and emotional shock persist for a long time.
- The mourner obsessively reconstructs events in an effort to both comprehend the death and prepare for it in retrospect.
- The mourner experiences a profound loss of security and confidence in the world and increasing anxiety.
- The loss cuts across experiences in the relationship and tends to highlight what was happening at the time of the death, predisposing to problems with unrealistic recollection and guilt.
- The death tends to leave mourners with relatively more intense emotions, along with a strong need to determine blame and affix responsibility for it.

GRIEVING ACROSS THE LIFE SPAN

Numerous authors have defined "tasks of mourning" as activities that facilitate the resolution of significant loss. Adults and children experience grief after a loss, but the manifestations are developmentally

Table 1: Manifestations of Grief

Affective	Behavioral
Despair	Agitation
Anxiety	Fatigue
Guilt	Crying
Anger	Social withdrawal
Hostility	
Loneliness	
Cognitive	**Physiological**
Decreased self-esteem	Anorexia
Preoccupation with image of deceased	Sleep disturbances
Helplessness	Energy loss and exhaustion
Hopelessness	Somatic complaints
Self-blame	Susceptibility to illness/disease
Problems with concentration	

determined (Table 2). It is important to recognize the different ways that children express grief; the age of the child is an important determinant and should be taken into account when information is shared and support provided.

Special attention should be paid to bereaved children because there is often confusion about age-appropriate information and support. In working with children, you must remember that a mature understanding of death is tied to the cognitive capacity to understand that death is permanent. This occurs in children at about the age of 5. The child's developmental needs help to define the significance of the loss.

Simple, clear information about the young child's reaction to the death should be given to the primary caregiver. Printed, easily understandable information should be given to caregivers to take home. Iverson has published a simple but complete list of adult behaviors that are helpful to young children. It is essential that the child be told the truth in words that he/she can understand. Real words should be used to describe what has happened, such as, "Your mom was in a terrible car crash. The doctors have worked real hard to try and fix her but her body just stopped working and she died." Children take their cues from their adult caregivers, and closely watch adults' reaction.

Some basic principles for grief in children follow:

- Children as young as 3 years can understand the concept of death.
- Do *not* tell children the dead person has gone away or is sleeping, as this will only confuse them.

- Use real words to describe the death.
- Answer the questions that the child asks. When a death occurs, children often worry about 3 issues: Did I make it happen? Will it happen to me? Who will take care of me?
- Give the child the opportunity to attend the family ritual surrounding death. If the child asks to attend, that usually means he/she is old enough to do so.

MANAGEMENT OF ACUTE GRIEF AFTER TRAUMATIC DEATH

The sudden and often violent nature of death from trauma can lead to complicated mourning as described previously. However, certain strategies for support and communication can and should be applied in the immediate situation that may facilitate long-term coping and bereavement. These can be divided into three time frames around the death of a patient: support for family contact with the dying patient *prior* to death, communication of bad news and death notification, and facilitation of postmortem rituals and time with the deceased. While the physician may not be primarily responsible for bereavement support immediately after death, he/she is usually called on to deliver bad news and can facilitate other members of the health care team to support the family.

Because the inability to say goodbye is associated with PTSD and complicated grief, the surgeon should offer the survivors an opportunity to see the patient *before* death if at all possible. Reliable research supports having family members attend resuscitation; of course, this applies only if they want to attend. They should be brought into the room two at a time and never left unattended. This process allows the family to witness attempts to save the patient's life and also prepares them for the eventual death. This process creates opportunities for the family to say goodbye. Not all families want to be present, and not all resuscitations are amenable to family presence. What is most important is that a bereavement support person who is not caring for the patient must be free to accompany the family. This can be a social worker, pastoral caregiver, bereavement counselor, nurse, or other experienced member of the team.

Communication of bad news or death of the patient to surviving family members is one of the most difficult tasks of the trauma surgeon. Research has demonstrated that the manner in which this is done is long remembered by families, and will affect their lifelong bereavement. However, several studies have revealed some simple, yet important skills for compassionate and effective communication in this setting. First, create an appropriate setting for delivering the news: it should be private, quiet, and secure. Prepare yourself as to the identity of the family members and their relationship to the patient. Do not assume that family members already know their loved one has died, even if they have witnessed the event. Your news

Table 2: Tasks of Mourning: Children versus Adults

Adult's Tasks of Mourning	Child's Tasks of Mourning
Accept the reality of the loss.	Understand that someone has died.
Experience the pain or emotional aspects of the loss.	Face the psychological pain of the loss. Cope with periodic resurgence of pain.
Adjust to an environment in which the deceased is missing.	Invest in new relationships. Develop a new sense of identity that includes experience of the loss.
Emotionally relocate the deceased (this relocation process still allows for continuing bonds to the deceased).	Reevaluate the relationship to the person who has died. Return to age-appropriate developmental tasks.

will come as a shock, so for this reason it is helpful to give a warning shot: "I am afraid I have bad news." Then follow with a clear, direct statement about the death of the patient. Avoid vague euphemisms such as "passed away," "passed on," or "we lost him"; instead, use the word "died" or "dead." Elaborate explanations of medical details at this time are confusing; time is needed for the news to sink in first. Listen and provide support by acknowledging the family's emotions. Then allow time for questions if they arise. Reassure family members that they can see and spend time with the deceased, and provide a plan for follow-up support and questions. Family-support personnel, social workers, and pastoral caregivers can and should be called in during this process (Table 3).

After sudden death, there is usually no chance for the family to say goodbye while the patient is alive or conscious. The only chance is in the immediate aftermath of the news, and this is often in the hospital or emergency room. As the ability to say goodbye to the deceased is correlated with a positive bereavement outcome, the opportunity to see, touch, and hold the deceased is especially important after trauma and should be provided as soon as possible. Many physicians are concerned about this in circumstances when there is mutilation or disfigurement. There is no research data in the grief literature to support the idea that family members are harmed by viewing the body of their dead loved one. One of the authors (PM) has been involved in family support in trauma services for more than 20 years. In all that time no family member ever reported an adverse reaction to viewing the body. It is important that the family be prepared for what they are going to see, that is, all physical trauma should be explained in advance, and the body cleaned and covered. Usually the family can and should decide how much they can handle. The worst thing that could happen, the death, has already happened! The role of the health care team is to support them as they cope with the tragedy. Do not leave them alone, unless they ask to be alone. Encourage them to cut a lock of hair, sit with the body, and ask if they want a clergy person to be with them. This is particularly important for parents after the death of a child, and they should be supported if they wish to hold the child. However, if the family continually declines to view the body, they should not be coaxed into doing so.

COMPLICATED GRIEF

There are many characteristics of acute traumatic grief that can lead to complicated grief. Death that is sudden and unexpected, violent, mutilating, and random can lead to complicated grief reactions.

Often the griever has some of the following complications: cognitive dissonance, murderous impulses and anger, guilt and blame, and emotional withdrawal.

Cognitive dissonance occurs because the mind is overwhelmed with events prior to, during, and after the event. There is a constant rehearsal of the event, and the person continually asks when, how, where, who did what, and the unanswerable "why(???)." The most helpful intervention involves giving the person whatever information you have and referring them to others who may have the answers to their questions. They may ask the same questions over and over, and sometimes the only answer is "I don't know." Often there is no answer to their questions, but they need to keep asking.

Many survivors have murderous impulses and anger toward whoever they think caused the death. If the death was caused by someone in the commission of a crime, such as an auto accident caused by a drunk driver, assault, and shooting, then the normal anger of grief is compounded by rage, and the desire to violently destroy whoever is perceived as the cause. It is in the venting and verbalizing of some of theses impulses that the anger begins to lose some of its intensity. It is important to remember that thoughts that can be expressed do not have to be acted out.

Guilt is intricately embodied with a sense of control and the search for a reason. The traumatic loss is internalized, and the barrage of "If only's" is endless. Human beings seek to blame others or themselves in order to make sense of the tragedy and to confirm a sense of control over their lives. Family members often blame each other. Immediately following the loss, this dynamic is expected and part of the process. If it persists for more than 3 months, professional help may be necessary to resolve the loss.

Emotional withdrawal often occurs as members of the family withdraw from each other. They nurse their own psychic pain and grief separately. Individuals may also withdraw from friends and activities that provide comfort and support because they believe that no one else could ever imagine their level of pain and despair. Often survivors have thoughts of suicide as an attempt to avoid the intense pain.

Complicated grief requires specialized interventions beyond the scope of this chapter and beyond the scope of practice of surgeons. What a surgeon must know is that there is help available and how to access that help. Every hospice program offers support groups for bereaved individuals that are open to all in the community. In addition, hospital pastoral care departments can be very helpful in complicated grief situations. Do not hesitate to reach out to other professionals for help.

Table 3: Cardinal Rules for Communication of Bad News

Include communication with the family and bereavement support in routine trauma care after death of the patient.
Provide timely and straightforward information.
Give families frequent updates, even if there is no significant new information.
If you have bad news, fire a "warning shot."
If you have inconclusive news, invite people to "hope for the best and plan for the worst."
Always pledge constancy: "I (we) will stick with you through this regardless of what happens."
Remember that people are usually tougher than we give them credit for.
Remember that good information enables most people.
Know your limits and get help.
Use the knowledge and skill of colleagues who specialize in bereavement work.
Avoid giving advice about what the family should do that is not based on evidence or best practices.
Remember that the more someone differs from you (age, ethnicity, religious orientation, etc.), the less you can rely on your empathy to know what they feel or want or value.

Suggested Readings

Buckman R: *How to Break Bad News: A Guide for Health Professionals.* Baltimore, Johns Hopkins University Press, 1992.

Iverson K: *Grave Words: Notifying Survivors about Sudden, Unexpected Deaths.* Tucson, AZ: Galen Press, 1999.

Jurkovich G, Pierce B, Pananen L, Rivara F: Giving bad news: the family perspective. *J Trauma* 48:865–873, 2000.

Mosenthal A, Murphy P: Trauma care and palliative care: time to integrate the two? *J Am Coll Surg* 197:509–516, 2003.

Murphy P, Price D: Dying and grieving in the inner city. In Doka K, Davidson J, editors: *Living with Grief: Who We Are, How We Grieve.* Wash-

ington, DC, Hospice Foundation of America; Philadelphia, Brunner/Mazel, 1998.

Oliver RC, Sturtevant JP, Scheetz, JP, et al: Beneficial effects of a hospital bereavement intervention program after traumatic childhood death. *J Trauma* 50:440–448, 2001.

Rando T: *Treatment of Complicated Mourning.* Champaign, IL, Research Press, 1993.

Redmond L: *Surviving When Someone You Love Was Murdered.* Clearwater FL: Psychological and Educational Services, 1990.

Stroebe M, Hansson R, Stroebe W, Schut H: *Handbook of Bereavement Research.* Washington DC, American Psychological Association, 2001.

Trauma Rehabilitation

Wayne Dubov, Michael M. Badellino, and Michael D. Pasquale

In 2002, unintentional injury was the most common cause of death between the ages of 1 and 44 years. There were 161,000 total injured deaths (56 per 100,000 population) that year. It was the fifth leading cause of death for all ages, after heart disease, malignant neoplasms, cerebrovascular events, and chronic respiratory disease. For males, it is the third leading cause of death, and seventh overall for females.[1] Motor vehicle collision (MVC) was the most common cause of death related to trauma.

There were many more nonfatal than fatal injuries. In 2004, there were 29,654,475 (~10,000/100,000) in the United States—involving all races, ages, and both sexes. Falls were most common (2756/100,000), followed by transportation-related injuries (1545/100,000). Violent nonfatal injuries occurred at a rate of 755/100,000.[1]

Trauma rehabilitation is the restoration of injured patients. Rehabilitation of patients who sustain traumatic injuries is unique compared to other types of rehabilitation. There is a large range of types and degree of diagnoses associated with trauma. Patients will therefore have many different medical, surgical, and rehabilitation needs.

Musculoskeletal injuries (such as fractures to limbs, pelvis, and spine) limit function and are the most common hospitalized injuries. Traumatic brain injuries, spinal cord injuries, peripheral nerve injuries, burns, and amputations are also common. Although patients with chest and abdominal injuries are frequently admitted, these conditions do not often lead to long-term disability.

The focus of this chapter is the assessment and rehabilitation of patients in a Level 1 trauma care setting. The role of a physiatrist (specialist in physical medicine and rehabilitation) is discussed, as well as the role of the trauma rehabilitation team.

TRAUMA REHABILITATION TEAM

The trauma rehabilitation team at our particular acute Level 1 trauma center consists of a physiatrist and departments of physical therapy (PT), occupational therapy (OT), and case management. The request for consultation by other team members is determined by the patient's needs and includes speech pathology and substance abuse counseling. A trauma rehabilitation consultation is initiated by the trauma service (the admitting service), and this provides an automatic consult to physiatry, PT, OT, and case management.

The physiatrist is the physician leader of the trauma rehabilitation team. This physician establishes rehabilitation needs and provides diagnostic evaluation after reviewing all available test results, assessing the patient's injuries, and determining any contraindications for early mobility. Emphasis is placed on detection and evaluation of neurological injuries. The physiatrist's examination is multisystem, with focus on orthopedic and neurological injuries such as traumatic brain injury (TBI), spinal cord injury (SCI), and peripheral nerve injury. The presence of a physiatrist allows a physician consultant to perform a tertiary survey, looking for any previously unrecognized injuries.

Team physical therapists perform an examination and assess the injuries. They then work with a patient in the acute care setting to improve functional mobility. They may also play a role in wound care. Occupational therapists assess the patient to determine how to facilitate basic activities of daily living and to maximize functional restoration of the upper extremities. They also fabricate splints and provide family teaching. Speech pathologists assess swallowing and make recommendations related to appropriate food consistency. They also assess for any cognitive and language deficits, particularly in patients sustaining TBI.

The case manager usually has a background in social service or nursing. Case managers play an integral role by assisting patients and their families with social and discharge planning issues. These managers are responsible for securing durable medical equipment, such as wheelchairs and modified commodes, for patients who are being discharged to home. See Figure 1 regarding rehabilitation screening of trauma patients.

ASSESSMENT OF PATIENTS WITH SPINAL CORD INJURY

Epidemiology of Traumatic Spinal Cord Injury in the United States

The incidence of SCI is estimated to be approximately 40 new cases per million population per year, or roughly 11,000. The estimated prevalence in the United States is 250 million persons.[2] SCI primarily affects young adults. The average age at the time of injury is 37.6 years. The percentage of persons older than 60 years at injury has increased from 4.7% in 1980 to 10.9% since 2000. Of the SCI reported to the national database, 79% has occurred among males. Since 2000, MVC have accounted for 47.5% of SCI cases reported. Falls are the next most common cause of SCI, followed by acts of violence and recreational activities. Since 2000, the most frequent neurological category is incomplete tetraplegia (34.5%), followed by complete

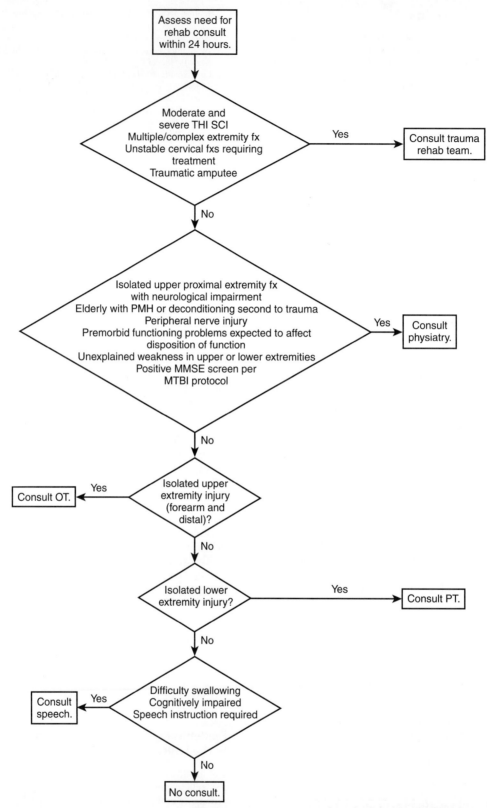

Figure 1 Rehabilitation screening of trauma patients (all ages). *fx*, Fracture; *MMSE*, mini mental state examination; *MTBI*, mild traumatic brain injury; *OT*, occupational therapy; *PMH*, past medical history; *PT*, physical therapy; *rehab*, rehabilitation; *SCI*, spinal cord injury; *TBI*, traumatic brain injury.

paraplegia (23.1%), complete tetraplegia (18.4%), and incomplete paraplegia (17.5%).[3]

Neurological Classification

Determining the neurological level and completeness of injury is the most accurate way of prognosticating recovery and functional outcome. Using the International Standards of Neurological and Functional Classification of Spinal Cord Injury, the examiner determines the motor and sensory level on the right and left and ascertains whether the injury is complete or incomplete.[4]

Using standard dermatomes and myotomes defined by the American Spinal Injury Association (ASIA), motor level is defined as the most caudal segment to have a muscle grade of 3. Five muscle groups are tested in the upper extremities, and five muscle groups are tested in the lower extremities. Each muscle group is supplied by two root levels, and each muscle group is graded from 0 to 5. Therefore, if the muscle grade is at least 3 of 5 the proximal root is believed to be intact. The sensory level is defined as the most caudal dermatome to have normal sensation to pin prick and light touch. Specific testing points are defined by ASIA[4] (Figure 2).

In addition to defining the neurological level, the completeness of injury must be determined. See the ASIA impairment scale in Figure 2. A complete injury results in no motor or sensory function preserved in the sacral segments (ASIA A). There are four incomplete levels of

ASIA: B, C, D, and E. *Incomplete* is defined as sparing of sensory and/or motor function below the neurological level that includes the sacral (S4-S5) segments.

There are a number of incomplete SCI syndromes, including central cord syndrome, Brown-Sequard syndrome, anterior cord syndrome, dorsal column syndrome, cauda equina syndrome, and conus medullaris syndrome. Central cord syndrome occurs in the cervical cord and produces greater weakness in the upper extremities than lower extremities. Brown-Sequard syndrome is a lesion that produces ipsilateral motor and proprioceptive loss and contralateral loss of pain and temperature perception. Anterior cord syndrome causes variable loss of motor function, pain, and temperature perception while sparing proprioception. This is usually seen with injury to the anterior spinal artery in the thoracic level. Dorsal column syndrome is rare and would produce abnormal proprioception but preserved motor function and pain and temperature sensation. In cauda equina syndrome, the lumbosacral roots are injured because the spinal cord ends at approximately the L1-L2 level. This causes lower motor neuron symptoms, such as areflexic bladder, bowel, and lower limbs. Conus medullaris syndrome involves injury to the end of the spinal cord. At this level, the lumbar and sacral roots are affected.

Acute Medical Management

All patients with acute traumatic SCI receive methylprednisolone. This is based on the National Acute Spinal Cord Injury Studies (NASCIS), the last being NASCIS 3. This study concluded that patients treated within 3 hours of injury should receive 24 hours of steroids, and those treated in 3–8 hours of injury should receive 48 hours of steroids.[5]

The degree of respiratory dysfunction after SCI is related to the neurological level and the completeness of injury. The level of pulmonary dysfunction increases concomitantly with the level of injury.

C1-C3 neurological levels will require ventilatory support. The phrenic nerve (supplied by C3-C5 nerve roots) will be intact in patients with a C5 neurological level and below. As the level descends from mid-cervical to lower cervical, and then to thoracic, there will be greater innervation to abdominal and intercostal muscles—thereby making the work of breathing easier. The primary objective in early pulmonary management in SCI is to minimize secondary complications, including preventing hypoxemia, preventing and treating atelectasis, reducing risk of aspiration, and providing aggressive pulmonary management to compensate for impaired clearing of secretions.[6]

During spinal shock (temporary loss of all or most spinal reflexic activity below the level of injury), sympathetic activity is reduced or absent. This leads to bradycardia and hypotension. After resuscitation, elastic stockings, abdominal binders, adequate hydration, and gradual upright positioning are used to reduce the effects of orthostatic hypotension.

Bladder management is usually accomplished with an indwelling catheter, as the bladder is often initially areflexic. The goals of team bladder management are to allow the bladder to empty, prevent urinary retention, minimize urinary tract infections, and determine which methods facilitate independent bladder management. Methods may include use of an indwelling Foley catheter or placement of a suprapubic tube. Intermittent catheterization is appropriate for patients with use of their upper extremities.

Male patients who have reflex voiding and detrusor hyperreflexia may require a sphincterotomy procedure or pharmacological agents to reduce outflow resistance and allow use of an external catheter. Some patients with incomplete spinal cord injuries will be incontinent. Urodynamic studies are useful at some point to help classify the neurogenic bladder, in order to select adequate bladder management methods.

ASIA IMPAIRMENT SCALE

☐ **A = Complete**: no motor or sensory function is preserved in the sacral segments S4–S5.

☐ **B = Incomplete**: sensory but not motor function is preserved below the neurological level and includes the sacral segments S4–S5.

☐ **C = Incomplete**: motor function is preserved below the neurological level, and more than half of key muscles below the neurological level have a muscle grade less than 3.

☐ **D = Incomplete**: motor function is preserved below the neurological level, and at least half of key muscles below the neurological level have a muscle grade of 3 or more.

☐ **E = Normal**: motor and sensory function are normal

CLINICAL SYNDROMES

☐ Central cord
☐ Brown-Sequard
☐ Anterior cord
☐ Conus medullaris
☐ Cauda equina

Figure 2 American Spinal Injury Association Impairment Scale. *(Adapted from American Spinal Injury Association: International Standards for Neurological Classification of Spinal Cord Injury, rev. 2006. Chicago, American Spinal Injury Association, 2006.)*

A bowel program should be established. Initially, a paralytic ileus is common. Patients may be placed on a stool softener and a daily or every-other-day suppository, with digital stimulation. This routine should be established about the same time each day. The goal is to prevent or minimize incontinence between bowel programs.

Deep venous thromboembolism (DVT) prevention is extremely important, as DVT and pulmonary embolism are major causes of morbidity and mortality in the SCI population. Sequential compression devices should be used, with or without elastic stockings, to improve lower extremity venous return. Such methods are contraindicated in patients with severe arterial insufficiency. Pharmacologic prophylaxis should be initiated within the first 72 hours, when not contraindicated. Low-molecular-weight heparin is the current recommendation. Anticoagulation should be continued for 8 weeks in patients with uncomplicated complete motor impairments, and for 12 weeks in complete motor injuries with other risk factors (lower limb fractures, history of thrombosis, cancer, heart failure, obesity, and age over 70). Vena cava filter placement is indicated in SCI patients with a contraindication for pharmacologic prophylaxis.[7]

ASSESSMENT OF PATIENTS WITH TRAUMATIC BRAIN INJURY

Epidemiology of Traumatic Brain Injury in the United States

There are 1.4 million people who sustain TBI in the United States annually. Approximately 50,000 will die, 235,000 are hospitalized, and 1.1 million are treated and released from the emergency department.[8] Between 80,000 and 90,000 people experience long-term disability associated with TBI.[9] According to the TBI Model System database, MVCs account for 48.3%—with the next most common cause of TBI being falls, followed by violence. The most common cause of death from MVCs is TBI. Approximately 5.3 million Americans (or about 2% of the population) currently live with disabilities caused by TBI.[10]

Pathophysiology of Traumatic Brain Injury

Primary injuries occur at the moment of impact and can be focal or diffuse. Focal injuries include skull fractures, contusions, or extraaxial hematomas. They may develop in the region of direct impact (coup) or at the opposite site of the skull (contrecoup), where the brain contacts the skull. In addition, there are acceleration-deceleration and rotational forces that produce diffuse axonal shearing at the white-gray borders. This is referred to as a diffuse axonal injury (DAI).

Secondary injuries are the biochemical and physiological result of the primary brain injury. These cause tissue hypoxia and cerebral ischemia. Attempts should be made to minimize hypoxemia, hypercarbia, hypotension, and acidosis. Development of intracranial hematomas and cerebral edema also causes secondary brain injury.

Initial Physiatric Consultation and Early Rehabilitation Intervention

The chart should be thoroughly reviewed, including all associated injuries, comorbid conditions, and diagnostic studies. It is important to document social information, including premorbid vocational and educational status, as well as the family and home situation.

Obtaining prehospital records documenting any loss of consciousness and Glasgow Coma Scale (GCS) prehospital and at admission will help determine the severity of brain injury. A GCS of 8 or less is considered severe, a GCS between 9 and 12 is considered moderate, and a GCS of 13–15 is a mild TBI (Table 1).

A thorough neurological examination includes a mental status evaluation and assessment of neurological recovery using the Rancho Los Amigos Scale of Cognitive Functioning (Table 2). The Rancho Los Amigos Scale is used for patients with moderate to severe TBI and spans from Level 1 to Level 8. Level 1 indicates no response to any stimuli. Level 8 is when all activities are purposeful and appropriate.[11]

Medical Considerations and Complications in Traumatic Brain Injury

Several potential medical complications unique to moderate to severe TBI must be assessed with emphasis on preventing disability. Spasticity is a motor disorder characterized by a velocity-dependent increase in tonic stretch reflexes (muscle tone). The degree of spasticity usually correlates with the severity of brain injury. It is one feature of the upper motor neuron picture. Treatment is indicated to improve positioning, prevent contractures, and sometimes to reduce pain. Physical modalities such as ice, stretching, splinting, inhibitive casting, and appropriate positioning can be used. Attempts should be made to position the patient with hips and knees flexed rather than in a supine position.

Medications can be used, but they provide varied results. Dantrolene acts directly on skeletal muscle and reduces muscle contraction by a direct effect on the excitation-contraction coupling mechanism. Dantrolene is effective for cerebral spasticity. It should not be used for people with liver dysfunction, and all those on Dantrolene should be given liver function tests. Baclofen inhibits monosynaptic and polysynaptic spinal reflexes, and is more effective for spinal spasticity. Sedation is a common side effect, and the dosage should be increased slowly. Tizanidine binds to central alpha2-

Table 1: Glasgow Coma Scale

Parameter	Score
Best Motor Response	
Normal	6
Localizes	5
Withdraws	4
Flexion	3
Extension	2
None	1
Best Verbal Response	
Oriented	5
Confused	4
Verbalizes	3
Vocalizes	2
None	1
Eye Opening	
Spontaneous	4
To command	3
To pain	2
None	1

Table 2: Rancho Los Amigos Scale of Cognitive Functioning

I	No response to any stimuli.
II	Generalized reflex response to pain.
III	Localized response. Blinks to light, tracks, inconsistent response to commands.
IV	Alert, but confused and agitated.
V	Confused, nonagitated. Social, but with inappropriate verbalizations.
VI	Inconsistent orientation. Impaired short-term memory. Goal-directed behavior, with assistance.
VII	Automatic appropriate behavior in familiar tasks and environment.
VIII	Purposeful, appropriate behavior allows functional independence. Social, emotional, intellectual levels may be decreased compared to pretraumatic brain injury.

adrenergic receptors, and therefore reduces spasticity by acting centrally. Tizanidine is more effective for spinal spasticity than cerebral spasticity. Hypotension and elevated liver function tests are common side effects. Diazepam and other benzodiazepines are also effective, but are sedating and usually should be avoided. Local injections using *Botulinum* toxin, phenol, or alcohol can be used for specific muscles. Intrathecal Baclofen may be considered if the previously cited measures do not work.

Central dysautonomia, sometimes referred to as *storming*, is problematic in patients with severe brain injury. There is an increase in circulating catecholamines, leading to tachycardia, diaphoresis, hypertension, hyperthermia, pupillary dilatation, and increased spasticity or posturing. Beta-blockers such as propranolol and clonidine, alpha2-adrenergic agonists, can be used to treat the cardiovascular symptoms of central dysautonomia. Opioids are used to reduce pain. Antispasticity drugs are effective in decreasing the dystonia; particularly tizanidine, which has the added benefit of being an alpha2-adrenergic agonist.

The risk of seizures is increased by brain injury severity, depressed skull fracture, intracranial hematoma, early seizure, penetrating injury, and prolonged unresponsiveness. According to practice guidelines of the American Academy of Physical Medicine and Rehabilitation, there is evidence for the use of antiepileptic drugs within the first week after TBI. However, there is no good evidence to support their use after the first week of injury.[12]

Patients with TBI are at high risk for DVT, and prophylaxis is needed. Early on, if there is concern about bleeding mechanical methods such as sequential compressive devices and thigh high compressive dressings should be used. Pharmacologic prophylaxis should be started, when it is deemed safe, usually within 1–2 weeks. If this needs to be delayed even further, insertion of an inferior vena cava (IVC) filter should be considered.

Heterotopic ossification (HO) may occur in patients with severe brain injury. HO is the formation of ectopic bone and most commonly occurs at the hips, shoulders, elbows, and knees. Early signs of contracture (a hard endpoint with range of motion, pain, and erythema) might suggest this diagnosis. Initially a plain x-ray will be normal, but a three-phase bone scan as well as elevated serum alkaline phosphatase levels can confirm the diagnosis of HO. Anti-inflammatory agents, diphosphonate, and localized irradiation have been used. However, sometimes surgical resection is needed. Prevention is best, by providing range of motion and proper positioning, reducing spasticity, and avoiding prolonged chemical paralysis.

Other potential medical consequences of TBI include neuroendocrine disorders. There is a syndrome of inappropriate antidiuretic hormone (SIADH), which leads to hyponatremia. Diabetes insipidus causes excessive water secretion due to diminished ADH (vasopressin) secretion. This leads to dilute urine and causes hypernatremia, polydipsia, polyuria, and possibly hypotension due to decreased intravascular volume.

ASSESSMENT OF PATIENTS WITH PERIPHERAL NERVE INJURY

Epidemiology of Peripheral Nerve Injuries

The estimated incidence of peripheral nerve injuries in patients admitted to a Level I trauma center, including plexus and root injuries, is about 5%.[13] The radial nerve is the most frequently injured nerve in the upper extremity due to mid-shaft humerus fractures, as the radial nerve travels around the spiral groove. Ulnar nerve injuries are associated with elbow fractures, with or without dislocations. The median nerve may also be injured at the level of the elbow or with supracondylar distal humerus fractures. Rarely, there may be peripheral nerve injuries due to forearm fractures—particularly in the rare case of compartment syndrome in the forearm.

In the lower extremity, the sciatic nerve is frequently injured. This is most often seen with acetabular fractures or femoral head dislocation because the sciatic nerve is directly posterior to the hip joint. When the sciatic nerve is injured, the common peroneal nerve is more prone to injury than the tibial nerve (these nerves are separate nerves, but are contiguous with each other as the sciatic nerve until they separate at the popliteal fossa). The common peroneal nerve lies more laterally, and there is less epineurium (connective tissue) protecting the common peroneal nerve than the tibial nerve. The peroneal nerve can be injured in the area of the fibula head, where it lies superficially. Compartment syndrome in the lower leg can also lead to tibial or peroneal nerve injuries, depending on the compartment affected.

Brachial plexus injuries occur largely as the result of MVCs or motorcycle crashes. They may be seen in patients with TBI, and there are signs upon examination in the unresponsive or minimally responsive patient. The absence of reflexes, flaccid tone, and poor movement compared to the other extremities suggests a brachial plexus injury. This is particularly true when there is no weakness of the ipsilateral lower extremity, and therefore a central etiology is less likely. Many times there will be an associated clavicle or scapular fracture on the same side as the brachial plexus injury, but fractures do not have to exist for brachial plexus injuries to be present. A careful neurological exam in the awake patient will usually differentiate a brachial plexus injury versus a central nervous system injury, such as a cervical SCI or effects of TBI.

Electrodiagnostic Testing and Classification of Peripheral Nerve Injury

A commonly used classification of peripheral nerve injury is the Seddon classification.[14] Neurapraxia is the most mild because there is no axonal degeneration (Wallerian degeneration). There is focal demyelination or ischemia causing partial or complete conduction block at the site of injury. The nerve distal to the injured segment functions normally. Recovery is usually good and takes weeks to months, but may be only hours or days if mild and localized. Axonotmesis occurs when there is Wallerian degeneration. For recovery to occur, there must be regeneration of the nerve. Both the axon and the myelin are disrupted. The extent of recovery will depend on the extent of disruption, including the surrounding connective tissue (endoneurium and perineurium) as well as the distance between the site of injury and the muscles it supplies. Neurotmesis is diagnosed when the axon and all connective tissue, including the most external (the epineurium), are disrupted. There will be no spontaneous recovery and only surgery may be helpful.

Many times, electrodiagnostic studies (electromyography [EMG], plus nerve conduction studies) are used to confirm and prognosticate the recovery of a nerve injury. Wallerian (axonal) degeneration takes up to 9 days for motor fibers, and 11 days for sensory fibers, postinjury.[15] This information is relevant in performing nerve conduction studies.

It may take up to 3 weeks to see axonal degeneration on needle EMG. When possible, waiting at least 3 weeks to perform EMG/nerve conduction studies will provide more valuable diagnostic information.

Rehabilitation of Nerve Injuries

The focus of early rehabilitation intervention is to improve function, control edema, decrease pain, and maintain range of motion. Elevation of the affected extremity, use of elastic sleeves or stockings, and providing massage are all helpful in decreasing and preventing swelling. Desensitization of the involved extremity, appropriate pain medications, and splints to maintain optimal positioning are all important.

Orthoses (splints) are also used to assist with function. In the upper extremities, the most common type of splint treats weakness or loss of finger and wrist extension due to radial nerve injuries. A static wrist cock-up splint retains some wrist extension, promoting more effective hand grip and finger flexion. A dynamic wrist and digit extension splint can also be used to encourage functional hand grip, while keeping the fingers and wrist extended. In the lower extremity, a resting foot drop splint is used when a patient has a sciatic nerve injury or a peroneal nerve injury causing weakness or absence of ankle dorsiflexion. For ambulation, a custom molded ankle foot orthosis (MAFO) is prescribed to allow toe clearance and ankle protection. If the patient is non weight bearing on the extremity due to an orthopedic injury, waiting to prescribe a custom MAFO is appropriate. An MAFO is not necessary while the patient is non weight bearing on the affected extremity, and the nerve may recover by the time weight bearing is allowed. It is important to maintain range of motion, so that if the nerve does recover the affected limb will have the best functional outcome.

Many medications have been used for neuropathic pain. They include tricyclic antidepressants, anticonvulsants, and topical agents. Anticonvulsant drugs, particularly Gabapentin, pregabalin, and carbamazepine, are commonly used. Topical agents such as transdermal lidocaine patches are also effective.

ASSESSMENT OF PATIENTS WITH MULTIPLE ORTHOPEDIC INJURIES: THE POLYTRAUMA PATIENT

Orthopedic injuries account for almost half of all trauma-related hospital and inpatient rehabilitation admissions annually in the United States. Patients with multiple orthopedic injuries, or poly-

trauma patients, account for approximately 10% of inpatient rehabilitation admissions.[16] The care of polytrauma patients in an acute care setting is extremely challenging, as they are often victims of high-speed decelerations with significant nonorthopedic-associated wounds. The hospital course of these patients is often complicated by the need for hemodynamic resuscitation, multiple surgical procedures, and the occasional delayed diagnosis of occult injuries. As noted, many of these patients will require intensive inpatient rehabilitation upon discharge. Early involvement of a well-trained physiatrist is critical to ensure the best possible rehabilitative potential and to prevent delays in care and avoidable long-term complications.

Acute Hospital Care

Following initial resuscitation and/or resuscitative surgery, most polytrauma patients can be expected to experience a significant ICU stay. Although care must first be directed to the diagnosis and treatment of life-threatening injuries, fixation of orthopedic injuries should occur without unnecessary delay. If attention must be paid to nonorthopedic injuries such as intracranial, thoracic, or intraabdominal injuries—or if a patient remains in a nonresuscitated state for several hours—simple splinting of extremity fractures, traction for long bone fractures, and/or the use of pelvic compression devices may be required as temporizing maneuvers. Time permitting, external fixation devices may be employed to better stabilize fractures in the more stable but still critical patient.

A careful and thorough head-to-toe tertiary survey to include a complete neurological exam should be performed by an experienced examiner as soon as practical to rule out potentially significant missed injuries and possible associated spinal cord injuries. All of these tasks are made more difficult in the intubated and unresponsive patient.

Once the polytrauma patient is resuscitated and all injuries have been properly addressed, early consultation with a physiatrist experienced in the care of trauma patients should occur. Although it may seem counterintuitive that significant rehabilitation can occur in an acute ICU setting, there are simple and effective rehabilitative modalities that can and should be initiated in the ICU. Passive range of motion exercises performed by experienced physical therapists may benefit patients by reducing complications such as joint contracture and muscle atrophy. Likewise, the use of pressure pads, functional bracing, and compressive dressings at amputation sites may promote healing and avoid long-term complications.

Proper wound care, especially at open fracture and amputation sites, and decubitus prevention will avoid unnecessary morbidity and shorten ICU stays. Because polytrauma patients are often significantly hypercatabolic, adequate nutritional support should be instituted early and markers of protein synthesis measured frequently to facilitate rapid wound healing. Although not traditionally considered as such, nutritional support is a vital part of acute rehabilitative care. Timely and proper application of these modalities may very well have a significant impact on rehabilitation potential and outcome.

Once the patient is transferred out of the ICU, rehabilitation should be continued with a goal of maximizing functional recovery. Early involvement of a physiatrist and a team of physical and occupational therapists is critical for the seamless transition of rehabilitation care from the ICU to the floor. A unified rehabilitation plan, designed by a well-trained physiatrist and carried out regularly and without interruption, is in the patient's best interest. The specific rehabilitative regimen for a particular patient is extremely variable, based not only on the pattern of orthopedic injuries present and the method of their repair but the presence or absence of significant associated injuries (especially TBI).

Generally, in-hospital rehabilitation will follow a logical progression from immobilization (occasionally with casts or braces) to passive range of motion exercises. If the patient is cooperative, this is followed by conditioning exercises—especially if the patient experienced significant deconditioning or muscle atrophy. Finally, varying degrees of weight bearing will be allowed—often aided by the use of crutches or walkers. The provision of adequate analgesia is absolutely critical during this early rehabilitative phase. Narcotics or nonsteroidal drugs must be timed properly to have maximum effect during periods of increased activity, yet not be dosed in a fashion to produce lethargy or foster dependency. For patients with low pain tolerances or previous drug dependency, early involvement of a pain management consultant may facilitate and shorten rehabilitation. Lack of appropriate participation in rehabilitation by a patient may be a sign of depression, and if so should trigger involvement of a psychologist or psychiatrist. Patients with significant TBI are particularly challenging because they may not be able to adequately participate in any meaningful active rehabilitation regimens.

As noted previously, polytrauma patients account for approximately 10% of all inpatient rehabilitation admissions. Because many insurance carriers will not certify an inpatient rehabilitation admission unless a patient can engage in a set amount of meaningful rehabilitation therapy activities daily, many polytrauma patients may need to be transferred first to a skilled nursing facility once inpatient acute care is complete.

LEVELS OF CARE AFTER ACUTE TRAUMA HOSPITAL STAY

When patients are medically stable and have completed any necessary surgeries, they are ready for discharge from the Level 1 trauma center. Determining the next step is an important role of the trauma rehabilitation team. Discharge settings include home, an acute inpatient rehabilitation unit, a subacute or skilled nursing rehabilitation facility, a long-term acute care hospital, or an assisted living/personal care facility.

Whenever possible, direct return to home is best. The patient must be able to function safely and have support systems in place. They should be capable of independent function. When their injuries prevent them from doing so, the appropriate services (including home care) need to be available. Outpatient rehabilitation services should be arranged if needed.

Many times acute inpatient rehabilitation is appropriate. Patients should be able to participate and require at least 3 hours a day of physical therapy, occupational therapy, and/or speech therapy. Rehabilitation settings also should provide psychological services, rehabilitation nursing, and case management. This setting is usually needed for patients with SCIs, traumatic brain injuries, and multiple orthopedic injuries. When patients are not able to function safely or independently but have the potential to do so, acute inpatient rehabilitation is indicated.

Subacute or skilled nursing rehabilitation is necessary when patients cannot be cared for at home, or when their injuries limit participation in rehabilitation. Examples include patients with limited ability to bear weight due to severe injuries and those who would not tolerate many hours of therapy, particularly the elderly. Long-term care may be needed if return to a home setting is not possible in the future.

Long-term acute care hospitals are appropriate for those patients requiring ventilator weaning, prolonged antibiotics, or wound care, or those with continued complex medical needs. An assisted living or personal care facility is necessary for those patients who are fairly independent but need supervision or some assistance with self-care, mobility, and meal preparation.

CONCLUSIONS

Early involvement of an interdisciplinary rehabilitation team is essential for a patient who has sustained trauma. The team promotes optimal mobility, maximizes functional outcome, educates family members, communicates with other health care professionals, and determines the best discharge environment for an individual.

REFERENCES

1. National Center for Injury Prevention and Control: WISQUARS (Web-based Injury Statistics Query and Reporting System) leading causes of nonfatal injury reports, 2006. www.cdc.gov/ncipc/wisquars.
2. Cardenas DD, Hoffman JM, Stockman PL: Spinal cord injury. In Robinson LR, editor: *Trauma Rehabilitation.* Philadelphia, Lippincott, Williams and Wilkins, 2005.
3. National Spinal Cord Injury Statistical Center: Facts and figures at a glance—June, 2005. www.spinalcord.uab.edu.
4. Marino RJ, editor: American Spinal Injury Association: *International Standards for Neurological and Functional Classification of Spinal Cord Injury,* rev. 2002. Chicago, American Spinal Injury Association, 2002.
5. Bracken MB, Shephard MJ, Holford TR, Leo-Summers L, Aldrich EF, Faz LM, et al: Administration of methylprednisolone for 24 or 48 hours or tirilizad mesylate for 48 hours in the treatment of acute spinal cord injury. Results of the Third National Acute Spinal Cord Injury Randomized Controlled Trial. National Acute Spinal Cord Injury Study. *JAMA* 277: 1597–1604, 1997.
6. Lanig IS, Peterson WP: The respiratory system in spinal cord injury. *Phys Med Rehabil Clin North Am* 11(1):29–43, 2000.
7. Consortium for Spinal Cord Medicine: *Clinical Practice Guidelines. Spinal Cord Medicine: Prevention of Thromboembolism in Spinal Cord Injury,* 2nd ed. Consortium for Spinal Cord Medicine, 1999. http://www.pva.org/publications/pdf/DVT.pdf.
8. Langlois JA, Rutland-Brown W, Thomas KE: *Traumatic Brain Injury in the United States: Emergency Department Visits, Hospitalizations, and Deaths.* Atlanta, GA, Centers for Disease Control and Prevention, National Center for Injury Prevention, Nation Center for Injury and Prevention and Control, 2004. http://www.cdc.gov/ncipc/pub-res/TBI_in_US_04/TBI-USA_Book-Oct1.pdf.
9. Thurman DJ, Alverson C, Dunn KA, Guerrero J, Sniezek JE: Traumatic brain injury in the United States: a public health perspective. *Head Trauma Rehabil* 14(6)602–615, 1999.
10. Traumatic Brain Injury National Data Center: *The Traumatic Brain Injury Model Systems.* West Orange, NJ, Kessler Medical Rehabilitation Research and Education Corporation. www.tbindc.org.
11. Nalkmus D, Booth BJ, Kodimer C: *Rehabilitation of the Head Injured Adult: Comprehensive Cognitive Management.* Downey, CA: Professional Staff Association of Rancho Los Amigos Hospital, 1980.
12. Brain Injury Special Interest Group of the American Academy of Physical Medicine and Rehabilitation: Practice parameter: antiepileptic drug treatment of posttraumatic seizures. *Arch Phys Med Rehabil* 79:594–597, 1998.
13. Noble J, Munro CA, Prasad VS, Midha R: Analysis of upper and lower extremity peripheral nerve injuries in a population of patients with multiple injuries. *J Trauma* 45(1):116–122, 1998.
14. Seddon HJ: *Surgical Disorders of the Peripheral Nerves,* 2nd ed. Edinburgh and New York, Churchill Livingstone, 1975.
15. Chaudhry V, Cornblath DR: Wallerian degeneration in human nerves: serial electrophysiological studies. *Muscle Nerve* 15(6):687–693, 1992.
16. Uniform Data System for Medical Rehabilitation: Annual Inpatient Rehabilitation Facilities Report, 2003–2004. Amherst, NY, Uniform Data System for Medical Rehabilitation, 2004.

TRAUMA OUTCOMES

Michael Rhodes and **Glen Tinkoff**

All surgeons who care for patients with injury are subject to increased scrutiny relative to the outcomes of their patients. In fact, all participatory physicians, nurses, technicians, hospitals, and state trauma systems should have a heightened interest in trauma outcomes. Not only does outcome analysis provide a platform for performance improvement and patient safety, but may have a significant impact on liability, cost, and reimbursement. As pay-for-performance initiatives emerge, the survival of trauma centers and systems may be at risk.

More importantly, measurement of outcomes allows comparative benchmarking of care and provides a measure of the effectiveness of current processes of care such as triage, diagnosis, treatment, and rehabilitation. Fortunately, venues for outcome analysis are maturing such as the work of the many trauma/critical care societies as well as the American College of Surgeons. Examples of this resource include the National Trauma Data Bank (NTDB) and the Office of Evidence Based Surgery at the American College of Surgeons.

OUTCOMES

Outcomes may be viewed differently from the perspective of the patient, provider, payer, and society. The standard outcome parameters are outlined in Table 1. Although survival (live/die) seems straightforward, the endpoint in time may vary considerably, including in hospital, 30 days, 6 months, 1 year, and time to death. These variations project imprecision into many of the existing severity scoring and mortality prediction models.

The use of morbidity as an outcome requires distinguishing between a complication and a pre-existing condition (i.e., a comorbidity) and providing a precise definition of a complication. A wound infection requires a precise diagnosis using the NISS classification; however, many of the infections are discovered and treated as outpatients and are never recognized by registries. Distinguishing between pre-existing renal or pulmonary disease and subsequent renal or pulmonary dysfunction after trauma can be challenging.

Hospital length of stay is a gross parameter of quality or outcome because of the variety of practices in institutions relative to the use of intensive care unit, step-down, floor, and outpatient care. The effect of early discharge is widely unknown relative to the effect on the patient's family, visiting nurses, physician's offices, and unanticipated hospital readmissions.

As with all outcome parameters, the cost of trauma care can be in the eye of the beholder. The payer is likely to know his/her cost with some precision, which usually reflects what he/she paid plus administrative costs. The patient usually perceives the cost as out-of-pocket expenses plus lost wages. However, the cost to the providers (i.e., emergency medical services, physician, and hospital) has many confounding variables, and is much less precise. The cost to society is even more abstract and studies have revealed substantial variation in estimates.

Quality of life has been recognized by researchers as desired outcome measures. The Functional Independence Measure (FIM), Glasgow Outcome Scale (GOS), Functional Capacity Index (FCI),

Quality of Well-Being Scale, Sickness Impact Profile (SIP), and the SF-36 Survey are among the most popular in trauma-related outcome studies. Some are labor intensive and become impractical except for focused studies.

Many commercially available survey tools are religiously utilized by hospital and system administrators as measures of patient satisfaction. Goals are frequently set to meet target scores, suggesting either improvement or decline in outcome.

Finally, measuring compliance with evidence-based guidelines can provide a measurement of outcomes. Studies of compliance with Advanced Trauma Live Support (ATLS) guidelines, as well as head injury guidelines, have provided several outcome studies. Using guideline compliance as an outcome itself assumes that the desired outcome is compliance, inferring improvement in other standard patient outcomes based on the evidence on which the guidelines were developed. Therefore, caution is required in interpreting this outcome parameter.

EVIDENCE-BASED MEDICINE

The discipline of evidence-based medicine has emerged over the past decade to allow investigators to quantify the power of scientific studies based on the certainty of the scientific methods employed. Although simplistic, a classification system has been well received by the medical community that allows dialog among investigators (Table 2). Fortunately, the trend of dominance of class III data in the world of trauma outcomes is slowly giving way to significant class II and class I outcome studies in trauma and critical care.

In general, class I and class II studies provide the fuel for the strongest evidence-based guidelines on which to base the processes of trauma care (Table 3). The value of class III studies is to point the researcher toward an area of need and to help formulate the appropriate null hypothesis for a higher-power study. However, there are many clinical questions that have prohibitive barriers that prevent class I and class II studies, thereby augmenting the value of class III evidence.

PERFORMANCE IMPROVEMENT AND PATIENT SAFETY

For over two decades, performance improvement (previously called quality assurance) has been a centerpiece of trauma care as promulgated by the American College of Surgeons Committee on Trauma. Recently, as a result of studies by the Institute of Medicine and the response to those studies by the Joint Commission on Accreditation of Health Care Organizations, patient safety has been added to the equation. Most health care organizations are under a mandate for demonstration of performance improvement and patient safety (PIPS) initiatives.

The Surgical Care Improvement Project (SCIP) is a national initiative to improve outcomes for patients having surgery. This project represents a coalition of 10 organizations, including the American College of Surgeons, Agency for Healthcare Research and Quality, Centers for Medicare and Medicaid Services, and Joint Commission on Accreditation of Healthcare Organizations. Although some of the initiatives are not specific to trauma care, many relate to critical care and general care of any patient, including those with injury (Table 4). Most of these initiatives are centered on evidence-based guidelines reflective of class I or II outcome studies. Therefore, it is important to understand the very strong link between trauma/critical care–related PIPS and outcome studies.

Table 1: Outcome Parameters in Medicine

Survival (mortality)

Complications (morbidity)

Length of stay

Cost

Quality of life

Patient satisfaction

Compliance with guidelines

Table 2: Evidence-Based Classification of Outcome Studies

Evidence	Description
Class I	Prospective, randomized, controlled trials—the gold standard of clinical trials. However, some may be poorly designed, lack sufficient patient numbers, or suffer from other methodological inadequacies.
Class II	Clinical studies in which the data were collected prospectively; retrospective analyses based on clearly reliable data. Types of study so classified include observational studies, cohort studies, prevalence studies, and case–control studies.
Class III	Most studies based on retrospectively collected data. Evidence used in this class indicates clinical series, databases, registries, case reviews, case reports, and expert opinion.
Technology assessment	The assessment of technology, such as devices for monitoring intracranial pressure, does not lend itself to classification in the format above. Thus, for technology assessment, devices were evaluated in terms of accuracy, reliability, therapeutic potential, and cost effectiveness.

Table 3: Trauma-Related Evidence-Based Guidelines

1. Resuscitation end points
2. Emergency department thoracotomy
3. Management of mild traumatic brain injury
4. Severe closed head injury
5. Identifying cervical spine injuries after trauma
6. Screening of blunt cardiac injury
7. Diagnosis and management of blunt aortic injury
8. Prophylactic antibiotic use for tube thoracostomy
9. Evaluation of blunt abdominal trauma
10. Nonoperative management of blunt injury to liver and spleen
11. Prophylactic antibiotic use in penetrating abdominal trauma
12. Penetrating intraperitoneal colon injuries
13. Pelvic fracture
14. Genitourinary injury
15. Optimal timing of long bone fracture stabilization in polytrauma patients
16. Prophylactic antibiotic use in open fractures
17. Management of penetrating trauma to lower extremity
18. Venous thromboembolism in trauma patients
19. Ventilator management of patients with respiratory failure
20. Nosocomial pneumonia
21. Weaning and extubation
22. Agitation and sedation
23. Alcohol withdrawal prophylaxis
24. Pain management
25. Stress ulcer prophylaxis
26. Infection control of invasive lines
27. Nutritional support of trauma patient
28. Albumin transfusion
29. Hyperglycemia
30. Geriatric trauma
31. Violence prevention programs

NATIONAL TRAUMA DATA BANK

In 1989, the Regents of the American College of Surgeons established the National Trauma Data Bank (NTDB) subcommittee under the aegis of the American College of Surgeons Committee of Trauma. The goal of this initiative was to develop a database that would serve as a national repository of data on trauma center care in the United States. After completing its preliminary work, including establishing the standard data set of 93 elements, the NTDB initiated a first call for data in 1997. It continues to do so annually, requesting data from the previous year. As of 2005, the NTDB has accrued over 1.4 million records from 405 U.S. trauma centers in 43 states, territories, and the District of Columbia, making it the largest aggregate of trauma data ever assembled. Table 5 outlines research studies that were at least in part based on the NTDB.

Although the sheer size of the NTDB makes it an attractive resource for trauma-related research and benchmarking, it has several significant limitations. The NTDB represents a convenience sample of trauma care provided by the participating hospitals, which are predominately trauma centers. Accordingly, it can not be used as a population-based assessment of U.S. trauma care.

The NTDB contains data originally collected using many different trauma registry programs. Because of the variability of the data definitions contained in the registry programs, there is significant data variability within the data set of the NTDB itself. In order to limit this variability, the data files are scanned to ensure that they are within valid ranges prior to entry. Presently, the NTDB Subcommittee with assistance from the U.S. Health Resources and Service Administration is engaged in a major effort to standardize the NTDB's data set for eventual distribution to the participating hospitals.

The NTDB's nonsystematic sampling also lends itself to a selection bias. This bias makes benchmarking problematic, as not all hospitals or trauma centers participate and certain injuries (e.g., hip fractures) are not uniformly reported. Furthermore, because of the voluntary and nonuniform nature of reporting, the NTDB participating hospitals can provide varying amounts of data within the data set. As many hospitals fail to report certain information such as complications or comorbidities, comparative analysis in these areas is impossible.

Table 4: Surgical Care Improvement Project: Process and Outcome Measures

Infection

Prophylactic antibiotic received within 1 hour prior to surgical incision

Prophylactic antibiotic selection for surgical patients

Prophylactic antibiotics discontinued within 24 hours after surgery end time (48 hours for cardiac patients)

Postoperative wound infection diagnosed during index hospitalization (OUTCOME)

Surgery patients with appropriate hair removal

Colorectal surgery patients with immediate postoperative normothermia

Cardiac

Noncardiac vascular surgery patients with evidence of coronary artery disease who received beta-blockers during the perioperative period

Surgery patients on a beta-blocker prior to arrival who received a beta-blocker during the perioperative period

Intraoperative or postoperative acute myocardial infarction diagnosed during index hospitalization and within 30 days of surgery (OUTCOME)

Venous Thromboembolism

Surgery patients with recommended venous thromboembolism prophylaxis ordered

Surgery patients who received appropriate venous thromboembolism prophylaxis within 24 hours prior to surgery to 24 hours after surgery

Intraoperative or postoperative pulmonary embolism diagnosed during index hospitalization and within 30 days of surgery (OUTCOME)

Intraoperative or postoperative deep vein thrombosis diagnosed during index hospitalization and within 30 days of surgery (OUTCOME)

Respiratory

Number of days ventilated surgery patients had documentation of the head of the bed being elevated from recovery end date (day 0) through postoperative day 7

Patients diagnosed with postoperative ventilator-associated pneumonia during index hospitalization (OUTCOME)

Number of days ventilated surgery patients had documentation of stress ulcer disease prophylaxis from recovery end date (day 0) through postoperative day 7

Surgery patients whose medical record contained an order for a ventilator weaning program (protocol or clinical pathway)

Global

Mortality within 30 days of surgery

Readmission within 30 days of surgery

Table 5: National Trauma Data Bank–Related Research

Epidemiology

George RL, et al: The association between gender and mortality among trauma patients as modified by age. *J Trauma*, 2003.

Hawkins A, et al: The impact of combined trauma and burns on patient mortality. *J Trauma*, 2005.

Ikossi DG, et al: Profile of mothers at risk: an analysis of injury and pregnancy loss in 1,195 trauma patients. *J Am Coll Surg*, 2005.

Kon AA, et al: The association of race and ethnicity with rates of drug and alcohol testing among US trauma patients. *Health Policy*, 2004.

Marcin JP, et al: Evaluation of race and ethnicity on alcohol and drug testing of adolescents admitted with trauma. *Acad Emerg Med*, 2003.

McGwin G Jr, et al: Pre-existing conditions and mortality in older trauma patients. *J Trauma*, 2004.

Minei JP, et al: Gender differences in survival may be due to a lower risk of complications in females: an analysis of the National Trauma Data Bank. Presented (poster) at annual meeting of American Association for the Surgery of Trauma, Maui, HI, September 2004.

Santaniello JM, et al: Ten year experience of burn, trauma, and combined burn/trauma injuries comparing outcomes. *J Trauma*, 2004.

Steljes TP, et al: Epidemiology of suicide and the impact on Western trauma centers. *J Trauma*, 2005.

Prevention

Eastridge B, et al: Economic impact of motorcycle helmets: from impact to discharge. Presented (oral) at the annual meeting of the American Association for the Surgery of Trauma, September 2004, Maui, HI. *J Trauma*, 2004.

Hundley JC, et al: Non-helmeted motorcyclists: a burden to society? A study using the National Trauma Data Bank. *J Trauma*, 2004.

Knudson MM, et al: Thromboembolism after trauma: an analysis of 1602 episodes from the American College of Surgeons National Trauma Data Bank. *Ann Surg*, 2004.

Nance ML, et al: Determining Injury Prevention Priorities in the United States. American Public Health Association Meeting, New Orleans, LA, November 2005.

System

Demetriades D, et al: The effect of trauma center designation and trauma volume on outcome in specific severe injuries. *Ann Surg*, 2005.

Esposito TJ, et al: Neurosurgical coverage: essential, desired, or irrelevant for good patient care and trauma center status. *Ann Surg*, 2005.

Scoring

Glance LG, et al: Evaluating trauma center quality: does the choice of the severity-adjustment model make a difference? *J Trauma*, 2005.

Healey C, et al: Improving the Glasgow Coma Scale score: motor score alone is a better predictor. *J Trauma*, 2003.

Kilgo PD, et al: A note on the disjointed nature of the Injury Severity Score. *J Trauma*, 2004.

Kilgo PD, et al: The worst injury predicts mortality outcome the best: rethinking the role of multiple injuries in trauma outcome scoring. *J Trauma*, 2003.

Meredith JW, et al: Independently derived survival risk ratios yield better estimates of survival than traditional survival risk ratios when using the ICISS. *J Trauma*, 2003.

Meredith JW, et al: A fresh set of survival risk ratios derived from incidents in the National Trauma Data Bank from which the ICISS may be calculated. *J Trauma*, 2003.

Millham FH, et al: Factors associated with mortality in trauma: re-evaluation of the TRISS method using the National Trauma Data Bank. *J Trauma*, 2004.

Prehospital

Shafi S, et al: Prehospital endotracheal intubation and positive pressure ventilation is associated with hypotension and decreased survival in hypovolemic trauma patients: an analysis of the National Trauma Data Bank. *J Trauma*, 2005.

Resuscitation

Kincaid EH, et al: Admission base deficit in pediatric trauma: a study using the National Trauma Data Bank. *J Trauma*, 2001.

Martin RS, et al: Injury-associated hypothermia: an analysis of the 2004 National Trauma Data Bank. *Shock*, 2005.

Nirula R, Gentilello LM: Futility of resuscitation criteria for the "young" old and the "old" old trauma patient: a National Trauma Data Bank analysis. *J Trauma*, 2004.

Shafi S, Gentilello L: Hypotension does not increase mortality in brain injured patients more than it does in the non–brain injured patients. *J Trauma*, 2005.

Shafi S, Gentilello L: Is hypothermia simply a marker of shock and injury severity or an independent risk factor for mortality? An analysis of a large national trauma registry (NTDB). *J Trauma*, 2005.

Operating Room

Acierno SP, et al: Is pediatric trauma still a surgical disease? Patterns of emergent operative intervention in the injured child. *J Trauma*, 2004.

Ahmed N, et al: The contribution of laparoscopy in evaluation of penetrating abdominal wounds. *J Am Coll Surg*, 2005.

Hemmila MR, et al: Delayed repair for blunt thoracic aortic injury: is it really equivalent to early repair? *J Trauma*, 2004.

Nance ML, et al: Timeline to operative intervention for solid organ injuries in children. Presented at meetings of American Association for the Surgery of Trauma, Atlanta, GA, September 2005.

Wright JL, et al: Renal and extrarenal predictors of nephrectomy from the National Trauma Data Bank (NTDB). *J Urol*, 2006.

Critical Care

Friese RS, et al: Pulmonary artery catheter is associated with reduced mortality in severely injured patients: a National Trauma Data Bank analysis of 53,312 patients. *J Trauma*, 2004.

NATIONAL SURGICAL QUALITY IMPROVEMENT PROGRAM

The National Surgical Quality Improvement Program (NSQIP) was developed by the Veterans Administration in response to a congressional mandate to demonstrate optimal outcomes in the VA Hospitals. The program was developed by surgeons for surgeons and represents the first attempt at measuring surgical outcomes from a clinical rather than an administrative database.

This program is sponsored by the American College of Surgeons and is currently being promulgated to nonmilitary health care organizations. The Committee on Trauma of the American College of Surgeons is working with NSQIP to provide a trauma-related outcome module. This will provide a much more robust tracking of morbidities and will allow validation of the definitions of complications.

SUMMARY AND FUTURE DIRECTION

The ability to demonstrate high-quality outcomes for all health care efforts will be essential for surgeons, including those caring for the injured. The quality of outcome data continues to improve, especially in the areas of the critical-care phase of trauma. The National Trauma Data Bank and the National Surgical Quality Improvement Program can provide platforms to benchmarking. There is a need for improvement in the precision of definitions of outcome parameters, especially in the area of complications. The electronic health record of the future will include a repository, clinical decision support, and an integrated concurrent data management system that will allow for much better local outcome assessment. National efforts to improve funding for trauma outcome studies will be necessary to improve the quality of outcome studies, especially in the prehospital, resuscitation, and operative phases of trauma care.

Suggested Readings

Eastern Association for the Surgery of Trauma: Home page. www.east.org/guidelines.

National Surgical Quality Improvement Project: Home page. https://acsnsqip.org.

National Trauma Data Bank: Home page. http://ntdb.org.

Rhodes M: Trauma outcomes. In Moore EE, et al., editors: *Trauma,* 5th ed. New York, McGraw-Hill, 2004.

Society of Critical Care Medicine: Home page. www.sccm.org.

Surgical Care Improvement Project: Home page. http://www.medqic.org/scip/.

U.S. Department of Health and Human Services: Medicare Website, CMS pay for performance measures. www.medicare.gov.